A Modern Atlas for Implantable Devices of the Spine, Brain, and Nerve

A Modern Atlas for Implantable Devices of the Spine, Brain, and Nerve

For Pain, Movement Disorders, and Nerve Dysfunction

Edited by

Timothy R. Deer
President and CEO, The Spine and Nerve Centers of the Virginias, Charleton, WV, United States

Jason E. Pope
President and CEO, Evolve Restorative Center, Santa Rosa, CA, United States

ELSEVIER

ACADEMIC PRESS
An imprint of Elsevier

Academic Press is an imprint of Elsevier
125 London Wall, London EC2Y 5AS, United Kingdom
50 Hampshire Street, 5th Floor, Cambridge, MA 02139, United States

ISBN: 978-0-443-36528-7

For information on all Academic Press publications visit our website at https://www.elsevier.com/books-and-journals

Publisher: Megan Ball
Acquisitions Editor: Simonetta Harrison
Editorial Project Manager: Vikrant Dixit
Production Project Manager: Gomathi Sugumar
Cover Designer: Mark Rogers

Typeset by TNQ Tech

Dedication

For more than 3 decades, I have treated many patients who suffer from pain and have their lives interrupted by this dark cloud. Working with my amazing clinical team and research team, we have salvaged many of those souls and made living worthwhile for the patients, their families, and the society. This book is dedicated to the patients, their loved ones, and those who took the chance on the research and development that I needed to do to advance the field.

Most importantly, I want to thank God for the blessings of good physical and mental health and my wonderful family for all the support for my complex career. In addition, a big thank you to my work family, who make it all possible, and my huge American Society of Pain and Neuroscience family, who are changing the world.

Timothy R. Deer, MD

Dedication

The specialty of pain management has been my professional life's work. This book captures the excitement and innovation of what the specialty of pain management is today: a specialty that requires expertise in anatomy, surgical skill, patient candidacy, and postoperative care, with vigilance for patient safety and efficacy.

I dedicate this book to my peers who are always seeking to refine their skills and care, to our patients to elevate their outcomes, and to my family.

I want to express a special thank you to Dr. Timothy Deer. His vision, through hard work, dedication, collaboration, and the development of an active physician community in professional organizations and beyond, is shaping the field and changing lives.

I welcome you to join the cause and grow our village. But, we are not finished. We need to continue to chase new treatments, acquire clinical data, and pursue collaboration to improve patient access and care.

Let's go.

Jason E. Pope, MD, FIPP, DABPM

Contents

Section 2
The spine anatomy

Section 3
Spinal cord stimulation

9. Cervical spinal cord stimulation

Jonathan M. Hagedorn, Boss Povieng, Benjamin Gill and Daniel A. Jimenez

10. Thoracic and lumbar spinal cord stimulation

Derron Keith Wilson, Kwasi K. Ampomah, Shashank Vodapally, Arti Ori and Israel Riley Pena

11. Neuromodulation for pelvic pain

Corey Hunter, Shawn K. Puri, Raj G. Patel and Iden M. Cowan

12. Complications of neuromodulation of the spine

Chau Vu, Andrew Dudas, Warren Grace, Harjot S. Bhandal and Jason E. Pope

Section 4
Dorsal root ganglion

13. Cervical dorsal root ganglion stimulation

Timothy Lubenow, Alexandra Moreira, Boss Povieng and Johnson S. Ho

14. Thoracic dorsal root ganglion stimulation

Tolga Suvar, Kristin Jarzombek, Chris Massey and Rosa Garcia

15. Dorsal root ganglion stimulation

Kenneth B. Chapman, Christopher J. Mallard, Christopher A. Paul and Ajax Yang

20. Surround inhibition

Nitish Aggarwal, Roshan Santhosh, Ajay Antony, Sayed E. Wahezi, Ugur Yener and James North

21. Differential target multiplexed (DTM)

Ricardo Vallejo, Melissa Murphy, Matthew Chung and Mark N. Malinowski

22. New waveform concepts for spinal cord stimulation

Vinicius Tieppo Francio, Lucas Bracero, Marco Lawandy, Daniel Pak, Marc Russo and Mitsukuni Yoshida

Section 6
Closed loop systems

23. Physiologic closed loop controlled spinal cord stimulation

Trishul Kapoor, Chau Vu, Chheany Ung, Timothy Deer and Jason E. Pope

24. Closed loop: Spinal cord stimulation

Michael Fishman, Melissa Murphy, Thomas Salazar, Harman Chopra and Nomen Azeem

Contributors

Daniel A. Jimenez, Physical Medicine and Rehabilitation, University of Michigan Health-Sparrow, Lansing, MI, United States

Alaa Abd-Elsayed, Department of Anesthesiology, University of Wisconsin School of Medicine and Public Health, Madison, WI, United States

Nitish Aggarwal, Pain Management, TriState Pain Institute, Fort Mohave, AZ, United States

Rohit Aiyer, Westside Pain Management, Long Beach, CA, United States

Latrice A. Akuamoah, Department of Anesthesiology, The Zucker School of Medicine at Hofstra/Northwell, New York, NY, United States; Visco Spine and Joint Center, Hoboken, NJ, United States

Tariq AlFarra, Department of Rehabilitation and Human Performance, Icahn School of Medicine at Mount Sinai, New York, NY, United States

Rushna Ali, Neurosurgery, Mayo Clinic, Rochester, MN, United States

Mansoor M. Aman, Endeavor Health, Evanston, IL, United States

Kwasi K. Ampomah, USA Rehab Services, Atlanta, GA, United States

Christopher Andriano, Georgia Pain Care, Atlanta, GA, United States

Ajay Antony, Pain Management, The Orthopaedic Institute, Gainesville, FL, United States

Nomen Azeem, Florida Spine & Pain Specialists, Tampa, FL, United States

Aydin Babakhani, Nervonik, Los Angeles, CA, United States; UCLA, Los Angeles, CA, United States

Jonathan Bao, Department of Neurosurgery, Vanderbilt University Medical Center, Nashville, TN, United States

Daniyal Bashir, Trinity Health West Michigan, Muskegon, MI, United States

Marshall D. Bedder, Wellstar/MCG Department of Psychiatry and Health Behavior, Chief of Pain Medicine, VA Augusta Health System, Addiction Medicine Fellowship Program, Augusta, GA, United States

Harjot S. Bhandal, MarinHealth, Larkspur, CA, United States

Sushanth Boda, Southern Pain and Spine, Newnan, GA, United States

Lucas Bracero, The Spine and Nerve Centers of the Virginias, Charleston, WV, United States

Mustafa Broachwala, Department of Anesthesiology and Pain Medicine, University of California, San Diego, CA, United States; Pain Anesthesia, University of California San Diego, San Diego, CA, United States

Patrick Buchanan, Pain Medicine, Spanish Hills Interventional Pain Specialists, Camarillo, CA, United States

Colin M. Buday, The Spine and Nerve Centers of the Virginias and West Virginia University, Morgantown, WV, United States

Tyler Burns, Endeavor Health, Evanston, IL, United States

Michael Cannone, Rocky Vista University, Montana College of Osteopathic Medicine, Billings, MT, United States

Kenneth B. Chapman, The Spine & Pain Institute of New York, New York, NY, United States; Department of Anesthesiology, NYU Langone Medical Center, New York, NY, United States; Department of Anesthesiology, The Zucker School of Medicine at Hofstra/Northwell, New York, NY, United States

Harman Chopra, Department of Physical Medicine & Rehabilitation, Johns Hopkins University, Baltimore, MD, United States; Weill Cornell Medicine, Department of Anesthesiology, Critical Care, and Pain Medicine, New York, NY, United States; Department of Pain, Weill Cornell Medicine, New York, NY, United States; Colorado Rehabiliation and Occupational Medicine, Denver, CO, United States

Matthew Chung, Department of Pain Medicine, Division of Critical Care Anesthesia and Pain Medicine, The

University of Texas MD Anderson Cancer Center, Houston, TX, United States

Iden M. Cowan, Interventional Spine Capitol Pain Institute, Greenwood Village, CO, United States

Daniel Cummins, Department of Neurosurgery, The Icahn School of Medicine at Mount Sinai, New York, NY, United States

Michael Danko, Premier Pain Treatment Institute, Loveland, OH, United States

Timothy Deer, The Spine and Nerve Centers of the Virginias and West Virginia University, Morgantown, WV, United States; Anesthesiology and Pain Medicine, WVU School of Medicine, American Society of Pain and Neuroscience, Charleston, WV, United States

Dirk De Ridder, University of Otago, Dunedin, New Zealand

Ramneek Dhillon, Evolve Restorative Center, Santa Rosa, CA, United States

David M. Dickerson, Endeavor Health, Evanston, IL, United States

Andrew Dudas, Mays & Schnapp Neurospine and Pain, Memphis, TN, United States; Mays & Schnapp Neuroscience and Spine, Memphis, TN, United States

Dario J. Englot, Department of Neurosurgery, Vanderbilt University Medical Center, Nashville, TN, United States

Steven Falowski, Neurosurgery, Neurosurgical Associates of Lancaster, Lancaster, PA, United States

Michael Fishman, Brixton Biosciences Cambridge, Cambridge, MA, United States

Derek Fitzgerald, Division of Pain Medicine, Department of Anesthesiology and Pain Medicine, University of California, Davis, Sacramento, CA, United States

Michael Flamm, Interventional Pain Physician, VA Harbor Health System, Rusk Institute of NYU Langone Health, New York, NY, United States

Vinny Francio, Division of Pain Medicine, Department of Anesthesiology, Washington University School of Medicine in St. Louis, Barnes-Jewish Hospital, Center for Advanced Medicine, St. Louis, MO, United States

Rosa Garcia, Department of Anesthesiology and Pain Medicine, University of Florida, Gainesville, FL, United States

Corey Gatewood, Department of Physical Medicine and Rehabilitation, University of California, Davis, Sacramento, CA, United States

Tony K. George, Division of Pain Medicine, Department of Physical Medicine and Rehabilitation, Hackensack Meridian Health – JFK University Medical Center, Edison, NJ, United States

Benjamin Gill, Nevada Advanced Pain Specialists, Reno, NV, United States

Christopher Gilmore, Carolinas Pain Institute, Winston-Salem, NC, United States

Brandon Gish, Lexington Clinic Interventional Pain, Lexington, KY, United States

Johnathan Goree, University of Arkansas for Medical Sciences, Little Rock, AR, United States

Chad Gorman, Partner at Physician Partners of America, Tampa, FL, United States

Warren Grace, Redefine Healthcare, Union, NJ, United States

Jay S. Grider, Div Interventional Pain, UofL Health, Louisville, KY, United States

Amit Gulati, Chronic Pain, Memorial Sloan Kettering Cancer Center, New York, NY, United States

Mayank Gupta, Kansas Pain Management, Overland Park, KS, United States

Christine Haddad, Innovative Pain and Wellness, Phoenix, AZ, United States

Jon Hagedorn, Mayo Clinic, Rochester, MN, United States

Robert Heros, Spinal Diagnostics, PC, Tualatin, OR, United States; Cascade Spine Center, LLC, Tualatin, OR, United States

Johnson S. Ho, Department of Interventional Pain Management, NJ Spine and Orthopedic, West Orange, NJ, United States

Corey Hunter, Montefiore Medical Center, Multidisciplinary Pain Program, Department of Physical Medicine & Rehabilitation at Albert Einstein College of Medicine, Bronx, NY, United States

Kristin Jarzombek, Greater Austin Pain Center, Austin, TX, United States

David S. Jevotovsky, NYU Langone Health, Department of Physical Medicine and Rehabilitation, New York, NY, United States

Shawn K. Puri, Integrated Pain Associates, Killeen, TX, United States

Hemant Kalia, Center for Research & Innovation in Spine & Pain, Rochester, NY, United States

Trishul Kapoor, Department of Pain Management, Cleveland Clinic Foundation, Cleveland, OH, United States

Leonardo Kapural, Carolinas Pain Institute and Best Opinion Doctorcom, Winston-Salem, NC, United States; Atrium Heath, Wake Forest Baptist Pain Center-Premier, Winston Salem, NC, United States

Marcin Karcz, The Spine and Nerve Centers of the Virginias, Charleston, WV, United States

Inamullah Khan, University of Missouri, Columbia, MO, United States

Nasir Khatri, Insight Health Systems, Flint, MI, United States

Ahmed Khawer, Department of Physical Medicine and Rehabilitation, Johns Hopkins University School of Medicine, Baltimore, MD, United States; Johns Hopkins University, Baltimore, MD, United States

Kevin Ko, SamWell Pain Institute, Colonia, NJ, United States

Brian Harris Kopell, Center of Neuromodulation, Neurology, Psychiatry, and Neuroscience, The Icahn School of Medicine at Mount Sinai, New York, NY, United States

Jeffery Kramer, Volta Research, Minneapolis, MN, United States; University of Illinois, Chicago, IL, United States; Nervonik, Los Angeles, CA, United States

Marco Lawandy, Department of Physical Medicine & Rehabilitation, Montefiore Medical Center, Bronx NY, United States

David Lee, Fullerton Orthopedics, University of California Irvine, Yorba Linda, CA, United States

Denise Lester, Department of Physical Medicine & Rehabilitation, Richmond VA Medical Center, Virginia Commonwealth University, Richmond, VA, United States

Timothy Lubenow, Midwest Anesthesia and Pain Specialists, Interventional Pain Management, Chicago, IL, United States

David M. Gallacher, Endeavor Health, Evanston, IL, United States

Jonathan M. Hagedorn, Anesthesiology and Perioperative Medicine, Mayo Clinic, Rochester, MN, United States

Warren Mackie-Jenkins, Interventional Pain Medicine, NOVA Orthopedic and Spine, Center for Advanced Orthopedics, Woodbridge, VA, United States

Ammar Mahmoud, Alleviate Pain & Spine, Bangor, ME, United States

Mark N. Malinowski, Ohio Health Hospital System, Columbus, OH, United States

Christopher J. Mallard, University of Kentucky, Department of Anesthesiology, Lexington, KY, United States

Chris Massey, Pain Specialists of America, Austin, TX, United States

Robin Mata, Rush University Medical Center, Chicago, IL, United States; University of Miami, Coral Gables, FL, United States

Justin McCarthy, Mary Free Bed Rehabilitation Hospital, Grand Rapids, MI, United States

Gladstone C. McDowell, II, Targeted Care Solutions, Columbus, OH, United States

Kai McGreevy, McGreevy NeuroHealth, St. Augustine, FL, United States

Robert Moghim, Interventional Spine and Pain, Denver, CO, United States; Colorado Pain Care, Denver, CO, United States

Alexandra Moreira, Southern Pain and Spine, Interventional Pain Management, Atlanta, GA, United States

Melissa Murphy, North Texas Orthopedics and Spine Center, Grapevine, TX, United States

Ramana Naidu, MarinHealth Spine Institute, Larkspur, CA, United States

Morad Nasseri, Boomerang Healthcare, Interventional Pain Medicine, Walnut Creek, CA, United States

Lee Nguyen, Division of Pain Medicine, Department of Anesthesiology and Pain Medicine, University of California, Davis, Sacramento, CA, United States

James North, Interventional Pain Management Department, The Center for Clinical Research, LLC, Winston −Salem, NC, United States

Arti Ori, Mass General Brigham, Harvard Medical School, Boston, MA, United States

Daniel Pak, Pain Medicine Division, University of Texas Health Science Center at Houston, Houston, TX, United States

Viktoras Palys, Department of Neurosurgery, University of Arkansas for Medical Sciences, Little Rock, AR, United States

Jonathan Paris, Center for Pain Management at Stony Brook Medicine, Stony Brook, NY, United States

Raj G. Patel, Capitol Pain Institute, Austin, TX, United States

Kiran V. Patel, Lenox Hill Hospital, Barbara and Donald School of Medicine at Hofstra/Northwell, New Hyde Park, NY, United States

Christopher A. Paul, University of Kentucky, Department of Anesthesiology, Lexington, KY, United States

Danika L. Paulo, Department of Neurosurgery, Henry Ford Hospital, Detroit, MI, United States

Israel Riley Pena, JPS Leuda Pain Management Clinic, JPS Health Network, Fort Worth, Texas, United States

Evan Peskin, Insight Health Systems, Flint, MI, United States

Edward Podgorski, III, Hawthorne Oncology Pain Experts (HOPE), Tampa, FL, United States

Jason E. Pope, Evolve Restorative Center, American Society of Pain and Neuroscience, Santa Rosa, CA, United States

Boss Povieng, Department of Anesthesiology, Rush University Medical Center, Chicago, IL, United States; Insight Medical Center Chicago, Interventional Pain Management, Chicago, IL, United States

Scott Pritzlaff, Division of Pain Medicine, Department of Anesthesiology and Pain Medicine, University of California, Davis, Sacramento, CA, United States

Hamzah Adel Ramawad, Center for Pain Medicine & Surgery Center, Fargo, ND, United States

Manish Ranjan, Neurosurgery and Neuroscience, West Virginia University, Morgantown, WV, United States

Dustin Reynolds, Ortho Alliance, Columbus, OH, United States

Christopher L. Robinson, Department of Anesthesiology, Perioperative & Pain Medicine, Harvard Medical School, Brigham & Women's Hospital, Boston, MA, United States

Jason D. Ross, Department of Anesthesiology, Northwestern University, Feinberg School of Medicine, Chicago, IL, United States

Qing Zhao Ruan, Warren Alpert Medical School, Brown University, Providence, RI, United States

Marc Russo, Hunter Pain Specialists, Broadmeadow, Australia

Harjot S. Bhandal, Evolve Restorative Center, Santa Rosa, CA, United States

Thomas Salazar, Colorado Rehabiliation and Occupational Medicine, Denver, CO, United States

Roshan Santhosh, Physical Medicine and Rehabilitation, Larkin Community Hospital, Miami, FL, United States

Michael E. Schatman, Department of Anesthesiology, Perioperative Care, and Pain Medicine, NYU Grossman School of Medicine, New York, NY, United States; Department of Population Health-Division of Medical Ethics, NYU Grossman School of Medicine, New York, NY, United States

Jayunkumar Shah, Center for Neuromodulation, The Icahn School of Medicine at Mount Sinai, New York, NY, United States

Anuj Shah, Department of Anesthesiology, Division of Pain Management, New York Presbyterian Hospital/Weill Cornell Medicine, New York, NY, United States

Amit Sharma, UPMC Pain Management, Department of Anesthesiology and Perioperative Medicine, University of Pittsburgh, Pittsburgh, PA, United States

Jonathan Silverman, Orthopedic Associates of SW Ohio, Dayton, OH, United States

Ioannis Skaribas, Expert Pain PA, Houston, TX, United States

Matthew Slitzky, Burke Rehabilitation Hospital, Montefiore Health System, White Plains, NY, United States

John-Allen Smith, University of California, Davis, School of Medicine, Sacramento, CA, United States

Lawson Smith, Endeavor Health, Evanston, IL, United States

Harry Soar, York and Scarborough Teaching Hospitals NHS Foundation Trust, Yorkshire, United Kingdom

Peter S. Staats, The Vagus Nerve Society and National Spine and Pain Centers, Atlantic Beach, FL, United States

Tolga Suvar, Rush University, Chicago, IL, United States

Vinicius Tieppo Francio, Division of Pain Medicine, Department of Anesthesiology, Washington University School of Medicine, St. Louis MO, United States

Carlos E. Trigo, Alivio Pain Center, Carolina, PR, United States

Chheany Ung, Virginia Interventional Pain and Spine Centers, Virginia Tech Carilion School of Medicine, INJX Group Purchasing Organization, Roanoke, VA, United States

Ali Valimahomed, Advanced Orthopedics and Sports Medicine Institute-Harvard Medical School, Freehold, NJ, United States

Ricardo Vallejo, CEO, CFLow Labs Inc., CMO, Capri-Medical Ltd, President Emeritus, MiVI, Madrid, Spain

Adelaide Viguri, Regenerative Pain & Spine, Chicago, IL, United States

Shashank Vodapally, Trinity Health Medical Group - Hauenstein Neurosciences, PM&R and Pain Management, Grand Rapids, MI, United States

Chau Vu, Evolve Restorative Center, Santa Rosa, CA, United States; Interventional Pain Specialist, Evolve Restorative Center, Santa Rosa, CA, United States

Sayed E. Wahezi, Montefiore Multidisciplinary Pain Program, Bronx, NY, United States

Daniel Wang, University of Miami Miller School of Medicine/Health System, Miami, FL, United States

Jacqueline Weisbein, Napa Valley Orthopaedic Medical Group, Napa, CA, United States

Donovan Wilcox, Mary Free Bed Rehabilitation Hospital, Grand Rapids, MI, United States

Derron Keith Wilson, Goodman Campbell Brain & Spine, Carmel, IN, United States

Ajax Yang, The Spine & Pain Institute of New York, New York, NY, United States; Department of Anesthesiology, NYU Langone Medical Center, New York, NY, United States; Department of Anesthesiology, The Zucker School of Medicine at Hofstra/Northwell, New York, NY, United States

Ugur Yener, Montefiore Multidisciplinary Pain Program, Bronx, NY, United States

Mitsukuni Yoshida, Division of Pain Medicine, Department of Anesthesiology, Washington University School of Medicine, St. Louis MO, United States

Preface

This book is a work that takes into account my 30-year practice and my commitment to advancing the field. Partnering with my very close friend and well-respected colleague, Jason Pope, who shares my passion for innovation, we created this book to educate and elevate the field. The highly satisfying part of this book is that we are now seeing neuromodulation become a concern of many different specialties. The movement of electroceuticals to treat a variety of conditions is just beginning, and most likely, this book will require a Second Edition in a few years. The pace is like a disruptive race car, weaving, sometimes crashing, but eventually breaking the course record. We will see more new ideas, a greater funding stream of investors, and more new patents with a focus on intellectual property advancement that will cross many current barriers.

In addition, our commitment to this book is to be comprehensive and to teach our friends and colleagues from basic knowledge to the most advanced methods and techniques. It is imperative that the reader takes this information and combines it with proper hands-on training, a review of the literature, and a carefully selected patient population.

It is our commitment to improve many patients' lives with the proper and judicious use of neuromodulating methods. This book that you now are bringing into your library of information is a tool for you to bring to your clinic, your operating room, and your community. We wish you great success and many successful outcomes. Go out there and make the world a better place.

Timothy Deer, MD

Section 1

General anatomy

Introduction to section 1 general anatomy

Maria Cecilia Guerrero[1] and Timothy Deer[2]

[1]Department of Physical Medicine & Rehabilitation, Larkin Hospital System, South Miami, FL, United States; [2]The Spine and Nerve Center of the Virginias, Charleston, WV, United States

Introduction

Over the past 4 decades, neuromodulation has evolved from an emerging therapy into a central pillar in the management of chronic pain and neurologic dysfunction. Modern systems now engage spinal, central, and peripheral circuits through refined waveforms and physiologic feedback. Yet, one principle remains unchanged: technology is only as good as its anatomical placement and the patient selection guiding the implant. Clinical experience and current evidence lead to the same conclusion—precise, anatomy-guided placement is what turns potential into outcomes [1,2,6].

A neuromodulation lead that sits even a few millimeters off target can miss its mark, cause side effects, or damage nearby structures. A solid grasp of the regional anatomy minimizes those risks and improves efficacy by aligning electrodes with the intended neural population and reducing avoidable complications [1,3,4]. In this field, anatomy is not about memorizing levels or nerve names—it is about *functional, three-dimensional neuroanatomy* that comes alive in real time. It means understanding the microanatomy of the dorsal columns, the position of the DRG within the foramen, the curvature of the epidural space, pedicle and facet relationships, and the fascicular pattern of the peripheral nerves. Knowing those details allows the clinician to navigate the complex terrain with purpose rather than hesitation. That is the art of anatomy—the ability to translate static structures into dynamic understanding [2,5,6].

The growth of the field

As the burden of chronic pain grows, neuromodulation has become increasingly selective, adaptable, and patient-specific. Closed-loop SCS, DRG stimulation, and targeted peripheral approaches reflect a larger shift toward anatomy-informed precision—delivering energy where it matters most. Despite advances in technology, success still depends on the operator's ability to see, interpret, and move precisely within structures that allow little room for error [1,2]. Every improvement in hardware or waveform design only reinforces that truth: precision placement begins with a precise understanding of the target.

Why anatomical mastery matters

Reducing risk through understanding

Recognizing vascular corridors, foraminal width and angle, and the root or DRG trajectories helps prevent complications that occur when the mental picture does not match the patient's anatomy. A few millimeters can be paramount in the difference between a great outcome and a troubling complication [3,4].

Enhancing efficacy through precision

Small deviations can alter coverage or comfort. Anatomical fluency supports deliberate, confident lead placement; fewer revisions; and more consistent results. In addition, the target in the brain, the hypoglossal nerve or vagal nerve, can be a life altering therapy that changes function, quality of life, and disease management. Understanding the surrounding tissues is also very important to aid in dissection, anchoring, and tissue sparing [1,2,6].

Seeing beyond the image

Fluoroscopy, CT, and MRI each tell part of the story. True mastery means reconstructing the anatomy beneath those projections—understanding how the bone, ligament, nerve, and vessel relate in three dimensions [5,6]. When you can visualize what lies beyond the image, it becomes an extension of your hands and judgment. This ability is often experience-based, and early in your career, you may want to err on the side of additional images, angles, and methods of imaging to better understand the "full anatomical picture."

Adapting in real time

No two patients are the same. Prior surgeries, scoliosis, congenital variants, and scar tissue can completely alter the landscape. Anatomical fluency lets you adjust entry points, trajectories, or depth with confidence—decisions grounded in structure, not guesswork. This may require live adjustment during an implant to change your normal method to one tailored to the patient [3–5].

Anatomy as the language of neuromodulation

Anatomy connects every domain of neuromodulation—spinal, central, and peripheral—and unites procedural technique with physiologic insight [6].

- **Spinal anatomy** provides the foundation: Vertebral landmarks, epidural compartments, dorsal columns, nerve roots, and vascular corridors define both access and constraints.
- **Central anatomy** integrates those signals through ascending and descending tracts, brainstem nuclei, anterior cingulate structures, thalamic areas, and cortical networks that transform stimulation into perception or into a change in perception.
- **Peripheral anatomy** bridges accessibility and specificity: Fascicular arrangements, branching patterns, and neural envelopes shape how energy is transmitted and interpreted. In addition, fascial planes, adjacent muscles, and the formation of scar tissue may impact the decision to revise a system, change an implant route, or defer a lead placement.

Together, these systems form a continuous network. To modulate one effectively, you must understand that area of medicine. You may not need to be proficient in all the areas to master one method or technique, but when venturing into new surgeries, you must be humble and learn each area extensively [2,5,6].

The roadmap of this chapter

The following pages move from spinal anatomy—the landscape of lead placement—to central structures that shape signal processing and, finally, to the peripheral nervous system, where targets are more accessible, but precision remains equally critical. Each section connects structure with function, showing how anatomical understanding informs intraoperative decisions and outcomes [1,2,5].

Before we continue, two guiding principles anchor this discussion:

1. Read your own imaging when appropriate.
   MRI, CT, and fluoroscopy often reveal more than a report conveys. Recognize canal caliber, pedicle integrity, DRG position, and the relationships among the facet, foramen, epidural fat, and vessels. Seeing those details is essential for safe, accurate targeting [5,6]. In some areas of the body, you may not have the proper training to read all the areas of implanting interest. In this situation, it is a good idea to speak directly with the radiologist is questions arise, or with a more senior physician who understands the procedure that is planned.
2. Make anatomically informed decisions in real time.

Adjustment from the initial plan is critical. This means a plan is made preoperatively to achieve the desired implant, revision, or explant. As situations occur, such as anatomical deviation, scar tissue, or bleeding, the plan should be adjusted. Fluency allows you to reangle, adjust depth, or redirect safely and efficiently [3–5].

Conclusion

Neuromodulation exists at the intersection of technology, anatomy, and clinical judgment. Devices and algorithms will continue to evolve, but anatomy remains the constant beneath every decision we make. Mastery means thinking in three dimensions, translating imaging into action, and respecting the structures that make this field possible. Spinal, central, and peripheral anatomies form the thread that ties safety, precision, and innovation together. Understanding them deeply allows us to practice with both confidence and humility [1,2,5,6].

References

[1] Mekhail N, Levy RM, Deer TR, et al. Long-term safety and efficacy of closed-loop spinal cord stimulation to treat chronic back and leg pain (Evoke): a double-blind, randomized, controlled trial. Lancet Neurol 2020;19(2):123–34. https://doi.org/10.1016/S1474-4422(19)30414-4.

[2] Esposito MF, Malayil R, Hanes M, Deer T. Unique Characteristics of the Dorsal Root Ganglion as a Target for Neuromodulation. Pain Med 2019;20 (Suppl 1):S23–30. https://doi.org/10.1093/pm/pnz012.

[3] Eldabe S, Buchser E, Duarte RV. Complications of Spinal Cord Stimulation and Peripheral Nerve Stimulation Techniques: A Review of the Literature. Pain Med 2016;17(2):325–36. https://doi.org/10.1093/pm/pnv025.

[4] Liem L, van Dongen E, Huygen FJ, Staats P, Kramer J. The Dorsal Root Ganglion as a Therapeutic Target for Chronic Pain. Reg Anesth Pain Med 2016;41(4):511–9. https://doi.org/10.1097/AAP.0000000000000408.

[5] Sdrulla AD, Guan Y, Raja SN. Spinal Cord Stimulation: Clinical Efficacy and Potential Mechanisms. Pain Pract 2018;18(8):1048–67. https://doi.org/10.1111/papr.12692.

[6] Zander HJ, Graham RD, Anaya CJ, Lempka SF. Anatomical and technical factors affecting the neural response to epidural spinal cord stimulation. J Neural Eng. 2020;17(3):036019. https://doi.org/10.1088/1741-2552/ab8fc4. Published 2020 Jun 12.

Chapter 1

Spinal anatomy regarding neuromodulation methods: An overview

Brandon Gish[1], Robin Mata[2], Roshan Santhosh[3] and Jon Hagedorn[4]

[1]Lexington Clinic Interventional Pain, Lexington, KY, United States; [2]Rush University Medical Center, Chicago, IL, United States; [3]Physical Medicine and Rehabilitation, Larkin Community Hospital, Miami, FL, United States; [4]Mayo Clinic, Rochester, MN, United States

Introduction

Understanding the relevant anatomy of the spine and neural networks is crucial to a successful neuromodulation practice. The extraspinal and intraspinal soft tissues and supportive structures form the landscape from which a neuromodulator must navigate safely to avoid injury and optimize success. Before one can begin placing leads, a specific target for neuromodulation must be identified and a plan for access and placement predetermined. Comorbid conditions, anatomical variations, and prior spinal intervention must be accounted before successful neuromodulation. Herein we endeavor to describe spinal anatomy as it pertains to neuromodulation. We will also depict and review confirmatory fluoroscopic imaging that, when used properly, can give confidence to the practitioner as challenging cases inevitably arise.

Key points

- Before beginning any procedure involving neurostimulation, the practitioner should have identified a pain generator and anatomically relevant target nerve.
- Simply placing a lead in the same location out of habit is likely to result in poor outcomes.
- Relevant imaging of the target for neurostimulation should be reviewed before procedure to mitigate risk of injury and facilitate smooth placement
- Comorbid conditions such as body habitus or other deviations from normal should be considered and plans for altered approach predetermined.
- Utilize fluoroscopy not only as a guide for placement but as a roadmap of anatomical landmarks and confirmation of proper placement.

Fascial planes and soft tissues

The epidural space is a fat filled potential space between the dura mater and the periosteum of the vertebral canal, bounded anteriorly by the posterior longitudinal ligament, posteriorly by the vertebral laminae and ligamentum flavum, and laterally by the vertebral pedicles and intervertebral foramina. During epidural access for spinal procedures, a needle traverses, from superficial to deep: skin, subcutaneous tissue, supraspinous ligament, interspinous ligament, and the ligamentum flavum (Fig. 1.1). As the needle traverses each layer the practitioner encounters varying degrees of resistance, culminating with passage through the highly resistant ligamentum flavum and finally the epidural space, which has no resistance and is thus termed loss of resistance [1]. Understanding these tissue planes and the impact of comorbid conditions (e.g., obesity, age, spinal stenosis, previous surgery) can reduce the risk of inadvertent dural puncture and other complications [2].

During implantation of spinal cord stimulator (SCS) systems the thoracolumbar fascia and nuchal fascia serve as crucial anchoring points for securing leads. The thoracolumbar fascia's (TLF) main attachments are the lumbar spinous process (L2-5), the iliac crest, the iliolumbar ligament and the medial crest of the sacrum [3]. The nuchal fascia has

A Modern Atlas for Implantable Devices of the Spine, Brain, and Nerve. https://doi.org/10.1016/B978-0-443-36528-7.00048-0

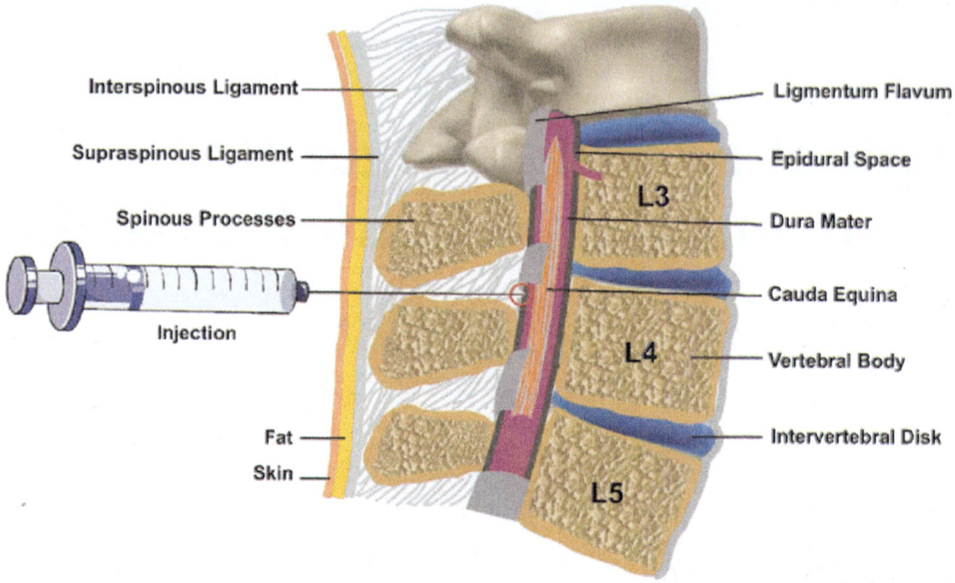

FIGURE 1.1 Illustration of soft tissue layers traversed during epidural access. Labeled superficial to deep: the skin, subcutaneous tissue, supraspinous ligament, interspinous ligament, and ligamentum flavum.

attachments at occipital protuberance (cephalad) and the lower cervical and upper thoracic spinous processes (caudad) [4]. The TLF in the thoracolumbar spine, and nuchal fascia in the cervicothoracic region provide robust anchoring points for SCS leads to reduce migration risk (Fig. 1.2) [5]. These fascial anchors are essential for the long-term effectiveness of SCS and dorsal root ganglion stimulation (DRGS) by ensuring leads remain in the optimal position for delivering electrical stimulation to the spinal cord.

Neuroanatomy

Dorsal column stimulation (cervical/thoracic)

Sensory and motor information are processed in distinct regions of the spinal cord, allowing for a refined and cohesive perception of the world around us. Dorsal horns receive sensory information and are divided into laminae, each with unique cellular architecture and function (Fig. 1.3). Laminae I and II are responsible for receiving and processing pain and temperature sensations (Fig. 1.4). Lamina I, also called the marginal zone, receives signals regarding peripheral tissue damage and temperature from the primary afferent fibers (PAFs) of the dorsal root ganglion (DRG). The most abundant PAF are C (slow, dull pain, heat, itch), A-delta (sharp pain, cold), and A-beta (light touch, mechanoreception of pressure) fibers (Fig. 1.3) [6]. Lamina II, (substantia gelatinosa (SG)), is minimally myelinated but rich in small interneurons and acts as a signal modulator. The SG spans the entire spinal cord extending rostrally into the medulla oblongata, where it eventually becomes the spinal nucleus of the trigeminal nerve. The SG serves a critical neurophysiological role in the gate control theory of pain integrating information from surrounding laminae and descending brain pathways to relay signals to other regions of the dorsal horn and ascending brain [6,7].

Laminae III and IV (nucleus proprius (NP)), are more heavily myelinated and contain a greater diversity of larger interneurons (Fig. 1.4). The SG relays information to the NP for further processing and integration [6]. The NP primarily processes nonnoxious sensory information about touch, pressure, and proprioception. Lamina III receives information from both A-beta and A-delta fibers, which carry pain and temperature signals. Lamina IV receives nonnoxious sensory information, such as light touch and proprioception. Like the SG, laminae III and IV contain interneurons that integrate and modulate incoming sensory information before being relayed to higher brain. The NP acts as a relay station for sensory information about the external environment and the body's internal state [6].

The spinal cord's deeper laminae contribute to motor control and integration. Lamina V acts as a bridge, receiving input from both nociceptors and low-threshold mechanoreceptors, thus processing a broad spectrum of sensory information, encompassing pain, temperature, and touch, and receives descending modulation from higher brain centers, integrating cognitive and emotional influences on sensory perception. Lamina VI receives proprioceptive input from

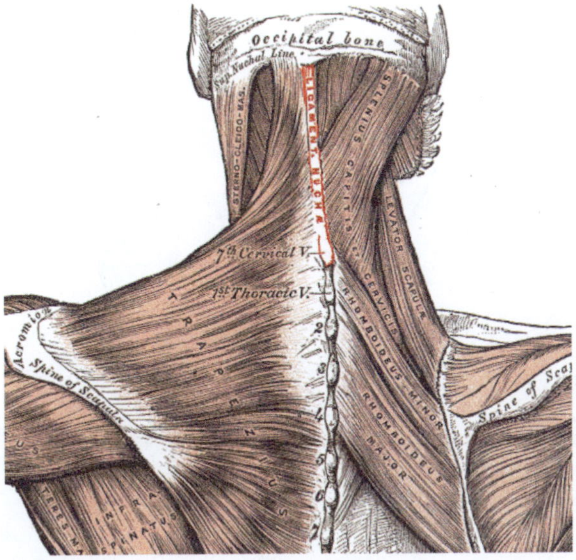

FIGURE 1.2 Anatomical illustration of nuchal fascia.

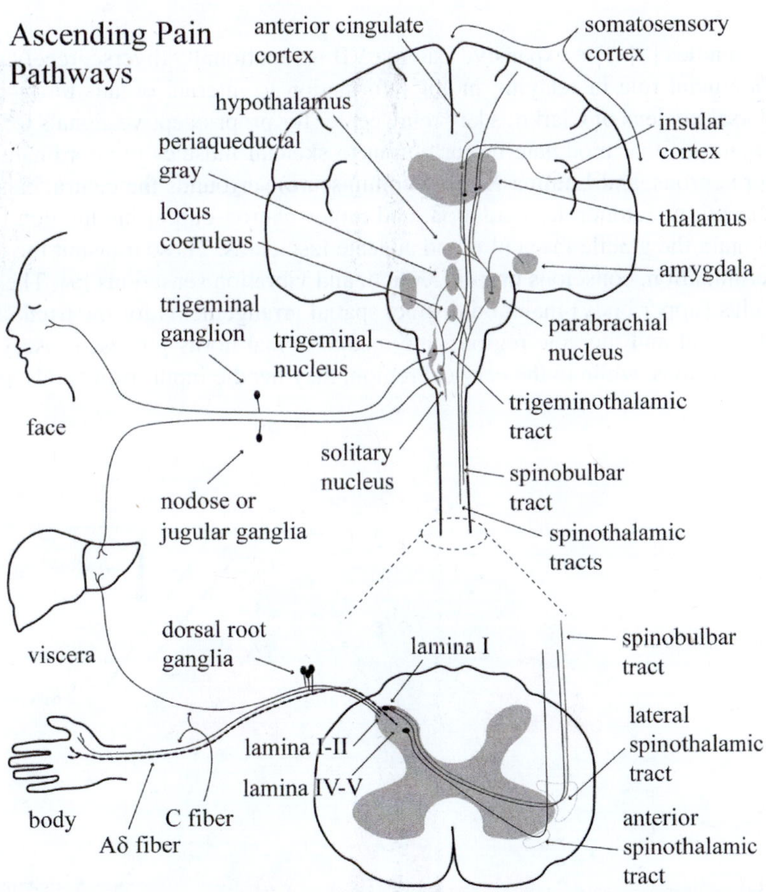

FIGURE 1.3 Illustrated ascending pain pathways with dorsal horn laminae receiving sensory input from somatic and visceral sources.

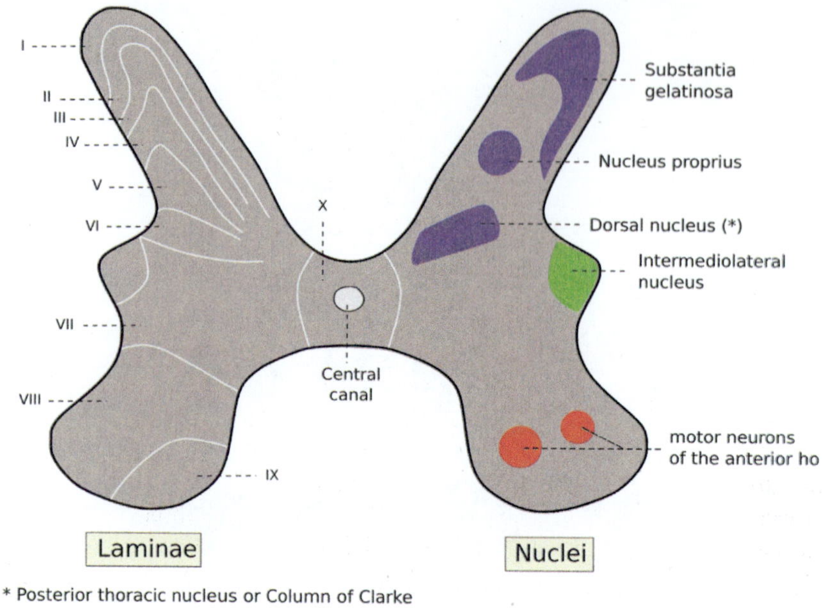

FIGURE 1.4 Illustrated ascending pain pathways with dorsal horn laminae receiving sensory input from somatic and visceral sources.

structures such as muscle spindles [8]. The expansive Lamina VII is functionally diverse, receiving input from laminae II-VI and viscera, playing a crucial role in relaying motor information to internal organs through the autonomic nervous system and housing the dorsal nucleus of Clarke, a key relay center for proprioceptive signals to the cerebellum (Fig. 1.4). Lamina VIII houses interneurons that modulate motor output to skeletal muscles to coordinate movement and reflexes. Lamina IX contains motor neurons, and Lamina X (gray commissure) surrounds the central canal and integrates sensory information, visceral nociception, autonomic regulation, and motor neuron output modulation [8].

The dorsal columns contain the gracile fasciculus and cuneate fasciculus. These transmit the conscious appreciation of fine touch, two-point discrimination, conscious proprioception, and vibration sensations [9]. The gracile fasciculus (lower body) and cuneate fasciculus (upper body) maintain distinct spatial arrangements for the trunk and extremities [9] (Figs. 1.5 and 1.6). In the lumbosacral and thoracic regions, the medial dorsal horns process sensory information from distal body parts such as the feet and toes, while in the cervical region, they handle input from hands and fingers (Fig. 1.6) [10].

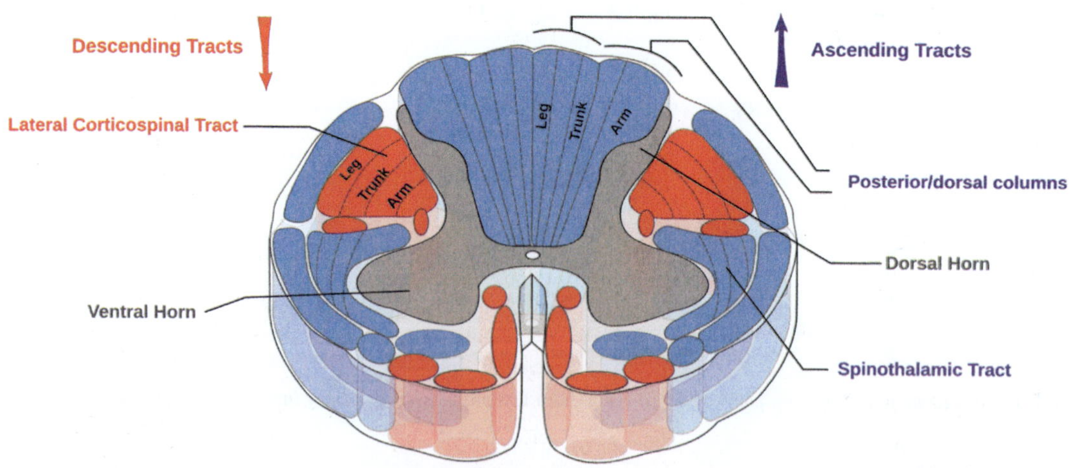

FIGURE 1.5 Illustrated spinal cord cross section with labeled somatotopy by trunk and extremities within the dorsal columns.

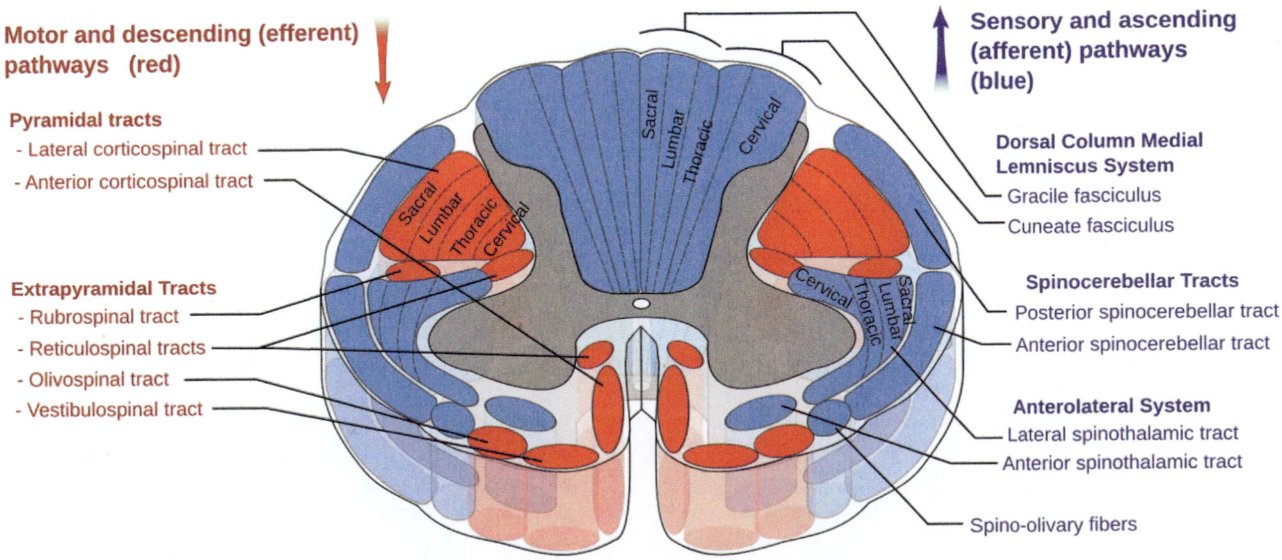

FIGURE 1.6 Detailed illustrated spinal cord cross-section with dorsal column somatotopy and ventral horn localization.

Spinal cord, dural sac, epidural fat

The spinal cord is the central conduit for neural signals, extending from the brainstem to the conus medularis at approximately L1. It is surrounded by a protective layer of membranes called the meninges (pia, arachnoid, and dura mater) and is divided into 31 segments, each of which gives rise to a pair of spinal nerves. Spinal nerve roots travel distally and terminate as peripheral sensory nerves to transmit sensory information along their respective dermatomes (Fig. 1.7) [11]. The organization of the spinal cord and peripheral nerves make it a prime target for neurostimulation therapies to alleviate chronic pain by altering neural activity in specific regions of the body.

The thecal sac contains cerebrospinal fluid, which is a low resistance conduit for neurostimulation to reach the underlying dorsal columns (Fig. 1.8) [12]. SCS leads reside in the fat-filled epidural space. Excessive fat content (epidural lipomatosis) and narrowing (degenerative or congenital spinal stenosis) can affect SCS lead placement and function [13] (Fig. 1.9). In some cases surgical laminectomy may be necessary to create space for SCS leads. When not addressed both conditions can cause cord compression and potentially neurologic deficits when SCS leads are placed [14].

Bones and ligaments of the spine

The bony spine is comprised of seven cervical vertebrae, 12 thoracic vertebrae with costal attachments, and five lumbar vertebrae [15,16]. Ligaments provide support to the spine, enabling function range of motion (Fig. 1.10). The anterior longitudinal ligament (ALL) spans the anterior vertebral bodies, resisting hyperextension, while the posterior longitudinal ligament (PLL) spans the posterior vertebral bodies and resists hyperflexion. The ligamentum flavum (LF) fills the posterior epidural space and attaches each successive laminae, maintaining congruity during different motions. Interspinous ligaments between spinous processes restrict flexion and shear forces, and the supraspinous ligament prevents excessive flexion.

In the cervical spine, the LF is notably thinner than in other spinal regions and must be accounted for during epidural access. Significant degenerative changes can affect LF thickness and contribute to spinal stenosis, which must be assessed before lead placement [17].

Confirmatory epidural placement

SCS and DRG leads are placed with the aid of fluoroscopic guidance [12]. After obtaining epidural access, leads are inserted at the desired spinal level [12]. Appropriate placement is confirmed with fluoroscopic views and confirmed by either paresthesia testing or asleep neuromonitoring. For dorsal column SCS leads are placed near over the dorsal columns to the desired laterality in the posterior epidural space. Anterior–Posterior (AP) and contralateral oblique or lateral

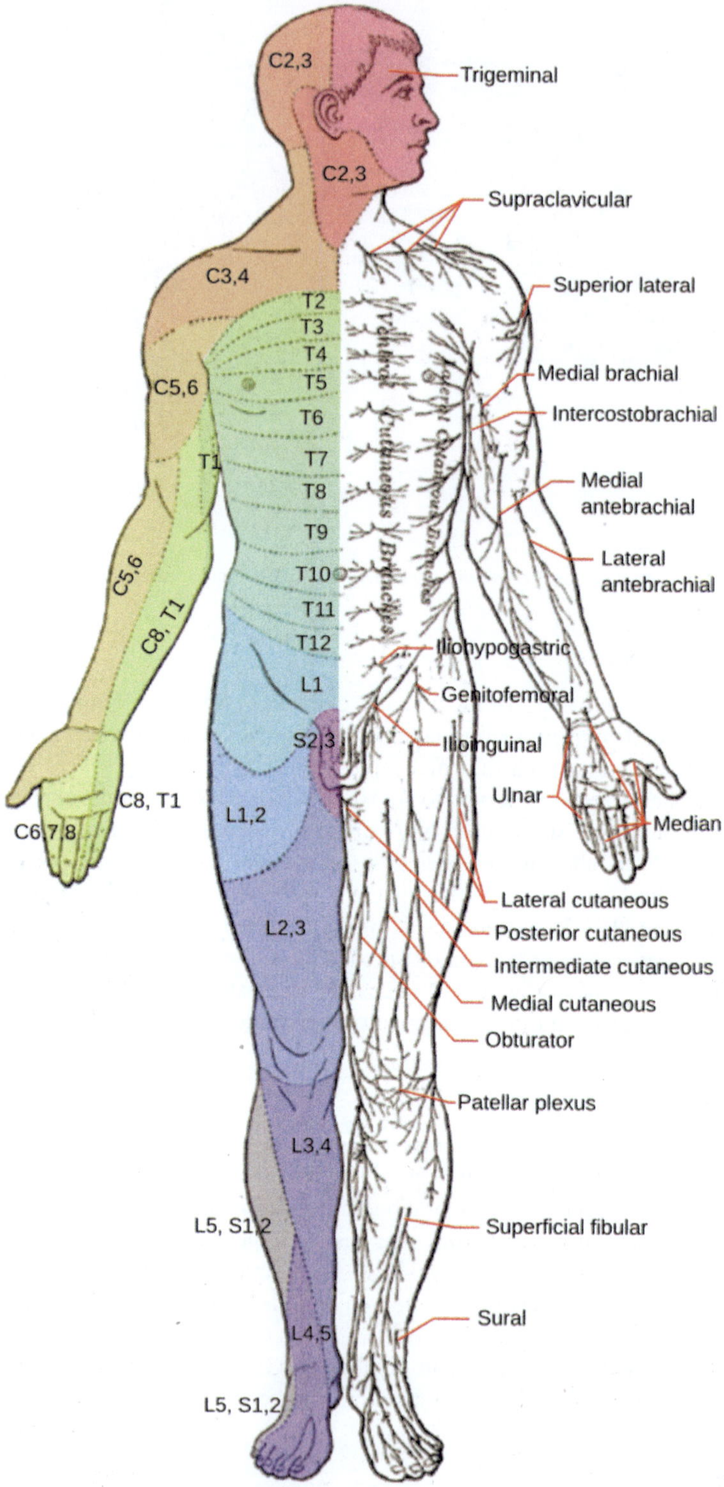

FIGURE 1.7 Anatomic illustration of dermatomes and respective peripheral nerves that derive from spinal nerves.

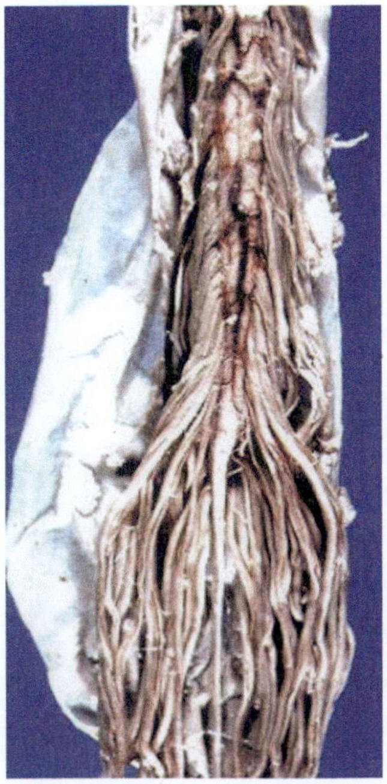

FIGURE 1.8 Cadaveric dissection of dural sac and spinal cord.

fluoroscopic views are used to confirm placement [18,19]. An example of proper posterior placement of dorsal column SCS leads is shown in Fig. 1.11 (thoracic) and Fig. 1.12 (cervical).

Prompt identification of lead malposition is imperative to avoid neurologic complications and poor outcomes. Proper lead placement is in the posterior epidural space as confirmed by fluoroscopy. If there is any question or suspicion, a quick image can ease any concerns. Anterior lead placement may occur when the lead is placed or migrates anterior to the spinal cord. This can occur due to intrathecal placement or when a lead is directed too far laterally, as can occur with steep needle entry. Anterior placement causes motor activation during testing due ventral motor horn stimulation [20,21]. Intrathecal placement can lead to cerebrospinal fluid (CSF) leaks, spinal cord trauma, and low impedance stimulation. Neither are effective or appropriate locations for SCS leads and steps should be taken to remedy this situation.

Proper DRG stimulator lead placement is also confirmed by both fluoroscopy and either awake paresthesia feedback or asleep neuromonitoring. The initial epidural access is through the epidural space, but the leads are smaller and placed directly over the targeted DRG. On AP imaging the middle contacts should be just beneath the 6 o'clock position of the

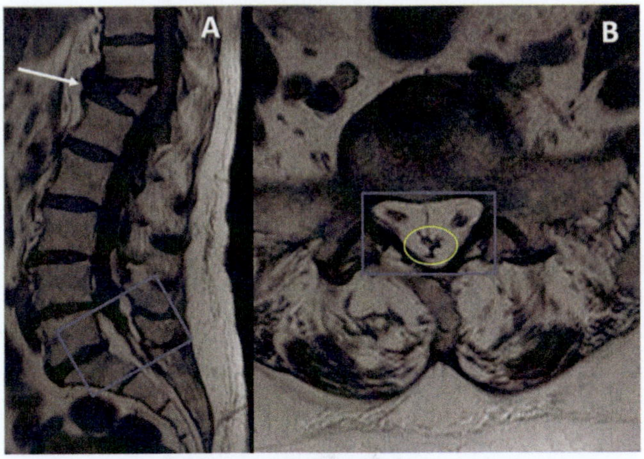

FIGURE 1.9 (A) Sagittal T1-weighted imaging (WI); (B) axial T1-WI. A marked vertebral body collapse of the T12 vertebra is detectable (white arrow). Moreover, a condition of spinal epidural lipomatosis at L5-S1 level (blue rectangles) with compression of the thecal sac resembling the letter "Y" (yellow oval) is found.

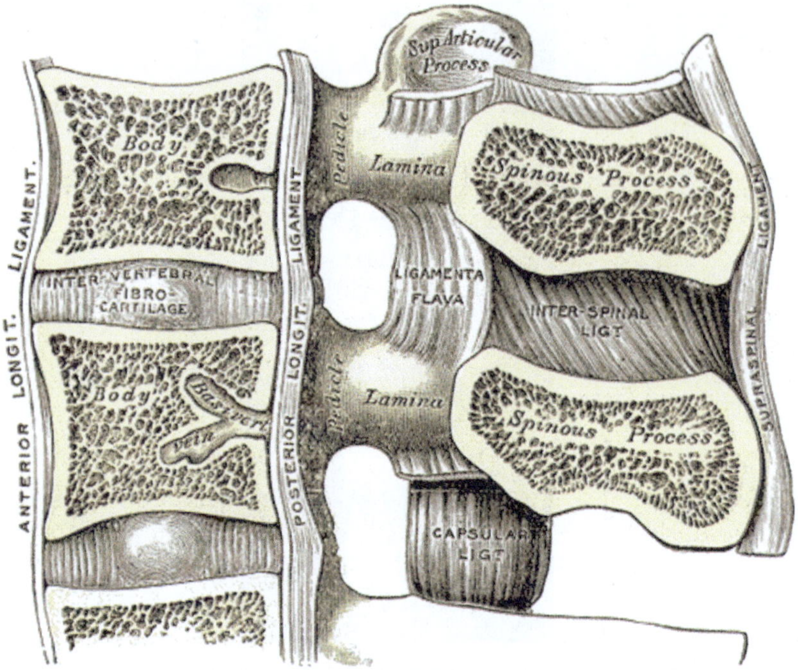

FIGURE 1.10 Lateral view of spinal ligaments including anterior/posterior longitudinal, interspinous, supraspinous ligaments, and ligamentum flavum.

pedicle. Some variances of this may exist as the location of the DRG within the foramen may vary individually and certainly varies based on the spinal level, as previously covered. Lateral fluoroscopic imaging can confirm placement such that the leads appear to be small circles as they are viewed in cross section (Fig. 1.13). For S1 placement, AP views will have an inferolateral trajectory along the S1 foramen, but more importantly the lateral view should show leads with the distal tip just anterior to the anterior sacral line (Fig. 1.14).

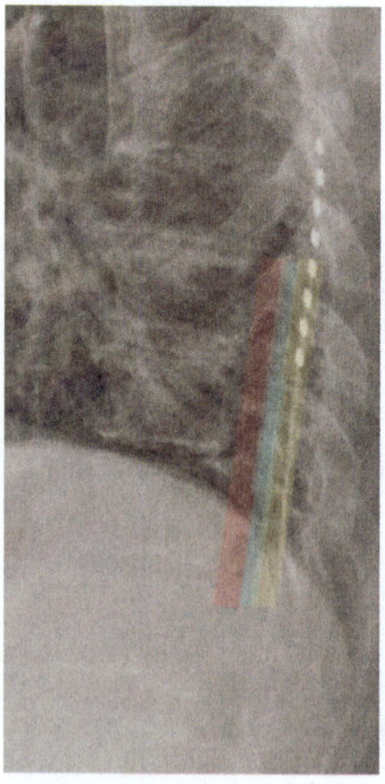

FIGURE 1.11 Lateral thoracic fluoroscopic image of posterior (yellow) percutaneous lead placement. Lateral (blue) and anterior (red) placement are noted.

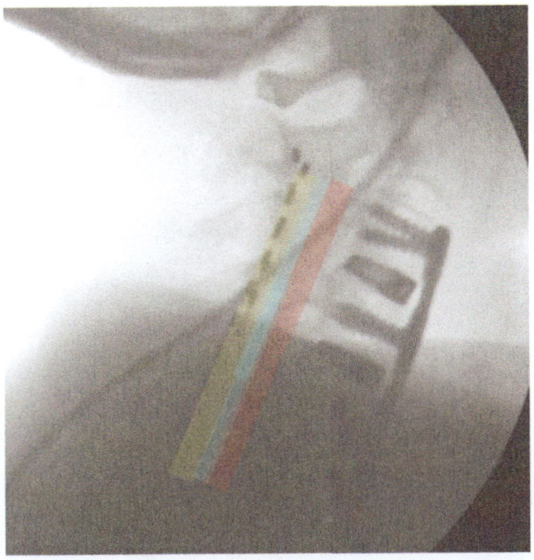

FIGURE 1.12 Lateral cervical fluoroscopic image of posterior (yellow) percutaneous lead placement. Lateral (blue) and anterior (red) placement are noted.

The dorsal root ganglion (DRG) consists of a collection of pseudouniploar neuron cell bodies, which carry sensory signals from A-beta, A-delta, and C type nerve fibers [22]. The DRG is circumferentially surrounded by supportive glial cells and is permeable to signaling molecules including cytokines [23]. The nerve fibers within the DRG are somatotopically organized in animal models, with specific peripheral nerve tracts having dorsal-ventral stratification [24]. The

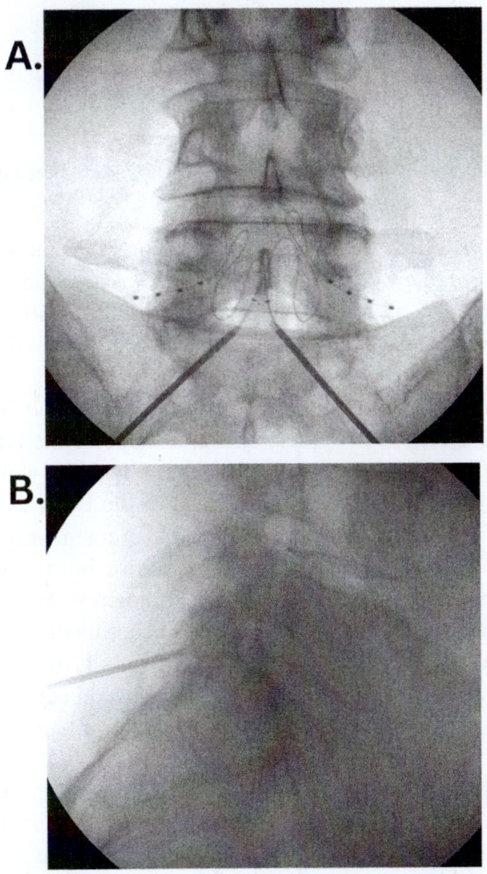

FIGURE 1.13 AP (A) and lateral (B) fluoroscopic views of DRG leads placed over the bilateral L5 DRG.

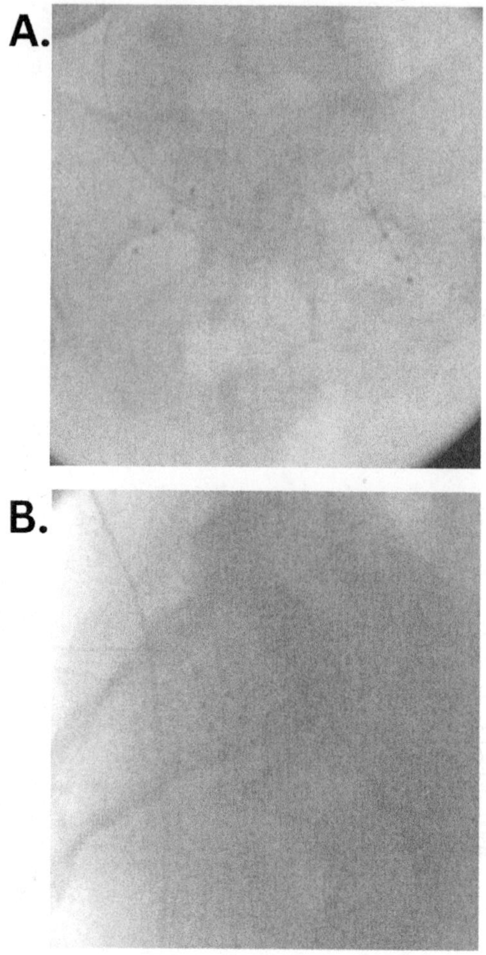

FIGURE 1.14 AP (A) and lateral (B) fluoroscopic views of DRG leads placed over the bilateral S1 DRG.

neuron cell bodies that reside in the DRG receive sensory information from the periphery and communicate this to the central nervous system in the spinal cord. This coordinated organization is theorized to include multiple pain processing mechanisms within the DRG that has made it a target for neuromodulation. Additionally, the limited CSF around the DRG allows for less impedance, more uniform and lower amplitude electrical stimulation of the nerve fibers when compared with dorsal column stimulation [22].

The DRG is located bilaterally within the spinal foramen, extending from the epidural space. There are 8 cervical, 12 thoracic, 5 lumbar, and 4 paired sacral DRGs. The typical size and shape of the DRG is variable and correlates with the number of neurons contained within. The DRG increases in size from C1–C8 as well as L1-L5, with larger DRGs found at lower levels of the spinal column [25]. Within the sacrum, the size of the DRG decreases from S1 to S4 [26]. The DRG and distal nerve root exit the spinal canal through the intervertebral foramen, which has anterior borders formed by the posterior aspects of the vertebral body and disc complex. The posterior border is formed by the superior and inferior articular processes and the facet joints. The roof and floor of the foramen is bound by adjacent pedicles. There are five major types of transforaminal ligaments including the superior corporopedicular, inferior corporopedicular, superior transforaminal, midtransforaminal, and inferior transforaminal ligaments [26]. Finer ligaments known as intraforminal ligaments suspend neural and vascular tissues and anchor them from contact with transforaminal ligaments and surrounding bony structures [27]. These are especially relevant to DRG stimulation for both placement and reducing lead movement (Fig. 1.15).

The DRG is located in the super portion of the foramen adjacent to the superior pedicle. There is variability in the location of the DRG within the intervertebral foramen, with more rostral DRGs at level of L1 found extraforaminally. The DRG is consistently in the foramen in the lumbar levels but tends to reside more laterally as you approach L5 [25]. The primary blood supply of the DRG arises from the spinal branch of the dorsal trunk of the segmental arteries [26].

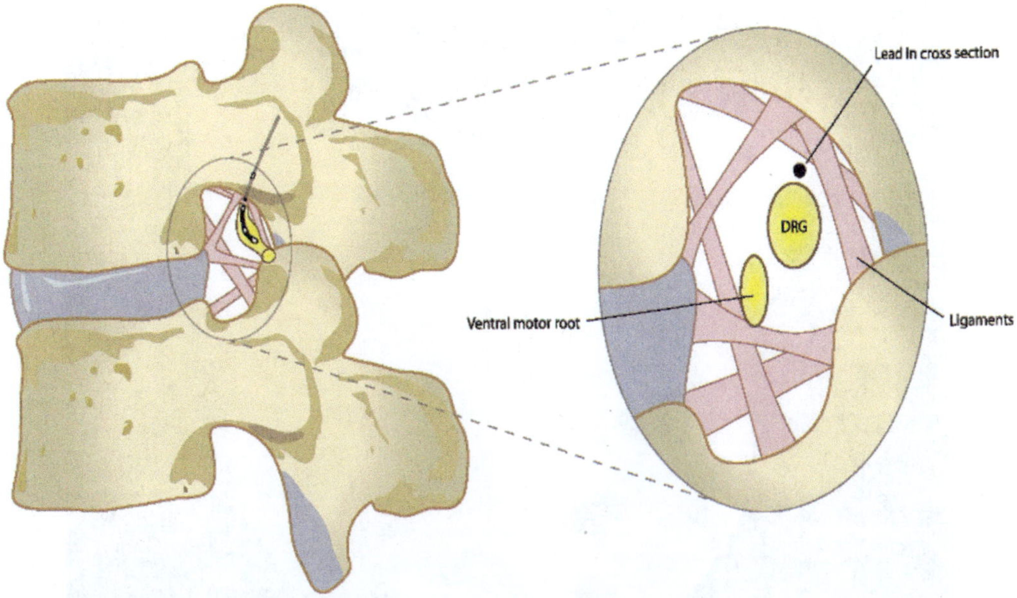

FIGURE 1.15 A sagittal view of the foramen with several transforaminal ligaments pictured in purple. Not depicted in this schematic are the intraforaminal suspensory ligaments supporting the DRG and spinal nerve, as well as vasculature.

The posterior radiculomedullary branch of the segmental arteries is found along the ventral aspect of the dorsal spinal nerve. Delicate placement of instruments and leads is necessary to avoid trauma to surrounding tissues and vasculature (Fig. 1.16).

A foundational understanding of sacral anatomy can alleviate many of the procedural challenges associated with sacral DRG lead placement. The sacrum is formed by the fusion of 5 sacral vertebrae. There are two ridges that run laterally to the midline sacral crest known as intermediate crests, most prominent at the S1 level. The intermediate crests are formed from the fused articular processes of the sacral vertebrae and extends caudally to form the sacral cornua, denoting the

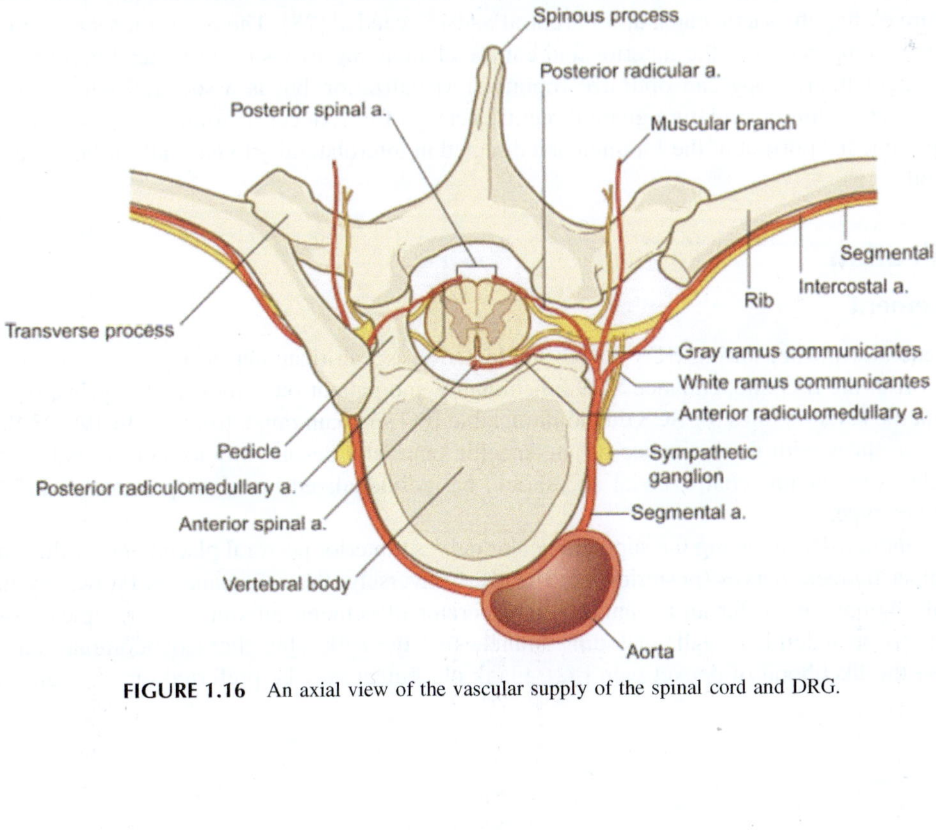

FIGURE 1.16 An axial view of the vascular supply of the spinal cord and DRG.

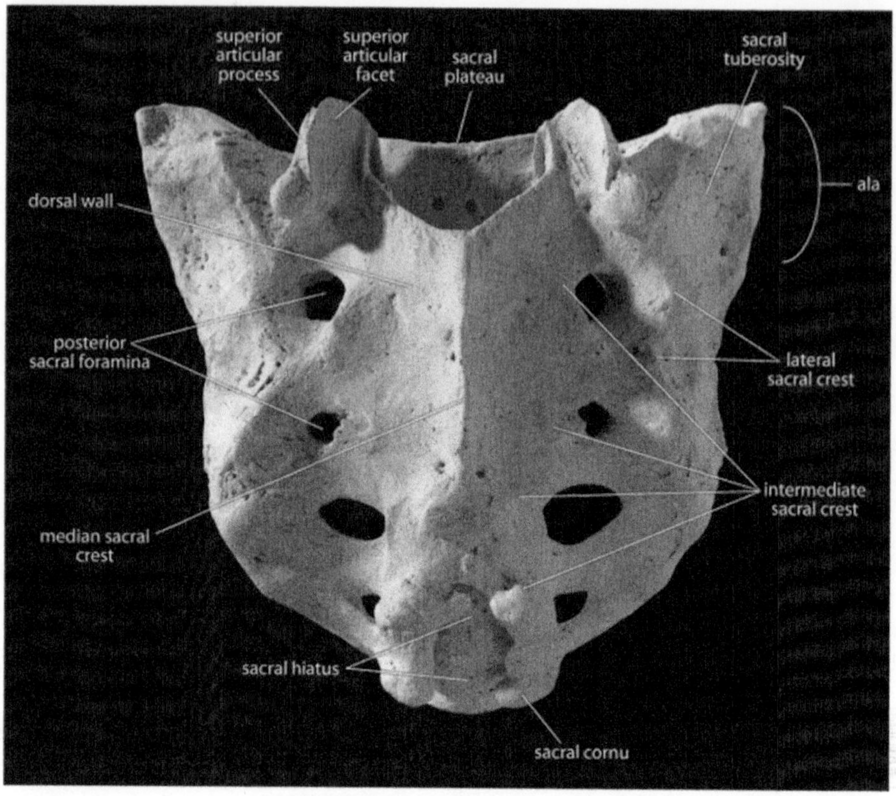

FIGURE 1.17 Sacral bony anatomy.

sacrococcygeal hiatus. At this level, these intermediate crests may partially obstruct the medial aspect of the S1 posterior sacral foramen. The sacral foramina are the sacral analogue to the intervertebral foramen and have both an anterior and posterior component. The anterior sacral foramen is bordered rostrally and caudally by the pedicles and laterally by the fused winged sacral transverse processes. The anterior sacral foramina projects inferolaterally with sacral DRG, nerve root, and vasculature exiting the sacral canal at 30° ventral and 15° caudad [28]. The posterior sacral foramina is typically smaller in size when compared with the anterior and can be challenging to visualize under fluoroscopy. An ipsilateral oblique approach under fluoroscopy can optimize foraminal visualization but is associated with an increased risk for damage to DRG or surrounding vasculature given direct trajectory of introducer instruments. It is best to enter the sacral foramen at the superomedial portion of the foramen and directed in inferolaterally to naturally follow the sacral nerve root [29] (Figs. 1.17 and 1.18).

Clinical application

Generator placement

Creation of the generator pocket during SCS device implantation is a critical step to minimize postoperative pain and long-term discomfort at the IPG site, enhance SCS functionality and patient outcomes, and improve overall satisfaction. Studies suggest that the revision rates for SCS due to intractable IPG site pain range from 1% to 19% [30]. The location of IPG implantation correlates with the incidence of site-specific pain, and despite biomechanical and computer modeling [31] the optimal IPG site remains controversial and should be individualized based on patient-specific factors, surgical technique, and device type.

Chest wall placement risks damaging the supraclavicular nerves (anterior pectoral placement) or the anterior cutaneous branches of the upper thoracic nerves (posterior chest wall). Conversely, the subcutaneous fat density in the abdominal and posterior flank regions may offer an advantage for generator placement, although the complex vascular and nerve structures in the anterior abdominal wall, including branches of the subcostal, thoracoabdominal, and iliohypogastric nerves can increase the likelihood of pocket pain [32]. Flank placement may be preferred due to reduced lead extension

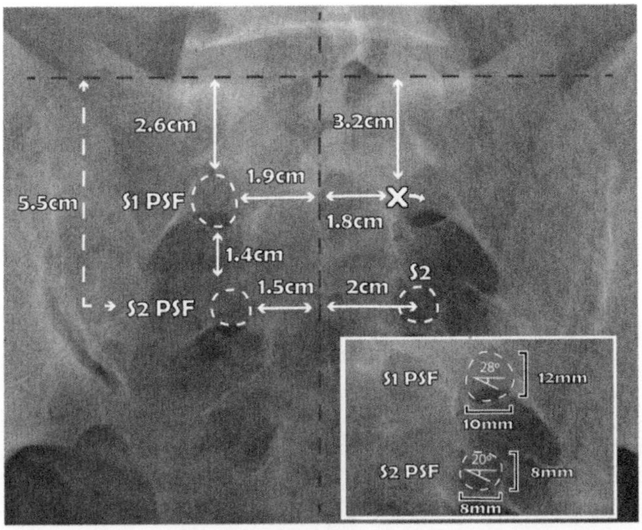

FIGURE 1.18 Sacral measurements under fluoroscopy with the sacral endplate aligned at 35 degrees. Gray dashed-lines represent the midline and the aligned sacral promontory. The inset box demonstrates the angle at which the dorsal root ganglion and nerve root exit the intervertebral foramen. *PSF*, posterior sacral foramen.

length, decreased risk of generator migration with proper anchoring, and improved patient comfort. Flank placement is generally either superficial or deep to the thoracolumbar fascia, which serves as the anchoring point. One should reference manufacturer requirements for tissue depth for charging and reprogramming. Blunt dissection can help mitigate the risk of injury to the lateral branches of the dorsal rami of the lower thoracic spinal nerves as they are cutaneous branches pierced through the thoracolumbar fascia (Fig. 1.19). Although buttock placement is commonly performed, it has been associated with a higher incidence of pocket pain and revision surgery, potentially due to the proximity to the posterior superior iliac spine and cluneal nerves, leading to cluneal neuralgia or periosteal irritation [33]. Moreover, generator placement in the buttock has been linked to higher revision rates compared with flank placement [34]. Several common generator implant sites for thoracic SCS and DRG are shown in Figs. 1.20 and 1.21.

Lead anchoring

Proper anchoring of the leads to the thoracolumbar or nuchal fascia is important to reduce the risk of migration. It is the authors opinion that anchoring devices are preferred over placing sutures directly on the leads as this may facilitate early lead deterioration and fracture due to having a single focal stress point. It is important that the distal lead anchor extend deep to the fascia into the deeper tissues (Figs. 1.22 and 1.23) and not reside on the fascial plane. Despite an anchor properly being adhered to fascia, if the tip does not extend deep to the fascial plane the leads can migrate and move within this plane, potentially leading to migration or fracture. The point at which the lead exits the anchor distally is a common fracture location due to the rigid nature of the lead anchor and the inherent movement of the surrounding tissues outside the anchor.

Scoliosis

Scoliosis is a challenging syndrome to treat. For a patient undergoing thoracic dorsal column stimulation with thoracic scoliosis, lead placement can be challenging. Proper fluoroscopic alignment is crucial to identify landmarks and safely enter the epidural space. Fluoroscopic alignment will need to be adjusted as the fluoroscope is moved cephalad to align the spinous processes in midline and square the vertebral endplates to accommodate for scoliotic changes. On table testing is highly recommended as paresthesia testing can reveal whether lead placement is too lateral. Visual landmarks may not account for the rotation of the spine and the position of the spinal cord relative to the bony landmarks. If leads are placed too far laterally the patient may experience flank or rib paresthesia, which is therefore not optimally aligned over the dorsal columns. A patient with scoliosis undergoing dorsal column SCS trial is shown in Fig. 1.24.

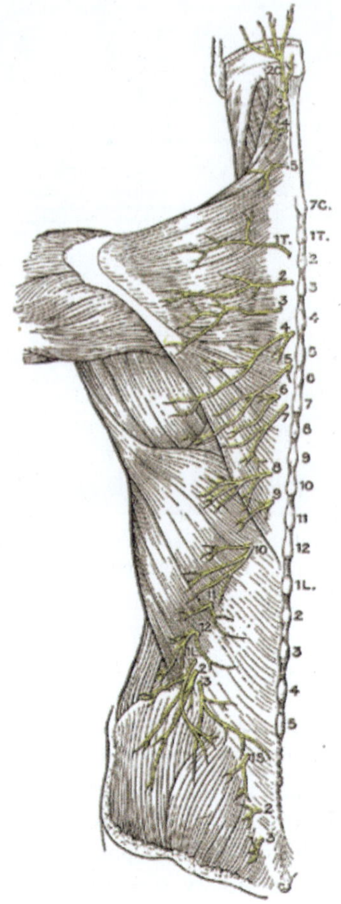

FIGURE 1.19 Anatomic illustration demonstrating cutaneous branches of the lateral branch of the dorsal rami of the lower thoracic spinal nerves as they traverse the thoracolumbar fascia.

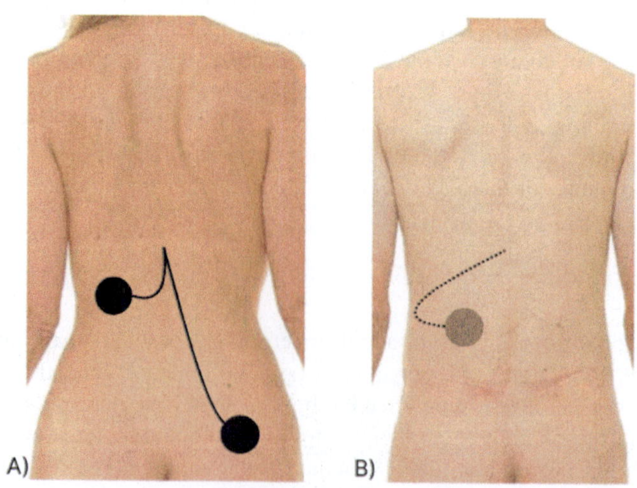

FIGURE 1.20 Typical locations for generator placement after thoracic SCS placement. (A) paraspinal and gluteal, (B) abdominal.

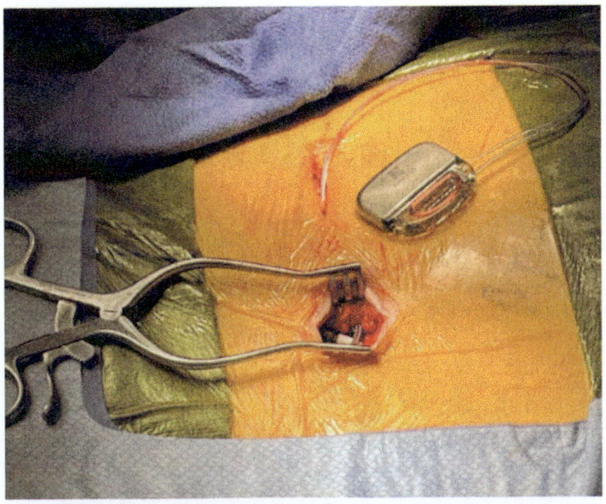

FIGURE 1.21 SCS leads placed near midline, anchored to thoracolumbar fascia and tunneled to the left flank for generator implantation.

Previous surgery

When evaluating a patient for neurostimulation with a previous history of spine surgery, it is important to have a thorough understanding of the previous surgical interventions, whether this included fusion, laminectomy, discectomy, and the levels treated. Preoperative magnetic resonance imaging (MRI) is useful for determining the degree of stenosis present as this may be exacerbated adjacent to fused levels. In the case of a prior laminectomy, needle entry for epidural access should not occur at these levels and it is not advised to drive the leads in the epidural space through a level that previously undergone a laminectomy as the dura is likely to have adhered to the ligamentum flavum and risk of dural tear is high. In the case of a previous pedicle fusion that extends into the thoracic spine, needle entry level will need to be cephalad to the fusion and there must be adequate distance within the epidural space to contain the leads. Levels adjacent to fusions are likely to develop stenosis when this may not otherwise be expected. This is relevant to epidural access and preoperative MRI should be utilized to evaluate this before needle entry (Fig. 1.25).

Obesity

In obese patients the depth from skin to ligamentum flavum is much greater depending on adipose distribution. To achieve a properly angled entry to the epidural space, the needle should begin at a more inferior position. This angle can be gauged with contralateral oblique or lateral views. A shallow needle angle helps prevent lateral lead displacement during entry into the epidural space. In the case of PNS, one should reduce the distance from lead contacts to generator as excessive body motion is expected due to abnormal body habitus.

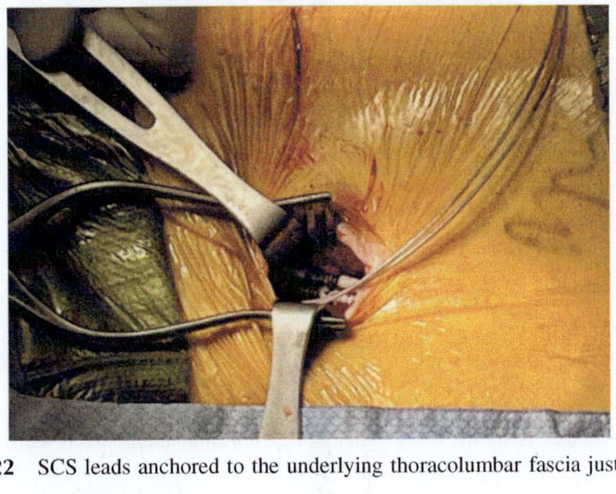

FIGURE 1.22 SCS leads anchored to the underlying thoracolumbar fascia just off midline.

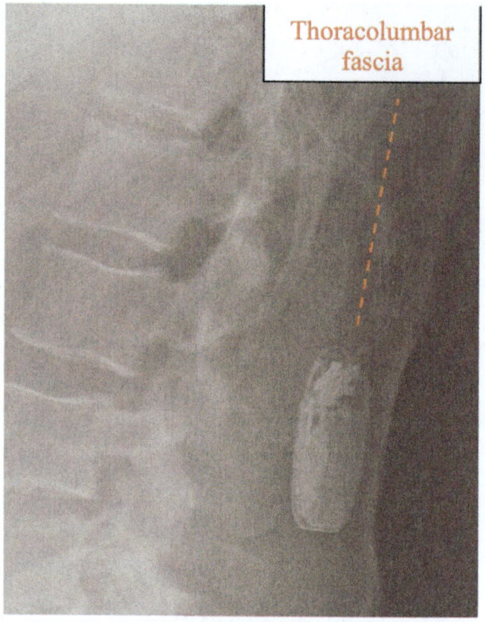

FIGURE 1.23 Lateral fluoroscopic view demonstrating percutaneous dorsal column thoracic spinal cord stimulator leads entering the epidural space at T12-L1, with lead anchoring devices anchored to the thoracolumbar fascia. Importantly, the distal tip of the anchors pierced tissues deep to the thoracolumbar fascia.

Lead migration

Lead migration can occur due to poor surgical anchoring technique or excessive movement of the patient in the early postoperative period. This risk can be mitigated by instituting appropriate postoperative protocols to limit aggressive twisting or bending at the waist for approximately 6 weeks. The use of anchoring devices sutured to the underlying fascia with nonabsorbable suture should be adequate to reduce the risk of migration.

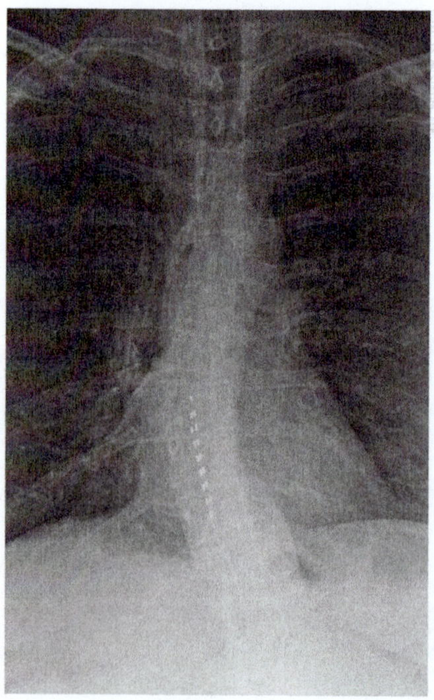

FIGURE 1.24 A patient with thoracic scoliosis is shown while undergoing a dorsal column percutaneous spinal cord stimulator trial with leads in midline.

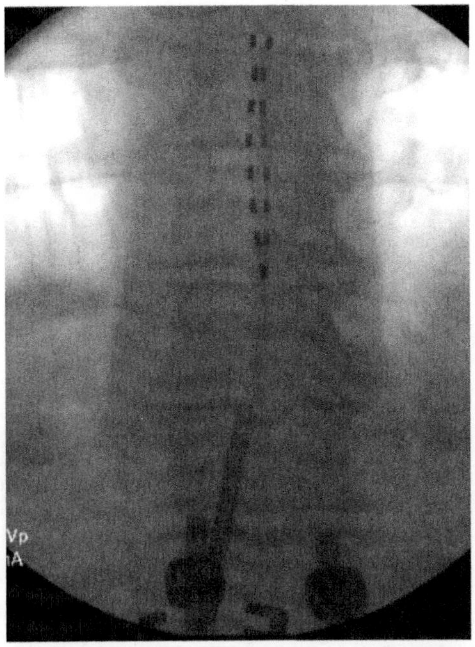

FIGURE 1.25 Percutaneous thoracic dorsal column lead placement is shown adjacent to a thoracolumbar fusion that extends to T11, with epidural access achieved at the T9-10 level and leads advanced to the superior portion of T7.

Lead fracture

Lead fracture can occur due to trauma of the leads, excessive shearing motion of surrounding tissues, and poor surgical technique. As previously mentioned, appropriate anchoring deep to the fascia can reduce stress on the leads as they exit the anchoring device. It is important to place the leads as close to midline as possible to avoid the shear effect of the lumbar extensor musculature. It is difficult to guard against all trauma, however patient should be advised of the fragile nature of the underlying lead system and the locations where they are most susceptible (Fig. 1.26).

Percutaneous versus paddle

The choice of percutaneous or surgical paddle leads depends on physician preference, experience, and anatomical considerations. In the cervical spine, if there has been posterior cervical laminectomy it is not advised to pass an epidural lead

A) B)

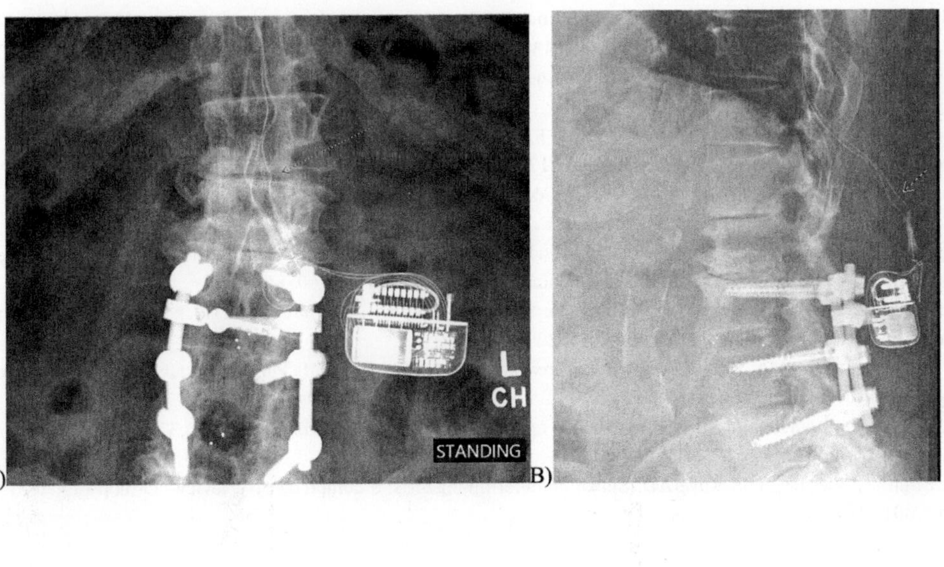

FIGURE 1.26 Thoracic SCS leads with lead fracture (arrow) as the lead exits the anchoring device shown in anterior–posterior (A) and lateral (B) views.

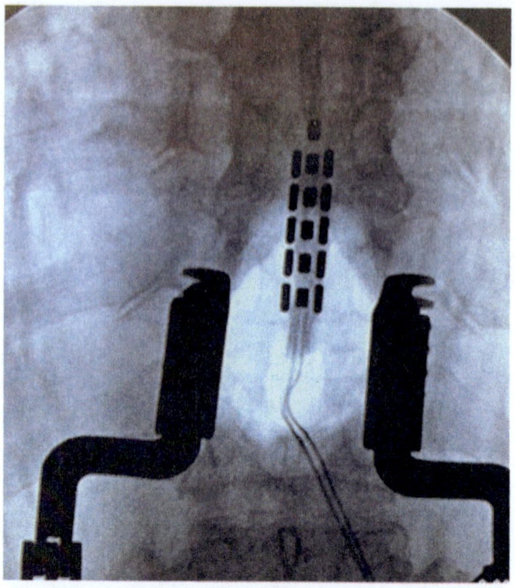

FIGURE 1.27 Fluoroscopic anterior–posterior view of intraoperative paddle lead placement in the thoracic spine.

through this laminectomy and would be preferred to place a retrograde paddle through the C2-3 space when appropriate. In patients that have had previous lead migration or are felt to be at high risk for lead migration (i.e., obesity) a paddle lead may be preferred, as it has demonstrated lower risk of migration [35]. The average spinal canal is large enough to support either a percutaneous or paddle lead place; however, congenital or degenerative stenosis can reduce the diameter of the canal and should be noted, particularly in the cervical spine. If the target level of stimulation has significant stenosis that would not safely support a percutaneous lead, paddle lead placement with decompressive laminectomy can create adequate space for lead placement and reduce the risk of cord compression (Fig. 1.27).

References

[1] Jane LA, Wray AA. Lumbar puncture. In: StatPearls [internet]. Treasure Island (FL): StatPearls Publishing; 2025. Available from: https://www.ncbi.nlm.nih.gov/books/NBK557553/.

[2] Deer TR, Stewart CD. Complications of spinal cord stimulation: identification, treatment, and prevention. Pain Med 2008;9(Suppl. 1). https://doi.org/10.1111/j.1526-4637.2008.00444.x.

[3] Bogduk N, Macintosh JE. The applied anatomy of the thoracolumbar fascia. Spine 1984;9(2):164–70. https://doi.org/10.1097/00007632-198403000-00006.

[4] Kadri PA, Al-Mefty O. Anatomy of the nuchal ligament and its surgical applications. Neurosurgery 2007;61(5 Suppl. 2):301–4. https://doi.org/10.1227/01.neu.0000303985.65117.ea.

[5] Chapman KB, Patel KV, van Helmond N, Chien GCC. Dorsal root ganglion stimulation lead fracture within the superficial fascial layers in 4 cases. A&A Pract 2020;14(11):e01307. https://doi.org/10.1213/XAA.0000000000001307.

[6] Sheikh NK, Dua A. Neuroanatomy, substantia gelatinosa. In: StatPearls [internet]. Treasure Island (FL): StatPearls Publishing; 2025. Available from: https://www.ncbi.nlm.nih.gov/books/NBK551522/.

[7] Wall PD. The role of substantia gelatinosa as a gate control. Res Publ Assoc Res Nerv Ment Dis 1980;58:205–31.

[8] Khalid S, Tubbs RS. Neuroanatomy and neuropsychology of pain. Cureus 2017;9(10):e1754. https://doi.org/10.7759/cureus.1754.

[9] Al-Chalabi M, Reddy V, Alsalman I. Neuroanatomy, posterior column (dorsal column). In: StatPearls [internet]. Treasure Island (FL): StatPearls Publishing; January 2025. Available from: https://www.ncbi.nlm.nih.gov/books/NBK507888/.

[10] Neuroscience. In: Purves D, Augustine GJ, Fitzpatrick D, et al., editors. Descending control of spinal cord circuitry: general information. 2nd ed. Sunderland (MA): Sinauer Associates; 2001 Available from: https://www.ncbi.nlm.nih.gov/books/NBK10978/.

[11] Ganapathy MK, Reddy V, Tadi P. Neuroanatomy, spinal cord morphology. In: StatPearls [internet]. Treasure Island (FL): StatPearls Publishing; January 2025. Available from: https://www.ncbi.nlm.nih.gov/books/NBK545206/.

[12] Dydyk AM, Tadi P. Spinal cord stimulator implant. In: StatPearls [internet]. Treasure Island (FL): StatPearls Publishing; January 2025. Available from: https://www.ncbi.nlm.nih.gov/books/NBK555994/.

[13] Zhang Y, Wood MJ, Gilligan C. Spinal cord stimulation in a patient with spinal epidural lipomatosis. Pain Med 2011;12(3):377–81. https://doi.org/10.1111/j.1526-4637.2011.01057.x.

[14] Walker PB, Sark C, Brennan G, Smith T, Sherman WF, Kaye AD. Spinal epidural lipomatosis: a comprehensive review. Orthop Rev 2021;13(2):25571. https://doi.org/10.52965/001c.25571.

[15] Kaiser JT, Reddy V, Launico MV, et al. Anatomy, head and neck: cervical vertebrae. In: StatPearls [internet]. Treasure Island (FL): StatPearls Publishing; January 2025. Available from: https://www.ncbi.nlm.nih.gov/books/NBK539734/.

[16] Waxenbaum JA, Reddy V, Futterman B. Anatomy, back, thoracic vertebrae. In: StatPearls [internet]. Treasure Island (FL): StatPearls Publishing; January 2025. Available from: https://www.ncbi.nlm.nih.gov/books/NBK459153/.

[17] Sayit E, Daubs MD, Aghdasi B, Montgomery SR, Inoue H, Wang CJ, Wang BJ, Phan KH, Scott TP. Dynamic changes of the ligamentum flavum in the cervical spine assessed with kinetic magnetic resonance imaging. Glob Spine J 2013;3(2):69–74. https://doi.org/10.1055/s-0033-1337121.

[18] Hayatsu K, Tomita M, Fujihara H, Baba H, Yamakura T, Taga K, Shimoji K. The placement of the epidural catheter at the predicted site by electrical stimulation test. Anesth Analg 2001;93(4):1035–9. https://doi.org/10.1097/00000539-200110000-00048.

[19] Zan E, Kurt KN, Yousem DM, Christo PJ. Spinal cord stimulators: typical positioning and postsurgical complications. AJR Am J Roentgenol 2011;196(2):437–45. https://doi.org/10.2214/AJR.10.4789.

[20] Olmsted ZT, Wu PB, Katouzian A, Dorsi MJ. Intrathecal placement of percutaneous spinal cord stimulation leads: illustrative cases. J Neurosurg Case Lessons 2024;8(13):CASE24275.

[21] Pope JE, Stanton-Hicks M. Accidental subdural spinal cord stimulator lead placement and stimulation. Neuromodulation J Int Neuromodul Soc 2011;14(1):30–3. https://doi.org/10.1111/j.1525-1403.2010.00299.x.

[22] Berger AA, Liu Y, Possoit H, et al. Dorsal root ganglion (DRG) and chronic pain. Anesthesiol Pain Med 2021;11(2). https://doi.org/10.5812/aapm.113020.

[23] Esposito MF, Malayil R, Hanes M, Deer T. Unique characteristics of the dorsal root ganglion as a target for neuromodulation. Pain Med June 2019;20(Suppl. _1):S23–30. https://doi.org/10.1093/pm/pnz012.

[24] Puigdellívol-Sánchez A, Prats-Galino A, Ruano-Gil D, Molander C. Sciatic and femoral nerve sensory neurones occupy different regions of the L4 dorsal root ganglion in the adult rat. Neurosci Lett July 31, 1998;251(3):169–72. https://doi.org/10.1016/s0304-3940(98)00518-7.

[25] Shen J, Wang HY, Chen JY, Liang BL. Morphologic analysis of normal human lumbar dorsal root ganglion by 3D MR imaging. AJNR Am J Neuroradiol 2006 ;27(10):2098–103.

[26] Gilchrist RV. Anatomy of the intervertebral foramen. Pain Phys 2002;5(4):372–8. https://doi.org/10.36076/ppj.2002/5/372.

[27] Akdemir G. Thoracic and lumbar intraforaminal ligaments: laboratory investigation. J Neurosurg Spine SPI 2010;13(3):351–5. https://doi.org/10.3171/2010.3.SPINE09799.

[28] Chapman KB, Sayed D, Lamer T, Hunter C, Weisbein J, Patel KV, Dickerson D, Hagedorn JM, Lee DW, Amirdelfan K, Deer T, Chakravarthy K. Best practices for dorsal root ganglion stimulation for chronic pain: guidelines from the American society of pain and neuroscience. J Pain Res 2023;16:839–79. https://doi.org/10.2147/JPR.S364370.

[29] Chapman KB, van Helmond N, Kallewaard JW, Vissers KC, Patel KV, Motivala S, Hagedorn JM, Deer TR, Dickerson DM. An anatomy-informed, novel technique for S1 dorsal root ganglion stimulation lead placement. Pain Med October 2022;23(10):1750–6. https://doi.org/10.1093/pm/pnac062.

[30] Dietvorst S, Decramer T, Lemmens R, Morlion B, Nuttin B, Theys T. Pocket pain and neuromodulation: negligible or neglected? Neuromodulation 2017;20(6):600–5.

[31] Henderson JM, Schade CM, Sasaki J, et al. Prevention of mechanical failures in implanted SCS systems. Neuromodulation 2006;9(3):183–91.

[32] Baranidharan G, Bretherton B, Richert G, et al. Pocket pain, does location matter: a single-center retrospective study of patients implanted with a spinal cord stimulator. Reg Anesth Pain Med 2020;45(11):891–7.

[33] Abd-Elsayed A, Gyorfi MJ. Peripheral nerve stimulation for the treatment of superior cluneal neuralgia: a cadaver demonstration of a novel technique for lead placement. J Pain Res March 20, 2024;17:1235–41. https://doi.org/10.2147/JPR.S450177.

[34] Mehta SH, et al. Implantable pulse generator site may Be associated with spinal cord stimulation revision surgeries. Neuromodulation 2021;24(8):1336–40.

[35] El Hadwe S, Wronowski F, Rehman S, Ansong SYO, Barone DG. Cylindrical vs paddle leads in spinal cord stimulation for the long-term treatment of chronic pain: a systematic review and meta-analysis. Neuromodulation February 2025;28(2):204–33. https://doi.org/10.1016/j.neurom.2024.10.007.

Further reading

[1] Basadonna PT, Gasparini D, Rucco V. Iliolumbar ligament insertions. In vivo anatomic study. Spine 1996;21(20):2313–6. https://doi.org/10.1097/00007632-199610150-00002.

[2] Chin KJ, Versyck B, Elsharkawy H, Rojas Gomez MF, Sala-Blanch X, Reina MA. Anatomical basis of fascial plane blocks. Reg Anesth Pain Med 2021;46(7):581–99. https://doi.org/10.1136/rapm-2021-102506.

[3] Hasoon J, Mahmood S, Nguyen A, Orhurhu V. Erector spinae plane block for chronic lumbosacral pain: a case report. Orthop Rev 2024;16:124769. https://doi.org/10.52965/001c.124769.

[4] He J, Zhang F, Pan Y, Feng Y, Rushmore J, Torio E, Rathi Y, Makris N, Kikinis R, Golby AJ, O'Donnell LJ. Reconstructing the somatotopic organization of the corticospinal tract remains a challenge for modern tractography methods. Hum Brain Mapp 2023;44(17):6055–73. https://doi.org/10.1002/hbm.26497.

[5] Kohara K, Hashimoto R, Maegawa T, Kubota M. A simple procedure of epidural electrode lead replacement through a tissue sheath in spinal cord stimulation. NMC Case Rep J 2024;11:33–6. https://doi.org/10.2176/jns-nmc.2023-0183.

[6] L. Kafshdooz, H. Kahroba, T. Kafshdooz, R. Sheervalilou & H. Pourfathi, CC BY 4.0, via Wikimedia commons.

[7] Saker E, Graham RA, Nicholas R, D'Antoni AV, Loukas M, Oskouian RJ, Tubbs RS. Ligaments of the costovertebral joints including biomechanics, innervations, and clinical applications: a comprehensive review with application to approaches to the thoracic spine. Cureus 2016;8(11): e874. https://doi.org/10.7759/cureus.874.

[8] Schleip R, Gabbiani G, Wilke J, Naylor I, Hinz B, Zorn A, Jäger H, Breul R, Schreiner S, Klingler W. Fascia is able to actively contract and may thereby influence musculoskeletal dynamics: a histochemical and mechanographic investigation. Front Physiol 2019;10:336. https://doi.org/10.3389/fphys.2019.00336.

[9] Pritzlaff SG, Kreis PG, Fishman SM. Permanent spinal cord stimulator placement. In: Kreis PG, others, editors. Spinal cord stimulation: percutaneous implantation techniques. 2 edn. New York: Oxford Academic; 2023. 1 June 2023.

[10] Henry Vandyke Carter - Henry Gray. Anatomy of the human body (see "book" section below)Bartleby.com: gray's anatomy, plate 801, public domain. 1918. https://commons.wikimedia.org/w/index.php?curid=541644.

[11] Taken at City Studios in Stockholm (www.stockholmsfotografen.se), September 29, 2011, with assistance from KYO (The organisation of life models) in Stockholm. Wikimedia Commons. https://commons.wikimedia.org/wiki/File:Posterior_view_of_human_female_and_male_backs_(cropped).jpg.

[12] Tubbs RS, Lobashevsky A, Oakes P, et al. Meningeal relationships to the spinal nerves and rootlets: a gross, histological, and radiological study with application to intradural extramedullary spinal tumors. Childs Nerv Syst 2015;31(5):675–81. https://doi.org/10.1007/s00381-015-2648-z.

[13] Pavel J, Kellerova E, Snopkova J. Spinal cord vasculature: general anatomy and physiology. In: Yaksh T, Hayek S, editors. Neuraxial therapeutics. Cham: Springer; 2023. https://doi.org/10.1007/978-3-031-39558-1_6.

[14] Chaitow L, DeLany J. The pelvis. Clin Appl Neuromusc Tech 2011;2:299–389. https://doi.org/10.1016/b978-0-443-06815-7.00011-5.

Chapter 2

Anatomy of the intervertebral disc

Patrick Buchanan[1], Roshan Santhosh[2], David Lee[3] and Robert Heros[4, 5]

[1]*Pain Medicine, Spanish Hills Interventional Pain Specialists, Camarillo, CA, United States;* [2]*Physical Medicine and Rehabilitation, Larkin Community Hospital, South Miami, FL, United States;* [3]*Fullerton Orthopedics, University of California Irvine, Yorba Linda, CA, United States;* [4]*Spinal Diagnostics, PC, Tualatin, OR, United States;* [5]*Cascade Spine Center, LLC, Tualatin, OR, United States*

Introduction

Intervertebral discs (IVD) are soft cushion like structures which support and offer flexibility to the surrounding bony anatomy of the spine. Low back pain is among the most common causes of chronic pain with an annual prevalence of 10%–30% and lifetime prevalence of 65%–80% in US adults [1]. Disc pathology is thought to contribute to axial, radicular, and referred pain presentations in patients with back and neck pain [1]. This section will discuss the anatomy of IVDs, their relevant supporting neurovasculature, pathophysiology seen in degenerative disc disease, and neuromodulation considerations for disc pathologies.

Disc anatomy

The intervertebral discs are cartilaginous structures found between bony vertebrae, contributing about 20%–30% of the height of the spine. There are 23 discs in total, found between all vertebrae except C1–C2 and the fused vertebral bodies of the sacrum and coccyx [2]. As seen in Fig. 2.1, each intervertebral disc is bounded anteriorly by the anterior longitudinal ligament, which spans vertically to connect the anterior aspects of adjacent vertebral bodies (Fig. 2.2).

The disc in its non-athological state should be contained within the footprint of the adjacent vertebral bodies. From a structural perspective, the disc is composed of the central nucleus pulposus surrounded by concentric collagen fibers known as the annulus fibrosus, and is bounded superiorly and inferiorly by the vertebral endplates [3]. The nucleus pulposus is a proteoglycan hydrogel with poorly organized collagen fibers and a high-water content, which is tightly contained by the annulus fibrosus [4]. The annulus fibrosus is composed of a highly organized matrix of concentric lamellae of largely type 1 collagen fibers with sparse elastin fibers oriented radially – preserving the annulus organization during loading and bending [5]. Studies have demonstrated that the IVD experiences diurnal changes in intradiscal pressure associated with increased loading from upright posture and load-bearing activities [6]. These higher loads are associated with increased hydrostatic pressures within the disc itself, leading to loss of fluid and increased proteoglycan concentration as well as oxygen concentration and pH levels [7].

The vertebral endplate consists of the ostium and hyaline cartilage tissue and prevents the nucleus pulposus from pushing into the adjacent vertebral bodies. Chondrocytes at the endplate produce a rich proteoglycan matrix, which modulates the flow of nutrients and maintains disc hydration [5]. The IVD is poorly vascularized, and the cells within the nucleus pulposus, especially, are highly adapted for this environment in which nutrients and oxygen must be delivered via diffusion from the interface at the vertebral endplates [8]. As noted in Fig. 2.3, the blood supply of the endplates can be traced back to segmental branches from the aorta, and interosseous arteries that feed rich capillary networks of vertebral endplates as well as outer annulus fibrosus [5,10]. Given this poor blood supply, the IVD is relatively isolated from the immune system, and as such, with herniation of the nucleus pulposus, a robust immune response is observed [4].

As outlined in Fig. 2.4, although typically portrayed as a poorly innervated structure, recent work has demonstrated that the sinuvertebral nerve, ventral rami of the spinal nerves, as well as derivatives of the gray rami communicans, may all carry nociceptive signals from the disk [12]. Although human studies are limited, animal models have demonstrated the presence of increased innervation into the inner layers of the annulus fibrosus in degenerative disc disease, with increased density of both mechanoreceptor transmitting via A-beta neurons as well as nociceptive A-delta and C neuron fiber types

A Modern Atlas for Implantable Devices of the Spine, Brain, and Nerve. https://doi.org/10.1016/B978-0-443-36528-7.00005-4

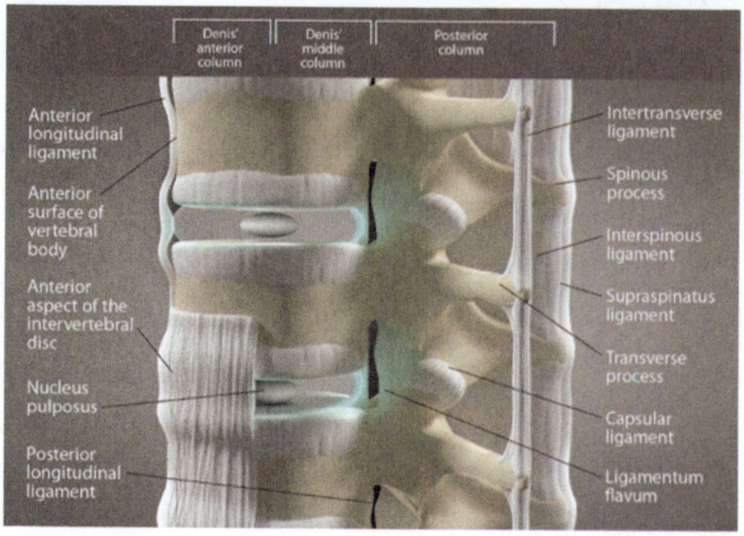

FIGURE 2.1 Denis three column model for spinal fracture classification outlining the surrounding ligamentous and bony anatomy of the intervertebral disc. *Reproduced with permission from Ref. [3]*

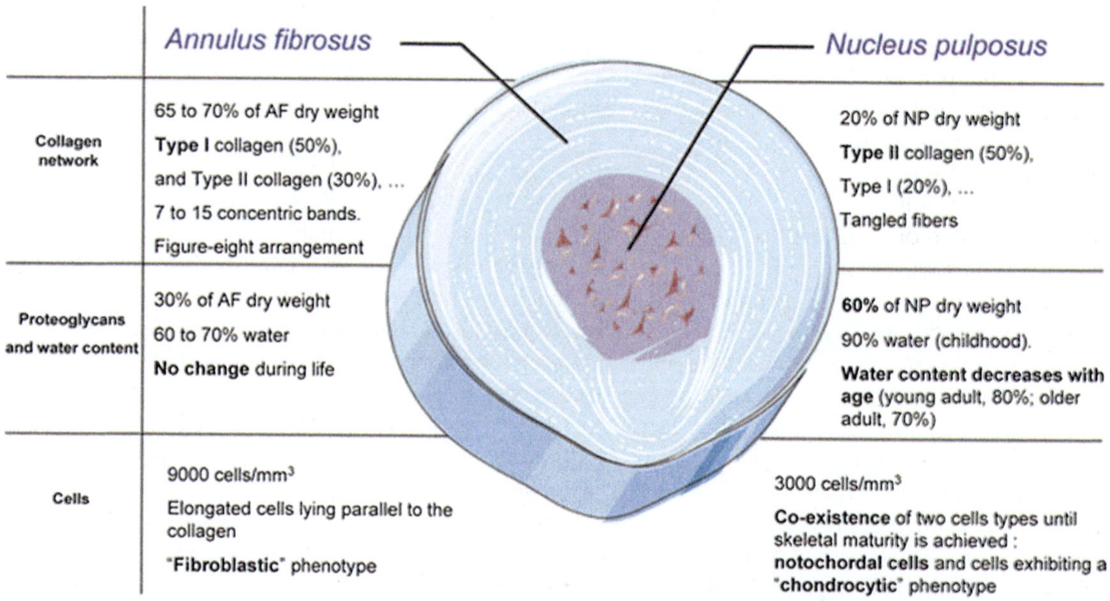

FIGURE 2.2 The intervertebral disc is composed of the annulus fibrosus and nucleus pulposus. *Reproduced with permission from Ref. [4]*

being noted [11,12]. The vertebral endplates interface with the disc and, as such, may play an important role in the transmission of discogenic pain [13]. The basivertebral nerve is a branch of the sinuvertebral nerve, which enters the vertebral body through the foramen in its posterior wall and arborizes to provide innervation to both superior and inferior endplates [14]. Recent models have suggested that "vertebrogenic pain" mediated via degenerative endplate changes may represent a continuum of discogenic disease [13,15].

Degenerative disc disease

The pathophysiology of degenerative disc disease (DDD) is multifactorial, with genetic, biomechanical and biochemical pathways contributing. A reduction in protective notochordal cells, which reduce inflammatory mediators including interleukin (IL)-1b, IL-6, and nerve growth factor in the nucleus pulposus, is observed as early as the first decade of life [16]. There are also notable changes in the homeostasis of extracellular matrix maintenance, leading to a loss of proteoglycans, including hyaluronic acid and type II collagen. This, in turn, leads to a loss of tissue hydration as well as the osmotic

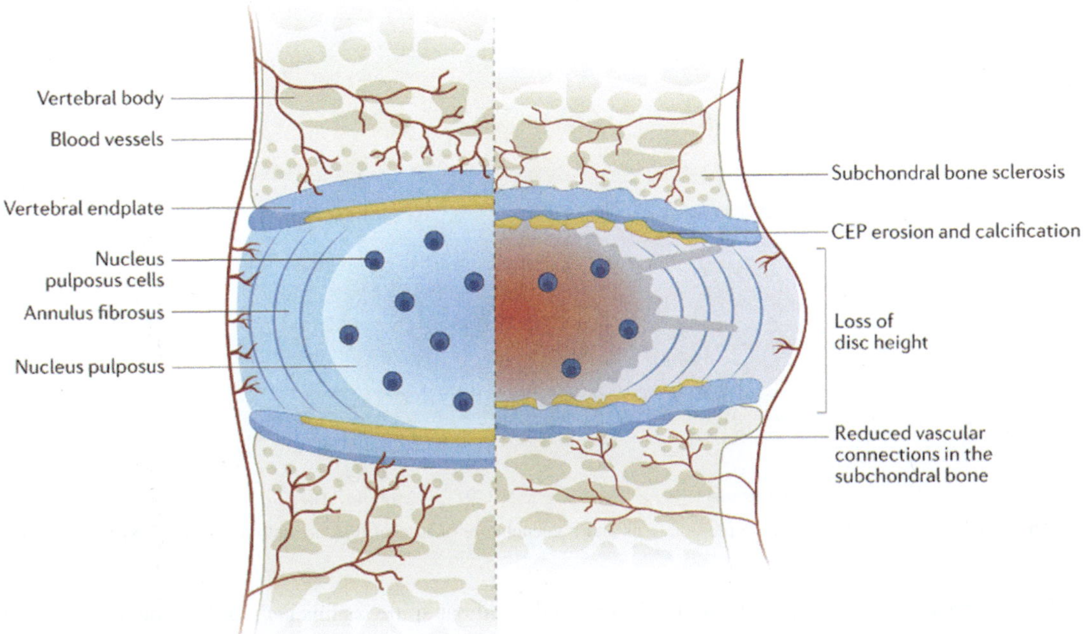

FIGURE 2.3 A model of the changes to the intervertebral disc and cartilaginous end plates (CEPs). *Reproduced with permission from [9].*

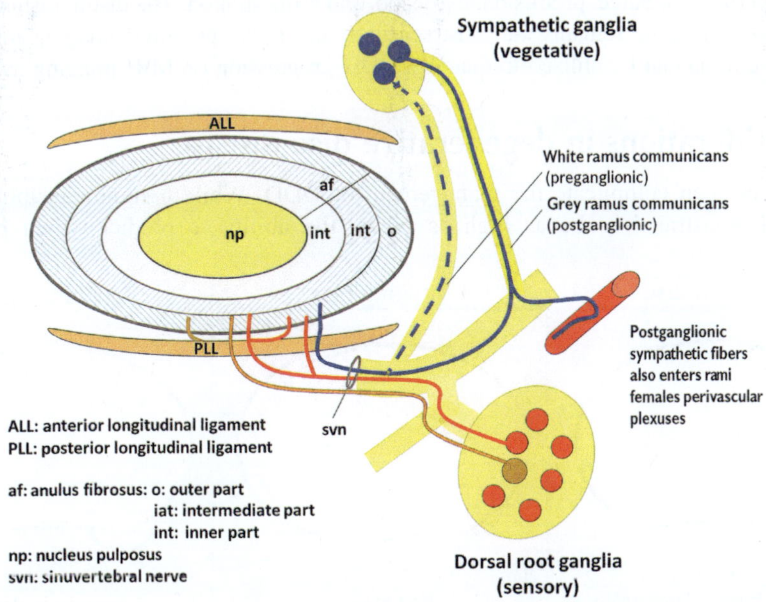

FIGURE 2.4 Schematic representation of the innervation of the intervertebral disc (IVD). Not pictured are nerve fibers from the nerve plexi contained within the anterior and posterior longitudinal ligaments, which also innervate the outer annulus fibrosus. *Reproduced with permission from Ref. [11]*

pressure of the IVD [17]. This ultimately contributes to reduced load-bearing capacity by the IVD, increasing pressure on the vertebral bodies, which subsequently develop osteophytes as the vertebral endplate begins to calcify [18]. Over time, the structural changes contribute to further disc breakdown, with fissure formation in the annulus fibrosus leading to exposure of the nucleus and subsequent immune response, which culminates in sensory nerve ingrowth and vascularization [18]. These degenerative sequelae can be characterized by the location at which the herniation occurs, as detailed in Fig. 2.5.

The incidence of disc herniations is about 5–20 cases per 1000 adults annually, most commonly occurring between the third and fifth decade of life [20]. Among these, symptomatic herniations are observed in a 2:1 ratio in men when compared to women, and are most common in the lumbar region and involve L4-L5 or L5-S1 [21]. Symptomatic herniations are frequently

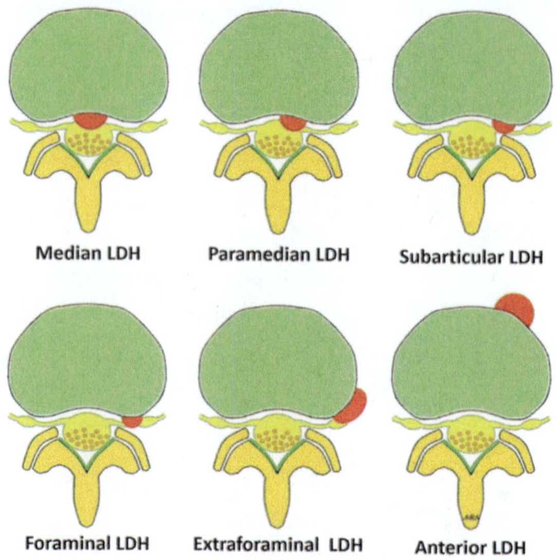

FIGURE 2.5 An illustrative depiction of common presentations and nomenclature of lumbar disc herniations (LDHs.). *Reproduced with permission from Ref. [19].*

observed in the posterolateral region of the annulus fibrosus in the lumbar spine, as this is thought to be the region in which the annulus fibrosus is weakest, with minimal reinforcement from the anterior and posterior longitudinal ligaments [20]. Disc degeneration may include such pathological changes as fissures (indicating disruption of the annulus fibrosus), desiccation, fibrosis, narrowing of the disc space, disc bulging, osteophyte formation, and endplate sclerosis [22]. Other nomenclature used to describe DDD include herniation, bulge, protrusion, extrusion, and sequestration. The distinguishing features of the same are highlighted in Fig. 2.6. MRI imaging remains the most sensitive and is the preferred imaging modality for detecting disc pathology [24]. Pfirmann criteria can be utilized to quantify DDD progression on MRI imaging as noted in Fig. 2.7.

Management considerations in degenerative disc disease

The natural disease process can complicate the management of DDD. While a significant portion of disc herniations spontaneously resorb (demonstrated to be as high as 66%), the ability to predict which patients will respond to

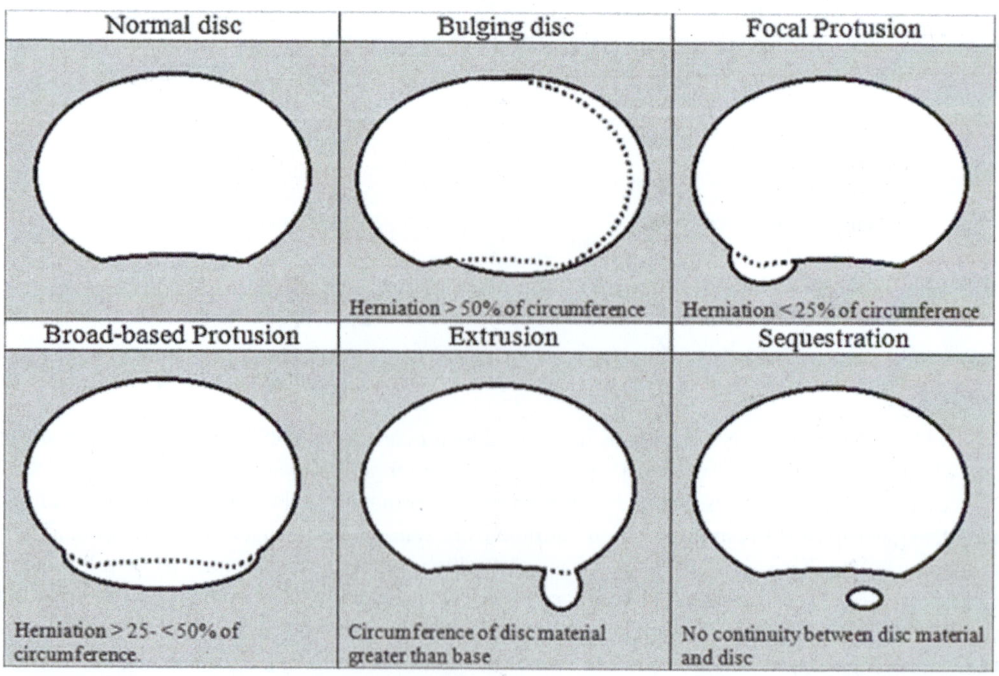

FIGURE 2.6 An illustrative depiction of the forms of degenerative disc disease presentations that may be observed as proposed by a multi-society working group [22]. *Reproduced with permission from [23].*

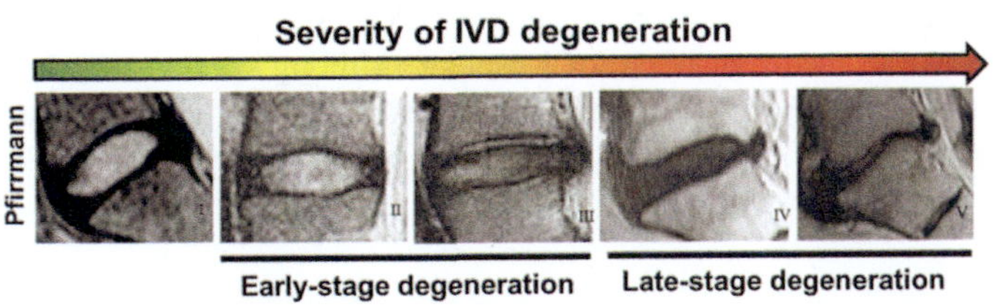

FIGURE 2.7 An illustrative representation of the progression of DDD observed in the original Pfirmann grading criteria. A modified Pfirmann criteria has been proposed which includes the addition of three more grades with 5-8 quantifying the degree of loss of disk height. *Reproduced with permissions from [25].*

conservative management remains quite poor [26,27]. In addition, not all pathologies seen on diagnostic imaging are clinically symptomatic [28]. They conducted a meta-analysis which found that MRI imaging of disc degeneration, including disc bulge, extrusion, protrusion, Modic one changes, and spondylosis are more prevalent in patients with low back pain. In part, this variability in the clinical data is due to numerous ways in which "discogenic pain" can present. As many as four distinct pain generators can be implicated with varying distributions and presentations of symptoms stemming from activation of nociceptive signaling via lumbosacral nerve roots, spinal nerves, dorsal rami, as well as the sinuvertebral nerves[29]. As outlined in Fig. 2.8, the vertebral endplates are also often implicated in DDD with observed Modic changes on MRI imaging, potentially modulating the transmission of discogenic pain [31].

Neuromodulation of the intervertebral disk

The current standard of care treatment modalities utilized for degenerative disc disease include pharmacological therapy, physical modalities including physical therapy, epidural, or, less commonly, intradiscal injections of local anesthetic or steroid versus regenerative modalities [32]. For patients with refractory symptoms or severe disease, particularly with evidence of instability, there is evidence for surgical interventions including minimally invasive discectomy, fusion, and or artificial disc replacement, depending on individual patient presentations and selection criteria [33]. Recently, radiofrequency ablation of the basivertebral nerve has emerged as a treatment modality for the management of vertebrogenic pain, mediated by degenerative endplate changes [15]. Neuromodulation therapies targeting the disc are currently limited,

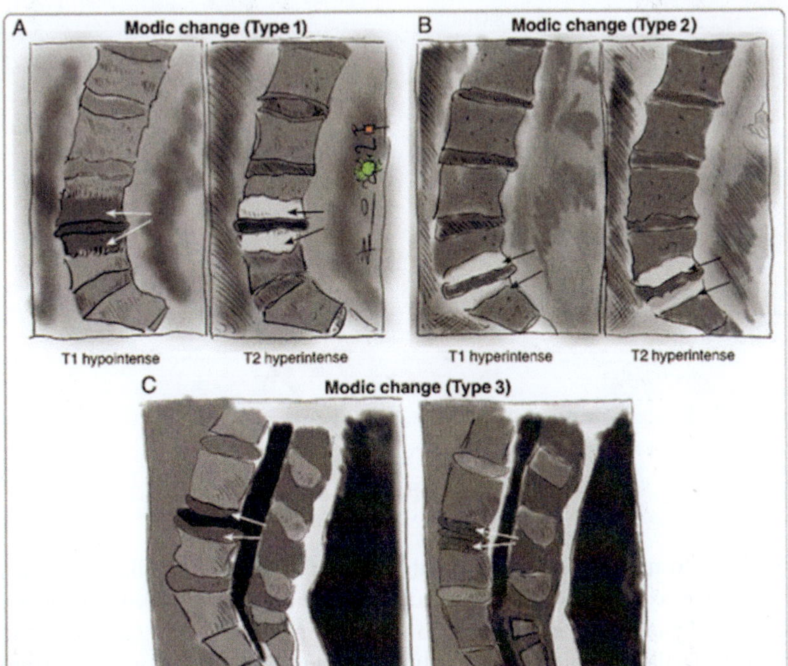

FIGURE 2.8 Modic changes type I are hypointense on T1 and hyperintense on T2, consistent with bone marrow edema. Modic changes type II are hyperintense on T1 and T2 weighted imaging, denoting fatty infiltration of the vertebral endplates. Modic changes type III are hypointense on both T1 and T2, indicating end plate sclerosis. *Reproduced with permission from [30].*

but there are clinical trials underway utilizing a system with an implantable pulse generator (IPG) as well as a lead to be placed targeting the sinuvertebral nerve, otherwise known as the recurrent nerve of Luschka. Although preclinical data appear promising, enrollment for clinical trials is still underway. Future neuromodulation technologies may play an important role in the management of discogenic pain, given the numerous nociceptive signaling pathways implicated [33].

Anatomy of the multifidus muscle

The muscles of the back are broadly arranged into three layers: superficial (extrinsic), intermediate (extrinsic), and deep (intrinsic). The deep, intrinsic back muscles themselves are further subdivided into superficial, intermediate, and deep layers. The superficial layer includes the splenius capitis and cervicis, which assist with shoulder and neck movement. The intermediate layer includes the erector spinae, further subdivided into iliocostalis, longissimus, and spinalis, from lateral to medial.

This deepest layer of the intrinsic back muscles, collectively known as the transversospinalis muscles are comprised of the semispinalis, multifidus, and rotatores. This deepest layer of back muscles play important role in stabilizing and supporting the spine [34]. The lumbar multifidus is the largest of the back muscles that traverses the lumbosacral junction. It is composed of deep, intermediate, and superficial fascicles, each of which serves a different function. The deep fascicles have the smallest muscle fiber bundle length and the lowest muscle volume; they are thought to provide intersegmental stability and proprioception from the lumbar spine. The intermediate fascicles have attachments to the lateral spinous processes and may assist in intersegmental movement. The superficial fascicles have the largest muscle volume and longest fibers, assisting in spinal rotation and extension [35].

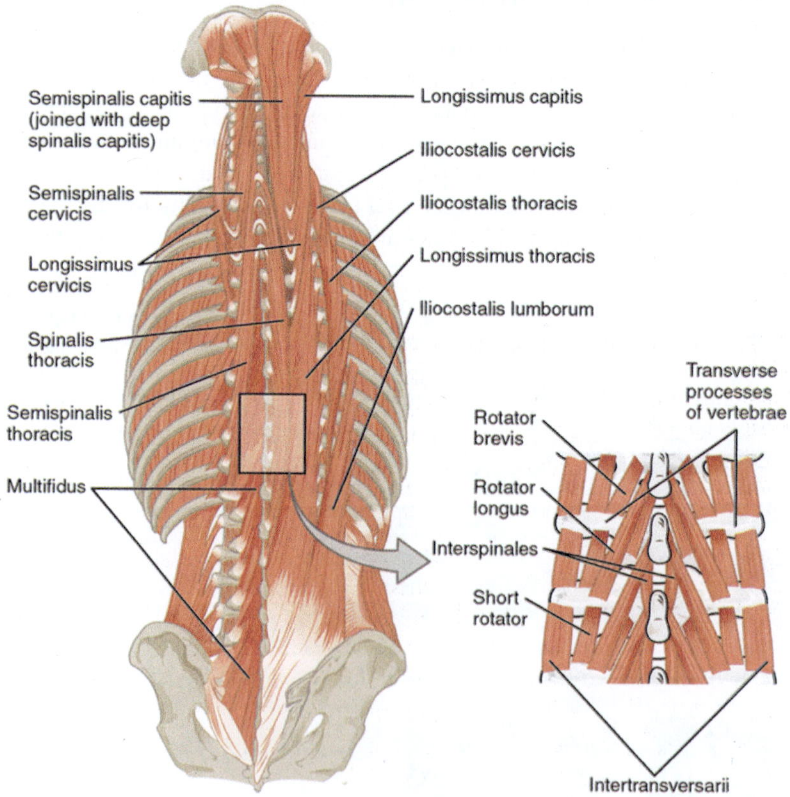

The deep fascicles provide proprioceptive feedback from single segments of the lumbar spine. Intermediate fascicles control intersegmental movement. Lastly, the superficial fascicles play a role in rotation and extension [36]. Pain signals from the spine (facet joints, intervertebral discs, spinal ligaments, etc) can lead to inhibited neuromuscular control in the brain and spinal cord, leading to a reduced neural drive to the multifidus muscle. Impaired neuromuscular control, in turn, can reduce spine stability and allow for overloading of the spinal column.

Innervation of the multifidus muscle

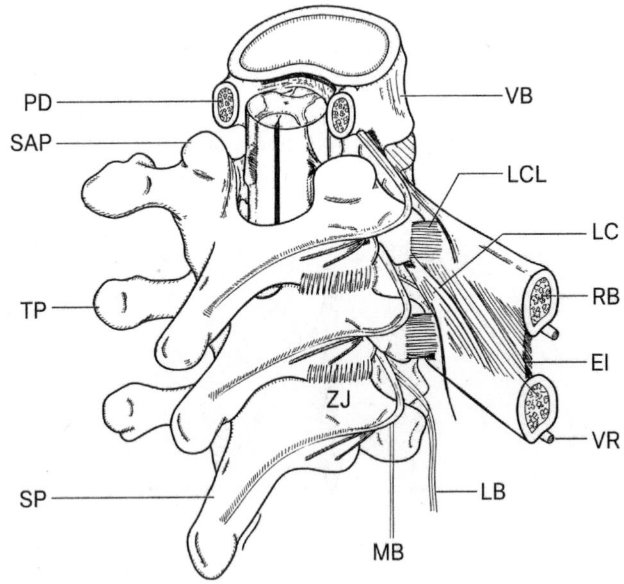

The multifidus segmentally derives motor innervation through the medial branch nerves, which also provide sensory innervation to the spinal zygaphophyseal or facet joints. The spinal nerve exits the intervertebral foramen and divides into the meningeal branch, communicating branch, ventral ramus, and dorsal ramus. The dorsal ramus is a small branch and runs dorsally on the medial aspect of the intertransversii muscles. The dorsal ramus then divides into the medial and lateral branches, forming a 30-degree angle at the superior border of the lower transverse process. The medial and lateral branches of the dorsal rami supply the surrounding skin and muscles. Specifically in the lumbar spine, lateral branches of the dorsal rami primarily innervate the iliocostalis lumborum muscle. Medial branches innervate facet joints and multifidus muscles, while intermediate branches supply the longissimus muscle. There are varied anastomoses seen between the adjacent medial and lateral branches, and dorsal rami. The medial branch is the most consistently targeted nerve located at the junction of the superior articular process and transverse process [37]. This has been shown in multiple studies for facet radiofrequency ablation [38].

The multifidus muscles, crucial for spinal stabilization, are primarily activated involuntarily during movements and various postures. Dysfunction or atrophy of the multifidus has been associated with chronic axial low back pain, making it a critical target for therapeutic interventions [39]. Arthrogenic inhibition is a reflexive neuromuscular response characterized by the decreased activation of muscles surrounding a joint following injury, inflammation, or pain. [40]. This phenomenon is often seen in the quadriceps muscle following a knee injury [41]. Change in joint sensory information (due to pain, inflammation, laxity) and thus integration in the central nervous system ultimately leads to a disconnect between central nervous signaling and muscle activation. The mechanism of arthrogenic inhibition explains the consequences of joint pain and the understanding of joint pain recurrence. This same mechanism of action can be applied to the multifidus muscle and low back pain [42]. Reflex inhibition of the multifidus is clinically supported by ultrasound and EMG, which has shown evidence of reduced neural drive and altered recruitment of the multifidus in back pain patients. Ultrasound has also shown impaired muscle thickness change with contraction.

Multifidus inhibition subsequently may lead to muscle atrophy if left untreated. Patients with chronic low back pain are found to have multifidus atrophy and/or fat infiltration/tissue remodeling. Similarly, in a recent sheep study, it was found that multifidus dysfunction was associated with increased connective tissue within the multifidus muscle [43].)

Neuromodulation: restorative multifidus stimulation

Patients with multifidus dysfunction typically report chronic mechanical lower back pain, which should be differentiated from neurogenic sources of low back pain (i.e., chronic lumbosacral radiculopathy, neurogenic claudication secondary to spinal stenosis). This specific type of chronic low back pain (CLBP) is often exacerbated by mild activities such as standing, walking, changing position, as well as many common activities of daily living (i.e., slight flexion while brushing teeth, washing dishes, etc.). Furthermore, light exercise and physical therapy (which require core stabilization) may exacerbate low back pain symptoms. Notwithstanding, there are no conclusive pathognomonic signs for multifidus dysfunction that presently exist.

Imaging allows for direct visualization of the multifidus muscle, and atrophy of the multifidus can be graded based on the amount of fatty infiltration noted. Axial reconstructions on magnetic resonance imaging are the most optimal view for evaluation. While imaging may be helpful in identifying multifidus atrophy, it is paramount to recognize that multifidus dysfunction may occur in the absence of atrophy or fatty infiltration, and like any other imaging pathology, atrophy alone may or may not be relevant clinically. As such, diagnosing multifidus dysfunction is based on a combination of history, imaging and physical examination.

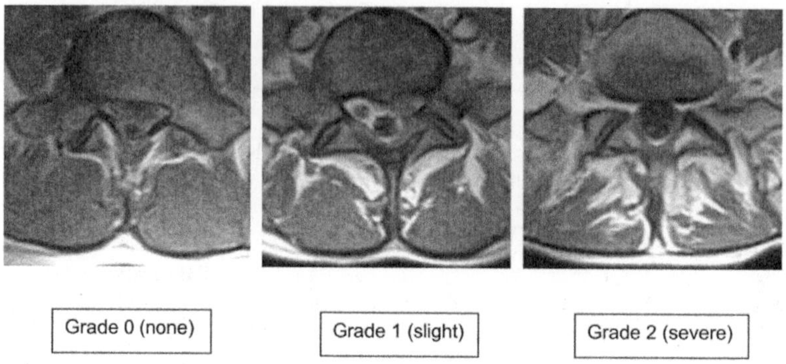

Physical examination of the multifidus dysfunction includes two well-reported provocative maneuvers; the Prone Instability Test (PIT) and the Multifidus Lift Test (MLT). Both maneuvers have been validated and have been shown to have a high interrater reliability, and are therefore reproducible. Detailed explanations and demonstrations of these examinations has been described elsewhere in the literature [42].)

When multifidus dysfunction has been diagnosed, interventions aimed at activating and restoring functionality to the multifidus muscle may be considered. Therapeutic interventions include targeted physical therapy exercises to activate the deep multifidus muscle, but isolated activation of the deep multifidi is often difficult due to nonvolitional control of the muscle. Reestablishing voluntary control of the multifidus muscle may not be feasible for every patient with physical therapy and exercise alone. In these instances, direct electrical stimulation of the multifidus may be a suitable alternative. Transcutaneous neuromuscular electrical stimulation (NMES) has already been used successfully to initiate contraction of the larger and more superficial muscle groups (i.e., quadriceps muscles in patients with knee osteoarthritis and subsequent arthrogenic inhibition of the quadriceps). However, transcutaneous electrical stimulation does not allow for targeted muscle stimulation, nor does it penetrate deeply enough to cause contraction of the deep multifidus fascicles. In addition, while research is ongoing, neither direct muscle stimulation nor transcutaneous stimulation has demonstrated reproducible long-term benefit for CLBP patients.

Restorative neurostimulation is a more recent therapeutic option for this patient population. This neuromodulation device stimulates the bilateral L2 medial branches at the L3 vertebral body level, inducing a physiologic contraction of the muscle to override inhibition and, over time, restore physiologic motor control. For properly selected patients with multifidus dysfunction, restorative neurostimulation has proven to be effective and safe, and is the only form of neuromodulation for lower back pain with published and sustainable long-term outcomes at 5 yrs [44].) Successful restoration of motor control and functional stability of the lumbar spine may allow for lifestyle changes and increased participation in treatments, including physiotherapy and exercises to prevent relapse or recurrence.

References

[1] Urits I, Burshtein A, Sharma M, Testa L, Gold PA, Orhurhu V, Viswanath O, Jones MR, Sidransky MA, Spektor B, Kaye AD. Low back pain, a comprehensive review: Pathophysiology, diagnosis, and treatment. Curr Pain Headache Rep 2019;23:23.

[2] Ghosh P. The biology of the intervertebral disc1. Boca Raton: CRC Press; 1988.

[3] Hauser RA, Matias D, Woznica D, Rawlings B, Woldin BA. Lumbar instability as an etiology of low back pain and its treatment by prolotherapy: A review. J Back Musculoskelet Rehabil 2022;35:701–12.

[4] Clouet J, Vinatier C, Merceron C, Pot-Vaucel M, Hamel O, Weiss P, Grimandi G, Guicheux J. The intervertebral disc: From pathophysiology to tissue engineering. Jt Bone Spine 2009;76:614–8.

[5] Tomaszewski KA, Saganiak K, Gładysz T, Walocha JA. The biology behind the human intervertebral disc and its endplates. Folia Morphol (Warsz) 2015;74:157–68.
[6] Chan SCW, Ferguson SJ, Gantenbein-Ritter B. The effects of dynamic loading on the intervertebral disc. Eur Spine J 2011;20:1796–812.
[7] Sivan S, Neidlinger-Wilke C, Würtz K, Maroudas A, Urban JPG. Diurnal fluid expression and activity of intervertebral disc cells. Biorheology 2006;43:283–91.
[8] Urban JPG, Smith S, Fairbank JCT. Nutrition of the intervertebral disc. Spine 2004;29:2700–9.
[9] Zehra U, Tryfonidou M, Iatridis JC, Illien-Jünger S, Mwale F, Samartzis D. Mechanisms and clinical implications of intervertebral disc calcification. Nat Rev Rheumatol 2022;18:352–62.
[10] Fournier DE, Kiser PK, Shoemaker JK, Battié MC, Séguin CA. Vascularization of the human intervertebral disc: A scoping review. JOR Spine 2020;3.
[11] García-Cosamalón J, Del Valle ME, Calavia MG, García-Suárez O, López-Muñiz A, Otero J, Vega JA. Intervertebral disc, sensory nerves and neurotrophins: who is who in discogenic pain? J Anat 2010;217:1–15.
[12] Takahashi Y, Ohtori S, Takahashi K. Peripheral nerve pathways of afferent fibers innervating the lumbar spine in rats. J Pain 2009;10:416–25.
[13] Conger A, Smuck M, Truumees E, Lotz JC, DePalma MJ, McCormick ZL. Vertebrogenic pain: A paradigm shift in diagnosis and treatment of axial low back pain. Pain Med 2022;23:S63–71.
[14] Bailey JF, Liebenberg E, Degmetich S, Lotz JC. Innervation patterns of PGP 9.5-positive nerve fibers within the human lumbar vertebra. J Anat 2011;218:263–70.
[15] Michalik A, Conger A, Smuck M, Maus TP, McCormick ZL. Intraosseous basivertebral nerve radiofrequency ablation for the treatment of vertebral body endplate low back pain: Current evidence and future directions. Pain Med 2021;22:S24–30.
[16] Tang S, Richards J, Khan S, Hoyland J, Gallego-Perez D, Higuita-Castro N, Walter B, Purmessur D. Nonviral transfection with brachyury reprograms human intervertebral disc cells to a pro-anabolic anti-catabolic/inflammatory phenotype: A proof of concept study. J Orthop Res 2019;37:2389–400.
[17] Sha'ban M, Yoon SJ, Ko YK, Ha HJ, Kim SH, So JW, Idrus RBH, Khang G. Fibrin promotes proliferation and matrix production of intervertebral disc cells cultured in three-dimensional poly(lactic-co-glycolic acid) scaffold. J Biomater Sci Polym Ed 2008;19:1219–37.
[18] Mohd Isa IL, Teoh SL, Mohd Nor NH, Mokhtar SA. Discogenic low back pain: Anatomy, pathophysiology and treatments of intervertebral disc degeneration. Int J Mol Sci 2022;24.
[19] Akhaddar A. Central and subarticular lumbar disk herniations. In: Atlas of sciatica. Cham: Springer International Publishing; 2023. p. 239–59.
[20] Dydyk A, Massa R, Mesfin F. Disc herniation. StatPearls; 2023.
[21] Jordan J, Konstantinou K, O'Dowd J. Herniated lumbar disc. BMJ Clin Evid 2009;2009.
[22] Fardon DF, Williams AL, Dohring EJ, Murtagh FR, Gabriel Rothman SL, Sze GK. Lumbar disc nomenclature: version 2.0. Spine J 2014;14:2525–45.
[23] Macki M, Hernandez-Hermann M, Bydon M, Gokaslan A, McGovern K, Bydon A. Spontaneous regression of sequestrated lumbar disc herniations: Literature review. Clin Neurol Neurosurg 2014;120:136–41.
[24] Li Y, Fredrickson V, Resnick DK. How should we grade lumbar disc herniation and nerve root compression? A systematic review. Clin Orthop Relat Res 2015;473:1896–902.
[25] Radek M, Pacholczyk-Sienicka B, Jankowski S, Albrecht Ł, Grodzka M, Depta A, Radek A. Assessing the correlation between the degree of disc degeneration on the Pfirrmann scale and the metabolites identified in HR-MAS NMR spectroscopy. Magn Reson Imaging 2016;34:376–80.
[26] Hornung AL, Baker JD, Mallow GM, Sayari AJ, Albert HB, Tkachev A, An HS, Samartzis D. Resorption of lumbar disk herniation: Mechanisms, clinical predictors, and future directions. JBJS Rev 2023;11.
[27] Zhong M, Liu J-T, Jiang H, Mo W, Yu P-F, Li X-C, Xue RR. Incidence of spontaneous resorption of lumbar disc herniation: A meta-analysis. Pain Physician 2017;20:E45–52.
[28] Brinjikji W, Diehn FE, Jarvik JG, Carr CM, Kallmes DF, Murad MH, Luetmer PH. MRI findings of disc degeneration are more prevalent in adults with low back pain than in asymptomatic controls: A systematic review and meta-analysis. Am J Neuroradiol 2015;36:2394–9.
[29] Bogduk N. The anatomy of the lumbar intervertebral disc syndrome. Med J Aust 1976;1:878–81.
[30] Herger N, Bermudez-Lekerika P, Farshad M, Albers CE, Distler O, Gantenbein B, Dudli S. Should degenerated intervertebral discs of patients with modic type 1 changes Be treated with mesenchymal stem cells? Int J Mol Sci 2022;23:2721.
[31] Dudli S, Fields AJ, Samartzis D, Karppinen J, Lotz JC. Pathobiology of modic changes. Eur Spine J 2016;25:3723–34.
[32] Simon J, McAuliffe M, Shamim F, Vuong N, Tahaei A. Discogenic low back pain. Phys Med Rehabil Clin N Am 2014;25:305–17.
[33] Zhao L, Manchikanti L, Kaye AD, Abd-Elsayed A. Treatment of discogenic low back pain: Current treatment strategies and future options—a literature review. Curr Pain Headache Rep 2019;23:86.
[34] Matheve T, Hodges P, Danneels L. The role of back muscle dysfunctions in chronic low back pain: State-of-the-art and clinical implications. J Clin Med 2023;12(17):5510.
[35] Rosatelli AL, Ravichandiran K, Agur AM. Three-dimensional study of the musculotendinous architecture of lumbar multifidus and its functional implications. Clin Anat 2008;21(6):539–46.
[36] Tieppo Francio V, Westerhaus BD, Carayannopoulos AG, Sayed D. Multifidus dysfunction and restorative neurostimulation: a scoping review. Pain Med 2023;24(12):1341–54.
[37] Liu Z, Chen J, Fang D, Xu Y, Zhou X, Zheng Z, Zhang Z, Fan C, Luo S, Liu Z, Li Q, Zhao Q. Anatomical observation and clinical significance of the medial branch of the lumbar dorsal rami. Spine 2024;49(11):E164–72.

[38] Schneider BJ, Doan L, Maes MK, Martinez KR, Gonzalez Cota A, Bogduk N, Standards Division of the Spine Intervention Society. Systematic review of the effectiveness of lumbar medial branch thermal radiofrequency neurotomy, stratified for diagnostic methods and procedural technique. Pain Med 2020;21(6):1122–41.

[39] Goubert D, Oosterwijck JV, Meeus M, Danneels L. Structural changes of lumbar muscles in non-specific low back pain: A systematic review. Pain Physician 2016;19(7):E985–1000.

[40] Russo M, Deckers K, Eldabe S, Kiesel K, Gilligan C, Vieceli J, Crosby P. Muscle control and non-specific chronic low back pain. Neuromodulation 2018;21(1):1–9.

[41] Hopkins JT, Ingersoll CD. Arthrogenic muscle inhibition: 20 Years on. J Sport Rehabil 2022;31(6):665–6.

[42] Chakravarthy K, Lee D, Tram J, Sheth S, Heros R, Manion S, Patel V, Kiesel K, Ghandour Y, Gilligan C. Restorative neurostimulation: A clinical guide for therapy adoption. J Pain Res June 20, 2022;15:1759–74.

[43] James G, Ahern B, Goodwin W, Goss B, Hodges P. ISSLS Prize in Basic Science 2025: Structural changes of muscle spindles in the multifidus muscle after intervertebral disk injury are resolved by targeted activation of the muscle. Eur Spine J 2025;34(5):1600–13. https://doi.org/10.1007/s00586-025-08744-w.

[44] Gilligan C, Volschenk W, Russo M, et al. Five-year longitudinal follow-up of restorative neurostimulation shows durability of effectiveness in patients with refractory chronic low back pain associated with multifidus muscle dysfunction. Neuromodulation 2024;27(5):930–43.

Chapter 3

Anatomy of the head and neck for neuromodulation

Kai McGreevy[1], Mustafa Broachwala[2], Peter S. Staats[3] and Morad Nasseri[4]

[1]*McGreevy NeuroHealth, St. Augustine, FL, United States;* [2]*Department of Anesthesiology and Pain Medicine, University of California, San Diego, CA, United States;* [3]*The Vagus Nerve Society, Atlantic Beach, FL, United States;* [4]*Boomerang Healthcare, Walnut Creek, CA, United States*

Introduction

As with any interventional procedure in medicine, it is essential to have a firm understanding of relevant anatomy for safety and efficacy of therapy. This is particularly true when targeting neural structures for neuromodulation. In this chapter and other chapters to follow, neuromodulation for pain, movement, and psychiatric disorders implicate many neural structures and pathways involving peripheral nerves and brain circuitry. Anatomical approaches for precise neural targeting and safety optimization, specifically for head and neck neuromodulation procedure technique, will be emphasized.

Brief Historical Perspective. The history of neuromodulation for painful and nonpainful conditions of the head and neck includes the development of spinal cord stimulation (SCS), peripheral nerve stimulation (PNS) and deep brain stimulation (DBS).

SCS was introduced by the foundational work of Norman Shealy in the late 1960s, aligning with the emerging gate control theory proposed by Melzack and Wall [1]. During the 1970 and 1980s, innovators began exploring cervical lead placements to manage craniofacial pain, discovering that carefully placed electrodes at higher spinal segments could significantly modulate orofacial symptoms. In 2014, Deer et al. demonstrated improvements in pain relief, quality of life, patient satisfaction and disability indices in a prospective, international, multicenter registry on the use of cervical SCS [2]. Since this landmark study, cervical SCS has become an invaluable therapeutic option for a myriad of refractory disorders.

PNS advancements, in parallel with SCS, further opened the door to targeted therapies for occipital neuralgia and severe headache disorders, enabling direct stimulation of peripheral nerves including the occipital and trigeminal nerves rather than relying solely on dorsal column pathways [3]. These early milestones set the stage for the modern field of neuromodulation of the head and neck, which now employs sophisticated imaging and evolving electrode technologies to refine safety and efficacy for both painful and nonpainful conditions.

DBS was successfully used in the 1970s to target the somatosensory thalamus for intractable facial pain [4]. However, heterogeneous studies pursuing various chronic pain syndromes resulted in a range of reported efficacy. As interest for DBS utilization for treatment of painful conditions declined in the 1980s, it began to be used for motor symptoms of movement disorders such as Parkinson's disease. This application has grown rapidly with continued research and technological developments. More recently, there has been a resurgence of interest in DBS for depression and chronic pain syndromes.

Suggested Specialty Training for Appropriate Intervention. Specialty training is essential to ensure both the safety and efficacy of interventional pain procedures, including neuromodulation in the head and neck region. ACGME-accredited fellowships, widely recognized as the gold standard for postresidency training, provide an intensive curriculum encompassing fluoroscopic guidance, ultrasound imaging, and advanced interventional and surgical techniques. As technology continues to evolve, graduates of ACGME-accredited fellowships are optimally positioned to integrate new imaging modalities into routine practice, refine procedure-based skillsets, and proactively address challenges or

A Modern Atlas for Implantable Devices of the Spine, Brain, and Nerve. https://doi.org/10.1016/B978-0-443-36528-7.00052-2

complications. In tandem with ongoing professional development—through workshops, cadaver labs, and accredited continuing medical education (CME) courses—this robust framework maintains and enhances the competence needed for successful neuromodulation interventions in the head and neck.

Surgical specialists, such as neurosurgeons, may also train to implant devices in the head and neck regions. Their surgical proficiency and anatomic understanding are developed through their respective surgical residencies, subspecialty training and subsequent postgraduate continuing education.

Key points

- Understanding head and neck anatomy is essential for safe and effective interventions as the field of neuromodulation evolves and gains acceptance for clinical use in painful and nonpainful disorders.
- Neuromodulatory treatments such as DBS, PNS and SCS have been effectively utilized for treating brain, craniofacial and craniocervical disorders.
- Anatomical and technical considerations for *craniofacial pain disorders* are reviewed, with an emphasis on trigeminal nerve stimulation (TNS), supraorbital nerve stimulation (SoNS), sphenopalatine ganglion stimulation (SPGS), occipital nerve stimulation (ONS), and high cervical spinal cord stimulation (hcSCS).
- Anatomical considerations for *nonpainful disorders* utilizing glossopharyngeal nerve stimulation (GNS) for obstructive sleep apnea, vagal nerve stimulation (VNS) for epilepsy and depression, and DBS for movement disorders are introduced.
- Understanding central processing mechanisms is becoming increasingly important for all forms of neuromodulation.

Anatomy

Anatomy System Scope. This chapter reviews pertinent head and neck anatomy for painful and nonpainful disorders amenable to neuromodulation, with an emphasis on the trigeminal, glossopharyngeal, vagus and occipital nerves. Anatomical considerations for TNS, SoNS, SPGS, ONS, and hcSCS will be emphasized for craniofacial pain, while anatomical considerations for GNS, VNS and DBS will be introduced for nonpainful conditions.

Relevant anatomy

Trigeminal nerve (CN V)

The great majority of craniofacial pain information is transmitted through the trigeminal nervous system, branches of the cervical plexus, and medial branches of the dorsal rami of the cervical spinal nerves, as illustrated in Fig. 3.1.

The trigeminal nerve is cranial nerve five (CN V). The trigeminal nerve exits the brainstem from the ventrolateral pons and travels through Meckel's cave, where the trigeminal (or Gasserian) ganglion gives rise to three dermatomal branches that innervate craniofacial structures.

The ophthalmic division (V1) travels through the inferior part of the cavernous sinus to exit the skull through the superior orbital fissure, and includes nociceptive afferents from the forehead, upper eyelid, eye, superior nasal cavity, nasal ridge, and mucosa of the frontal, sphenoid and ethmoid sinuses, as well as pial, arachnoid and dural vasculature and other large cerebral arteries [5]. The major V1 branches for neuromodulation have included the supraorbital and supratrochlear nerves [6].

The maxillary division (V2) exits the skull through the foramen rotundum, and includes nociceptive afferents from the lower eyelid, upper cheek, and upper lip, lower nasal cavity, mucosa and upper teeth and palate, gingiva, and skin associated with the maxilla, palatine, and zygomatic bone [5]. The major V2 branch for neuromodulation has included the infraorbital nerve that immediately enters the infraorbital foramen [6].

The mandibular division (V3) exits the skull through the foramen ovale, and includes nociceptive afferents from the lower lip, lower teeth and oral floor, chin and muscles of mastication. The major branches of V3 includes the inferior alveolar, lingual, buccal and auriculotemporal nerves [5].

Orthodromic sensory pathway of CN V. Primary nociceptive afferents in each of the three divisions of CN V are composed of small-diameter, unmyelinated C-fibers responsible for slow, dull burning pain, and thinly-myelinated A-delta fibers responsible for quick, sharp shooting pain. Both extracranial and intracranial trigeminal sensory neurons express calcitonin gene-related peptide, substance P, vasointestinal peptide and neuronal nitric oxide synthase. The cell bodies of these afferents reside within the trigeminal ganglion, whose central axons project toward the brainstem to

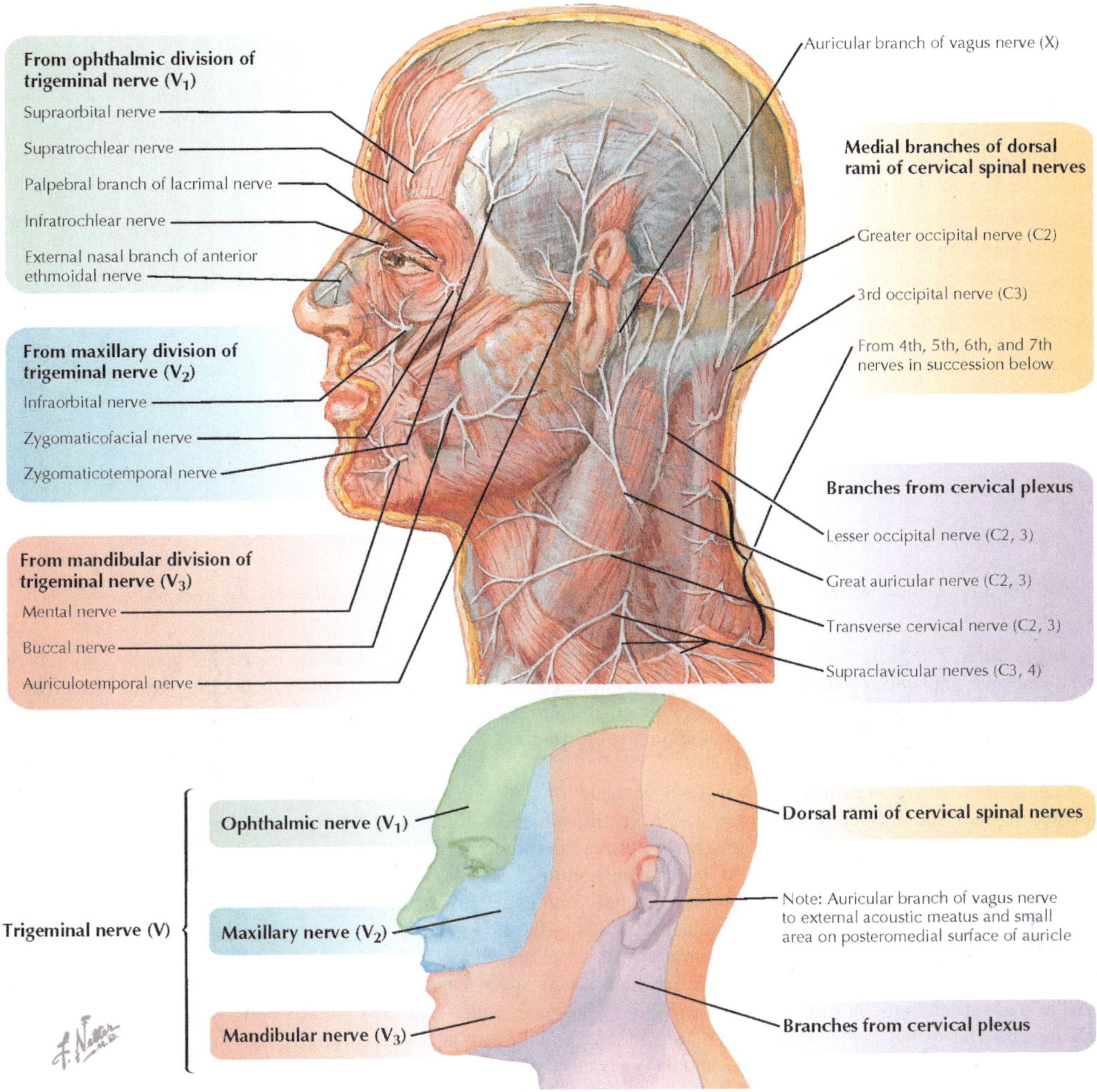

FIGURE 3.1 Craniofacial pain dermatomes including trigeminal and cervical nerve branches. *Netter illustration from www.netterimages.com*

mainly synapse on the spinal trigeminal nucleus, specifically on trigeminal nucleus caudalis (TNC) in the caudal medulla. There is anatomical overlap of trigeminal afferent with cervical and occipital afferent nociceptive information at these nuclei, a location known as the trigeminocervical complex (TCC) [7], as illustrated in Fig. 3.2.

Procedure-related considerations for trigeminal nerve stimulation (TNS)

TNS has been utilized for trigeminal neuralgia [8], atypical facial pain [9] and other craniofacial disorders [10].

External TNS. Transcutaneous stimulation devices that use electrical currents to stimulate the supraorbital nerves have been successfully used for the treatment of facial pain and headaches. These devices are described in more detail in Section 11, Chapter 40 (External Devices for Pain and Depression) and Chapter 41 (External Peripheral Nerve Devices).

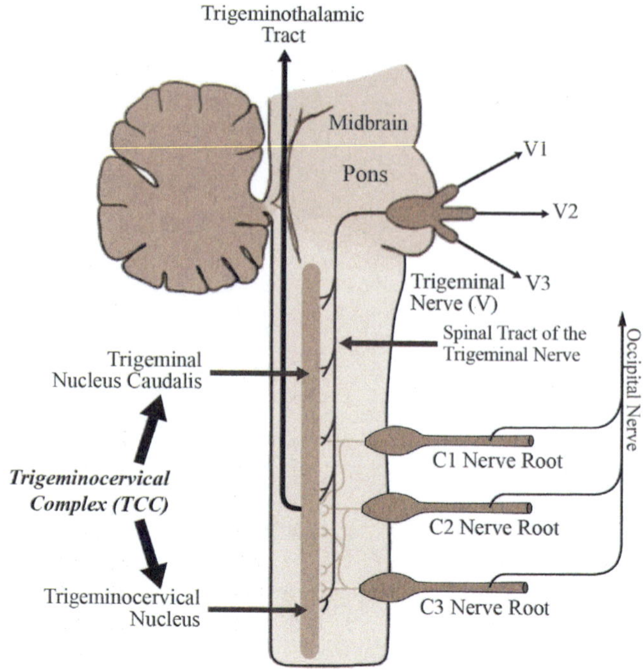

FIGURE 3.2 Schematic representation of the trigeminocervical complex. *Reproduced with permission,* Pain Physician, *ASIPP Publishing.*

Implantable TNS. Fluoroscopy or frameless stereotaxy may be utilized to place the trigeminal ganglion stimulator. Trial leads are implanted on the trigeminal ganglion through a percutaneous Hartel approach, but often results in masseter contraction. Alternatively, the trigeminal ganglion stimulation permanent implants may involve placing a grid electrode over Meckel's cave through subtemporal craniotomy, offering selective stimulation of desired trigeminal nerve branches without muscular (V3) side effects [11].

Supraorbital nerve stimulation (SoNS). PNS implantation for trigeminal nerve branches have been reported and often involve supraorbital and infraorbital branches [6], as illustrated in Fig. 3.3. SoNS technique has been described in the literature [12]. Most often, the implant procedure utilizes fluoroscopy to ensure that lead placement is identical to the trial leads. General anesthesia is often used for patient comfort, especially during tunneling of the lead cables to the implantable pulse generator (IPG). Preparation and positioning are similar for trial and implant, with careful attention to accessing the IPG site and the ability to tunnel the leads to the IPG pocket.

Lead Entry Technique. The skin is infiltrated with local anesthetic at the entry point, and then a small entry stab incision is made in the lateral forehead, approximately 1.5 cm superolateral to the tip of eyebrow. A Tuohy or introducer needle is advanced in the subcutaneous space overlying the nerve with a trajectory parallel to the nerve or at an angle to it. The inner stylet of the Tuohy needle is withdrawn, and a guidewire is advanced guided by fluoroscopic imaging. The Tuohy needle is withdrawn, and a plastic cannula is advanced over the guidewire. The guidewire is withdrawn. The lead is threaded through the cannula and its position is confirmed under fluoroscopy. The cannula is withdrawn.

Lead Anchoring, Tunneling, and IPG Placement. The leads are anchored to the fascia using a nonabsorbable stitch or with the available anchors with the stimulation system itself. A strain-relief loop can minimize the risk of migration or fracture due to lead kinking. Skin incision is performed and a subcutaneous pocket is prepared for the IPG. Possible sites are the flank, abdominal, axillary, subscapular, and infraclavicular areas. The leads are tunneled from the anchor site to the generator pocket, using extension cables where required, and connected to the IPG. Impedance must be checked on the whole system to assess technical integrity, function of the system, and proper alignment of the contact points of the leads to their compatible points at the IPG. Antibiotic irrigation is performed at the incision sites. The IPG pocket and tunneling site and then the incisions are closed and dressed [6].

Sphenopalatine ganglion (SPG)

The sphenopalatine ganglion (SPG) lies in the pterygopalatine fossa, immediately posterior to the maxilla, and is the location where V2 emerges from the cranial cavity. The SPG receives somatosensory, parasympathetic, and sympathetic

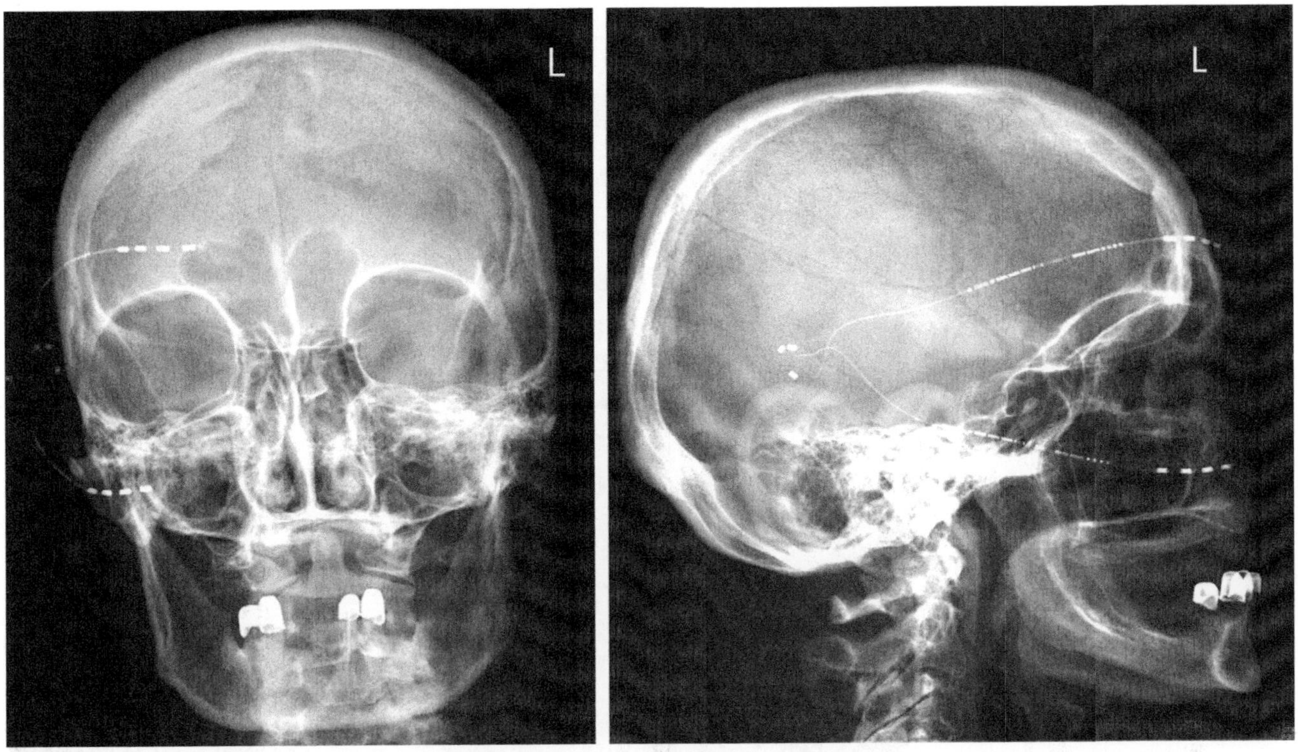

FIGURE 3.3 Fluoroscopic image of supraorbital and infraorbital lead placement for the treatment of facial pain. *Reproduced with permission, Wireless Subcutaneous Trigeminal Nerve Field Stimulation for Refractory Trigeminal Pain: A Single Center Experience,* Neuromodulation: Technology at the Neural Interface, *Elsevier 2021.*

input. The SPG has somatosensory connections to the facial nerve, lesser occipital nerve (LON), and the cutaneous cervical nerves. Sympathetic fibers from the superior cervical ganglion pass through the SPG and enter branches of V2. Postganglionic parasympathetic branches from the SPG have been shown to course superomedially into the orbital cavity, providing parasympathetic innervation to the meningeal and cerebral blood vessels, which upon activation lead to neuropeptide release that cause vasodilation or activation of trigeminal nociceptors in the meninges, and potentially headache pain. The SPG is a key structure responsible for cranial and facial autonomic symptoms in conditions such as migraine [13], trigeminal neuralgia [14], cluster headache [15] and trigeminal autonomic cephalalgias (TACs) and has been the site for a variety of clinical interventions due to its involvement in the trigeminal-autonomic pain reflex including sphenopalatine ganglion stimulation [14].

Procedure-related considerations for sphenopalatine ganglion stimulation (SPGS)

SPGS has been reviewed for various headache disorders including migraine [13], trigeminal neuralgia [14] and cluster headache [15]. Different approaches can be used to access the SPG, including transnasal, infrazygomatic, or suprazygomatic routes, depending on the desired target and patient anatomy [16,17].

Fluoroscopy or frameless stereotaxy may be utilized to place the sphenopalatine ganglion stimulator, as illustrated in Fig. 3.4. Patients are initially trialed before implantation. Leads are implanted in the pterygopalatine fossa near the SPG through a transpterygoid (lateral-medial, infrazygomatic) approach described elsewhere [11].

When considering SPGS, key anatomical points for the SPG include its location within the pterygopalatine fossa, its close proximity to V2, the need to access it through the sphenopalatine foramen, and surrounding bony landmarks such as the pterygoid plates, which can guide needle placement during a block or stimulation procedure; precise localization within the fossa is critical for effective stimulation and reducing potential complications. Incorrect needle placement could result in inadvertent V2 stimulation, causing facial pain or paresthesia. CT angiography has been supported for preoperative localization of the SPG before microstimulator implantation [18].

A randomized, sham-controlled study of 32 patients was performed to evaluate the use of SPGS for the acute treatment of chronic cluster headache [19]. In this study, the SPG neurostimulator (Autonomic Technologies Inc, Redwood City,

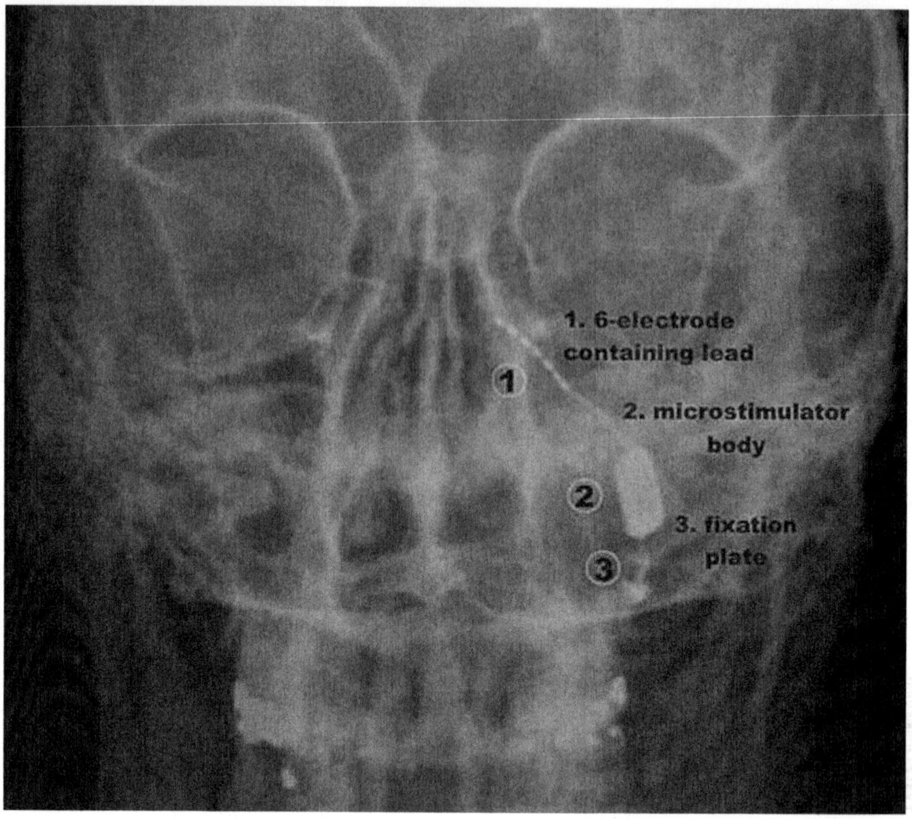

FIGURE 3.4 Fluoroscopic view of sphenopalatine ganglion stimulator implantation. *Reproduced with permission,* Pain Physician, *ASIPP Publishing.*

CA, USA) was implanted using a minimally invasive gingival buccal incision. The neurostimulator contained an integral lead that was placed within the pterygopalatine fossa approximating the SPG. The body of the neurostimulator, which contained no battery, was placed along the maxilla and was powered on demand by the patients using an external hand-held remote controller [19].

Potential Pitfall of PNS involving the face. The cavernous sinus, a dural venous sinus, drains blood from the face. Due to this connection, superficial facial infections from the nose, sinuses, ears, or teeth may spread to the cavernous sinus to cause cavernous sinus thrombosis [20], a potential life-threatening condition. Symptoms may include proptosis, periorbital edema, decrease or loss of vision, headaches, and possible cranial neuropathy, specifically abducens palsy. Therefore, the importance of preoperative planning, sterile technique, procedure duration, intraoperative risk reduction and postoperative monitoring cannot be overstated for implantable systems involving the face.

Glossopharyngeal nerve (CN IX)

The glossopharyngeal nerve is cranial nerve nine (CN IX), and its course is illustrated in Fig. 3.5. It has several branches. Pain sensation arising from the posterior third of the tongue, pharynx and ear is transmitted by CN IX, whose sensory ganglia reside in the superior ganglion at the exit point of the jugular foramen, with projections to the TNC in the caudal medulla, indirectly impacting the TCC for craniofacial pain sensation. CN IX also connects with V3, primarily through the otic ganglion, allowing for functional interplay between these two nerves, particularly related to sensory information from the throat and oral cavity. Due to this connection, conditions affecting one nerve (as with glossopharyngeal neuralgia) can manifest with symptoms that mimic those of the other nerve (as with trigeminal neuralgia) [21].

CN IX is also responsible for a variety of other functions including motor innervation of the stylopharyngeus muscle, which elevates the pharynx and larynx during swallowing and provides airway stability. This is relevant to emerging therapies including glossopharyngeal nerve stimulation for obstructive sleep apnea [22].

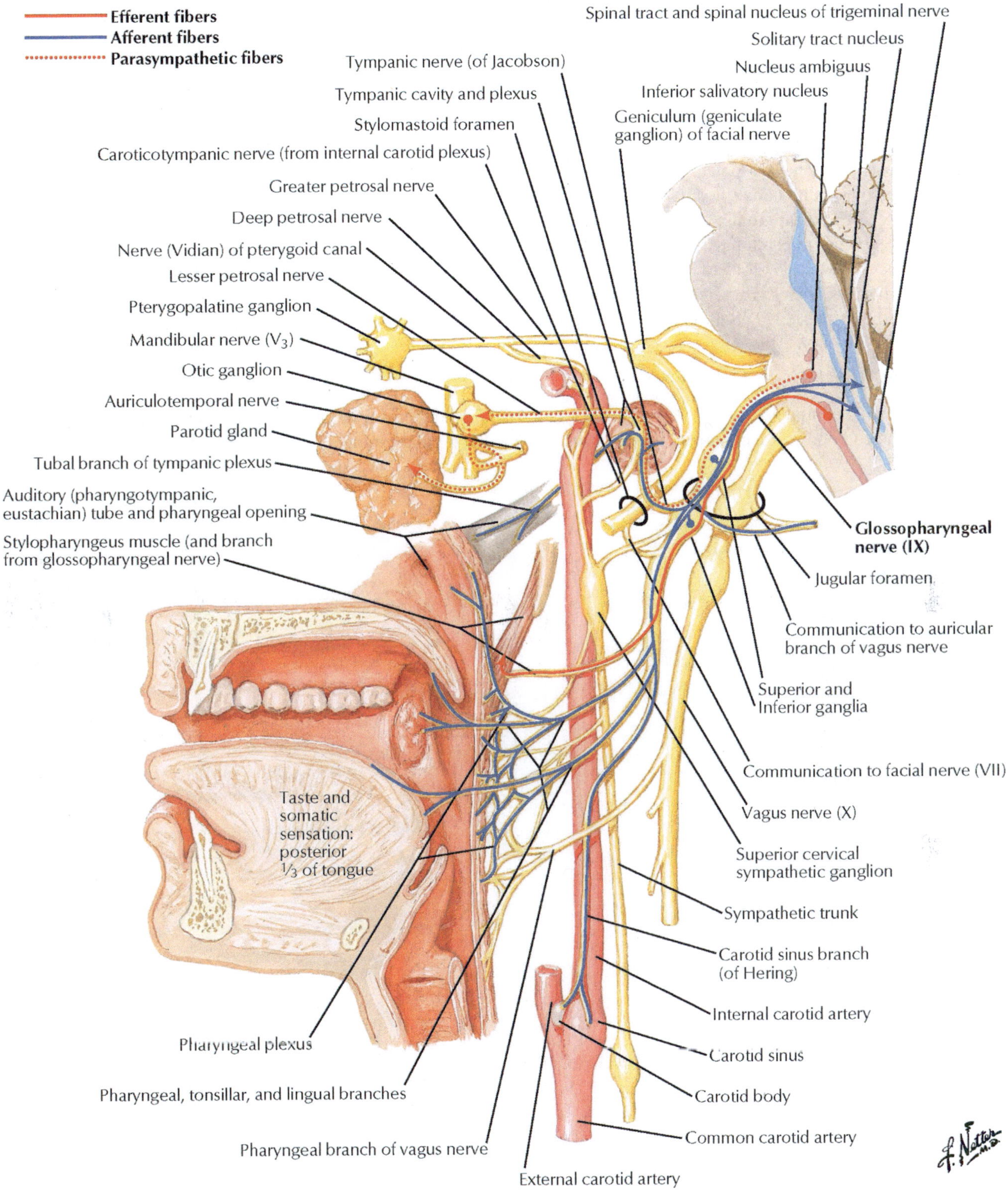

FIGURE 3.5 Glossopharyngeal nerve anatomy. *Netter illustration from www.netterimages.com © Elsevier Inc. All rights reserved.*

Procedure-related considerations for glossopharyngeal nerve stimulation (GNS)

Clinical applications of GNS include the treatment of obstructive sleep apnea (OSA) and glossopharyngeal neuralgia, a condition characterized by severe pain in the throat and ear. When considering GNS, key anatomical points include its deep location within the neck, close proximity to the carotid sinus, from which the carotid sinus branch of CN IX receives sensory information during the baroreceptor reflex for monitoring blood pressure, its involvement in swallowing function through the stylopharyngeus muscle, whereby stimulation can potentially cause unwanted side effects such as gagging, salivation, or changes in heart rate, and the potential for variability in its branching pattern, making precise targeting crucial during implant placement; additionally, the close proximity of the CN IX to CN X near the jugular foramen, as demonstrated in Fig. 3.5, can lead to potential unintended vagal stimulation during procedures and affect stimulation efficacy.

For OSA, evolving research has shown the potential of GNS in improving upper airway muscle tone and reducing sleep apnea episodes. Anatomical considerations for GNS include the base of the styloid process, the base of the styloid pyramid, and the transverse process of the atlas, serving as the three main landmarks of CN IX in the extracranial region in the infratemporal fossa [22]. Further details on GNS for OSA is discussed in Section 10, Chapter 37 (Glossopharyngeal Nerve for Sleep Apnea).

Vagus nerve (CN X)

The vagus nerve is cranial nerve 10 (CN X) and in addition to CN IX, exits through the jugular foramen, again illustrated in Fig. 3.6. The cell bodies are contained inside or just outside the jugular foramen in the inferior and superior ganglia. CN

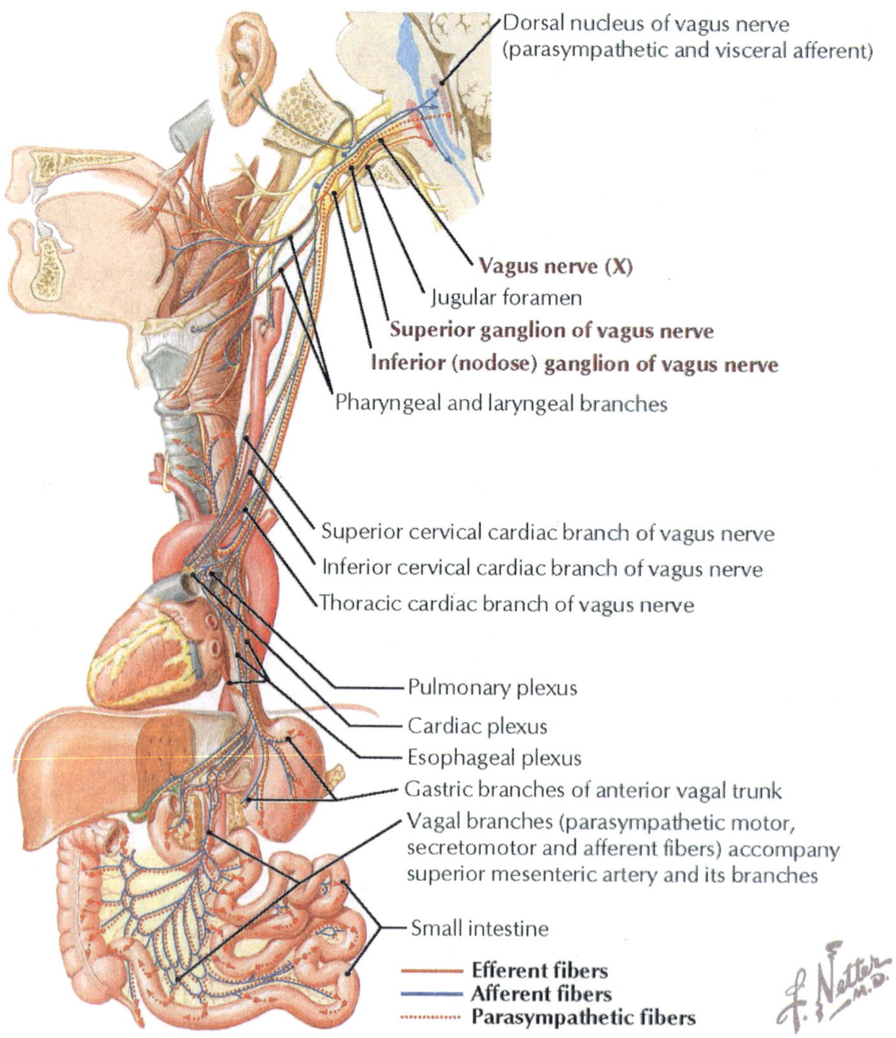

FIGURE 3.6 Vagus nerve anatomy. *Netter illustration from www.netterimages.com © Elsevier Inc. All rights reserved.*

X transmits general sensation from the auricle, external acoustic meatus, and dura mater of the posterior cranial fossa [5]. CN X also interacts with CN V, which is responsible for facial sensation, allowing for potential pain referral to the face. Studies in animal models have demonstrated that stimulating CN X can suppress nociceptive activity of trigeminocervical neurons in the TCC involved in pain perception, particularly in the head and neck region; this connection is often cited as a potential mechanism for treating headaches and other facial pain conditions through VNS [23]. VNS has been shown to reduce seizure propagation [24] and depression [25], implicating central nervous system influences on neuronal processing. Because of this broad coverage, many studies have targeted this nerve to treat a multitude of disorders.

Procedure-related considerations for vagus nerve stimulation (VNS)

A transcutaneous noninvasive VNS device has been used for the treatment of migraine and cluster headaches, and will be discussed elsewhere in Section 10, Chapter 38 (Vagal Nerve Stimulation: Implanted and External). Implantable VNS is primarily used to treat epilepsy, treatment-resistant depression, and stroke recovery [26].

The surgical implantation of a cervical VNS requires a detailed understanding of neck anatomy to ensure safe and effective placement. CN X descends within the carotid sheath, positioned between the internal jugular vein laterally and the common carotid artery medially [5]. Surgeons typically access the nerve through a transverse incision along the anterior border of the sternocleidomastoid muscle, usually at the level of the cricoid cartilage (C5–C7 vertebral levels). Careful dissection is essential to avoid injury to adjacent structures, including the recurrent laryngeal nerve, which branches off CN X and innervates the vocal cords. Injury to this nerve can result in hoarseness or voice changes. Additionally, preserving the ansa cervicalis, a loop of the cervical plexus that runs near CN X, is crucial to prevent postoperative motor deficits [27].

Proper electrode placement around the vagus nerve is critical for effective stimulation without causing unwanted side effects. Surgeons typically use helical electrodes, which gently wrap around the nerve without compressing it, to maintain nerve integrity and function. It is important to identify and avoid the cervical sympathetic trunk, located posterior to the carotid sheath, as damage can cause Horner's syndrome. Meticulous hemostasis is required to prevent hematoma formation, which could compress the airway. The lead from the electrode is tunneled subcutaneously to the pulse generator, which is typically implanted in a subpectoral or infraclavicular pocket, as illustrated in Fig. 3.7. Surgeons must ensure a secure connection and proper strain relief to prevent lead migration or fracture. Overall, a comprehensive understanding of cervical anatomy and careful surgical technique are paramount to achieving a successful VNS implantation and minimizing complications [28].

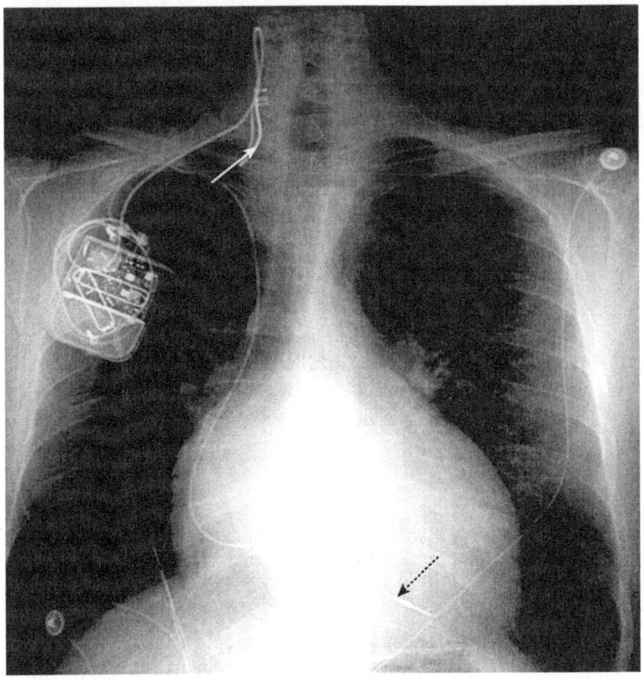

FIGURE 3.7 AP Chest X-ray illustrating vagal nerve stimulator implantation. *Reproduced with Permission, Clinical Cardiac Pacing, Defibrillation, and Resynchronization Therapy, Fifth Edition, Fig. 24.2. Elsevier 2017.*

When implanting a VNS, surgeons consider the anatomical location of CN X and the potential risks of stimulating it. The VNS is usually implanted around the left vagus nerve, which innervates the atrioventricular node, while the right vagus nerve innervates the sinoatrial node. Stimulating the right vagus nerve could cause cardiac side effects, such as bradycardia and asystole. Implantation can result in a peri-incisional hematoma, dyspnea, and localized infection around the wound site [28]. Refer to Section 10, Chapter 38 (Vagal Nerve Stimulation: Implanted and External) for further details.

Occipital nerves

The nerves that innervate the occipital area include the greater (GON), lesser (LON) and third (TON) occipital nerves, as illustrated in Fig. 3.8. The GON provides sensation to the middle and upper back of the scalp, while the LON innervates the lateral posterior scalp and the upper part of the ear (pinna), primarily along the posterior border of the sternocleidomastoid muscle. The TON provides sensory innervation to a small area of the medial occipital scalp, specifically just below the superior nuchal line, overlapping with the distribution of the GON and LON; it primarily supplies the skin in the midline region of the posterior neck and upper occipital area [5].

GON course. The GON is derived from the medial branch of the dorsal primary rami of C2 with some contribution from C3 nerve roots. The GON originates below the atlas's posterior arch, emerges between the first and second cervical vertebrae, passes between the inferior oblique and semispinalis capitis muscles, crosses the roof of the suboccipital triangle, turns dorsally and pierces the semispinalis capitis muscle, runs laterally and rostrally, deep to the trapezius muscle, piercing it and the sternocleidomastoid muscle, and becomes subcutaneous below the superior nuchal line, supplying sensation to the skin on the posterior scalp to the vertex. The GON has multiple branches that innervate the scalp in the occipital region. A significant feature of GON anatomy is its close relationship with the occipital artery, a branch of the external carotid artery at the exit site. This artery frequently crosses the GON at multiple points along its course, which has important implications for both vascular compression syndromes as well as inadvertent arterial compromise. In fact, in

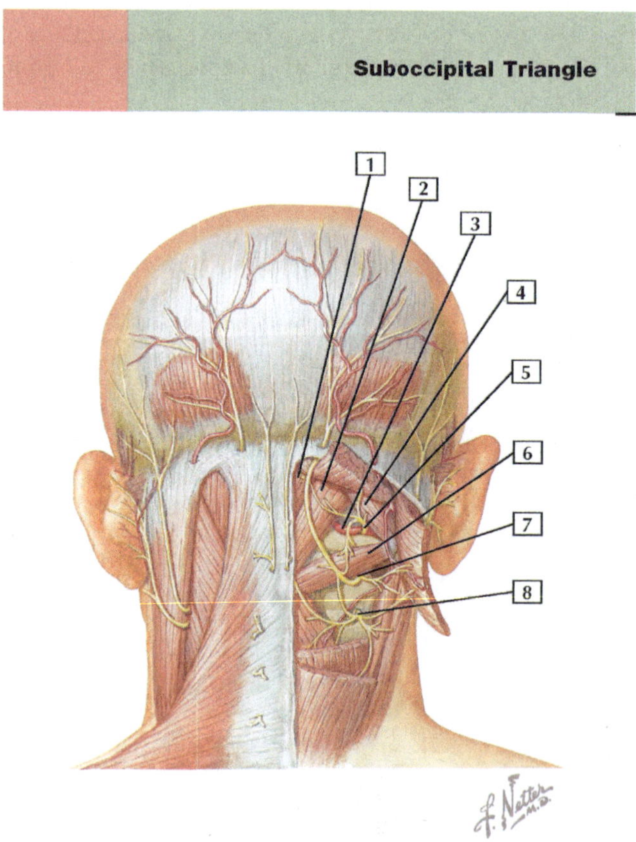

Suboccipital Triangle

1. Rectus capitis posterior minor m.
2. Rectus capitis posterior major m.
3. Vertebral a.
4. Obliquus capitis superior m.
5. Suboccipital n.
6. Obliquus capitis inferior m.
7. Greater occipital n.
8. 3rd occipital n.

Borders of the suboccipital triangle:
- Obliquus capitis superior
- Obliquus capitis inferior
- Rectus capitis posterior major

The roof of the suboccipital triangle is composed of dense connective tissue, whereas the floor of the suboccipital triangle is composed of:
- Posterior atlantooccipital membrane
- Posterior arch of the atlas

Suboccipital triangle is paired.

Contents

ARTERY	VEIN	NERVE	STRUCTURE

FIGURE 3.8 Suboccipital triangle including anatomic relationships between muscles, vasculature and the occipital nerves. *Netter illustration from www.netterimages.com © Elsevier Inc. All rights reserved.*

some patients, pulsatile irritation from the occipital artery has been identified as a contributing factor to vascular-related occipital neuralgia [29].

LON course. The LON originates from the anterior rami of C2 and C3 spinal nerve roots, runs superiorly along the sternocleidomastoid muscle, pierces the deep cervical fascia and emerges onto the occipital bone. The LON is a cutaneous branch that provides sensory innervation to the skin of the upper and posterior part of the auricle [30].

TON course. The TON, also known as the least occipital nerve, originates as the superficial medial branch of C3 spinal nerve root, lies medial to the greater occipital nerve, travels along the lateral and dorsal aspects of the C2–C3 zygapophyseal joint, supplies the joint, and pierces the part of semispinalis capitis and splenius capitis muscles before emerging on the skin of the suboccipital region, running medial to the GON and communicating with it. It courses along the posterior neck and supplies sensation to the lower part of the occiput [30].

Suboccipital triangle. The "suboccipital triangle" (SOT) is a small anatomical region at the base of the skull where the GON originates and passes through. The SOT serves as a key anatomical reference point for accessing the GON and adjacent structures during ONS implantation. The triangle is bounded by Ref. [31].

- Superomedial border: The rectus capitis posterior major (RCPMaj), spanning from C2 to the occipital bone.
- Superolateral border: The obliquus capitis superior (OCS), which originates from C1 and inserts onto the occipital bone.
- Inferolateral border: The obliquus capitis inferior (OCI) muscle, which extends from the spinous process of C2 to the transverse process of C1.

Sites of GON entrapment. Cadaveric studies have identified six potential sites of GON entrapment, which can affect both natural nerve function and response to ONS therapy [29].

1. At the emergence from the suboccipital region, where the nerve crosses beneath the OCI.
2. At the semispinalis capitis muscle, where fibrous bands may compress the nerve.
3. At multiple potential intersections with the occipital artery, leading to vascular irritation.
4. At the trapezius aponeurosis, where connective tissue constriction is common.
5. At additional crossing points with the occipital artery, leading to repeated pulsatile compression.
6. Along its terminal branches, particularly in patients with anatomical variations that predispose them to neural entrapment.

Procedure-related considerations for occipital nerve stimulation (ONS)

ONS is a form of PNS with mounting evidence for its use in craniofacial pain disorders including migraine, cluster headache, occipital neuralgia and other cervicogenic headache disorders [32]. ONS implantation techniques have varied widely, and as of this writing, head and neck neuromodulation including implantable ONS approaches and technical advances continue to evolve. Nonetheless, successful surgical technique is predicated on the basics of optimizing electrode positioning, lead anchoring, and IPG placement. Fluoroscopy is traditionally used for lead placement, although the use of ultrasound guidance alone or in addition to fluoroscopy allows for precise mapping of the GON, LON and TON, as well as identifying adjacent vascular structures that should be avoided during implantation [33].

The technique of ONS implantation was introduced by Weiner and Reid in 1999. Variations on this technique have since been described [34]. General anesthesia for ONS implantation is usually preferred to reduce patient discomfort especially since subcutaneous tunneling is a noxious stimulus, and to maximize sterility.

Patient positioning. Before permanent implantation, a stimulation trial should be performed to assess the optimal electrode placement and stimulation parameters. For ONS implantation, the recommended patient positioning is typically prone (face down) with the head resting on a horseshoe-shaped headrest to allow for proper access to the occipital nerve area and optimal visualization under fluoroscopy; the cervical spine should be slightly flexed during the procedure.

Traditional lead entry technique. The approach to skin entry using a midline versus lateral incision has been debated, and the rationale for either approach has been described. With the more traditional medial-to-lateral approach, a 2–3 cm horizontal midline incision is made 1–2 cm below the superior nuchal line or over C1, with careful dissection down to the occipital fascia. Generous local anesthetic infiltration creates a wheal along the proposed path of the 14 gauge introducer needle. The introducer is advanced under AP fluoroscopy in a medial to lateral trajectory. The mastoid process is the lateral-most fluoroscopic landmark for placement of the needle tip. The stylet is removed, and the lead is inserted through the introducer needle until resistance is met at the tip of the needle. At this point, the most proximal electrode should be confirmed by AP fluoroscopy at or slightly lateral to the midline. Once lead position is satisfactory, the introducer is removed under live fluoroscopy, taking care to keep the lead tip at its desired location. Lead placement should overlap the

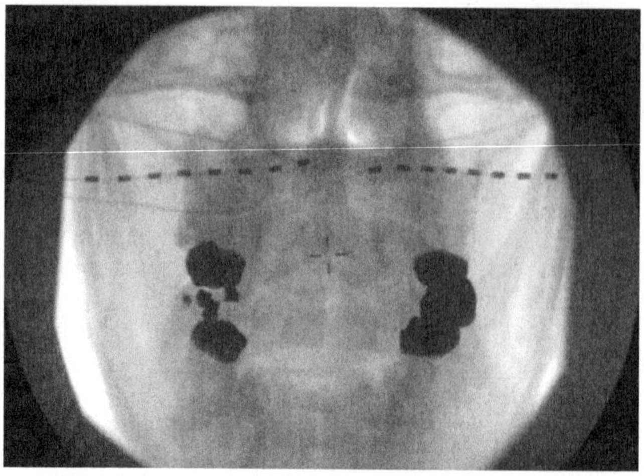

FIGURE 3.9 Fluoroscopic image of bilateral occipital nerve stimulator lead placement. *Reproduced with permission, Techniques in Regional Anesthesia and Pain Management, Central neurostimulation techniques for primary headaches, Elsevier 2012.*

GON and LON over the occipital ridge, as illustrated in Fig. 3.9. Intraoperative test stimulation is conducted to confirm that paresthesia coverage aligns with the patient's pain distribution [35].

Alternative lead entry techniques. A lateral retromastoid approach has been described [35], and involves lateral decubitus positioning, and making a retromastoid incision with leads tunneled horizontally across the nuchal ridge, either with a single lead from a lateral to medial trajectory, or advanced across the occipital midline in an effort to provide bilateral stimulation coverage. A singular lead can be placed across the occiput, spanning 10–15 cm between the mastoid processes, ensuring coverage of the GON, LON and TON. Leads with more electrodes (12 contacts) can be placed past midline to obtain bilateral coverage. A subcutaneous pocket is created by undermining the incision. The purpose is two-fold; the pocket creates an area large enough for anchoring the lead, and allows for a strain relief loop of the lead, both of which are designed to prevent LM.

The rationale for the midline approach for bilateral transformed migraine and the lateral approach for unilateral occipital neuralgia has been described [36]. Still, other techniques have been described with the incision starting more caudally and advancing the lead into the soft tissues of the neck over the SOT. As the nerve transitions from a deep muscular course to a more superficial trajectory, lead placement within this zone can significantly impact stimulation efficacy [37]. Advantages include avoiding those complications seen with the traditional midline approach. Disadvantages include placement of the lead in a 'high traffic' region of the upper neck with muscle groups with the potential for intolerable muscle spasm, lead integrity compromise or migration.

Lead Anchoring, Tunneling, and IPG Placement. Once lead placement is achieved, a silicone anchor can be secured to the lead, and the lead-anchor complex sutured to the occipital fascia using nonabsorbable sutures at the lead exit site in the occipital pocket. Additionally, medical grade silicone glue can be administered between the lead and the anchor to form a bond. Strain relief loops are utilized. The lead is then tunneled toward the IPG pocket. One or more counter-incisions with strain relief loops may be used along the path of the tunneled lead to the IPG pocket. There is no consensus as to the preferred anchor configurations, suture materials, or suture techniques. However, leads are typically tunneled subcutaneously toward a pocket in the infraclavicular, posterior flank, buttock, abdomen, or midaxillary line depending on patient preference and habitus. However, one must take into consideration longer lead pathways can increase the risk of hardware fatigue, lead migration and other complications [38].

Final Testing and Closure. Once the leads and IPG are secured, intraoperative test stimulation is conducted to confirm that paresthesia coverage aligns with the patient's pain distribution. Then, surgical incisions are copiously irrigated and closed in layers, and a fluoroscopic image should be obtained to document final lead position. Patients are advised to minimize excessive neck movement for at least 6 weeks postoperatively to facilitate lead encapsulation and stabilization.

Pearls and pitfalls of ONS

Lead migration has traditionally been a primary concern in ONS implantation. Percutaneous cylindrical electrodes are preferred over paddle leads due to their flexibility, adaptability, and broader stimulation coverage, though they carry a slightly higher risk of migration. The highly mobile neck region places stress on system components, favoring the alternative lateral approach. Methods to avoid forces that lead to migration depend on an understanding of upper neck muscle anatomy and physiology. Robust fixation techniques to optimize long-term stability is paramount for avoiding loss of effective stimulation coverage and symptom recurrence. Strategies such as anchoring leads at a 45-degree angle, strain relief loops and silicone sheath anchoring to dense occipital or cervical fascia, and minimizing tension during tunneling have been developed to mitigate this risk [39].

Identification of lead migration starts with clinical suspicion followed by fluoroscopic evaluation. Loss of paresthesia coverage in the LON but preservation of GON coverage should raise suspicion for lead migration in patients undergoing midline technique due to lateral to medial migration. Loss of GON coverage with preservation of LON coverage would suggest the possibility of lateral lead migration, which may occur if initial introducer placement is overzealous toward the mastoid process. An understanding of GON and LON anatomy and sensory distribution is critical for troubleshooting [40].

Hardware failure, including electrode breakage, lead fractures, and IPG malfunctions, has been reported, and require revision surgery or replacement of malfunctioning components [40]. There is theoretical risk of injury to both the occipital nerve and lead fracture given the superficial nature of the placement, should there be occipital head trauma as with a fall.

Infection has been a postoperative concern, most commonly caused by Staphylococcus aureus; superficial infections can often be managed with antibiotics, but deep infections typically necessitate complete system explantation [41]. Meticulous hemostasis is especially important as the occipital scalp region is a highly vascular area, and this helps to protect against the risk of hematoma and subsequent infection. Safety considerations when dissecting and placing leads for surgical implantation include the occipital artery, which juxtaposes next to the GON in the scalp. Careful use of blunt tip introducers should be considered to avoid injury, and a flexible introducer with a bend to the contour of the occipital cranium should be considered to ensure parallel orientation of the lead with the scalp contour. The 'danger area of the scalp' refers to the layer of loose areolar connective tissue as it contains the valveless emissary veins that connect the superficial veins in the subaponeurotic space with the intracranial venous sinuses. This connection could potentially allow a deeper infection to spread from the scalp to the meninges [42].

Skin erosion has been described in some ONS case reports, a disadvantage of the midline approach. It is important to place the introducer and subsequently, the lead, in the subcutaneous fat, superficial to the fascia. This prevents direct muscle stimulation if the lead is placed too close to the fascia. Conversely, care must be taken to prevent lead placement from being too superficial, with risk of skin erosion [43].

Some patients have experienced unintended paresthesia, dysesthesia, or hypersensitivity, usually related to improper lead positioning or excessive stimulation intensity; while many of these symptoms could be managed with device reprogramming, refractory cases required lead repositioning or surgical revision [44].

Many of these challenges are based on studies utilizing older devices and leads. Continued advancements in lead design, implantation techniques, and device programming, and PNS systems that do not require an IPG are expected to enhance long-term safety and efficacy, reducing these complications, surgical revisions and improving patient outcomes.

Procedure-related considerations for high cervical spinal cord stimulation (hcSCS) and C2 dorsal root ganglion stimulation (DRG)

There is emerging evidence that hcSCS with lead placement at the C2 vertebral level, as illustrated in Fig. 3.10, may provide benefit for chronic migraines, cluster headache, TACs, trigeminal neuropathic pain and cervicogenic headaches, particularly when more conservative treatments are ineffective. hcSCS delivered to the dorsal column at C2-3 directly targets the TCC through electrical current delivered by the implanted lead, which could result in analgesic activity and significantly reduce the frequency and intensity of migraine headaches in some patients [45]. Randomized, double-blind, sham-controlled trials are needed to demonstrate efficacy. Procedural technique for implanting dorsal column stimulator leads into the cervical epidural space is demonstrated in Section 3, Chapter 9 (Cervical Spinal Cord Stimulation). It is also conceivable that C2 cervical dorsal root ganglion (DRG) stimulation may treat craniofacial disorders including migraine [46], however, further research on this topic is necessary. Procedural technique for implanting cervical DRG stimulator leads is demonstrated in Section 4, Chapter 13 (Cervical Dorsal Root Ganglion Stimulation).

Central processing of craniofacial nociceptive afferents

First-order neurons of the trigeminal and cervico-occipital primary afferents, along with contributions from vagus and glossopharyngeal nerves, form a network known as the TCC in an area in the upper cervical and medullary dorsal horn, as

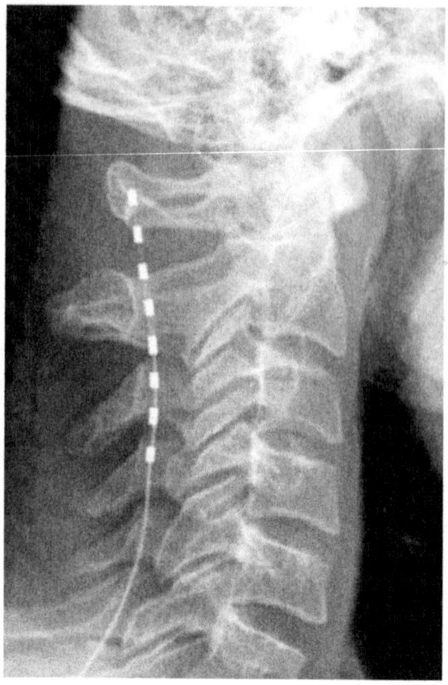

FIGURE 3.10 Lateral fluoroscopic image of high cervical spinal cord stimulator lead placement at C2 for the treatment of headache. *Reproduced with permission, Techniques in Regional Anesthesia and Pain Management, Central neurostimulation techniques for primary headaches, Elsevier 2012.*

previously illustrated in Fig. 3.2. The TNC is considered the primary nucleus within the TCC where the sensory pathway from CN V converges with the upper cervical spinal cord neurons from C2 [47].

Second-order neurons from the TNC/TCC decussate, sending pain and temperature information through a central pathway, as illustrated in Fig. 3.11, through the trigeminothalamic tract, and synapsing on multiple contralateral thalamic nuclei, the most important of which is the ventral posteromedial nucleus (VPM) of the thalamus. While en route to the thalamus, collateral projections also terminate at the rostral ventromedial medulla, locus coeruleus, periaqueductal gray (PAG), and hypothalamus. Sensitization of these neurons help explain the spread and referral of pain in patients with headache disorders and can lead to amplification of all convergent inputs, which may explain the hypersensitivity seen in various headache syndromes. Due to the convergence of trigeminal and cervical inputs within the TCC, this structure plays an important role in the pathogenesis of the pain component of headaches, and serves as a potential site for neuromodulation with hcSCS.

Third-order neurons carrying nociceptive information from craniofacial structures project from the thalamus to somatosensory cortices and the posterior insula for sensory processing and integration through the *lateral pain pathway*. Further pain processing occurs in the anterior insula and dorsal anterior cingulate cortex, which project to limbic system structures, assigning the affective component of the pain experience through the *medial pain pathway*. The prefrontal cortex, in combination with the pregenual anterior cingulate cortex, participates in the *descending modulatory pain pathway*, with projections to the periaqueductal gray and rostral ventromedial medulla, synapsing onto the dorsal raphe nucleus to inhibit facial pain, and onto superficial laminae of the cervical dorsal horn to inhibit neck pain [48].

Neuromodulatory effects on brain circuitry, as with supraspinal influences of SCS waveforms on the lateral, medial and descending pain pathways [49], may also lead to analgesia for craniofacial pain disorders. SCS waveforms are discussed in detail later in Section 5, Chapter 18 (Burst Waveforms), Chapter 19 (High Frequency Stimulation), Chapter 20 (Fast Waveforms and Stimulation), Chapter 21 (DTM), and Chapter 22 (New Waveform Concepts for Spinal Cord Stimulation).

Deep brain stimulation (DBS)

DBS has been utilized for movement disorders [50], mood disorders [51] and chronic pain [52]. The precise placement of DBS electrodes depends on the disorder being treated, and the approach to these targets relies on applying knowledge of the relevant anatomy.

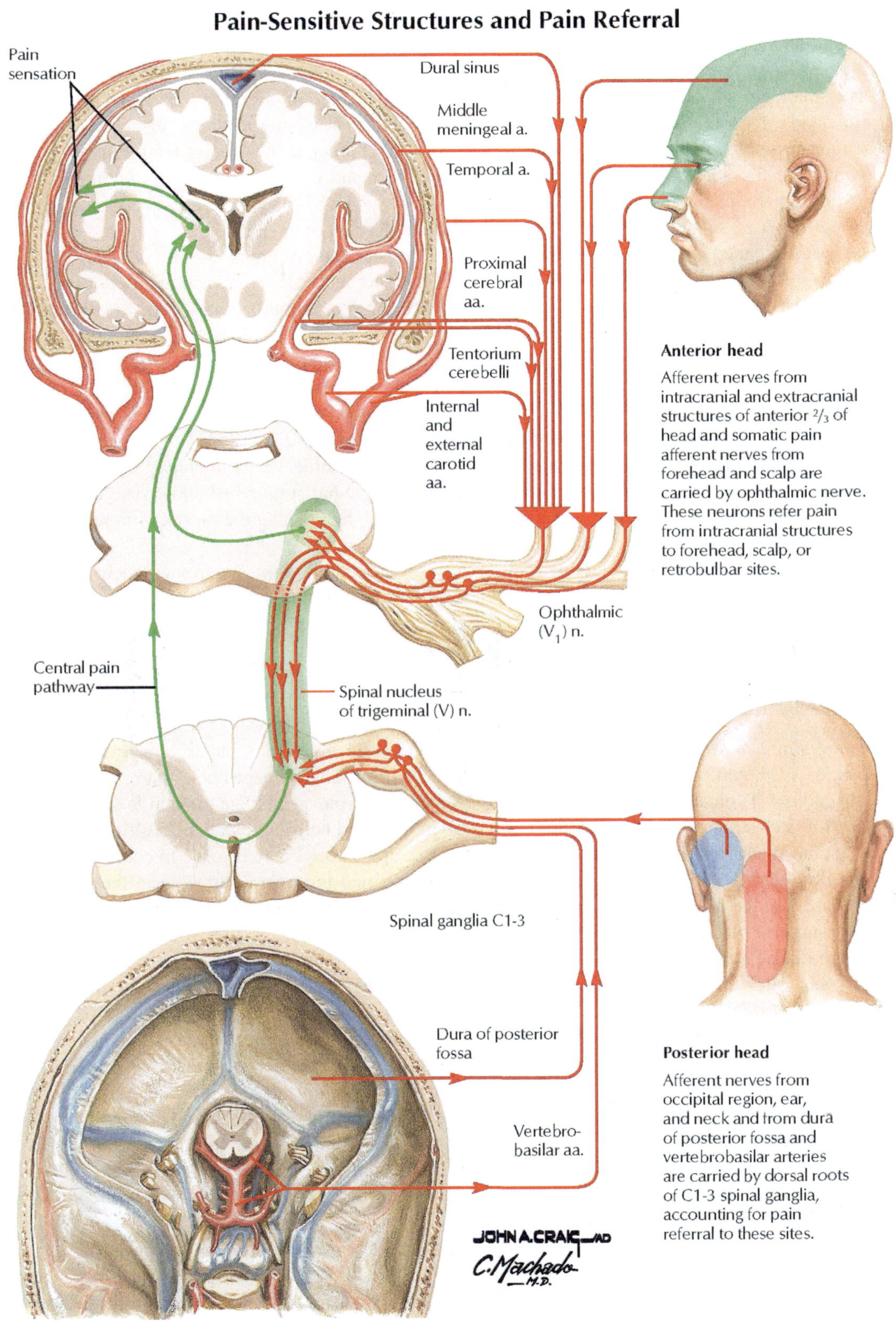

FIGURE 3.11 Pain-sensitive structures and central mechanisms for craniofacial pain. *Netter illustration from www.netterimages.com © Elsevier Inc. All rights reserved.*

DBS for Movement Disorders. Important targeted structures for Parkinson's disease [50] include the globus pallidus internus (GPi) and subthalamic nucleus (STN), and for essential tremor [50] include the ventral intermedius nucleus (VIM) of the thalamus, among other targets, as illustrated in Fig. 3.12.

The STN is a small, glutamatergic nucleus involved in the subcortical motor circuitry, measuring approximately 7 × 5 × 3 mm in dimension. It resides ventrally below the thalamus and zona incerta at the level of the red nucleus in the midbrain. It's anterior border is the cerebral peduncle and posterior border is the medial lemniscus. The STN receives excitatory inputs from the cerebral cortex through the hyperdirect pathway and inhibitory inputs from the external segment of the globus pallidus (GPe) as a part of the indirect pathway. The STN sends its excitatory projections to the GPi and substantia nigra pars reticularis, also known as the basal ganglia output nuclei [53].

The GPi is a wedge-shaped nucleus that is a main inhibitory output center of the motor circuit in the basal ganglia. It's lateral border is the GPe and medial border is posterior limb of the internal capsule, and resides superiorly above the optic tract. The GPi receives input from the striatum, GPe, and STN and has inhibitory projections to the motor thalamus through the ansa lenticularis and lenticular fasciculus [53].

The VIM is roughly 4 mm in the anterior–posterior dimension and approximately 10–12 mm in the rostral–caudal dimension. It is anterior to the ventrolateral caudalis nucleus, which receives somatosensory input from the medial lemniscus, and is posterior to the ventralis oralis posterior nucleus, which receives input from the basal ganglia. The VIM also receives unconscious proprioceptive fibers from the dentatorubrothalamic tract [54].

DBS for Mood Disorders. Important targeted structures for mood disorders have included the subcallosal cingulate gyrus (SCG), ventral capsule/ventral striatum, nucleus accumbens, medial forebrain bundle, lateral habenula, inferior thalamic peduncle, and the bed nucleus of the stria terminalis, with the SCG being the most commonly studied target for treatment-resistant depression [51].

DBS for Pain Syndromes. Important targeted structures for intractable pain syndromes such as poststroke pain, phantom limb pain, and neuropathic pain, have included the PAG, periventricular gray matter, thalamic ventral posterior lateral (VPL) and ventral posterior medial (VPM) nuclei, orbitofrontal cortex, primary motor cortex, and dorsolateral prefrontal cortex, among others [52].

Procedure-related considerations for DBS

DBS planning, mapping and targeting. High-resolution MRI or CT scans are used to identify anatomical landmarks, such as the STN, GPi, or VIM, and plan the trajectory of electrode insertion. These images help map the brain and determine the optimal entry points. Typically, the target structure is located based on specific anatomical landmarks, with standard coordinates used for each structure. A stereotactic frame is often used and helps with patient positioning and targeting for precise electrode placement. In some cases, intraoperative fluoroscopy or MRI may be used to confirm the position of the electrode in real-time during surgery. The electrode is typically inserted through a burr hole in the skull, and the entry point is chosen based on the brain structure being targeted and the patient's brain anatomy. Microelectrode recording is often used during surgery to detect neuronal firing patterns to confirm the precise location of the target structure, providing real-time feedback during electrode placement. Modern DBS systems often use directional leads, which allow for more precise targeting and can help limit side effects by modulating specific regions of the brain more effectively [55].

Anatomic Safety Considerations. The surgeon must plan the trajectory to minimize damage to critical structures such as the motor cortex, sensory cortex, and blood vessels, and avoid disruption of white matter tracts involved in cognition, speech and vision. Each patient's brain anatomy may differ slightly, and therefore, individual factors including age, head shape and prior surgery should be considered. Brain atrophy in elderly patients or those with neurodegenerative diseases can alter the size and location of brain structures. In addition to structural imaging, functional mapping techniques may be employed to avoid regions of the brain responsible for critical functions such as motor control, speech, and cognition. The brain's vasculature must be carefully considered to avoid large blood vessels (e.g., anterior cerebral artery) during electrode placement. After implantation, patients are carefully monitored for any signs of complications, such as infections, bleeding, or hardware malfunction [56].

In summary, DBS implantation requires careful consideration of the target structure, brain anatomy, and patient-specific factors to ensure precise electrode placement and minimize risks. Advanced imaging and intraoperative monitoring techniques are essential to guide the surgery and confirm correct placement. Detailed procedural approaches to some of these targets are described in detail in Section 10, Chapter 34 (Deep Brain Stimulation: Movement Disorders), Chapter 35 (Deep Brain Stimulation: Depression and Psychological Issues), and Chapter 36 (Deep Brain Stimulation: Pain).

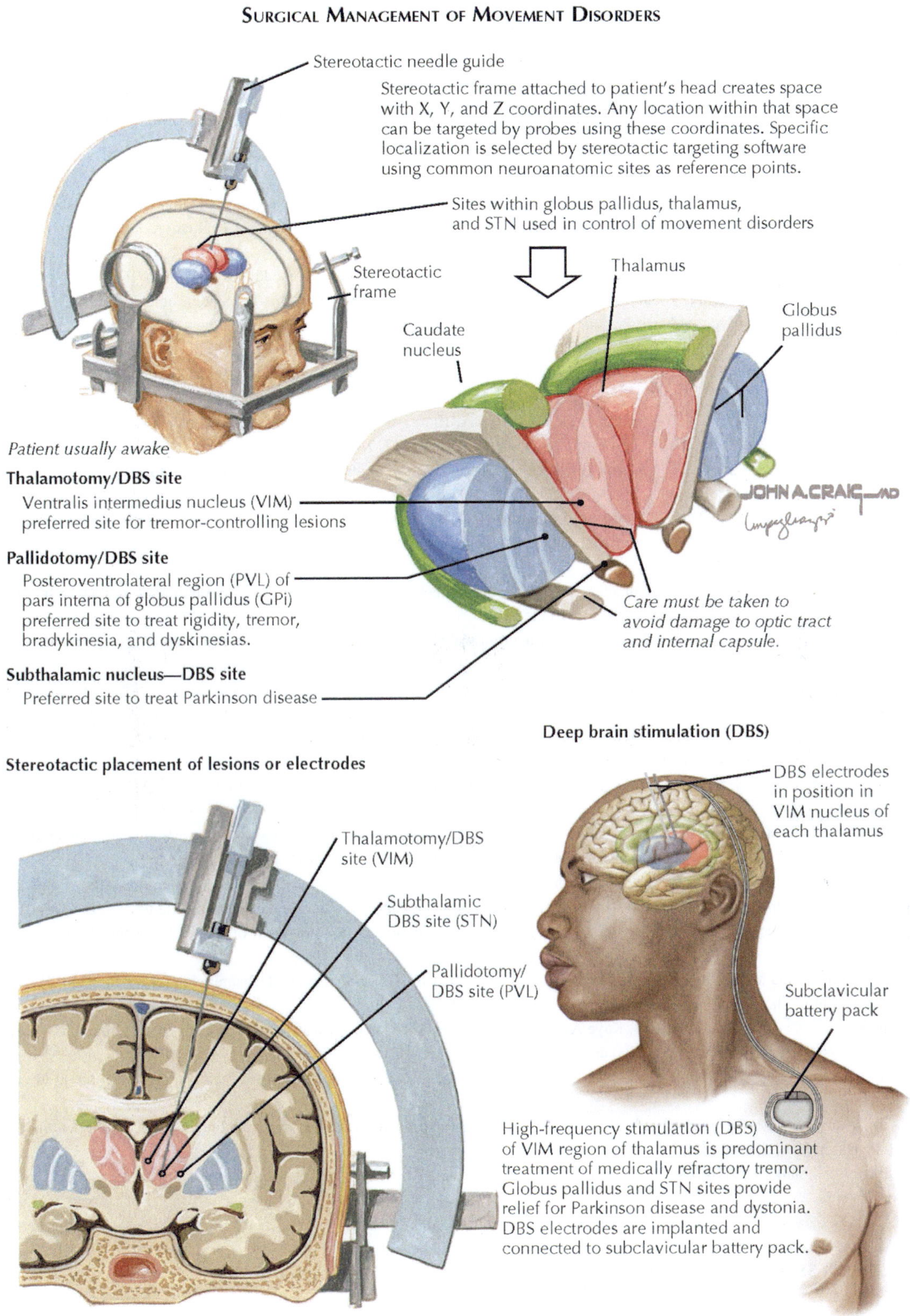

FIGURE 3.12 Schematic representation of anatomical sites for deep brain stimulation for movement disorders. *Netter illustration from www.netterimages.com © Elsevier Inc. All rights reserved.*

References

[1] Melzack R, Wall PD. Pain mechanisms: A new theory. Science 1965;150(3699):971–9. https://doi.org/10.1126/science.150.3699.971.

[2] Deer TR, Skaribas IM, Haider N, Salmon J, Kim C, Nelson C, Tracy J, Espinet A, Lininger TE, Tiso R, Archacki MA, Washburn SN. Effectiveness of cervical spinal cord stimulation for the management of chronic pain. Neuromodulation 2014;17(3):265–71.

[3] Strand N, D'Souza RS, Hagedorn JM, Pritzlaff S, Sayed D, Azeem N, Abd-Elsayed A, Escobar A, Huntoon MA, Lam CM, Deer TR. Evidence-based clinical guidelines from the American society of pain and neuroscience for the use of implantable peripheral nerve stimulation in the treatment of chronic pain. J Pain Res 2022;15:2483–504.

[4] Ben-Haim S, Mirzadeh Z, Rosenberg WS. Deep brain stimulation for intractable neuropathic facial pain. Neurosurg Focus 2018;45(2):E15.

[5] Grisold W, Struhal W, Grisold A. The cranial nerves in neurology: A comprehensive and systematic evaluation of cranial nerves, pathology and specific conditions. 2023.

[6] Pak RJ, Ku JB, Abd-Elsayed A. Neuromodulation for craniofacial pain and headaches. Biomedicines December 16, 2023;11(12):3328.

[7] Goadsby PJ, Bartsch T. The anatomy and physiology of the trigeminocervical complex. In: Fernández de las Peñas C, Arendt-Nielsen L, Gerwin RD, editors. Tension-type and cervicogenic headache: pathophysiology, diagnosis and treatment. Sudbury: Jones and Barlett; 2010. p. 109–16.

[8] Abd-Elsayed AA, Grandhi R, Sachdeva H. Effective management of trigeminal neuralgia by neurostimulation. Ochsner J. Summer 2015;15 (2):193–5.

[9] McMahon JT, Tora MS, Bentley JN, Texakalidis P, Campbell MA, Keifer Jr OP, Boulis NM. Percutaneous trigeminal nerve stimulation for persistent idiopathic facial pain: A case series. World Neurosurg 2019;126:e1379–86.

[10] Ellis JA, Mejia Munne JC, Winfree CJ. Trigeminal branch stimulation for the treatment of intractable craniofacial pain. J Neurosurg 2015;123 (1):283–8.

[11] William A, Azad TD, Brecher E, Cherry T, Bernstein I, Bruce DM, Rohrer S, Smith Z, William M, Sabelman E, Heit G, Pezeshkian P, Sedrak M. Trigeminal and sphenopalatine ganglion stimulation for intractable craniofacial pain–case series and literature review. Acta Neurochir 2016;158 (3):513–20.

[12] Hajiabadi MM, Jakobs M, Unterberg A, Ahmadi R. Wireless subcutaneous trigeminal nerve field stimulation for refractory trigeminal pain: A single center experience. Neuromodulation 2021;24(6):1115–20.

[13] Khan S, Schoenen J, Ashina M. Sphenopalatine ganglion neuromodulation in migraine: What is the rationale? Cephalalgia 2014;34(5):382–91.

[14] Qin L, Chen D, Li X, Gao Y, Xia W, Dai H, Qiu L, Yang J, Zhang L. Sphenopalatine ganglion stimulation: A comprehensive evaluation across diseases in randomized controlled trials. Front Neurol 2024;15:1352145.

[15] Goadsby PJ, Sahai-Srivastava S, Kezirian EJ, Calhoun AH, Matthews DC, McAllister PJ, Costantino PD, Friedman DI, Zuniga JR, Mechtler LL, Popat SR, Rezai AR, Dodick DW. Safety and efficacy of sphenopalatine ganglion stimulation for chronic cluster headache: A double-blind, randomised controlled trial. Lancet Neurol 2019;18(12):1081–90.

[16] Ho KWD, Przkora R, Kumar S. Sphenopalatine ganglion: Block, radiofrequency ablation and neurostimulation—A systematic review. J Headache Pain 2017;18:118.

[17] Mehta DG, Gurianov R, Gombolevskiy VA, et al. A computerized tomographic and cadaveric study of sphenopalatine ganglion block via the pterygomaxillary fissure: anatomical considerations of the suprazygomatic approach. Ann Head Med 2021;04(02).

[18] Siakallis L, Connor SEJ. Localization of the sphenopalatine ganglion within the pterygopalatine fossa on computed tomography angiography-A potential role in the setting of sphenopalatine ganglion microstimulator implantation. Neuromodulation 2021;24(8):1422–8.

[19] Láinez MJ, Puche M, Garcia A, Gascón F. Sphenopalatine ganglion stimulation for the treatment of cluster headache. Ther Adv Neurol Disord 2014;7(3):162–8.

[20] Plewa MC, Tadi P, Gupta M. Cavernous sinus thrombosis [Updated 2023 Jul 3]. In: StatPearls. Treasure Island (FL): StatPearls Publishing; 2025. https://www.ncbi.nlm.nih.gov/books/NBK448177/.

[21] Han A, Montgomery C, Zamora A, Winder E, Kaye A, Carroll C, Aquino A, Kakazu J, Kaye AD. Glossopharyngeal neuralgia: epidemiology, risk factors, pathophysiology, differential diagnosis, and treatment options. Health Psychol Res 2022;10(5):36042.

[22] Ozveren MF, Türe U, Ozek MM, Pamir MN. Anatomic landmarks of the glossopharyngeal nerve: A microsurgical anatomic study. Neurosurgery 2003;52(6):1400–10.

[23] Hawkins JL, Cornelison LE, Blankenship BA, Durham PL. Vagus nerve stimulation inhibits trigeminal nociception in a rodent model of episodic migraine. Pain Rep 2017;2(6):e628.

[24] Pérez-Carbonell L, Faulkner H, Higgins S, Koutroumanidis M, Leschziner G. Vagus nerve stimulation for drug-resistant epilepsy. Pract Neurol 2020;20(3):189–98.

[25] Austelle CW, O'Leary GH, Thompson S, Gruber E, Kahn A, Manett AJ, Short B, Badran BW. A comprehensive review of vagus nerve stimulation for depression. Neuromodulation 2022;25(3):309–15.

[26] Austelle CW, Cox SS, Wills KE, Badran BW. Vagus nerve stimulation (VNS): Recent advances and future directions. Clin Auton Res 2024;34 (6):529–47.

[27] Giordano F, Zicca A, Barba C, Guerrini R, Genitori L. Vagus nerve stimulation: Surgical technique of implantation and revision and related morbidity. Epilepsia 2017;58(Suppl. 1):85–90.

[28] Mandalaneni K, Rayi A. Vagus nerve stimulator [Updated 2023 Aug 7]. In: StatPearls. Treasure Island (FL): StatPearls Publishing; 2025.

[29] Sağlam L, Gayretli O, Coşkun O, Kale A. Morphological features of the greater occipital nerve and its possible importance for interventional procedures. J Anat 2023;244(3):312–24.

[30] Yu M, Wang SM. Anatomy, head and neck, occipital nerves [Updated 2022 Oct 31]. In: StatPearls. Treasure Island (FL): StatPearls Publishing; 2025.

[31] Hacking C, Kanagarajah A. Occipital triangle. Published Radiopaedia.Org 2017. [Accessed 5 February 2025].

[32] Paemeleire K, Bartsch T. Occipital nerve stimulation for headache disorders. Neurotherapeutics 2010;7(2):213–9.

[33] Eldrige JS, Obray JB, Pingree MJ, Hoelzer BC. Occipital neuromodulation: Ultrasound guidance for peripheral nerve stimulator implantation. Pain Pract 2010;10(6):580–5.

[34] Trentman TL, Zimmerman RS. Occipital nerve stimulation: technical and surgical aspects of implantation. Headache 2008;48(2):319–27.

[35] McGreevy K, Hameed H, Erdek MA. Updated perspectives on occipital nerve stimulator lead migration: case report and literature review. Clin J Pain 2012;28(9):814–8.

[36] Meier K, Fogh-Andersen IS, Sørensen JCH. Occipital nerve stimulation: A detailed description of a surgical approach and a discussion on implantation techniques. Pain Pract 2025;25(1):e13444.

[37] Fabry A, Nedunchelian M, Stacoffe N, et al. Review of craniofacial pain syndromes involving the greater occipital nerve: Relevant anatomy, clinical findings, and interventional management. Neuroradiology 2023;66(2):161–78.

[38] Trentman TL, Mueller JT, Shah DM, Zimmerman RS, Noble BM. Occipital nerve stimulator lead pathway length changes with volunteer movement: An in vitro study. Pain Pract 2010;10(1):42–8.

[39] Zimmerman RS, Dodick DW, Weaver L, Cunniff B, Mayer J, Rothrock JF. Occipital nerve stimulation for chronic intractable headache: long-term safety and efficacy. Cephalalgia 2012;32(16):1165–73.

[40] Mueller OM, Oertel JM, Korinthenberg R, Weigel R, Boecher-Schwarz HG. Occipital nerve stimulation for the treatment of chronic headaches: Long-term follow-up in a small series. Acta Neurochir 2013;155(11):1859–66.

[41] Veilleux C, Khousakoun C, Kwon C, Amoozegar F, Girgis F. Efficacy of occipital nerve stimulation in trigeminal autonomic cephalalgias: A systematic review. Neurosurgery 2023;93(4):755–63.

[42] Germann AM, Jamal Z, Al Khalili Y. Anatomy, head and neck, scalp veins [Updated 2023 Jan 13]. In: StatPearls. Treasure Island (FL): StatPearls Publishing; 2025.

[43] Zhou L, Ashkenazi A, Smith JW, Jen N, Deer TR, Zhou C. Long-term clinical outcome of peripheral nerve stimulation for chronic headache and complication prevention. Anesth Pain Med 2016;6(4):e35983.

[44] Montenegro MM, Kissoon NR. Long-term outcomes of occipital nerve stimulation. Front Pain Res (Lausanne) 2023;4:1175678.

[45] (a) De Agostino R, Federspiel B, Cesnulis E, Sandor PS. High-cervical spinal cord stimulation for medically intractable chronic migraine discussion 296. Neuromodulation 2015;18(4):289–96. https://doi.org/10.1111/ner.12236. Epub 2014 Sep 23. PMID: 25250943.
(b) Towne BV, Girgiss CB, Schuster NM. Use of spinal cord stimulation in treatment of intractable headache diseases. Pain Med 2023;24(Suppl. 2):S6–296.

[46] Boos A, Nader A. Ultrasound-guided percutaneous peripheral nerve stimulation of C2 dorsal root ganglion for the treatment of refractory atypical facial pain: A technical report and case series. Neuromodulation 2024;27(1):130–4.

[47] Bartsch T, Goadsby PJ. Increased responses in trigeminocervical nociceptive neurons to cervical input after stimulation of the dura mater. Brain 2003;126(8):1801–13.

[48] Ossipov MH, Dussor GO, Porreca F. Central modulation of pain. J Clin Investig 2010;120(11):3779–87. https://doi.org/10.1172/JCI43766.

[49] De Ridder D, Vanneste S, Smith M, Adhia D. Pain and the triple network model. Front Neurol 2022;13:757241. https://doi.org/10.3389/fneur.2022.757241.

[50] Weaver FM, Follett KA, Stern M, Luo P, Harris CL, Hur K, et al. Randomized trial of deep brain stimulation for Parkinson disease: Thirty-six-month outcomes. Neurology 2012;79(1):55–65.

[51] Holtzheimer 3rd PE, Mayberg HS. Deep brain stimulation for treatment-resistant depression. Am J Psychiatry 2010;167(12):1437–44.

[52] Boccard SG, Pereira EA, Aziz TZ. Deep brain stimulation for chronic pain. J Clin Neurosci 2015;22(10):1537–43.

[53] Dallapiazza RF, De Vloo P, Fomenko A, et al. Considerations for patient and target selection in deep brain stimulation surgery for Parkinson's disease. In: Stoker TB, Greenland JC, editors. Parkinson's disease: pathogenesis and clinical aspects [internet]. Brisbane (AU): Codon Publications; 2018.

[54] Vaillancourt DE, Sturman MM, Verhagen Metman L, Bakay RA, Corcos DM. Deep brain stimulation of the VIM thalamic nucleus modifies several features of essential tremor. Neurology 2003;61(7):919–25.

[55] Campbell BA, Machado AG, Baker KB. Electrophysiologic mapping for deep brain stimulation for movement disorders. Handb Clin Neurol 2019;160:345–55.

[56] Cook R, Chennell Dutton N, Silburn PA, Meagher LJ, Fracchia G, Anderson N, Cooper G, Dinh HM, Cook SJ, Silberstein P. Minimising the rate of vascular complications in deep brain stimulation surgery for the management of Parkinson's disease: A single-centre 600-patient case series. BMJ Neurol Open 2024;6(2):e000793.

Chapter 4

Anatomy of the peripheral nervous system

Jeffery Kramer[1], Robert Moghim[2], Melissa Murphy[3], Timothy Deer[4] and Christopher Gilmore[5]

[1]*Volta Research, Minneapolis, MN, United States;* [2]*Colorado Pain Care, Denver, CO, United States;* [3]*North Texas Orthopedics and Spine Center, Grapevine, TX, United States;* [4]*The Spine and Nerve Centers of the Virginias, Charleston, WV, United States;* [5]*Carolinas Pain Institute, Winston-Salem, NC, United States*

Peripheral nervous system overview

- Nerves in the peripheral nervous system send efferent signals to end organs and transmit afferent sensory information to the central nervous system
- Sensory nerves innervate distinct anatomical regions and travel to the CNS via distinct spinal levels; this allows specific therapeutic targeting
- Nerves can be primarily sensory, motor or mixed function and this understanding helps plan therapy approaches and avoid complications

Apart from the central nervous system (CNS), which comprises the brain and spinal cord, the peripheral nervous system (PNS) lies outside the CNS. Generally, the PNS contains the efferent nerves projecting from the CNS that innervate end organs, as well as the afferent projections that send encoded neural signals from various somatic and visceral tissues [1]. Anatomically, the PNS follows an innervation pattern that is related to regions of the body, in that specific efferent motor nerves consistently control various functions (e.g., skeletal muscle contraction, autonomic motor outflow, etc.) and sensory nerves do the same. Anatomically, the motor and sensory nerves exit and enter the CNS via specific pathways through the spinal column (Fig. 4.1). In this way, nerves and their corresponding motor and sensory regions correspond to a myotomal (for motor) or dermatomal (for sensory) innervation pattern [2,3]. These maps demonstrate the rough innervation patterns that are observed relative to spinal level. Nerves that sequentially branch from the original spinal nerve roots then innervate the more distal tissues in a standard and predictive fashion. This specificity of nerve innervation patterns, and therefore functional concordance, allows for a precise anatomical and physiological means by which to target therapies to restricted anatomical areas [1].

Nerves in the PNS are defined in several ways, including innervation region, size, pre- or post-ganglionic and functionally. Nerves in the PNS are comprised of nerve fibers that conduct specific forms of efferent or afferent signals, and are grossly defined by size, myelination and function. These fibers are divided into categories including (from largest to smallest in diameter): Aα (motor neurons), Aβ (large diameter, myelinated sensory fibers), B (autonomic fibers), Aδ (small, finely myelinated sensory fibers) and C (unmyelinated, sensory fibers). Visceral fibers transmit various information such as organ function, metabolic status, pain and other internal organ functions. The somatic sensory fibers convey specific types of information from the periphery such as light touch, proprioception, deep pressure, cold, hot, pain, etc. The size, myelination and other physiologic characteristics allow for selective modulation of function both therapeutically and diagnostically. For example, electrical fields can selectively activate or block different fiber types based upon the "size principle". This can be tailored for the specific fiber types by controlling specific components of the electrical stimulation pulses being delivered.

In many cases nerves contain both motor and sensory fibers as well as autonomic fibers. While this is anatomically efficient, it can pose challenges for electrically targeting a nerve therapeutically, since the mixed components might lead

A Modern Atlas for Implantable Devices of the Spine, Brain, and Nerve. https://doi.org/10.1016/B978-0-443-36528-7.00006-6

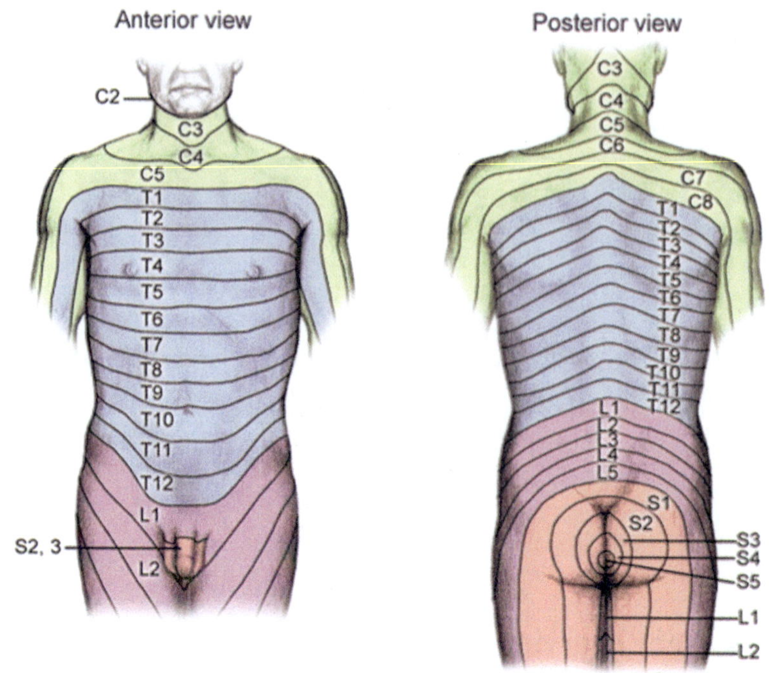

FIGURE 4.1 Dermatomal distributions by spinal level. Peripheral nerves enter the spinal cord with predictable receptive field distributions [26].

to unwanted side effects [4]. Solutions can be to target a different nerve or area of the nervous system without this overlap or be selective in the application of therapy to avoid unwanted effects and complications.

Anatomy of the head and neck

There are multiple cranial and neck nerve targets that are useful in the treatment of chronic pain conditions. In many cases, cephalalgia or facial neuropathic pain conditions are the primary indications for targeting these nerve structures. Sensory innervation of the head and neck are accomplished by both somatic and cranial nerve afferent fibers which then project to the CNS. In some cases there is heavy integration of these sensory fibers in spinal and brain regions indicating the potential for therapeutic synergies [5]. In other cases, motor fibers are activated to produce desired therapeutic effects.

There are several primary anatomic targets in the head and neck for neuromodulation therapies including the occipital nerve(s) and several cranial nerves:

- **Occipital Nerves.** The lesser and greater occipital nerves originate, primarily in the occipital region of the skull and more superficial tissues, although recent work suggests that sensory afferents innervating the dura also travel in the occipital nerves [6]. The nerves travel sagitally along the back of the head with primary landmarks being the external occipital protuberance (Fig. 4.2a) [7]. The travel through the C2 and C3 nerve roots to the spinal cord synapsing in the trigeminocervical complex [5].
- **Trigeminal Nerves (CNV).** The fifth cranial nerve (CNV) has three branches (I-III) each originating in different areas of the facial region (Fig. 4.2b). Superficial nerves such as the supraorbital or infraorbital nerves provide access to the branches of the trigeminal system. These project to the spinal cord transmitting various forms or sensory information. Anatomical distribution of facial (e.g., periorbital, jaw, etc.) and deeper structures such as a brain dura by CNV branch allow for a more precise anatomic understanding for therapeutic targeting.
- **Vagus Nerve (CNX).** The vagus nerve has several branches, although for implantable neuromodulation therapies the primary target is the cervical vagus. This bilateral nerve runs in parallel with the carotid artery and contains multiple efferent and afferent autonomic nerve fibers projecting to multiple end organs and brainstem structures [8].
- **Hypoglossal Nerve (CNXII).** The hypoglossal nerve is a purely somatic motor nerve projecting from the brainstem to various muscles in the tongue which control such movements as protrusion which is being used to treat obstructive sleep apnea [9].

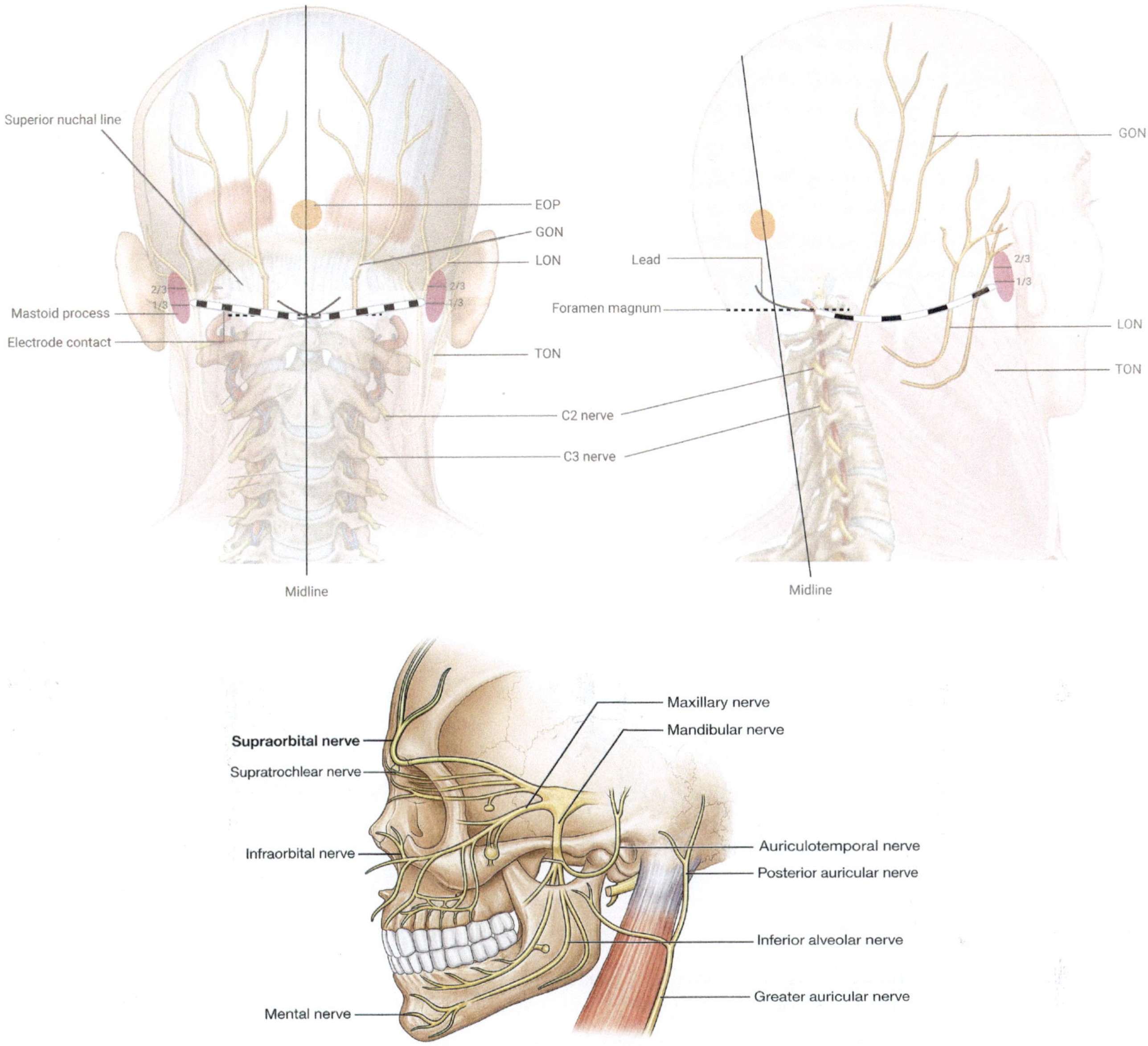

FIGURE 4.2 Panel A. Anatomical distribution of the greater and lesser occipital nerves and external occipital protuberance landmark [27]. Panel B. Branches of the trigeminal nerve in the head and face [28].

- **Sphenopalatine Ganglia.** This intracranial nerve structure situated in the pterygopalatine fossa, integrates inputs from both sympathetic and parasympathetic nerves innervating periorbital, nasal and deeper cranial structures.
- **Cochlear Nerve (CNVIII).** The cochlear nerve is a branch of the Vestibulocochlear Nerve, also known as cranial nerve VIII. This nerve originates from the spiral ganglion within the cochlea and projects to the brainstem. It is primarily responsible for hearing, carrying signals about pitch, volume and localization of external sounds [10].

Anatomy of the shoulder and upper extremities

The nerves of the upper extremity may be targeted as proximally as the trunks of the brachial plexus or as distally as the smaller individual branches in the distal forearm. The patient's anatomy, pain distribution, device selection, and implanter skillset all contribute to choice of target site(s) (Fig. 4.3).

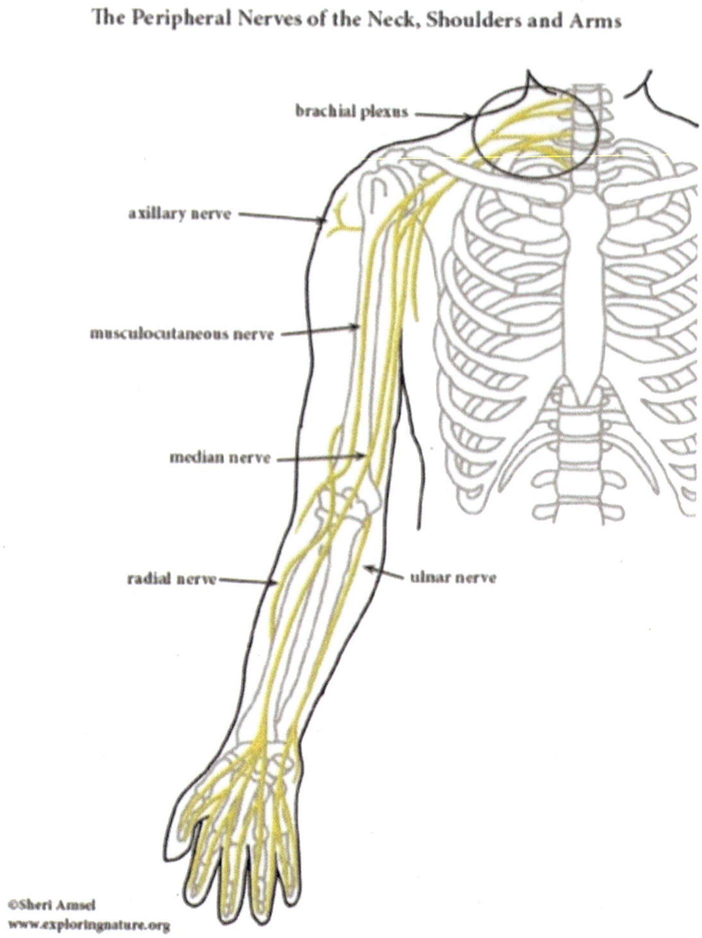

FIGURE 4.3 Main nerve branches of the shoulder and arm [29].

Brachial plexus

- Divided into Roots, Trunks, Divisions, Cords, and Branches [11].
- Originates from the ventral rami of the C5-T1 spinal nerves (Roots) [12].
- Interscalene Brachial Plexus
  - Composed of Superior, Middle, and Inferior Trunks derived from the C5 and six roots, C7 root, and C8 and T1 roots respectively
  - Located between the anterior and middle scalene muscles
  - Prime target location for shoulder pain [13]. This structure is quite superficial, so skin entry for introducer placement is typically in the posterolateral neck.
- Supraclavicular Brachial Plexus
  - Continuation of the Trunks before they split into Anterior and Posterior Divisions
  - Easily visualized laterally and posteriorly to the subclavian artery
  - Targeting here may be ulnar sparing due to location of the Inferior Trunk relative to the remainder of the nerve bundle based on regional anesthesia studies
- Infraclavicular Brachial Plexus
  - Lateral, Medial, and Posterior Cords named relative to the axillary artery
  - Deep to fascia of the pectoralis minor
  - Site sometimes chosen for its relative stability compared to the interscalene and supraclavicular sites

Suprascapular nerve

- Arises from the Superior Trunk of the Brachial Plexus (C5 and six roots)
- Provides sensory and proprioceptive innervation to the glenohumeral and acromioclavicular joints
- Provides motor innervation to the supraspinatus and infraspinatus muscles
- Often targeted at the suprascapular notch and/or spinoglenoid notch

Axillary nerve

- Arises from the Posterior Cord of the Brachial Plexus
- Provides sensory innervation to the posterolateral aspect of the shoulder and upper arm [14].
- Provides motor innervation to the deltoid and teres minor muscles
- Courses with the posterior circumflex humeral artery in the quadrangular space, a region bordered by the teres minor, teres major, long head of the triceps, and surgical neck of the humerus

Median nerve

- Originates from the Lateral and Medial Cords of the Brachial Plexus (C5-T1)
- Runs in the medial arm lateral to the brachial artery before crossing anteriorly to the medial side of the artery before entering the forearm anterior to the medial epicondyle of the humerus
- Found between the Flexor Digitorum Superficialis and the Flexor Digitorum Profundus distal to the elbow
- Before passing through the carpal tunnel, it courses between the tendons of the Flexor Carpi

Ulnar nerve

- Branches from the Medial Cord of the Brachial Plexus in the axilla (C8-T1)
- After initially lying on the medial side of the brachial artery in the anterior compartment of the arm, it enters the posterior compartment and arrives in the forearm posterior to the medial epicondyle of the humerus in the ulnar groove
- Provides innervation to the ventral medial forearm as well as the ring and little fingers
- Targeted 9–13 cm proximal to the medial epicondyle

Radial nerve

- Distal continuation of the Posterior Cord of the Brachial Plexus
- Provides innervation to the dorsal skin and musculature of the arm, forearm, and hand
- Targeted proximal to the elbow at the radial (spiral) groove of the humerus 10–14 cm superior to the lateral epicondyle

Anatomy of the truck, abdomen and low back (Fig. 4.4)

Key nerve targets in the upper trunk

- The Intercostal nerve is a major nerve target in the trunk, a part of the somatic nervous system innervating the skin and parietal pleura [15].
- Important landmarks include the inferior border of the scapula and the 12th rib.
- The nerve is external to the parietal pleura and the innermost intercostal muscle. The nerve dives between the innermost intercostal and internal intercostal muscles, traveling inferior to the intercostal artery and vein [16].
- The intercostal nerves are implicated in post-thoracotomy syndrome, post-mastectomy syndrome, and intercostal neuralgia, all of which involve significant pain and sensory alterations in the ribs, chest wall, and abdomen.

Key targets in the low back

- **Medial Branch Nerves**
    - The medial branch of the spinal dorsal ramus innervates the facet joints, multifidus muscles, interspinous ligament, and supraspinous ligament [17].
    - The medial branch of the spinal dorsal ramus runs posteriorly, medially, and caudally at the lateral border of the superior articular process of the inferior vertebra.
    - Each facet joint is innervated by the medial branches from two adjacent dorsa rami.

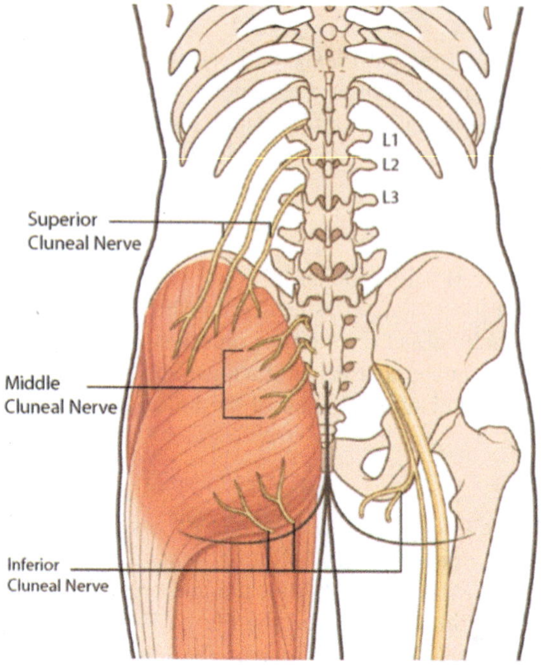

FIGURE 4.4 Cluneal nerve distributions in the lower back [30].

- **Cluneal Nerves**
  - Cluneal nerves are branches of the posterior rami of the lumbar L1- L3 spinal nerves (Superior), S1-3 (Middle and Inferior).
  - The three sets of cluneal nerves- Superior, Middle, and Inferior-innervate the lateral low back and upper buttock, sacral region, and inferolateral gluteal region and perineum respectively

Key targets in the abdomen

- The iliohypogastric, ilioinguinal, and genitofemoral nerves are derived from the T12 to L2 lumbar plexus.
- The ilioinguinal nerve arises from the lateral border of the psoas major and enters the transversus abdominis at the anterior iliac crest [18].
- It supplies the skin of the superomedial thigh, root of the penis, anterior scrotum in men and pubis and labium majus in women [18].
- Ilioinguinal neuralgia can result from herniorrhaphy surgery.

Anatomy of the lower extremities

Key nerve targets in the upper leg (Fig. 4.5)

The lower extremity is primarily innervated by the lumbosacral plexus, which originates from the anterior rami of L1-S4 spinal nerves [11]. In the upper leg, key peripheral nerve targets include the sciatic nerve, the femoral nerve, the obturator nerve, and the lateral femoral cutaneous nerve.

- **Sciatic Nerve (L4-S3):** The sciatic nerve derives its fibers from the ventral rami of spinal nerves L4 through S3. Both anterior and posterior divisions of the lumbosacral plexus are involved [19]. The convergence of these fibers exits the pelvis as a single nerve through the greater sciatic foramen, most commonly, deep to the piriformis muscle, though there are a number of variations of this relationship. The nerve subsequently traverses the posterior compartment of the thigh situated deep to the long head of the biceps femoris muscle, superficial to adductor magnus and short head of the biceps femoris muscle, and laterally to semitendinosus and semimembranosus muscles. The sciatic nerve is the main motor and sensory nerve supply to the posterior thigh, leg, and foot.

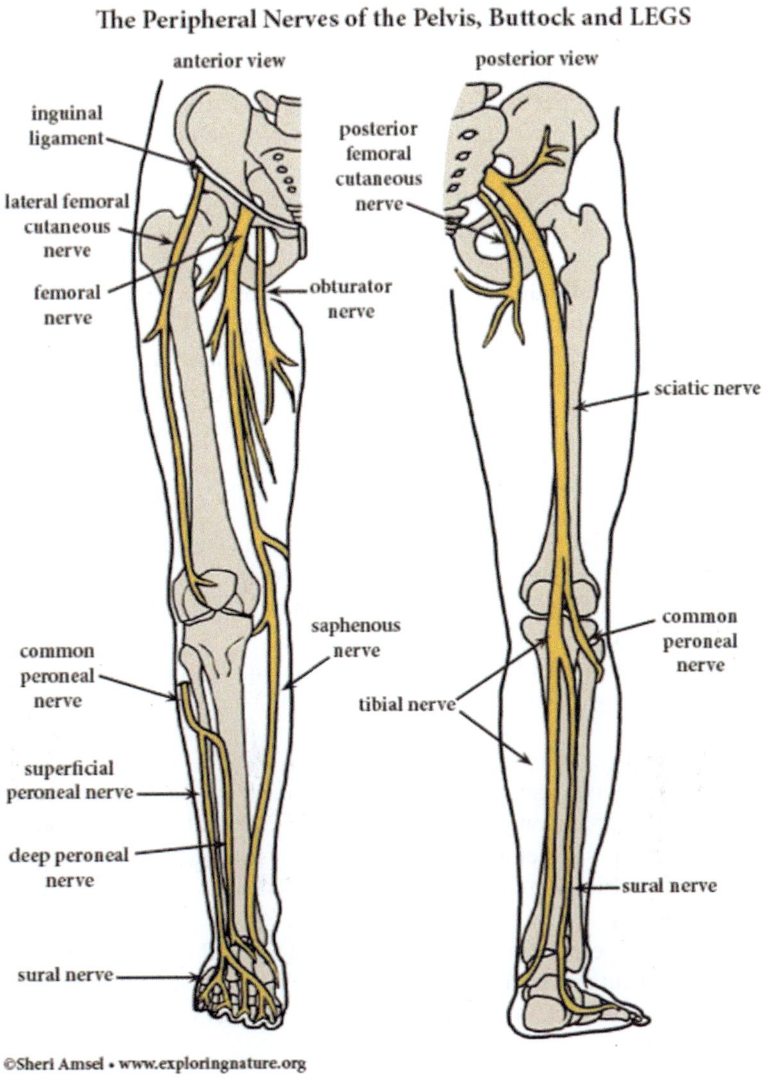

FIGURE 4.5 Main nerve branches of the upper and lower leg [29].

- **Femoral Nerve (L2-L4):** The femoral nerve emerges from the posterior division of the lumbosacral plexus and descends through the psoas major muscle. It exits the pelvis beneath the inguinal ligament, lateral to the femoral artery, and provides motor innervation to the anterior thigh muscles, including the quadriceps, and sensory innervation to the anterior thigh and medial lower leg via the saphenous nerve [20].
- **Obturator Nerve (L2-L4):** The obturator nerve exits the pelvis through the obturator foramen and innervates the medial thigh muscles, including the adductors. It also provides sensory input to the medial thigh. Its anatomical course makes it a critical target for interventions addressing spasticity or chronic pelvic pain.
- **Lateral Femoral Cutaneous Nerve (L2-L3):** This purely sensory nerve emerges from the lumbar plexus, passing medial to the anterior superior iliac spine (ASIS) and beneath the inguinal ligament. It provides sensation to the anterolateral thigh. Compression at the inguinal ligament can result in meralgia paresthetica, a condition often targeted by nerve blocks [21].

Nerve targets in the knee and lower leg

The lower leg is innervated by the saphenous nerve and branches of the sciatic nerve, which bifurcates into the tibial and common peroneal nerves near the popliteal fossa nerve, the termination of the femoral nerve. Key nerves include the posterior tibial nerve, superficial peroneal nerve, deep peroneal nerve, sural nerve, and saphenous nerve.

- **Posterior Tibial Nerve:** The tibial nerve (L4-S3) travels along the posterior compartment of the leg, passing posterior to the medial malleolus through the tarsal tunnel. It provides motor innervation to the calf muscles and plantar flexors and sensory innervation to the sole of the foot via the medial and lateral plantar nerves [22].
- **Superficial Peroneal Nerve:** Originating from the common peroneal nerve, this nerve courses along the lateral compartment of the leg and provides motor innervation to the peroneus longus and brevis muscles. It also supplies sensation to the dorsum of the foot, excluding the first web space [23].
- **Deep Peroneal Nerve:** This branch of the common peroneal nerve innervates the anterior compartment of the leg, including the tibialis anterior and extensor digitorum muscles. It provides sensory input to the first web space of the foot and articular branches to the ankle joint [23].
- **Sural Nerve:** The sural nerve is a sensory nerve formed by contributions from the tibial and common peroneal nerves. It travels along the posterior aspect of the leg and supplies sensation to the lateral foot and ankle [24].
- **Saphenous Nerve:** As the longest branch of the femoral nerve, the saphenous nerve supplies sensation to the medial aspect of the lower leg and foot. It can be accessed for diagnostic or therapeutic blocks to manage chronic pain conditions [25].

Key anatomical landmarks

- **Inguinal Ligament:** A critical reference point for locating the femoral and lateral femoral cutaneous nerves.
- **Anterior Superior Iliac Spine (ASIS):** Used to identify the lateral femoral cutaneous nerve.
- **Popliteal Fossa:** The bifurcation of the sciatic nerve into tibial and common peroneal nerves occurs here.
- **Medial Malleolus:** The posterior tibial nerve passes posteriorly through the tarsal tunnel.
- **Fibular Head:** The common peroneal nerve winds around the fibular neck, making it susceptible to injury.

Pearls and pitfalls

- Scan Beforehand- It is imperative to become familiar with your patient's particular anatomy very early in the procedural planning process as there may be non-native or aberrant anatomy in play. If you plan to use ultrasound guidance for implantation, it is recommended that you scan the patient's target nerve and surrounding structures along its entire course prior to implant date in order to identify the optimal target point and any potential alternates. If using fluoroscopic guidance, review imaging studies prior to implant.
- Give Yourself Enough Runway- The site of skin entry for percutaneously implanted leads should be remote enough from the target so that at least 4–5 cm of lead is in the subcutaneous tissue. Plan to tunnel an additional length of lead under skin if necessary. Skin entry site selection should also take into account the ability to accommodate a subcutaneous anchor if non-tined leads are being used.
- Fascial Planes are Your Friends- Fascial planes are useful connective tissue pathways for percutaneously placed needles and trocars, which allow for stimulator arrays to be placed without crossing through muscular fibers, which may help to mitigate against migration and discomfort. Similarly, perineural fat is a useful structure in which tines can be anchored.
- Look Around- Always be aware of sensitive structures that surround the target nerve and lead trajectory, i.e., lung, vasculature, hollow organs, etc.

References

[1] Goldstein B. Anatomy of the peripheral nervous system. Phys Med Rehabil Clin N Am 2001;12(2):207–36.

[2] Lee MW, McPhee RW, Stringer MD. An evidence-based approach to human dermatomes. Clin Anat 2008;21(5):363–73.

[3] Sonoo M. Recent advances in neuroanatomy: the myotome update. J Neurol Neurosurg Psychiatry 2023;94(8):643–8.

[4] Boezaart AP, Smith CR, Chembrovich S, et al. Visceral versus somatic pain: An educational review of anatomy and clinical implications. Reg Anesth Pain Med 2021;46(7):629–36.

[5] Mehnert J, Basedau H, Sturm LM, et al. Functional brainstem representations of the human trigeminal cervical complex. Cephalalgia 2023;43 (5):3331024231174862.

[6] Schueler M, Neuhuber WL, De Col R, Messlinger K. Innervation of rat and human dura mater and pericranial tissues in the parieto-temporal region by meningeal afferents. Headache 2014;54(6):996–1009.

[7] Lefel N, van Suijlekom H, Cohen SPC, et al. 11. Cervicogenic headache and occipital neuralgia. Pain Pract 2025;25(1):e13405.

[8] Baquiran M, Bordoni B. Anatomy, head and neck: Anterior vagus nerve. Treasure Island (FL): StatPearls; 2025.

[9] Kim SY, Naqvi IA. Neuroanatomy, cranial nerve 12 (hypoglossal). Treasure Island (FL): StatPearls; 2025.

[10] Peterson DC, Reddy V, Launico MV, Hamel RN. Neuroanatomy, auditory pathway. Treasure Island (FL): StatPearls; 2025.
[11] Standring S. In: Standring S, editor. Gray's anatomy: the anatomical basis of clinical Practice. 42nd ed. Elsevier; 2021.
[12] Okwumabua E, Black AC, Thompson JH. Anatomy, shoulder and upper limb, nerves. Treasure Island (FL): StatPearls; 2025.
[13] Bouche B, Manfiotto M, Rigoard P, et al. Peripheral nerve stimulation of brachial plexus nerve roots and supra-scapular nerve for chronic refractory neuropathic pain of the upper limb. Neuromodulation 2017;20(7):684–9.
[14] Mansfield JT, Desai MJ. Axillary peripheral nerve stimulation for chronic shoulder pain: a retrospective case series. Neuromodulation 2020;23 (6):812–8.
[15] Glenesk NL, Rahman S, Lopez PP. Anatomy, thorax, intercostal nerves. Treasure Island (FL): StatPearls; 2025.
[16] Mayes J, Davison E, Panahi P, et al. An anatomical evaluation of the serratus anterior plane block. Anaesthesia 2016;71(9):1064–9.
[17] Shuang F, Hou SX, Zhu JL, et al. Clinical anatomy and measurement of the medial branch of the spinal dorsal ramus. Medicine (Baltim) 2015;94 (52):e2367.
[18] Reinpold W, Schroeder AD, Schroeder M, et al. Retroperitoneal anatomy of the iliohypogastric, ilioinguinal, genitofemoral, and lateral femoral cutaneous nerve: Consequences for prevention and treatment of chronic inguinodynia. Hernia 2015;19(4):539–48.
[19] Giuffre BA, Black AC, Jeanmonod R. Anatomy, sciatic nerve. Treasure Island (FL): StatPearls; 2025.
[20] Tubbs RSSM, Loukas M. Bergman's comprehensive encyclopedia of human anatomic variation. Wiley-Blackwell; 2016.
[21] Chalk C, Namiranian D. Meralgia paresthetica. Handb Clin Neurol 2024;201:195–201.
[22] Dellon A. Tarsal tunnel syndrome: A multiple etiology syndrome. Clin Podiatr Med Surg 2021;38(2):285–300.
[23] Fortier LM, Markel M, Thomas BG, et al. An update on peroneal nerve entrapment and neuropathy. Orthop Rev 2021;13(2):24937.
[24] Miniato MA, Nedeff N. Anatomy, bony pelvis and lower limb: Sural nerve. Treasure Island (FL): StatPearls; 2025.
[25] Mathew K, Varacallo MA. Anatomy, bony pelvis and lower limb: Saphenous nerve, artery, and vein. Treasure Island (FL: StatPearls; 2025.
[26] Patel S. Human dermatomes. In: Sea T, editor. Nerves and nerve injuries, 1. Academic Press; 2015. p. 477–83.
[27] Kurt E, Kollenburg L, van Dongen R, et al. The untold story of occipital nerve stimulation in patients with cluster headache: Surgical technique in relation to clinical efficacy. Neuromodulation 2024;27(1):22–35.
[28] Justiz R, Trescot AM. Supraorbital nerve entrapment. In: Trescot AM, editor. Peripheral nerve Entrapments. Springer; 2016.
[29] Amsel S. Peripheral nervous system - nerves (advanced). 2024. http://www.exploringnature.org/db/view/Peripheral-Nervous-System-Nerves-Advanced.
[30] Kalia H. Inferior cluneal nerve. In: Abd-Elsayed A, Trescot AM, editors. Peripheral nerve stimulation. Elsevier; 2023. p. 142–5.

Section 2

The spine anatomy

Introduction to section 2 the spine anatomy

It has been nearly 60 years since the first successful spinal cord stimulator implant in a human. Over the past several decades, there have been great advances in our understanding of neurophysiology, anatomy, and technology that have greatly expanded our ability to modulate pain. Perhaps the most basic and fundamental requirement for successful neuromodulation is a detailed understanding of the anatomy of the nervous system. This allows practitioners to identify the precise location along the neural pathways to alter the transmission of pain. Failure to understand the anatomy can contribute to ineffective therapy, neural injury, damage to surrounding structures, or unintended effects of stimulation. While an understanding of general spinal anatomy provides a basic map, patient-specific anatomy based on image findings must be considered for successful personalized treatment. Several patient-specific factors, including spinal degenerative pathology, neoplastic or infectious processes, prior surgeries, and spinal deformity, greatly alter the anatomy and pose challenges by compromising the patency of the epidural space or neural foramina or the relative location of the spinal cord within the canal. Optimal application of neuromodulation requires practitioners to combine clinical diagnosis with diagnostic studies to match technology to the patient. Advanced imaging modalities (MRI and CT) serve as an invaluable resource for identifying the neural, bony, and adjacent anatomy as well as recognizing pathology that may be contributing to symptoms or may pose specific challenges to the application of neuromodulation devices. The safety and accuracy of neuromodulation are greatly enhanced when there is a preoperative understanding of the anatomy that can be correlated with the standard intraoperative imaging modalities (fluoroscopy, ultrasound) used to aid in device placement. Advances in spinal navigation and augmented reality will likely emerge as additional tools to enhance neuromodulation.

The following chapters provide detailed descriptions of spinal anatomy with an emphasis on the relative anatomy for safe and effective placement of spinal cord and dorsal root ganglion stimulators. As our understanding of the pathophysiology underlying pain continues to grow and new technologies are developed and implemented, these essential fundamental teachings on anatomy will continue to serve as a reference for current and future generations of neuromodulators.

Chapter 5

Cervical spine anatomy

David S. Jevotovsky[1], Harman Chopra[2], Mustafa Broachwala[3] and Morad Nasseri[4]

[1]NYU Langone Health, Department of Physical Medicine and Rehabilitation, New York, NY, United States; [2]Weill Cornell Medicine, Department of Anesthesiology, Critical Care, and Pain Medicine, New York, NY, United States; [3]Department of Anesthesiology and Pain Medicine, University of California, San Diego, CA, United States; [4]Boomerang Healthcare, Interventional Pain Medicine, Walnut Creek, CA, United States

Introduction

Brief historical perspective

The earliest known descriptions of cervical spine injuries and their management date back to the Egyptians (c.17th century BC), which differentiated between cervical sprain, fracture, and dislocations. By the time of Hippocrates (fourth century BC), rudimentary cervical treatments such as traction and local pressure were employed, although these were based on limited anatomic and biomechanical knowledge. The Renaissance prompted the first serious attempts at understanding spinal anatomy and biomechanics, during which Leonardo da Vinci (1452–1519) described the anatomy of the spine and investigated spinal stability [1].

In the 16th century, Andreas Vesalius provided foundational anatomical descriptions of the cervical spine in his seminal work "De Humani Corporis Fabrica" that laid the groundwork for future anatomic studies. Anatomists in the 17th and 18th centuries, such as Thomas Willis and Albrecht von Haller, continued to develop understanding of the cervical vertebral structures [2].

By the 1960s, Sir Frank Holdsworth proposed a two-column model of the spine, which was later refined into the modern three-column model by Francis Denis, supported by sophisticated biomechanical testing [3,4].

The 20th century brought the development of advanced imaging techniques, such as X-ray, MRI and CT scans, revolutionizing the visualization and diagnosis of cervical spine pathologies. These advancements, coupled with innovations in surgical interventions, techniques, and instrumentation, have significantly improved the management of cervical spine disorders.

Suggested specialty training for appropriate intervention

Comprehensive education, which includes a hands-on component, is essential for the implantation of devices into the cervical spine. Given the complex pathophysiology of pain, treating cervical pain requires a multidisciplinary approach. Training typically follows an apprenticeship model and can be obtained through various subspecialties.

Interventional pain management physicians are trained to perform cervical injections and advanced neuromodulatory techniques such as spinal cord stimulation (SCS) and dorsal root ganglion (DRG) stimulation. These physicians may come from diverse backgrounds, including anesthesiology, physiatry, neurology, psychiatry, or emergency medicine.

Surgical specialists, such as orthopedic surgeons and neurosurgeons, may also train to implant devices in the cervical spine. Their surgical proficiency and anatomic understanding is developed through their respective surgical residencies and subsequent practices.

A Modern Atlas for Implantable Devices of the Spine, Brain, and Nerve. https://doi.org/10.1016/B978-0-443-36528-7.00059-5

Key points

1. Cervical spine anatomy may be limited by surface area but is dense with several key structures, serving the role of mobility and protection of vital neurovascular structures
2. Understanding and respecting the critical portions of cervical anatomy, allows for safe and efficient minimally invasive procedures
3. Knowledge of anatomical landmarks and various imaging modalities (X-ray, CT, MRI, ultrasound, and fluoroscopy) is important, accounting for patient-specific anatomical variations and pathologies.
4. The overlapping nerve distributions of the cervical spine make diagnosis difficult, as the corresponding targets differ, emphasizing the importance of a thorough history and physical, to ensure procedure success

Cervical spine anatomy

Cervical spine anatomy scope

The cervical spine is a highly specialized part of the axial skeleton that provides stability and mobility for the head that typically weights 10–12 pounds, while protecting critical neural and vascular structures within. Its seven vertebrae (C1–C7) that lie with normal sagittal lordosis and 37 joints allow for mobility unparalleled compared with other spinal levels. A complex network of musculature enables the multidirectional range of motion of the cervical spine including flexion-extension, axial rotation, and lateral bending. Axial rotation is particularly dynamic at the C1–C2 level; however, this extensive mobility comes with an increased risk of injury and degeneration due to significant mechanical stress on the intervertebral discs and zygapophyseal joints [5,6]. As such, the cervical spine is designed to strike a balance between providing sufficient mobility for dynamic movements while ensuring adequate support to protect the critical structures within the neck.

The cervical spine protects the spinal cord, exiting spinal nerves and the vertebral arteries, ensuring smooth motor control, sensory feedback and cerebral blood flow. The central spinal canal houses the spinal cord, which transmits fine touch, proprioception and vibration signals through the dorsal column-medial lemniscus pathway, as well as pain, temperature, crude touch, and voluntary movement signals through the more anterior or laterally located spinothalamic and corticospinal tracts, respectively. [7]. The vertebral arteries, traversing through the transverse foramina from C6 to C1, branch to form the anterior and posterior spinal arteries in the cervical spine. Each cervical nerve root exits above its corresponding vertebra, aside from the C8 nerve root, which exits between the C7 and T1 vertebrae [8]. The C5–C8 nerves join the T1 nerve to contribute to the brachial plexus, providing innervation to the upper limbs, shoulders and neck. Comprehensive insight into this anatomy is crucial for assessment of potential pain generators and potential safe planning of further intervention (Fig. 5.1).

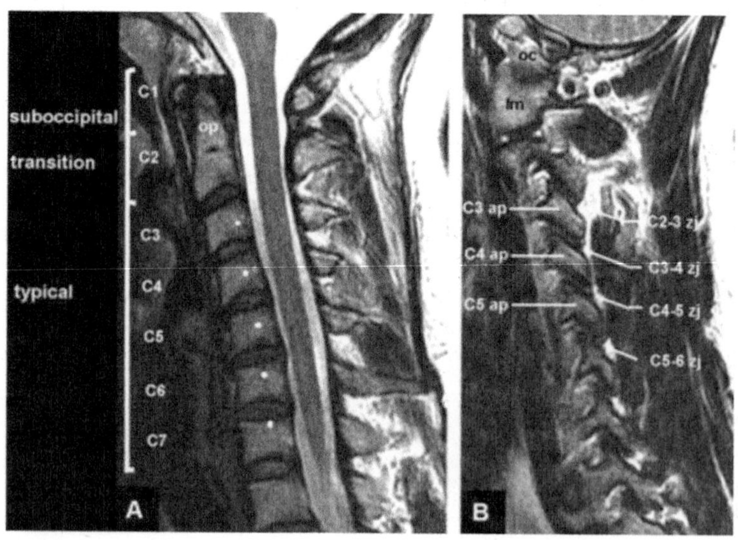

FIGURE 5.1 A sagittal view MRI of the cervical spine.

Relevant anatomy in the cervical spine

Vertebrae

Compared with the rest of the spine, the cervical vertebrae are small and consist of a higher proportion of trabecular bone, which facilitates a balance of flexibility and strength in the neck [9]. The C3–C6 cervical vertebrae exhibit a relatively uniform structure, whereas the C1, C2, and C7 vertebrae present more nuanced anatomies.

The first cervical vertebrae, also known as the atlas, is unique from other cervical vertebrae in its ring shape and lack of a vertebral body, spinous process, and inferior disc. Through its articulation with the occiput at the atlanto-occipital (AO) joints and the C2 vertebrae at the atlantoaxial (AA) joint, the atlas supports the skull and contributes to a head posture and many cervical movements. Two superior concave facet joints articulate with the occipital condyles and contribute to around half of neck flexion and extension [10]. The posterior arch joins the anterior arch to complete the ring, with anterior and posterior tubercles serving as attachment points for supporting musculature. The arches converge at the lateral masses, whose superior surfaces articulate with the occiput and form the AO joints. At the midline of the anterior arch's inner aspect, an indentation articulates with the dens of C2, forming the AA joint.

The second cervical vertebrae, known as the axis, is unique due to the peg-like odontoid process (dens) that projects cranially and articulates with the anterior arch of C1 described above. This AA joint enables the head's rotational movement and is stabilized primarily by the transverse ligament of the atlas. Unlike the atlas, the axis has a vertebral body and a posterior bifid spinous process that serve as attachment points for cervical musculature. Laterally, the transverse processes contain articular surfaces for adjacent vertebrae, as well as transverse foramen through which the vertebral arteries pass. Steel's rule of thirds describes the spatial relationship of the AA joint, dividing the spinal canal into thirds: one third containing the dens, another third with the spinal cord itself, and the remainder with free space to buffer against cord compression [11].

The subaxial cervical vertebrae (C3–C7) share a largely uniform structure, with C7 distinguished by a few unique anatomical features. Their vertebral bodies are smaller than the more robust thoracic or lumbar vertebral bodies, with a larger spinal canal to allow for more dynamic movements without compression [12]. Distinct to the cervical spine, the lateral superior aspects of the body have a small cranial projection (i.e., uncinate process) that articulates with the inferior aspect of the adjacent superior body. This uncovertebral joint, or Joint of Luschka, is important to prevent posterolateral hypertranslation and limit lateral side-bending [13]. The uncovertebral joint serves as a useful lateral landmark during cervical interventions. Laterally, the bilateral transverse processes and pedicles encircle the transverse foramen through which the vertebral vasculature passes from C6 to C1. Grooves on the superior surface of the transverse processes carry the exiting spinal nerves after they pass through the neural foramen. Dorsolateral to the pedicles, the lateral masses articulate cranially and caudally as the cervical facet joints before continuing on dorsomedially as the laminae. The lateral mass is often a preferred site for surgical screw fixation due to the relatively small pedicle size in the cervical spine. The orientation of the superior articular facets of the subaxial cervical spine transitions from a posteromedial direction at C3 to a posterolateral direction at C7, allowing for greater flexibility in axial rotation and lateral bending [14]. The bilateral laminae converge to form the spinous processes, which are bifid at levels C3–C6. In contrast, the nonbifid spinous process of C7 is easily palpable, making it an important landmark for physical examination and interventional procedures. C7 is also unique in that the vertebral arteries do not travel through the transverse foramina in most individuals [15] (Fig. 5.2).

Ligaments (Fig. 5.3)

The ligamentous structures in the cervical spine place a crucial role in maintaining the stability and alignment of its bony components. Similar to the thoracic and lumbar regions, the anterior and posterior longitudinal ligaments (ALL and PLL) run along the anterior and posterior surfaces of the vertebral bodies, respectively, extending caudally to the sacrum to provide anterior and posterior stability. The ligamentum flavum connects adjacent laminae. Its higher elastin content in the cervical spine allows for greater flexibility and range of motion without impinging on the spinal cord or nerve roots [16]. The ligamentum nuchae extends from the occipital protuberance to the spinous process of C7 to limit neck flexion and provide posterior stability. The alar ligaments and transverse ligament of the atlas stabilize the AA join. The transverse ligament secures the dens of C2 against the anterior arch of C1 to prevent anterior odontoid displacement, while the alar ligaments connect the dens laterally to the occipital condyles to limit rotation and lateral bending. Capsular ligaments that surround the cervical facet joints to limit excessive movement, protecting spinal nerves as they exit the spinal canal.

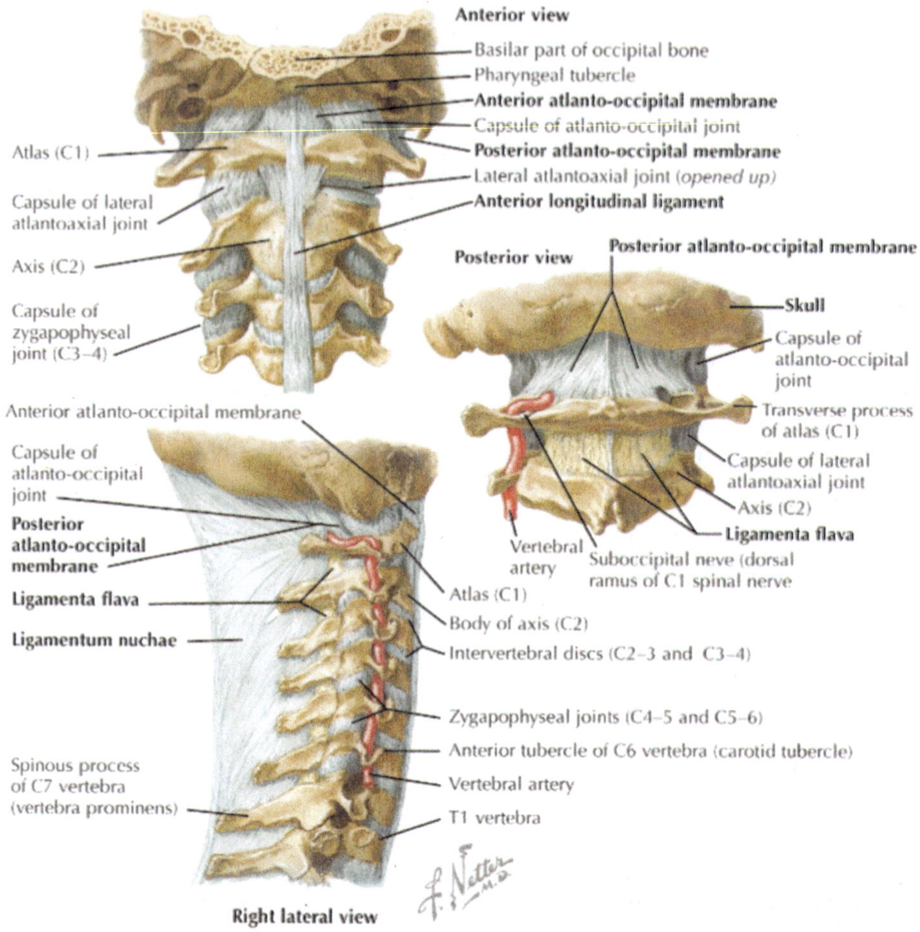

FIGURE 5.2 Bony anatomy of the cervical spine.

Intervertebral discs (Fig. 5.1)

In addition to the stability provided by facet joints, the intervertebral discs serve as an additional point of articulation, effectively distributing mechanical forces and acting as shock absorbers. In the cervical spine, the first intervertebral discs lies between C2 and C3. The intervertebral discs are composed of three primary components: the inner nucleus pulposus, outer annulus fibrosus and the adjacent superior and inferior cartilaginous endplates [17]. The gelatinous inner nucleosus pulposus, composed primarily of type II collagen, proteoglycans and water, facilitates the dissipation of compressive forces on the spine. In contrast, the outer annulus fibrosus relies on the tensile strength of its type I collagen to stabilize the vertebrae. Beyond serving as an attachment point for the annulus fibrosus, the cervical endplates also buffer mechanical forces by distributing axial loads.

Musculature (Fig. 5.4)

The ventral muscles of the neck are divided into superficial and deep layers. Most superficially, the thin platysma extends from the mandible to the second rib and acromion, contributing to facial expression. Below this, the sternocleidomastoid (SCM) runs obliquely from the clavicle and sternum to the mastoid and occiput to aid in head rotation, neck flexion-extension and side-bending. The deep muscular layer of the anterior neck contains the infrahyoid, scalene and longus groups. The infrahyoid group, which includes the mylohyoid, stylohyoid, geniohyoid, digastric, and omohyoid muscles, attach to the hyoid bone. The anterior, medial, and posterior scalene muscles originate from various cervical transverse processes and insert on the ribs. The longus muscles are found within the prevertebral fascia, including the longus colli, longus capitis, and rectus lateralis and assist in cervical flexions and stability.

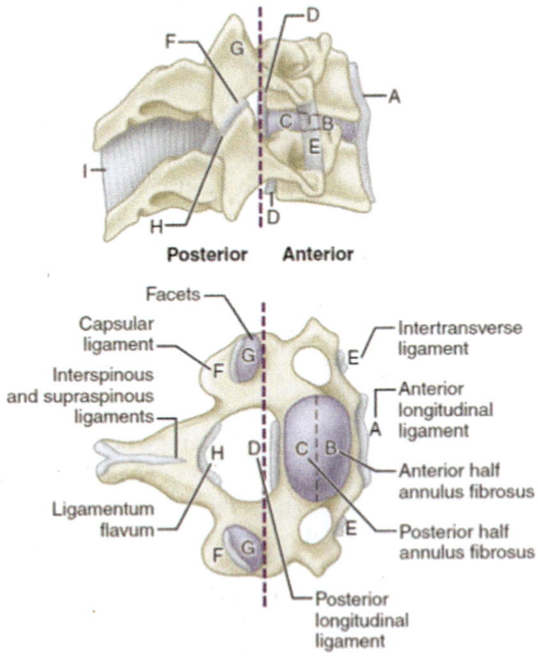

FIGURE 5.3 Detailed anatomy of cervical spine vertebrate.

The dorsal cervical muscles can be split into superficial, intermediate, and deep layers, and provide vertebral tension to maintain upright positioning and balance. The superficial layer contains the trapezius, splenius and levator scapulae muscles, which work synergistically to rotate, extend, and laterally bend the cervical spine. Most superficially, the trapezius interacts with the occipital protuberance, lateral clavicle and spinous processes inferiorly into the thoracic region. The splenius group consists of both the splenius capitus and splenius cervicis. The intermediate layer consists of the iliocostalis, longissimus and semispinalis muscles (listed lateral to medial), also known at the erector spinae. These muscles originate at the iliac crest, sacrum and lumbar spinous processes and work together to extend and side-bend the cervical spine. The deep multifidus and rotator muscles make up the transversospinalis group and are innervated by the dorsal rami of the cervical spinal nerves.

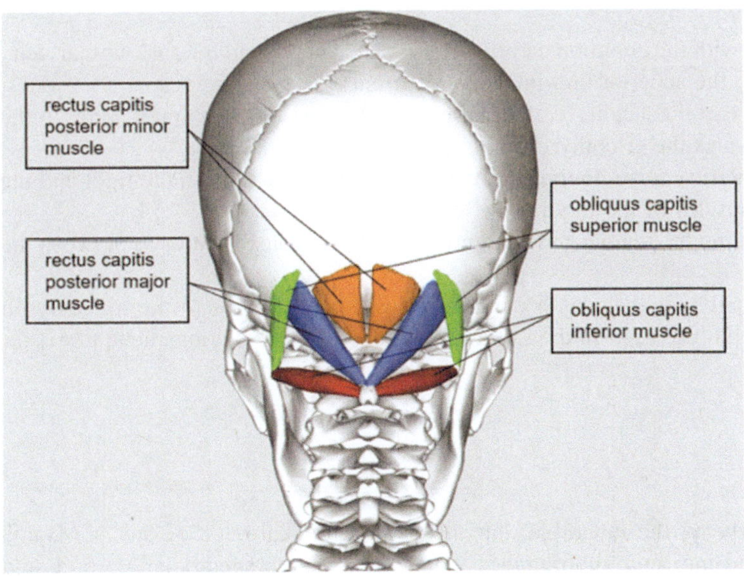

FIGURE 5.4 Muscle attachments in the posterior occiput.

Neurovascular (Fig. 5.2)

The spinal cord travels caudally after exiting the foramen magnum through the spinal canal, terminating around the L1-L2 level. Transverse sections of the cord reveal the inner gray matter, which houses the nerve cell bodies, surrounded by the outer white matter. Cervical gray matter is divided into anterior and posterior horns, with alpha motor neurons located anteriorly and sensory neurons posteriorly. The circumferential white matter of the spinal cord contains myelinated axons. Laterally, the lateral corticospinal tract houses efferent motor neurons that aid in ipsilateral extremity movement. In addition, the lateral spinothalamic tract transmits afferent sensory signals related to pain and temperature from the contralateral limb. Posteriorly, the dorsal column contains the gracilis and cuneatus fasciculi, which transmit contralateral afferent proprioceptive, vibration, and fine touch signals. An anterior spinothalamic tract is responsible for crude touch afferent signal transmission.

Encasing the spinal cord, the meninges are composed of the pia, arachnoid and dura mater. The pia lies directly above the spinal cord and is encased by the web-like arachnoid. Between the two layers, cerebrospinal fluid flows in the subarachnoid space. The most superficial meningeal layer is the dura.

The eight cervical nerve roots exit the intervertebral foramen above the pedicle of their corresponding spinal levels, except the C8 nerve roots, which exit inferior to the C7 pedicles. Exiting nerve roots take up about one-third of the space of the Neuroforamen. Cervical flexion-extension changes the size of the Neuroforamen, which may compress or alleviate compression of the roots. The C5 to C8 nerve roots, along with contributions from T1, converge to form the brachial plexus that controls the motor and sensory function of the upper extremities.

Blood flow to the cervical spine stems from the vertebral arteries after branching off the subclavian artery. As the vertebral arteries course through the transverse foramen of C6 to C1, collateral branches sprout to form the anterior and posterior spinal arteries. The anterior spinal artery supplies the anterior two-thirds of the cord, leaving the posterior one-third to the posterior spinal artery. Around C1, the bilateral vertebral arteries enter the foramen magnum and join together to form the basilar artery. There are three anterior and three posterior veins around the spinal cord.

External features

Prominent peripheral nerves originating from the cervical spine include the greater and lesser occipital nerves (GON and LON), the third occipital nerve (TON) and the great auricular nerve (GAN). Often implicated in occipital neuralgia, migraine and cervicogenic headaches, these nerves are often targeted for intervention.

The GON stems from the dorsal ramus of C2 and ascends superolaterally between the obliquus capitis inferior and semispinalis capitis to innervate the posterior scalp up to the vertex.

The TON branches off the dorsal ramus of C3 and ascends the semispinal capitis muscle to innervate the inferior aspect of the occiput.

The LON arises from the ventral rami of C2 and C3 and courses along the posterior SCM to innervate the posterolateral aspect of the occiput.

The GAN is formed by the ventral rami of C2 and C3 to innervate the posterior auricular area, as well as the skin over the parotid gland and mastoid process.

The carotid sheath lies nearby the cervical spine with the common carotid artery, vagus nerve and internal jugular vein. The vagus nerve gives off two important branches: the superior and inferior (recurrent) laryngeal nerves.

The superior laryngeal nerve runs medial to the carotid sheath. Its internal branch provides sensory innervation to the laryngeal mucosa, while the external branch innervates the cricothyroid muscle.

The recurrent laryngeal nerve follows an asymmetric course, looping around the subclavian artery on the right and the aortic arch on the left. It innervates the intrinsic muscles of the larynx.

The hypoglossal nerve is responsible for innervating the tongue and strap muscles and is typically situated between the carotid artery and internal jugular vein.

The cervical sympathetic chain runs longitudinally for the length of the cervical spine, medial to the longus colli muscle. The inferior cervical and first thoracic ganglia fuse to form the stellate ganglion, a frequent sympathetic target for intervention located at the level of C7-T1.

Procedure-related considerations

The cervical triangles

The anterior cervical triangle is bordered superiorly by the mandible, laterally by the medial edge of the SCM, and medially by the neck's midline. It is further divided into four subtriangles: the submental, submandibular, carotid, and muscular triangles. Understanding these relationships is crucial for surgical planning.

The submental triangle, bordered by the anterior bellies of the digastric muscles, hyoid bone and mylohyoid muscle, is the smallest and most central anterior cervical triangle. Adjacent to the submental triangle, the submandibular triangle is formed by the mandible, anterior belly of the digastric muscle and stylohyoid muscle, containing the submandibular gland, lymph nodes, the hypoglossal nerve, and the facial and lingual vasculature. The carotid triangle, delineated by the posterior belly of the digastric muscle, the SCM, and omohyoid muscle houses vital structures such as the common carotid's bifurcation point, the internal jugular vein, the vagus nerve, and hypoglossal nerve. Finally, the muscular triangle is defined by the hyoid bone, midline of the neck and laterally by the SCM and superior belly of the omohyoid muscle. It contains the infrahyoid muscles, thyroid and parathyroid glands, larynx, trachea, and esophagus.

Imaging guidance (Fig. 5.1)

Despite advances in imaging technology, plain radiography remains the initial modality of choice for cervical spine evaluation due to its simplicity and excellent visualization of bone structures. Flexion and extension radiographs can provide valuable insights into spinal stability. While limited in soft tissue assessment, radiographs serve as foundational anatomical maps, often complemented by computed tomography (CT) or magnetic resonance imaging (MRI) for more detailed evaluation.

CT is particularly used to assess fractures, ligament injuries, and dislocations, oftentimes offering superior bone detail compared with radiographs. The ionizing radiation employed during CT captures data through X-ray attenuation, which is then reconstructed into 2D and 3D images. CT imaging is often chosen when MRI is contraindicated, such as in patients with non-MRI-compatible implants. However, CT is limited in soft tissue visualization, and its associated radiation exposure necessitates careful consideration, especially in vulnerable populations such as pregnant patients.

MRI is the gold standard for evaluating soft tissue structures in the cervical spine, including intervertebral discs, spinal cord, nerve roots, and ligaments. Its contrast resolution and nonionizing radiofrequency technology make it invaluable for identifying disc herniations, spinal cord compression, and neural involvement. Unlike CT, MRI is highly sensitive to soft tissue abnormalities and is particularly advantageous for repeated imaging, as it avoids radiation exposure. However, its sensitivity to incidental findings unrelated to clinical symptoms—such as asymptomatic disc bulges—requires careful interpretation and clinical correlation to avoid overdiagnosis.

Ultrasound is an emerging modality for evaluating more superficial structures in real-time, particularly the cervical musculature, ligaments, and vasculature. Given its noninvasive nature, portability, and lack of ionizing radiation, ultrasound is an excellent choice for real-time needle placement during procedures such as cervical nerve blocks or injections. Additionally, ultrasound can detect superficial pathologies such as muscle tears or hematomas. However, its penetration depth and operator dependence restrict its utility for deeper structures such as the spinal cord or intervertebral discs.

Similarly, fluoroscopy provides real-time X-ray imaging and is widely used for needle placement in procedures requiring precise visualization of bony landmarks, such as cervical spine procedures. However, fluoroscopy carries a risk of radiation exposure, which should be carefully managed to minimize potential harm to both the patient and healthcare provider.

A fluoroscopic contralateral oblique (CLO) view of the cervical spine is often utilized to enhance localization of anatomic landmarks and to avoid injury to critical structures, particularly in cervical epidural steroid injections (CESI). A CLO at 50° provides a clear view of the interlaminar spaces and has demonstrated superior needle tip visualization for accessing the epidural space compared with the lateral view, reducing risks of complications such as dural puncture [18–20]. Like the "Scottie Dog" sign used in the lumbar region, the CLO view in the cervical spine similarly optimizes the delineation of bony structures and neural foramina.

Pathologic variations

Patient-specific pathological variations can influence cervical anatomy and impact the procedural approach and placement of neuromodulatory devices. These variations may be congenital (e.g., congenital cervical spinal stenosis), degenerative (e.g., disc herniation, facet hypertrophy), or iatrogenic (e.g., cervical fusions).

Congenital cervical spinal stenosis, or the reduced spinal canal diameter at multiple levels without degenerative changes, may alter the ratio of which the spinal cord occupies the spinal canal. Careful preoperative assessment with imaging should be taken to ensure adequate space is available for safe epidural placement of neuromodulatory hardware.

Degenerative changes may impact the stability and alignment of the cervical spine or narrow neural foramina. Significant obstruction to neural foramina may complicate procedural approach and placement of any implants. Hence, preoperative planning should include precise imaging studies in order to identify any such anatomical obstacles.

Cervical fusions require significant hardware installment that may complicate subsequent procedural approaches. Furthermore, surgical fusions of the cervical vertebrae may increase stress at adjacent spinal levels. Some clinicians may perform laminotomies cephalad to the targeted levels, which can bypass scarring and instrumentation from previous surgeries [21].

Implant targets

Optimal lead placement of implantable devices is essential to optimize therapeutic efficacy and safety of the procedure. SCS leads target the dorsal column of the spinal cord for best modulation of pain signals. In addition, it is critical to choose the appropriate spinal level that will best address the patient's symptoms. Anatomic parameters, including the length and diameter of the cervical spinal canal, may also influence lead stability and the risk of migration, ultimately affecting outcomes [22].

Some of the target levels for specific indications are listed below:

- SCS leads placed at C1–C2 have been shown to improve level of consciousness in patients with disorders of consciousness [23]. These reports, however, are restricted to case series level of evidence. Electrode deviations greater than 30 degrees can reduce the maximum tolerable stimulation intensity and lead to poorer outcomes in this population [22]. Neuromodulation at C2-3 is particularly useful for treating refractory headaches and trigeminal neuralgia due to the proximity to the trigeminal nucleus caudalis, which transmits nociceptive signals to the head and face [24,25]. More peripherally, the Q2-approach has been used to target intractable headaches more peripherally at the C2 DRG [26].
- SCS or DRG lead placement at the C5–C6 level is commonly used in treatment of postlaminectomy syndrome, cervical radiculopathy, complex regional pain syndrome (CRPS), and Raynaud's disease [23,27–29].
- Evidence for Cervical neuromodulation evidence for vascular disease is largely based on case series, but stimulation may impact sympathetic tone and improve blood flow [30,31].
- There may also be a role for peripheral nerve stimulation (PNS) in the treatment of cervical facetogenic pain syndromes, as this technology has been explored in the lumbar spine [32].
- Due to the sympathetic involvement in the pathophysiology of CRPS, the stellate ganglion has also been studied as a treatment target and holds promise as a focus for future implantable treatments [33,34].

Landmark assignments

Palpation of the neck, both anteriorly and posteriorly, can help approximate the cervical spinal level. Posteriorly, the C7 spinous process is typically the most prominent and easily palpable cervical vertebra, making it a reliable reference point for counting vertebral levels during clinical and surgical procedures [35]. Anteriorly, many palpation landmarks are used to identity cervical levels, including the angle of the mandible (C2–C3 interspace), hyoid bone (C3 body), thyroid cartilage (C4–C5 disc), cricoid cartilage (C6 body), and the carotid tubercle (C6 body) [36]. These approximations, however, may vary with different sex, age, and height [37].

Under fluoroscopy, identifying the attachment point of the first rib indicates the first thoracic vertebra, with C7 lying directly superior to it. Each superior body can be counted cranially from there, using it as a reference point. Alternatively, levels can be counted caudally from C2. Recall that the interface between the C1–C2 is referred to as the atlantoaxial joint, while the atlanto-occipital joint describes the interaction between C1 and the occipital bone.

In the anterior-posterior (AP) fluoroscopic view, the transverse processes project laterally from the vertebral bodies. A "true" lateral view may be obtained by lining up the lateral masses. The transverse foramina is easily identified within the transverse processes on CT/MRI, through which the vertebral arteries pass. Oblique fluoroscopic views of the cervical spine allow for better visualization of the intervertebral foramina, where the spinal nerve exits and the DRG resides. The DRG typically lies within the lateral foramen dorsal to vertebral artery. Understanding this relationship during DRG stimulation is crucial to avoid injury to the vasculature, which could lead to stroke or death.

The inferior and superior articular processes of adjacent vertebral bodies articulate bilaterally to form the zygapophyseal (or facet) joints. The cervical facet joints are located posterior to the transverse processes.

The spinous processes are easily identifiable as the most posterior bony structures of the cervical spine. To obtain an accurate anteroposterior view of the cervical spine, alignment of the spinous processes must be achieved.

The interlaminar space between the lamina of adjacent vertebrae provides an access point for many posterior cervical interventional procedures.

Pearls and pitfalls

Vertebral artery segments

V1 (Preforaminal Segment): Originates from the subclavian artery and ascends until it enters the transverse foramen, typically at the level of C6.

V2 (Foraminal Segment): Travels vertically upward through the transverse foramina of the cervical vertebrae, usually from C6 through C2.

V3 (Extracranial/Atlantoaxial Segment): Emerges from the transverse foramen of C2, then takes a tortuous, looping course around the atlas (C1) in the sulcus arteriosus before approaching the cranial cavity.

V4 (Intradural Segment): Enters the cranial vault through the foramen magnum and courses along the ventrolateral surface of the brainstem, ultimately converging with its contralateral counterpart to form the basilar artery.

On a lateral fluoroscopic view of the cervical spine, the structures are typically visualized in the following order from anterior to posterior:

- **Prevertebral Soft Tissues:** This includes the soft tissue shadow of the trachea and esophagus.
- **Anterior Vertebral Cortex:** The front edge of the vertebral bodies, often outlining the anterior longitudinal ligament.
- **Intervertebral Disc Spaces:** Appearing as radiolucent gaps between the vertebral bodies.
- **Posterior Vertebral Cortex:** The posterior margin of the vertebral bodies can sometimes identify posterior longitudinal ligament, especially if ossified.
- **Vertebral Foramen:** Contains the spinal cord and is useful for visualizing contrast spread
- Intervertebral Foramen: Exit point for the dorsal root ganglion and target for transforaminal
- **Facet Joints**: Iconic Scottie's dog can be visualized for targeting medial branches
- **Lamina (Spinolaminar Line):** The converging laminae create a distinct line that indicates the beginning of the posterior bony elements.
- **Spinous Processes:** The most posterior elements, seen as the terminal bony projections.

On a standard anterior-posterior (AP) fluoroscopic view of the cervical spine, the structures are typically visualized in the following order from lateral to medial) (Fig. 5.5).

Transverse Processes/Foramen Transversarium: These are the most lateral structures visible on an AP view, where the foramen transversarium houses the vertebral arteries.

Lateral Masses: Immediately medial to the transverse processes, the lateral masses include the facets and articular processes, serving as key landmarks in AP imaging.

Pedicles: These narrow bony bridges connect the lateral masses to the central vertebral body, visible as distinct radiopaque structures.

Vertebral Body and Intervertebral Disc Spaces: Centrally located, the vertebral bodies form the main bony block, with disc spaces appearing as radiolucent gaps between them.

Spinous Processes: Representing the most medial elements, the spinous processes form the posterior midline, often superimposed on the vertebral bodies in an AP view.

Quick tips

Know Your Landmarks! The prominent C7 spinous process is a reliable starting point for identifying cervical levels during physical exams and lies directly superior to the thoracic levels that articulate with the ribs on imaging.

Patient-Specific Factors: Age, gender, height, and weight may impact the use of surface landmarks, so be mindful of individual anatomical variations.

Patient-Specific Pathology: Conditions such as congenital stenosis, disc herniation, facet hypertrophy, or postsurgical changes may complicate access and placement of neuromodulation device components.

C1–C2 (Atlantoaxial) Joint: Remember, the C1–C2 joint is the primary site of cervical spine rotation. Any procedures in this area should consider the unique anatomy and stabilization provided by the transverse ligament.

Uncovertebral Joints (C3–C7): These joints limit lateral side-bending and prevent hypertranslation. Understanding their role is crucial for accessing or manipulating the cervical spine.

SCS Electrode Level Choice: Carefully consider your patient's symptoms when selecting the appropriate level for spinal cord stimulation (SCS) lead placement. Targeting the correct level can optimize outcomes.

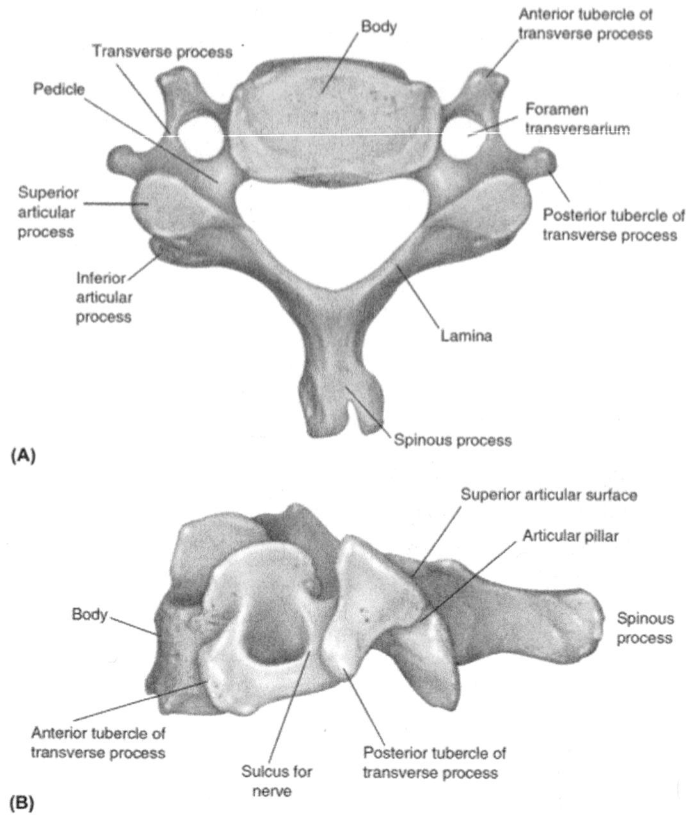

FIGURE 5.5 Relevant anatomy of cervical spine vertebrate.

Protect the Vertebral Artery: Be extra cautious around the vertebral arteries, which pass through the transverse foramina, especially during cervical procedures involving the DRG. Injury to these arteries can result in serious complications.

Cervical Flexion-Extension and Nerve Root Compression: Cervical flexion and extension can dynamically alter the size of the intervertebral foramina, leading to nerve root compression. Be aware of these changes when performing diagnostic injections or other interventions and be prepared to adjust patient positioning as needed to alleviate or exacerbate compression.

References

[1] Sanan A, Rengachary SS. The history of spinal biomechanics. Neurosurgery 1996;39:657–68. discussion 668-9.

[2] Boukebous B, Baker JF, Fanchette J, Rousseau MA. A long gestation: spine anatomy from the medieval age to the end of the 19th century. An analytical historical review. J Neurosurg Spine 2025;42:110–9.

[3] Holdsworth F. Fractures, dislocations, and fracture-dislocations of the spine. J Bone Joint Surg Am 1970;52:1534–51.

[4] Denis F. The three column spine and its significance in the classification of acute thoracolumbar spinal injuries. Spine 1983;8:817–31.

[5] Lindenmann S, Tsagkaris C, Farshad M, Widmer J. Kinematics of the cervical spine under healthy and degenerative conditions: a systematic review. Ann Biomed Eng 2022;50:1705–33.

[6] Anderst WJ, Donaldson WF, Lee JY, Kang JD. Cervical motion segment contributions to head motion during flexion\extension, lateral bending, and axial rotation. Spine J 2015;15:2538–43.

[7] Tan S, Faull RLM, Curtis MA. The tracts, cytoarchitecture, and neurochemistry of the spinal cord. Anat Rec 2023;306:777–819.

[8] Tanaka N, Fujimoto Y, An HS, Ikuta Y, Yasuda M. The anatomic relation among the nerve roots, intervertebral foramina, and intervertebral discs of the cervical spine. Spine 2000;25:286–91.

[9] Yoganandan N, Pintar FA, Stemper BD, Baisden JL, Aktay R, Shender BS, Paskoff G. Bone mineral density of human female cervical and lumbar spines from quantitative computed tomography. Spine 2006;31:73–6.

[10] Hurley RW, Adams MCB, Barad M, Bhaskar A, Bhatia A, Chadwick A, Deer TR, Hah J, Hooten WM, Kissoon NR, Lee DW, Mccormick Z, Moon JY, Narouze S, Provenzano DA, Schneider BJ, Van Eerd M, Van Zundert J, Wallace MS, Wilson SM, Zhao Z, Cohen SP. Consensus

practice guidelines on interventions for cervical spine (facet) joint pain from a multispecialty international working group. Reg Anesth Pain Med 2022;47:3–59.
[11] Ebraheim NA, Lu J, Yang H. The effect of translation of the C1-C2 on the spinal canal. Clin Orthop Relat Res 1998:222–9.
[12] Wang TY, Mehta VA, Dalton T, Sankey EW, Rory Goodwin C, Karikari IO, Shaffrey CI, Than KD, Abd-El-Barr MM. Biomechanics, evaluation, and management of subaxial cervical spine injuries: a comprehensive review of the literature. J Clin Neurosci 2021;83:131–9.
[13] Kotani Y, Mcnulty PS, Abumi K, Cunningham BW, Kaneda K, Mcafee PC. The role of anteromedial foraminotomy and the uncovertebral joints in the stability of the cervical spine. A biomechanical study. Spine 1998;23:1559–65.
[14] Rong X, Liu Z, Wang B, Chen H, Liu H. The facet orientation of the subaxial cervical spine and the implications for cervical movements and clinical conditions. Spine 2017;42:E320–e325.
[15] Wakao N, Takeuchi M, Kamiya M, Aoyama M, Hirasawa A, Sato K, Takayasu M. Variance of cervical vertebral artery measured by CT angiography and its influence on C7 pedicle anatomy. Spine 2014;39:228–32.
[16] Ivancic PC, Coe MP, Ndu AB, Tominaga Y, Carlson EJ, Rubin W, Dipl-Ing FH, Panjabi MM. Dynamic mechanical properties of intact human cervical spine ligaments. Spine J 2007;7:659–65.
[17] Chan WC, Sze KL, Samartzis D, Leung VY, Chan D. Structure and biology of the intervertebral disk in health and disease. Orthop Clin N Am 2011;42:447–64 [vii].
[18] Gill JS, Aner M, Nagda JV, Keel JC, Simopoulos TT. Contralateral oblique view is superior to lateral view for interlaminar cervical and cervicothoracic epidural access. Pain Med 2015;16:68–80.
[19] Kwon HJ, Kim CS, Kim J, Kim S, Shin JY, Choi SS, Shin JW, Kim DH. Contralateral oblique view can prevent dural puncture in fluoroscopy-guided cervical epidural access: a prospective observational study. Reg Anesth Pain Med 2023;48:588–93.
[20] Sim JH, Kwon HJ, Kim CS, Kim EH, Kim DH, Choi SS, Shin JW. Comparison of contralateral oblique view with the lateral view for fluoroscopic-guided cervical epidural steroid injection: a randomized clinical trial. Reg Anesth Pain Med 2022;47:171–6.
[21] Awad AJ, Murray MM, Morris JL, Pahapill PA. The retrograde approach of surgical paddle-lead placement for spinal cord stimulation. Neuromodulation 2025;28:323–30.
[22] He Q, Han B, Xia X, Dang Y, Chen X, He J, Yang Y. Related Factors and outcome of spinal cord stimulation Electrode deviation in disorders of consciousness. Front Neurol 2022;13:947464.
[23] Piedade GS, Vesper J, Chatzikalfas A, Slotty PJ. Cervical and high-thoracic dorsal root ganglion stimulation in chronic neuropathic pain. Neuromodulation 2019;22:951–5.
[24] Towne BV, Girgiss CB, Schuster NM. Use of spinal cord stimulation in treatment of intractable headache diseases. Pain Med 2023;24:S6–s10.
[25] Velásquez C, Tambirajoo K, Franceschini P, Eldridge PR, Farah JO. Upper cervical spinal cord stimulation as an alternative treatment in trigeminal neuropathy. World Neurosurg 2018;114:e641–6.
[26] Chen Q, Qian X. The Q2 approach for percutaneous peripheral neuromodulation stimulator implantation targeting the C2 dorsal root ganglion at the C2 lamina for treatment of intractable headache: a technical note. Pain Med 2025;26:140–5.
[27] Hunter CW, Carlson J, Yang A, Deer T. Spinal cord stimulation for the treatment of failed neck surgery syndrome: outcome of a prospective case series. Neuromodulation 2018;21:495–503.
[28] Chivukula S, Tempel ZJ, Weiner GM, Gande AV, Chen CJ, Ding D, Moossy JJ. Cervical and cervicomedullary spinal cord stimulation for chronic pain: efficacy and outcomes. Clin Neurol Neurosurg 2014;127:33–41.
[29] Graca MJ, Lubenow TR, Landphair WR, Mccarthy RJ. Efficacy and safety of cervical and high-thoracic dorsal root ganglion stimulation therapy for complex regional pain syndrome of the upper extremities. Neuromodulation 2023;26:1781–7.
[30] Chapman KB, Kloosterman J, Schor JA, Girardi GE, Van Helmond N, Yousef TA. Objective improvements in peripheral arterial disease from dorsal root ganglion stimulation: a case series. Ann Vasc Surg 2021;74. 519.e7-519.e16.
[31] Benyamin R, Kramer J, Vallejo R. A case of spinal cord stimulation in Raynaud's Phenomenon: can subthreshold sensory stimulation have an effect? Pain Phys 2007;10:473–8.
[32] Deer TR, Gilmore CA, Desai MJ, Li SC, Depalma MJ, Hopkins TJ, Burgher AH, Spinner DA, Cohen SP, Mcgee MJ, Boggs JW. Percutaneous peripheral nerve stimulation of the medial branch nerves for the treatment of chronic axial back pain in patients after radiofrequency ablation. Pain Med 2021;22:548–60.
[33] Gibbs GF, Drummond PD, Finch PM, Phillips JK. Unravelling the pathophysiology of complex regional pain syndrome: focus on sympathetically maintained pain. Clin Exp Pharmacol Physiol 2008;35:717–24.
[34] Kim ED, Yoo WJ, Kim YN, Park HJ. Ultrasound-guided pulsed radiofrequency treatment of the cervical sympathetic chain for complex regional pain syndrome: a retrospective observational study. Medicine (Baltim) 2017;96:e5856.
[35] Albuquerque P, Da Silva EPC, Melo TMS, Montenegro EJN, De Oliveira DA, Guerino MR, De Siqueira GR. Inter-rater accuracy and reliability of a palpation protocol of the C7 spinous process comprising a combination of 3 traditional palpation techniques. J Manip Physiol Ther 2022;45:227–34.
[36] Johnson MD, Schwieterman W, Bugada M, Garner RM, Na J, Prestigiacomo CJ. History of cervical spine localization: surface landmarks. World Neurosurg 2025;193:191–8.
[37] Oh CH, Ji GY, Yoon SH, Hyun D, Choi CG, Lim HK, Jang AR. Surface landmarks do not correspond to exact levels of the cervical spine: references according to the sex, age and height. Korean J Spine 2014;11:178–82.

Chapter 6

Thoracic spine anatomy

Rohit Aiyer[4], Kenneth B. Chapman[1, 2, 3], Tony K. George[5], Latrice A. Akuamoah[3, 6] and Ajax Yang[1, 2, 3]

[1]*The Spine & Pain Institute of New York, New York, NY, United States;* [2]*Department of Anesthesiology, NYU Langone Medical Center, New York, NY, United States;* [3]*Department of Anesthesiology, The Zucker School of Medicine at Hofstra/Northwell, New York, NY, United States;* [4]*Westside Pain Management, Long Beach, CA, United States;* [5]*Division of Pain Medicine, Department of Physical Medicine and Rehabilitation, Hackensack Meridian Health – JFK University Medical Center, Edison, NJ, United States;* [6]*Visco Spine and Joint Center, Hoboken, NJ, United States*

Introduction

The thoracic spine is generally defined as the region between thoracic levels T1-T12 and across the posterior side of the trunk. The International Association for the Study of Pain (IASP) refers to nonspecific thoracic spine pain (TSP) as pain in the most lateral margins of the erector spinae muscles [1].

Thoracic spine pain, compared to neck and low back pain, has a relatively low prevalence. The literature suggests that the lifetime prevalence of thoracic pain is between 13% and 17%, compared to neck (40%) and low back pain (57%) [2]. Furthermore, thoracic pain has been shown to coexist with other chronic pain conditions in different anatomical regions, such as neck, elbow, shoulder and low back.

TSP can arise from a variety of sources, including the thoracic spine, cervical spine, thorax, renal, cardiopulmonary and gastrointestinal systems. The thoracic spine is often a site for metabolic, infective, and neoplastic conditions. It can be associated with comorbid conditions, such as osteoporosis, vertebral fractures, osteoarthritis and Scheuermann's disease [3].

This chapter has the goals of explaining in detail the anatomy of the thoracic spine and how it plays a role with regard to treating chronic pain conditions, as well as utilization of neuromodulation techniques.

Thoracic spine

The thoracic spine is a kyphotic segment with sharp, angulated spinous and transverse processes and lateral rib reinforcements protecting the thoracic cavity. Consisting of 12 thoracic vertebral segments, which are grouped into three sections: upper thoracic (T1–T4), mid thoracic (T5–T8) and lower thoracic (T9–T12). Its transitional zones in the superior and inferior thoracic spine segments have unique features, including the presence of a complete rib articulating facet at the T1 vertebral level and floating ribs of the T11 and T12 ribs. The upper and mid thoracic segments have raised transverse processes and downward sloping spinous processes unique to this region. Its kyphotic curvature protects vital organs, absorbing shock and evenly distributing weight in case of impact. Its role as a stabilizer overshadows its role as a mobilizer, key functions of the cervical and lumbar spines.

Vertebral structure

As a whole, its vertebrae are intermediate in size and shape. T1 is the smallest of the 12 vertebrae, with subsequent descending vertebrae circumferentially increasing in size. The thoracic vertebrae appear heart-shaped and connect to the posterior vertebral arch through pedicles on each side.

The vertebral segment encloses a spinal canal dimensionally narrower than the cervical and lumbar canals. The vertebral bodies of the anterior column have demifacets, excavations on the vertebral surface serving as rib articulating junctions.

Unique to the thoracic spine, demifacets are located posterior and lateral toward the superior and inferior junctions of the vertebral bodies, with secondary attachments to the transverse processes. Ribs attach to the inferior vertebral demifacets at one level with the superior vertebral demifacets one level below, with an intervertebral disc nestled in between.

A Modern Atlas for Implantable Devices of the Spine, Brain, and Nerve. https://doi.org/10.1016/B978-0-443-36528-7.01006-2

Each vertebral body has six facet articulations, including four demifacets and two rib articulations on either side of the transverse process. Exceptions include the 1st, 10th, 11th, and 12th ribs, which are attached to their corresponding T1, T10, T11, and T12 vertebral bodies, respectively, with some outliers to this rule.

The posterior vertebral arch has articular processes: two superior and two inferior. These interlock with the processes of the segment above and below, forming the facet joints. In the thoracic segments, facet orientation shifts from a coronal to a sagittal plane moving down from upper to lower segments, where the superior segments' coronal orientation aligns with adjacent cervical segments and at the inferior segments, sagittal orientation aligns with adjacent lumbar segments. Coronal facet orientation enhances rotational motion in the upper facet segments, which transitions to flexion and extension agility at the sagittal-oriented lower facet segments. In addition, rib articulation limits flexion and extension by reinforcing rigidity, yet thoracic rotation is preserved by upper and middle facets. See Fig. 6.1.

Thoracic intervertebral discs

Thoracic discs are fibrocartilaginous structures composed of an inner nucleus pulposus and an outer annulus fibrosus. The annulus, composed of collagen and the nucleus of hyaline, maintains its structural integrity through the annular rings and nuclear gelatinous core. Its annular rings expand circumferentially away from the central nucleus, redistributing axial forces horizontally and maintaining its segmental stability by absorbing shock. The annular fibers absorbing shear rotational forces are active in the upper and mid thoracic segments, and flexion-extension forces are active in the lower thoracic segments. Thoracic discs are thinner, located more centrally, and have the lowest heights compared to the cervical and lumbar segments. Although uncommon, disc herniations have a higher incidence in the lower thoracic levels, including T10, T11, and T12, due to their increased mobility coming from their lumbar type configurations and the movement in the thoracolumbar junction.

Costovertebral and costotransverse joints

Costovertebral and costotransverse joints are junctions for rib articulations. They anchor ribs on each side and circumvent anteriorly around the thoracic cavity to attach centrally to the sternum. In addition, it stabilizes the thoracic spine through minor contributions in segmental spine stability, rib stability and rib motion. The costotransverse and costovertebral joints increase thoracic stability and limit disc motion, making the segments less prone to disc herniations. The costotransverse rib articulations at the transverse process permit these motions for the ribs with the exception of the T11 and T12 ribs, which lack costotransverse facets.

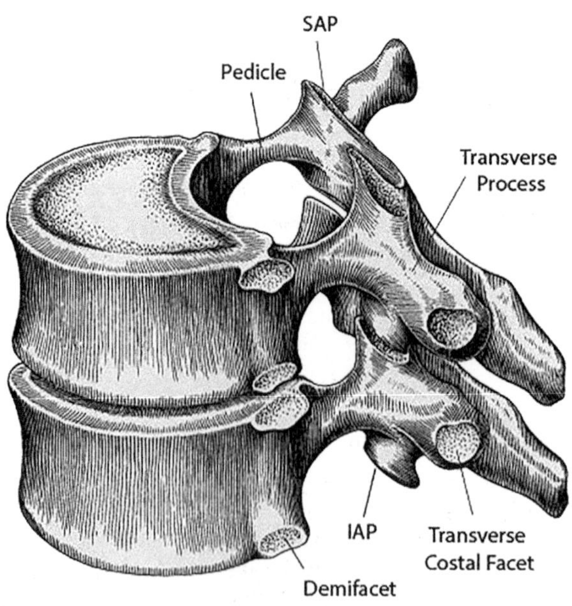

FIGURE 6.1 The thoracic spine has articulations for the rib known as demifacets, from the level above and below. The rib also articulates with the transverse process at the transverse costal facet. The angulation of the thoracic spinous processes is steeper to protect the contents of the spinal canal. The superior articular processes (SAP) and inferior articular processes (IAP) form the thoracic facet joint.

Ligamentous and muscular anatomy

Ligaments

The thoracic spine is supported by a complex network of ligaments that provide structural stability and limit excessive movement. These include: Anterior Longitudinal Ligament (ALL): A thick, broad ligament running along the anterior surface of the vertebral bodies, preventing hyperextension. Severe ALL injuries can lead to spinal instability [4].

Posterior Longitudinal Ligament (PLL): Positioned along the posterior vertebral bodies inside the spinal canal. Segmentally, PLL has an hour-glass shaped appearance, i.e., wider on the top and bottom with the narrowest portion at the mid vertebral level. PLL resists hyperflexion and reinforces the intervertebral discs [5].

Ligamentum Flavum: A highly elastic ligament connecting adjacent laminae, contributing to spinal flexibility while protecting the spinal cord.

Interspinous ligament: Located between the spinous processes of adjacent vertebrae. It plays a role in stabilization and limiting excessive spinal flexion [6].

Supraspinous Ligament: Running along the tips of the spinous processes, it provides additional support against flexion forces, especially in the upper thoracic spine. Disruption of this ligament in trauma cases can indicate significant instability.

Muscles

The musculature of the thoracic spine can be categorized into intrinsic and extrinsic groups, both of which play a critical role in movement, posture, and stabilization.

Intrinsic muscles

Multifidus: Deep stabilizer of the spine, providing segmental control and proprioceptive feedback. Fatty infiltration of the multifidus has been associated with chronic thoracic pain and postural dysfunction.

Rotators: Originate from the transverse process and insert onto the spinous process of the vertebra one ("short rotatores") or two levels ("long rotatores") cephalad. These small, paired muscles assist in segmental rotation and proprioception. They are often implicated in myofascial pain syndromes of the thoracic spine.

Semispinalis Thoracis: it is made up of five muscle fascicles originating from the transverse processes of five consecutive vertebrae (T6–T10). These muscle fibers conjoin to form a single muscle belly cranially. Semispinalis Thoracis supports extension and rotational movement, commonly assessed in cases of whiplash-associated disorders.

Extrinsic muscles

Trapezius: Large superficial muscle involved in scapular movement and spinal stabilization. The upper and middle fibers are common sites for trigger points treated with dry needling or botulinum toxin injections.

Rhomboids: Act to retract the scapula, contributing to upper back stability. Dysfunction in this muscle group is often linked to chronic postural pain and shoulder dysfunction.

Serratus Posterior Superior and Inferior: Assist in respiratory function by elevating and depressing the ribs. These muscles may be involved in rib dysfunction syndromes and intercostal neuralgia.

Neural anatomy

The spinal cord carries vital information between the body and the brain. It is divided into cervical, thoracic, lumbar, sacral, and coccygeal regions. The thoracic spine is smaller in caliber relative to the cervical and lumbar spines because it contains less gray matter. In the thoracic region, there are 12 spinal segments (T1–T12), and each segment contains paired spinal nerves composed of dorsal sensory fibers and ventral motor fibers.

The dorsal root is thicker than the ventral root and contains neuronal cell bodies of the dorsal root ganglion [7]. At each segment, afferent branches from the dorsal root relay sensory information from a specific section of skin, called a dermatome, to the brain. Anatomic landmarks allow for approximation of dermatomal levels. For example, T1 correlates with the forearm, T4 with the level of the nipples, T6 with the xyphoid process, and T10 with the umbilicus [8]. The ventral roots are composed of efferent somatic motor fibers as well as autonomic preganglionic motor neurons. The cell bodies are contained within the medial gray matter of the anterior horn.

The dorsal and ventral roots connect to form the spinal nerve in the intervertebral foramen. The spinal nerve splits into dorsal and ventral rami. The dorsal rami branch into medial and lateral nerves supplying the sensory and motor innervation of the back, and the ventral rami supply the sensory and motor innervation of the anterior and lateral trunk after branching to become the intercostal nerves [9].

Thoracic canal and spinal cord

The thoracic spinal cord contains input from the trunk and lower extremities. Input from the lumbar spinal nerves forms the lumbar enlargement, creating a wider, more ellipsoid SC at the T11–T12 vertebral levels. The thoracic cord then remains relatively stable in diameter until approximately the T2 level, where the cervical enlargement of the cord begins. Within the thoracic SC is significantly less gray matter as compared to the cervical and lumbar spinal segments. Within this gray matter is the lateral gray column, where the intermediolateral nucleus resides, containing sympathetic and preganglionic sympathetic fibers from the trunk and lower extremities.

Thoracic spinal canal diameter can vary in normal adults, with studies demonstrating AP diameters at T1, T8, and T12 ranging from 15.0 to 16.1 mm, 14.6–16.6 mm, and 16.7 to 17.2, respectively [10]. Spinal cord diameter measurements from T1 to T12 range from 5 to 9 mm, with the spinal cord diminishing in size from T1 to T8 and increasing in size from T8 to T12 [11].

Spinal canal stenosis is defined by having a canal AP diameter of <10 mm, and $<$ 5m deemed critical. As paddle electrodes typically measure 2 mm in depth, a >12 mm AP canal diameter is a recommended threshold for implantation. Smaller diameters would necessitate more extensive laminotomy or the placement of an SCS lead, which measures approximately 1.25 mm in diameter. Compressive complications range from thoracic radiculopathies, abdominal pain, to lower extremity paresthesias [12].

Cerebrospinal Fluid (CSF) has a far lower impedance than the surrounding intracanicular structures [13]. This allows for diffusion of the majority of the current from an electrical pulse and generates heat in the CSF. Dorsal CSF thickness generally decreases from rostral to caudal levels [14]. The SC is suspended within the canal and moves within the subarachnoid space with changes in posture, leading to postural fluctuations in stimulation intensity on the SC. Paresthesia-free waveforms and closed-loop technology have relatively overcome this challenge. See Fig. 6.2.

These anatomic variations led the Neuromodulation Appropriateness Consensus Committee (NACC) to recommend a preoperative thoracic spine MRI prior to lead placement to evaluate for thoracic stenosis [15].

Vascular anatomy

A single anterior spinal artery (ASA) branches from the vertebral arteries, and two posterior spinal arteries (PSA) branch from the vertebral arteries or the posterior inferior cerebellar artery. The ASA supplies the anterior two-thirds of the spinal cord by giving off central sulcal branches. The surface of the spinal cord is supplied by the pial plexus, a circumferential vascular network created by branches of the ASA and PSA. As the ASA and PSA descend along the thoracic spinal cord, they are supplied by posterior intercostal arteries.

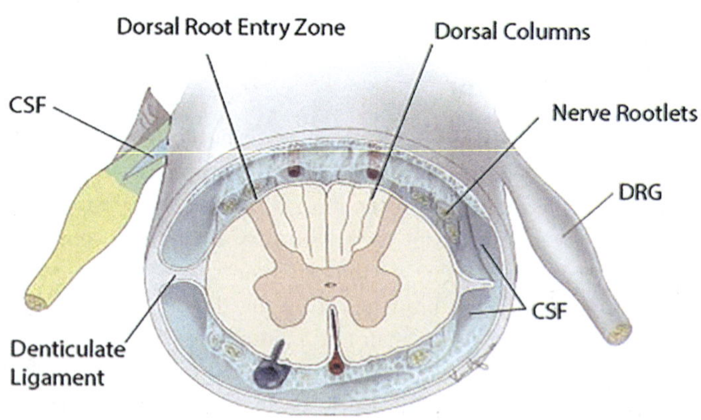

FIGURE 6.2 Cross-section of the thecal sac. The spinal canal is suspended by ligaments, including the denticulate ligament. Cerebrospinal fluid (CSF) surrounds the spinal cord and nerve rootlets. The dura extends beyond the DRG and continues as the epineurium. The CSF ends at the medial portion of the DRG. A single anterior spinal artery (ASA) and two posterior spinal arteries (PSA) supply the blood to the cord. Nerve rootlets travel within the CSF prior to entering the cord.

The lower nine posterior intercostal arteries arise from the thoracic aorta, and the upper two arise from the supreme intercostal artery. The dorsal division of these segmental arteries splits into a vertebral branch and a spinal branch before continuing to supply the dorsal musculature and skin.

The spinal branch enters the intervertebral foramen prior to branching into anterior and posterior radicular arteries, which travel and terminate along the anterior and posterior ramus of the spinal nerves, respectively [16]. Some radicular arteries continue their course to supply the ASA and PSA and are designated as anterior and posterior radiculomedullary arteries (RMA) relative to which they supply. The number of RMAs is highly variable, ranging from 2 to 14 anterior RMAs and 11 to 16 posterior RMAs [17].

The largest anterior RMA is the artery of Adamkiewicz (AKA), which in 81% of cases arises from a left-sided radicular artery at T9-L1 but has been documented at higher and lower levels in the spine [18]. The AKA enters the neuroforamen and then traverses several levels up the spinal cord before combining with the ASA. The AKA is the major blood source to the lower two-thirds of the spine, and if interrupted, can cause anterior spinal artery syndrome (ASAS), an ischemic injury to the spinal cord. ASAS can result in varying degrees of neurological deficits, including paraplegia, bowel and bladder dysfunction, and bilateral loss of pain and temperature sensation. The PSA is more resistant to ischemia than the ASA because of the robust anastomoses between the paired arteries.

Injury to the AKA in the neuroforamen during transforaminal epidural steroid injection is a concern. Debated mechanisms of injury include direct dissection, vasospasm, hematoma, and vascular occlusion by particulate steroid. Since the course of the AKA is variable, the use of nonparticulate steroid is recommended, and contrast should be used to avoid intravascular injection [18].

There are six tortuous longitudinal veins that drain into the internal (Batson Plexus) and external vertebral venous plexus, which ultimately drain into the azygous system. The internal vertebral plexus is a low-pressure network of valveless veins that allows bidirectional flow. The system helps maintain homeostasis of intracranial and thoracic pressure during postural changes, straining, and respiration. The lack of valves in the Batson Plexus may also allow the system to act as a conduit for metastases from the breast and pelvis, as well as for the spread of infection [19].

Pain pathways

Nociception begins with the activation of specialized peripheral sensory receptors called nociceptors, which respond to mechanical, thermal, or chemical stimuli. These receptors initiate electrical impulses that travel via primary afferent fibers—myelinated Aδ fibers (fast-conducting, sharp pain) and unmyelinated C fibers (slow-conducting and dull pain)—toward the spinal cord. Upon entering the spinal cord through the dorsal root, these fibers may ascend or descend one or two spinal segments in Lissauer's tract before synapsing in the dorsal horn [20].

Second-order neurons in the dorsal horn relay nociceptive information to higher centers. The spinothalamic tract (STT), part of the anterolateral system, is the principal ascending pathway for pain and temperature sensation. After crossing to the contralateral side within the spinal cord, STT fibers ascend to synapse on the thalamus, where third-order neurons then project to the primary somatosensory cortex, contributing to the conscious perception of pain [21].

While not primarily responsible for pain, the dorsal column-medial lemniscus (DCML) pathway, composed mainly of large-diameter Aβ fibers, transmits touch, vibration, pressure, and proprioception. These fibers synapse in the dorsal column nuclei of the brainstem and continue via the medial lemniscus to the thalamus and somatosensory cortex. However, Aβ fibers can modulate pain at the spinal level via inhibitory interneurons—a mechanism exploited in neuromodulatory therapies [22].

Lissauer's tract, a thin bundle of transmitting fibers adjacent to the dorsal horn, plays a key role in segmental pain processing. Its fibers contribute to the spread of pain signals across multiple spinal levels and are thought to participate in diffuse pain syndromes such as visceral or axial pain through a process called convergence, where somatic and visceral afferents share spinal pathways [23,24].

Understanding these pathways is essential for surgical pain interventions, particularly those targeting segmental or supraspinal modulation. See Fig. 6.3.

Imaging modalities

X-ray

Primarily used as a first-line imaging modality for assessing vertebral alignment, fractures, scoliosis, and degenerative changes. X-rays offer limited sensitivity for soft tissue structures but provide essential information on spinal stability, e.g., dynamic flexion-extension views.

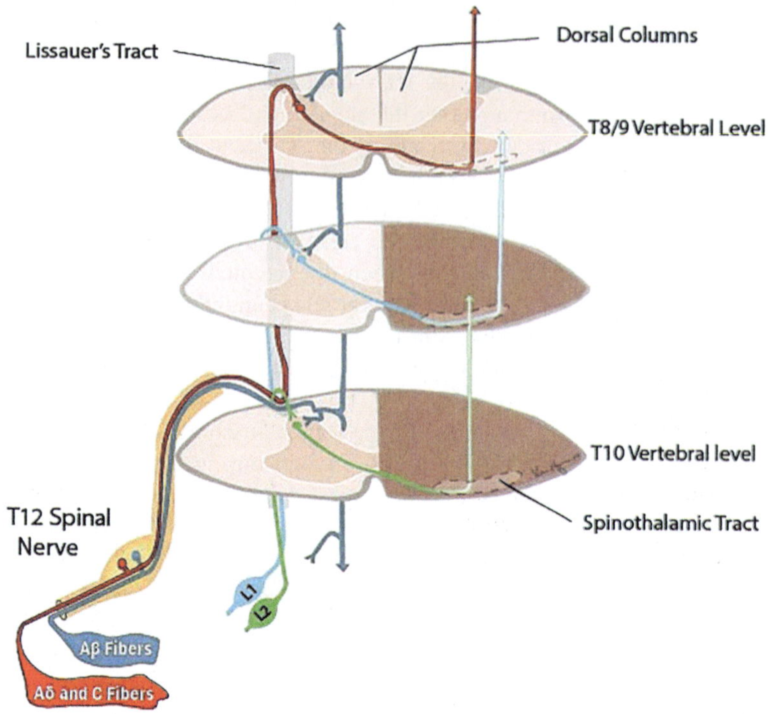

FIGURE 6.3 Brown Sequard syndrome: A hemisection of the spinal cord causes loss of pain and temperature 2 levels above the transection. Aδ and C-fibers enter Lissauer's tract and travel rostrally two levels before entering the spinal dorsal horn to synapse. The sensation then crosses the anterior white commissure to enter the spinothalamic tract and travel rostrally. Aβ fibers (dark blue) enter the dorsal horn at their corresponding level, enter the dorsal columns, and then form collaterals at multiple levels. Both of these spinal pathways travel to the somatosensory cortex for the localization of pain.

Magnetic Resonance Imaging

Magnetic Resonance Imaging (MRI) has become the gold standard for evaluating soft tissue structures of the spine, including intervertebral discs, the spinal cord, nerve roots, and ligaments. The spinal cord and nerve roots are highly sensitive to compression, inflammation, and neoplastic changes, therefore, MRI's ability to provide high-resolution and high contrast between soft tissues make it indispensable in the diagnosis and management of spinal pathologies.

T2-weighted and Short Tau Inversion Recovery (STIR) sequences are used to detect inflammation and conditions involving swelling, such as syrinx, disc herniations, spinal cord edema, acute vertebral compression fracture, and abscesses. Water molecules move more freely in pathological areas, such as regions affected by inflammation or tumor infiltration. Mechanistically, T2-weighted sequences are sensitive to the transverse relaxation time (T2), which is prolonged in tissues with increased water content. Intervertebral discs are primarily composed of water, collagen fibers, and proteoglycans. Therefore, a healthy nucleus pulposus is visible on T2-weighted imaging [25]. Hyperintensity in T2 sequencing allows for superior detection of herniated discs and associated nerve root compression by leveraging the differences in tissue water content and proton density, highlighting areas and severity of degeneration (which typically have reduced water content) and herniation [26]. The STIR sequence, which suppresses the signal from fat, further enhances the visibility of soft tissues affected by inflammation, such as abscesses, discitis, osteomyelitis or spondylitis [27].

CT scan

Provides superior bony detail, useful in evaluating fractures, hardware-bone loosening, ossification of ligaments, and congenital anomalies. On occasion, a CT myelography is beneficial for assessing nerve root compression in cases where an MRI is contraindicated.

Ultrasound

A dynamic and nonionizing modality is gaining traction in musculoskeletal assessments.

Useful for evaluating muscle thickness, detecting atrophy, and guiding various percutaneous nerve blocks of the chest wall [28].

Anatomical variations

Recognizing anatomical variations is critical in procedural planning and optimizing patient outcomes. Scoliosis alters normal spinal biomechanics, contributing to asymmetric degenerative changes and requiring adjusted fluoroscopic imaging angles during interventions. Scoliosis can lead to pain through facet-related pain and/or nerve impingement.

Congenital Variations such as hemivertebrae (results from incomplete development of one side of the vertebra) or spina bifida occulta (small gap or split in the vertebrae) may present challenges in spinal instrumentation and procedural planning.

Tethered spinal cord: can result in abnormal tension on the spinal column, leading to symptoms such as pain, weakness, or developmental delays. Although the spinal cord is not directly part of the vertebrae, this condition can be associated with vertebral malformations in the thoracic region.

Role of the thoracic spine in neuromodulation

The thoracic spine provides structural support and stability for the torso while protecting the thoracic segment of the spinal cord, which contains neurons that innervate the trunk and lower extremities. Although pain originating from the thoracic vertebral column is less common, the thoracic spinal cord remains a key anatomical target for neuromodulation, particularly for managing pain in the back, legs, and trunk. This anatomical overview lays the foundation for understanding the thoracic region's critical role in neuromodulation—including lead placement techniques—which will be explored in detail throughout this book.

References

[1] Risetti M, Gambugini R, Testa M, Battista S. Management of non-specific thoracic spine pain: a cross-sectional study among physiotherapists. BMC Muscoskelet Disord May 19, 2023;24(1):398.

[2] Heneghan NR, Gormley S, Hallam C, Rushton A. Management of thoracic spine pain and dysfunction: a survey of clinical practice in the UK. Musculoskeletal Sci Pract February 2019;39:58–66.

[3] Louw A, Schmidt SG. Chronic pain and the thoracic spine. J Man Manip Ther July 2015;23(3):162–8.

[4] Ivancic PC, Pearson AM, Panjabi MM, Ito S. Injury of the anterior longitudinal ligament during whiplash simulation. Eur Spine J February 2004;13(1):61–8.

[5] Aryal V, Black AC, Jimenez A. Anatomy, back, posterior longitudinal ligament [Updated 2023 Jul 30]. In: StatPearls. Treasure Island (FL): StatPearls Publishing; January 2025. https://www.ncbi.nlm.nih.gov/books/NBK560691/.

[6] Merter A, Karaca MO, Yazar T. Biomechanical effects of sequential resection of the posterior ligamentous complex on intradiscal pressure and resistance to compression forces. Acta Orthop Traumatol Turcica November 2019;53(6):502–6. https://doi.org/10.1016/j.aott.2019.08.016.

[7] Ganapathy MK, Reddy V, Tadi P. Neuroanatomy, spinal cord morphology [Updated 2024 Sep 10]. In: StatPearls. Treasure Island (FL): StatPearls Publishing; January 2025. https//www.ncbi.nlm.nih.gov/books/NBK545206/.

[8] Lee MW, McPhee RW, Stringer MD. An evidence-based approach to human dermatomes. Clin Anat July 2008;21(5):363–73.

[9] Ishizuka K, Sakai H, Tsuzuki N, Nagashima M. Topographic anatomy of the posterior ramus of thoracic spinal nerve and surrounding structures. Spine June 15, 2012;37(14):E817–22.

[10] Fradet L, Arnoux PJ, Ranjeva JP, Petit Y, Callot V. Morphometrics of the entire human spinal cord and spinal canal measured from in vivo high-resolution anatomical magnetic resonance imaging. Spine February 15, 2014;39(4):E262–9. https://doi.org/10.1097/BRS.0000000000000125.

[11] Frostell A, Hakim R, Thelin EP, Mattsson P, Svensson M. A review of the segmental diameter of the healthy human spinal cord. Front Neurol December 23, 2016;7:238. https://doi.org/10.3389/fneur.2016.00238.

[12] Ragel BT, Riedman T, McGehee M, Raslan AM. Analysis of spinal canal diameter in the placement of thoracic spinal cord stimulator paddle leads. Pain Pract January 2024;24(1):91–100. https://doi.org/10.1111/papr.13289.

[13] Molnar G, Barolat G. Principles of cord activation during spinal cord stimulation. Neuromodulation June 2014;17(Suppl. 1):12–21. https://doi.org/10.1111/ner.12171.

[14] Hines K, Tran C, Koka A, Mouchtouris N, Hafazalla K, Hattar E, Wu C, Sharan A. Thoracic canal morphology on preoperative magnetic resonance imaging in spinal cord stimulation patients. Pain Pract November 2024;24(8):1035–41. https://doi.org/10.1111/papr.13398.

[15] Westrup AM, Conner AK. Percutaneous thoracic spinal cord stimulator placement. Cureus March 16, 2021;13(3):e13916.

[16] Bosmia AN, Hogan E, Loukas M, Tubbs RS, Cohen-Gadol AA. Blood supply to the human spinal cord: part I. Anatomy and hemodynamics. Clin Anat January 2015;28(1):52–64.

[17] Perez Perez VH, Hernesniemi J, Small JE. Anatomy of the great posterior radiculomedullary artery. AJNR Am J Neuroradiol December 2019;40(12):2010–5.

[18] Alvernia JE, Simon E, Khandelwal K, Ramos CD, Perkins E, Kim P, Mertens P, Messina R, Luzardo G, Diaz O. Anatomical study of the thoracolumbar radiculomedullary arteries, including the Adamkiewicz artery and supporting radiculomedullary arteries. J Neurosurg Spine September 23, 2022;38(2):233–41.

[19] Johnson JN, Teton ZE, Lee JE, Bergsneider M, Srinivasan VM, Colby GP, Wang AC, Kan P. The human craniospinal venous system and its influence on postural intracranial pressure: a review. J Neurosurg July 19, 2024;141(6):1484–93.
[20] Waxman SG. Clinical neuroanatomy. McGraw-Hill Education; 2017.
[21] Willis WD, Westlund KN. Neurons involved in the transmission and modulation of pain. In: McMahon SB, Koltzenburg M, editors. Wall and Melzack's textbook of pain. 6th ed. Elsevier; 2013.
[22] Fields HL, Basbaum AI. Central nervous system mechanisms of pain modulation. In: McMahon SB, Koltzenburg M, editors. Wall and Melzack's textbook of pain. 6th ed. Elsevier; 2013.
[23] Al-Chaer ED. Visceral pain pathways: the anatomy of somatovisceral convergence. Curr Pain Headache Rep 2004;8(4):277–82. https://doi.org/10.1007/s11916-004-0049-7.
[24] Chapman KB, Groenen PS, Vissers KC, van Helmond N, Stanton-Hicks MD. The pathways and processes underlying spinal transmission of low back pain: observations from dorsal root ganglion stimulation treatment. Neuromodulation June 2021;24(4):610–21.
[25] Smith MR, et al. Cervical myelopathy: clinical and MRI European spine. Journal 2015;24(10):2334–43.
[26] Zhao X, et al. T2-weighted MRI sequences for assessing herniated discs. NeuroRadiol J 2013;26(6):697–703.
[27] Benkhaled F, et al. STIR imaging in inflammatory spinal diseases. Eur Radiol 2011;21(8):1773–81.
[28] Yang A, Nadav D, Legler A, Chen GH, Hingula L, Puttanniah V, Gulati A. An interventional pain algorithm for the treatment of postmastectomy pain syndrome: a single-center retrospective review. Pain Med March 18, 2021;22(3):677–86.

Further reading

[1] Grant R. Physical therapy of the cervical and thoracic spine. 2nd ed. London: Churchill Livingstone; 1988 [Google Scholar].

Chapter 7

Lumbar spine anatomy

Corey Gatewood[1], Derek Fitzgerald[2], Lee Nguyen[2] and Scott Pritzlaff[2]
[1]Department of Physical Medicine and Rehabilitation, University of California, Davis, Sacramento, CA, United States; [2]Division of Pain Medicine, Department of Anesthesiology and Pain Medicine, University of California, Davis, Sacramento, CA, United States

Introduction

Neuromodulation has rapidly evolved, expanding beyond traditional pain management to include innovative treatments for a range of chronic pain conditions. Advances in spinal cord stimulation (SCS), dorsal root ganglion stimulation (DRG-S), and neurorestorative therapies have transformed the landscape of interventional pain medicine. These innovations have been driven by improved device technology, expanded indications, and a deeper understanding of neural anatomy.

Historical perspective

Developed initially for post-laminectomy syndrome—now termed persistent spinal pain syndrome type 2 (PSPS-2)—SCS has expanded to treat painful diabetic neuropathy (PDN), axial low back pain (non-surgical), and other chronic pain syndromes [1–3]. DRG-S has emerged as a transformative therapy for complex regional pain syndrome (CRPS) and peripheral neuropathic pain syndromes, providing precise targeting with minimal unwanted paresthesia [4]. Meanwhile, neurorestorative stimulation, focuses on multifidus muscle activation to restore function in patients with refractory lumbar pain, with promising long-term data. Newer technology has revolutionized neuromodulation, including remote programming and closed-loop systems that use evoked compound action potentials (ECAPs) for real-time therapy adjustments. Closed-loop stimulation aims to both advance the precision and effectiveness of spinal cord stimulation.

Suggested specialty training for appropriate intervention

As neuromodulation techniques become increasingly sophisticated, the need for specialized training in lumbar spinal anatomy is more important than ever. Pain medicine fellowship programs play a critical role in developing this expertise, offering in-depth education on lumbar spine structures, epidural space navigation, and imaging interpretation—particularly MRI. Proficiency in fluoroscopic and ultrasound-guided procedures is essential, and hands-on experience through cadaver-based training further enhances technical skill, promotes procedural accuracy, and helps reduce complications.

Key points

- The **lumbar spine (L1–L5)** serves as a key entry point and anatomical landmark for neuromodulation procedures such as SCS, DRG-S, and multifidus stimulation.
- Each vertebra consists of a vertebral body and arch (pedicles, laminae, spinous and transverse processes, articular processes), forming the **vertebral canal** which houses the spinal cord and cauda equina.
- **Intervertebral discs** provide cushioning and load-bearing support, with the L4-L5 disc being the thickest and L5-S1 most prone to degeneration.
- The **epidural space**, located just beneath the ligamentum flavum, contains fat and veins and is the primary target for lead placement in SCS and DRG-S.
- **Neuroforamina** contain the spinal nerves, dorsal root ganglion (DRG), arteries (including the artery of Adamkiewicz), and venous plexuses, which are critical for precise lead placement in DRG-S.
- **MRI imaging** is essential for planning procedures due to variations in epidural space size, ligament thickness, and DRG location.

A Modern Atlas for Implantable Devices of the Spine, Brain, and Nerve. https://doi.org/10.1016/B978-0-443-36528-7.00054-6

Anatomy

Anatomy system scope

The lumbar spine is an important anatomical landmark for neuromodulation and often serves as the entry point for many procedures. It also provides structural support and houses the neural elements essential for neuromodulation interventions, including SCS, DRG-S, and multifidus stimulation.

A discussion of the lumbar spine begins with the lumbar vertebrae located between the thoracic vertebrae and the sacrum. There are five total lumbar vertebrae, numbered L1 to L5. Each lumbar vertebrae consists of a vertebral body and a vertebral arch. The vertebral body is an anterior bony element that supports the spinal column. The vertebral arch includes the pedicles, laminae, transverse and spinous processes, and superior and inferior articular processes [5]. Each vertebral body is connected posteriorly to the vertebral arch via pedicles, forming the lamina [6]. The laminae extend medially to form the spinous processes, which serve as attachment points for spinal muscles that function as levers for posture and movement, including the multifidus muscle [5,6]. The transverse processes project laterally to from the pediculolaminar junction, providing attachment sites for muscles involved in rotation and lateral flexion. Arising from the pediculolaminar junction are the superior and inferior articular processes forming the zygapophyseal joints [6].

The vertebral foramen is a circular opening formed by the vertebral body, pedicles, laminae, and spinous processes. Collectively, the vertebral foramina form the vertebral canal, also called the spinal canal, which houses the neural elements. These include the spinal cord which terminates commonly at L1 or L2 to become the cauda equina [6]. The vertebral canal also contains vasculature, lymphatics, and adipose tissue. The openings where the spinal nerve roots exit are called neuroforamina and are bordered superiorly and inferiorly by pedicles [5].

Between the vertebral bodies are intervertebral discs, which facilitate spinal flexibility and absorb axial load [7]. The height of the intervertebral discs increases caudally, with the most significant height at L4-L5. However, the L5-S1 disc has a smaller load-bearing surface, possibly contributing to its higher susceptibility to degeneration [7]. Disc degeneration is associated with vertebral endplate changes; however, a detailed discussion of these changes is beyond the scope of this chapter. The vertebrae and intervertebral discs form the spinal column and provide structural support to the spine.

The lumbar spine is richly vascularized. The arterial supply originates from the aorta, which gives rise to bilateral lumbar intersegmental arteries that course posteriorly and laterally to enter the neuroforamen. Within the neuroforamen, the intersegmental arteries branch further. Most notably, the medial branch becomes the radicular artery, which supplies the nerve root. The radicular artery is commonly located at the anterosuperior aspect of the neuroforamen along the dorsal nerve root [8]. The radicular artery pierces the dura to become the anterior and posterior radiculomedullary arteries. The radiculomedullary arteries join the anterior and posterior spinal arteries to supply the spinal cord [8]. Notably, the most dominant anterior radiculomedullary artery is the artery of Adamkiewicz, a major supplier of the anterior spinal cord. Its location is highly variable, though predominantly arises from the left side of the aorta and most commonly arises between T8 and L3 [9]. Other branches of the lumbar intersegmental artery include an anterolateral branch, which supplies the vertebral body, and a branch that supplies the posterior elements, including the epidural adipose tissue.

The venous drainage of the lumbar spine is complex and consists of multiple interconnected networks. The external vertebral venous plexus surrounds the vertebral bodies and vertebral canal, while the internal vertebral venous plexus is present within the vertebral canal. The external and internal venous plexuses are connected by the intervertebral veins, which pass through the superior and inferior aspects of each neuroforamen. The superior intervertebral veins accompany the dorsal root ganglion and exiting nerve roots [6].

Relevant anatomy

A thorough understanding of the lumbar spine's anatomical structures is essential to apply neuromodulation techniques safely and effectively. This section will specifically highlight the spinal ligaments, epidural space, neuroforamen, and dorsal root ganglion, as they serve as key targets in neuromodulation procedures.

Numerous ligamentous structures are relevant to neuromodulation. From superficial to deep, these include the supraspinous ligaments, which run along the posterior aspect of the spinous processes, followed by the interspinous ligaments that connect adjacent spinous processes. Located deep to the interspinous ligament is the ligamentum flavum, which connects adjacent laminae and forms the posterior boundary of the spinal canal. Directly beneath the ligamentum flavum lies the epidural space.

Additional ligaments of note include the posterior longitudinal ligament, which lines the posterior aspect of the vertebral bodies and intervertebral discs, and the anterior longitudinal ligament, which connects the anterior surfaces of the vertebral bodies and intervertebral discs [7]. The intertransverse ligaments further contribute to spinal stability by connecting adjacent transverse processes. The ligaments within the neuroforamen will be discussed in a subsequent section.

The epidural space is of particular importance in spinal neuromodulation. It typically measures between 4 and 6 mm in depth, though this can vary based on gender and has a positive correlation with height and weight [6]. Within the epidural space, there is epidural adipose tissue along with a network of veins. Beneath the epidural space lie the meninges, which enclose the spinal cord. The meninges consist of three layers, arranged from superficial to deep: the dura mater, arachnoid mater, and pia mater [6]. The spinal cord is enveloped by these protective layers.

Another critical landmark for neuromodulation, particularly for DRG-S, is the neuroforamen. Within the foramen are the spinal nerves and their associated dural root sleeves, the radicular artery, communicating veins between the vertebral venous plexuses, recurrent meningeal nerves, and lymphatics. These structures are all surrounded by adipose tissue.

The spinal nerves are composed of the dorsal and ventral nerve roots, which converge within the neuroforamen before exiting and dividing into dorsal and ventral rami [10]. Additionally, a network of transforaminal ligaments is present within the neuroforamen [10]. Functionally, the neuroforamen serves as the transition point between the central and peripheral nervous systems. This transition is marked by the dorsal root ganglion (DRG), an enlargement of the dorsal nerve root present at every vertebral level. The DRG contains the cell bodies of up to 15,000 sensory neurons and is surrounded by glial cells at an approximate 8:1 ratio to sensory neurons [11]. The DRG is most commonly positioned beneath the pedicle within the vertebral body and is typically located intraforaminally [12]. By recognizing the spatial relationships of these anatomical landmarks, clinicians can optimize neuromodulation procedures, enhancing both precision and patient outcomes.

Appropriate images, drawings, X-rays

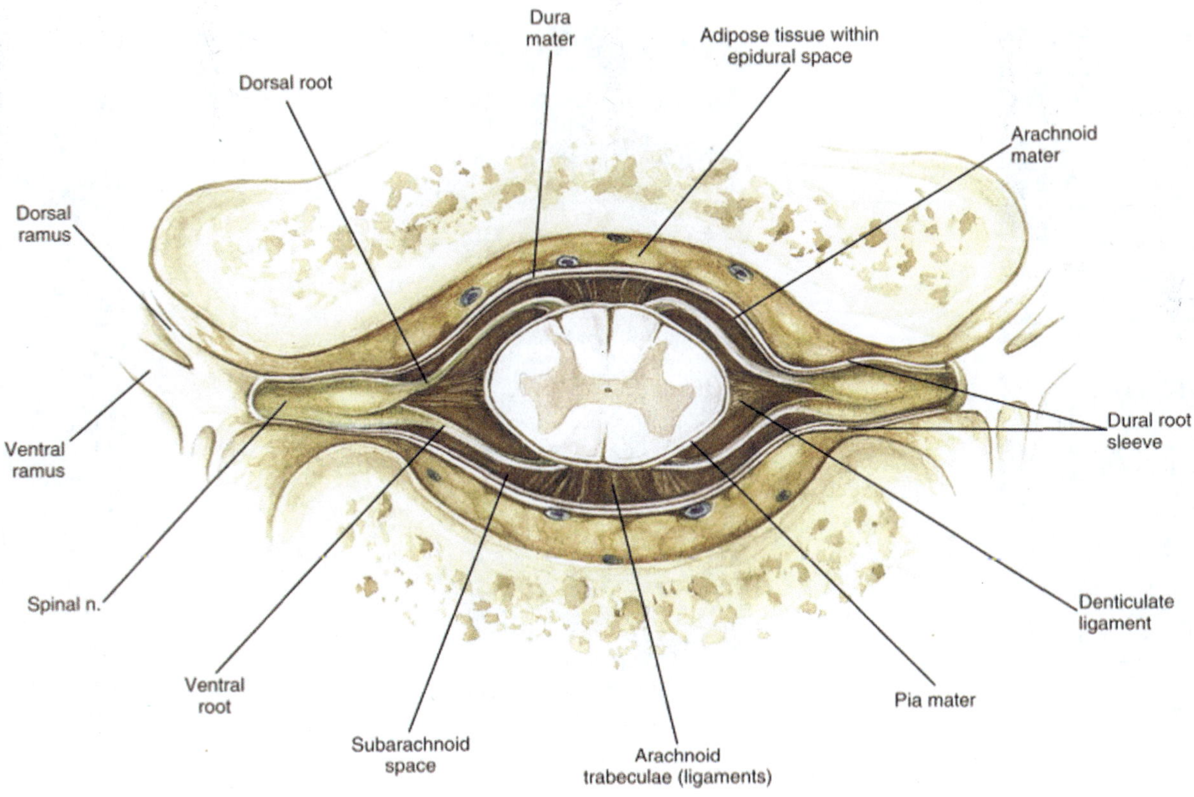

SCHEMATIC DIAGRAM OF SPINAL CANAL IN CROSS SECTION.

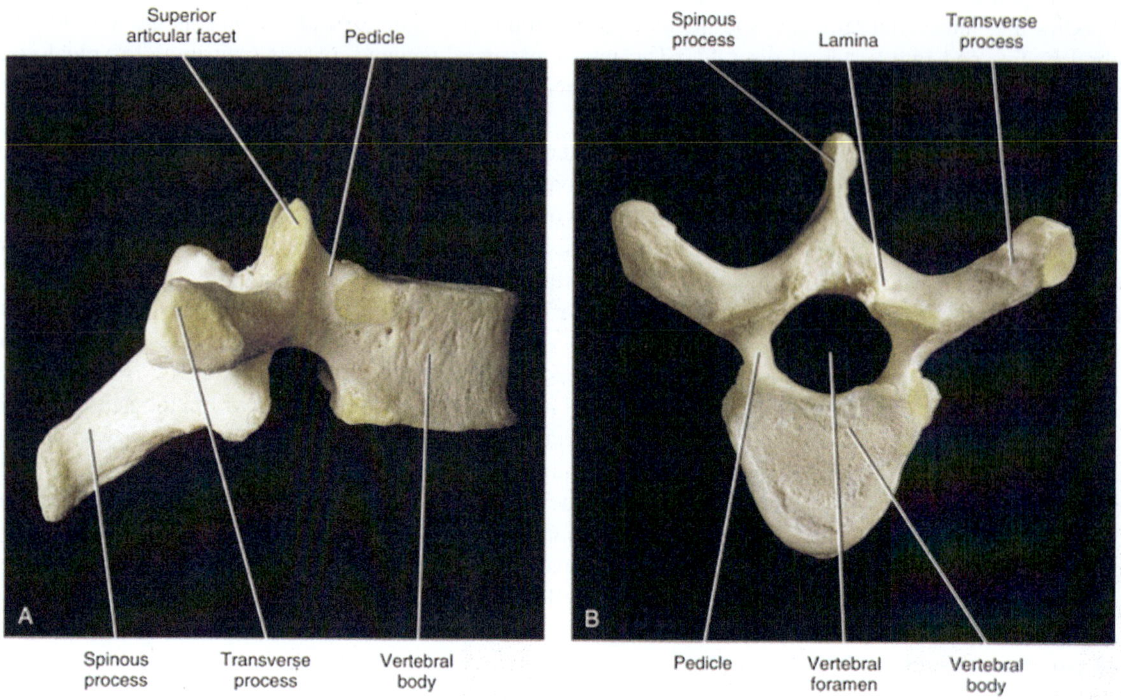

LUMBAR VERTEBRA BONY ANATOMY.

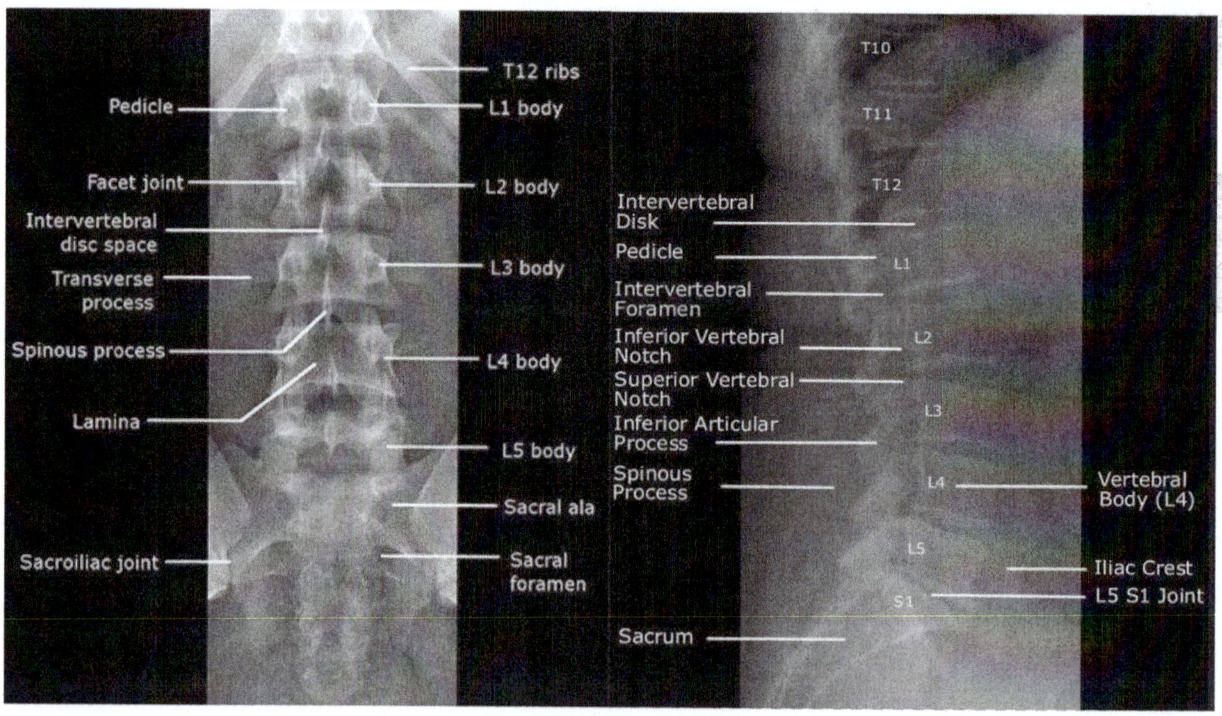

RADIOGRAPHIC FILMS DEPICTING LUMBAR ANATOMY IN THE LATERAL AND ANTERIOR POSTERIOR VIEWS.

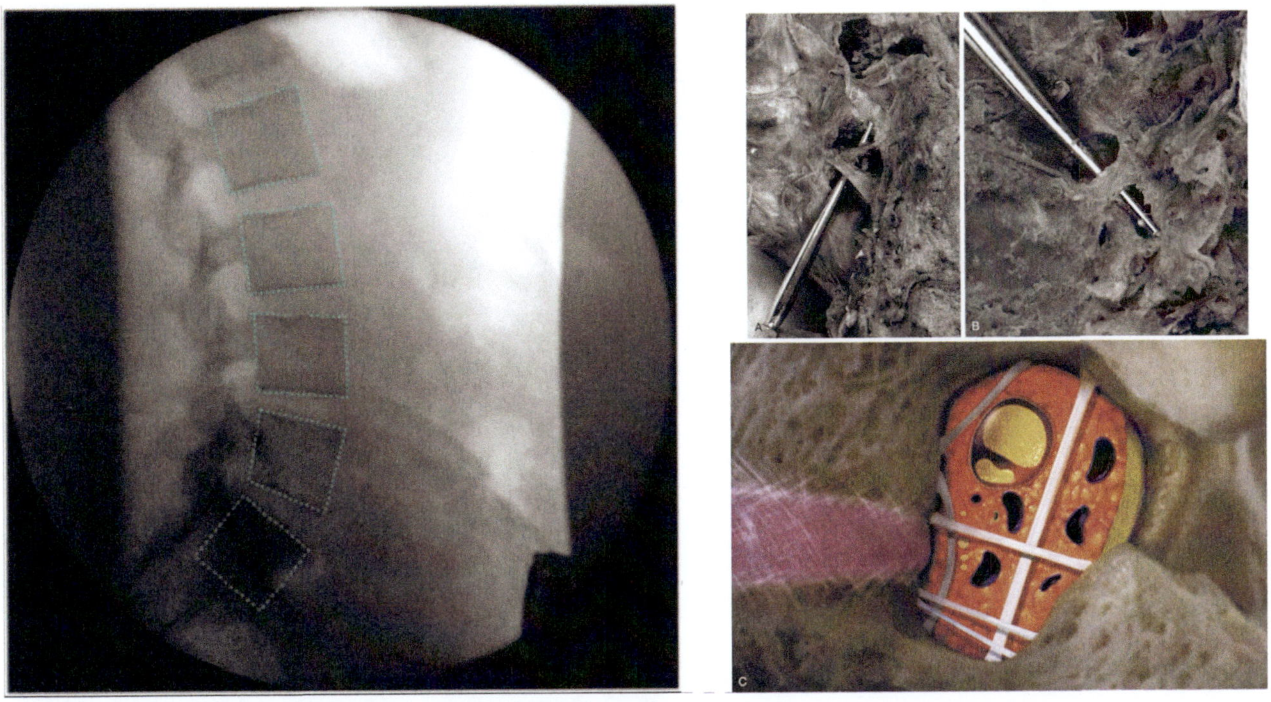

LUMBAR SPINE LATERAL FLUOROSCOPIC IMAGE; CADAVERIC DISSECTION OF TRANSFORAMINAL LIGAMENTS.

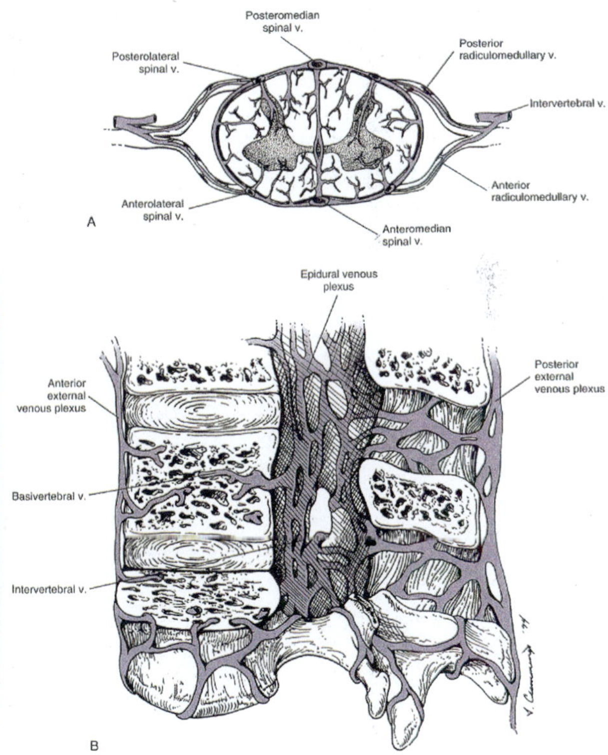

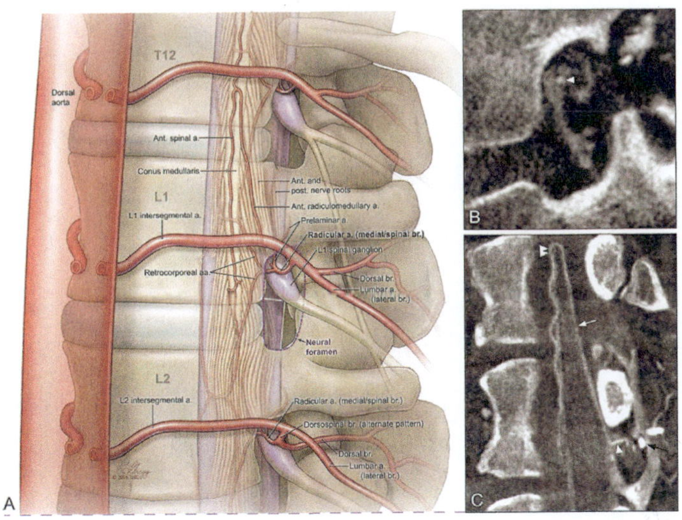

SCHEMATIC DEPICTION OF NEUROFORAMINAL BLOOD SUPPLY.

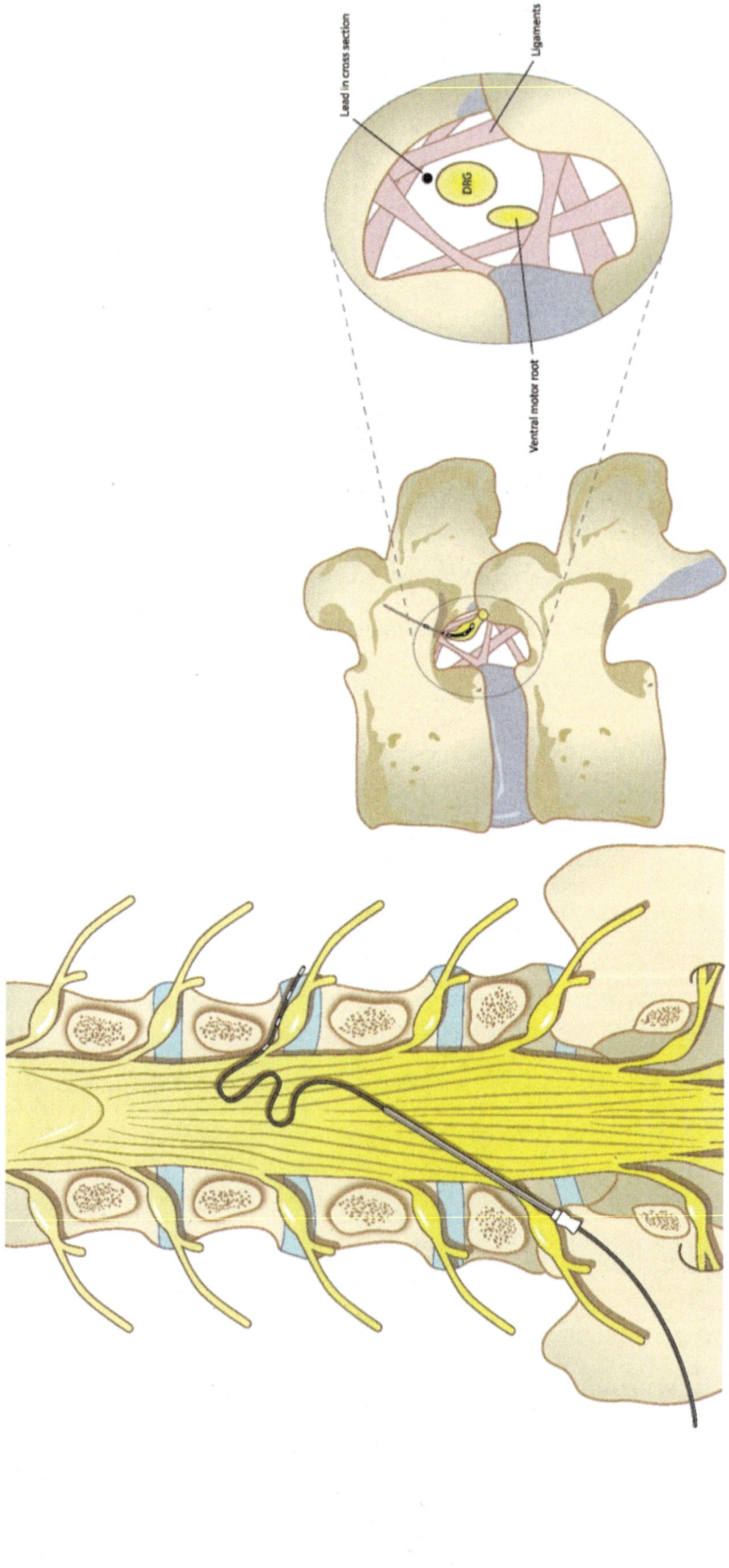

SCHEMATIC DEPICTION OF DRG-S WITHIN THE NEUROFORAMEN AND DRG STIMULATOR LEAD PLACEMENT.

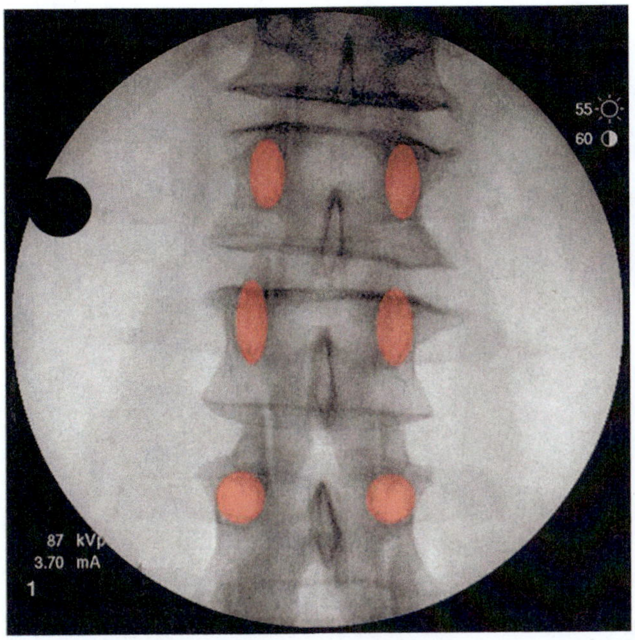

Lumbar: Alignment of the vertebral endplates.

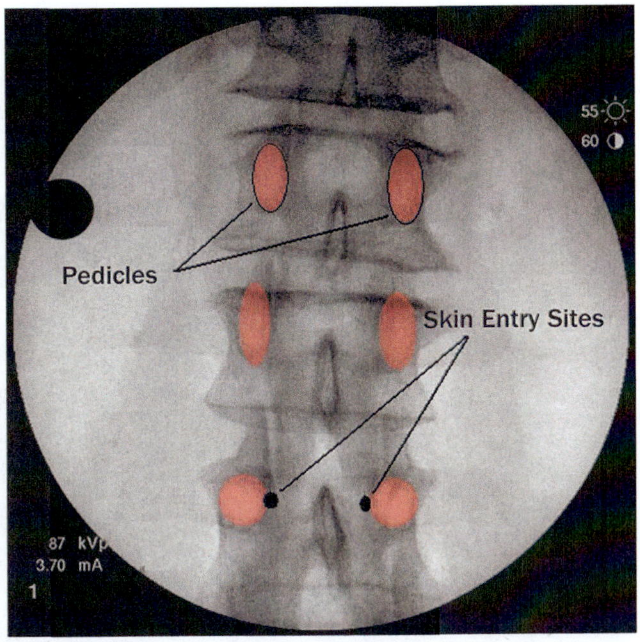

Lumbar: Selection of skin entry points.

FLUOROSCOPIC ALIGNMENT OF VERTEBRAL ENDPLATES AND SKIN ENTRY SITES FOR SPINAL CORD STIMULATOR.

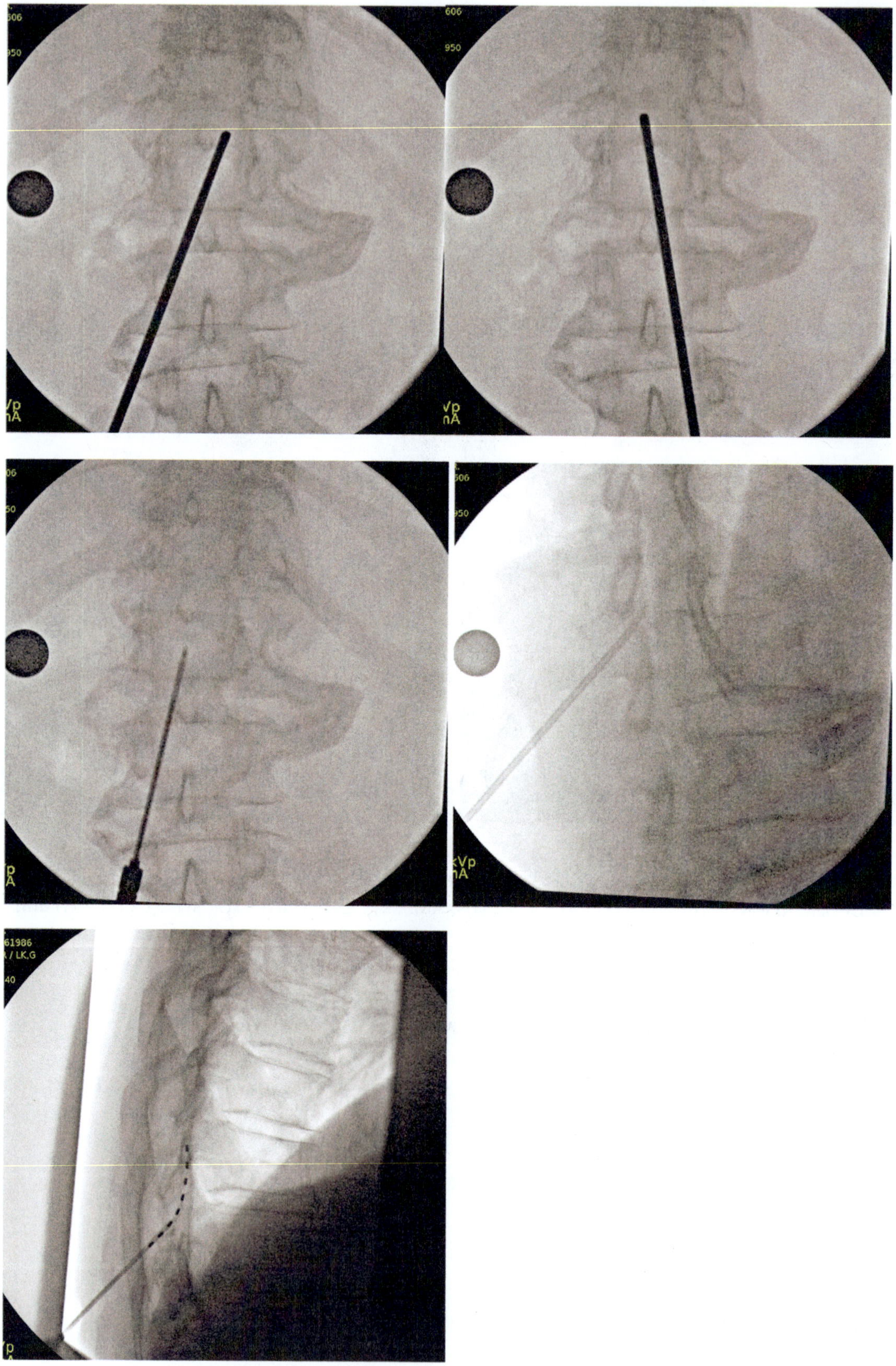

FLUOROSCOPIC IMAGES OF EPIDURAL ENTRY AND LEAD INSERTION FOR SCS (DEIDENTIFIED PHOTOS).

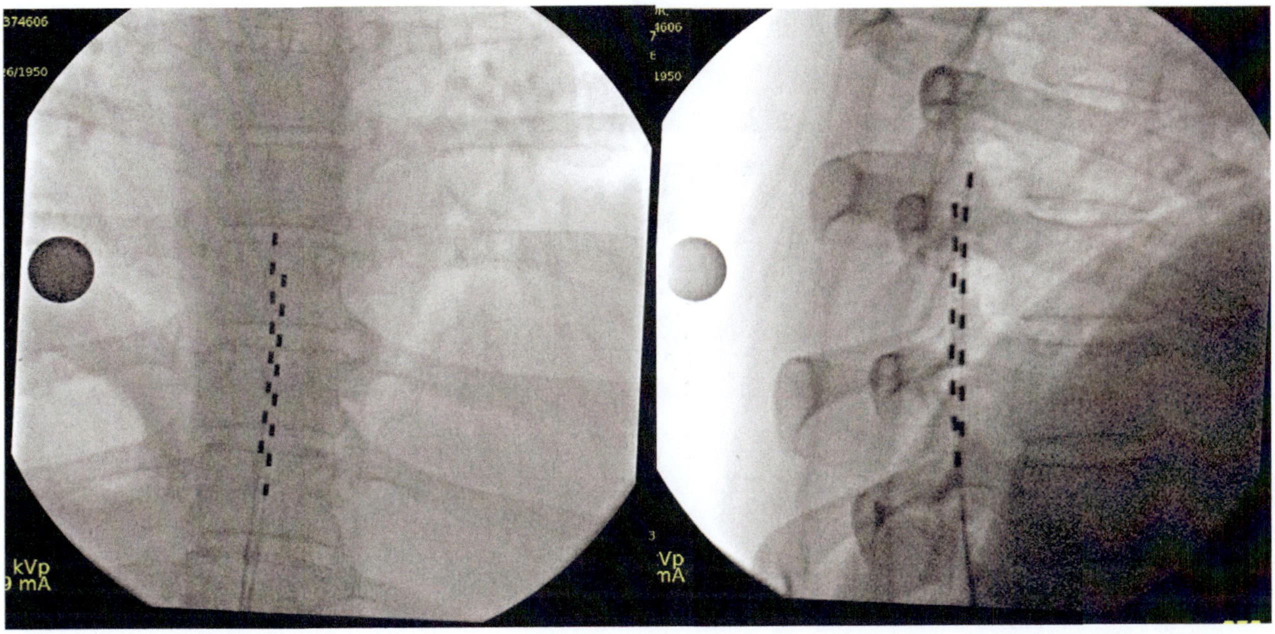

FLUOROSCOPIC IMAGES OF SPINAL STIMULATOR LEADS (DEIDENTIFIED PHOTOS).

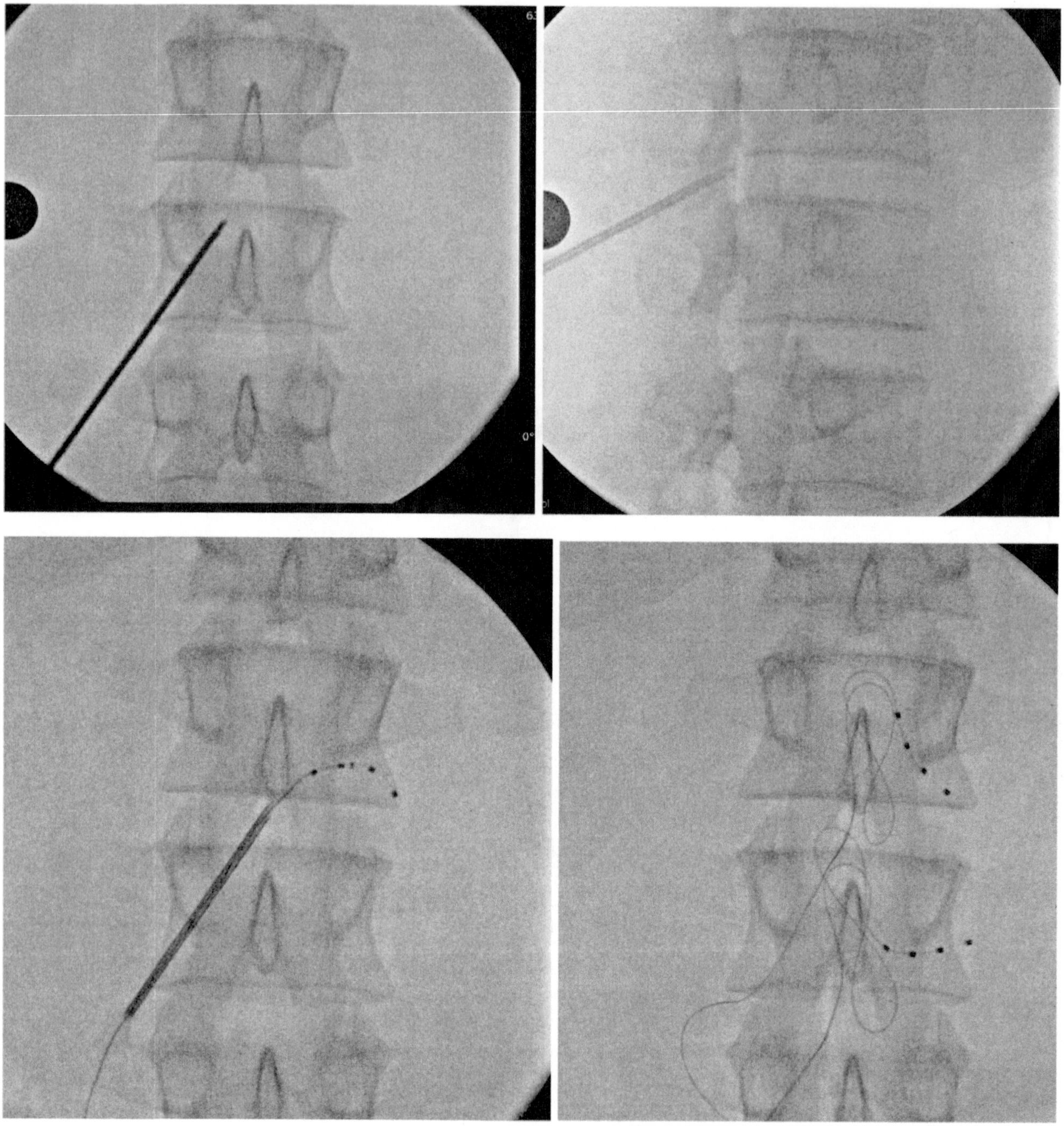

RADIOGRAPHIC IMAGES OF EPIDURAL ENTRY AND LEAD INSERTION (FOR DRG-S) (DEIDENTIFIED PHOTOS).

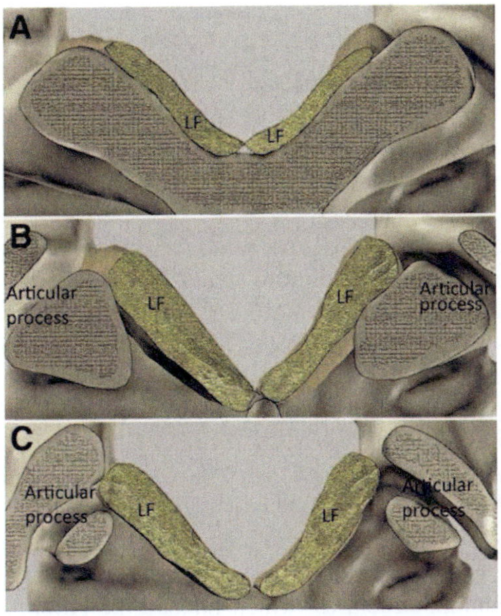

Three-dimensional reconstruction of human lumbar ligamentum flavum. A, B, and C, Successive transverse sections from rostral to caudal zone of same ligamentum flavum (LF).

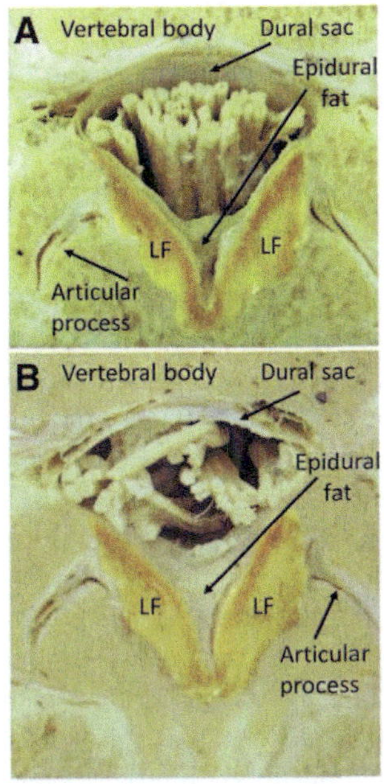

Transverse section of human lumbar spine. A and B, At L_3 vertebral level. LF = ligamentum flavum.

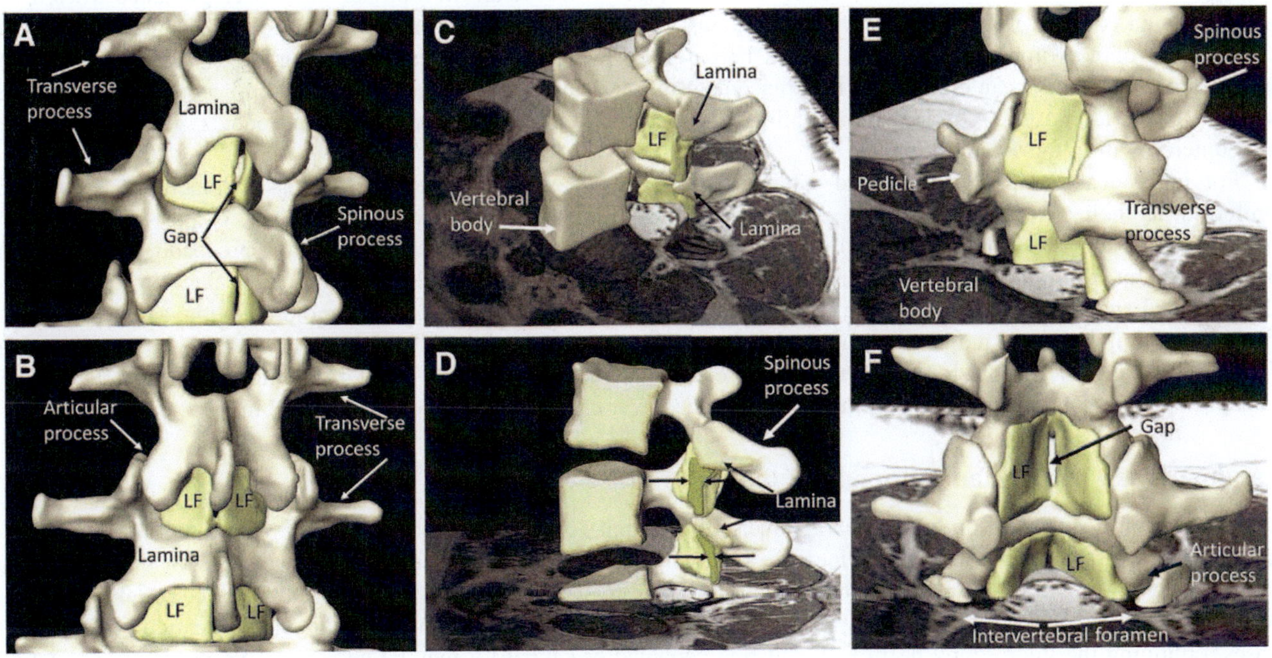

Three-dimensional reconstruction of human lumbar ligamentum flavum (LF). A, Posterior-lateral view. B, Posterior view. C and D, Lateral view with sagittal section. E, Anterior lateral view. F, Anterior view.

RECONSTRUCTIONS AND CADAVERIC DISSECTION DEPICTING LIGAMENTUM FLAVUM.

Procedure related considerations

Targeting the lumbar epidural space, dorsal root ganglion, or intrathecal space

The lumbar epidural space is a potential space within the rigid spinal canal that expands to accommodate neuromodulating devices [13]. The size of the epidural space varies at each lumbar vertebral level due to factors such as spinal stenosis, osteophyte formation, disc protrusions, and ligamentum flavum hypertrophy [14]. Prior imaging, such as 3-Tesla MRI imaging, is crucial for identifying lumbar epidural levels with sufficient space for SCS, DRG-S, and intrathecal pump placement [15].

For SCS, common interlaminar epidural entry points include the T12-L1, L1-L2, and L2-L3 interlaminar spaces, which provide an optimal angle and track for lead insertion into the thoracic epidural space. The L2-L3 interlaminar space can be a safer target as the conus medullaris is positioned more cephalad [15,16]. MRI evaluation is essential to assess for spinal stenosis, which may impede epidural access and lead placement. Reviewing MRI imaging for epidural space dimensions and ligamentum flavum hypertrophy is critical, as a thick ligamentum flavum may significantly increase resistance upon the needle tip when it engages [15]. There is also a potential for a false loss of resistance (LOR) before the needle tip engages the ligamentum flavum [16,17]. Additionally, once the leads are inserted and driven cephalad along the dorsal columns, ventral lead migration may result in pain or motor stimulation [16].

The location of the DRG can be variable, and MRI imaging should be utilized for procedural planning. Typically, the DRG is found inferior to the pedicle in the lumbar spine, but it may be positioned intraspinally, intraforaminally, or extraforaminally [4]. Physicians must also consider the neuroforaminal structures, which include the Artery of Adamkiewicz, sympathetic fibers, intervertebral arteries, veins, fatty tissue, and intraforaminal ligaments [18]. Additionally, ganglionic and spinal branches of the lumbar artery reside within the foramen.

For DRG-S, the preferred approach is the intraspinal method, requiring lumbar epidural access before passing the lead into the neuroforamen adjacent to the DRG. Midline epidural access allows optimal introducer guidance toward the neuroforamen [4]. The intervertebral foramen contains multiple ligaments that may impede lead placement [19]. A patient's level of neuroforaminal stenosis should be carefully evaluated preoperatively using MRI. Moderate to severe neuroforaminal stenosis can complicate lead placement into the neuroforamen, and alternative procedures, such as SCS, should be considered [4]. A guidewire or saline injection can help form a track for the introducer when resistance is encountered within the foramen [4].

For intrathecal pump placement and subarachnoid access, pencil-point needles such as Whitacre or Sprotte are preferred, as their rounded tips separate dural fibers rather than cutting them, reducing the risk of post-dural puncture headache (PDPH) [20]. Proper confirmation assessments are critical for both approaches. Before proceeding with epidural lead placement, aspiration should be performed to rule out unintended subarachnoid or intravascular entry [21]. A test dose of local anesthetic with epinephrine can help detect inadvertent vascular or subarachnoid injection, as an unexpected rapid increase in heart rate may indicate intravascular placement. In subarachnoid targeting, the free flow of cerebrospinal fluid (CSF) from the needle hub confirms proper entry into the subarachnoid space [22]. Mastering these techniques enhances accuracy and safety in neuromodulation procedures, ensuring effective patient outcomes.

Landmark assignments and procedural localization

Accurate identification of lumbar vertebral levels is essential for neuromodulation device implantation. To enhance procedural accuracy, clinicians should identify key bony landmarks using fluoroscopy, marking skin entry sites, the interlaminar space entry site, and vertebral levels [16]. Counting from the 12th thoracic rib aids in determining vertebral levels, particularly when scoliosis, compression fractures, or osteophytes obscure standard identification [16]. In such cases, obliquing the fluoroscopy beam and adjusting cephalad or caudal tilt may be necessary to optimize visualization.

Vertebral bodies and intervertebral disc spaces are primary reference points, with two pedicles corresponding to each vertebral level [16]. Fluoroscopic visualization of intervertebral disc spaces is particularly useful in patients with degenerative changes, ensuring precise electrode placement and minimizing complications. Under fluoroscopy, the lumbar interlaminar spaces are typically inferior to the corresponding vertebral body's spinous process.

Other critical bony landmarks include the iliac crests, which typically align with the L4 vertebral level or L4-L5 disc space, serving as a helpful landmark [23]. Posterior spinous processes provide midline reference points, often corresponding to the S1 or S2 vertebral levels (Fig. 7.1) [24].

The red circles depict two common interlaminar spaces used for epidural access in SCS. The topmost red circle is the T12-L1 interspace, and the bottom circle is the L1-L2 interspace.

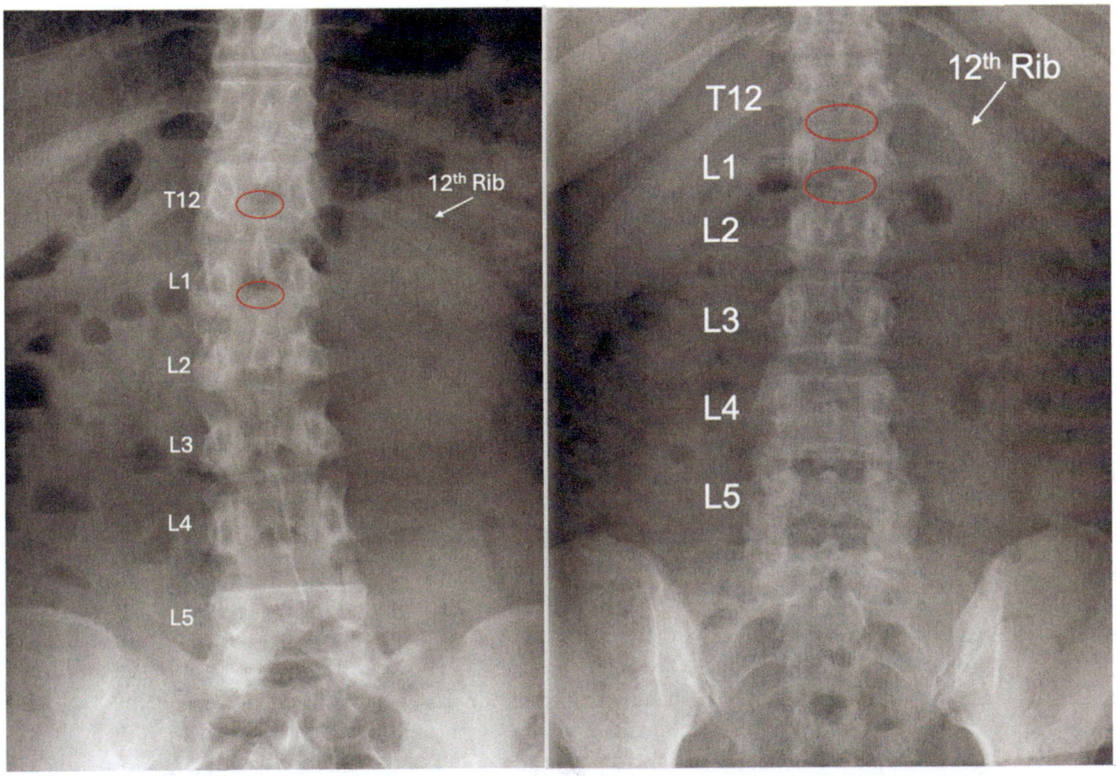

FIGURE 7.1 Lumbar spine X-ray depicting common sites of epidural access (original photos).

Pearls and pitfalls

Anatomic variations such as scoliosis, degenerative changes, obesity, and prior surgical alterations significantly impact neuromodulation procedures. Scoliosis alters vertebral alignment, shifting midline structures and requiring fluoroscopic recentering of the spinous processes between the pedicles to achieve an accurate midline epidural approach. Degenerative changes, including disc protrusions, ligamentum flavum hypertrophy, facet hypertrophy, and osteophyte formation, can reduce spinal canal and epidural space volume, affecting electrode placement and injectate spread. The ligamentum flavum, which is typically fused, may be unfused at the midline in up to 22.2% of lumbar cases, increasing dural puncture risk [25]. Preoperative imaging helps identify these variations and optimize procedural planning.

Obesity further complicates access due to increased body fat, which reduces fluoroscopic image clarity, prolongs fluoroscopy time, and increases radiation exposure. Despite these challenges, SCS implantation is safe in patients with BMI >40, with no increased risk of infection, wound dehiscence, or neurologic deficits compared to patients with lower BMI [26].

Congenital abnormalities such as spina bifida may increase dural puncture risk, while post-surgical changes like epidural fibrosis and spinal hardware can obscure visualization of anatomical landmarks. Patients with prior laminectomy or implanted hardware may require alternative approaches and fluoroscopic imaging must be carefully adjusted at each vertebral level during cephalad lead advancement to optimize visualization.

Imaging considerations

Multiplanar fluoroscopic guidance is essential for procedural accuracy. Contralateral oblique (CLO) views enhance visualization of the spinolaminar line, facilitating precise epidural access [27]. Lateral views help confirm needle depth for epidural and foraminal lead placement while detecting anterior lead migration during SCS implantation. In cases of spinal deformity, axial rotation of vertebral bodies in kyphoscoliosis introduces technical challenges that require tailored fluoroscopic positioning [28]. For patients with a history of spinal surgery, preoperative imaging plays a critical role in determining epidural space patency and identifying optimal lead placement. Entry at L1-L2 or L2-L3 must be approached cautiously to avoid injury to the conus medullaris, ensuring safe lead advancement. In some cases, a tunneled trial may be indicated, in which an externally connected permanent lead is used during the trial phase before final implantation [29].

By integrating thorough preoperative imaging with intraoperative adjustments tailored to anatomical variations, clinicians can enhance procedural safety and optimize neuromodulation outcomes.

Quick tips

1. Ensuring patient safety during neuromodulation device implantation requires meticulous technique and adherence to key precautions to minimize the risk of neural injury. Gentle tissue handling reduces trauma to muscles, ligaments, and nerves. At the same time, careful needle advancement should be performed with controlled movements, maintaining awareness of changes in resistance that may indicate proximity to critical structures. Although neurologic injury is rare, it can occur due to direct trauma from the needle or lead. Intraoperative neuromonitoring can help mitigate this risk by providing real-time feedback on neural integrity.
2. For epidural placement, the loss of resistance (LOR) technique using air or saline is commonly employed, and a sudden drop in resistance signals entry into the epidural space. The hanging drop technique, where a drop of saline at the needle hub is drawn inward upon epidural entry, may serve as an additional confirmation method. The epidural space should be accessed incrementally (1–2 mm at a time) while using contralateral oblique (CLO) views for guidance to ensure proper lead placement. The final position of the lead introducer needle tip should be just ventral to the ventral interlaminar line in CLO views or just sublaminar in lateral views. Once positioned, the spinal cord stimulator lead is inserted through the introducer needle and advanced approximately 1–2 cm (or 2–4 electrode contacts), ensuring it remains in the posterior epidural space [1].
3. Successful neuromodulation procedures require adapting to anatomical variations to ensure precise lead placement and minimize complications. Patient body mass index (BMI) significantly influences procedural adjustments; individuals with a low BMI may require a more cephalad needle angle, while those with a higher BMI often necessitate a more caudal approach. In such cases, adjusting the needle placement approximately 1 cm above or below the medial aspect of the target, two levels below the intended interlaminar space can help optimize lead positioning.
4. Additionally, understanding the MRI conditionality of neuromodulation systems is essential, as most devices are MRI-conditional with specific restrictions. Practitioners must know these limitations to ensure patient safety during postoperative imaging. By effectively employing fluoroscopy and intraoperative navigation tools while minimizing radiation exposure, clinicians can enhance procedural accuracy and safety in neuromodulation interventions.
5. Advanced imaging techniques enhance procedural accuracy. High-resolution ultrasound is particularly valuable for peripheral nerve stimulation (PNS) lead placement; however, its effectiveness may be limited by bony structures or patient body habitus. In such instances, combining ultrasound with fluoroscopy improves visualization and guidance. The American Society of Pain and Neuroscience recommends utilizing ultrasound whenever possible to enhance precision. Fluoroscopy remains essential for real-time X-ray imaging, allowing for continuous visualization of anatomical structures and needle trajectory.
6. Intraoperative neuromonitoring (IONM) is critical in ensuring safe spinal cord stimulator (SCS) lead placement, particularly in anaesthetized patients. By utilizing somatosensory evoked potentials (SSEPs) and electromyography (EMG), IONM helps detect potential neurological complications, optimize electrode placement, and reduce the risk of postoperative deficits. SSEPs monitor sensory pathway integrity within the spinal cord, while motor evoked potentials (MEPs) assess motor pathway function. EMG further enhances safety by monitoring the activity of specific muscles, providing real-time feedback on potential nerve irritation or compression. Incorporating these techniques into neuromodulation procedures improves patient safety and procedural success by accommodating each patient's unique anatomical considerations.
7. For dorsal root ganglion stimulation (DRG-S), when challenges arise with access or lead placement using the traditional anterograde approach, a transgrade approach may be considered. This technique has demonstrated efficacy in cases where concerns about lead dislodgement exist or when prior surgical interventions—such as discectomies, laminectomy syndrome, minimally invasive interbody fixation, or epidural adhesions—affect anatomical access [30].

References

[1] Yue JJ, Gilligan CJ, Falowski S, Jameson J, Desai MJ, Moeschler S, et al. Surgical treatment of refractory low back pain using implanted BurstDR spinal cord stimulation (SCS) in a cohort of patients without options for corrective surgery: findings and results from the DISTINCT study, a prospective randomized multi-center-controlled trial. N Am Spine Soc J September 2024;19:100508. https://doi.org/10.1016/j.xnsj.2024.100508.

[2] Petersen EA, Stauss TG, Scowcroft JA, Jaasma MJ, Edgar DR, White JL, et al. High-frequency 10-kHz spinal cord stimulation provides long-term (24-month) improvements in diabetes-related pain and quality of life for patients with painful diabetic neuropathy. J Diabetes Sci Technol January 2026;20(1):124–33. https://doi.org/10.1177/19322968241268547.

[3] van de Minkelis J, Peene L, Cohen SP, Staats P, Al-Kaisy A, Van Boxem K, et al. 6. Persistent spinal pain syndrome type 2. Pain Pract Off J World Inst Pain. September 2024;24(7):919–36. https://doi.org/10.1111/papr.13379.

[4] Chapman KB, Sayed D, Lamer T, Hunter C, Weisbein J, Patel KV, et al. Best practices for dorsal root ganglion stimulation for chronic pain: guidelines from the American society of pain and neuroscience. J Pain Res 2023;16:839–79. https://doi.org/10.2147/JPR.S364370.

[5] Levy RM. Anatomic considerations for spinal cord stimulation. Neuromodul J Int Neuromodul Soc June 2014;17(Suppl. 1):2–11. https://doi.org/10.1111/ner.12175.

[6] Cramer GD. The lumbar region. In: Clinical anatomy of the spine, spinal cord, and ans [internet]. Elsevier; 2014. p. 246–311. https://doi.org/10.1016/B978-0-323-07954-9.00007-4. Available from: https://linkinghub.elsevier.com/retrieve/pii/B9780323079549000074.

[7] Hashmi SS, Seifert KD, Massoud TF. Thoracic and lumbosacral spine anatomy. Neuroimaging Clin November 2022;32(4):889–902. https://doi.org/10.1016/j.nic.2022.07.024.

[8] Gregg L, Gailloud P. Neurovascular anatomy: spine. Handb Clin Neurol 2021;176:33–47. https://doi.org/10.1016/B978-0-444-64034-5.00007-9.

[9] Lindeire S, Hauser JM. Anatomy, back, artery of Adamkiewicz. In: StatPearls [internet]. Treasure Island (FL): StatPearls Publishing; 2026 [cited 2026 Apr 22]. Available from: http://www.ncbi.nlm.nih.gov/books/NBK532971/PubMed PMID: 30422566.

[10] Cramer GD. General characteristics of the spine. In: Clinical anatomy of the spine, spinal cord, and ans [internet]. Elsevier; 2014. p. 15–64. https://doi.org/10.1016/B978-0-323-07954-9.00002-5. Available from: https://linkinghub.elsevier.com/retrieve/pii/B9780323079549000025.

[11] Esposito MF, Malayil R, Hanes M, Deer T. Unique characteristics of the dorsal root ganglion as a target for neuromodulation. Pain Med June 1, 2019;20(Suppl. 1):S23–30. https://doi.org/10.1093/pm/pnz012.

[12] Hasegawa T, Mikawa Y, Watanabe R, An HS. Morphometric analysis of the lumbosacral nerve roots and dorsal root ganglia by magnetic resonance imaging. Spine May 1, 1996;21(9):1005–9. https://doi.org/10.1097/00007632-199605010-00001.

[13] Malinowski MN, Kim CH, Deer TR. Relevant anatomy for spinal drug delivery. In: Neuromodulation [internet]. Elsevier; 2018. p. 793–801. https://doi.org/10.1016/B978-0-12-805353-9.00064-4. Available from: https://linkinghub.elsevier.com/retrieve/pii/B9780128053539000644.

[14] Genevay S, Atlas SJ. Lumbar spinal stenosis. Best Pract Res Clin Rheumatol April 2010;24(2):253–65. https://doi.org/10.1016/j.berh.2009.11.001.

[15] Deer TR, Mekhail N, Provenzano D, Pope J, Krames E, Leong M, et al. The appropriate use of neurostimulation of the spinal cord and peripheral nervous system for the treatment of chronic pain and ischemic diseases: the neuromodulation appropriateness consensus committee. Neuromodul Technol Neural Interf August 2014;17(6):515–50. https://doi.org/10.1111/ner.12208.

[16] Pritzlaff SG, Kreis PG, Fishman SM. Percutaneous trial of spinal cord stimulation. In: Kreis PG, Pritzlaff SG, Copenhaver DJ, Fishman SM, editors. Spinal cord stimulation [internet]. 2nd ed. Oxford University Press; 2023. 79–C7P69. https://doi.org/10.1093/med/9780190095086.003.0007 Available from: https://academic.oup.com/book/46587/chapter/409015480.

[17] Lawrence S, Llewellyn S, Hunt H, Cowin G, Sturgess DJ, Reutens D. Anatomy of the lumbar interspinous ligament: findings relevant to epidural insertion using loss of resistance. Reg Anesth Pain Med December 2021;46(12):1085–90. https://doi.org/10.1136/rapm-2021-103014.

[18] Boggan JE. In: Kreis PG, Pritzlaff SG, Copenhaver DJ, Fishman SM, editors. Spinal cord stimulation: percutaneous implantation techniques [internet]. 2nd ed. Oxford University Press; 2023. https://doi.org/10.1093/med/9780190095086.001.0001 Available from: https://academic.oup.com/book/46587.

[19] Umeh R, Fisahn C, Burgess B, Iwanaga J, Moisi M, Oskouian RJ, et al. Transforaminal ligaments of the lumbar spine: a comprehensive review. Cureus October 2, 2016;8(10):e811. https://doi.org/10.7759/cureus.811.

[20] Halpern S, Preston R. Postdural puncture headache and spinal needle design: metaanalyses. Anesthesiology December 1, 1994;81(6):1376–83. https://doi.org/10.1097/00000542-199412000-00012.

[21] Schultz DM. Needle manipulation techniques. In: Manchikanti L, Kaye AD, Falco FJE, Hirsch JA, editors. Essentials of interventional techniques in managing chronic pain [internet]. Cham: Springer International Publishing; 2018. p. 125–39. https://doi.org/10.1007/978-3-319-60361-2_10. Available from: http://link.springer.com/10.1007/978-3-319-60361-2_10.

[22] Furnish T, Wallace MS. Intrathecal drug delivery. In: Practical management of pain [internet]. Elsevier; 2014. p. 953–65. https://doi.org/10.1016/B978-0-323-08340-9.00070-0. e1. Available from: https://linkinghub.elsevier.com/retrieve/pii/B9780323083409000700.

[23] Kim JT, Jung CW, Lee JR, Min SW, Bahk JH. Influence of lumbar flexion on the position of the intercrestal line. Reg Anesth Pain Med 2003;28(6):509–11. https://doi.org/10.1016/j.rapm.2003.08.027.

[24] Chakraverty R, Pynsent P, Isaacs K. Which spinal levels are identified by palpation of the iliac crests and the posterior superior iliac spines? J Anat February 2007;210(2):232–6. https://doi.org/10.1111/j.1469-7580.2006.00686.x.

[25] Lirk P, Moriggl B, Colvin J, Keller C, Kirchmair L, Rieder J, et al. The incidence of lumbar ligamentum flavum midline gaps. Anesth Analg April 2004:1178–80. https://doi.org/10.1213/01.ANE.0000101486.41355.35.

[26] Sommer TW, Ivankovic S, McCall TD. Effect of body mass index on paddle lead spinal cord stimulator safety implantation for chronic pain management. World Neurosurg February 2023;170:e712–5. https://doi.org/10.1016/j.wneu.2022.11.101.

[27] Gill JS, Nagda JV, Aner MM, Keel JC, Simopoulos TT. Contralateral oblique view is superior to the lateral view for lumbar epidural access. Pain Med May 2016;17(5):839–50. https://doi.org/10.1093/pm/pnv031.

[28] Bowens C, Dobie KH, Devin CJ, Corey JM. An approach to neuraxial anaesthesia for the severely scoliotic spine. Br J Anaesth November 2013;111(5):807–11. https://doi.org/10.1093/bja/aet161.

[29] Pritzlaff SG, Kreis PG, Fishman SM. Tunneled trial of spinal cord stimulation. In: Kreis PG, Pritzlaff SG, Copenhaver DJ, Fishman SM, editors. Spinal cord stimulation [internet]. 2nd ed. Oxford University Press; 2023. 92–C8P51. https://doi.org/10.1093/med/9780190095086.003.0008 Available from: https://academic.oup.com/book/46587/chapter/409015566.

[30] Smith GL, Petersen EA, Paul C, Goree JH. Transgrade dorsal root ganglion stimulation as a salvage technique for three different anatomical barriers: a case series. Neuromodul J Int Neuromodul Soc. June 2021;24(4):763–8. https://doi.org/10.1111/ner.13276.

Chapter 8

Sacral spine anatomy

Amit Sharma[1], John-Allen Smith[2] and Scott Pritzlaff[3]

[1]UPMC Pain Management, Department of Anesthesiology and Perioperative Medicine, University of Pittsburgh, Pittsburgh, PA, United States; [2]University of California, Davis, School of Medicine, Sacramento, CA, United States; [3]Division of Pain Medicine, Department of Anesthesiology and Pain Medicine, University of California, Davis, Sacramento, CA, United States

Introduction

The sacrum plays a key role in spinal stability and neural function. As a fused structure of five vertebrae, it connects the spine to the pelvis and helps support the body's weight during standing and walking. Its wide shape and strong bony architecture reflect adaptations for upright posture and load bearing [1].

Embryologically, the sacrum develops through both primary and secondary neurulation. Variations or disruptions in development can lead to congenital abnormalities such as sacral agenesis. The sacral vertebrae progressively fuse as individuals grow, typically completing in early adulthood. This process is influenced by weight-bearing forces [1].

Anatomical features such as the sacral foramina, sacral canal, and sacroiliac joints are essential landmarks for interventions. Understanding these structures and normal variations is critical for procedures like sacral neuromodulation, where precise lead placement can affect outcomes. Advancements in imaging—particularly fluoroscopy and CT—have improved the safety and accuracy of sacral procedures, allowing better visualization of bony and neural anatomy.

Suggested specialty training for appropriate intervention

Clinicians performing sacral interventions should have a background in interventional pain management, radiology, orthopedic spine, neurosurgery, or urology for bladder-related procedures. Hands-on cadaveric lab experience is essential for developing proficiency in sacral access and electrode placement. Fluoroscopy-guided techniques are critical for accurate needle and lead positioning, enhancing procedural safety, and improving clinical outcomes.

Key points

- The sacrum serves as a **structural and neurological bridge** between the spine and pelvis. It is formed **by five fused vertebrae with key landmarks like the sacral promontory, foramina, and hiatus**, which are crucial for interventions such as neuromodulation and caudal injections.
- Embryologic development and common variants, such as **lumbosacral transitional vertebrae and sexual dimorphism**, can significantly affect clinical presentation, procedural anatomy, and pain syndromes (e.g., Bertolotti syndrome, SIJ dysfunction).
- Sacral neuroanatomy is complex and clinically relevant, with DRG positions varying from **intraforaminal (S1–S2) to intracanalar (S3–S5), informing safe and effective targeting** during sacral neuromodulation procedures.
- The **sacral venous plexus and lateral sacral arteries pose important procedural risks** due to their proximity to common target sites, especially at S3 and S4. This highlights the need for precise, image-guided interventions to avoid bleeding complications.
- The sacroiliac joints, pelvic musculature, and ligamentous structures play central roles in **load transfer, shock absorption, and pain generation.** Disruptions in SIJ biomechanics are implicated in a significant portion of chronic low back pain cases.

A Modern Atlas for Implantable Devices of the Spine, Brain, and Nerve. https://doi.org/10.1016/B978-0-443-36528-7.00056-X

- Fluoroscopy-guided access techniques, including **midline, paramedian, and Taylor's approaches, and caudal epidural entry via the sacral hiatus,** require a detailed understanding of anatomical variability to minimize complications and maximize therapeutic efficacy.

Anatomy system scope

The following sections will explore the bony and neurovascular anatomy of the lumbosacral spine, including pertinent anatomic variations. Relevant musculoskeletal biomechanics, nerve, muscle, and ligamentous functions will be reviewed to understand better pain pathologies related to these structures. A summary of epidural and caudal procedural anatomy will follow before focusing on imaging modalities, procedure-related considerations, and landmark assignments for neuromodulation in the sacral spine.

Bony anatomy of the sacral spine

The sacrum is usually formed from five fused vertebral segments, a process that begins during embryonic development and continues throughout young adulthood [2]. The sacrum is broad at the L5-S1 spinal level, with wing-like lateral projections at S1 called **sacral ala**, which meet the ilium of the pelvis to form the **sacroiliac joints (SIJs)** [2]. As the sacrum descends, it tilts posteriorly and tapers to a point at the inferior border of S5, where it articulates with the coccyx. The sacrum has a kyphotic curve, like the thoracic spine, which increases intracavitary volume to accommodate the pelvic structures [2].

The sacrum has an inverted triangle shape, with the superior aspect at L5-S1 known as the **sacral base** and the inferior-most point called the **sacral apex** [2]. Along the anterosuperior rim of the S1 vertebra is the sacral promontory, a dense ring-like projection of bone that demarks the superior boundary of the pelvis [3,4].

Since the sacral vertebrae are fused, the sacral foramina are true foramina and are easily visualized with standard radiographs. The sacral hiatus is a caudally oriented, ovoid-shaped opening formed by the incomplete fusion of lamina and spinous processes in the sacral spine [5]. The exact number of unfused spinal segments varies between patients, determining the sacral apex's location and its overall diameter [6]. The sacral hiatus is flanked inferolaterally and bilaterally by sacral cornu, bony prominences derived from the inferior articular processes of S5 that serve as important surface anatomy landmarks during caudal anesthetic blocks [5]. The sacral hiatus is an important caudal access point for SCS lead placement (Fig. 8.1).

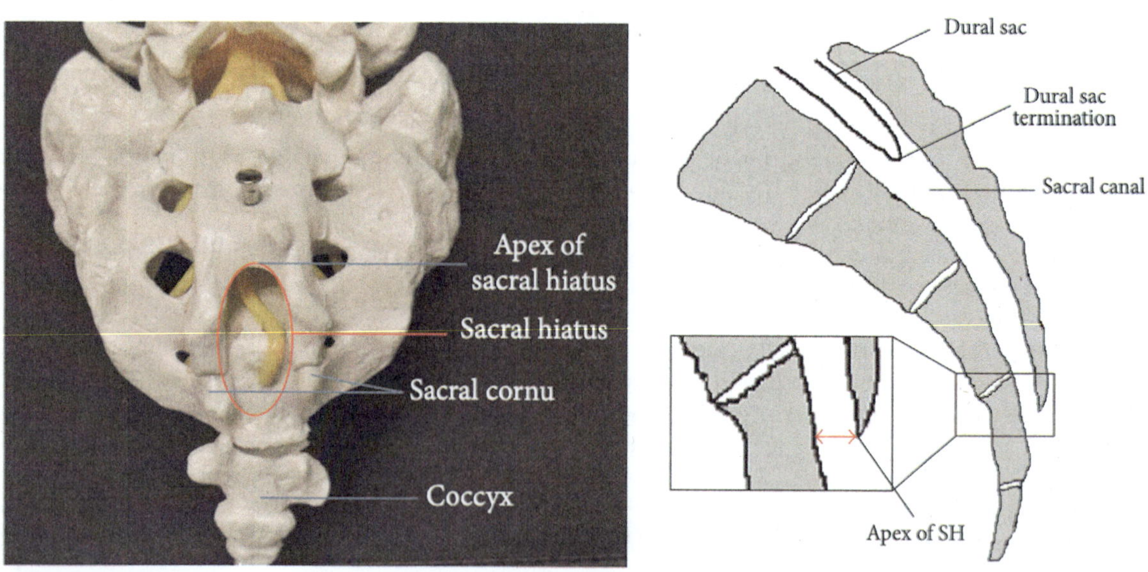

FIGURE 8.1 Left: Posterior view of sacrum; Right: Sagittal view of sacrum. *SH*, sacral hiatus. *Reproduced from Ref. [5], BioMed Research International, CC BY 4.0.*

Clinically relevant anatomic variation in the sacral spine

Lumbosacral transitional vertebrae

While having a sacrum composed of five vertebrae is most common, anatomic variants with differing numbers of vertebrae are found in an estimated 12.3% (4%–35%) of patients [7]. These variants, termed lumbosacral transitional vertebrae (LSTV), can occur in unilateral or bilateral fashion, arising during embryonic development when the process of vertebral differentiation is altered. LSTV may alter the biomechanics of intervertebral discs and facet joints, predisposing patients to lumbosacral pain pathophysiology, termed Bertolotti syndrome [8].

Sacralization of L5 (7.5%): the transverse processes of L5 broaden and fuse along with the S1–S5 vertebrae to form a six-vertebrae sacrum. The intervertebral disc space is sacralized, and the first pair of sacral foramina contain the nerve roots of L5 [7] (Fig. 8.2).

Lumbarization of S1 (5.5%): the S1 vertebra does not fuse with S2–S5 to form the sacrum, instead maintaining a more lumbar-like appearance, including transverse processes, an S1–S2 intervertebral disc space, and non-sacralized neural (false) foramina. Therefore, the first pair of sacralized foramina contain the S2 nerve root, and the sacrum is comprised of only four vertebral segments [7] (Fig. 8.3).

Sexual dimorphism of the sacrum

Sex-linked differences in the morphology of the sacrum are clinically relevant in understanding normal variations of anatomy and considering possible etiologies of pain (i.e., SIJ dysfunction, deformity). Compared to the male sacrum, the female sacrum tends to be wider, shorter, and broader, increasing the diameter of the pelvic outlet. These differences

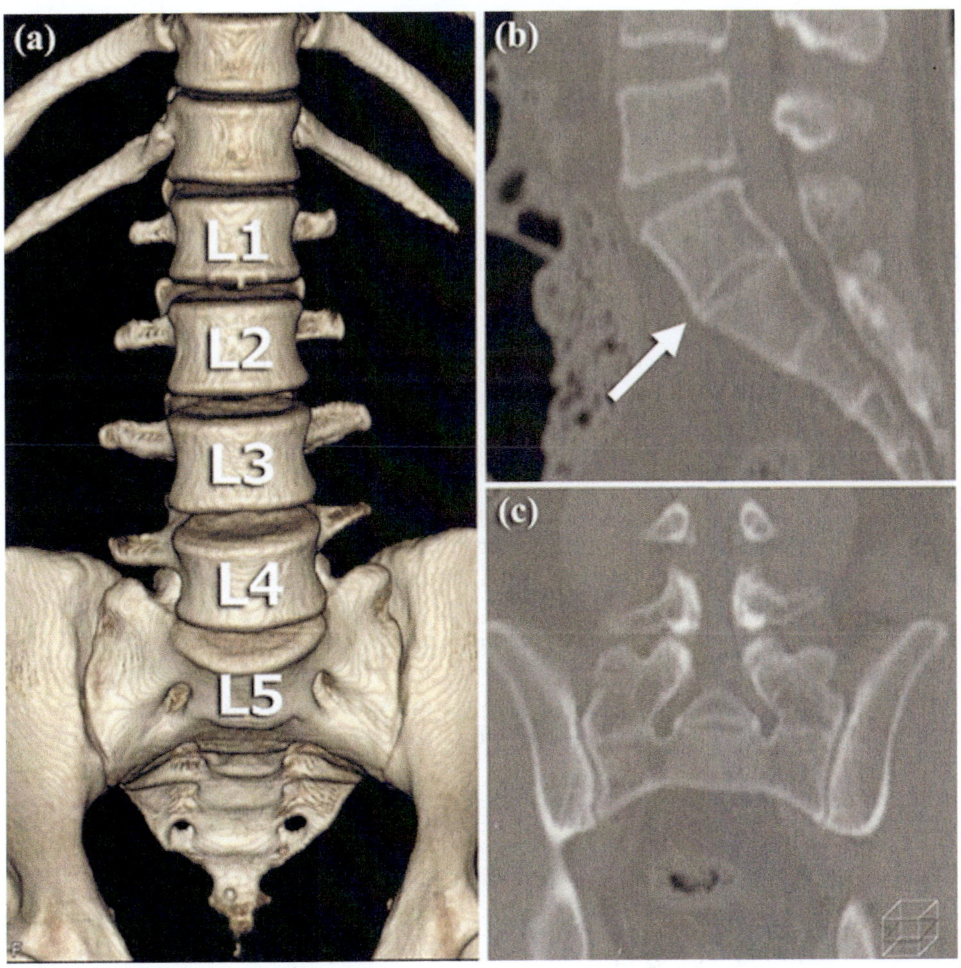

FIGURE 8.2 Sacralization of L5. **a.** VR image of the lumbar vertebrae and sacrum showing anomalous fusion of the transverse processes of L5 with the sacrum. **b.** Sagittal MPR image of sacralized L5 vertebral body. There is no disk between L5 and S1 (*white arrow*). **c.** Coronal MPR image of L5. Anomalous fusion of the transverse processes of L5 with the sacrum. *Reproduced from Ref. [7], Insights into Imaging (CC BY 4.0).*

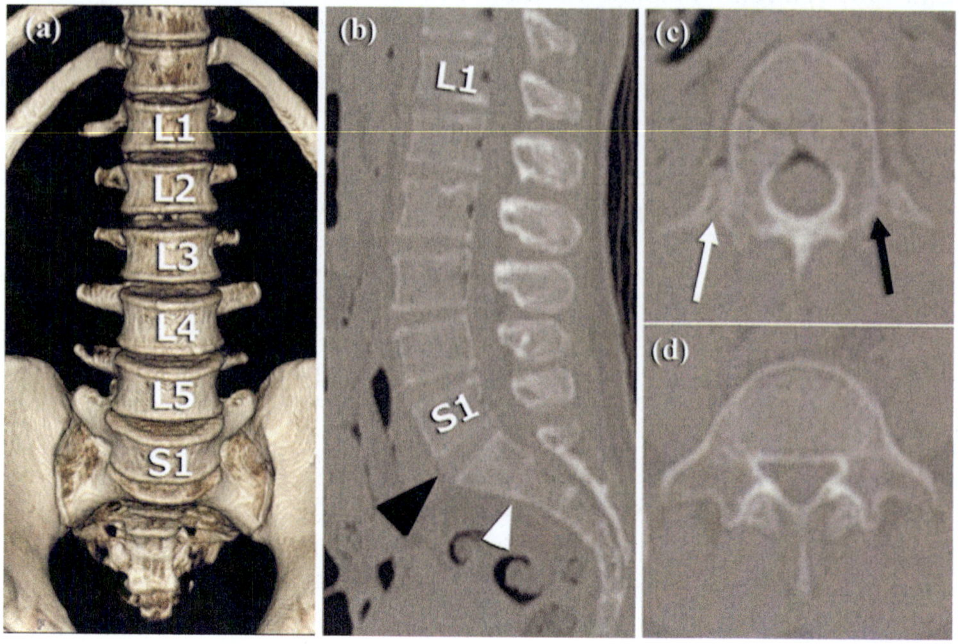

FIGURE 8.3 Lumbarization of S1. **a.** VR image of the anterior aspect of the lumbar vertebrae showing lumbarization of S1. **b.** Sagittal MPR image of the lumbar vertebrae showing a lumbar-type disk at S1–S2 (black arrowhead) and a sacrum-type disk at S2–S3 (white arrowhead). **c.** Axial MPR image of L1 vertebra showing an articulated lumbar rib on the right side (white arrow) and a non-articulated transverse process on the left side (black arrow). **d.** Axial MPR image of S1 with transverse processes, resembling L5. *Reproduced from Ref. [7], Insights into Imaging (CC BY 4.0).*

contribute to pelvic adequacy for pregnancy but consequently also affect the dynamics of the female sacroiliac joints; female SIJs tend to have greater mobility and encounter larger shearing stresses, predisposing women to greater ligamentous strain compared to male SIJs [9].

Neuroanatomy of the sacral spine

Though the spinal cord terminates at the L2 spinal level, tracts descending below this level continue as the **cauda equina**, extending into the sacral spine through the central (sacral) canal. Dura mater ensheathes the cauda equina through the S2 spinal level. The pia mater continues as the **filum terminale (coccygeal ligament)**, anchoring the spinal cord caudally to the dorsum of the first coccygeal segment. The S1–S4 nerve roots exit the central canal laterally through bilateral **sacral foramina**, while the S5 nerve root, coccygeal nerve roots, and filum terminale exit inferomedially through the **sacral hiatus** [10].

Lumbosacral nerve plexus

The **lumbosacral nerve plexus** is a complex network of nerve roots spanning the T12-S4 spinal levels that provides innervation of the lower extremities, pelvic organs, and anogenital region. Anatomic variations in this region are common, and pain-related pathophysiology often results from disturbance of normal anatomy (i.e., endometriosis, neoplastic lesions) [11].

The **lumbar plexus** is found integrated within or posterior to the *psoas muscle* and is formed from the union of T12-L4 nerve roots bilaterally [10] (Table 8.1).

The **lumbosacral trunk** is formed by the peroneal contribution of the L4 nerve root and the ventral rami of L5, which descend over the sacral ala and coalesce with the ventral rami of S1–S4 to form the **sacral plexus**, overlying the anterior aspect of the *piriformis muscle* bilaterally [10] (Table 8.2).

The **pudendal nerve** plays a central role in bladder and bowel control, and neuromodulation targeting the S3 nerve root is an effective treatment for bowel and bladder dysfunction [12,13].

Coccygeal nerve plexus

The S5 nerve root and coccygeal nerve exit through the sacral hiatus, where contributions of S3–S4 join to form the **coccygeal nerve plexus (CNP)**, which lays within the *coccygeus muscle*. The CNP provides innervation to the pelvic

TABLE 8.1 Nerves originating from the lumbar plexus [10].

Nerve *and Branches*	Roots	Structures supplied	Sensory functions
Nerves exiting the psoas muscle laterally:			
Iliohypogastric n.	L1	Internal oblique transverse abdominus	Gluteal, labia majora
Ilioinguinal n.	L1		Inner thigh/groin, scrotum, labia majora
Genitofemoral n.	L1-L2	Cremaster muscle (males)	Anterior thigh, scrotum, labia majora
Femoral n. *- saphenous n.*	L2-L4	Hip flexors, quadriceps	Anterolateral thigh, medial knee/leg
Lateral femoral cutaneous n.	L2-L3	–	Lateral thigh
Nerves exiting the psoas muscle medially:			
Obturator n.	L2-L4	Thigh adductors, obturator externus	Medial thigh
Lumbosacral trunk	L4-S4		

TABLE 8.2 Nerves originating from the sacral plexus [10].

Nerve	Roots	Structures supplied	Sensory functions
Sciatic n. *- tibial n.* *- common peroneal n.*	L4-S3	Hamstrings, gastrocnemius, soleus, plantar- and dorsi-flexors	Posterior thigh, anterior and lateral leg, plantar and dorsal foot
Pudendal n.	S2–S4	Voluntary bowel and bladder control (external sphincters), pelvic floor muscles	External genitals, anus, perineum
Superior gluteal n.	L4-S1	Hip abductors (gluteus medius, minimus), tensor fascia lata	–
Inferior gluteal n.	L5-S2	Gluteus maximus	

floor muscles (i.e., levator ani, coccygeus), contributes to anal tone and regulation of bowel movements, and provides for superficial sensation over the tailbone [14].

Coccydynia is a clinical condition of pain over the "tailbone", usually worse when seated. It may be caused by trauma (i.e., GLF), unfused coccygeal vertebrae, hypermobile joints, and other etiologies affecting typical anatomy adjacent to the coccygeal nerve plexus [14].

Dorsal root ganglia of the sacral spine

The DRG of the sacrum are responsible for the sensory transduction of the pelvis and lower extremities and are clinically important targets for the treatment of chronic neuropathic pain, including complex regional pain syndromes type I and II [15].

At the S1 and S2 spinal levels, DRGs are intraforaminal in about half of studied patients. By comparison, all S3–S4 spinal levels are intracanalar (within the sacral canal) [16]. The S5 DRG are also intracanalar at the sacral hiatus. The S3 foramen is the most common site of lead implantation for DRG-SCS, usually located 15–25 mm lateral to the S3 spinous process, 0–25 mm caudal to the SI joint line, and angled approximately 60 degrees relative to the skin [17,18].

The sacroiliac joints

The SIJs are the largest axial joints in the human body yet possess no transarticular musculature to coordinate movement. Instead, SIJs are gliding-type joints braced indirectly by muscles joining the trunk and pelvis to the lower extremities and by a network of ligaments that hold the SIJs under tension [9]. This configuration allows the SIJs to resist shearing loads while acting as shock absorbers for the spine. Compressive loads and bending moments from the trunk exert a downward force on the sacrum, while the normal force exerts an upward compressive load through the lower extremities onto the pelvis that varies with bipedal motion. These forces are balanced across the SIJs through subtle micromotions occurring within the SIJs, stabilizing the pelvis and spine. When the mobility of SIJs is compromised (i.e., hypermobility, ankylosing spondylitis), these biomechanical stresses may coordinate abnormally onto adjacent structures, with studies suggesting that as many as 15%–30% of cases of chronic LBP may originate from underlying SIJ pathology [9].

Muscular structures

The sacrum serves a crucial biomechanical role in several motions of the hip. Anterior to the sacrum lie the posterior pelvic musculature; some iliacus fibers originate from the lateral wing of the sacrum and join the descending psoas to form the **iliopsoas complex**. The iliopsoas attaches to the lesser trochanter of the femur and works as a primary hip flexor and secondary external rotator of the hip. The **piriformis muscle** originates from the anterolateral border of the sacrum, travels through the greater sciatic notch, and attaches to the greater trochanter of the femur, contributing to lateral rotation of the hip [9]. Parts of the **gluteus maximus** originate on the posterior sacrum; they insert onto the gluteal tubercles bilaterally, acting as primary lateral rotators and extensors of the hip [19].

Ligamentous structures

Intrinsic (capsular) ligaments bracing the SIJs include the interosseous (axial) ligaments, and the anterior and short/long posterior sacroiliac ligaments [9,20]. **Extrinsic (accessory) ligaments** include the sacrotuberous, sacroiliac, and iliolumbar ligaments [20].

The **sacrotuberous ligament (STL)** arises broadly from S2 through the second coccygeal segment, travels inferolaterally, and attaches to the ischial tuberosity [9,20]. The STL plays a limited role in SIJ stability but is commonly implicated in **pelvic girdle pain** [21]. The anterior and posterior **sacroiliac ligaments** (SIL) are broad fibrous bands that overly the SIJs, contributing to joint stability. The **sacrospinous ligament** originates at the caudal sacrum and first coccygeal segment, crosses the STL posterolaterally, and attaches to the ischial spine. The intersection of these ligaments forms the **greater and lesser sciatic foramina**, where **pudendal nerve entrapment** can occur [9]. Finally, the **iliolumbar ligament** arises from the transverse process of L5 and attaches to the iliac crest posteriorly [9] (Fig. 8.4).

The spine's anterior and posterior longitudinal ligaments taper at the sacrum and are contiguous with the **anterior and deep posterior sacrococcygeal ligaments,** which attach to the coccyx. The ligamentum flavum attaches to the sacrum and, due to ossification of intervening segments of the sacral spine, is noncontiguous with its sacral counterpart, the **superficial sacrococcygeal ligament,** which originates at the sacral hiatus and attaches to the coccyx [22].

Procedural anatomy: Spinal and caudal epidural access

Spinal epidural anatomy

The contents of the epidural space include the dural sac, spinal nerves, blood vessels, lymphatics, connective tissue, and cerebrospinal fluid. The epidural space is bounded anteriorly by the posterior longitudinal ligament (PLL), laterally by the pedicles and intervertebral foramina, and posteriorly by the ligamentum flavum (LF), a structure densely packed with elastin (Fig. 8.5). Thus, as a Tuohy needle advances anteriorly and encounters the LF, a **loss of resistance technique** can indicate entry into the epidural space. However, during embryonic development, the LF grows from lateral to medial and fuses at the midline, a process that is commonly incomplete in patients at varying spinal levels. Thus, with a **midline technique**, an advancing needle may not encounter the expected resistance, and dural puncture risk is therefore higher. The needle passes through skin, fat, subcutaneous tissue, the supraspinous and interspinous ligaments, and finally, the ligamentum flavum into the epidural space [23].

A **paramedian technique** may also be performed, angling the needle mediocranially, using a walk-off technique to guide the needle beneath the lamina until the ligamentum flavum is pierced and the epidural space entered. With the paramedian approach, the supraspinous and interspinous ligaments are not encountered [23].

Lastly, **Taylor's approach** can be used at the L5-S1 spinal level, with a needle placed 1 × 1 cm caudomedial to the posterior superior iliac spine (PSIS) and angled mediocranially, walking off the sacrum until the ligamentum flavum is pierced. Like the paramedian approach, the supraspinous and interspinous ligaments are not encountered. Both paramedian and Taylor's approach methods reduce the risk of dural puncture compared to the midline technique [23].

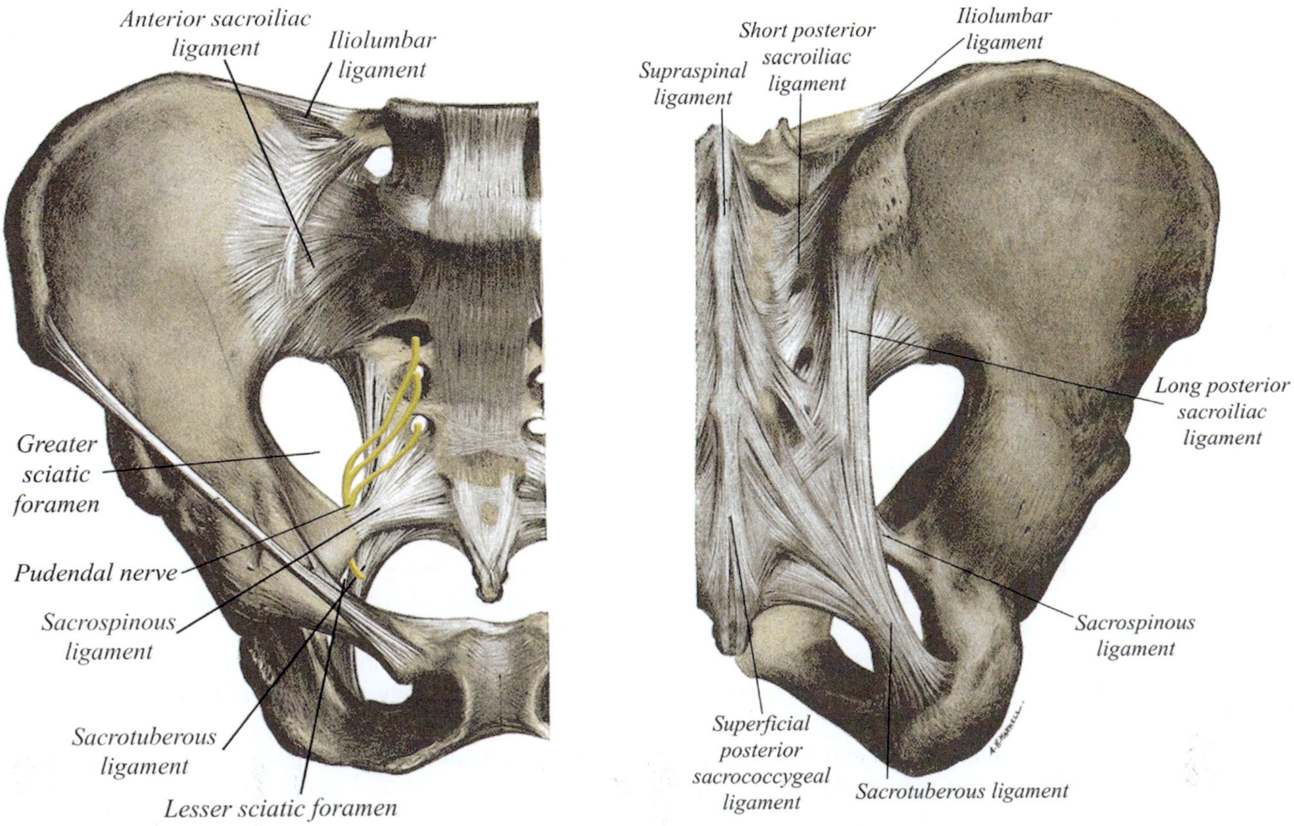

FIGURE 8.4 Ligamentous anatomy of the hip. Left, anterior view. Right, posterior view. *Adapted from Gray's Anatomy (20th ed., 1918), Plates 319 and 320. Public domain.*

Caudal block anatomy

Procedural anatomy: Caudal interventions are performed by accessing the sacral hiatus, which is bounded inferolaterally by the sacral cornu and superiorly by the sacral apex. The needle tract passes through skin, subcutaneous fat, the sacrococcygeal ligaments, then into the CSF space at the sacral hiatus. When the sacral apex is located above the S4 spinal level, there is an increased risk of dural puncture; when it is located at the S5 spinal level, it is more technically challenging to perform by blind technique, given the shorter window through the sacrococcygeal ligament [5].

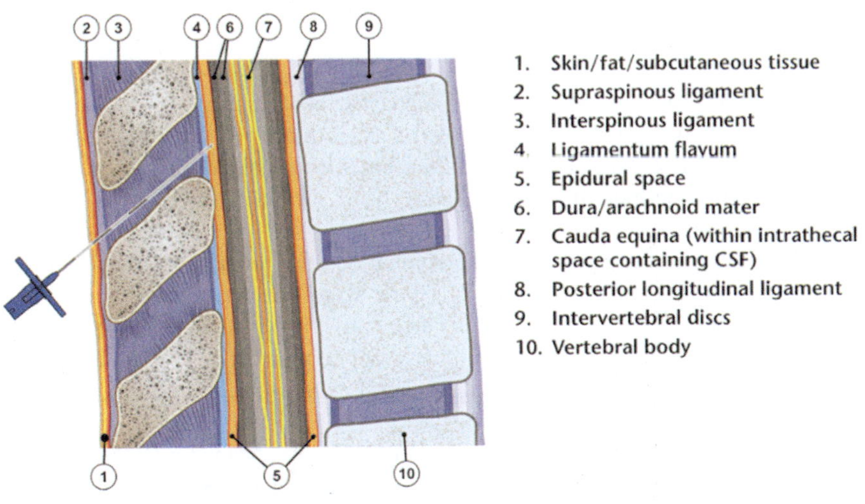

FIGURE 8.5 Spinal epidural anatomy. *Reproduced from Ref. [23] (© 2022 Elsevier Inc.; used with permission).*

Surface anatomy: When palpable bilaterally, the sacral cornu are landmarks for performing a caudal anesthetic block with blind technique. However, the sacral cornu are impalpable in a significant fraction of patients [5].

Appropriate imaging modalities

Patients following the typical referral pathway for SCS placement will have typically failed multiple conservative therapies, and >70% present after at least one prior laminectomy or fusion of the lumbar spine [24]. With extensive histories, >60% of patients in the United States present with at least one MRI performed within a year of referral for SCS [25]. Understanding the role of various imaging modalities in the evaluation, planning, and post-implantation care for patients referred for sacral neuromodulation (SNM) is therefore nuanced and requires careful consideration (Table 8.3). In most cases, it is important to obtain updated radiographs and advanced imaging prior to SNM implantation when existing studies have not been performed within the last 12 months [26].

X-ray

X-ray imaging plays an important role in all phases of care for SNM patients. Prior to SNM implantation, it is important to obtain baseline radiographs to evaluate bony anatomy and surgical hardware and to identify transitional morphology if not already known [26]. The information obtained from these studies guides the types and extent of advanced imaging to follow as part of preprocedural planning. For instance, when transitional morphology is present, it may be necessary to order full-spine advanced imaging to ensure correct identification of spinal levels prior to SNM implantation to avoid wrong-level implantation [26,27].

Immediately post-implantation, AP and lateral X-rays are recommended to determine lead positioning and to provide for future comparison in cases where lead migration may be suspected. Initial early follow-up visits may benefit from additional radiographs to assess for early lead migration, even when no loss of efficacy is reported, as this provides documentation for programming maps and may indicate a need for programming adjustments to maintain efficacy. In longer term follow-up, plain film radiographs are the first-line modality for assessing loss of efficacy and paresthesia shift, which may suggest lead migration or fracture [26].

Magnetic resonance imaging (MRI)

Non-contrast MRI remains the gold standard for preoperative planning prior to SNM implantation. It gives excellent soft tissue detail, important for assessing central canal adequacy, visualizing neurologic structures such as the spinal cord and nerve roots, evaluating interlaminar windows, and for patients with altered coagulation assesses vascular anatomy for entry-site planning to reduce the risk of epidural hematoma [26,28].

MRI is not part of routine post-implantation surveillance, but it may be indicated when patients report new neurologic deficits or when tumor or infection is suspected. Physical exam alone is not usually sufficient to reliably distinguish between superficial and deep infections, so when clinical concern for infection exists, it is imperative to obtain MRI studies to rule out epidural abscess. In all of these cases, obtaining both contrast and non-contrast studies is recommended [26].

Computed tomography (CT) scans

CT scans are a reasonable alternative to MRI when MRI is contraindicated. MRI may be contraindicated when a patient has an implanted device not known to be MRI-compatible (i.e., older/unknown cardiac implants, orthopedic devices, some intracranial and cochlear implants, etc.), when MRI may cause interaction between multiple implanted devices (even if each are independently MRI-compatible), or when metallic foreign bodies (retained bullet fragments, shrapnel) are present [29,30].

In these cases, selecting the appropriate CT study is guided by the specific clinical question or purpose for which the study is being ordered. For preoperative planning, a non-contrast CT (NCCT) gives excellent detail of bony anatomy including target foramina, ossified ligaments, osteophytes, and central canal narrowing. However, when central canal stenosis may be present, NCCT does not visualize the degree of thecal sac or nerve root compression. In these cases, CT myelograms should be considered to assess central canal adequacy and visualize neural elements prior to SCS placement [28].

IV-contrast CT scans are rarely utilized in SCS management but have a role in identifying enhancing lesions such as tumors, and for distinguishing epidural abscesses (enhancing) from hematomas (non-enhancing) when MRI cannot be

TABLE 8.3 Summary of imaging selection [24,26,28–33,35,36].

Study	Indications	Structures visualized	Downsides/Notes
XR (AP and lateral)	• First-line for initial workup • First-line for post-implantation monitoring	Osseous structures Hardware	• Minimal radiation exposure
Non-contrast MRI	• First-line for initial workup • Evaluates vasculature for those with altered coagulation • Evaluates epidural hematoma when infection not suspected	Soft tissues: Neurovascular structures and central canal adequacy	• May be contraindicated in patients with older implanted devices or retained metallic foreign bodies
Contrast MRI	• New neurologic deficits • Rules out epidural abscess when clinical concern for infection is present • Tumors	Enhancing lesions (tumors, abscesses)	• Gadolinium contrast exposure • May be contraindicated in patients with older implanted devices or retained metallic foreign bodies • Should be obtained with non-contrast MRI as well
Non-contrast CT	• Preoperative evaluation when MRI contraindicated • First-line for evaluation of lead fracture when XR equivocal • Evaluates epidural hematoma when abscess not suspected and MRI is contraindicated	Bony structures	• All CT scans expose patients to radiation
CT myelogram	• Assesses central canal adequacy and neural structures prior to implantation when MRI is contraindicated	Neural structures	• Invasive, requires LP • Iodinated contrast exposure • Strictly contraindicated if patient has space-occupying intracranial lesion
IV-contrast enhanced CT	• Identifies tumors, and • Differentiates epidural abscess from hematoma when MRI is contraindicated	Enhancing lesions (tumors, abscesses)	• Iodinated contrast exposure
Fluoroscopy	• Fundamental imaging modality for SNM implantation • Immediately post-operatively may be used when dural puncture or lead misplacement are suspected	Bony anatomy, instruments, needles, leads	• Typical radiation exposure = 100–300 chest X-rays • Risk is reduced by limiting live fluoroscopy exposure

safely performed [31,32]. When epidural abscess is not suspected and MRI cannot be performed, NCCT is an appropriate alternative for assessing epidural hematomas [31].

Lastly, NCCT is the first-line advanced imaging modality for detailed hardware evaluation when lead fracture is suspected but plain film radiographs are equivocal [33].

Fluoroscopy

Fluoroscopy is the primary imaging modality utilized during SNM implantation and revision. Using a continuous or pulsed X-ray beam, fluoroscopy visualizes bony anatomy, instruments and injected contrast in real-time to guide needle advancement, confirm entry into the epidural space, and track lead advancement, positioning, and laterality using AP, lateral and oblique views [26,34]. The average SCS trial exposes patients to ~133 seconds of radiation (equivalent to 100–300 chest X-rays), so disclosing this exposure to patients is an important element of informed consent [35]. Additionally, ALARA (as low as reasonably achievable) principles have been recommended to minimize radiation exposure [36].

ALARA principles for fluoroscopic imaging [36]

1. Minimize Time
   a. Use pulsed instead of continuous fluoroscopy
   b. Use low-dose setting on C-arm
   c. Use "last image hold"
2. Maximize Distance
   a. Use leaded booms, positioning devices, and extended controls
   b. Maximize patient distance from X-ray tube when possible
3. Utilize Shielding
   a. Use lead aprons, thyroid shields, and leaded glasses
   b. Install ceiling-suspended and table-skirting shields
   c. Collimate the beam

Though fluoroscopy is not routinely used in follow-up, when intraoperative complications such as dural puncture or misplacement are suspected, immediate post-operative fluoroscopy may be performed to evaluate for such complications [26,34].

Procedure-related considerations

Sacral neuromodulation (SNM) applications

Chronic refractory pelvic pain syndromes (i.e., pudendal neuralgia, coccydynia, sacral radiculopathy, perineal pain) are the most common indications for neuromodulation in the sacral spine. In patients with CRPS type 1 or causalgia in the lower limbs, the 2017 ACCURATE trial compared L5/S1 DRG stimulation to traditional SCS for patients with these conditions, finding a higher treatment success rate (74% vs. 53%) at 12 months in the DRG cohort compared to traditional SCS [37]. Overactive bladder, urinary retention, sexual dysfunction, and fecal incontinence have also been successfully treated with SNM therapies [11–13,38–40].

Sacral access points for neuromodulation

Parasympathetic outflow from the sacral spine is carried predominately by the S3 sacral roots, with S2 and S4 providing additional parasympathetic fibers [41,42]. The S3 sacral roots supply the perineum, pelvic floor, anal region, and coccyx with minor contributions from S4, while the S2 sacral root provides greater supply to the lateral buttocks and groin [42].

Though the S3 foramen is the ideal target for most cases of focal pelvic and coccygeal pain, if there is inadequate response to trial therapy, it may be reasonable to trial up and/or down a level prior to converting to a dorsal SCS modalities [40]. At the S2 foramen patients sometimes report undesirable lower extremity muscle recruitment, while the S4 foramen sometimes produces weaker response, despite more specific localization to the coccygeal and perineal regions [12,40,43].

For treatment of CRPS type 1 and causalgia, the L5 and S1 dermatomes map quite well to typical pain patterns, covering the dorsal and plantar foot, posterior thigh and leg [37,44]. The S1 DRG is commonly targeted when pain is isolated to the foot, with L5 DRG being additionally targeted when pain extends more proximally into the leg [37,44].

When sacral DRG stimulation is not technically feasible due to unfavorable foraminal anatomy, surgical hardware, or dense scarring/fibrosis due to prior interventions, neuromodulation access may also be achieved via an epidural approach at the sacral hiatus [45–47]. This should also be considered for patients whose pain remains refractory to DRG stimulation therapy and may be preferred when pain complaints are more diffuse (i.e., coccygeal pain with gluteal spread) [44,48].

Dorsal column stimulation via this approach has the benefit of covering multiple spinal levels, potentially providing broader dermatomal coverage [49].

Challenges of lead placement and migration

Sacral foramina are highly variable in morphology, and contralateral asymmetry is commonly seen within patients. Foraminal AP diameters average 2–6 mm and decrease in size from S1–S4, and foraminal angles vary as much as 20–30 degrees between individuals. S3 and S4 are also more susceptible to closure with age due to degenerative sclerosis and osteophyte formation [50,51].

Additionally, sacral foramina are obliquely oriented, and the posterior sacral foramina are narrower than their anterior counterparts, making visualization in the AP plane a practical challenge. Various techniques have been described to overcome this challenge: the "tunnel view" utilizes a 20–30 degrees ipsilateral oblique view with the C-arm, but this risks placing the Tuohy needle directly in the path of the DRG; utilizing cephalad tilt has been proposed as an alternate means of foraminal visualization that may reduce this risk [24].

Sacral foramina tend to angle anteromedially toward the pelvic cavity, with S3 having the most favorable AP trajectory for less difficult sheath passage. By comparison, S2 foramina tend to be more craniolaterally oriented. S4 foramina tend to be steep and anteriorly directed, making access more technically challenging and increasing the risk of lead kinking and poor anchoring [40,50].

The S1 foramina by comparison are quite large and more easily cannulated. However, DRG are intraforaminal in approximately one-half of studied patients at the S1 and S2 spinal levels and are highly sensitive to both mechanical and chemical stimulation, so it is especially important to avoid instrumentation within the foramina at these levels [16,51].

The lead trajectory should be carefully planned utilizing a paramedian or medialized approach, avoiding sharp bends at the fascia and foramen, and tunneling deep to Scarpa's fascia. A tension-free strain-relief "S-loop" should be incorporated between the anchor and tunnel to the pocket. Primary fixation should be achieved via deep fascial anchoring, with secondary fixation with measured slack at the pocket using a pocket tie-down or integrated anchor to secure the lead proximal to the implantable pulse generator (IPG) [24,52]. These considerations reduce risk of lead fracture, and anchor placement is critical for reducing risk of lead migration into the epidural space [53].

Landmark assignments for interventional procedures

Surface landmarks for needle and lead placement for the sacrum

The key surface landmarks for sacral needle and lead placement include:

Posterior Superior Iliac Spines (PSIS)—The PSIS appear as distinctive surface depressions bilaterally in the lower lumbar region of many patients. These anatomical markers serve as reference points for proceduralists seeking to identify sacral levels. An imaginary line can be drawn between the bilateral PSIS, which typically intersects the S2 vertebral level. This reliable anatomical relationship provides interventionalists with a valuable external landmark that facilitates accurate needle placement and improves procedural precision when targeting sacral structures [54].

Sacral Hiatus—This is a significant anatomical opening located at the inferior end of the sacrum between the sacral cornua. It results from the failure of the fusion of the lamina and the spinous process of the lower sacral vertebrae. The average diameter of the sacral canal is 6.0 ± 1.9 mm. This landmark is significant for caudal epidural injections as it provides access to the sacral canal [6].

Sacral Cornua—Bony prominences can be palpated on either side of the sacral hiatus. The cornua can be felt through the skin, providing tactile guides for locating the sacral hiatus. Proper identification of the cornua significantly improves the accuracy of needle placement, especially in caudal approaches to the epidural space [5].

To visualize proper landmarks via fluoroscopy, start by confirming the level on AP view. Count down from the 12th rib to ensure the correct vertebral bodies. Once the correct level is identified, tilt the fluoroscope 35 degrees cephalad. This maneuver compensates for the lumbosacral junction and convex sacrum, allowing optimal visualization of the sacral promontory and dorsal S1 foramen [24]. The needle target is the dorsal S1 foramen, located just inferior to the S1 pedicle. A slight ipsilateral oblique tilt can help better visualize the dorsal S1 foramen. The needle should be aimed at the superolateral aspect of the foramen as the nerve runs inferolateral. After the needle is in trajectory view, aiming at the dorsal S1 foramen on AP view, a lateral image, also known as the safety view, is used to determine the depth of the needle tip relative to the sacral canal. An accurate lateral view has the iliopectineal line as a single straight line, which can be optimized using wag on the C-arm (Fig. 8.6).

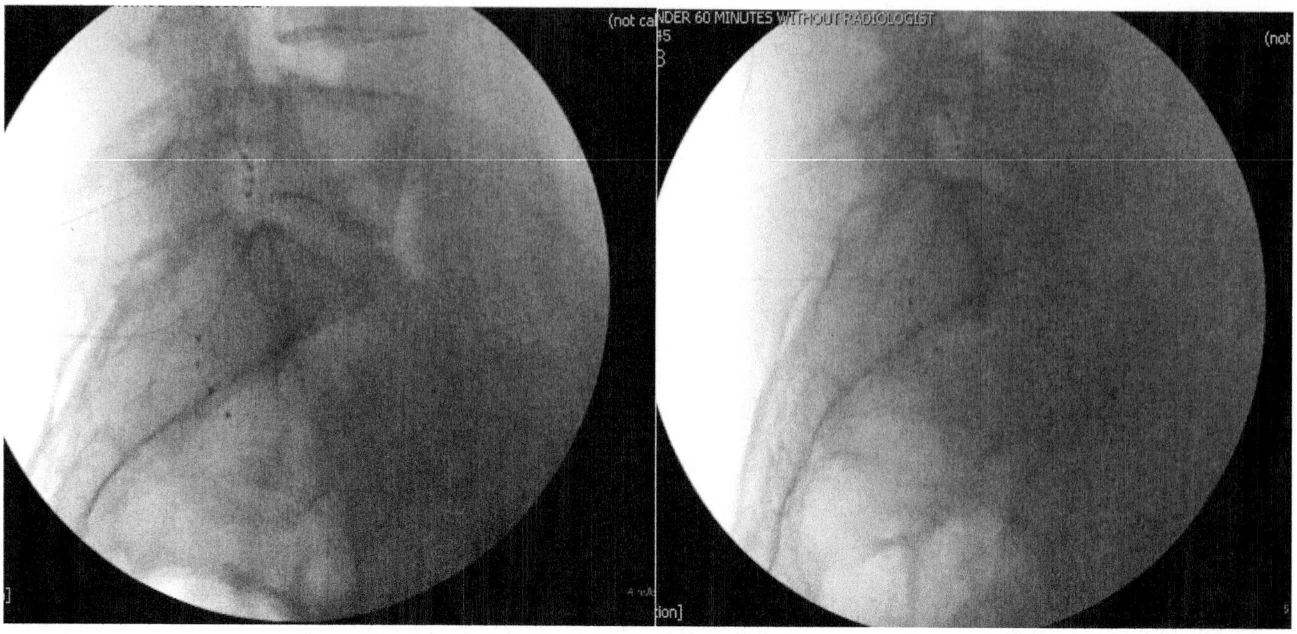

FIGURE 8.6 Lateral views of L5 and S1 DRG lead placement. The image on the left shows poor alignment of the iliopectineal line whereas this has been corrected on the right, indicating a true lateral image of the sacrum. *Images: Scott Pritzlaff MD.*

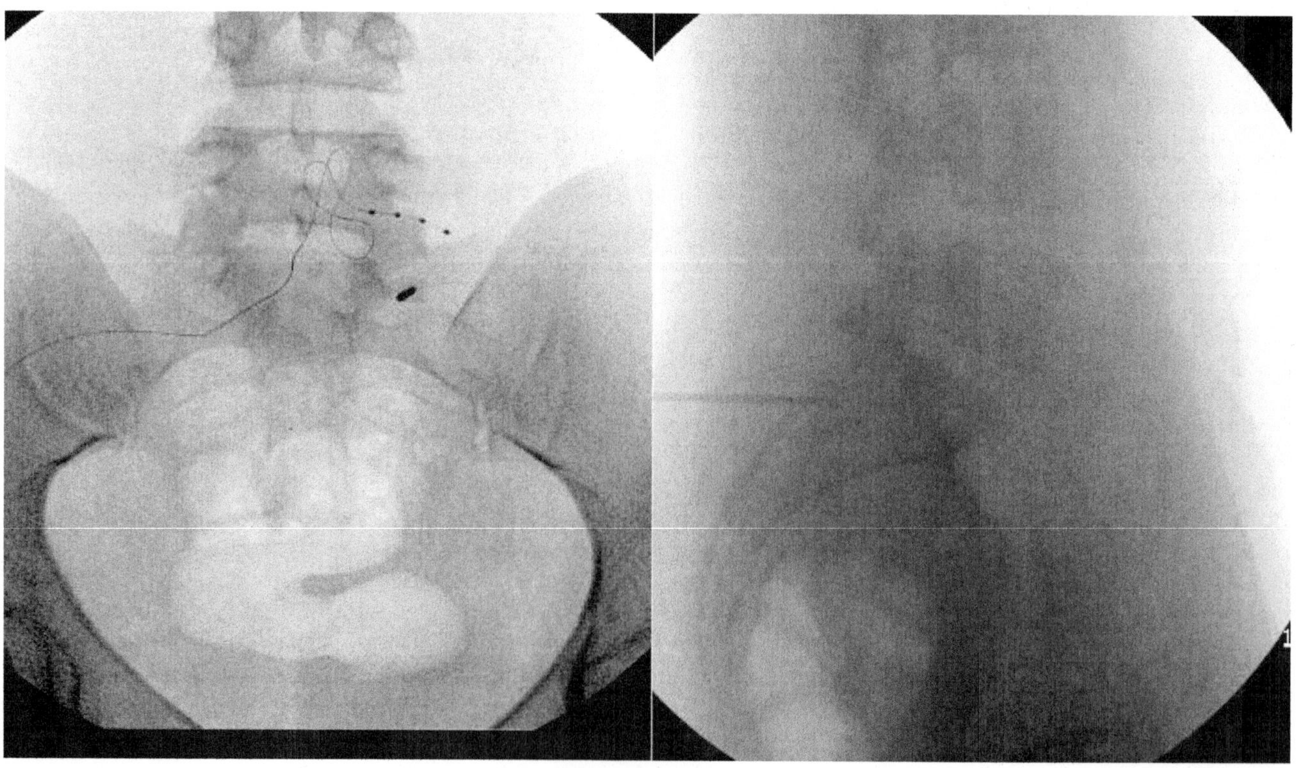

FIGURE 8.7 AP (left) and lateral (right) fluoroscopic images showing the right S1 neuroforamen and the needle trajectory for DRG lead placement. *Images: Scott Pritzlaff MD.*

Pearls and pitfalls

Procedural considerations for localization

For DRG implantation, a transforaminal approach described above is used to advance a 14-gauge Tuohy needle until it touches down on bone just superolateral to the opening of the right S1 foramen. The Tuohy needle is then walked medially until the S1 foramen is accessed. The Tuohy needle is advanced to the posterior portion of the sacral canal in the lateral view (Fig. 8.7). At this point, the lead is placed into the introducer and passed into Tuohy. The ideal final position of the lead is within the foramen along the ventral aspect of the sacrum. At least three out of the four electrodes usually remain in the foramen. Distinct from thoracic and lumbar DRGs, sacral DRGs demonstrate a progressive anatomical transition from an intraforaminal position to an intracanalar location with caudal progression from S1 to S4, with 100% of S3 and S4 DRGs were located in the intracanalar region [55]. This represents a significant topographical variation that must be considered during procedural planning.

The placement of dorsal root ganglion (DRG) stimulation leads, particularly for sacral DRG procedures, requires optimal lead positioning. Several intraoperative neuromonitoring modalities offer complementary information, each contributing to the procedure's success, including electromyography (EMG), somatosensory evoked potentials (SSEPS), and motor evoked potentials (MEPS). These provide essential real-time feedback that ensures proper lead positioning and helps prevent neural injury, especially in patients that are asleep under general anesthesia. A lead placement in an awake patient with only local anesthesia allows for clear confirmation of appropriate lead placement by asking the patient for feedback. If light or moderate sedation is used, it is important to be aware that the anesthetic agents used can affect the intraoperative recordings such as SSEPS and MEPS. EMG is highly sensitive in detecting neural contact, though it can occasionally produce false positives from muscle stimulation. Currently, there is insufficient data to determine the use of intraoperative neuromonitoring influences the overall success rate or safety of DRG implantation [56].

References

[1] Cheng JS, Song JK. Anatomy of the sacrum. Neurosurg Focus August 15, 2003;15(2):E3. https://doi.org/10.3171/foc.2003.15.2.3.

[2] Clinical anatomy of the spine, spinal cord, and ans. https://doi.org/10.1016/c2009-0-42801-0; 2014.

[3] Florian-Rodriguez ME, Hamner JJ, Corton MM. First sacral nerve and anterior longitudinal ligament anatomy: clinical applications during sacrocolpopexy. Am J Obstet Gynecol November 2017;217(5):607.e1–4. https://doi.org/10.1016/j.ajog.2017.07.008.

[4] Giraudet G, Protat A, Cosson M. The anatomy of the sacral promontory: how to avoid complications of the sacrocolpopexy procedure. Am J Obstet Gynecol April 2018;218(4):457.e1–3. https://doi.org/10.1016/j.ajog.2017.12.236.

[5] Kao SC, Lin CS. Caudal epidural block: an updated review of anatomy and techniques. BioMed Res Int 2017;2017:9217145. https://doi.org/10.1155/2017/9217145.

[6] Sekiguchi M, Yabuki S, Satoh K, Kikuchi S. An anatomic study of the sacral hiatus: a basis for successful caudal epidural block. Clin J Pain 2004;20(1):51–4. https://doi.org/10.1097/00002508-200401000-00010.

[7] Nastoulis E, Karakasi MV, Pavlidis P, Thomaidis V, Fiska A. Anatomy and clinical significance of sacral variations: a systematic review. Folia Morphol 2019;78(4):651–67. https://doi.org/10.5603/FM.a2019.0040.

[8] McGrath K, Schmidt E, Rabah N, Abubakr M, Steinmetz M. Clinical assessment and management of Bertolotti Syndrome: a review of the literature. Spine J August 2021;21(8):1286–96. https://doi.org/10.1016/j.spinee.2021.02.023.

[9] Kiapour A, Joukar A, Elgafy H, Erbulut DU, Agarwal AK, Goel VK. Biomechanics of the sacroiliac joint: anatomy, function, biomechanics, sexual dimorphism, and causes of pain. Int J Spine Surg February 2020;14(Suppl. 1):3–13. https://doi.org/10.14444/6077.

[10] Gasparotti R, Shah L. Brachial and lumbosacral plexus and peripheral nerves. In: Hodler J, Kubik-Huch RA, von Schulthess GK, editors. Diseases of the brain, head and neck, spine 2020–2023: diagnostic imaging [internet]. Cham (CH). Springer; 2020 [cited 2026 Mar 30]. (IDKD Springer Series). Available from: http://www.ncbi.nlm.nih.gov/books/NBK554335/.

[11] Zhang X, Li M, Guan J, Wang H, Li S, Guo Y, et al. Evaluation of the sacral nerve plexus in pelvic endometriosis by three-dimensional MR neurography. J Magn Reson Imag April 2017;45(4):1225–31. https://doi.org/10.1002/jmri.25435.

[12] Katuwal B, Bhullar J. Current position of sacral neuromodulation in treatment of fecal incontinence. Clin Colon Rectal Surg January 2021;34(1):22–7. https://doi.org/10.1055/s-0040-1714247.

[13] Bartley J, Gilleran J, Peters K. Neuromodulation for overactive bladder. Nat Rev Urol September 2013;10(9):513–21. https://doi.org/10.1038/nrurol.2013.143.

[14] Woon JTK, Stringer MD. Redefining the coccygeal plexus. Clin Anat March 2014;27(2):254–60. https://doi.org/10.1002/ca.22242.

[15] Rowe J, Deer TR, Mehta P, Pope JE, Patterson DG, Baksh J, et al. Sacral dorsal root ganglion spinal stimulation. In: Deer TR, Pope JE, Lamer TJ, Provenzano D, editors. Deer's treatment of pain [internet]. Cham: Springer International Publishing; 2019. p. 599–605. https://doi.org/10.1007/978-3-030-12281-2_73. Available from: http://link.springer.com/10.1007/978-3-030-12281-2_73.

[16] Ebraheim NA, Lu J. Morphometric evaluation of the sacral dorsal root ganglia. A cadaveric study. Surg Radiol Anat 1998;20(2):105–8.

[17] Matzel KE, Chartier-Kastler E, Knowles CH, Lehur PA, Muñoz-Duyos A, Ratto C, et al. Sacral neuromodulation: standardized electrode placement technique. Neuromodulation December 2017;20(8):816–24. https://doi.org/10.1111/ner.12695.

[18] McCullough MC, Decker S, Ford J, Downes K, Hilbelink D, Ordorica R, et al. Third sacral foramina morphometry for sacral neuromodulation. Female Pelvic Med Reconstr Surg 2013;19(1):23–30. https://doi.org/10.1097/SPV.0b013e31827bfdb1.

[19] Barker PJ, Hapuarachchi KS, Ross JA, Sambaiew E, Ranger TA, Briggs CA. Anatomy and biomechanics of gluteus maximus and the thoracolumbar fascia at the sacroiliac joint. Clin Anat March 2014;27(2):234–40. https://doi.org/10.1002/ca.22233.

[20] Poilliot AJ, Zwirner J, Doyle T, Hammer N. A systematic review of the normal sacroiliac joint anatomy and adjacent tissues for pain physicians. Pain Physician July 2019;22(4):E247–74.

[21] Aldabe D, Hammer N, Flack NAMS, Woodley SJ. A systematic review of the morphology and function of the sacrotuberous ligament. Clin Anat April 2019;32(3):396–407. https://doi.org/10.1002/ca.23328.

[22] Woon JTK, Stringer MD. Clinical anatomy of the coccyx: a systematic review. Clin Anat March 2012;25(2):158–67. https://doi.org/10.1002/ca.21216.

[23] Macpherson D, Quondamatteo F, Broom M. Update on applied epidural anatomy. BJA Educ May 2022;22(5):182–9. https://doi.org/10.1016/j.bjae.2021.12.006.

[24] Chapman KB, Sayed D, Lamer T, Hunter C, Weisbein J, Patel KV, et al. Best practices for dorsal root ganglion stimulation for chronic pain: guidelines from the American society of pain and neuroscience. J Pain Res 2023;16:839–79. https://doi.org/10.2147/JPR.S364370.

[25] Desai MJ, Hargens LM, Breitenfeldt MD, Doth AH, Ryan MP, Gunnarsson C, et al. The rate of magnetic resonance imaging in patients with spinal cord stimulation. Spine May 1, 2015;40(9):E531–7. https://doi.org/10.1097/BRS.0000000000000805.

[26] Hagedorn JM, Misercola B, Comer A, Tari-Blake J, Hoffmann CM, Mehta P, et al. The team approach to spinal cord and dorsal root ganglion stimulation: a guide for the advanced practice provider. Mayo Clin Proc Innov Qual Outcomes. June 2021;5(3):663–9. https://doi.org/10.1016/j.mayocpiqo.2021.05.002.

[27] Lian J, Levine N, Cho W. A review of lumbosacral transitional vertebrae and associated vertebral numeration. Eur Spine J May 2018;27(5):995–1004. https://doi.org/10.1007/s00586-018-5554-8.

[28] Expert Panel on Neurological Imaging, Hutchins TA, Peckham M, Shah LM, Parsons MS, Agarwal V, et al. ACR appropriateness criteria low back pain: 2021 update. J Am Coll Radiol November 2021;18(11S):S361–79. https://doi.org/10.1016/j.jacr.2021.08.002.

[29] Pedrosa I, Altman DA, Dillman JR, Hoff MN, McKinney AM, Reeder SB, et al. American college of radiology manual on MR safety: 2024 update and revisions. Radiology April 2025;315(1):e241405. https://doi.org/10.1148/radiol.241405.

[30] Russo RJ, Costa HS, Silva PD, Anderson JL, Arshad A, Biederman RWW, et al. Assessing the risks associated with MRI in patients with a pacemaker or defibrillator. N Engl J Med February 23, 2017;376(8):755–64. https://doi.org/10.1056/NEJMoa1603265.

[31] Tatagari V, Simons D. Spinal epidural hematoma following placement of a thoracic spinal cord stimulator. Interv Pain Med September 2022;1(3):100117. https://doi.org/10.1016/j.inpm.2022.100117.

[32] Katz JN. Lumbar disc disorders and low-back pain: socioeconomic factors and consequences. J Bone Joint Surg Am April 2006;88(Suppl. 2):21–4. https://doi.org/10.2106/JBJS.E.01273.

[33] Kim GU, Chang MC, Kim TU, Lee GW. Diagnostic modality in spine disease: a review. Asian Spine J December 2020;14(6):910–20. https://doi.org/10.31616/asj.2020.0593.

[34] Rekatsina M, Peng PWH. The importance of image guidance in common spine interventional procedures for pain management: a comprehensive narrative review. Pain Ther June 2025;14(3):841–63. https://doi.org/10.1007/s40122-025-00731-9.

[35] Deer TR, Mekhail N, Provenzano D, Pope J, Krames E, Leong M, et al. The appropriate use of neurostimulation of the spinal cord and peripheral nervous system for the treatment of chronic pain and ischemic diseases: the Neuromodulation Appropriateness Consensus Committee. Neuromodulation August 2014;17(6):515–50. https://doi.org/10.1111/ner.12208. ; discussion 550.

[36] Ali S, Hurdle MF, Ghazi SM, Gupta S. Boosting confidence: enhancing spinal cord stimulator needle and lead placement through simulation training. Cureus March 2024;16(3):e55550. https://doi.org/10.7759/cureus.55550.

[37] Deer TR, Levy RM, Kramer J, Poree L, Amirdelfan K, Grigsby E, et al. Dorsal root ganglion stimulation yielded higher treatment success rate for complex regional pain syndrome and causalgia at 3 and 12 months: a randomized comparative trial. Pain April 2017;158(4):669–81. https://doi.org/10.1097/j.pain.0000000000000814.

[38] Vogel K, Nakib N. Off-label but on-target: sacral neuromodulation for neurogenic bladder dysfunction. Curr Urol Rep June 23, 2025;26(1):52. https://doi.org/10.1007/s11934-025-01280-6.

[39] Alsannan B, Banakhar M, Hassouna M. Updates in pelvic neuromodulation: the role of pelvic neuromodulation in pelvic disorders. Front Urol 2024;4:1329305. https://doi.org/10.3389/fruro.2024.1329305.

[40] Brill SA, Margolin DA. Sacral nerve stimulation for the treatment of fecal incontinence. Clin Colon Rectal Surg February 2005;18(1):38–41. https://doi.org/10.1055/s-2005-864079.

[41] Goidescu OC, Dogaru IA, Enyedi M, Enciu O, Mutu DEG, Filipoiu FM. The pelvic and sacral splanchnic nerves - identification by dissection, trajectory. Maedica September 2022;17(3):571–5. https://doi.org/10.26574/maedica.2022.17.3.576.

[42] Aurore V, Röthlisberger R, Boemke N, Hlushchuk R, Bangerter H, Bergmann M, et al. Anatomy of the female pelvic nerves: a macroscopic study of the hypogastric plexus and their relations and variations. J Anat September 2020;237(3):487–94. https://doi.org/10.1111/joa.13206.

[43] Kohli N, Patterson D. InterStim therapy: a contemporary approach to overactive bladder. Rev Obstet Gynecol 2009;2(1):18–27.

[44] Huygen FJPM, Kallewaard JW, Nijhuis H, Liem L, Vesper J, Fahey ME, et al. Effectiveness and safety of dorsal root ganglion stimulation for the treatment of chronic pain: a pooled analysis. Neuromodulation February 2020;23(2):213–21. https://doi.org/10.1111/ner.13074.

[45] Lee DW, Lai A. Sacral burst neuromodulation via caudal approach as a treatment for chronic coccydynia. Neuromodulation December 2019;22 (8):992–4. https://doi.org/10.1111/ner.12808.

[46] Richter EO, Abramova MV, Aló KM. Percutaneous cephalocaudal implantation of epidural stimulation electrodes over sacral nerve roots–a technical note on the importance of the lateral approach. Neuromodulation January 2011;14(1):62–7. https://doi.org/10.1111/j.1525-1403.2010.00293.x. ; discussion 67.

[47] Mironer YE, Hodge PJ, Parrott JT, Lal S, LaTourette PC. A unique approach to neurostimulation in patients with previous two-segment spine surgery and obstruction of epidural access for spinal cord stimulation: a case series. Neuromodulation 2012;15(3):204–9. https://doi.org/10.1111/j.1525-1403.2011.00397.x. ; discussion 209.

[48] Caylor J, Reddy R, Yin S, Cui C, Huang M, Huang C, et al. Spinal cord stimulation in chronic pain: evidence and theory for mechanisms of action. Bioelectron Med June 28, 2019;5:12. https://doi.org/10.1186/s42234-019-0023-1.

[49] Surges G, Paulus J, Blaß T, Mendryscha K, Bettag M, Rotte A. Efficacy and safety of 10 kHz spinal cord stimulation using cervical and thoracic leads: a single-center retrospective experience. Pain Ther December 2021;10(2):1255–68. https://doi.org/10.1007/s40122-021-00287-4.

[50] Saluja S, Agarwal S, Tuli A, Raheja S, Tigga SR, Paul S. Morphometric analysis of the sacrum and its surgical implications. JCDR; 2018. https://doi.org/10.7860/jcdr/2018/33991.11661.

[51] Chapman KB, van Helmond N, Kallewaard JW, Vissers KC, Patel KV, Motivala S, et al. An anatomy-informed, novel technique for S1 dorsal root ganglion stimulation lead placement. Pain Med September 30, 2022;23(10):1750–6. https://doi.org/10.1093/pm/pnac062.

[52] Chapman KB, Spiegel MA, Dickerson DM, Billet B, Patel KV, Hunter C, et al. A paramedian approach for dorsal root ganglion stimulation placement developed to limit lead migration and fracture. Pain Pract November 2021;21(8):991–1000. https://doi.org/10.1111/papr.13063.

[53] Chapman KB, Mogilner AY, Yang AH, Yadav A, Patel KV, Lubenow T, et al. Lead migration and fracture rate in dorsal root ganglion stimulation using anchoring and non-anchoring techniques: a multicenter pooled data analysis. Pain Pract November 2021;21(8):859–70. https://doi.org/10.1111/papr.13052.

[54] Chakraverty R, Pynsent P, Isaacs K. Which spinal levels are identified by palpation of the iliac crests and the posterior superior iliac spines? J Anat February 2007;210(2):232–6. https://doi.org/10.1111/j.1469-7580.2006.00686.x.

[55] Esposito MF, Malayil R, Hanes M, Deer T. Unique characteristics of the dorsal root ganglion as a target for neuromodulation. Pain Med June 1, 2019;20(Suppl. 1):S23–30. https://doi.org/10.1093/pm/pnz012.

[56] Deer TR, Pope JE, Lamer TJ, Grider JS, Provenzano D, Lubenow TR, et al. The neuromodulation appropriateness consensus committee on best practices for dorsal root ganglion stimulation. Neuromodulation January 2019;22(1):1–35. https://doi.org/10.1111/ner.12845.

Section 3

Spinal cord stimulation

Introduction to section 3 spinal cord stimulation

By Peter Staats, MD, MBA, FIPP

I have long been captivated by the role of electricity in medicine—a force as fundamental to life as chemistry itself. Human physiology depends on electrical signals to drive essential functions, from nerve impulses to heartbeats. This understanding dates back to the late 18th century when Italian scientist Luigi Galvani observed a dissected frog's leg twitch when touched with a metal scalpel. He identified "animal electricity," recognizing that electrical impulses within nerves cause muscle contraction. His work laid the foundation for modern fields such as neuroscience, electrophysiology, and neuromodulation, inspiring therapies like spinal cord stimulation (SCS) and vagus nerve stimulation (VNS).

Benjamin Franklin was also an early pioneer in exploring electricity's effects on the human body. In the mid-18th century, Franklin conducted experiments using electricity to treat various ailments, including paralysis and pain. He applied electric currents to patients and documented cases where individuals reported temporary relief or improved function. Though rudimentary by modern standards, Franklin's work contributed to the growing scientific curiosity about bioelectricity, laying the groundwork for future therapeutic applications. Other notable early experimenters in electrical stimulation for pain treatment include Jean-Alban Bergonié (1857–1925), a French physician who studied the therapeutic effects of electrical stimulation in various medical conditions; Giovanni Aldini (1762–1834), Luigi Galvani's nephew, who expanded on his uncle's discoveries by applying electrical currents to human cadavers; Michael Faraday (1791–1867), whose contributions to electromagnetism influenced later medical applications; Duchenne de Boulogne (1806–1875), a French neurologist who pioneered localized electrical stimulation to diagnose and treat neuromuscular disorders; and Robert Bartholow (1831–1904), who conducted one of the earliest documented cases of direct electrical brain stimulation in a living human, demonstrating the link between electrical currents and neurological responses.

The development of practical electrical devices was essential for the advancement of neuromodulation. The Leyden jar, invented in 1746, could store charge and produce a spark of electricity, but continuous electrical current was not available until Alessandro Volta's invention of the electric pile in 1800, the forerunner of the modern battery. These innovations laid the groundwork for today's spinal cord stimulation.

These early explorations ultimately paved the way for modern neuromodulation therapies, which harness controlled electrical impulses to modulate nerve activity. The evolution from Franklin's crude electrical applications to modern spinal cord stimulation highlights the remarkable progress in utilizing bioelectricity to improve human health. Today, the role of electricity in treating cardiac arrhythmias with pacemakers, epilepsy with VNS, and incontinence with sacral nerve stimulators is unquestioned. Yet, despite numerous controlled clinical trials demonstrating its efficacy, spinal cord stimulation's role in pain management remains unfairly challenged. SCS emerged in the late 1960s when Norman Shealy implanted the first dorsal column stimulator, inspired by Melzack and Wall's gate control theory of pain. Since then, technological advances—ranging from fully implantable pulse generators to high-frequency, burst, and closed-loop stimulation—have expanded SCS's efficacy and applications. The therapy is now a standard of care for conditions such as failed back surgery syndrome (PSPS2), complex regional pain syndrome, and neuropathic pain.

My personal journey with SCS began as a fellow, revising an early two-contact electrode array. The profound experience of turning off pain signals with a percutaneous electrode placement fueled my lifelong fascination with neuromodulation. Over the years, advancements in electrode design, programming algorithms, novel waveforms, and closed-loop stimulation have led to personalized approaches, improving patient outcomes and broadening the scope of conditions treatable with SCS. The progress over the last 3–4 decades has been nothing short of astounding. We have moved from hoping to help half of our patients with half of their leg pain (the 50-50 club) to resolving more than 80% of total pain (back and leg) in 70% of patients.

Yet, the most exciting chapter lies ahead. The integration of artificial intelligence, machine learning, remote monitoring, and real-time feedback mechanisms promises to further optimize therapy delivery. Research into novel indications, such as ischemic pain and movement disorders, signals a future rich with possibilities.

As a physician dedicated to advancing neuromodulation, I believe the future of SCS depends on blending technological breakthroughs with patient-centered care. Incorporating advanced imaging, biometrics, and precision medicine will refine patient selection, streamline therapy titration, and maximize long-term outcomes. This textbook serves as both a comprehensive resource and a forward-looking guide, bridging the rich history of SCS with its emerging applications. The story of SCS is ultimately one of hope—hope for patients who have endured years of suffering and hope for a future where pain no longer controls lives.

Chapter 9

Cervical spinal cord stimulation

Jonathan M. Hagedorn[1], Boss Povieng[2], Benjamin Gill[3] and Daniel A. Jimenez[4]

[1]*Anesthesiology and Perioperative Medicine, Mayo Clinic, Rochester, MN, United States;* [2]*Department of Anesthesiology, Rush University Medical Center, Chicago, IL, United States;* [3]*Pain Medicine, Nevada Advanced Pain Specialists, Reno, NV, United States;* [4]*Physical Medicine and Rehabilitation, University of Michigan Health-Sparrow, Lansing, MI, United States*

Introduction

Cervical spinal cord stimulation (cSCS) has evolved significantly since its inception in the 1960s [1,2]. Similar to its application in other spinal regions, neuromodulation in the cervical spine may be used to modulate chronic and intractable pain associated with complex regional pain syndrome (CRPS) types I and II, persistent spinal pain syndrome pain (PSPS, formally failed back surgery syndrome (FBSS)), and neuropathic pain such as with diabetic neuropathy, trigeminal neuralgia, or migraines [3–5]. Approaches to cSCS include percutaneous cylindrical leads or surgically implanted paddle leads, and the use of paresthesia or sub-paresthesia waveforms [3]. Despite its promise, cSCS has often remained a last-resort therapy, typically considered only after more conservative treatments fail. However, ongoing research suggests an earlier role in the pain management continuum, highlighting the need for further trials to optimize patient outcomes and expand indications.

Key points

- **Mechanism of Action:** cSCS delivers electrical impulses to the dorsal aspects of the spinal cord, modulating pain signal transmission to the brain via interference with wide dynamic range (WDR) neurons and subsequently reducing the perception of chronic pain.
- **Clinical Indications**: cSCS is primarily used to treat chronic intractable pain conditions affecting the head, neck, shoulders, and upper extremities, including CRPS, neuropathic pain, and PSPS.
- **Historical Perspective**: The concept of spinal cord stimulation was introduced in the 1960s, evolving from the Gate Control Theory of pain proposed by Melzack and Wall, which suggested that electrical stimulation of the dorsal columns could inhibit pain signal transmission to the brain.
- **Advancements and Efficacy**: Modern innovations in cSCS include new stimulation patterns which may provide superior pain relief with reduced paresthesia. Studies have demonstrated significant improvements in pain reduction, functional outcomes, and patient quality of life with long-term therapy.

Anatomic considerations

Cervical spinal cord

The cervical spinal cord and the affiliated nerve root pairs C1–C8 are protected within the vertebral column spanning from C1 to the cephalad aspect of T1. cSCS applies electroceutical therapy to the dorsal column and dorsal horn as well as downstream targets such as the nucleus caudalis to confer relief for a variety of intractable pain conditions [6]. The volume of cord tissue is not ubiquitous through the cord length. Due to the dense afferent and efferent fibers necessary for complex innervation of the upper extremities there is an expansion of cord volume that exists between C5-T1 [7]. Furthermore, the shape of the cervical cord itself is not uniform with the mid-cervical cord being oblong in shape while the high cervical and cervico-thoracic segments are known to be round in shape [8]. An estimated normal anteroposterior diameter of the cervical spinal canal is between 17 and 18 mm with diameters of 13 mm or less suggestive of cervical canal stenosis [9]. Despite the

A Modern Atlas for Implantable Devices of the Spine, Brain, and Nerve. https://doi.org/10.1016/B978-0-443-36528-7.00001-7

cord being suspended in cerebrospinal fluid and protective meningeal tissue, the smaller dimensions of the dura and overlying epidural space merit further caution and precision with interventional therapies directed in the cervical spine.

Cervical epidural space

The cervical epidural space is triangular extending caudally from the foramen magnum to the lower margin of C7 [8]. The posterior epidural space contains blood vessels and epidural fat with which cSCS leads must traverse to arrive at their target location. Myodural bridges exist at the suboccipital segment that effectively collapse the posterior epidural space thereby limiting positioning of leads more cephalad or lateral at C1–C2. (10) Given cannulation of the cervical epidural space is inherently necessary for cSCS, an understanding of the subtle anatomic differences between cervical epidural space segments is critical to maximize safety during the procedural approach. For example, the anteroposterior depth of the posterior epidural space is reported to be 1.5–2 mm at C6 while increasing in depth to 2–3 mm at C7-T1 [11,12]. In the thoracic spine, the posterior epidural depth increases further to 2.5–3 mm at T6 [13]. Importantly, cervical posture will also influence posterior epidural space parameters with neck flexion favoring an increase in posterior epidural space depth to 3–4 mm at C7 [10,11,14]. With an understanding of the dynamic nature of the posterior epidural space volume and expected cervical cord expansion at C5-T1, epidural cannulation with patients positioned in cervical flexion will optimize a safe approach to implementing cSCS.

Procedure

Indications

cSCS on-label indications pertain to conditions that may relate to "chronic intractable pain" syndromes such as PSPS, CRPS in the cervical or high thoracic dermatomes, chronic cervical or high thoracic radicular pain syndrome, and associated pain in the setting of degenerative cervical or thoracic disc disease, arachnoiditis, epidural fibrosis, and other neuropathic conditions such as painful neuropathy and phantom limb pain [15–17]. There have also been cases of cSCS for treatment of chronic headaches, peripheral arterial disease, post-stroke facial pain, post-herpetic neuralgia, and refractory angina pectoris [5,18–22].

Patient selection considerations

An ideal cSCS candidate is an adult with at least 6 months of a focal intractable pain syndrome that imparts substantial functional debility and pain despite thorough conservative treatment and pathology not otherwise amenable to surgery. (See Table #1) (European Consensus Recommendations Table 2020) Candidates should also have a thorough review for identification of contraindications to this therapy or mitigation of complicating factors (Table 9.1).

TABLE 9.1 Proposed inclusion and exclusion patient selection criteria for spinal cord stimulation from the European Consensus Recommendations and E-Health Tool.

Inclusion criteria	Exclusion criteria

• Age ≥18 years
• Chronic pain with a duration of least 6 months
• One of the following primary indications:
  • Chronic low back/leg pain
  • Complex regional pain syndrome
  • Neuropathic pain syndrome
  • Ischemic pain syndrome
• Pain severity at least moderate (VAS ≥5) having a substantial impact on daily functioning and quality of life
• Insufficiently responding to appropriate trials of medication and/or minimally invasive treatments (such as local anesthetic nerve blocks) and/or experiencing intolerable side effects of these treatments
• No clear benefits of surgery expected
	• Unwilling to have an implant
	• Unable to manage the device
	• Absolute contra-indications for active treatment (e.g., unfit for undergoing SCS, pregnancy, spine infection, coagulation disorder)
	• Uncontrolled disruptive psychological or psychiatric disorder
	• Ongoing alcohol and drug misuse
	• Widespread pain

Absolute criteria for the consideration of SCS, selected by the expert panel.
Thomson S, Huygen F, Prangnell S et al. Appropriate referral and selection of patients with chronic pain for spinal cord stimulation: European consensus recommendations and e-health tool. *Eur J Pain*. 2020; 24(6):1169–1181. https://doi.org/10.1002/ejp.1562.

Training recommendations

Completion of an interventional pain fellowship recognized by the Accreditation Council for Graduate Medical Education is recommended for physicians in the United States seeking to utilize applied neuromodulation techniques. cSCS should be reserved for skilled interventionalists experienced with SCS targeting the thoracolumbar segments. Some facilities may require a proctor for initial cases. There are no current requirements at the society or industry level, but proposals and suggestions have been published in the literature [24].

Procedural technique

Patient positioning

Positioning should be carefully planned to ensure ease of percutaneous epidural access and necessary fluoroscopic views. The patient is placed in a prone position with elimination of cervical extension by using a patient positioning device, supportive foam, or folded blankets placed under the patient's chest. The patient's arms should be tucked at the sides, sometimes with retraction of the shoulders to facilitate unobstructed fluoroscopic lateral and contralateral oblique safety views.

Anesthesia considerations

Perioperative anesthesia strategies balance patient comfort and procedural safety. Some interventionalists use local anesthetic only for trials or mild intravenous sedation, while adding monitored anesthetic care for permanent implantation. Regardless, monitoring for neurological injury during cSCS is crucial, whether that is from patient feedback of paresthesia coverage, discomfort or motor activation, or via intraoperative neuromonitoring (IONM) [8]. If IONM is pursued, the concomitant administration of neuromuscular blocking agents may depress motor evoked potentials (MEPs) while volatile anesthetics may depress MEPs and somatosensory evoked potentials (SSEPs) [25].

Operating room time estimate

Operating room time estimate would typically be similar to that of thoracolumbar SCS trial and permanent procedures which one may anticipate a block time of at least 30 min for trials and an hour for permanent implants. Timing of these procedures will vary with the proceduralist. Additional allotted time is anticipated with neuromonitoring.

Relevant vendor support

The vendor representative should be physically present in the room when implementing cSCS therapies. Furthermore, vendor representatives may provide valuable expertise with periprocedural and postprocedural stimulation mapping. Interventionalists should be familiar with all the components of the cSCS trial or implantation kit.

Procedure

While cSCS may be accomplished with paddle electrode leads, which require open surgery for placement, the focus of this chapter will be on the use of percutaneous cylindrical electrodes.

First, the epidural introducer needle is positioned approximately one level caudad to the target interlaminar space at the ipsilateral pedicle for a paramedian trajectory. For permanent implantation of percutaneous cylindrical leads, the introducer needles may be placed within the midline or paravertebral vertical incisions. The selected level of lead entry for cSCS is often in the mid-to high-thoracic spine depending on patient anatomy. The needle tip may contact the lamina caudad to the target interlaminar space and incrementally advanced off the laminar surface to engage in the ligamentum flavum. Loss of resistance technique may be used with the assistance of either a fluoroscopic lateral or contralateral oblique to safely access the epidural space (Fig. 9.1A and B). Either the lead or guidewire is advanced and fluoroscopically confirmed to be within the dorsal aspect of the epidural space. The lead is then advanced to the target level of interest in anteroposterior fluoroscopic visualization (Fig. 9.2A and B). Under live fluoroscopy, the introducer needle are carefully retracted, ensuring the leads remain in their desired target position. The leads are then secured (either subcutaneously with an implant or to the skin with a trial). For a trial, the leads are connected to an external pulse generator. During implantation, a pocket for the implantable pulse generator (IPG) may be created in the preferred flank between the

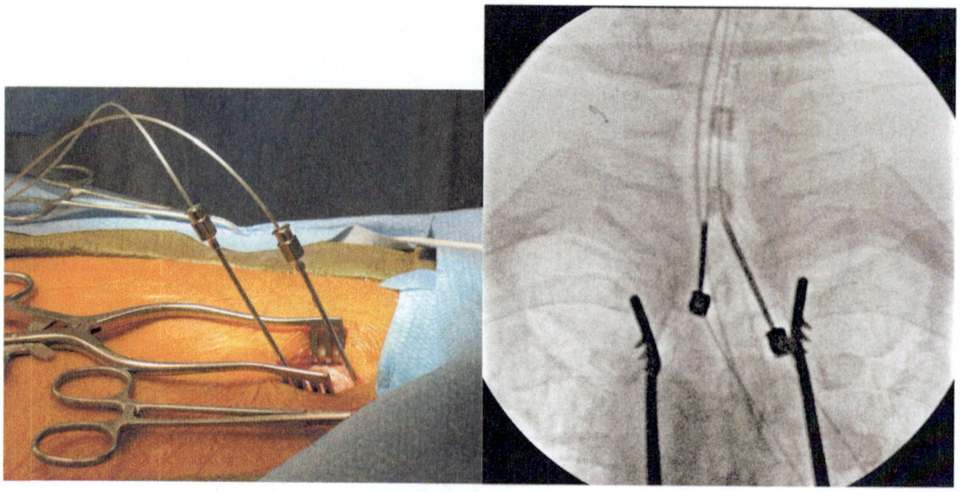

FIGURE 9.1 Cannulation of the epidural space in the cervical and high thoracic spine require a steep angulation of needle entry as depicted in Figure 9.1A. Fluoroscopic correlation is demonstrated in Figure 9.1B.

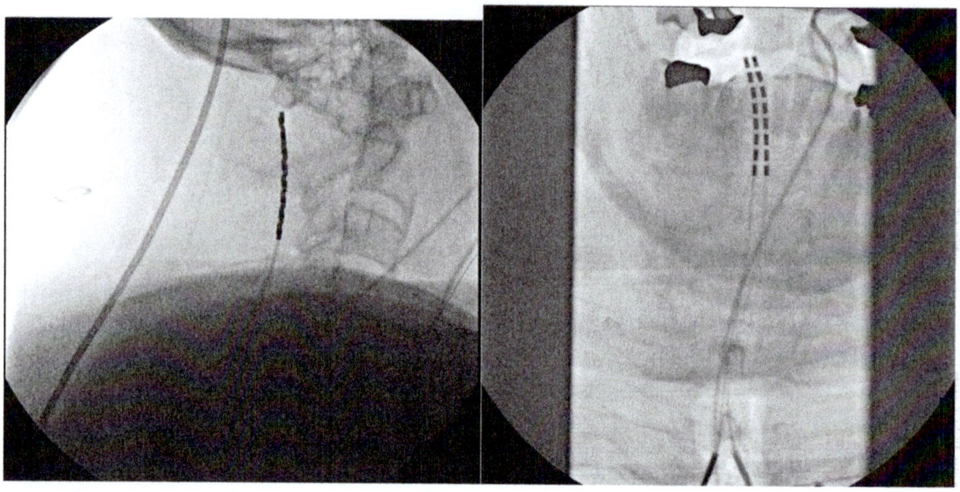

FIGURE 9.2 Appropriate placement of dual eight contact leads in the midline using lateral view to ensure dorsal positioning is depicted in Figure 9.2A as well as in anteroposterior view in Figure 9.2B.

12th rib and iliac crest. Using a tunneling tool of appropriate length, the leads are advanced from the anchor site to the pocket with a small loop for tension relief. After the leads are connected to the pulse generator and a device analysis for impedance is satisfactory, the remaining leads should be coiled in a circular fashion and placed under the IPG which is finally placed within the pocket (Fig. 9.3). The pocket and midline incision are thoroughly irrigated and closed in multilayer fashion. An overlying sterile dressing should be applied in the operating room. Table 9.2

Post-operative considerations

Pearls and Pitfalls

1. **Patient Selection** – Optimal candidates are patients who have chronic, refractory pain despite conservative management. Ideal patients should also undergo psychological screening in order to identify untreated mood disorders that may negatively impact outcomes [26,30–32].
2. **Preoperative Imaging** – MRI or CT imaging should be utilized in order to identify contraindications such as severe spinal stenosis, instability, or other structural pathology [26,30–32].

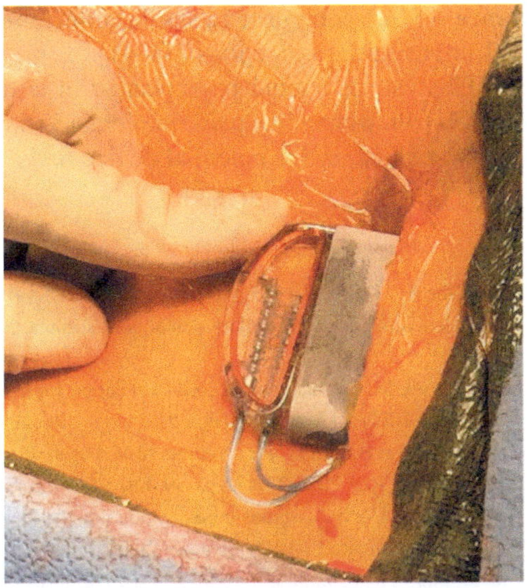

FIGURE 9.3 The internal pulse generator is placed in the flank pocket. The generator surface demarcated with intellectual property branding, should face ventrally and the leads should be coiled behind the back surface of the generator.

TABLE 9.2 Highlights of post-operative considerations in cSCS.

Postoperative considerations in cervical spinal cord stimulation	
Recovery	• Patients typically experience a short recovery period, with initial management focused on pain control and adjustment to device function. • Postoperative pain should be managed with short-term analgesics. Patients should be closely monitored for complications such as infection, hematoma, or cerebrospinal fluid leakage [26,27].
Bracing	• Routine bracing is not required postoperatively, but it may be recommended in select cases in order to minimize excessive cervical movement and reduce the risk of lead migration. • Prolonged immobilization should be avoided to prevent muscular atrophy and maintain cervical spine function. (30, 31)
Activity limitations	• Patients should avoid excessive cervical flexion, extension, and rotation for 4–6 weeks post-implantation. • Strenuous activities and heavy lifting should be limited to reduce lead migration risk, with gradual reintroduction of physical activity. • Patients should refrain from high-impact activities with repetitive cervical motion, as these may increase lead displacement risk [28,29].
Device Programming	• Programming adjustments (amplitude, frequency, pulse width) should be made in order to optimize pain relief while simultaneously minimizing undesired stimulation.
Monitoring and follow-up	• Routine follow-ups should occur at 2 weeks, 6 weeks, 3 months, and every 6–12 months thereafter. • Patients should be educated on monitoring for signs of postoperative infection (e.g., fever, worsening pain, drainage), which would require prompt evaluation.

3. **Lead Placement** – SCS lead placement should be guided fluoroscopically. Neuromonitoring may also be employed in order to prevent iatrogenic spinal cord injury [33–37].
4. **Lead Migration Prevention** –Leads should be securely anchored, and excessive cervical movement should be restricted for 6 weeks postoperatively.

5. **Infection Prevention and Surveillance** – Strict adherence to sterile surgical technique and appropriate perioperative antibiotic administration are essential in preventing infections [38–41].
6. **Indications for Device Removal** – SCS systems should be explanted in cases of deep-seated infections involving hardware or the epidural space. Persistent or worsening pain, intolerable dysesthesias, device malfunction, or loss of therapeutic efficacy may also warrant evaluation for potential device revision or removal [42–44].

References

[1] Melzack R, Wall PD. Pain mechanisms: A new theory. Science. 1965;150(699):971–9.

[2] Chivukula S, Tempel ZJ, Weiner GM, et al. Cervical and cervicomedullary spinal cord stimulation for chronic pain: Efficacy and outcomes. Clin Neurol Neurosurg 2014;127:33–41.

[3] Gupta M, Chitneni A, Ghorayeb J, Schnetzer B, Klusek M. Cervical spinal cord stimulation for trigeminal neuralgia: A narrative review. Curr Pain Headache Rep 2022;26(8):639–45. https://doi.org/10.1007/s11916-022-01066-2.

[4] Krog L, Maloney J, Pew S, Adeleye O, Johnson B, Glenn B, Gill B, Tieppo Francio V, Pagan-Rosado R, Whitney M, Sinha N, Strand N. Cervical spinal cord stimulation: A review. Curr Pain Headache Rep 2024;28(4):239–49. https://doi.org/10.1007/s11916-023-01200-8.

[5] Finnern MT, D'Souza RS, Jin MY, Abd-Elsayed AA. Cervical spinal cord stimulation for the treatment of headache disorders: A systematic review. Neuromodulation 2023;26(7):1309–18. https://doi.org/10.1016/j.neurom.2022.10.060.

[6] Lau JC. Nucleaus caudalis stimulation for facial pain. Neuromodulation 2022;25(6):S10. https://doi.org/10.1016/j.neurom.2022.04.018.

[7] Purves D, Augustine GJ, Fitzpatrick D, et al. The external anatomy of the spinal cord. In: Neuroscience. 2nd ed. Sinauer Associates; 2001. [Accessed 9 February 2025].

[8] Deer TR, Russo M, Grider JS, et al. The neurostimulation appropriateness consensus committee (NACC): Recommendations on best practices for cervical neurostimulation. Neuromodulation 2022;25(1):35–52. https://doi.org/10.1016/j.neurom.2021.10.013.

[9] Wolf BS, Khilnani M, Malis L. The sagittal diameter of the bony cervical spinal canal and its significance in cervical spondylosis. J Mt Sinai Hosp New York 1956;23(3):283–92. https://pubmed.ncbi.nlm.nih.gov/13320096/. [Accessed 13 March 2021].

[10] Enix DE, Scali F, Pontell ME. The cervical myodural bridge, a review of literature and clinical implications. J Can Chiropr Assoc June 2014;58 (2):184–92.

[11] Hogan Q. Distribution of solution in the epidural space: examination by cry- omicrotome section. Reg Anesth Pain Med 2002;27:150–6. https://doi.org/10.1053/rapm.2002.29748.

[12] Benzon HT, Huntoon MA, Rathmell JP. Improving the safety of epidural steroid injections. JAMA - J Am Med Associat. U S: Am Med Associat 2015;313(17):1713–4. https://doi.org/10.1001/jama.2015.2912.

[13] Macpherson D, Quondamatteo F, Broom M. Update on applied epidural anatomy. BJA Education 2022;22(5):182–9. https://doi.org/10.1016/j.bjae.2021.12.006.

[14] Figley CR, Stroman PW. Investigation of human cervical and upper thoracic spinal cord motion: implications for imaging spinal cord structure and function. Magn Reson Med 2007;58:185–9. https://doi.org/10.1002/mrm.21260.

[15] LCD - Spinal Cord Stimulators for Chronic Pain (L36204). Accessed March 31, 2025. https://www.cms.gov/medicare-coverage-database/view/lcd.aspx?LCDId=36204.

[16] https://www.ncbi.nlm.nih.gov/books/NBK11160/FDA Summary of Safety and Effectiveness Data (PMA P030017-S275). Accessed March 31, 2025. https://www.accessdata.fda.gov/cdrh_docs/pdf3/P030017S275B.pdf.

[17] Aiyer R, Barkin RL, Bhatia A, Gungor S. A systematic review on the treatment of phantom limb pain with spinal cord stimulation. Pain Manag 2017;7(1):59–69. https://doi.org/10.2217/pmt-2016-0041.

[18] Asimakidou E, Matis GK. Spinal cord stimulation in the treatment of peripheral vascular disease: a systematic review - revival of a promising therapeutic option? Br J Neurosurg 2022;36(5):555–63. https://doi.org/10.1080/02688697.2021.1884189.

[19] Tomycz ND, Deibert CP, Moossy JJ. Cervicomedullary junction spinal cord stimulation for head and facial pain. Headache 2011;51(3):418–25. https://doi.org/10.1111/j.1526-4610.2010.01829.x.

[20] Zhao L, Song T. Case report: short-term spinal cord stimulation and peripheral nerve stimulation for the treatment of trigeminal postherpetic neuralgia in elderly patients. Front Neurol 2021;12:713366. https://doi.org/10.3389/fneur.2021.713366.

[21] Kurklinsky S, Palmer SC, Arroliga MJ, Ghazi SM. Neuromodulation in postherpetic neuralgia: Case reports and review of the literature. Pain Med 2018;19(6):1237–44. https://doi.org/10.1093/pm/pnx175.

[22] Deer TR, Raso LJ. Spinal cord stimulation for refractory angina pectoris and peripheral vascular disease. Pain Physician 2006;9(4):347–52.

[23] Thomson S, Huygen F, Prangnell S, et al. Appropriate referral and selection of patients with chronic pain for spinal cord stimulation: European consensus recommendations and e-health tool. Eur J Pain 2020;24(6):1169–81. https://doi.org/10.1002/ejp.1562.

[24] Pritzlaff SG, Goree JH, Hagedorn JM, et al. Pain education and knowledge (peak) consensus guidelines for neuromodulation: a proposal for standardization in fellowship and training programs. J Pain Res 2023;16:3101–17. https://doi.org/10.2147/JPR.S424589.

[25] Rao S, Kurfess J, Treggiari MM. Basics of neuromonitoring and anesthetic considerations. Anesthesiol Clin 2021;39(1):195–209. https://doi.org/10.1016/j.anclin.2020.11.009.

[26] Deer TR, Krames ES, Mekhail N, et al. Comprehensive consensus statement on intrathecal drug delivery and spinal cord stimulation for the treatment of chronic pain and severe spasticity. Pain Med 2014;15(S1):S1–33.

[27] North RB, Cutchis PN, Goddard M, et al. Spinal cord stimulation for chronic, intractable pain: Experience over two decades. Neurosurgery 1993;32(3):384–95.

[28] Liem L, Russo M, Huygen F, et al. One-Year outcomes of spinal cord stimulation of the dorsal root ganglion in the treatment of chronic neuropathic pain. Neuromodulation 2015;18(1):41–8.

[29] Deer TR, Pope JE, Hayek SM, et al. Spinal cord stimulation for the treatment of chronic pain: Evolving indications and mechanism-based therapy. Pain Med 2019;20(Suppl. 1_1):S41–8.

[30] Kumar K, Hunter G, Demeria DD. Spinal cord stimulation in treatment of chronic benign pain: Challenges in treatment planning and present status, a 22-year experience. Pain Med 2006;7(Suppl. 1):S139–46.

[31] Martinson T, Pergolizzi Jr JV. Smoking, chronic pain, and opioid use: A complex triad in the context of spinal cord stimulation. Pain Pract 2016;16 (5):665–75.

[32] Turner JA, Loeser JD, Deyo RA, Sanders SB. Spinal cord stimulation for chronic pain: Systematic review and meta-analysis of randomized controlled trials. Pain 2004;108(1–2):137–47.

[33] Kapural L, Peterson E, Provenzano D. Spinal cord stimulation for chronic pain: Mechanisms of action and clinical effectiveness. Pain Med 2020;21(5):1030–42.

[34] Falowski S, Celii A, Sharan A. Spinal cord stimulation: Mechanisms of action, current technologies, and clinical effectiveness. Neurosurg Clin N Am 2014;25(4):631–45.

[35] Van Buyten JP, Al-Kaisy A, Smet I, Palmisani S, Smith T. High-frequency spinal cord stimulation: Efficacy and safety for chronic pain management. Pain Med 2013;14(4):552–60.

[36] Anderson WS, Pilitsis JG. Surgical considerations in spinal cord stimulator placement: Complication avoidance and risk management. Neurosurgery 2022;89(3):E98–103.

[37] Lamer TJ, Deer TR, Pope JE. Spinal cord stimulation safety considerations: Hemorrhagic complications and mitigation strategies. Clin J Pain 2019;35(3):208–14.

[38] Hayek SM, Veizi E, Hanes M. Treatment-limiting complications of percutaneous and surgical spinal cord stimulator leads: A review of available evidence. Pain Med 2015;16(11):2022–31.

[39] Eldabe S, Buchser E, Duarte RV. Spinal cord stimulation: A review of complications and management strategies. Pain Med 2016;17(2):325–36.

[40] Engle AM, Cameron T, Nagle J. Infection rates and risk factors following spinal cord stimulator implantation: A retrospective analysis. Pain Med 2019;20(5):1048–55.

[41] Cameron T. Safety and efficacy of spinal cord stimulation for the treatment of chronic pain: A 20-year literature review. J Neurosurg Spine 2004;100(3):254–67.

[42] Buvanendran A, Lubenow T. Predictors of success in spinal cord stimulation for chronic pain management: A clinical review. Pain Pract 2008;8 (1):54–65.

[43] Kumar K, Wilson JR, Taylor RS, Gupta S. Complications of spinal cord stimulation: Risk factors, prevention, and management. J Neurosurg Spine 2016;24(3):452–8.

[44] Deer TR, Lamer TJ, Pope JE, et al. The neurostimulation appropriateness consensus committee (NACC) recommendations for infection prevention and management. Neuromodulation 2017;20(1):31–50.

Chapter 10

Thoracic and lumbar spinal cord stimulation

Derron Keith Wilson[1], Kwasi K. Ampomah[2], Shashank Vodapally[3], Arti Ori[4] and Israel Riley Pena[5]

[1]Goodman Campbell Brain & Spine, Carmel, IN, United States; [2]USA Rehab Services, Atlanta, GA, United States; [3]Trinity Health Medical Group - Hauenstein Neurosciences, PM&R and Pain Management, Grand Rapids, MI, United States; [4]Mass General Brigham, Harvard Medical School, Boston, MA, United States; [5]JPS Leuda Pain Management Clinic, JPS Health Network, Fort Worth, Texas, United States

Introduction

Spinal cord stimulation (SCS) is a well-established neuromodulation technique designed to manage chronic, intractable pain [1,2]. By delivering low-voltage electrical impulses to the dorsal columns of the spinal cord, SCS modulates pain signal transmission and alters the patient's perception of pain.

Scope of procedure

Specific on-label indications encompass a wide spectrum of debilitating pain conditions, including failed back surgery syndrome (FBSS)—the most common indication in the United States [3–6]—refractory low back pain in patients unsuitable for corrective surgical intervention [7], radicular pain syndromes [8], post-laminectomy pain, degenerative disc disease (DDD) and herniated disc pain, complex regional pain syndrome (CRPS), reflex sympathetic dystrophy (RSD), peripheral causalgia, arachnoiditis, epidural fibrosis, and diabetic peripheral neuropathy [9]. SCS is also used off-label to address other chronic pain conditions—including postherpetic neuralgia, refractory angina, peripheral vascular disease, and visceral abdominal pain—highlighting its versatility in managing diverse pain syndromes [1,3,8–11].

Historical perspective

The origins of SCS date back to when early civilizations used electric fish—such as torpedo rays—to alleviate pain, indicating an early awareness of electricity's medicinal potential [12,13]. A major paradigm shift occurred in the 1960s with the introduction of Melzack and Wall's gate control theory of pain, which proposed that the spinal cord contains a neurological "gate" capable of modulating pain signals [14]. In 1967, Shealy, Mortimer, and Reswick performed the first SCS implant on a patient with intractable cancer pain—a landmark procedure that not only provided a new avenue for managing severe, previously untreatable pain but also established neuromodulation as a distinct and promising clinical discipline [15].

Procedure innovation

SCS technology has evolved significantly through continuous innovation in surgical technique, hardware, and stimulation paradigms. Early approaches involved open surgical procedures that relied on anatomical landmarks and trial-and-error lead placement, often resulting in prolonged recovery periods and higher complication rates [7,16]. A shift occurred in the 1980s with the introduction of percutaneous lead placement using minimally invasive techniques and fluoroscopic guidance, dramatically reducing surgical risks, shortening hospital stays, and improving patient comfort [17]. A randomized, double-blinded crossover study by Washburn et al. (2014) demonstrated that 70% of patients preferred constant-current (CC) SCS over constant-voltage (CV) stimulation—reporting significantly greater pain relief with CC systems [18]. The advent of rechargeable implantable pulse generators (IPGs) in the early 2000s marked a significant advancement by extending device longevity (up to 9 years) and reducing the frequency and cost of replacement surgeries, thereby

A Modern Atlas for Implantable Devices of the Spine, Brain, and Nerve. https://doi.org/10.1016/B978-0-443-36528-7.00018-2

enhancing the long-term cost-effectiveness of SCS therapy [19,20]. Furthermore, advancements in stimulation paradigms—such as high-frequency (10 kHz) and burst stimulation—have broadened therapeutic options beyond traditional tonic stimulation [21,22].

Relevant advancements

Recent advancements have enhanced the efficacy, safety, and personalization of SCS therapy. A key breakthrough is the FDA-approved closed-loop SCS systems, including Medtronic's Inceptiv (2024) [23,24] and Saluda Medical's Evoke (2020) [25,26], which optimize pain relief by automatically adjusting stimulation based on neural activity, evoked compound action potentials (ECAPs) [27,28]. Lead designs now feature up to 32 contacts for precise targeting, while multichannel devices enable refined modulation [29–32]. Innovations such as spatiotemporal neuromodulation, burst, and kilohertz stimulation further improve outcomes [22,33]. A battery-free miniaturized SCS system has shown promise in reducing pain and complications. Ongoing research, including differential target multiplexed (DTM) stimulation, continues to drive progress [29,34].

Key points

- **SCS Overview:** SCS is a minimally invasive neuromodulation technique that manages chronic, intractable pain by delivering low-voltage electrical impulses to the dorsal columns of the spinal cord.
- **Paresthesia Versus Paresthesia-Free:** Traditional SCS induces paresthesia to alleviate pain, whereas modern modalities can provide effective pain relief without this sensation, thereby improving patient comfort.
- **Scope of Application:** SCS is FDA-approved for managing refractory pain of the trunk and limbs, addressing conditions such as low back pain, FBSS, radicular pain, and neuropathic pain, with off-label applications including post-herpetic neuralgia, refractory angina, peripheral vascular disease, and visceral abdominal pain.
- **Recent Innovations:** Advancements include closed-loop systems, refined lead designs with increased contacts, rechargeable and miniaturized devices, and novel stimulation paradigms—all contributing to more personalized and effective pain management.

Relevant anatomy

a. Summary of Relevant Anatomy:
Spinal cord stimulation involves implanting electrodes in the epidural space to regulate pain signals. Situated between the dura mater and the vertebral wall, this space contains fat, small blood vessels, and nerve roots. Electrodes are typically positioned over the dorsal columns of the spinal cord, which play a crucial role in transmitting sensory information, including pain. The dorsal columns contain large-diameter A-beta fibers, which are preferentially activated by SCS to induce paresthesia and provide pain relief.

b. Editor's note: Reference appropriate Anatomy Chapters

Procedure

Diagnosis (with ICD-10 codes)

Thoracic and lumbar spinal cord stimulation is an elective procedure and is usually performed in the outpatient setting. Sterile technique is utilized during trial and permanent implant is of utmost importance as this is a device implant procedure. Full availability of cardiopulmonary resuscitation equipment is necessary. Spinal Cord Stimulation is indicated for various chronic pain conditions.

Common diagnoses associated with SCS include:

ICD-10 code	Condition [35]
G89.4 G90.50	Chronic pain syndrome Complex regional pain syndrome
M54.16	Lumbar radiculopathy (sciatica)
G57.10	Sciatic nerve disorders
M54.5	Low back pain
M79.2	Chronic neuropathic pain, neuralgia and neuritis
M96.1	Post-laminectomy syndrome

Emerging Indications
Angina
Limb ischemia
Abdominal and Visceral Pain
Pelvic Pain disorders
Phantom limb pain
Spinal cord Injury

c. Patient Selection Considerations

a. Age - The ideal age range 18–75. Older patients would need further preprocedural planning and anesthesia evaluation [36].

b. SCS therapy is contraindicated in patients with active infections, severe spinal deformities, which may interfere with lead placement, and bleeding disorders. Untreated psychiatric disorders are usually a contraindication, and patients usually undergo psychiatric evaluation before device trial and implantation.

c. Maintenance concerns- Maintenance concerns include concerns for battery longevity, MRI compatibility, lead migration and the need for revision surgery. Regular adjustments remain a practical concern as device reprogramming can be needed to optimize patient outcomes; therefore, regular follow-ups may also be needed [37].

Maintenance consideration	Source
Battery longevity (rechargeable vs. nonrechargeable)	ASIPP, Medtronic, Boston Scientific, Nevro
Lead migration risk (need for revision surgery)	INS, Boston Scientific, peer-reviewed literature (Deer et al. [7])
MRI compatibility (newer devices are MRI-safe)	Medtronic, Nevro, ASIPP
Device reprogramming (regular follow-ups needed)	ASIPP, INS, Medtronic, Deer et al. [7]

d. Training Recommendations- Physicians, having completed an ACGME-accredited pain fellowship, neurosurgery residency, MSK interventional radiology, or have attended other cadaveric workshops for training on SCS can perform the procedure. According to ASIPP guidelines for interventional pain management training, minimum volumes for trial placement [38] and permanent implantation [21] are a suggested baseline for competency procedure [39]. Hands on training and proctoring is suggested for first 10–15 cases [37,40].

e. Case Peer Review- The international neuromodulation society (INS) along with ASIPP and NANS recommend SCS case reviews by multidisciplinary team consisting of pain management, neurosurgery, and anesthesiology care providers [41]. This can help with tracking patient pain relief and device effectiveness. Furthermore, education about SCS can be enhanced with a standardized registry for SCS related outcomes [42].

Technique

a. Patient positioning: For thoracic spinal cord stimulator placement, the patient is placed in the prone position, which allows access to the spine as well as flank and buttock region for placement of the implantable pulse generator. Ideally a Wilson frame and Jackson table help to open up the interspinous spaces to facilitate percutaneous needle entry. Gel rolls or pillows under the abdomen may also be used (see Fig. 10.1).

The surgical field should be marked using clear polyethylene plastic drapes with an adhesive strip, ensuring a wide field to accommodate the spine incision and IPG pocket. Meticulous sterile technique is observed. The skin is prepped using ChloraPrep swabs, and the patient draped with sterile blue towels. An antimicrobial iodine-impregnanted drape is then placed over the skin and a surgical drape over the buttock and legs. Next, split drapes or a laparotomy drape can be used, and the c-arm draped with a sterile cover and a drape to allow for lateral fluoroscopic images to be taken without contamination of the field.

b. Anesthesia considerations:

Placement of trial leads or an implant is typically performed under monitored anesthesia care for sedation. Once leads are in place the patient is awakened to confirm coverage of the painful distribution of pain. General anesthesia with neuromonitoring is also commonly performed and has been shown to increase the safety and efficiency of these procedures. Falowski showed that operative time was shorter for the patients under general anesthesia compared with the

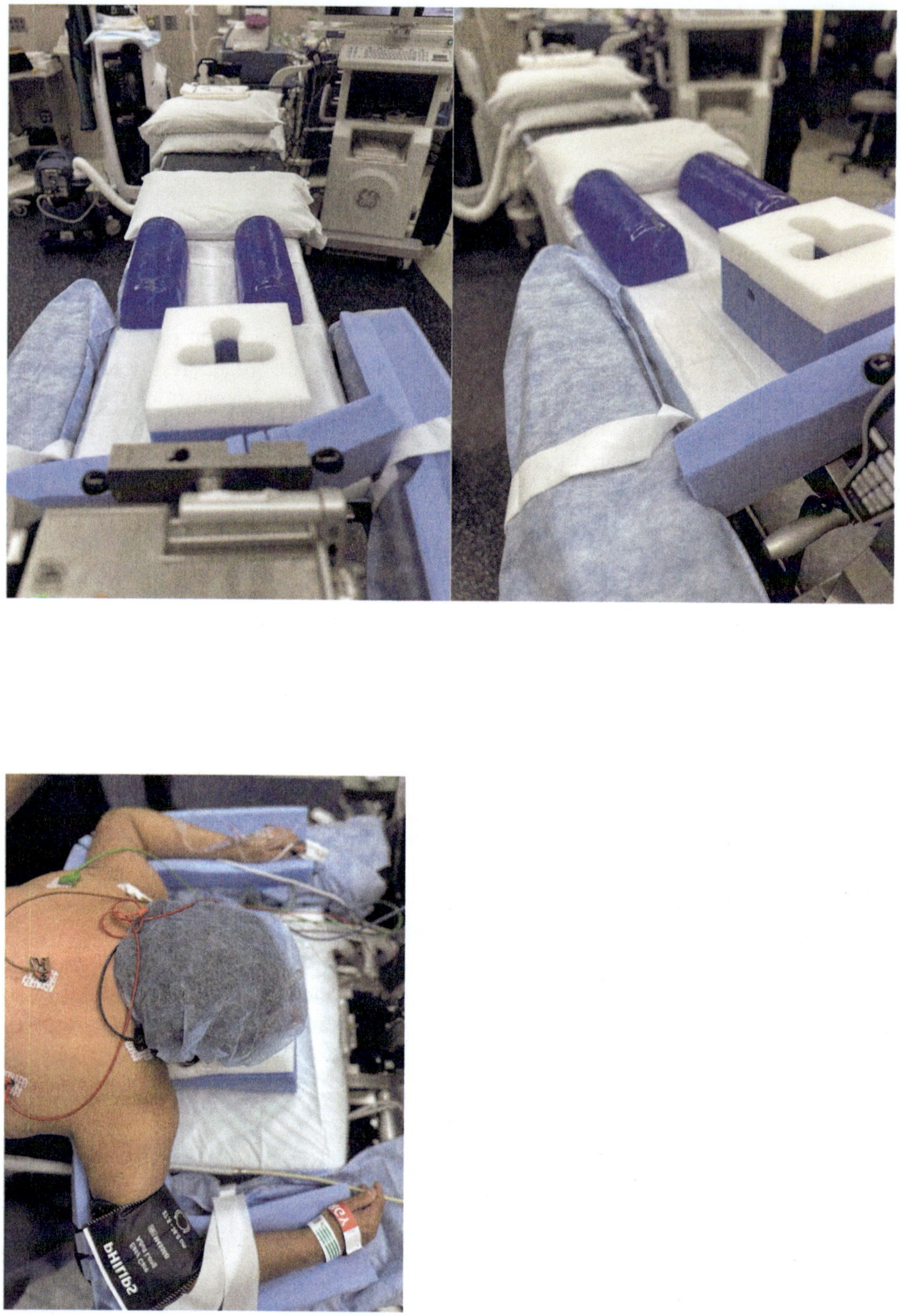

FIGURE 10.1 Patient positioning options.

awake patients [43]. With neuromonitoring, SSEPs and EMGs are elicited and CMAPs allowed us to optimize the left–right placement of the lead.

c. **Operating room time estimate:**

The estimated operative time a percutaneous spinal cord stimulator varies based on several factors including the specific technique and the patient's characteristics. In general, it could take 15 min to place a single lead in an anatomically non challenging spine, up to 90–120 min for two leads and IPG implantation.

d. Relevant Vendor Support:

Having a vendor representative in the operating room is important in ensuring adequate implant inventory and having back-up implants available for example different lengths of epidural needles [44], leads, and appropriate batteries i.e., rechargeable versus nonrechargeable. However, the patient's consent for vendor representative presence should be obtained as otherwise this could be construed as invasion of patient privacy.

e. Procedure:

Step 1: Lead placement:

The first step is to obtain a true AP view of the spine by flattening the endplates and ensuring the spinous process is in the center of the pedicles. While L1-2 is the most commonly used interspace, the most "open" interspace should be used, and this could be T12-L1 or even L2-3. When placing two leads it is best to place the lead furthest from you first. A marking pen can be used to mark the epidural space to be entered as well as the entry point in the skin. A Coude tip needle as compared with a straight tip needle facilitates passage of the lead dorsally. The skin and subcutaneous tissues is then anaesthetized. Using paramedian approach with the medial border of the pedicle as a starting point, the epidural

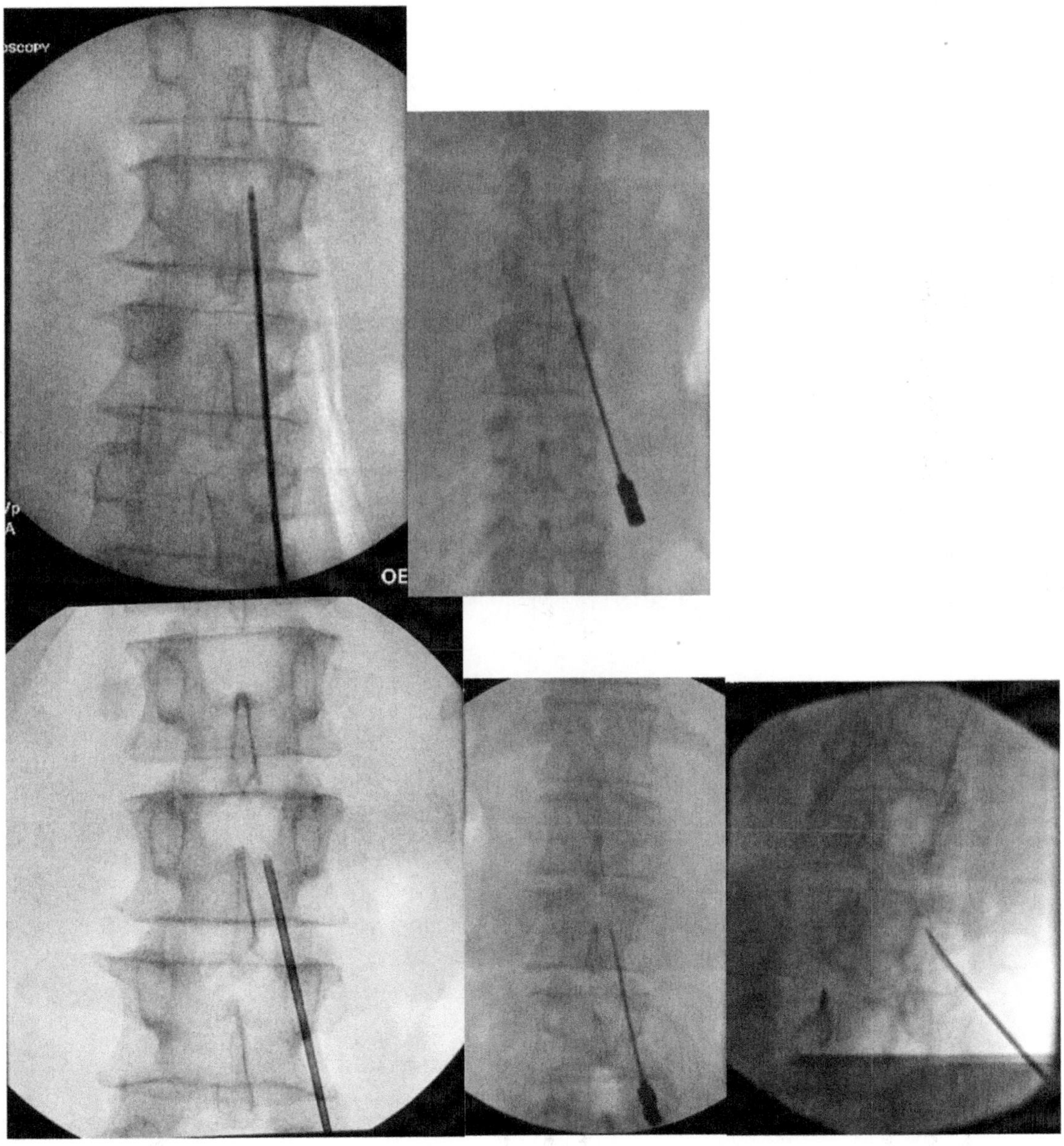

FIGURE 10.2 Fluoroscopic spine scans.

needle is advanced at a shallow angle of 30–45° to facilitate dorsal placement of the leads. Fig. 10.2 (choose best pictures).

The bevel faces dorsal and is advanced to land on the edge of the laminar of the desired epidural entry space. Then, a contra-lateral oblique fluoroscopic view is obtained to gauge the depth of the needle. The needle is advanced carefully using loss of resistance technique and the epidural space is entered. If the loss is equivocal, a guidewire can be used to check if the epidural space has been entered (Fig. 10.3).

The leads are then steered to the targeted level using an AP view, ensuring that they do not fall into the lateral gutter. The ideal technique is to advanced the lead with the left hand close to the hub of the needle, and steer the stylet with the right hand, which is grasped with the thumb and index finger. Lateral fluoroscopy confirms dorsal placement of the leads. At this point, when performing a trial, the epidural needle is then removed ensuring that the lead does not move from the targeted location. For low back and leg pain the target is T7-T9 and for thoracic pain, T4-T6. The leads are then secured using a catheter fixation device or steri-strips and Tegaderm (Fig. 10.4- choose best pictures).

When performing an implant, it is advisable to make the incision over the spine first, which is often a more facile technique than performing a cut down around the epidural needle. A vertical incision is marked in the midline, between the spinous process of the vertebral level to be entered and the level below, depending on the patient's body habitus. After the skin and subcutaneous tissues are anaesthetized, dissection is carried out down to the thoraco-lumbar fascia. The epidural needle is then placed using the technique described above, ensuring a shallow angle while accounting for the shorter distance to travel to the epidural space from the thoracodorsal fascia.

Step 2: Anchoring:

An anchor stitch is placed on either side of the epidural needle in the fascia with nonabsorbable suture. These can then be clamped with a snap or mosquito forceps and placed out of the way. The needle is then removed from the epidural space taking care not to move the Lead from the targeted location. The anchor is gently advanced over the lead and the tip of the anchor buried in the fascia. Each stitch is then tied down securely to fascia using a surgeon's knot. A final X-ray picture of the location of the leads should be obtained after anchoring has been performed.

Step 3: Tunneling and Pocket:

The pocket has been premarked in the preoperative area and the skin and subcutaneous tissues are anaesthetized. Using a scalpel, an incision is made and using blunt dissection the pocket is formed. Consult with your vendor representative as

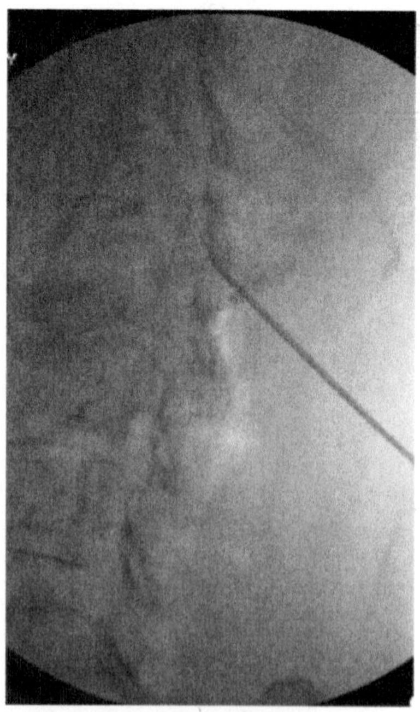

FIGURE 10.3 Lateral fluoroscopic scan.

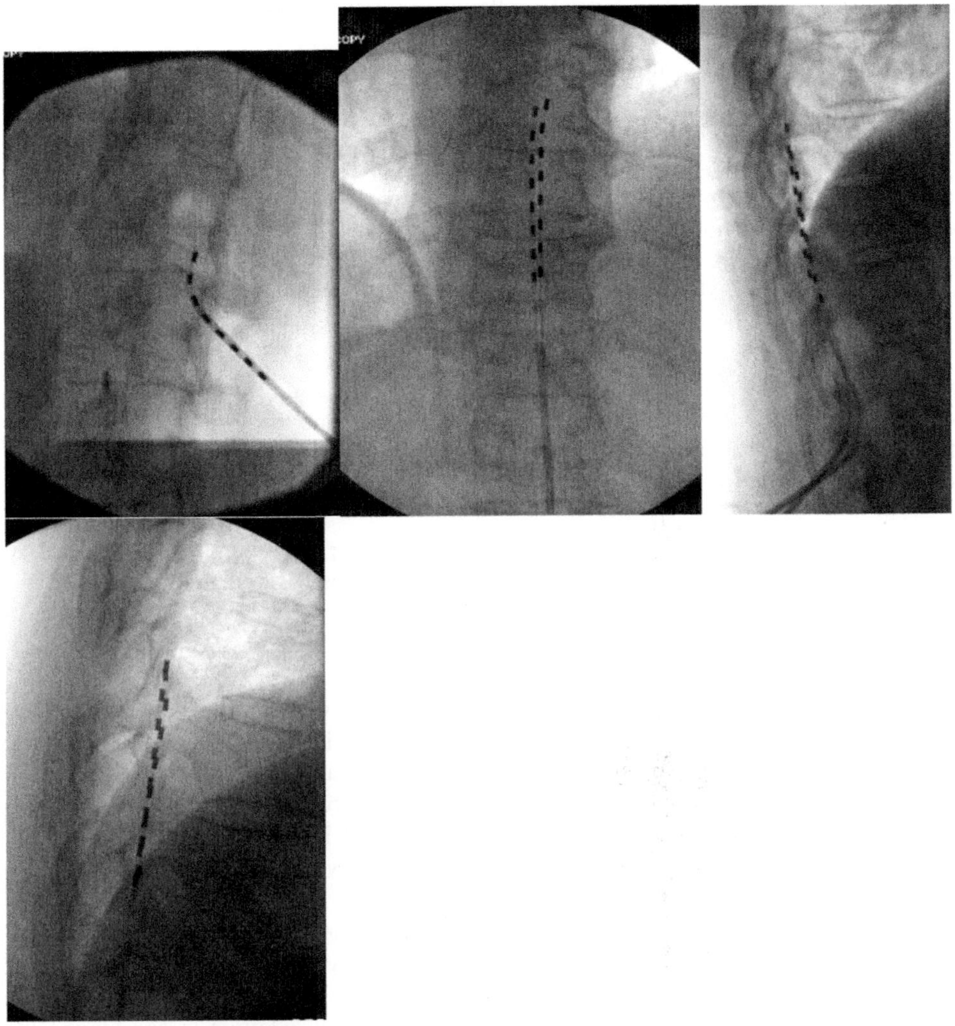

FIGURE 10.4 Fluoroscopic scans demonstrating segmented catheter tracking.

to the appropriate depth for battery replacement to allow for charging. The tunneling tool is then passed from the lead site toward the IPG pocket with continuous control over the tip of the tunneling tool ensuring that the plane is not too superficial or too deep. The leads are threaded into the tunneling tool after the stylet has been removed with care to leave a strained relief loop in the back, and connected to the battery. Impedances are checked by the representative. The battery can then be placed in an antimicrobial pouch with excess lead curled around the battery posteriorly and placed in the pocket with the label facing out. Hemostasis Is then ensured and both incisions irrigated with antibiotic solution. Both incisions are closed with a three layer closure using and absorbable suture such as 2/0 Vicryl on a CT2 needle. For the deep dermal layer, a barbed suture such as 3–0 Vloc can be used or an absorbable suture such as 3–0 Monocryl. For the skin, skin staples may be used or 4–0 monocryl for a running subcuticular closure.

Once the pt has recovered from anesthesia initial programming can be carried out in the recovery area.

Postoperative considerations

- **Recovery:** Recovery following thoracic and lumbar spinal cord stimulation implantation is dependent on several factors including patient comorbidities, surgical technique, and also adherence to postoperative recommendations.

Generally, it follows a structured timeline, where the first 6 weeks following the implantation are critical for wound healing, scar formation, and mitigation of lead migration.

- Primary focus during these first 2 weeks after SCS implantation is preventing infections, lead migration, and hardware/device complications.
- Surgical site pain is common during the first 2 weeks. Using multimodal medications such as acetaminophen, NSAIDs, gabapentinoids, and muscle relaxants for optimizing pain management during this phase is common. In spine surgery, implantation of enhanced recovery after surgery (ERAS) protocols have been found to accelerate postoperative patient recovery by decreasing hospitalization times, potentially decreasing complication rates, and overall optimizing functional recovery [38].
- Occlusive dressings should be maintained for 24–48 h after the surgery and patient and/or family education about appropriate incision care as well as signs/symptoms of surgical site infections (SSI) should be appropriately undertaken [44].
- Patients should follow up within the first 10–14 days for staples or nonabsorbable sutures to be removed [45].
- To mitigate risk of lead migration/fractures, strict limitations on twisting, bending, and lifting should be adhered to and patients should be educated before implantation **(See Image #)** [44]. These restrictions can be gradually lifted over time, but considering that remodeling and scar formation can occur for up to 14 weeks post implant, early adherence is critical.
- Initial device programming can occur within the first 2 weeks as swelling decreases, but patients should expect that fine-tuning and adjustments may be required periodically as scar tissue continues to form during the first 2–3 months.
- Periodic device and patient checkups every 3–6 months can be helpful in optimizing patients' pain control and device functionality.

- **Efficacy Estimates:** Spinal cord stimulation's efficacy in patients with chronic pain, who have had successful trials with greater than 50% reduction in their pain, has been well-documented, particularly in those with neuropathic pain, postsurgical pain syndrome type II, peripheral polyneuropathy and complex regional pain syndrome (CRPS). A recent systematic review and meta-analysis looked at the overall efficacy of SCS for these chronic pain states versus conventional medical management (CMM) at 6-month follow-up. A total of 13 studies and 1561 patients were included in this review. They found that SCS therapies, when compared with CMM, not only had improved pain but also decreased disability and improved quality of life [46].
- **Bracing Considerations:** Currently, there are no universal established bracing recommendations specifically for patients undergoing spinal cord stimulator implantation. Nonetheless, an important consideration post implantation is preventing postoperative fluid collections such as seromas. Garments such as abdominal binders may be considered to provide compression, which in turn can help reduce local swelling after surgery. In addition to considering the use of an abdominal binder, appropriate surgical technique involving sparing use of electrocautery and appropriately sizing of the IPG pocket, are important factors. Despite the use of a compressive garment, small amount of fluid collection/seroma formation can be expected and typically resolves within the first 8 weeks. Close monitoring is critical, because if fluid accumulates and there is no concern for underlying infection, then sterile aspiration may be considered [44]. There are no current recommendations about the use of bracing for patients who undergo laminotomy/laminectomy for paddle lead implantation, but may be considered on a case-by-case basis.
- **Activity Limitations:** Setting clear postoperative instructions regarding initial activity limitations to best facilitate healing and limit complications is essential for long-term success following SCS implantation. As monitoring continues during the healing process, these restrictions can gradually be lifted while combining with targeted physical therapy to provide better outcomes [47]. Per NACC guidelines, there is moderate consensus agreement regarded gradual return to physical activity during the initial 16 weeks following implantation decrease risk of lead migration, fractures, or displacements. A more detailed description of these activity limitations during each phase of the recovery process following SCS implantation, per the NACC guidelines, can be seen in **[Image #]** [44]. Following 16 weeks, a restriction in AROM of BUE and BLE can be lifted with a focus on developing functional independence when performing activities of daily living. Developing a sustainable long term exercise program that incorporates cardiovascular exercise is also recommended.

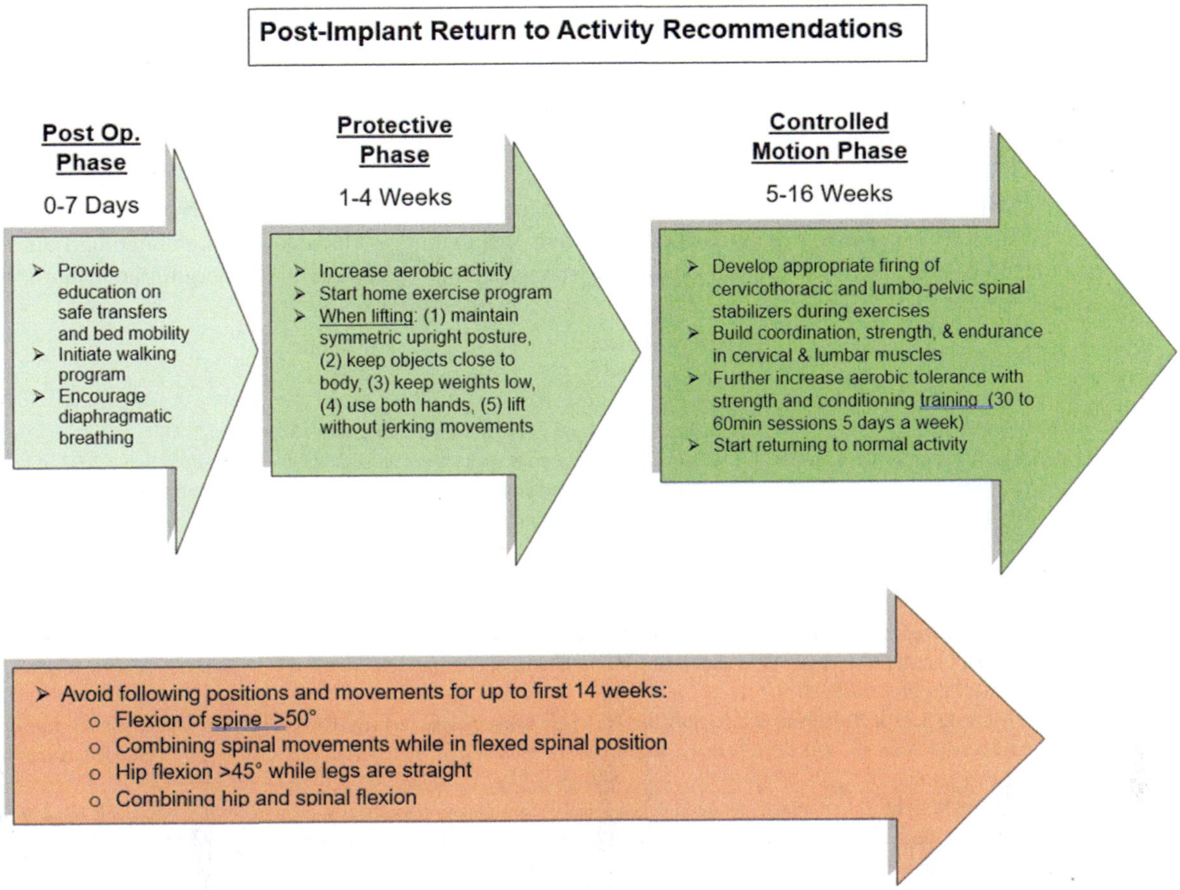

- **Maintenance Considerations:** Routine follow up every 3–6 months will facilitate early identification and work-up of amendable device related issues. Those with rechargeable IPGs should be educated about proper manufacturer specific charging practices to prevent battery depletion. Primary cell IPGs, which are nonrechargeable, can function anywhere from 5 to 10 years depending on programming parameters and usage. Periodic office visits with these patients allows for monitoring battery depletion alerts to better optimize a timely replacement rather than waiting for complete battery failure. If a return of baseline pain or periodic lapses in pain coverage is experienced, evaluation of the leads for migration or damage may be one of the first steps, particularly in the early months. Updated imaging of the region can help confirm this further, and although reprogramming may help some cases of lead migration, in other patients both lead migration and fractured leads require surgical revision. As the area heals and scars and neural plasticity evolves following the implant, periodic office follow ups with the patient allows stimulation parameters to be optimized by ensuring the IPG's firmware is up to date and various waveforms/stimulation parameters are available for the patient if needed. Additionally. patients should be educated on recognizing red flag symptoms that would prompt immediate evaluation, such as sudden stimulation loss, new neurological deficits, or persistent wound pain. Proper maintenance and patient follow-up care will likely impact long-term device efficacy and patient satisfaction.

Pearls and pitfalls

Pearls and Pitfalls in thoracic and lumbar spinal cord stimulation begin with **preoperative** considerations, where proper patient selection is critical—detailed assessments of comorbidities, psychological readiness, and functional goals help optimize outcomes. During the **intraoperative** phase, paying meticulous attention to patient positioning, target-specific lead placement, and real-time imaging and placing strong consideration to performing intraoperative testing can help prevent complications such as lead migration or suboptimal stimulation coverage. It is advisable to seek out additional surgical technique training should this be a deficit following formalized medical training. Pitfalls often arise post-operatively when activity restrictions are inadequately communicated, possibly leading to hardware displacement, infection, or delayed wound healing. Monitoring device functionality and providing thorough patient education regarding follow-up needs, activity modifications, and signs of device malfunction are essential **postoperative** steps. Finally, as the **scope** of this procedure evolves with on- and off-label indications, maintaining proficiency through ongoing training and adherence to evidence-based guidelines can help clinicians navigate both traditional and emerging applications while minimizing adverse events.

References

[1] Deer TR, Mekhail N, Provenzano D, et al. Spinal cord stimulation: state of the art. Pain Med 2007;8(Suppl. 1):S3–11.

[2] Kumar K, Hunter CW, Yampolsky C, et al. Spinal cord stimulation for chronic pain: a systematic review. J Neurosurg Spine 2007;6(3):204–21.

[3] White T, Justiz R, Almonte W, et al. 12-Month results from a randomized controlled trial comparing differential target multiplexed spinal cord stimulation and conventional spinal cord stimulation in subjects with chronic refractory axial low back pain not eligible for spine surgery. N Am Spine Soc J 2024;19. https://doi.org/10.1016/j.xnsj.2024.100528.

[4] North RB, Kidd DH, Zahurak M, et al. Spinal cord stimulation for chronic, intractable pain: experience over two decades. Neurosurgery 1993;32:384.

[5] Donnini RM. Use and effectiveness of spinal cord stimulation. Pract Pain Manag 2010;1:29.

[6] Lamer TJ, Moeschler SM, Gazelka HM, et al. Spinal stimulation for the treatment of intractable spine and limb pain: a systematic review of RCTs and meta-analysis. Mayo Clin Proc 2019;94:1475.

[7] Deer T, Gilligan C, Falowski S, et al. Treatment of refractory low back pain using passive recharge burst in patients without options for corrective surgery: findings and results from the DISTINCT study, a prospective randomized multicenter controlled trial. Neuromodulation 2023;26 (7):1387–99.

[8] White T, Justiz R, Fishman M, et al. Differential target multiplexed spinal cord stimulation for the treatment of chronic intractable upper limb pain: 12-month results from a prospective, multicenter study. Neuromodulation 2024 [Epub ahead of print]. S1094-7159(24)00628-7.

[9] van Beek M, Geurts JW, Slangen R, et al. Severity of neuropathy is associated with long-term spinal cord stimulation outcomes in painful diabetic peripheral neuropathy: five-year follow-up of a prospective two-center clinical trial. Diabet Care 2018;41(1):32–8. https://doi.org/10.2337/dc17-0983.

[10] Eldabe S, et al. Spinal cord stimulation in chronic pain: systematic review and meta-analysis of individual patient data. Pain 2016;157(4):852–61.

[11] van Beek M, Geurts JW, Verhagen S, Weber WE. Spinal cord stimulation for the treatment of refractory angina pectoris: a systematic review. Pain Pract 2018;18(2):259–74.

[12] Kellaway P. The William Osler Medal Essay. The story of the use of electric fishes in the treatment of disease. Bull Hist Med 1946;20(2):112–37.

[13] Steger HF. Ancient use of electric fish. JAMA 1982;247(2):256.

[14] Melzack R, Wall PD. Pain mechanisms: a new theory. Science 1965;150(3699):971–9.

[15] Shealy CN, Mortimer JT, Reswick JB. Electrical inhibition of pain by stimulation of the dorsal columns: preliminary clinical report. Anesth Analg 1967;46(4):489–91.

[16] Deer TR, et al. The appropriate use of neurostimulation: spinal cord stimulation and peripheral nerve stimulation for the treatment of chronic pain and peripheral vascular disease. Neuromodulation 2014;17(6):515–32.

[17] North RB. Spinal cord stimulation for chronic pain: fifty years. Pain 2017;158(Suppl. 1):S29–37.

[18] Washburn S, Catlin R, Bethel K, Canlas B. Patient-perceived differences between constant current and constant voltage spinal cord stimulation systems: a randomized controlled trial. Neuromodulation 2014;17(1):28–35. discussion 35–36.

[19] Wallace MS, et al. Cost-effectiveness analysis of spinal cord stimulation for failed back surgery syndrome. Pain Pract 2014;14(1):34–44.

[20] Deer TR, Pope JE, Falowski SM, Pilitsis JG, Hunter CW, Burton AW, Connolly AT, Verrills P. Clinical longevity of 106,462 rechargeable and primary cell spinal cord stimulators: real world study in the Medicare population. Neuromodulation 2023;26(1):131–8.

[21] Kapural L, et al. Novel 10-kHz high-frequency therapy (HF10 therapy) is superior to traditional low-frequency spinal cord stimulation. Anesthesiology 2015;123(4):851–60.

[22] De Ridder D, et al. Burst spinal cord stimulation: clinical evidence and basic mechanisms. Brain Stimul 2013;6(5):729–39.

[23] Medtronic. Medtronic receives FDA approval for Inceptiv closed-loop spinal cord stimulator [Press release]. April 26, 2024.

[24] Food and Drug Administration. Premarket approval (PMA) database: Inceptiv. 2024. Available from: [FDA Website].

[25] Saluda Medical. Evoke Spinal Cord Stimulation (SCS) System. Available from: FDA Recently Approved Devices.

[26] Food and Drug Administration. Premarket approval (PMA) database: Evoke. 2020. Available from: [FDA Access Data].

[27] Mekhail N, et al. Spinal cord stimulation for chronic pain: are we using the right targets? Pain Med 2022;23(4):689–701.

[28] Falowski S, et al. Closed-loop spinal cord stimulation: a review of the technology and its potential role in pain management. Pain Phys 2022;25 (7):595–608.

[29] Lee D, Bradley K, Syed ZA, Gillespie E, Esterly D. Improved stimulation targeting with a novel 16-contact percutaneous SCS lead: a computational model. In: Presented at: Abstracts of the 15th Annual Meeting of the North American Neuromodulation Society; December 2011; Las Vegas, NV; 2011.

[30] Gage E, et al. Rapid onset of analgesia during trial period utilizing fast-acting sub-perception therapy SCS [Abstract]. In: NANS 2023 Annual Meeting; January 12–15, Las Vegas, NV; 2023.

[31] Anitescu M, et al. Prospective, multicenter outcomes utilizing an SCS-system designed to engage surround inhibition using fast-acting sub-perception therapy [Abstract]. In: Sixteenth World Congress of the International Neuromodulation Society; May 11–16, 2024; Vancouver, BC, Canada; 2024.

[32] Ferro R, et al. Personalized spinal cord stimulation therapy via automated neural dosing (FAST AutoDose) [Abstract]. In: Sixteenth World Congress of the International Neuromodulation Society; May 11–16, 2024; Vancouver, BC, Canada; 2024.

[33] Lempka SF, Malone DA, Bendahmane M, et al. Next-generation neurostimulation systems. Expet Rev Med Dev 2021;18(6):605–15.

[34] Fishman MA, Cordner K, Justiz DR, Bolash R, Patel M, Hoelzer B, et al. Differential target multiplexed (DTM) spinal cord stimulation improves pain relief and psychological distress in patients with chronic pain: results of a prospective, open-label, multi-center trial. Pain Ther 2023:1–17.

[35] Meier K. Spinal cord stimulation: background and clinical application. Scand J Pain July 1, 2014;5(3):175–81. https://doi.org/10.1016/j.sjpain.2014.03.001.

[36] Deer T, Masone RJ. Selection of spinal cord stimulation candidates for the treatment of chronic pain. Pain Med May 2008;9(Suppl. 1):S82–92.

[37] Krames ES. Neuromodulation training: a structured approach for interventional pain specialists. Neuromodulation Technol Neural Interf 2021;24(5):765–75.

[38] Pennington Z, Cottrill E, Lubelski D, Ehresman J, Theodore N, Sciubba DM. Systematic review and meta-analysis of the clinical utility of Enhanced Recovery after Surgery pathways in adult spine surgery. J Neurosurg Spine 2020;34(2):325–47. https://doi.org/10.3171/2020.6.SPINE20795. Published 2020 Nov 6.

[39] Kapural L. Spinal cord stimulation: past, present, and future. Pain Med 2017;18(Suppl. 1):S1–4.

[40] Deer TR, Krames E, Mekhail N, Pope J, Lamer T, Rosenow J. Best practices in spinal cord stimulation: training, patient selection, and outcomes. Pain Med 2020;21(4):775–86.

[41] International Neuromodulation Society. INS guidelines on best practices for spinal cord stimulation. Retrieved from https://www.neuromodulation.com.

[42] Grider JS, et al. Effectiveness of spinal cord stimulation: a review of long-term outcome tracking. J Pain Res 2022;15:1123–35. https://doi.org/10.2147/JPR.S342312.

[43] Falowski SM, Sharan A, McInerney J, Jacobs D, Venkatesan L, Agnesi F. Nonawake vs awake placement of spinal cord stimulators: a prospective, multicenter study comparing safety and efficacy. Neurosurgery 2019;84(1):198–205. https://doi.org/10.1093/neuros/nyy062.

[44] Deer TR, Russo MA, Sayed D, et al. The neurostimulation appropriateness consensus committee (NACC): recommendations for the mitigation of complications of neurostimulation. Neuromodulation 2024;27(6):977–1007. https://doi.org/10.1016/j.neurom.2024.04.004.

[45] Deer TR, Douglas Stewart C. Complications of spinal cord stimulation: identification, treatment, and prevention. Pain Med May 2008;9(Suppl. 1):S93–101. https://doi.org/10.1111/j.1526-4637.2008.00444.x.

[46] Huygen FJPM, Soulanis K, Rtveladze K, Kamra S, Schlueter M. Spinal cord stimulation vs medical management for chronic back and leg pain: a systematic review and network meta-analysis. JAMA Netw Open 2024;7(11):e2444608. https://doi.org/10.1001/jamanetworkopen.2024.44608. Published 2024 Nov 4.

[47] Desai MJ, Ingraham MJ. Rehabilitation perspectives of neuromodulation. Curr Pain Headache Rep 2014;18(2):393. https://doi.org/10.1007/s11916-013-0393-0.

Further reading

[1] North RB. Spinal cord stimulation: fifty years after the gate control theory. Pain 2016;157(Suppl. 1):S3–9.

[2] Linderoth B, Foreman RD. Conventional and novel spinal stimulation algorithms: hypothetical mechanisms of action and comments on outcomes. Neuromodulation 2017;20(6):525–33.

[3] Deer TR, Mekhail N, Provenzano D, et al. The appropriate use of neurostimulation of the spinal cord and peripheral nervous system for the treatment of chronic pain and ischemic diseases: the Neuromodulation Appropriateness Consensus Committee. Neuromodulation 2014;17:515.

[4] Russo M, Cousins MJ, Brooker C, et al. Effective relief of pain and associated symptoms with closed-loop spinal cord stimulation system: preliminary results of the Avalon study. Neuromodulation 2018;21:38.

[5] Vallejo R, Kramer J, Benyamin R. Neuromodulation of the cervical spinal cord in the treatment of chronic intractable neck and upper extremity pain: a case series and review of the literature. Pain Phys 2007;10:305.

[6] Barolat G, Massaro F, He J, et al. Mapping of sensory responses to epidural stimulation of the intraspinal neural structures in man. J Neurosurg 1993;78:233.

[7] Salmon J, et al. Early experience with a novel miniaturized spinal cord stimulation system for the management of chronic intractable pain of the back and legs. Neuromodulation 2023;26(1):172–81.

Chapter 11

Neuromodulation for pelvic pain

Corey Hunter[3], Shawn K. Puri[1], Raj G. Patel[2] and Iden M. Cowan[4]
[1]*Integrated Pain Associates, Killeen, TX, United States;* [2]*Capitol Pain Institute, Austin, TX, United States;* [3]*Montefiore Medical Center, Multidisciplinary Pain Program, Department of Physical Medicine & Rehabilitation at Albert Einstein College of Medicine, Bronx, NY, United States;* [4]*Interventional Spine Capitol Pain Institute, Greenwood Village, CO, United States*

Introduction

Chronic pelvic pain (CPP) is estimated to affect 5.7%–26% of the world's female population [1,2]. It affects women more frequently than men, and its socioeconomic burden is substantial — healthcare costs for women alone approach $3 billion annually in the United States [3,4]. CPP is a complex and multifaceted condition defined as nonmalignant pain in the pelvic region persisting for at least 6 months, often considered a diagnosis of exclusion. CPP syndrome can result from a variety of underlying conditions (see Table 11.1) [5,6]. This broad classification reflects the difficulty in pinpointing a single cause—visceral pain, in particular, can be challenging to diagnose [7]. The diagnostic process is typically prolonged, with many patients waiting up to a decade for a definitive diagnosis. This delay, coupled with ineffective initial treatments, often exacerbates emotional distress and leads to excessive and unnecessary medical interventions like hysterectomies [3,8].

One of the greatest challenges in managing CPP lies in understanding its underlying mechanisms. In many cases, no clear pathology or identifiable pain generator emerges, and conventional imaging often fails to provide answers [5,9,10]. In some patients, CPP develops following identifiable triggers such as childbirth, surgery, or infections, while in others, it arises spontaneously. The elusive nature of its pathophysiology has led researchers to hypothesize that CPP may share similarities with complex regional pain syndrome (CRPS) [11]. This theory suggests a "wind-up" phenomenon, where pelvic neurons become hypersensitized to pain, similar to what occurs in CRPS but localized to the pelvic region.

Given this potential overlap with CRPS, neuromodulation techniques have been explored as treatment options. Spinal cord stimulation (SCS) has proven effective in other neuropathic and sympathetically mediated pain conditions, which initially made it a promising approach for CPP. However, the outcomes have been less successful than anticipated. The primary hurdle is the complex and overlapping innervation of the pelvic region. The pelvic area is served by multiple spinal levels, from T12/L1 levels to sacral levels, making it difficult to achieve consistent coverage of the painful areas. Patients frequently report incomplete relief or experience painful paresthesias in unaffected regions, leading to high explant rates—up to 33.3%, the highest among conditions treated with SCS [12].

To address these limitations, researchers and clinicians have experimented with alternative neuromodulation targets [2,3,5–7]. Dorsal root ganglion (DRG) stimulation has shown promise by allowing for more precise targeting of individual nerves, while peripheral nerve stimulation (PNS) has been explored to directly stimulate affected nerves.

Despite the current limitations, ongoing research continues to refine neuromodulation techniques for CPP. Although a definitive solution remains elusive, these evolving techniques offer hope for better managing this debilitating condition.

Relevant anatomy

A thorough understanding of pelvic pain anatomy and neuroanatomy is essential for accurate diagnosis and treatment. This will be a brief overview of the relevant structures of innervation that contribute to chronic pelvic pain.

The pelvis consists of the bony structure that includes the sacrum, coccyx, ileum, and pubis symphysis. Various muscles and ligaments are located within this bony ring to provide support to the skeletal system and the pelvic organs. The posterior ligaments are related to the muscles of the back, abdomen, and extremities, while the anterior ligaments are

A Modern Atlas for Implantable Devices of the Spine, Brain, and Nerve. https://doi.org/10.1016/B978-0-443-36528-7.00026-1

TABLE 11.1 Chronic Pelvic Pain (CPP) common causes.

Genitourinary	Endometriosis, dysmenorrhea, dyspareunia, vaginal pain (vulvodynia, vulvitis, vaginitis), interstitial cystitis, chronic-prostatitis, scrotal/testicular pain syndrome, chronic pelvic inflammatory disease, cancer pain/post-radiation pain
Vascular	Pelvic congestion syndrome, pelvic venous disease
Neurologic	Nerve entrapment (post surgical, surgical scar), post-surgical (adhesions, nerve injury), post-herniorrhaphy pain, postorchiectomy pain, pudendal neuralgia, ilioinguinal/Iliohypogastric neuralgia, genitofemoral neuralgia, sympathetically-mediated pain
Musculocutaneous	Pelvic floor dysfunction, myofascial pain, coccygodynia
Gastrointestinal	Irritable bowel syndrome, hernia, inflammatory bowel disease, anorectal pain

linked to the abdominal muscles and some of the lower extremities. Dysfunction in these muscles or ligaments can lead to pain or discomfort. The pelvis and the pelvic viscera are innervated by both somatic and autonomic systems.

Chronic pain can arise from various structures in the pelvis, including the vulva, vagina, cervix, uterus, fallopian tube, ovary, uterine ligaments, bowel, bladder, or perineum (see Fig. 11.1).

Anterior cutaneous innervation is banded by the mid to upper lumbar spinal nerves (T7-L1). These are arranged in a superioposterior to inferoanterior orientation. Four cutaneous nerves-the lateral branches of T12, the lateral femoral cutaneous nerve, the terminal branches of the ilioinguinal nerve, and the femoral branches of the genitofemoral nerve form dermatome bands from lateral to medial across the anterior thigh.

The posterior cutaneous innervation to the pelvis is innervated by the lumbar plexus, which is made up of the ventral rami of the L4 and L5 and directly from the dorsal primary rami. The lumbosacral trunk then joins with the ventral rami of S1, S2, and S3. The cutaneous innervation consists of the superior cluneal nerve (L1-L3 dorsal lumbar rami); middle cluneal nerve (S1–S3 dorsal rami), and the S1–S3 inferior cluneal nerve (S1–S3 posterior cutaneous nerve).

The primary nociceptive pathways of the pelvis consist of the pudendal, ilioinguinal nerve, iliohypogastric, genitofemoral nerve, lateral femoral cutaneous nerve, femoral nerve, and obturator nerve (see Fig. 11.2).

The pelvis is sympathetically innervated by the hypogastric plexus (superior, middle, and inferior).

The pudendal nerve consists of the anterior divisions of S2, S3, and the entire S4. It provides sensory innervation to the external genitalia, skin around the anus, anal canal and perineum. It also provides motor innervation for various pelvic muscles and sphincters. The nerve courses from the pelvic cavity through the greater sciatic foramen, then hooks around the ischial spine, enter perineum through the lesser sciatic foramen and proceeds anteriorly through Alcock's canal. The terminal branches are called the inferior anal nerve, the perineal nerve, and the dorsal nerve of the penis/clitoris.

The ilioinguinal nerve is a mixed sensory and motor nerve which is a continuation of the inferior branch of the anterior ramus of L1. There is also a possibility of contribution from T12 or L2. It provides sensory innervation to the skin of the upper anterior medial thigh and partially to the external genitalia. Motor innervation consists of the internal abdominal oblique and transversus abdominis muscles. The nerve initially starts posterior to psoas major and then emerges anteriorly to the quadratus lumborum, travelling obliquely into the inguinal canal and exiting through the superficial inguinal ring.

The iliohypogastric nerve also arises from the anterior ramus of the L1 spinal nerve. It provides sensory innervation to the external oblique, transversus abdominis, internal abdominal oblique, skin of the suprapubic region and posterolateral aspect of the gluteal region. The motor innervation consists of the transversus abdominus, internal abdominal oblique. It emerges from the psoas muscle, passing inferolaterally, piercing the abdominal obliques, and coursing anteriorly.

The genitofemoral nerve is a branch from the lumbar plexus that carries fibers from the anterior rami of L1 and L2. It is primarily sensory, innervating the upper thigh in males and females and the anterior scrotum in males and the mons pubis and labia majora in females. It supplies motor innervation to the cremaster muscle. It originates in the psoas major, emerging anteriorly and then descends retroperitoneally toward the inguinal ligament. Before reaching the inguinal ligament, the nerve bifurcates into terminal branches: the genital and femoral branches.

The obturator is a mixed nerve from the anterior rami of L2, L3, and L4. It provides sensory innervation to the skin over the proximal medial thigh and the articular branches for the hip and knee joints. It provides motor innervation to all the medial muscles of the thigh except for a portion of the adductor magnus. It originates from the iliac crest, travelling through the psoas major and then along the lateral wall and exiting the pelvis through the obturator canal to the anterior thigh.

The pelvis also contains sympathetic and parasympathetic innervation via the superior hypogastric plexus (see Fig. 11.3). The sympathetic contribution is from the L3, L4 lumbar splanchnic nerves. The superior hypogastric plexus consists of the union of the aortic plexus with the L3 and L4 splanchnic nerves. This site is a common target for

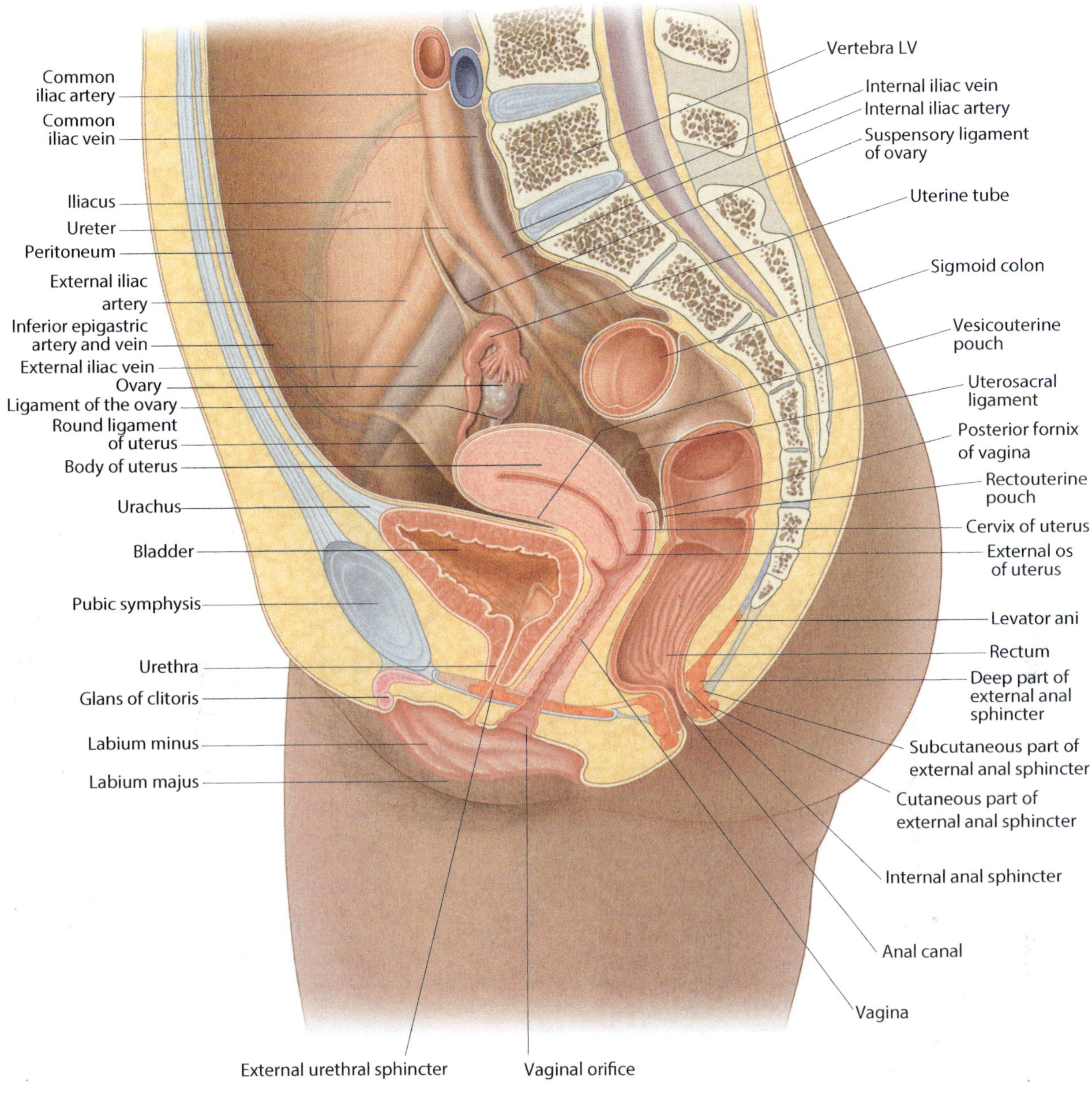

FIGURE 11.1 Pelvic anatomy. *From Drake RL, Wayne Vogl A, Mitchell AWM. Pelvis and perineum. In: Gray's Atlas of Anatomy. 3rd ed. Elsevier; 2020.*

interventional treatment such as nerve blocks or radiofrequency ablation. The superior hypogastric plexus is located anterior to the aortic bifurcation and the L5 vertebral body. The superior hypogastric plexus divides into the right and left hypogastric plexus descend into the pelvis. The superior hypogastric plexus provides innervation to a portion of the rectum, distal ureter, urinary bladder, reproductive tract, and blood vessels.

Another important sympathetic ganglion implicated in pelvic pain conditions is the ganglion impar. The ganglion impar is the terminal fusion of the two sacral sympahathetic chain. It is the only unpaired autonomic ganglion in the body. While there is anatomic variability in its location, which may contribute to variability in response to blockade, it is most commonly located anterior to the sacrococcygeal junction. At the ganglion impar, visceral afferents innervating the perineum, distal rectum, anus, distal urethra, vulva and distal third of the vagina unite. Therefore, this target may be useful

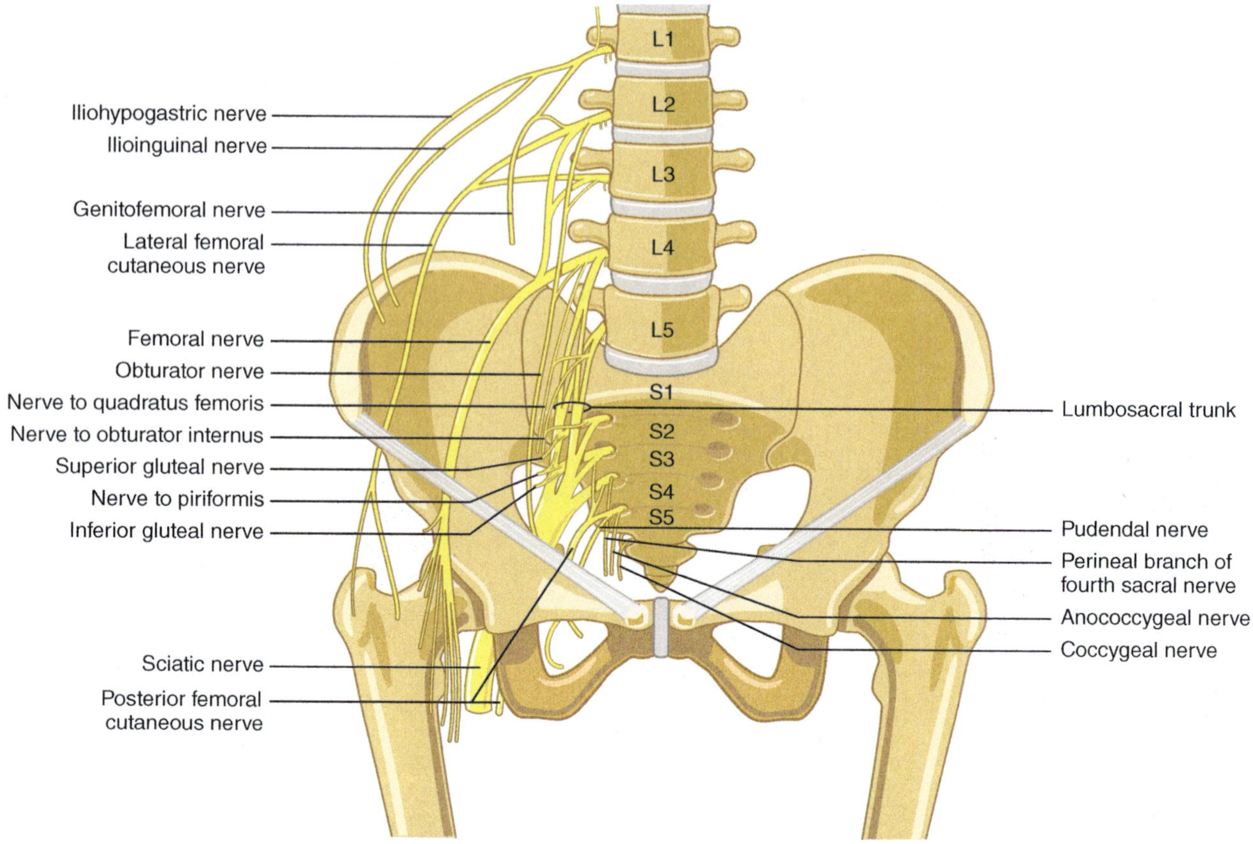

FIGURE 11.2 Nociceptive neural pathways of the pelvis.

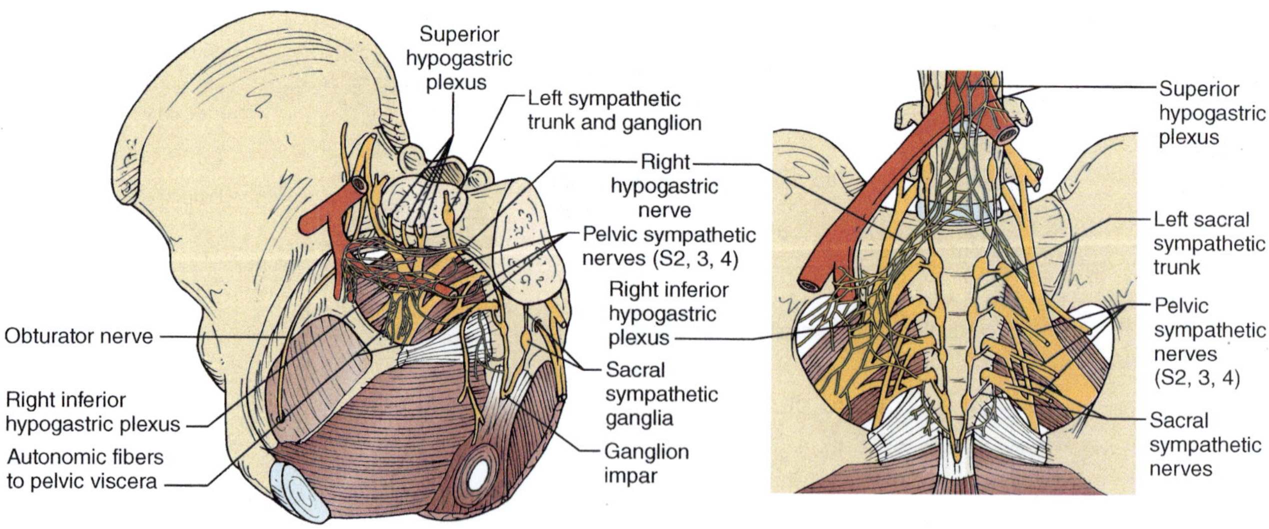

FIGURE 11.3 Pelvic sympathetic and parasympathetic innervation via the superior hypogastric plexus.

in the treatment of these painful conditions. Blockage is usually performed via the trans coccygeal approach under fluoroscopic guidance (see Fig. 11.4).

Another key anatomical consideration for the treatment of pelvic pain and some of the difficulties that lie therein are secondary to the somatotopic organization of the dorsal column of the spinal cord. The dorsal column is responsible for the transmission of fine touch, proprioception, and vibration sensation. Pelvic and sacral fibers are located most medially and "deep" within the spinal cord and, therefore, are more difficult to target with neuromodulation. This can either make it difficult to capture the sacral nerves to optimize pain control, or patients may feel unpleasant sensations in nonpainful

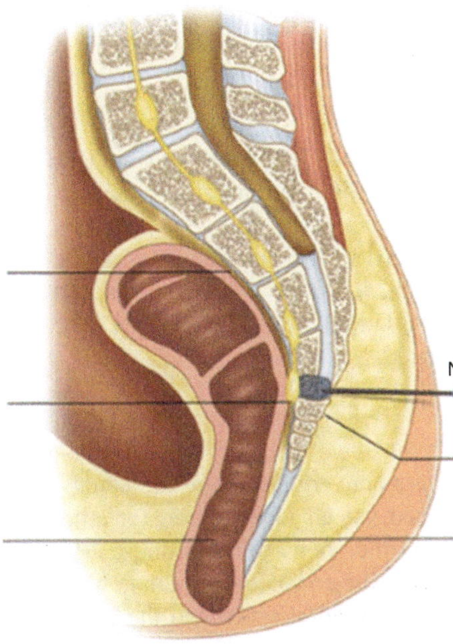

FIGURE 11.4 Ganglion of impar block via trans coccygeal approach.

areas due to stimulation of these areas or overstimulation secondary to high amplitudes necessary to target the intended targets.

Spinal cord stimulation

Given the potential overlap of the pathophysiology of CRPS and CPP, SCS was initially a promising approach for the treatment of CPP. However, there have been several challenges with the successful application of this technique, primarily stemming from the complex innervation of the pelvis. In turn, consistent coverage of the painful areas with SCS has remained elusive. There have been several techniques described for the placement of SCS.

Sacral stimulation

Placement of SCS leads within the sacrum to target the sacral nerves can be performed via a retrograde approach or an anterograde (transsacral hiatus or caudal) approach [5].

Retrograde technique

The retrograde approach was first described by Alo et al. [13]. In this approach, the epidural needle is inserted into the skin at a level superior to the target interlaminar epidural space and then advanced in a caudal and paramedian fashion into the epidural space. Leads are then steered in a cephalad to caudal direction for placement within the sacrum. While this approach is more technically challenging with an increased risk of dural puncture, this remains the preferred technique for placement of SCS leads within the sacrum. This approach allows for the typical SCS surgical and lead anchoring technique in the thoracolumbar fascia to be deployed.

Anterograde technique

While initial needle placement for the anterograde approach is more straightforward, this technique contains its own unique set of challenges [5]. Steering and placement of the lead is more difficult due to the paucity of epidural fat within the sacral canal, as well as the relatively short distance the leads will travel from the needle tip to their final position. There are also several surgical concerns. Considering the scarce fascial and soft tissue composition of the region overlying the sacral hiatus, there is often increased difficulty with anchoring the leads securely. Furthermore, this placement frequently poses the risk of patient discomfort and complications. The leads and anchors will remain in a very superficial position below the skin, in an area that will be subjected to considerable body weight when the patient is seated. This, in turn, poses an increased risk of skin erosion and infection.

Midthoracic stimulation

Placement of SCS leads from the T5-7 region has also been used to successfully target pelvic pain [7]. Given that visceral pain fibers have a complex path which does not adhere to known dermatomal patterns, it is proposed that placement of leads in this region may neuromodulate visceral/sympathetic fibers from the pelvis that would not be captured by sacral stimulation [7]. Furthermore, the caudal-most fibers exiting the spinal cord (i.e., sacral fibers) are arranged in the medial-most position in the dorsal column [14]. Based on this anatomic fact, it stands to reason that sacral fibers may be stimulated at any point along their progression through the spinal cord. Ultimately, the exact mechanism of midthoracic stimulation may be multifactorial; however, it is not yet fully elucidated.

Conus stimulation

The conus medullaris, usually present around the L1-2 region, serves as a convergence point for signals transmitted to and from the pelvis through the cauda equina [7]. Theoretically, this makes it an ideal region for stimulation. However, historically, there have been several challenges with the use of SCS at the conus for targeting CPP. First, the conus is relatively mobile within the spinal canal, resulting in difficulty with achieving consistent stimulation targeting and dosing. Second, there is an increased volume of cerebrospinal fluid between the epidural space and the conus, compared to the thoracic spine. This equates to higher voltages potentially being required to stimulate the appropriate dorsal column, in turn, leading to inadvertent stimulation of segmental roots. Ultimately, this may lead to patient discomfort and dissatisfaction with the therapy [7].

Novel waveforms and use in CPP

Closed-loop stimulation

With the advent of closed-loop stimulation (CLS) in recent years, there is growing evidence to suggest that this novel stimulation paradigm may overcome the aforementioned challenges of conus stimulation [15]. CLS allows for a more consistent stimulation dose by constant monitoring of the evoked compound action potential (ECAP) produced by stimulation, and thereafter adjusting the following stimulation impulse's amplitude as needed [16]. This type of stimulation theoretically addresses the difficulties of neuromodulation in an area with such positional variability of the neural target. A case series of patients targeted with conus CLS for CPP demonstrated an average of 77.38% pain reduction at a mean postimplant time of 6.7 months [10].

10 kHz SCS

High-frequency stimulation delivered at a frequency of 10 kHz has been demonstrated to be an effective long-term treatment of CPP. A single-arm, prospective multicenter study by Tate et al. demonstrated a 72% reduction in mean VAS scores 1 year postimplant [17]. There was also an average reduction in mean short-form McGill Pain Questionnaire-2 scores by 29 points at the 1-year mark. In this study of 21 patients, leads were placed in a staggered position to span from the T8 to T12 vertebral levels.

Dorsal root ganglion stimulation

Why the DRG?

When a peripheral nerve is injured, the corresponding dorsal root ganglion undergoes significant changes, including altered expression of ion channels, inflammation due to macrophage infiltration, an increase in the number of glial cells, and potential neuronal loss. This can lead to hyperexcitability of the neurons and contribute to the development of neuropathic pain that persists after initial tissue damage has healed [18,19]. Stimulating the appropriate DRG is an attractive treatment option to mitigate the painful sequelae.

The DRG is situated in the epidural space of the neuroforamen and is found at the junction of the dorsal root and the spinal cord. Each spinal nerve has its own DRG. It is a collection of cell bodies of primary sensory neurons and serves as a critical structure in sensory transduction and modulation. As part of the anatomical pathway involved in pain transmission, electrical stimulation of the DRG has been explored as a treatment for chronic pain [20]. For patients with refractory chronic pelvic girdle pain, DRG leads placed at L1 and S2 offer a promising neuromodulation modality delivering safe, reliable and targeted stimulation to focal areas and without relying on paresthesia testing [3,21].

The sympathetic nerve fibers run parallel to the spinal cord on both sides of the vertebral column and arise from the spinal cord segments between T1 and L2. Since the sympathetic outflow ends at L2, there are no preganglionic fibers exiting the spinal cord below this level. Spinal nerves T1-L2 carry sympathetic innervation for the trunk wall, as well as participating in forming the splanchnic nerves for innervation of the abdominopelvic viscera [22]. Sacral stimulation of the DRG alone would fail to capture the sympathetic component as these signals ascend on the sympathetic chain, and therefore, DRG lead placement at L1 is also critical for adequate coverage for CPP [3,21].

Two separately conducted case series with a total of 22 patients by Hunter et al. and Patel with DRG leads configured at L1 and S2 reported an improvement in ODI, a decrease in NRS, and decreased opioid use [3,21]. Patients reported improved symptoms and less interference of pain with ADLs [21]. Not one of the implanted patients reported loss of efficacy after 1 year of the initial implant [3,21]. Fifteen patients were followed at 6, 9, 12, and 18 months, respectively, and the decrease in modified ODI and NRS remained consistent or displayed further improvement [21]. While larger prospective studies would be helpful to elucidate which patients with CPP may benefit most from DRGS, and a large RCT would offer the gold standard for evaluating the efficacy of DRGS for CPP, ostensibly, DRGS with lead placement at L1 and S2 may provide a reproducible, targeted and effective treatment for patients with CPP syndromes who have previously failed conservative management.

When considering an advanced interventional treatment option, it is imperative to appropriately individually work up each patient, and when evaluating thoracic or lumbar DRG candidacy, to independently review recent MRI imaging in a T2-weighted sagittal view to ensure neuroforaminal adequacy to accommodate the corresponding DRG lead.

Peripheral nerve neuromodulation

Chronic pelvic pain localized to the genitals, groin, or anorectum may be a direct result of nerve injury, inflammation, or entrapment. The pudendal nerve supplies efferent motor innervation to the external genitalia, perineum, rectum, and anus and carries afferent sensory information from the posterior labia majora and scrotum, labia minora, vestibule, lower fifth of the vaginal canal, and the clitoris and penis. It is involved with clitoral and penile erections and innervates the external urethral and external anal sphincters [23,24]. Additionally, the ilioinguinal, genitofemoral, and iliohypogastric nerves provide overlapping innervation of the skin in the groin/pubic region and are also important nerves to consider for potential peripheral nerve targets [25]. Patients who suffer from CPP and are not candidates for a neuraxial treatment strategy (DRGS or SCS) because of anesthetic concerns, critical central or neuroforaminal stenosis or inability to safely withhold anticoagulation therapy, peripheral nerve neuromodulation may be a viable option. In this method, percutaneous electrodes may be introduced under a combination of ultrasound and or fluoroscopic guidance, depending on which specific peripheral nerve is being targeted.

In the following section, we will focus on pudendal nerve neuromodulation (PNN) as a potential target for patients with CPP as a result of pudendal neuralgia. Under fluoroscopic and or ultrasound guidance, a transgluteal approach may be utilized to place the percutaneous lead close to the pudendal nerve, just medial to the ischial spine, or alternatively accessing the pudendal nerve at the S3 nerve root [5,26,27]. While there is no extensive evidence for the use of PNN in the treatment of pudendal neuralgia, there are several case reports and case series illustrating significant improvement in symptoms [28,29]. Peters et al. conducted a retrospective review in which 19 patients who had undergone pudendal neuromodulation at a single center, of which 84% reported significant improvement in symptoms [29]. In a case series of three patients, Carmel et al. reported favorable outcomes, each with significantly reduced symptoms at their 2-year follow-up [28]. A retrospective study on 84 patients found that PNN could be recommended in patients who are refractory to sacral neuromodulation: 93% of patients who had previously failed sacral neuromodulation responded to pudendal stimulation [29,30]. Further studies are necessary to establish long-term treatment outcomes, efficacy and safety for this treatment option. It also appears that there could be an opportunity to foster greater collaboration with our urology colleagues to identify and treat CPP more expeditiously.

References

[1] Lamvu G, Carrillo J, Ouyang C, Rapkin A. Chronic pelvic pain in women: a review. JAMA June 15, 2021;325(23):2381–91. https://doi.org/10.1001/jama.2021.2631.

[2] Gish B, Langford B, Sobey C, Singh C, Abdullah N, Walker J, Gray H, Hagedorn J, Ghosh P, Patel K, Deer T. Neuromodulation for the management of chronic pelvic pain syndromes: a systematic review. Pain Pract February 2024;24(2):321–40. https://doi.org/10.1111/papr.13295.

[3] Hunter CW, Yang A. Dorsal root ganglion stimulation for chronic pelvic pain: a case series and technical report on a novel lead configuration. Neuromodulation January 2019;22(1):87–95. https://doi.org/10.1111/ner.12801.

[4] Stones RW, Selfe SA, Fransman S, Horn SA. Psychosocial and economic impact of chronic pelvic pain. Baillieres Best Pract Res Clin Obstet Gynaecol June 2000;14(3):415–31. https://doi.org/10.1053/beog.2000.0071.

[5] Hunter CW, Falowski S. Neuromodulation in treating pelvic pain. Curr Pain Headache Rep February 3, 2021;25(2):9. https://doi.org/10.1007/s11916-020-00927-y.

[6] Kothari SN. Neuromodulation approaches to chronic pelvic pain and coccydynia. Acta Neurochir Suppl 2007;97(Pt 1):365–71. https://doi.org/10.1007/978-3-211-33081-4_42.

[7] Hunter CW, Davé N, Diwan S, Deer T. Neuromodulation of pelvic visceral pain: review of the literature and case series of potential novel targets for treatment. Pain Pract January 2013;13(1):3–17. https://doi.org/10.1111/j.1533-2500.2012.00558.x.

[8] Green IC, Cohen SL, Finkenzeller D, Christo PJ. Interventional therapies for controlling pelvic pain: what is the evidence? Curr Pain Headache Rep February 2016;20(2):10. https://doi.org/10.1007/s11916-016-0540-4.

[9] Hunter C, Stovall B, Chen G, Carlson J, Levy R. Anatomy, pathophysiology, and interventional therapies for chronic pelvic pain: a review. Pain Phys March 2018;21(2):147–67.

[10] Ploteau S, Labat JJ, Riant T, Levesque A, Robert R, Nizard J. New concepts on functional chronic pelvic and perineal pain: pathophysiology and multidisciplinary management. Discov Med March 2015;19(104):185–92.

[11] Janicki TI. Chronic pelvic pain as a form of complex regional pain syndrome. Clin Obstet Gynecol December 2003;46(4):797–803. https://doi.org/10.1097/00003081-200312000-00014.

[12] Hayek SM, Veizi E, Hanes M. Treatment-limiting complications of percutaneous spinal cord stimulator implants: a review of eight years of experience from an academic center database. Neuromodulation October 2015;18(7):603–8. https://doi.org/10.1111/ner.12316. discussion 608–608.

[13] Alo KM, Yland MJ, Redko V, Feler C, Naumann C. Lumbar and sacral nerve root stimulation (NRS) in the treatment of chronic pain: a novel anatomic approach and neuro stimulation technique. Neuromodulation January 1999;2(1):23–31. https://doi.org/10.1046/j.1525-1403.1999.00023.x.

[14] Barolat G. Epidural spinal cord stimulation: anatomical and electrical properties of the intraspinal structures relevant to spinal cord stimulation and clinical correlations. Neuromodulation April 1998;1(2):63–71. https://doi.org/10.1111/j.1525-1403.1998.tb00019.x.

[15] Jain E, Smith Z, Hunter CW. Targeting the Conus medullaris with closed loop stimulation for chronic pelvic pain: a case series. In: Poster presented at: North American Neuromodulation Society Annual Meeting; January 2024; Las Vegas, NV; 2024.

[16] Mekhail N, et al. Long-term safety and efficacy of closed-loop spinal cord stimulation to treat chronic back and leg pain (Evoke): a double- blind, randomised, controlled trial. Lancet Neurol February 2020;19(2):123–34. https://doi.org/10.1016/S1474-4422(19)30414-4.

[17] Tate JL, Stauss T, Li S, Rotte A, Subbaroyan J. A prospective, multi-center, clinical trial of a 10-kHz spinal cord stimulation system in the treatment of chronic pelvic pain. Pain Pract January 2021;21(1):45–53. https://doi.org/10.1111/papr.12932.

[18] Delibaş B, Elamin AAE, Kaplan S. Neuronal plasticity in dorsal root ganglia following sciatic nerve injury. Explor Neuroprot Ther 2024;4:148–57. https://doi.org/10.37349/ent.2024.00076.

[19] Inoue K, Tsuda M. Microglia in neuropathic pain: cellular and molecular mechanisms and therapeutic potential. Nat Rev Neurosci 2018;19:138–52. https://doi.org/10.1038/nrn.2018.2.

[20] Liem L, Russo M, Huygen FJPM, van Buyten JP, Smet I, Verrils P, Cousins M, Brooker C, Levy R, Deer T, Kramer J. A Multicenter, Prospective trial to assess the safety and performance of the spinal modulation dorsal root ganglion neurostimulator system in the treatment of chronic pain. Neuromodulation 2013;16:471–82. https://doi.org/10.1111/ner.12072.

[21] Patel KV. Dorsal root ganglion stimulation for chronic pelvic pain [39T]. Obstet Gynecol May 2019;133:223S. https://doi.org/10.1097/01.AOG.0000559141.59342.5f.

[22] Alshak MN. Neuroanatomy, sympathetic nervous system. 2019. Available from: https://www.ncbi.nlm.nih.gov/books/NBK542195/.

[23] Kinter KJ, Newton BW. Anatomy, abdomen and pelvis, pudendal nerve. In: StatPearls. Treasure Island, FL: StatPearls Publishing; 2023.

[24] Graziottin A, Gambini D. Anatomy and physiology of genital organs–women. Handb Clin Neurol 2015;130:39–60. https://doi.org/10.1016/B978-0-444-63247-0.00004-3.

[25] Elkins N, Hunt J, Scott KM. Neurogenic pelvic pain. Phys Med Rehabil Clin 2017;28:551–69. https://doi.org/10.1016/j.pmr.2017.03.007.

[26] Spinelli M, Giardiello G, Gerber M, Arduini A, van den Hombergh U, Malaguti S. New sacral neuromodulation lead for percutaneous implantation using local anesthesia: description and first experience. J Urol November 2003;170(5):1905–7. https://doi.org/10.1097/01.ju.0000092634.64580.9a.

[27] Gregory NS, Terkawi AS, Prabhakar NK, Tran JV, Salmasi V, Hah JM. Peripheral nerve stimulation for pudendal neuralgia: a technical note. Pain Med 2020;21(Suppl. 1):S51–5. https://doi.org/10.1093/pm/pnaa171.

[28] Carmel M, Lebel M, Tu le M. Pudendal nerve neuromodulation with neurophysiology guidance: a potential treatment option for refractory chronic pelvi-perineal pain. Int Urogynecol J 2010;21(5):613–6. https://doi.org/10.1007/s00192-009-1054-zPubMed.

[29] Peters KM, Killinger KA, Boguslawski BM, Boura JA. Chronic pudendal neuromodulation: expanding available treatment options for refractory urologic symptoms. Neurourol Urodyn 2010;29(7):1267–71. https://doi.org/10.1002/nau.20823.

[30] Armstrong GL, Vancaillie TG. Combined site-specific sacral neuromodulation and pudendal nerve release surgery in a patient with interstitial cystitis and persistent arousal. BMJ Case Rep 2016. https://doi.org/10.1136/bcr-2015-213513.

Chapter 12

Complications of neuromodulation of the spine

Chau Vu[1], Andrew Dudas[2], Warren Grace[3], Harjot S. Bhandal[1] and Jason E. Pope[1]

[1]*Evolve Restorative Center, Santa Rosa, CA, United States;* [2]*Mays & Schnapp Neurospine and Pain, Memphis, TN, United States;* [3]*Redefine Healthcare, Union, NJ, United States*

Introduction

Spinal Cord Stimulation (SCS) has revolutionized the field of interventional pain space offering a minimally invasive, opioid free solution for patients who have failed conservative medical management. Over the years, the field of neuromodulation has seen remarkable growth with innovations in hardware, waveforms, techniques such as dorsal root ganglion stimulation and peripheral nerve stimulation, and technology such as closed loop. These advancements enhance outcomes and improve quality of life [1]. Although there has been much innovation, the fundamental SCS procedure remains unchanged: a temporary trial is conducted to establish efficacy, and if successful, is followed by implantation of SCS leads and an impulse generator.

Although SCS is considered safe, complications can still occur. Large retrospective reviews and society guidelines, such as those from the Neuromodulation Appropriateness Consensus Committee (NACC), have improved awareness and provided consensus statements to guide therapy. However, it remains imperative that implanters be both knowledgeable of the potential risks and complications, but also be proficient in preventing, managing, and treating these complications effectively.

SCS-related complications can arise at any stage of the neuromodulation journey, from patient selection, the SCS trial, device implantation, or long-term management and follow-up. This chapter examines a variety of SCS-related complications in an effort to provide physicians and medical practitioners with the knowledge and potential strategies necessary to optimize outcomes and ensure the safe and effective use of SCS therapies.

A summarized list of the NACC guidelines for risk mitigation in SCS therapy is included at the end of the chapter.

Hardware-related complications

Lead migration

Lead migration is one of the most common complications leading to loss or change in coverage, which can result in inadequate pain relief or stimulation in unwanted areas. Lead migration is less common in dorsal root ganglion (DRG) stimulation compared to traditional dorsal column stimulation (DCS). This is one reason some physicians may prefer DRG stimulation over DCS for appropriate diagnoses. Lead migration rates are improved even further with the addition of lead anchoring. However, lead migration can still occur in both settings and remains the most common device-related complication occurring between 0% and 13.6% [2–7].

If a patient has a loss of coverage or a change in pain relief, a lead migration may be suspected. Lead migration can be diagnosed by comparing updated spinal X-rays to intraoperative images. The initial management is to attempt to program around the new position of the migrated lead. Many times, this will correct the problem. If this does not improve the stimulation coverage adequately, or if the lead is outside the epidural space, a lead revision must be performed. This entails opening the previous surgical incision, disengaging the anchor, and attempting to reposition the lead to a more appropriate location. If this cannot be done, the original lead must be removed and then replaced with a new lead. This can

A Modern Atlas for Implantable Devices of the Spine, Brain, and Nerve. https://doi.org/10.1016/B978-0-443-36528-7.00007-8

be difficult due to scar tissue formation around the initial site, which can make epidural and foraminal access more challenging.

Lead migration risk can be minimized by anchoring the leads to the supraspinous ligament, creating tension relief loops, and securing the implantable impulse generators (IPG) pocket. Postoperative precautions such as limiting twisting, bending, and lifting, or using bracing, may also help stabilize leads as they heal in place. Paddle leads should be considered for patients at high risk of migration.

Lead fracture

Lead fracture can occur due to mechanical stress, trauma, repetitive movement, or excessive tension on the leads, and occurs at a rate of 1.2%–9% [2,7]. Like lead migration, patients may experience loss of or a change in therapy. On device interrogation, impedances will be high in the setting of lead fracture. An X-ray can also be obtained to assess for a lead fracture. A microfracture (internal) will likely not be apparent on XR. If a lead fracture is suspected, it is reasonable to try to reprogram on the remaining lead. If coverage is lost, the lead must be surgically revised. This is done as per the previously described method; however, much care should be taken in order to avoid retention of the fractured lead. If there is any retained lead, it is typically left in place; however, surgical referral can be made for surgical extraction of the lead. Of note, if the lead is retained, the MRI compatibility of the device is lost even if the previously implanted system was MRI compatible. Lead fracture can be minimized by using tension relief loops, anchoring, and activity limitations in the postoperative period when leads have not healed in place.

Impulse generator failure or end of life

The expected lifespan of an IPG ranges from 5 to 10 years, with a median lifespan of 8–9 years, depending on manufacturer and energy usage [8].

End of life (EOL) of the IPG occurring before the expected lifespan is considered an IPG failure and may result from battery depletion, device malfunction, internal component defect, or possible trauma to the IPG. This occurs at a rate of ~1.7% [2]. Newer waveforms and high-energy programs can accelerate battery depletion, particularly in nonrechargeable IPGs and should be taken into account when programming patients.

With IPG failure, patients may notice more frequent recharging requirements, that the IPG is unable to hold a charge, or the device simply doesn't turn on. There may be a history of direct trauma to the battery or electricity/electrocautery that was applied to the IPG, causing the device to malfunction. IPG failure necessitates IPG replacement.

High lead impedances

High lead impedances render an electrode unusable and can alter pain relief or therapy. This can be detected through interrogation of the device by a representative. Often, reprogramming around the lead is possible. If not, the lead may need to be revised. Of note: high impedances can sometimes render a device MRI incompatible, and device and MRI compatibility labeling should be reviewed.

Surgical site complications

Surgical site infections

Surgical site infection (SSI) is among the most serious complications of SCS therapy and has been estimated between 3.4% and 10% [2,7]. The data, however, are mixed on this and fortunately newer studies have found a significant decrease in the rate as the procedure is used more often and newer recommendations for infection prevention have been presented and can be as low as 1.9%–2.88% [7,9].

SSI can lead to significant morbidity and healthcare costs, including hospitalizations, device explants, neurological complications, sepsis, etc. Early recognition and prompt treatment are crucial to prevent severe outcomes, while adherence to preventative measures can reduce infection risk.

The IPG pocket site is the most common location for infection; however, the infection can also track back to the midline incision and into the epidural space, leading to an epidural abscess, discitis, meningitis, vertebral osteomyelitis, or even neurologic deficits/paralysis [10]. Infections are typically characterized as superficial or deep, with superficial infections involving the skin and subcutaneous tissue and deep infections involving the muscle and fascia. According to the

CDC, superficial infections occur within 30 days of surgery, while deep infections occur within 1 year of surgery [11]. Deep infections can track back to the neuroaxis, and epidural abscesses involve the neuroaxis itself.

NACC guidelines recommend in-person evaluation of the surgical sites within 7–10 days of surgery. The incision should be inspected for signs of infection. These include warmth, erythema, induration, dehiscence, fever, and pus formation or drainage. The surgical site may be extremely tender to touch, with even slight pressure causing significant discomfort. Systemic signs of infection such as nausea, vomiting, fevers, chills, hypo or hypertension may or may not be encountered may or may not be encountered [2].

If an infection is suspected:

Labs such as CBC, ESR, and CRP should be sent and trended. It should be noted that these labs are often elevated due to a surgical response or stress. Upward trends can help diagnose infection. Empiric antibiotics should be initiated to cover the most common bacteria, typically skin flora, including *Staphylococcus aureus*, *Staphylococcus epidermidis*, *Escherichia coli, and Pseudomonas aeruginosa* [9,10]. Target antibiotic therapy should be instituted if/when cultures and sensitivities are available. Ultrasound can also be used to look for an indolent abscess, and a CT/MRI scan can be considered to rule out proximal tracking of infection.

Some superficial infections may be able to be managed conservatively using antibiotics with gram-positive coverage for 7–10 days. Superficial infections can track more proximally into the epidural space, and therefore vigilance and caution should be taken when managing conservatively. The patient should be followed at regular intervals (recommended at least weekly) until the infection has resolved. If at any time the infection appears to have worsened, the device should be removed, and the patient should be evaluated for a deeper infection. Failure to aggressively treat a superficial infection can lead to a deeper infection, including an epidural abscess and paralysis [10].

If a deep infection is suspected or if the patient develops new or worsening neurologic deficits, back pain, meningeal signs, an incision and drainage should be performed with cultures of the site fluid should be sent for cytological examination. The device should be explanted. If Empiric antibiotics should be started and adjusted based on cultures and sensitivity, usually for 7–10 days [10].

More complicated infections include discitis, osteomyelitis, meningitis, or epidural abscesses; these require an infectious disease consult to help guide treatment. If meningitis is suspected, a lumbar puncture is necessary.

An epidural abscess can present as back pain with localized tenderness, progressing to radicular pain, fever, neck stiffness, then motor, sensory, and reflex deficits, and ultimately paralysis. Once neurologic symptoms begin, emergent decompression should be performed. Neurologic recovery is unlikely if paralysis has been present for more than 12 h. Epidural abscesses are associated with high mortality and morbidity, especially if not recognized or treated appropriately [2,12,13].

Prevention is always the best treatment for infection. Table 12.1 is a summary of the NACC guidelines for infection mitigation [9].

Epidural hematoma

Epidural hematoma is the most feared complication of spinal cord stimulation and is treated as a surgical emergency. Evacuation of the hematoma is recommended within 8 h of neurologic deficit. Fortunately, estimated incidences of epidural hematoma are low (0.3%–0.75%) [2,7]. There are many bridging vessels in the epidural space, and there is a risk of violating one of these while accessing the epidural space. The presence of anticoagulants, antiplatelet therapies, and inherent clotting disorders greatly increases this risk. American Society for Regional Anesthesia (ASRA) guidelines should always be consulted for appropriate holding of anticoagulation therapy prior to neuraxial manipulation and for restarting after the procedure. Fortunately, small amounts of blood in the epidural space do not always lead to space-occupying lesions; however, if the bleeding leads to compression of the spinal cord, signs and symptoms of cauda equina syndrome can be elicited. Other signs of compression include new paresthesia (even when the device is turned off), weakness, and severe back and leg pain. If a hematoma is suspected, an emergent MRI is indicated, or a CT scan with and without contrast should be ordered if an MRI is contraindicated or not readily available, and surgical consultation should be initiated for decompression and hematoma evacuation [2].

Seroma/superficial hematoma

Seroma and hematoma are both postprocedural fluid collections that can occur at any incision site. Seromas involve the accumulation of clear or straw-colored fluid, while hematomas involve the accumulation. Seroma formation is estimated to occur in approximately 2%–3% of patients and is most commonly seen at the IPG site [2].

TABLE 12.1 Summary of the recommendations for infection control by the North American Neuromodulation Society (NACC) guidelines.

Preoperative	Identify and treat all remote infections before trials and implants
	Optimize glucose control
	Discontinue tobacco
	Decolonize MSSA/MRSA carriers with mupirocin nasal ointment and chlorhexidine washes
	Use weight-based preoperative antibiotics 1 hour prior to incision.
	Remove hair with electric clippers immediately before surgery.
	Perform a surgical scrub for at least 2–5 min with an antiseptic.
	Keep nails short; avoid artificial nails, hand or arm jewellery.
Intraoperative	Wear a sterile gown, gloves, a surgical mask, and fully cover your hair with a cap or hood.
	Use chlorhexidine gluconate as a skin antiseptic.
	If using an incise drape, choose iodophor-impregnated drapes.
	Maintain laminar airflow and HEPA filters in the OR.
	Keep procedure doors closed and limit traffic in and out of the room.
	Minimize tissue trauma, maintain hemostasis, eradicate dead space, and avoid electrocautery at the tissue surface.
	Irrigate with saline before wound closure.
	Limit operative time
Postoperative	Avoid topical antimicrobials
	Apply an occlusive dressing for 24–48 h
	Do not continue antibiotics beyond 24 h postoperatively.
	Wash hands before and after dressing changes, and use sterile technique for dressing changes
	Educate patients and families on incision care, SSI symptoms and when to report concerns.
	Keep procedure doors closed and limit traffic in and out of the room.
	Recognize deep surgical site infections within 1-year postimplant
	When SSI is suspected, prescribe antibiotics covering likely causative agents, considering local resistance patterns and culture results.

On physical exam, they present with edema and fluctuation on palpation without overt signs of infection such as erythema, high fever, leukocytosis, CRP, or ESR. On CT or MRI, they will appear as a fluid collection without rim enhancement, which is seen with an abscess.

Seromas and hematomas are typically managed with conservative measures, including compression, such as an abdominal binder, as most will reabsorb over time. In cases where they fail to reabsorb, cause significant discomfort, drainage of the fluid collection can relieve pressure, alleviate pain, and confirm the diagnosis. However, fluid will often reaccumulate, and drainage carries the risk of introducing bacteria to the site; therefore, risks versus benefits must be weighed before drainage is considered. If the site is drained, continued use of an abdominal binder can help reduce the risk of fluid reaccumulation. In some instances, revision may be required. While seromas and hematomas can be uncomfortable, hematomas, in particular, can create an environment for bacterial growth, increasing the risk of infection. Left untreated, an expanding or even stagnant fluid collection could affect tissue healing and lead to wound dehiscence.

The use of postoperative abdominal binders can limit the risk of seroma and hematoma formation. Following guidelines to discontinue anticoagulation, achieve adequate hemostasis, and minimize tissue manipulation during dissection can decrease the risk of hematoma formation [2,9].

IPG site pain

Discomfort at the IPG site is a common postprocedural issue and can result from direct pressure, device migraine, localized inflammation, or patient weight loss, causing the device to become more superficial. While this is typically self-limited, it can be managed with ice, compression, nonopioid medications, lidocaine patches, and managing patient expectations.

Strategies to mitigate IPG site pain include careful pocket creation, proper device positioning, avoid electrocautery in the superficial tissue layers when possible. If the pain is due to anatomical pressure over the rigid IPG, consider external padding or soft wrap, i.e., abdominal binder or gauze, to prevent or minimize external forces from rubbing or pushing the IPG. If pain persists, the patient may need a revision.

Poor wound healing or dehiscence

Patients with diabetes, smokers, those with peripheral vascular disease, or poor nutritional status are at higher risk for poor wound healing or dehiscence. Optimizing these conditions preoperatively, such as smoking cessation, glucose control, optimizing nutrition, along with meticulous wound closure, can help to mitigate the risk of these complications.

Revision and explant considerations

Indications include loss of efficacy, infection, hardware failure, or patient dissatisfaction. The decision to revise or explant a system should be individualized to the patient, weighing risk versus benefit.

Neurological and biological complications

Post dural puncture headache/dural puncture

Postdural puncture headache (PDPH) can be seen in up to 11% of cases; however, as with other risks, this has been much lower in newer studies [7]. The constellation of symptoms associated with PDPH is positional headache (worse with standing or sitting upright, improved with lying down), light sensitivity, nystagmus, nausea, neck pain, and improvement of symptoms with lying flat. This is a clinical diagnosis and is treated initially with caffeine, NSAIDs, and fluids. If these do not resolve the symptoms, an epidural blood patch can be employed. Some physicians perform a preemptive blood patch if they know they have violated the dura during trial or implantation; however, this is not generally recommended due to the increased risk of infection. If CSF is observed during needle placement, it is recommended to either abort the procedure or to attempt epidural access at a level above initial access. In cases where there is a persistent CSF leak, surgical consultation should be requested.

Nerve injury

There is a risk of direct nerve root damage or spinal cord damage with manipulation of the leads, as well as with epidural or transforaminal access, particularly with multiple attempts at needle or electrode placement. Patients may present with new or worsening pain, paresthesia, weakness, paralysis, or bowel or bladder dysfunction. If significant nerve injury is suspected, a thorough neurological exam should be performed along with an emergent CT scan with contrast to rule out other etiologies, such as hematoma, which can present similarly. Neurosurgery and Neurology should be consulted. In the setting of spinal cord injury or nerve compression from the lead, the device should be explanted.

To minimize the risk of nerve or spinal cord injury, it is recommended to either keep the patient awake or responsive on epidural access and lead placement or to use neuromonitoring if the patient is under general anesthesia. These interventions can help reduce but do not eliminate risk. Risk of nerve compression due to hardware can be reduced by reviewing preoperative MRI and exercising caution or avoiding areas with severe central or foraminal stenosis.

For DRG placement, a postoperative neuritis can occur more commonly due to manipulation of the lead within the foramen. This can be mitigated by keeping the patient awake or using neuromonitoring. An electromyogram (EMG), and nerve conduction studies (NCS) can be used to more fully diagnose persistent symptoms. The timing of these tests must be assessed, as it can take time to demonstrate nerve damage on EMG/NCS. Fortunately, radiculitis associated with DRG lead placement will typically resolve on its own.

In both instances of direct spinal cord damage or nerve root damage, steroids and neuropathic pain medications can be employed to help with the pain.

Allergic reaction

Allergic reactions to device hardware or intraoperative medications can mimic infection, leading to erythema, pain, and drainage from the incision. Obtaining lab work to rule out infection, as well as cytological testing, can differentiate the two pathologies; however, ultimate device removal may be necessary if the allergy is to the device itself. For patients with known allergy to a potential component of the device, some manufacturers offer allergy test kits that can be used prior to trial or implantation.

Patient specific and psychological complications

Patient specific factors: placebo versus nocebo effects

Spinal cord stimulation (SCS), like many medical interventions, is susceptible to both placebo and nocebo effects. The placebo effect, where patients experience improvement due to the expectation of benefit rather than the treatment itself, can be substantial in SCS trials. A meta-analysis by Duarte et al. (2020) suggests a larger treatment effect in RCTs using a placebo control than a sham control, highlighting the importance of sham-controlled trials [14]. This underscores the challenge of isolating the true therapeutic effect. Conversely, the nocebo effect, where negative expectations lead to adverse outcomes, can also play a role. It can also be influenced by genetic variants, conscious and nonconscious learning processes, personality traits, and psychological factors, all potentially causing increased pain or other negative symptoms due to their apprehension about the procedure or device. In addition, physician behaviors, environmental cues and the appearance of medical devices can induce negative expectations that dramatically influence pain perception and processing [15]. This interplay between expectation and experience necessitates careful patient counseling and management of expectations.

Patient selection and therapy outcomes

A critical factor impacting SCS success is appropriate patient selection. Patients with significant psychological comorbidities often experience poorer outcomes. Sparkes et al. (2015) observed that depression and autonomous coping (control over pain, ability to reduce pain, and catastrophizing) may impact sensory aspects such as pain intensity and disability scores, affecting the outcome of SCS treatment. It was also noted that age at time of implant and duration of pain prior to implant were also found to impact SCS efficacy [16]. These patients may struggle with device management, have difficulty interpreting sensory changes associated with stimulation, or exhibit behaviors that hinder effective therapy. Furthermore, unrealistic expectations regarding pain relief can lead to disappointment and dissatisfaction. Patients should be counseled to expect a reduction in pain intensity and improved function rather than complete pain elimination.

Device programming and management

In addition to patient selection, SCS effectiveness relies heavily on appropriate device programming and patient engagement. Noncompliance with recommended stimulation parameters can lead to suboptimal pain relief and device disuse. Patients may struggle to understand the complexities of programming, generator charging, and forget instructions. Clear and repeated education about device operation, including how to adjust stimulation settings and troubleshoot common issues, is essential. Simplifying the programming interface and providing easy-to-understand instructions can improve patient compliance. Some vendors offer virtual services to directly connect with patients without having to make an appointment with the implanting physician. Others have simple engagement applications installed on the patient's mobile device, giving them the ability to optimize SCS therapy under their own control.

In some cases, patients may find SCS ineffective in treating their pain. This can lead to device disuse and dissatisfaction. Some literature has explored the concept of virtual explants, where patients effectively stop using the device and discontinue follow-up, even though the device remains implanted. This highlights the importance of ongoing assessment and support to ensure patients are receiving optimal benefit from SCS. The Neurostimulation Appropriateness Consensus Committee (NACC) recommends that after a system has definitively failed to meet the pain relief objectives and has failed a troubleshooting paradigm, the decision to either leave the system in situ or seek to have it explanted should be made. Several aspects may influence this decision, including any local discomfort or restriction in activities (favoring explant) or whether the system is software/hardware upgradable (favoring retention) [17].

Proactive care, artificial intelligence, and data collection

To improve patient satisfaction and adherence, some SCS vendors offer simple and complex proactive care. This remote patient monitoring allows clinicians to track patient progress, identify potential compliance or device issues, and adjust stimulation parameters remotely. Remote monitoring can improve access to care, reduce the need for in-person visits, and enhance patient engagement [18]. Furthermore, the use of artificial intelligence (AI) and cloud data collection has optimized therapy outcomes in SCS. AI algorithms can analyze patient data to personalize stimulation therapy and predict potential complications. Cloud-based platforms can store and analyze large datasets to identify trends and improve treatment protocols. Lastly, the identification of patient unique physiologic biomarkers known as evoked compound action potentials (ECAPs) paired with an automatic programming workflow has optimized patient experience by providing faster, consistent programming and reducing clinic inefficiencies [19].

These advancements hold promise for improving patient outcomes and satisfaction with SCS.

Quality of life impact

Device limitations (MRI access)

MRI conditionality is a significant consideration for patients undergoing SCS. Desai et al. (2015), reported 82%–84% of SCS implanted patients are expected to need at least 1 MRI within 5 years of implant [20]. While newer MRI conditional SCS are available, they still require specific protocols and precautions, which can oftentimes be problematic for patients who require MRI scans for other medical conditions. Open communication between the patient, SCS vendor, implanting physician, and radiology facility is crucial to ensure safe and appropriate MRI procedures.

Long-term satisfaction

While some patients experience sustained pain relief and improved quality of life for years from SCS therapy, others may experience a decline in effectiveness over time. Habituation is described as "a behavioral response decrement that results from repeated stimulation, and that does not involve sensory adaptation/sensory fatigue or motor fatigue." It has been reported to occur in 13%–34% of patients treated with SCS [21]. Additional factors affecting loss of efficacy include disease progression, neural target changes, pain generator changes, and device malfunctions [17].

It's essential to provide patients with realistic expectations about the long-term benefits of SCS and emphasize the importance of ongoing management. Regular reassessment of pain, device function, and quality of life is crucial to optimize outcomes and addressing any emerging challenges.

Remote management and its impact on long-term satisfaction

Remote management of SCS devices has emerged as a promising approach to improve long-term satisfaction and outcomes. As highlighted in the expert recommendations by Staats et al. (2023), remote management offers several potential benefits [22]. It allows for more frequent monitoring of patients, enabling timely identification and management of issues such as changes in pain patterns, device malfunctions, or the need for programming adjustments. This proactive approach can potentially prevent minor issues from escalating and leading to device disuse or dissatisfaction.

Furthermore, remote management can enhance patient engagement and empowerment. By providing patients with a greater sense of control over their therapy and facilitating communication with their healthcare providers, remote management can foster a stronger therapeutic alliance. This can lead to improved adherence to treatment recommendations and increased satisfaction with SCS therapy.

The expert recommendations also emphasize the importance of proper utilization of remote management tools. This includes providing adequate training to patients and clinicians on how to use the technology effectively, establishing clear communication protocols, and ensuring data security and privacy. Future considerations include the integration of remote management data with electronic health records and the development of standardized protocols for remote programming and troubleshooting.

Psychological factors play a critical role in the success of SCS. Addressing these factors through careful patient selection, management of expectations, comprehensive education, and ongoing support is essential for optimizing treatment outcomes and maximizing patient satisfaction. Further research is needed to better understand the complex interplay between psychological factors and SCS outcomes to develop more effective strategies for improving patient care.

Programming, technological, and ethical challenges

Programming and device optimization challenges

Spinal cord stimulation (SCS) programming involves adjusting device settings to deliver electrical impulses to the dorsal column of the spinal cord by selecting the optimal combination of parameters. The four primary programming parameters include contact (electrode) selection, amplitude, pulse width, and frequency [23]. The expanding use of SCS for various pain conditions has led to the development of multiple waveforms. Traditionally, only tonic, or conventional, stimulation was available. However, newer waveforms such as high frequency, burst, differential target multiplexed, and multiphase stimulation have since been introduced.

Conventional stimulation is characterized by lower frequency, between 40 and 80 Hz, higher pulse width, ranging from 200 to 500 μS, and higher amplitude, typically between 3.5 and 8.5 mA, all of which result in a higher charge per pulse [24]. This increased charge generates an action potential at the stimulation site, which is necessary for pain relief. Several studies suggest that paresthesia overlapping the area of pain is essential for effective pain relief in conventional SCS [25]. This is achieved through waveform amplitude adjustments and electrode selection via intraoperative paresthesia mapping and postoperative programming. Although newer waveforms, such as high-frequency SCS, offer paresthesia-free stimulation, they still rely on the same fundamental principles of electrode targeting and waveform adjustments for optimal pain relief.

During the initial programming phase, multiple programs can be created based on patient preferences and activity levels. The selection of electrodes is based on patient anatomy and the location of pain. Typically, two percutaneous leads or one paddle lead are implanted. The shape of the electrical field generated by the device is determined by lead separation and is further modified by the arrangement of the cathode and anode. When leads are placed with less separation, the electrical field is larger, resulting in broader paresthesia coverage [26].

Amplitude controls the intensity of electrical stimulation delivered to the spinal cord. A higher amplitude activates more nerve fibers, but excessive stimulation can cause discomfort [26]. High-frequency SCS is an exception, as it allows for higher amplitudes without causing paresthesia. Conversely, a lower amplitude may fail to activate enough fibers, leading to inadequate pain relief. Additionally, higher amplitudes consume more energy, reducing battery life and requiring more frequent charging or replacement.

Pulse width refers to the duration of each electrical pulse and influences the depth of neural activation. Shorter pulse widths, typically less than 200 μS, activate small, superficial Aβ fibers, leading to more precise stimulation but often requiring higher amplitudes to reach deeper nerves. Longer pulse widths, generally greater than 200 μS, activate larger nerve fibers, resulting in broader pain coverage at lower amplitudes [27]. Patients with focal pain, such as radiculopathy, may benefit from shorter pulse widths, while those with more diffuse pain, such as failed back surgery syndrome, often require longer pulse widths for broader coverage [28]. A wider pulse width also utilizes more energy, necessitating a balance between energy conservation and therapy effectiveness, particularly for primary cell generators.

Frequency, defined as the number of electrical pulses delivered per second, influences neuronal firing rates and may contribute to axonal blocking at higher levels [29]. Lower frequencies are used in paresthesia-based SCS systems, while high-frequency systems, operating above 1000 Hz, enable paresthesia-free pain relief but require significantly more energy.

Given the number of systems and variables involved in programming, improper device settings can lead to suboptimal therapy outcomes or adverse effects. Inadequate pain relief may result from incorrect lead placement, lead migration, or suboptimal parameter settings. In some cases, the stimulation may fail to cover the intended pain area due to improper electrode activation. Amplitude, pulse width, and frequency settings must be carefully adjusted to improve pain control. Overstimulation can cause discomfort, often due to excessive amplitude or pulse width, and may be mitigated by adjusting these parameters while increasing frequency to smooth out the stimulation [23].

Device representatives play a critical role in SCS programming, troubleshooting, and optimization. However, reliance on representatives varies across clinical settings, and delays may occur when a representative is unavailable. To improve efficiency, physicians should be well-versed in SCS programming and work collaboratively with representatives. Newer automated programming platforms aim to address variations in training and expertise. These systems use biomarker-based automation, measuring evoked compound action potentials (ECAPs) to tailor stimulation to a patient's unique neural response [30]. Additionally, closed-loop SCS has emerged as a promising technology, automatically adjusting parameters in real-time based on ECAP measurements. Unlike traditional open-loop SCS systems, which require manual adjustments based on subjective patient feedback, closed-loop systems may improve patient satisfaction and lead to more durable outcomes while reducing the need for frequent reprogramming visits [31].

Emerging technology concerns

As SCS technology evolves, concerns arise regarding safety, optimization, long-term efficacy, and patient accessibility. AI-driven SCS systems are increasingly utilizing machine learning algorithms, raising challenges related to data privacy, security, patient safety, and regulatory oversight [32].

The use of AI in neuromodulation may reduce physician control over therapy settings. Some automated algorithms override manual adjustments made by clinicians, which could limit the ability to tailor therapy based on patient-reported feedback. Additionally, AI models used in SCS are typically trained on specific populations and may not generalize well to all patients. Biases in AI training could lead to reduced efficacy in underrepresented populations or inaccurate adjustments for diverse pain responses.

Patient data privacy is another emerging concern. SCS systems that rely on remote monitoring and cloud-based data storage increase the risk of cybersecurity threats, including unauthorized access to patient medical data and device settings. Current HIPAA regulations protect electronic health records but may not fully extend to AI-driven neuromodulation data. If security vulnerabilities are exploited, patients could face unauthorized changes to their stimulation parameters, potentially leading to harmful effects [33]. Future developments in AI-integrated SCS must prioritize robust encryption, multi-factor authentication, and transparency in AI decision-making to ensure patient safety.

Ethical considerations

Informed consent is a critical ethical requirement for any medical intervention, particularly for SCS, which involves a trial phase, permanent implantation, and ongoing programming adjustments. Patients must have a clear understanding of the risks, benefits, alternatives, and long-term expectations before proceeding with treatment [34].

Several challenges exist in obtaining truly informed consent for SCS. Some patients may misinterpret SCS as a guaranteed cure rather than a tool for managing chronic pain. Psychological factors, such as depression and anxiety, which are common among chronic pain patients, may impair rational decision-making [35]. Additionally, cognitive impairments from opioid therapy, gabapentinoids, or tricyclic antidepressants can further impact a patient's ability to provide informed consent.

To improve patient understanding, clinicians should use clear, nontechnical language and provide decision aids such as visuals, models, or videos to explain the procedure. Multiple discussions should take place before obtaining consent to ensure patients fully comprehend the process. A psychological screening should also be conducted before the SCS trial to assess the patient's ability to make informed decisions. The risks associated with AI-driven closed-loop SCS, and remote monitoring systems should also be disclosed as part of the informed consent process.

The cost-effectiveness of SCS remains a significant ethical consideration. While the initial investment in SCS implantation is substantial, numerous studies indicate that it provides long-term financial benefits. A systematic review by Niyomsri et al. analyzed 14 studies and found that SCS is cost-effective over extended periods, particularly for failed back surgery syndrome and complex regional pain syndrome [36]. Despite higher upfront costs, improvements in quality of life and reductions in ongoing medical expenses make SCS a financially viable option for appropriate candidates [37].

Spinal cord stimulation offers substantial benefits in pain relief, opioid reduction, and overall quality of life. However, to maximize its potential, clinicians must address ethical concerns related to informed consent, AI-driven automation, and cybersecurity. By ensuring that patients are well-informed and protected, SCS can be a highly effective tool in chronic pain management.

Risk mitigation strategies

Below is a summary of recommendations for complication/risk mitigation from the Neuromodulation Appropriateness Consensus Committee of the Internal Neuromodulation Society [2]:

1. **Training & Credentialing**: Implanters should be trained in accredited interventional pain or surgical programs and follow community standards for perioperative care.
2. **Surgical Environment**: Procedures should be performed with trained personnel in accredited sterile environments.
3. **Patient Selection & Evaluation**:
    - Neuromodulation should be considered before long-term opioid therapy.
    - Patients should be selected based on pain characteristics
    - Psychological evaluations should be performed by a credentialed psychologist
    - Treatment should be interdisciplinary, addressing pain, emotional well-being, and function.
4. **Preoperative Planning**:
    - Patients' cosmetic preferences, implant choice, and surgery timing should be considered.
    - A thorough preoperative discussion, informed consent, and coordination with other physicians are required.
    - Preoperative checklists, lab tests, and risk assessments (e.g., for anticoagulation) should be completed.
    - Anticoagulation risks should be assessed and held if appropriate
5. **Trialing & Implantation**: A trial for tolerability and efficacy should precede permanent implantation.
6. **Procedure Considerations**:
    - Anesthesia should allow real-time patient interaction when possible; otherwise, general anesthesia with monitoring is an option.
    - Perioperative antibiotics must be given within an hour before incision.
7. **Postoperative Care & Device Management**:
    - Inspection of the wound within 7–10 days postoperatively
    - Device programming should be done by trained professionals with appropriate monitoring.
    - Physicians should monitor outcomes and complications for quality control

Conclusion

While neuromodulation is not without risk, it remains a cornerstone of therapy for chronic pain patients. Innovations in SCS therapy, research and knowledge related to complications, as well as multi-disciplinary and society-driven guidelines have improved outcomes. Proper patient selection, meticulous surgical technique, and proactive device monitoring are essential in minimizing risk and optimizing outcomes. By recognizing and addressing these challenges, we enhance SCS therapies' safety, efficacy, and viability as a long-term pain management solution.

References

[1] Rauck RL, Loudermilk E, Thomson SJ, et al. Long-term safety of spinal cord stimulation systems in a prospective, global registry of patients with chronic pain. Pain Manag 2023;13(2):115–27. https://doi.org/10.2217/pmt-2022-0091.

[2] Deer TR, Mekhail N, Provenzano D, et al. The appropriate use of neurostimulation: avoidance and treatment of complications of neurostimulation therapies for the treatment of chronic pain. Neuromodulation Appropriateness Consensus Committee. Neuromodulation 2014;17(6):571–98. https://doi.org/10.1111/ner.12206.

[3] Deer TR, Stewart CD. Complications of spinal cord stimulation: identification, treatment, and prevention. Pain Med 2008;9(Suppl. 1):S93–101. https://doi.org/10.1111/j.1526-4637.2008.00444.x.

[4] Turner JA, Loeser JD, Deyo RA, Sanders SB. Spinal cord stimulation for patients with failed back surgery syndrome or complex regional pain syndrome: a systematic review of effectiveness and complications. Pain 2004;108(1–2):137–47.

[5] Kumar A, Felderhof C, Eljamel MS. Spinal cord stimulation for the treatment of refractory unilateral limb pain syndromes. Stereotact Funct Neurosurg 2003;81(1–4):70–4.

[6] Hagedorn JM, Misercola B, Comer A, Tari-Blake J, Hoffmann CM, Mehta P, Deer TR. The team approach to spinal cord and dorsal root ganglion stimulation: a guide for the advanced practice provider. Mayo Clin Proc Innov Qual Outcomes 2021;5(3):663–9. https://doi.org/10.1016/j.mayocpiqo.2021.05.002.

[7] Ho JS, Glicksman M, Kang K, Zhang EX, Phung AT, Thérond A, Fonseca AC, Bulat E, Schatman ME, Kaye AD, Hasoon J, Yazdi C, Gill J, Ruan Q, Robinson CL, Simopoulos T. Spinal cord stimulator complication rates: a single-institution, 22-year study (1999-2021). Pain Physician 2024;27(8):E909–17.

[8] Deer TR, Pope JE, Falowski SM, et al. Clinical longevity of 106,462 rechargeable and primary cell spinal cord stimulators: real world study in the medicare population. Neuromodulation 2023;26(1):131–8. https://doi.org/10.1016/j.neurom.2022.04.046.

[9] Deer TR, Provenzano DA, Hanes M, Pope JE, Thomson SJ, Russo MA, McJunkin T, Saulino M, Raso LJ, Lad SP, Narouze S, Falowski SM, Levy RM, Baranidharan G, Golovac S, Demesmin D, Witt WO, Simpson B, Krames E, Mekhail N. The Neurostimulation Appropriateness

Consensus Committee (NACC) recommendations for infection prevention and management. Neuromodulation 2017;20(1):31–50. https://doi.org/10.1111/ner.12565.

[10] Esquer Garrigos Z, Farid S, Bendel MA, Sohail MR. Spinal cord stimulator infection: approach to diagnosis, management, and prevention. Clin Infect Dis 2020;70(12):2727–35. https://doi.org/10.1093/cid/ciz994.

[11] Centers for Disease Control and Prevention. In: Guideline for prevention of surgical site infection; 1999. http://www.cdc.gov/hicpac/pdf/SSIguidelines.pdf.

[12] Van Zundert A. The epidural abscess: diagnosis and treatment. Highlights in regional anaesthesia and pain therapy IX. Barcelona, Spain: Permanyer Pub.; 2000. p. 159–62.

[13] Ameer MA, Knorr TL, Munakomi S, et al. Spinal epidural abscess. In: StatPearls. Treasure Island (FL): StatPearls Publishing; 2025. https://www.ncbi.nlm.nih.gov/books/NBK441890/.

[14] Duarte RV, Nevitt S, McNicol E, Taylor RS, Buchser E, North RB, Eldabe S. Systematic review and meta-analysis of placebo/sham controlled randomised trials of spinal cord stimulation for neuropathic pain. Pain 2020;161(1):24–35.

[15] Blasini M, Corsi N, Klinger R, Colloca L. Nocebo and pain: an overview of the psychoneurobiological mechanisms. Pain Rep 2017;2(2):e585.

[16] Sparkes E, Duarte RV, Mann S, Lawrence TR, Raphael JH. Analysis of psychological characteristics impacting spinal cord stimulation treatment outcomes: a prospective assessment. Pain Physician 2015;18(3):E369–77.

[17] Deer T, Russo M, Grider J, Sayed D, Lamer T, Dickerson D, Hagedorn J, Petersen E, Fishman M, FitzGerald J, Baranidharan G, Ridder D, Chakravarthy K, Al-Kaisy A, Hunter C, Buchser E, Chapman K, Gilligan C, Hayek S, Robert Md. The Neurostimulation Appropriateness Consensus Committee (NACC): recommendations for spinal cord stimulation long-term outcome optimization and salvage therapy. Neuromodulation 2024;27. https://doi.org/10.1016/j.neurom.2024.04.006.

[18] Naidu RK, Kapural L, Li S, Tourjé C, Rutledge J, Dickerson D, Lubenow TR. A review of the prospera spinal cord stimulation system with multiphase stimulation and proactive care. Curr Pain Headache Rep 2025;29(1):25.

[19] Antony A, Pope J, Goree J, Smith G, Petersen E, Sayed D, Lam C, Gilmore C, Kapural L. Novel automated platform to upgrade SCS programming experience from subjective to objective - results from a prospective, dose-controlled closed-loop clinical study. In: Presented at: 2025 North American Neuromodulation Conference; 2025.

[20] Desai MJ, Hargens LM, Breitenfeldt MD, Doth AH, Ryan MP, Gunnarsson C, Safriel Y. The rate of magnetic resonance imaging in patients with spinal cord stimulation. Spine 2015;40(9):E531–7.

[21] Levy RM, Mekhail N, Kramer J, et al. Therapy habituation at 12 months: spinal cord stimulation versus dorsal root ganglion stimulation for complex regional pain syndrome type I and II. J Pain 2020;21:399–408.

[22] Staats P, et al. Remote management of spinal cord stimulation devices for chronic pain: expert recommendations on best practices for proper utilization and future considerations. Neuromodulation 2023;26(7):1295–308.

[23] Sheldon B, Staudt MD, Williams L, Harland TA, Pilitsis JG. Spinal cord stimulation programming: a crash course. Neurosurg Rev 2021;44(2):709–20. https://doi.org/10.1007/s10143-020-01299-y.

[24] Lam CM, Latif U, Sack A, Govindan S, Sanderson M, Vu DT, Smith G, Sayed D, Khan T. Advances in spinal cord stimulation. Bioengineering 2023;10(2):185. https://doi.org/10.3390/bioengineering10020185.

[25] North RB, Kidd DH, Zahurak M, James CS, Long DM. Spinal cord stimulation for chronic, intractable pain: experience over two decades. Neurosurgery 1993;32(3):384–95. https://doi.org/10.1227/00006123-199303000-00008.

[26] Sammartino F, Jain E, Asaad F, Ericson T. Approach to spinal cord stimulation programming: a problem-based learning discussion. ASRA Pain Medicine 2024. https://asra.com/news-publications/asra-updates/blog-landing/legacy-b-blog-posts/2024/02/13/approach-to-spinal-cord-stimulation-programming-a-problem-based-learning-discussion.

[27] Yearwood TL, Hershey B, Bradley K, Lee D. Pulse width programming in spinal cord stimulation: a clinical study. Pain Physician 2010;13(4):321–35.

[28] Crosby ND, Goodman Keiser MD, Smith JR, Zeeman ME, Winkelstein BA. Stimulation parameters define the effectiveness of burst spinal cord stimulation in a rat model of neuropathic pain. Neuromodulation 2015;18(1):1–8. https://doi.org/10.1111/ner.12221.

[29] Miller JP, Eldabe S, Buchser E, Johanek LM, Guan Y, Linderoth B. Parameters of spinal cord stimulation and their role in electrical charge delivery: a review. Neuromodulation 2016;19(4):373–84. https://doi.org/10.1111/ner.12438.

[30] Pope JE, Antony A, Petersen EA, Rosen SM, Sayed D, Hunter CW, Goree JH, Vu CM, Bhandal HS, Shumsky PM, Bromberg TA, Smith GL, Lam CM, Kalia H, Lee JM, Khurram A, Gould I, Karantonis DM, Deer TR. Identifying SCS trial responders immediately after postoperative programming with ECAP dose-controlled closed-loop therapy. Pain Ther 2024;13(5):1173–85. https://doi.org/10.1007/s40122-024-00631-4.

[31] Mekhail NA, Levy RM, Deer TR, Kapural L, Li S, Amirdelfan K, Pope JE, Hunter CW, Rosen SM, Costandi SJ, Falowski SM, Burgher AH, Gilmore CA, Qureshi FA, Staats PS, Scowcroft J, McJunkin T, Carlson J, Kim CK, Yang MI, Stauss T, Petersen EA, Hagedorn JM, Rauck R, Kallewaard JW, Baranidharan G, Taylor RS, Poree L, Brounstein D, Duarte RV, Gmel GE, Gorman R, Gould I, Hanson E, Karantonis DM, Khurram A, Leitner A, Mugan D, Obradovic M, Ouyang Z, Parker J, Single P, Soliday N, EVOKE Study Group. ECAP-controlled closed-loop versus open-loop SCS for the treatment of chronic pain: 36-month results of the EVOKE blinded randomized clinical trial. Reg Anesth Pain Med 2024;49(5):346–54. https://doi.org/10.1136/rapm-2023-104751.

[32] Hagedorn JM, George TK, Aiyer R, Schmidt K, Halamka J, D'Souza RS. Artificial intelligence and pain medicine: an introduction. J Pain Res 2024;17:509–18. https://doi.org/10.2147/JPR.S429594.

[33] Zhong T, William HM, Jin MY, Abd-Elsayed A. A review of remote monitoring in neuromodulation for chronic pain management. Curr Pain Headache Rep 2024;28(12):1225–33. https://doi.org/10.1007/s11916-024-01302-x.

[34] Cocanour CS. Informed consent-It's more than a signature on a piece of paper. Am J Surg 2017;214(6):993–7. https://doi.org/10.1016/j.amjsurg.2017.09.015.

[35] Sheng J, Liu S, Wang Y, Cui R, Zhang X. The link between depression and chronic pain: neural mechanisms in the brain. Neural Plast 2017;2017:9724371. https://doi.org/10.1155/2017/9724371.

[36] Niyomsri S, Duarte RV, Eldabe S, Fiore G, Kopell BH, McNicol E, Taylor RS. A systematic review of economic evaluations reporting the cost-effectiveness of spinal cord stimulation. Value Health 2020;23(5):656–65. https://doi.org/10.1016/j.jval.2020.02.005.

[37] McClure JJ, Desai BD, Ampie L, You W, Smith JS, Buchholz AL. A systematic review of the cost-utility of spinal cord stimulation for persistent low back pain in patients with failed back surgery syndrome. Glob Spine J 2021;11(Suppl. 1):66S–72S. https://doi.org/10.1177/2192568220970163.

Section 4

Dorsal root ganglion

Introduction to section 4 dorsal root ganglion

Timothy R. Deer, MD

The development of new therapies is typically driven by the unmet needs of specific patient populations. This is true for the therapy known as dorsal root ganglion stimulation (DRG-S). Spinal cord stimulation (SCS), developed in the 1960s, has been increasingly used for various painful conditions but shows specific failures based on pain patterns and diagnosis. These failures of therapy include neuropathic foot pain, focal nerve pain after surgery, and complex regional pain syndrome. Based on this unmet need, DRG-S was developed [1].

The process involved a focus on the known neurophysiology of the DRG and the role it plays in the sensitization of the peripheral nervous system when a neural injury occurs. Much work had been done in neurolytic processes to destroy the DRG or the DRG region of initial synapse in the cord. These destructive procedures often led to pain relief or reduction, but were complicated by severe and permanent complications, deafferentation syndromes, and failures. In animal models, it was determined than the application of current to the DRG led to a reduction of the transmission of the pain signal without an irreversible surgical procedure. It was this work that led to the development of the lead configuration that led to the current system known as the DRG-S [2,3]. This required extensive work on a sheath to deliver the lead and a generator that could deliver current in micro doses.

Once the lead system was developed, the next step was to develop a clinical evidence portfolio that would lead to patient access and reimbursement. The steps included a first in human publication, a multicenter international study, and, eventually, an investigational device exemption Food and Drug Administration-regulated approval study in the United States [4]. These data were positive, leading to the United States approval in 2016. This approval is important because for the past several years an extensive experience has led to very good data on the treatment of the foot, knee, and other areas where focal nerve pain exists. In addition, ongoing research may lead to improved indications and the salvage of many other failed therapies in this complex patient group. Safety analyses have shown that DRG-S is safe and effective as compared to other forms of neurostimulation [5]. The following sections will cover the indications, targets, methods, and best practices for DRG-S.

References

[1] Deer TR, Levy RM, Kramer J, Poree L, Amirdelfan K, Grigsby E, Staats P, Burton AW, Burgher AH, Obray J, Scowcroft J, Golovac S, Kapural L, Paicius R, Kim C, Pope J, Yearwood T, Samuel S, McRoberts WP, Cassim H, Netherton M, Miller N, Schaufele M, Tavel E, Davis T, Davis K, Johnson L, Mekhail N. Dorsal root ganglion stimulation yielded higher treatment success rate for complex regional pain syndrome and causalgia at 3 and 12 months: a randomized comparative trial. Pain 2017;158(4):669–81. https://doi.org/10.1097/j.pain.0000000000000814.

[2] Guha D, Shamji MF. The dorsal root ganglion in the pathogenesis of chronic neuropathic pain. Neurosurgery 2016;63(Suppl 1):118–26. https://doi.org/10.1227/NEU.0000000000001255.

[3] Kent AR, Min X, Hogan QH, Kramer JM. Mechanisms of dorsal root ganglion stimulation in pain suppression: a computational modeling analysis. Neuromodulation 2018;21(3):234–46. https://doi.org/10.1111/ner.12754.

[4] Deer TR, Pope JE, Lamer TJ, Grider JS, Provenzano D, Lubenow TR, FitzGerald JJ, Hunter C, Falowski S, Sayed D, Baranidharan G, Patel NK, Davis T, Green A, Pajuelo A, Epstein LJ, Harned M, Liem L, Christo PJ, Chakravarthy K, Gilmore C, Huygen F, Lee E, Metha P, Nijhuis H, Patterson DG, Petersen E, Pilitsis JG, Rowe JJ, Rupert MP, Skaribas I, Sweet J, Verrills P, Wilson D, Levy RM, Mekhail N. The neuromodulation appropriateness consensus committee on best practices for dorsal root ganglion stimulation. Neuromodulation 2019;22(1):1–35. https://doi.org/10.1111/ner.12845.

[5] Deer T, Pope J, Hunter C, Falowski S, Kapural L, Kramer J, Levy R. Safety analysis of dorsal root ganglion stimulation in the treatment of chronic pain. Neuromodulation 2020;23(2):239–44. https://doi.org/10.1111/ner.12941.

Chapter 13

Cervical dorsal root ganglion stimulation

Timothy Lubenow[1], Alexandra Moreira[2], Boss Povieng[3] and Johnson S. Ho[4]

[1]*Midwest Anesthesia and Pain Specialists, Interventional Pain Management, Chicago, IL, United States;* [2]*Southern Pain and Spine, Interventional Pain Management, Atlanta, GA, United States;* [3]*Insight Medical Center Chicago, Interventional Pain Management, Chicago, IL, United States;* [4]*Department of Interventional Pain Management, NJ Spine and Orthopedic, West Orange, NJ, United States*

Introduction

Because of a variable degree of efficacy for focal neuropathic pain with traditional spinal cord stimulation (SCS) coupled with the advancement in technology and identification of new targets, dorsal root ganglion stimulation (DRG-S) has emerged as a refinement in the application of neuromodulation. The DRG-S system employs a unique lead, distinct from those of conventional SCS systems. DRG-S has been shown to reduce focal lower extremity pain and trunk pain as well as to treat lower extremity chronic neuropathic pain, including phantom limb pain (PLP) and complex regional pain syndrome (CRPS) types I and II. The safety and effectiveness trial of spinal cord stimulation of the DRG for chronic lower limb pain, known as the ACCURATE study, demonstrated that DRG-S was superior in achieving greater than or equal to 50% reduction in pain relief compared to low-frequency tonic SCS in patients with lower extremity chronic pain [1]. The study included patients with CRPS Type I and Type II of the lower extremities, which, as of 2016, are the sole Federal Drug Administration (FDA) approved indications for DRG stimulation therapy in the US. Cervical and upper thoracic DRG stimulation remains an off-label indication in the United States. CRPS occurs more commonly in the upper extremities than the lower extremities [2,3]. A retrospective review from a single center including 20 patients with upper extremity CRPS demonstrated a similar degree of positive outcomes, with 85% of patients experiencing 50% or greater pain relief, supporting the use of DRG-S in the upper extremities [4,5]. The only other publication in the literature is a multicenter case series of successful use of DRG-S in the upper thoracic and cervical vertebral levels of 20 patients with a variety of chronic neuropathic pathologies, five of which were CRPS [6]. This chapter will discuss the important procedural considerations using DRG stimulation for pain conditions in cervical and high thoracic dermatomes.

Key points

- The cell bodies of primary sensory nerves are located within the DRG, which can be found in the neuroforamina bilaterally.
- Approximately 72% of the time, the C1 level does not contain a DRG.
- The C2–C8 DRGs are consistently located underneath the pedicles of C2–C7.
- Sensory innervation exhibits a form of duplicity due to arborization of the brachial plexus and the presence of Lissauer's tract within the cord, allowing the stimulation of specific DRG to confer downstream effects that may exist beyond the expected boundaries of the respective dermatome.
- Cervical and high thoracic DRG-S is promising but currently characterized as off-label for chronic painful conditions, including CRPS types I and II of the upper extremities by the FDA.
- DRG-S of the cervical and high thoracic dermatomes is an inherently more complex and challenging procedure than the lower thoracic and lumbosacral segments.
- There is an inherent increased risk of neurologic injury in the cervical and high thoracic spine due to the presence of natural cervical cord enlargement, which contributes to the smaller distance between the ligamentum flavum and the dura.

A Modern Atlas for Implantable Devices of the Spine, Brain, and Nerve. https://doi.org/10.1016/B978-0-443-36528-7.00037-6

Relevant anatomy

Summary of relevant anatomy

The formation of the dorsal root ganglia (DRG) is a complex process that involves coordinated migration, differentiation, and maturation of neural crest cells, influenced by intricate genetic and molecular mechanisms. This development is crucial for establishing the sensory pathways that enable the perception of external stimuli. As the neural tube closes, neural crest cells begin to migrate laterally and ventrally along specific pathways. These cells are highly migratory and differentiate into a variety of cell types, including neurons and glial cells of the peripheral nervous system [7]. The anatomy of the cervical and thoracic spine is outlined in the previous Anatomical chapters of this text (See the Anatomy Chapters on Cervical and Thoracic Spine Anatomy). For this chapter, we will expand on the anatomy of the dorsal root and neuroforamen.

The Dorsal root

The primary sensory nerve soma of the pseudounipolar neuron, as well as supporting glial and immune cells, constitute the cellular unit of the DRG. At the intersection of the T-junction, the DRG has an afferent axonal sensory limb from the periphery as well as an efferent projection into the central nervous system by means of the dorsal horn of the spinal cord, as demonstrated in Fig. 13.1 [8]. There is a diversity of neuronal fiber types pertaining to the DRG, with such elements as A-beta and A-delta fibers having associations with allodynic response [9]. In the cervical region, sensory innervation exhibits a form of duplicity due to two main factors: the arborization of the brachial plexus and the presence of Lissauer's tract. The brachial plexus, a network of nerves, contributes to this duplicity by distributing sensory fibers to the upper limb, allowing overlapping sensory territories. Additionally, Lissauer's tract, located in the spinal cord, facilitates the spread of sensory signals across multiple spinal segments. Together, these structures create a complex and overlapping sensory map, enhancing redundancy and ensuring robust sensory input from the cervical region. This capacity to allow for cross-talk has been reported and may allow for coverage beyond the anticipated boundaries of a respective DRG's anticipated dermatome [10]. The DRG itself is surrounded by cerebrospinal fluid and is sheathed in dura mater extending peripherally from the spinal cord, terminating in the lateral area in the furrow inferior to each segment's transverse process, as depicted in Fig. 13.2 [11]. There are seven pairs of cervical DRG and 12 pairs of thoracic DRG that belong to the exiting nerve roots. The cervical and thoracic spinal canals house the spinal cord proper. The presence of spinal cord and cervical cord expansion occurs in the segments of C5-T1 [12]. Due to this anatomy, there is an inherently greater risk of neurologic injury from inadvertent forces during the procedure when compared to dorsal root ganglion stimulation (DRG-S) in the lumbar spine. Further, the dorsal depth of the cervical spine epidural space has been reported to range between 1 and 1.5 mm (C5) mm compared with 2.5–3 mm in the thoracic spine (T6) and 5–6 mm in the lumbar spine (L2)

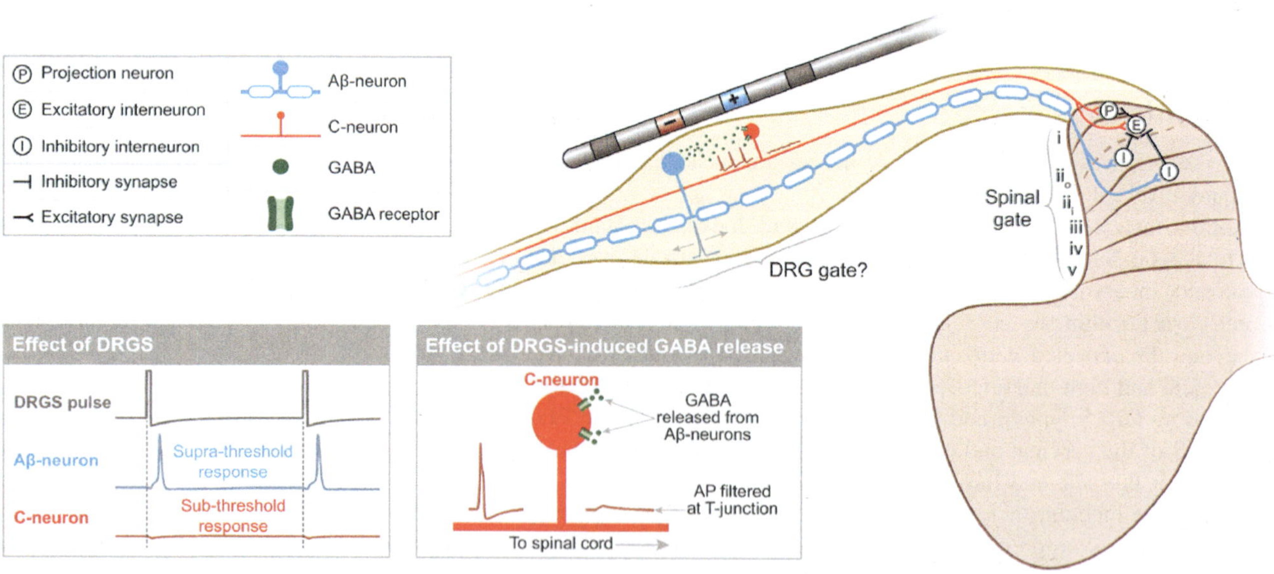

FIGURE 13.1 A depiction of the pseudounipolar neurons that constitute the DRG. DRGS applies trains of electrical pulses which induce APs in Aβ-neurons, which activate inhibitory interneurons in lamina iii and iii in the dorsal horn. Concurrently, Aβ-neurons may release GABA within the DRG, which can act on C-neurons and potentially prevent ectopic APs from propagating to the spinal cord. *From [8]; 23(2):196–211. https://doi.org/10.1016/j.jpain.2021.07.008*

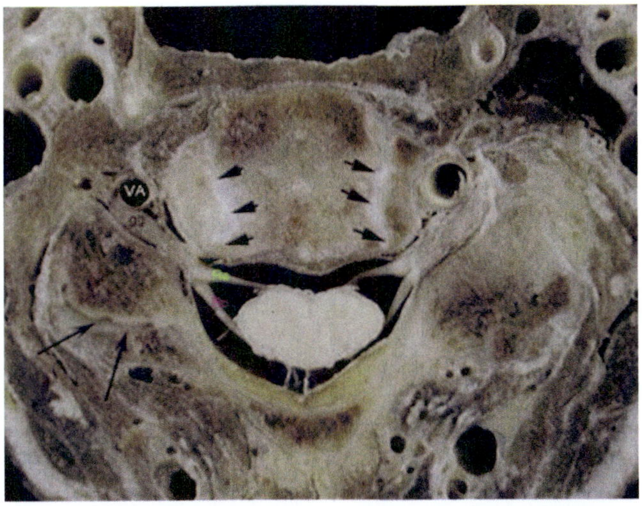

FIGURE 13.2 Horizontal midcervical slice, showing the relations of the nerve roots in the intervertebral foramen. Ra: anterior root; Rp: posterior root; gg: spinal ganglion; VA: vertebral artery; short arrow: uncus; long arrows: Posterior facet joint. *From [11]; 93(9):690–697. https://doi.org/10.1016/j.diii.2012.07.008.*

[13]. For this reason, the highest cephalad segment of epidural access is recommended to be C6–C7 at most [14]. In addition to depth, the smaller diameter of the cervical epidural space merits careful consideration, as there may be less margin to accommodate the S-loops created to anchor the leads. It has been recommended in a previous publication to avoid placing hardware in a region within the cervical spine where the anterior-posterior diameter is less than 13 mm [4]. It remains important to note that there exists intrinsic variability in cervical spinal canal diameters, given factors such as height, sex and ethnicity that should be considered [15].

The Neuroforamen

The neuroforamina themselves are formed superiorly and inferiorly by the pedicles of the adjacent vertebra, by the vertebral uncovertebral joint anteriorly, and by the facet joint posteriorly. The cervical neuroforamina have a smaller area and shallower dimension than their counterparts in the lumbar spine. This increases procedural complexity in placing cervical and high thoracic DRG-S leads. The osseous borders of the neuroforamina house the DRG as well as closely associated radicular arteries and venous components.

There is a variable vascular supply to the cervical cord. The upper and middle cervical cord are fed by two anterior spinal arteries and two to three anterior radiculomedullary arteries. Due to anatomic variation there C7 and upper thoracic cord segments may be vascularized by a single anterior radiculomedullary artery [11]. The few anatomical studies examining the foraminal ligaments of the cervical spine suggest that cervical DRG and vascular bundle tend to be suspended within the foramen by numerous thin intraforaminal ligaments [16], and unlike the lumbar spine, the DRG tends to be more closely tethered to venous components rather than epidural fat [11]. The spinal nerve is further supported by extraforaminal ligaments in the lateral furrow under the respective transverse process, namely the transforaminal ligament, costotransverse ligament, and anterior superior costotransverse ligament, which have similar counterparts within the thoracic spine. [17]. The anatomy of the neuroforamen in sagittal views from cadaveric and radiographic display is depicted in Fig. 13.3. In this chapter, we will discuss the technical aspects of placing the needle, introducer sheath and the electrode. It is important to understand the significant differences in neuroforaminal area in the various levels of the cervical spine when in flexed position compared to extended and neutral positions [18]. This is significant when performing preoperative planning, as seen in Fig. 13.4.

Procedure

Indications

DRG-S is a type of neuromodulation therapy used to manage chronic pain. It is particularly effective for certain conditions where traditional spinal cord stimulation might not be as successful. DRG-S is currently approved by the US Food and

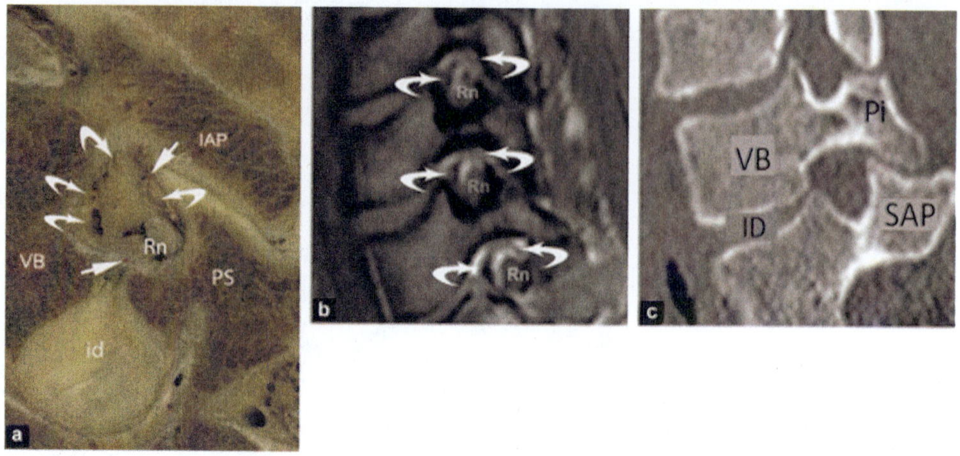

FIGURE 13.3 Midportion of a cervical intervertebral foramen studied in an oblique sagittal plane perpendicular to the axis of the transverse processes: a: Anatomical slices; b: MRI T1-weighted sagittal slice; c: CT slice, constant. CV: Vertebral body; id: intervertebral disc; IAP: Inferior articular process; SAP: Superior articular process; Rn: nerve roots; curved arrows: Foraminal veins; arrows: Arteries. *From [11]; 93(9):690–697. https://doi.org/10.1016/j.diii.2012.07.008.*

Drug Administration for the treatment of neuropathic pain associated with complex regional pain syndrome (CRPS) and/or causalgia in the groin and lower extremity [19,20]. The following diagnoses are considered on-label indications: Complex regional pain syndrome type 1 (G90.52), and Complex regional pain syndrome type 2 (G57.7). Other off-label indications include: posthernia [21], postarthroplasty [22], phantom limb [23], postabdominal surgery [24], pelvic pain [25], postthoracotomy pain [26], peripheral diabetic neuropathy [27], Postherpetic neuralgia [28], Persistent Postsurgical Pain Syndrome [24] and mononeuropathies [29].

Patient selection considerations

There are many factors to consider when selecting patients for cervical dorsal root ganglion stimulation. DRG-S has been demonstrated as superior to treating focal neuropathic pain conditions in the lower extremities. Cervical DRG stimulation may be as successful in treating upper extremity neuropathic pain conditions. The anatomy of the cervical canal is important to understand for patient safety and optimal outcomes using this therapy. The normal anteroposterior dimension of the cervical canal is 15 mm or greater. Congenital spinal canal stenosis is described when the canal diameter is 13 mm. This procedure is contraindicated in patients with a cervical canal less than or equal to 12 mm in AP diameter [4]. Elderly patient populations may make DRG-S placement more technically challenging due to the associated comorbid condition

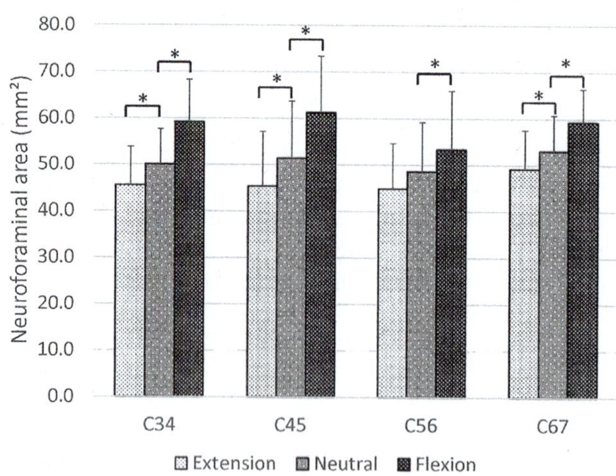

FIGURE 13.4 Neuroforaminal width of the four segments in three positions during dynamic flexion-extension. * there were significant differences between the neutral position and flexion or extension ($P < 0.05$). Error bars represent the standard deviations. Differences in area in neuroforamen by cervical spine level in extension, neutral and flexion positions. *From [18]; 16(4):540–546. https://doi.org/10.1016/j.spinee.2015.11.052.*

of degenerative arthritis. On the other end of the age spectrum, teenagers and above do not necessarily serve as a contraindication to neuromodulation, including cervical DRG [30].

Maintenance concerns

Cervical DRG stimulation to focal neuropathic painful areas in the upper extremities permits the use of lower electrical dose delivery to the central nervous system with a nonrechargeable battery pack that should last more than 5 years. Maintenance of this therapy is the same as DRG-S limitations in the lumbar region, which is dictated by battery life, reprogramming parameters, and potential revisions.

Training recommendations and suggested case volume for competence

Implanting physicians should have completed an ACGME pain medicine fellowship and must have sufficient skill and experience in performing lower extremity DRG before contemplating using this technique in the cervical region. The senior author has recommended that one should not attempt cervical DRG until one has demonstrated a proficiency in DRG-S in the lumbar spine region, performing a volume of at least 80 DRG-S implants.

Case peer review

Certain local hospital systems may require that you have a proctor available to you when you do your first several cervical DRG-S cases. There are no requirements currently at the society or industry level.

Technique

Patient positioning

As with the implantation of other neuromodulation devices, proper patient positioning is paramount, especially when it comes to cervical DRG-S. With the patient placed in a prone position with arms tucked at the sides, it is critical to minimize or eliminate cervical lordosis while maintaining patient comfort, to maximize posterior interlaminar space opening, neuroforaminal width, and optimise setup for smooth and successful lead placement.

Anesthesia considerations

Patient-specific anesthetic considerations rely on the balance between patient comfort, safety and efficiency [1]. It is important that patients can interact and provide real-time clinical feedback during procedures that carry the risk of injury to neural structures, as the primary monitor of neurological function. Therefore, it is optimally preferable for patients to be fully awake and conversant, and responsive to painful stimuli, to be able to detect and minimize likelihood of nerve injury. However, placement of cervical DRG electrodes in an awake patient with local anesthesia only is usually possible only in select patients. Because there are portions of the procedure that can be associated with transient pain such as navigating of intraforaminal ligaments, with nerves nearby that are usually already hypersensitized, it is important to be able to offer appropriate analgesia as needed, such as with light or medium sedation with careful monitoring and titration of medications, including midazolam, fentanyl, propofol, and/or dexmetomidine. General anesthesia is also an option; however, in these instances, intraoperative neuromonitoring (IONM) would be recommended to detect potential abnormalities in real time. Electrophysiological monitoring factors to monitor include changes in latency or amplitude of somatosensory evoked potentials (SSEPs), or findings of neurotonic discharges with motor evoked potentials (MEPs) that, when detected, may be suggestive of neural insult or injury. When using neuromonitoring, it is important to also be aware of the influence that anesthetic agents have on recordings, such as the fact that neuromuscular blockages and benzodiazepines depress MEPs, while volatile anesthetics and propofol depress MEPs, and additionally increase latency and decrease amplitude of SSEPs [1].

Operating room time estimate

Operating room time estimate would typically be similar to that of traditional spinal cord stimulator trial and permanent procedures, with a difference of more time buffer recommended to account for the additional leads and finesse required for placement of DRG leads, especially to the cervical region, and depending on anesthesia and use of neuromonitoring considerations.

Relevant vendor support

The vendor representative should be physically present in the room when performing cervical DRG stimulation procedures. In addition to the support they give, it is important to be familiar with the hardware provided within the kit, including a 14-gauge modified Tuohy needle, large introducer sheaths, stylet, guidewire, and electrode leads.

Procedure appropriate intraoperative imaging

Regarding the technique of performing the procedure itself, there are two primary approaches. First is the traditional approach that uses a contralateral paramedian technique that places leads via an oblique angle contralateral to the target foramen, along a line drawn between the target foramen below the pedicle, epidural entry at the midpoint of the vertebral interbody interspace preferably at one level below, and skin entry point that is typically 1.5 to two levels below the interlaminar target.

The difference with DRG stimulation application to the cervical region compared to lower lumbar levels is a slightly more medial and steeper angle taken for entry. After midline needle entry to the epidural space preferably along the inferior 1/3 point of the space in AP view, and confirming depth on lateral fluoroscopy view, needle bevel and introducer sheath are pointed toward the foramen, with care taken to gently advance the introducer sheath and lead combination into superior aspect of the target foramen along the seven o'clock (left) and five o'clock (right) borders of the pedicle, until lead contacts are parked with the two middle contacts immediately underneath the pedicle in the vertical interpedicular zone, noting to avoid directing the needle and introducer sheath too medially and avoid advancing the sheath itself into the foramen. A lateral view is taken to confirm the lead position in the neural foramen. Leads can be tested for impedance at this point, with position confirmed by radiology, neuromonitoring or mapping.

Figure 13.5 and 13.6 are examples of final AP and lateral views of DRG leads placed to the left C6 and C7 neural foramen via contralateral paramedian technique, with epidural access obtained at the C7-T1 interspace for the C6 DRG lead so as not to enter the epidural space above C7-T1 for safety considerations, and T1-T2 interspace accessed for C7 DRG lead. Here, after entering the epidural space, the introducer sheath was advanced up to the C5-6 level and passed through the neuroforamina at the C5-6 level. Figure 13.7 and 13.8 are AP and lateral views of DRG leads placed to Left

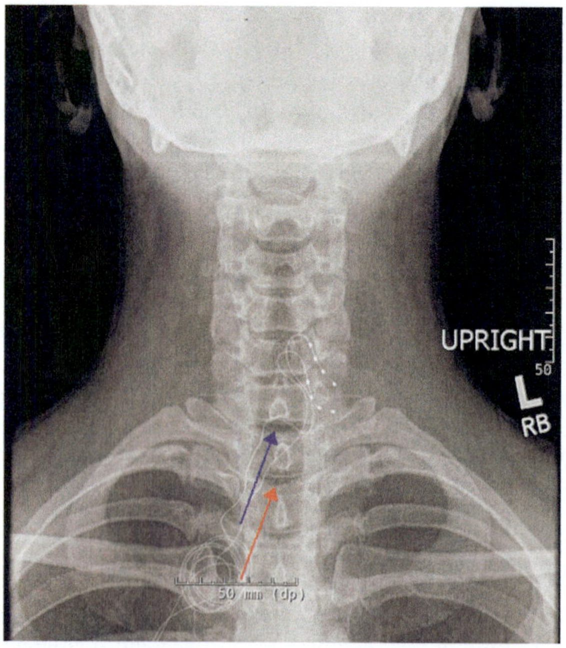

FIGURE 13.5 Epidural needle entrance and trajectory for DRG leads in Left C6 (blue arrow) and C7 (red arrow) neural foramen AP view; epidural access was obtained at the C7 – T1 interspace for C6 DRG lead, and T1 – T2 interspace for C7 DRG lead.

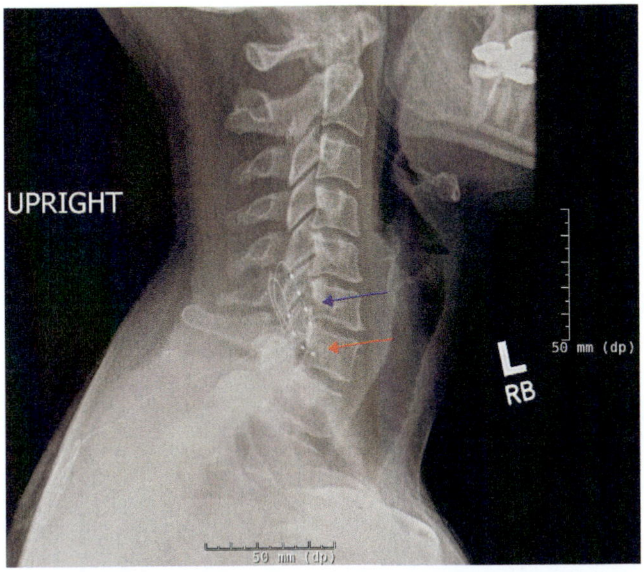

FIGURE 13.6 DRG leads in C7 (blue arrow) and C8 (red arrow), neural foramen lateral view.

C8 and T1 neural foramen, also via the contralateral paramedian technique, where the epidural space was accessed at T1-T2 for the C8 lead, and at T2-T3 for the T1 lead.

Following placement of DRG leads, an intraepidural curve creation with an S-shaped strain-relief loop is made for redundancy to reduce migration and to serve as final anchors. This is created by directing the needle and introducer sheath first to a 12 o'clock position to create the cephalad loop not above the inferior endplate of the immediately adjacent cephalad vertebral body, followed by an approximate 8-9 o'clock (left) or 3-4 o'clock position (right) for the inferior loop, followed by back to 12 o'clock. Determination of the height position of the superior loop would be considered to avoid especially areas that would have a narrowing of the canal diameter below 13 mm. After creation of the loops, the needle and sheath are removed while maintaining lead stabilization. If with concern for a limited sufficient epidural strain-relief

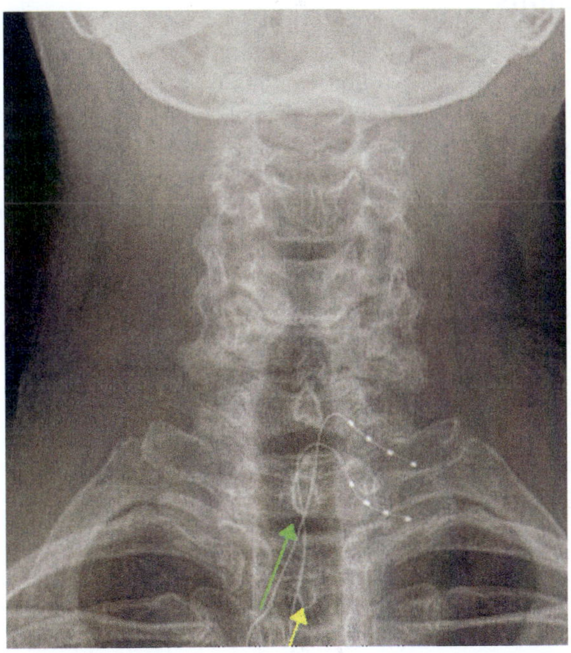

FIGURE 13.7 Six months post placement. Epidural needle entrance and trajectory for dorsal root ganglion stimulation at Left C8 (green arrow) and T1 (yellow arrow) nerve roots, AP view; epidural space accessed at T1 and T2 for C8 lead, and T2 and T3 for T1 lead. Here, the inferior portion of the S loops had pulled out subsequent to the initial placement.

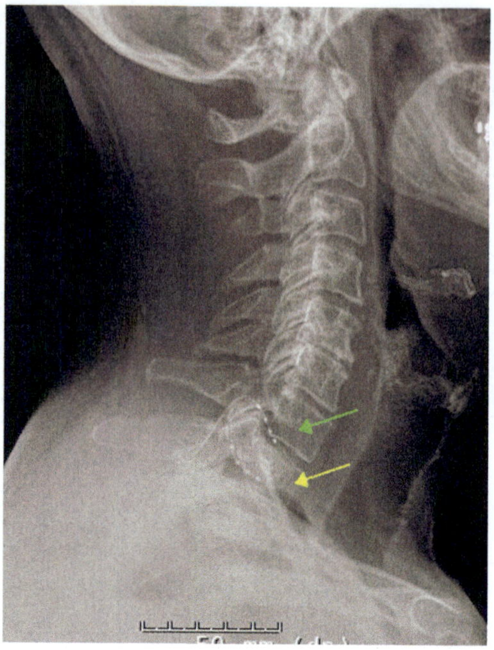

FIGURE 13.8 Dorsal root ganglion stimulation at Left C8 (green arrow) and T1 (yellow arrow) nerve roots, lateral view.

curve, additional extraspinal anchoring with a 1–2 cm loop in the lead wound is recommended. If the trialling method of a staged trial with permanent trial leads was preplanned, followed by a plan for subsequent permanent insertion of the implantable pulse generator, a tunneled trial approach may be used, with placement of temporary extension wires exteriorized to an external pulse generator. Otherwise, for final implantation, tunneling and implantable pulse generator placement, including pocket creation, would be accomplished as per careful preoperative planning, according to steps as with implantation of other neuromodulation devices.

Postoperative considerations

Recovery after placement of cervical DRG stimulation is similar to postoperative considerations of DRG stimulation. Efficacy estimates specific to cervical DRG stimulation are thus far primarily based on small uncontrolled studies. For example, Graca et al. published a retrospective study of 20 patients with upper extremity CRPS of which 17 proceeded to implant, and at 6 months postimplant, all the patients had experienced ≥50% pain reduction, with a mean NRS pain reduction of 5.5, that with updated data from a 12-month follow up, demonstrated mean pain reduction of 6.0 with opioid use remaining lower than baseline [5]. Immobilization with a soft cervical collar may be used. One should limit bending, lifting, minimizing overhead reaching activities above 90° shoulder abduction and twisting activities for 2 to 4 weeks after surgery. Otherwise, consistent with postoperative considerations for implantation of other neuromodulation devices, such as no excessive bending or twisting, lifting of heavy objects, or bathing or soaking, for the duration of anticipated recovery period. As per maintenance, medications, and programming considerations, they are the same as with other modulation devices, to be addressed at every post op visit within the first 12 months.

Pearls and pitfalls

Preoperative

Preoperative evaluation of MRI or CT scans should be reviewed to measure for the absence of clinically significant spinal canal stenosis or foraminal stenosis at the intended levels to be treated. Factors, including the degree or severity of foraminal stenosis, previous hardware, and epidural scarring, can impact outcomes and affect surgical approach. Measurement of the cervical canal diameter is the most important measurement in this regard. The potential for spinal cord injury exists either from the introducer or electrode as it is introduced or from the space occupied by the S loops once advanced inside the canal, which may compromise the spinal cord because of their physical presence. When making S loops, care should be taken to ensure that the cephalad loop does not ascend too high within the cervical epidural space. The implanter should understand the cervical spinal anatomy and be aware of any significant cervical spinal stenosis above the targeted DRG level, and be wary of that when advancing and making the S loop. Evaluation of relevant patient factors and foreseeable procedural challenges influences the specific sedation and anesthesia plan for individuals undergoing DRG-S placement. Choice of anesthetic and monitoring should be discussed prior to the day of the procedure, and the implanter and patient preferences should be aligned. Discussions regarding patient positioning, procedural pain tolerance, and reinforcement in your confidence in the patient's ability to tolerate the experience are paramount. Given the incidence of spinal surgery and central stenosis in the lumbar spine, the traditional anterograde placement of DRG-S leads may not be possible. Such anatomical variations may exclude DRG-S as a modality using the anterograde approach. DRG best practices article. Cervical SCS would be more appropriate in treating patients with neuropathic pain whose pain pattern involves a wider distribution of pain. Patients who have had any posterior cervical spine surgery would not be considered appropriate candidates for cervical DRG.

Intraoperative

The use of intraoperative neuromonitoring is used to optimize immediate repositioning of the lead to reduce any possible postoperative neurologic deficits. Improving outcomes and decreasing complications with implantable therapies is a necessary and vital process [31]. The need for intraoperative paresthesia mapping is at the discretion of the provider. A lead placed with two contacts within the foramen in the AP and lateral fluoroscopic view is often adequate. Minimize foraminal instrumentation with the semirigid introducer sheath and rotating its bevel ventrally in the canal. Consider repositioning the introducer sheath or reaccessing the epidural space at a different location rather than making multiple repeated failed attempts at foraminal passage.

The use of electrocautery and radiofrequency energy can render the IPG unable to connect to the programming device. "Surgery mode" was designed to limit this potential. Traditional precautions include limiting electrocautery use, placement of the grounding pad adjacent to the procedural site, and use of bipolar cautery devices. In addition to losing the ability for device connection, there is a possibility that motor or painful stimulation may occur if the device remains in the "on mode".

Postoperative

Initial postoperative programming should be delayed until any anesthetic effects have dissipated. Waiting this period also allows any fluid in the epidural space and foramen to dissipate as well. Saline, heme, or serous fluid increases impedance and can lead to overstimulation if the patient is programmed before these fluids dissipate. Patient's may complain of initial pocket site pain postoperatively. In addition, other postoperative considerations are lead migration and loss of efficacy of the therapy. These are all variables that need to be proactively addressed by following the NACC guidelines carefully.

References

[1] Deer TR, Levy RM, Kramer J, et al. Dorsal root ganglion stimulation yielded higher treatment success rate for complex regional pain syndrome and causalgia at 3 and 12 months: A randomized comparative trial. Pain 2017;158(4):669–81. https://doi.org/10.1097/j.pain.0000000000000814.

[2] Teichmüller K, Rose N, Dreiling J, et al. Incidence and treatment of complex regional pain syndrome after surgery: Analysis of claims data from Germany. Pain Rep 2024;9(6):e1210. https://doi.org/10.1097/PR9.0000000000001210.

[3] de Mos M, de Bruijn AGJ, Huygen FJPM, Dieleman JP, Stricker BHC, Sturkenboom MCJM. The incidence of complex regional pain syndrome: A population-based study. Pain 2007;129(1):12–20. https://doi.org/10.1016/j.pain.2006.09.008.

[4] Graca MJ, Lubenow TR, Landphair WR, McCarthy RJ. Efficacy and safety of cervical and high-thoracic dorsal root ganglion stimulation therapy for complex regional pain syndrome of the upper extremities. Neuromodulation 2023;26(8):1781–7. https://doi.org/10.1016/j.neurom.2022.09.007.

[5] Graca MJ, Lubenow TR. Update to "efficacy and safety of cervical and high-thoracic dorsal root ganglion stimulation therapy for complex regional pain syndrome of the upper extremities." Neuromodulation 2024;27(3):593–5. https://doi.org/10.1016/j.neurom.2023.08.005.

[6] Piedade GS, Vesper J, et al. Cervical and high-thoracic dorsal root ganglion stimulation in chronic neuropathic pain. Neuromodulation 2019;22(8):951–5. https://doi.org/10.1111/ner.12916.

[7] Gilbert SF. Developmental biology. 6th ed. Sunderland (MA): Sinauer Associates; 2000. https://www.ncbi.nlm.nih.gov/books/NBK10065/.

[8] Graham RD, Sankarasubramanian V, Lempka SF. Dorsal root ganglion stimulation for chronic pain: Hypothesized Mechanisms of action. J Pain 2022;23(2):196–211. https://doi.org/10.1016/j.jpain.2021.07.008.

[9] Crawford LK, Caterina MJ. Functional anatomy of the sensory nervous system: Updates from the neuroscience bench. Toxicol Pathol 2020;48(1):174–89. https://doi.org/10.1177/0192623319869011.

[10] Lee J, Hunter C. ID: 204856 DRG stimulation modulates sympathetic pathways allowing cross-talk between levels: A case series and technical report. Neuromodulation 2023;26(4):S161. https://doi.org/10.1016/j.neurom.2023.04.284.

[11] Demondion X, Lefebvre G, Fisch O, Vandenbussche L, Cepparo J, Balbi V. Radiographic anatomy of the intervertebral cervical and lumbar foramina (vessels and variants). Diagn Interv Imaging 2012;93(9):690–7. https://doi.org/10.1016/j.diii.2012.07.008.

[12] Purves D, Augustine GJ, Fitzpatrick D, et al. The external anatomy of the spinal cord. In: Neuroscience. 2nd ed. Sinauer Associates; 2001. https://www.ncbi.nlm.nih.gov/books/NBK11160/. [Accessed 9 February 2025].

[13] Macpherson D, Quondamatteo F, Broom M. Update on applied epidural anatomy. BJA Educ 2022;22(5):182–9. https://doi.org/10.1016/j.bjae.2021.12.006.

[14] Deer TR, Russo M, Grider JS, et al. The neurostimulation appropriateness consensus committee (NACC): Recommendations on best practices for cervical neurostimulation. Neuromodulation 2022;25(1):35–52. https://doi.org/10.1016/j.neurom.2021.10.013.

[15] Goddard-Hodge D, Boukebous B, Baker JF. Anteroposterior cervical spine canal diameter: Exploring ethnic variation between European and Polynesian populations. ANZ J Surg November 2024;94(11):1963–70. https://doi.org/10.1111/ans.19186.

[16] Yang Y, Shi B, Duan Y, Qiu S, Liu Z. Anatomic morphology and clinical significance of intraforaminal ligaments of the cervical spine. Clin Anat 2019;32(5):654–60. https://doi.org/10.1002/ca.23364.

[17] Nonthasaen P, Nasu H, Kagawa E, Akita K. A morphological comparison of the extraforaminal ligament between the cervical and thoracic regions. Surg Radiol Anat 2018;40(5):571–80. https://doi.org/10.1007/s00276-017-1963-3.

[18] Mao H, Driscoll SJ, Li JS, Li G, Wood KB, Cha TD. Dimensional changes of the neuroforamen in sub-axial cervical spine during in vivo dynamic flexion-extension. Spine J 2016;16(4):540–6. https://doi.org/10.1016/j.spinee.2015.11.052.

[19] Deer TR, Pope JE. Dorsal root ganglion stimulation approval by the Food and Drug Administration: advice on evolving the process. Expert Rev Neurother 2016;16(10):1123–5. https://doi.org/10.1080/14737175.2016.1206817.

[20] Chapman KB, Sayed D, Lamer T, Hunter C, Weisbein J, Patel KV, et al. Best practices for dorsal root ganglion stimulation for chronic pain: guidelines from the American society of pain and neuroscience. J Pain Res 2023;16:839–79. https://doi.org/10.2147/JPR.S364370.

[21] Liem L. Stimulation of the dorsal root ganglion. In: Slavin KV, editor. Stimulation of the peripheral nervous system. The neuromodulation frontier. Basel: Karger; 2016. p. 213–24.

[22] Hunter CW, Sayed D, Lubenow T, et al. DRG focus: A multicenter study evaluating dorsal root ganglion stimulation and predictors of trial success. Neuromodulation 2019;22:61–79.

[23] Eldabe S, Burger K, Moser H, et al. Dorsal root ganglion (DRG) stimulation in the treatment of phantom limb pain (PLP). Neuromodulation 2015;187:610–6.

[24] Schu S, Gulve A, ElDabe S, et al. Spinal cord stimulation of the dorsal root ganglion for groin pain—a retrospective review. Pain Pract 2015;15(4):293–9. https://doi.org/10.1111/papr.12194.

[25] Rowland DCL, Wright D, Moir L, FitzGerald JJ, Green L. Successful treatment of pelvic girdle pain with dorsal root ganglion stimulation. Br J Neurosurg 2016;306:685–6.

[26] Ali R, Epstein L, Khelemsky Y. Successful treatment of chronic post thoracotomy pain syndrome with dorsal root ganglion (DRG) stimulation. Paper presented at: 20th Annual North American Neuromodulation Society. NV: Las Vegas; 2017. p. 19–22.

[27] Eldabe S, Espinet A, Wahlstedt A, et al. Retrospective case series on the treatment of painful diabetic peripheral neuropathy with dorsal root ganglion stimulation. Neuromodulation 2018;21(8):787–92. https://doi.org/10.1111/ner.12767.

[28] Kim JH, Apigo A, Fontaine C. Dorsal root ganglion stimulation for refractory post-herpetic neuralgia. Pain Pract 2021;21(7):794–8. https://doi.org/10.1111/papr.13017.

[29] Morgalla MH, Bolat A, Fortunato M, Lepski G, Chander BS. Dorsal root ganglion stimulation used for the treatment of chronic neuropathic pain in the groin: a single-center study with long-term prospective results in 34 cases. Neuromodulation 2017;20(8):753–60. https://doi.org/10.1111/ner.12713.

[30] Graca, M.J., et al. *Dorsal root ganglion stimulation therapy in pediatric patients: Acase series.* (2021).

[31] Deer TR, Pope JE, Lamer TJ, Grider JS, Provenzano D, Lubenow TR, FitzGerald JJ, Hunter C, Falowski S, Sayed D, Baranidharan G, Patel NK, Davis T, Green A, Pajuelo A, Epstein LJ, Harned M, Liem L, Christo PJ, Chakravarthy K, Gilmore C, Huygen F, Lee E, Metha P, Nijhuis H, Patterson DG, Petersen E, Pilitsis JG, Rowe JJ, Rupert MP, Skaribas I, Sweet J, Verrills P, Wilson D, Levy RM, Mekhail N. The neuromodulation appropriateness consensus committee on best practices for dorsal root ganglion stimulation. Neuromodulation 2019;22(1):1–35. https://doi.org/10.1111/ner.12845.

Chapter 14

Thoracic dorsal root ganglion stimulation

Tolga Suvar[1], Kristin Jarzombek[2], Chris Massey[3] and Rosa Garcia[4]

[1]*Rush University, Chicago, IL, United States;* [2]*Greater Austin Pain Center, Austin, TX, United States;* [3]*Pain Specialists of America, Austin, TX, United States;* [4]*Department of Anesthesiology and Pain Medicine, University of Florida, Gainesville, FL, United States*

Introduction

Neuromodulation has been shown to be an effective pain-treatment modality for refractory pain conditions that negatively impact the quality of life [1]. Dorsal root ganglion stimulation (DRG-S) is an innovative neuromodulatory therapy that provides electrical stimulation to a focal area of neuropathic pain. This therapy places an electrical field in close proximity to the pseudo-unipolar cells of the DRG, which contains primary sensory neurons that relay signals from the periphery to the central nervous system instead of targeting the dorsal column like conventional spinal cord stimulation (SCS) [2]. Although both systems use a tonic waveform, DRG operates with lower therapeutic power demands attributable to its more focal targeting of sensory neurons. Additionally, DRGS has been shown to be efficacious even when delivered intermittently in a subthreshold, paresthesia-free manner at lower frequencies, optimizing the patient experience and device efficiency [2]. The concept of modulating neural activity via the cell bodies of sensory neurons emerged in the early 2000s when investigators acknowledged its distinct role in pain processing. DRG-S was introduced in the European Union in 2011 and later in 2016 in the United States (US) [3]. Initial investigations in Europe demonstrated that DRG-S processed less positional sensitivity, possessing more stability with the potential for reduced risk of lead migration compared to SCS. In addition, it provided other benefits such as greater than 50% pain relief compared to baseline through 6 months, coverage of painful areas without generating large unwanted areas of paresthesia, and improved quality of life [3].

The ACCURATE study demonstrating the preeminence of DRG-S in Complex Regional Pain Syndrome (CRPS) of the lower extremities compared to conventional SCS at 3 and 12 months was the landmark that resulted in the Food and Drug Administration (FDA) approval in the USA in February 2016 [4], with lead placement from T10 to S2. However, despite its early application focused on lumbosacral pain syndromes, its use has broadened to include cervical and thoracic applications with the evolving technology [1]. Certain pathologies, such as post-herpetic neuralgia, post-surgical neuropathic pain, CRPS of the upper extremity, and intercostal neuralgia, are commonly seen in the thoracic region and may benefit from this therapy [5]. Innovations in electrode designs and implantation techniques are under investigation. DRG-S with paddle leads are being studied to allow access to complex spinal segments and aid in challenging revisional cases [6,7]. Other innovations include the use of wireless neurostimulation systems using an implantable passive electrode contact array, microprocessor receiver and an embedded antenna within the electrode wire that couples with an external transmitting antenna and external pulse generator (EPG), which have the potential to diminish procedural invasiveness, leading to lower complication rates [8,9]. However, these technologies are still undergoing testing and have not yet been approved by the Food and Drug Administration (FDA). In conclusion, thoracic DRG-S is an innovative modality that is rapidly evolving and has the potential to improve chronic pain conditions. Although data on procedural techniques, efficacy, and outcomes are still emerging, ongoing research into its mechanisms, applications, and technological innovations continue to enhance its potential and refine its role in pain medicine.

Key points

1. Thoracic Dorsal Root Ganglion Stimulation (DRG-S) is a relatively new target for neuromodulation.
2. Typical targets include low back and groin pain (e.g., post-herniorrhaphy pain syndrome)

A Modern Atlas for Implantable Devices of the Spine, Brain, and Nerve. https://doi.org/10.1016/B978-0-443-36528-7.00043-1

3. It is currently only FDA-approved for T10-T12 and is most commonly used in conjunction with Lumbar DRG.
4. Thoracic DRG is technically more difficult than Lumbar DRG due to a smaller spinal canal diameter, steeper needle entry angle, and presence of the spinal cord.

Relevant anatomy

The DRG is a neural structure that houses primary sensory neurons that convey sensory information from the periphery to the dorsal column of the spinal cord. Anatomically, it is a pseudo-unipolar neuron with an incorporated T-junction that assists with the transmission of action potentials from the nerve cell endings to the dorsal root entry zone [10]. The T-junctions judiciously inhibit information from the periphery to the central nervous system, thereby serving as a low filter for electrical information [10]. Following a nociceptive input, the DRG undergoes a sequence of events that induce the release of excitatory neurotransmitters and pro-inflammatory cytokines, which result in reduced neural membrane and, ultimately, DRG neuron hyperexcitability, leading to neuropathic pain [11]. Upon discussing its anatomic location, it is habitually confined superolateral in the intervertebral foramina at high vertebral levels and centrally in lower levels. Still, it may also be found adjacent to the foramina [12]. The thoracic DRG, in particular, is located within the neural foramen of the thoracic spine (T1-T12), roughly proximal to the vertebral pedicle [13]. It tends to have a smaller size, with sensory variations compared to lumbar levels [13,14]. This could be attributable to the thoracic region primarily housing internal organs with less complex sensory needs [15]. At the same time, the lower limbs require detailed sensory information for distinct movements and balance, thus requiring a more significant number of sensory fibers in the lumbar DRGs. Table 14.1 outlines key differences in DRG anatomy across various spinal levels. The thoracic DRG is perfused through superficial and deep plexuses originating from radicular-medullary branches of the segmental arteries [12]. Venous drainage occurs through the peri-ganglionic venous plexus by intervertebral veins [16]. Understanding the thoracic DRG structure guides the provider during the imaging review, as essential features should be assessed pre-operatively. These may include foraminal patency, nerve root alignments, or anatomical variations such as aberrant nerve configurations [6]. In addition, providers should evaluate structural alterations from prior surgeries, as these may require a tactical entry point to achieve adequate contact. It's paramount to note that DRG leads should not be inserted at levels with pre-existing hardware in post-surgical patients [6]. These anatomical insights promote advancements in neuromodulation, enhancing the efficacy and safety of this therapy.

Procedure

Diagnosis

The current diagnosis codes most commonly used for DRG stimulation are CRPS 1 and CRPS 2 (causalgia). Below are other currently acceptable ICD-10 codes for thoracic DRG stimulation.

ICD code	Description
G90.52, G90.521, G90.512, G90.513	Complex regional pain syndrome (CRPS) of the lower extremity
G57.7, G57.71, G57.72, G57.73	Causalgia of the groin or lower extremity

Indications

On label	Off label
Complex regional pain syndrome of the lower extremities	CRPS of the chest wall (NOS) (non-FDA approved levels)
Causalgia of the lower extremities	Axial low back pain
Causalgia of the groin	Localized chronic pain conditions refractory to conventional medical therapy
	Pelvic floor pain (in combination with sacral DRG)

TABLE 14.1 Key differences in DRG anatomy across spinal levels y.

Spinal level	Average foramen size	Average spinal canal diameter (mm)	DRG size in relation to the foramen
Cervical level [2, 17]	• Height: 11.08 mm • Width: 5.69 mm	17	DRG size at cervical levels increases from the very small and absent in >70% at level C1 to the largest at the C8 level. The C8 DRG has a larger volume (177 mm^3).
Thoracic level [2, 18]	• Height: 19.4 mm • Width: 8.4 mm	15–18	DRG size in thoracic levels is approximately 144 mm^3 at the T1 level.
Lumbar level [19, 20]	• Height: 19.4 mm • Width: 8.8 mm	17.5	DRG size at lumbar levels gradually increases from L1 to L5, from approximately 4 × 4.5 mm at L1 to 5.5 × 10 mm at L5.
Sacral level [21,22]	• Height: 20–23 mm • Width: 8–10 mm		DRG size at sacral levels gradually decreases from S1 to S4, with the S1 DRG measuring roughly 6.5 × 13 mm compared to 5 × 3 mm at S4.

Patient selection considerations

When considering DRG stimulation as a possible treatment modality, one must consider the appropriate patient selection criteria. Patients afflicted with CRPS can range from the pediatric population to the elderly. DRG therapy is supposed to be more invasive than pharmacologic therapy but less invasive than amputation [13]. All patients are more likely to benefit from early implementation of dorsal root ganglion stimulation to allow for appropriate neuronal remodeling in the earlier disease process. When considering patient selection, however, physicians new to the therapy may choose to select younger patients with less degeneration in their spinal column as the anatomy may be more amenable to placement of a DRG electrode in the neural foramen. Thoracic DRG stimulation is currently FDA-approved at the levels of T10-T12, which are used to cover the lower abdomen, groin, and lower back. Newer techniques for targeting refractory axial low back pain include targeted DRG stimulation of the bilateral T12 dorsal root ganglia.

Contraindications to neuromodulation, in general, include pregnancy, coagulopathy, active infection, active addiction to psychoactive substances, and severe cognitive impairment that may limit the patient's ability to cooperate with the therapy. Contraindications to DRG stimulation, in particular, would include spinal cord damage at the target level (especially when considering thoracic dorsal root ganglion stimulation given the presence of cord at this level) and severe foraminal stenosis at the target foramen.

Training recommendations

DRG stimulation can be performed by any physician familiar with epidural access and neuromodulation in general. This can include pain management specialists, spine surgeons, and interventional radiologists. The American Board of Anesthesiologists accredits the majority of interventional pain specialists with dual board certification in pain management. However, many pain specialists have other medical backgrounds, including but not limited to physical medicine and rehabilitation, emergency medicine, neurology, and psychiatry.

The commonly requested DRG stimulation case volume is between 5 and 20 cases. It is not uncommon to request proctoring for a physician's first 5 cases to ensure confidence in the technique and competence with lead placement and loop formation. However, physicians more accustomed to accessing the epidural space may feel comfortable providing this therapy with fewer cases, and physicians lacking a background in pain interventions may feel more competent with a more extended period of proctoring in general.

As above, proctoring should be considered, at the very least, for a physician's initial trial and/or implant. It is recommended that proctoring be considered for a more extended period for physicians less experienced in neuromodulation and for new levels (i.e., L5 DRG lead placement or sacral DRG lead placement).

Many physicians new to the therapy should consider providing case peer reviews to more experienced clinicians for the initial period of providing DRG stimulation to their patient populations.

Technique

The technique for performing a DRG trial and implant in the Thoracic spine is very similar to that in the Lumbar spine. Differences in the anatomy of the thoracic and lumbar spines must be understood to prevent nerve root irritation since all levels of the Thoracic spine are narrower than their corresponding Lumbar levels, and the spinal cord is present (Table 14.1).

Patient positioning

Patients are positioned prone on the operating table, using pillows or a Wilson frame to exaggerate thoracic kyphosis. Arms should be abducted to less than 90° with shoulders relaxed forward to prevent excess pressure on the joints and prevent stretching of peripheral nerves. Straps and/or belts can be utilized to prevent patients from falling during the procedure.

Anesthesia considerations

Anesthetic techniques vary from Monitored Anesthesia Care (MAC) to General Endotracheal Anesthesia (GETA). The DRG-S Physician Implant Manual states: “The patient must be awake and conversant during portions of the procedure to minimize the likelihood of nerve damage.” Patients who are otherwise relatively healthy, without significant heart or lung-related comorbidities, can generally tolerate MAC sedation without any issue. However, patients who are obese, have airway difficulties or have gastroesophageal reflux disease (GERD) may pose a risk of obstruction or aspiration during MAC and would likely benefit from GETA. For these patients, neuromonitoring with SSEPs and EMG is required to monitor for nerve root irritation and appropriate lead placement [6].

Operating room time estimate

Operating room times vary based on the clinician’s experience level and patient considerations, making gaining access to the desired level more challenging. In general, 15–30 min per level is a good rule of thumb when planning for these cases.

Relevant vendor support

Representatives from the device company should always attend trial and implant procedures to aid the physician and guide patients throughout the trial and implant process. They can educate patients on the technical details of the procedure and answer any questions the patient may have. They will be the point of contact during the trial and postoperative period. Once the implanted leads are attached to the trial or permanent battery, the representative will turn the device on to ensure it works correctly before closing. If desired, they can facilitate intraoperative testing by turning on the prosecution or implant leads. They can also provide adequate coverage in the postoperative period.

Procedure

The target vertebral body is identified with fluoroscopy and adjusted to center the spinous processes and align the superior endplates. A Tuohy needle is placed overlying the contralateral (or ipsilateral) pedicle two levels below the target vertebral body [6]. The Tuohy needle is advanced toward the spinous process one level below the target body. Once contact with the lamina is made, the Tuohy is advanced into the epidural space using a loss of resistance technique (LOR), to either saline or air. The DRG lead is advanced into the epidural space and “driven” under fluoroscopic guidance underneath the target pedicle. Care must be taken to prevent the lead from coming into direct contact with the DRG, which can cause paresthesias. The appropriate position of the lead is the anterosuperior quadrant of the foramen on the lateral view, with two contacts crossing the pedicle on the AP view. Once correctly placed, the stylet is carefully withdrawn to the hub of the introducer. The strain-relieving S-loop is created by turning the introducer cephalad, advancing the lead upward to the top of the vertebral body above. Once the top loop is placed, the stylet is again withdrawn back into the hub of the introducer. The introducer is then oriented to the caudad, creating the second half of the S-loop. The stylet is carefully withdrawn into the introducer, and the Tuohy and introducer are removed without withdrawing the distal end of the lead. If performing a trial, the lead can be anchored to the skin with either steri-strips or sutures. The leads are attached to the trial battery and secured with steri-strips, gauze, Tegaderm, and tape.

When performing a permanent lead placement, the leads can be anchored to the fascia underneath the skin using the provided anchors and secured with a non-absorbable suture such as Ethibond. Anchoring the leads has been shown to reduce lead migration rates to approximately 1.4% and lead fracture rates to 1.9% [23].

With the leads secure, a pocket for the stimulator battery is created on the ipsilateral flank [6]. Dissection occurs down to Scarpa's fascia, no further than 4 cm, allowing the battery to communicate with the remote [24]. Once the desired depth is achieved, the pocket is created using blunt or instrument dissection. The battery should sit beneath the incision site, with approximately one-third above and two-thirds below the incision. The leads are tunneled from their corresponding exit sites to the pocket beneath the fascia using the available tunneling tool. Once the leads are attached to the battery and impedances are normal, the battery is placed into the pocket with the leads tucked behind it.

The pocket is irrigated with saline infused with Vancomycin. The incision is closed in a three-layered fashion: the fascial layer, followed by the deep dermal layer, and finally, the dermal layer. Sterile dressings are placed over the incisions.

Postoperative considerations

Recovery (Chris Massey)

The recovery process for Thoracic DRG implantation is the same as for Lumbar DRG. In general, recovery after a DRG trial is minimal. Patients usually report soreness at the needle insertion site or lamina sites contacted by the needle. Generous use of local anesthetic during the procedure can mitigate post-procedural pain. The same is true during the permanent implant. After the implant, patients usually complain of more pain for a longer duration due to pocket creation, tunneling, and lead anchoring.

Efficacy estimates

Due to a lack of Level 1 data and Randomized Control Trials, the efficacy of Thoracic DRG cannot be determined. Several case studies and series describe successful uses of Thoracic DRG, but there is no data beyond a retrospective review [25–27].

Bracing considerations and activity limitations

Following thoracic dorsal root stimulation, activity modification is essential to ensure proper lead stability and prevent migration. Patients are generally instructed to avoid activities such as bending, twisting, and lifting objects over 2 kg (5 lbs) for at least 6 weeks following implantation [24]. In addition, activities involving excessive stretching of the thoracic spine, such as yoga and certain contact sports, should also be limited. These activities may occasionally lead to movement, ultimately resulting in overstimulation or understimulation for the patient. Patients may be advised to wear a soft thoracic brace-such as the thoracic, lumbar spinal orthosis (TLSO) for low-mid thoracic regions or cervical brace at T1-T3 levels, which is commonly recommended for use up to 6–12 weeks following spinal procedures. Repeated surgery may be needed for lead replacement in cases of excessive migration [28]. In contrast, patients who feel unwanted paresthesias attributable to postural changes should not climb ladders or make abrupt movements such as running or jumping, which could alter stimulation intensity perceptions and cause falls or loss of equipment control [24].

Maintenance considerations

Patients who do well after a DRG implant must remember that DRG stimulation does not cure the pathology causing their pain. Instead, it is designed to mask and reduce pain symptoms to give patients back their freedom and improve their quality of life. Patients must be diligent in maintaining control of their pain by staying active, eating healthy, and utilizing other conservative methods to treat their pain.

Patients should also take care not to damage their stimulator. Trauma, such as falls or motor vehicle collisions, can cause lead fracture or migration. Any subtle migration can significantly reduce the stimulator's efficacy, requiring revision or a complete explanation. For those who experience reduced coverage or efficacy, the DRG-S can be reprogrammed as necessary.

Many patients will need advanced imaging, including MRIs, in their lifetime. The current Proclaim IPG is MRI conditional when used on-label at T10 or below [24]. It must be placed in MRI mode prior to the MRI. Like most other SCS devices, lead fracture or battery depletion renders the device MRI incompatible.

Pearls and pitfalls

Thoracic dorsal root ganglion (DRG) stimulation effectively treats focal neuropathic pain conditions such as complex regional pain syndrome (CRPS) and post-herpetic neuralgia. While it offers precise targeting of painful dermatomes, successful implementation depends on careful patient selection, intraoperative techniques, and postoperative management.

Preoperatively, patient selection remains a cornerstone of success. Ideal candidates include those with well-localized neuropathic pain, particularly unilateral pain syndromes. Imaging studies, including MRI or CT scans, are essential. These can aid in assessing foraminal patency and identifying anatomical variations, such as spinal canal stenosis in the painful dermatome, that may complicate lead placement. However, poor patient selection, particularly in individuals with widespread pain, central sensitization, or significant psychological comorbidities, can lead to suboptimal outcomes. Furthermore, failing to recognize foraminal stenosis or osteophytes preoperatively can increase the risk of difficult lead placement, postoperative migration, and radiculitis associated with DRG placement [4,29].

Intraoperative success hinges on precise lead placement and technique. High-quality fluoroscopic guidance using anteroposterior, lateral, and oblique views ensures accurate lead positioning at the targeted DRG. A key technical pearl is using an "S-curve" technique to gently advance the lead while minimizing tension. Intraoperative paresthesia mapping through test stimulation can confirm adequate coverage of the painful dermatome; this is mainly done with a moderate amount of sedation and can also be done with the use of intraoperative neuromonitoring. DRG stimulation and dorsal column stimulation include the risks of lead migration due to improper anchoring, potential risk of dural puncture resulting in post-dural puncture headaches, dural tears leading to cerebrospinal fluid leaks, and hemorrhagic complications if vascular structures within the foramen are inadvertently injured and anticoagulation medications are not adequately held. Additionally, poor steering techniques can lead to difficulty in maneuvering properly into the epidural space and desired neuroforamina, potentially resulting in abandoned procedures or suboptimal outcomes [6,30].

Postoperative care plays a critical role in ensuring long-term efficacy. Patients should adhere to activity restrictions, which include avoiding excessive twisting, bending, and lifting for at least 4–6 weeks to allow for fibrous encapsulation of the leads. Reprogramming of stimulation parameters can optimize pain relief while minimizing discomfort. However, common pitfalls include over-tightening suture anchors, which can cause lead fractures or micromotion, leading to inconsistent stimulation. Additionally, without multidisciplinary care, overlooking the psychological components of chronic pain may result in patients requiring adjunct cognitive-behavioral therapy to maximize their treatment outcomes [31].

From a broader scope perspective, the role of thoracic DRG stimulation is expanding beyond CRPS to encompass post-thoracotomy pain, post-mastectomy, and intercostal neuralgia pain syndromes. While cost-effectiveness studies suggest significant benefits in reducing opioid reliance and improving quality of life, challenges remain. One major limitation is the relative lack of long-term data compared to spinal cord stimulation, necessitating further research to establish durability. Additionally, a steep learning curve exists for new practitioners, as thoracic DRG procedures require advanced training that is not widely available in standard pain fellowship curricula [32].

In conclusion, thoracic DRG stimulation is an evidence-based modality for treating focal neuropathic pain, provided meticulous attention is given to patient selection, procedural technique, and postoperative management. Future studies should aim to refine best practices, address training gaps, and expand indications to optimize patient outcomes further.

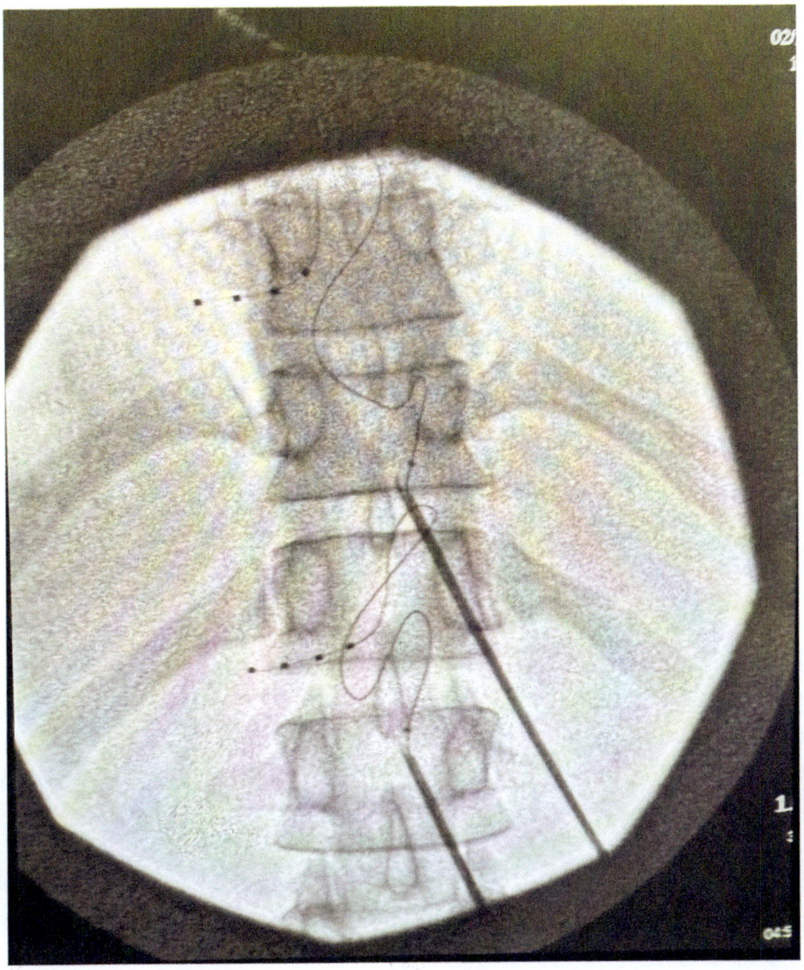

Left T10 and T12 DRG trial, contralateral approach

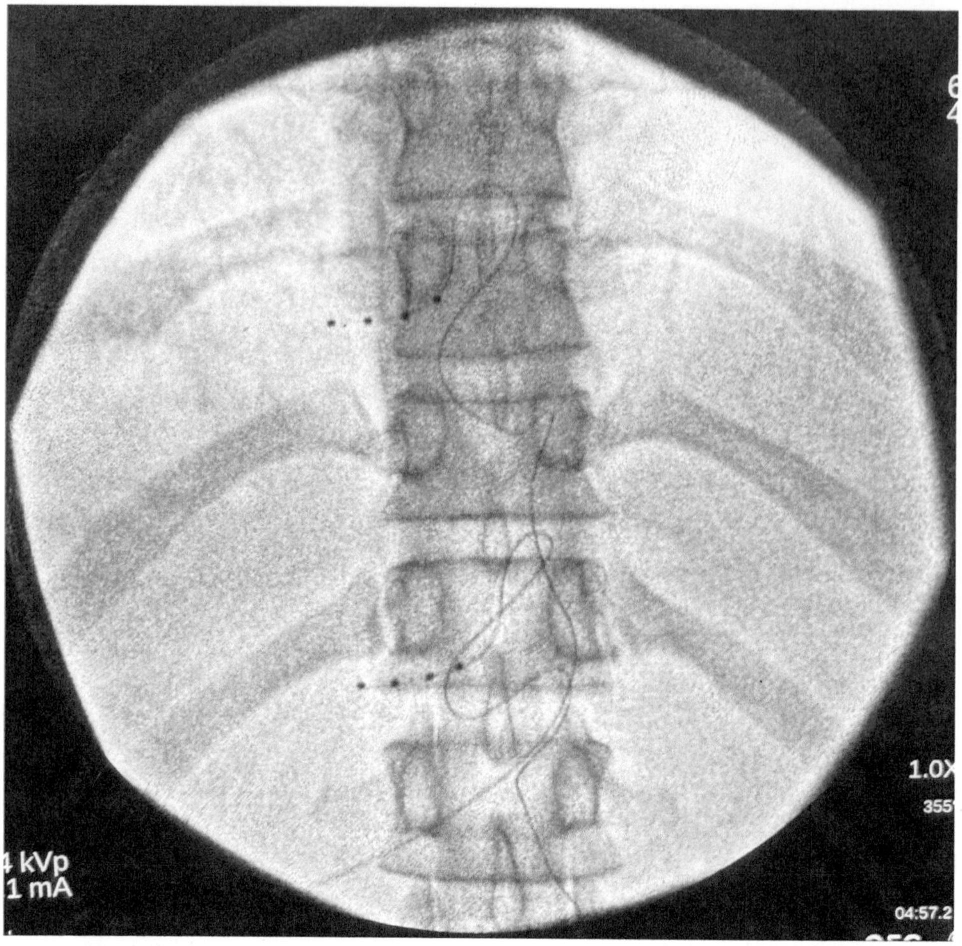

Left T10 and T12 DRG trial

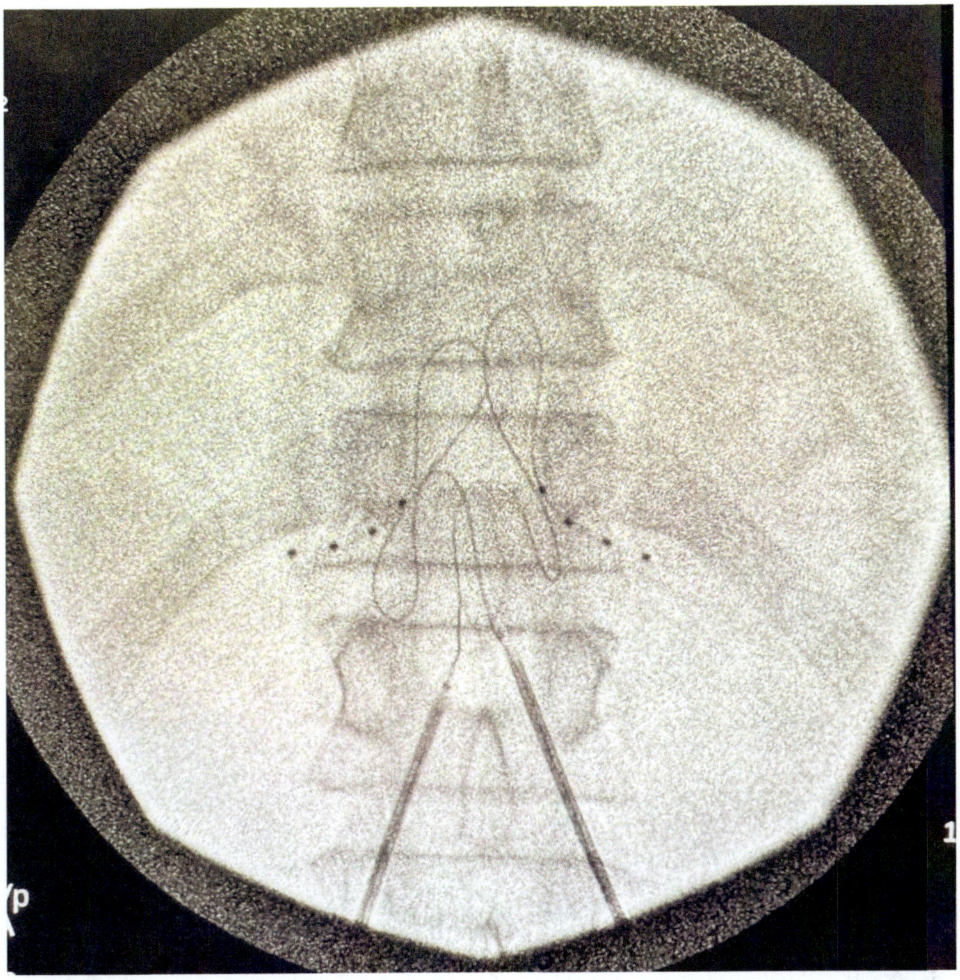

Bilateral T12 DRG trial

References

[1] Deer TR, Grigsby E, Weiner RL, Wilcosky B, Kramer JM. A prospective study of dorsal root ganglion stimulation for the relief of chronic pain. Neuromodulation Technol Neural Interf 2013;16(1):67–72.

[2] Chapman KB, Sayed D, Lamer T, Hunter C, Weisbein J, Patel KV, Dickerson D, Hagedorn JM, Lee DW, Amirdelfan K, Deer T. Best practices for dorsal root ganglion stimulation for chronic pain: guidelines from the American Society of Pain and Neuroscience. J Pain Res 2023:839–79.

[3] Liem L, Russo M, Huygen FJ, Van Buyten JP, Smet I, Verrills P, Cousins M, Brooker C, Levy R, Deer T, Kramer J. A multicenter, prospective trial to assess the safety and performance of the spinal modulation dorsal root ganglion neurostimulator system in the treatment of chronic pain. Neuromodulation Technol Neural Interf 2013;16(5):471–82.

[4] Deer TR, Levy RM, Kramer J, Poree L, Amirdelfan K, Grigsby E, Staats P, Burton AW, Burgher AH, Obray J, Scowcroft J. Dorsal root ganglion stimulation yielded higher treatment success rate for complex regional pain syndrome and causalgia at 3 and 12 months: a randomized comparative trial. Pain 2017;158(4):669–81.

[5] Piedade GS, Vesper J, Chatzikalfas A, Slotty PJ. Cervical and high-thoracic dorsal root ganglion stimulation in chronic neuropathic pain. Neuromodulation Technol Neural Interf 2019;22(8):951–5.

[6] Deer TR, Jain S, Hunter C, Chakravarthy K. Neurostimulation for intractable chronic pain. Brain Sci 2019;9(2):23.

[7] Manfield J, Vajramani G. Burst dorsal root ganglion stimulation with paddle leads: report of two cases. Neuromodulation 2024;27(8):1479–82. https://doi.org/10.1016/j.neurom.2024.06.500. Epub 2024 Aug 12. PMID: 39140935.

[8] Billet B, Wynendaele R, Vanquathem NE. Wireless neuromodulation for chronic back pain: delivery of high-frequency dorsal root ganglion stimulation by a minimally invasive technique. Case Rep Med 2017;2017(1):4203271.

[9] Zhong T, William HM, Jin MY, Abd-Elsayed A. A review of remote monitoring in neuromodulation for chronic pain management. Curr Pain Headache Rep 2024:1–9.

[10] Hunter CW, Sayed D, Lubenow T, Davis T, Carlson J, Rowe J, Justiz R, McJunkin T, Deer T, Mehta P, Falowski S, Kapural L, Pope J, Mekhail N. DRG FOCUS: a multicenter study evaluating dorsal root ganglion stimulation and predictors for trial success. Neuromodulation January 2019;22(1):61–79. https://doi.org/10.1111/ner.12796.

[11] Esposito MF, Malayil R, Hanes M, Deer T. Unique characteristics of the dorsal root ganglion as a target for neuromodulation. Pain Med 2019;20(Suppl. 1):S23–30.

[12] Haberberger RV, Barry C, Dominguez N, Matusica D. Human dorsal root ganglia. Front Cell Neurosci 2019;13:271. https://doi.org/10.3389/fncel.2019.00271.

[13] Abd-Elsayed A, Vardhan S, Aggarwal A, Vardhan M, Diwan SA. Mechanisms of action of dorsal root ganglion stimulation. Int J Mol Sci 2024;25(7):3591.

[14] Cramer GD, Darby SA. Clinical anatomy of the spine, spinal cord, and ANS. 2013.

[15] Guzzi G, Della Torre A, Bruni A, Lavano A, Bosco V, Garofalo E, La Torre D, Longhini F. Anatomo-physiological basis and applied techniques of electrical neuromodulation in chronic pain. J Anesth Analg Crit Care 2024;4(1):29.

[16] Parke WW, Whalen JL. The vascular pattern of the human dorsal root ganglion and its probable bearing on a compartment syndrome. Spine 2002;27:347–52.

[17] Sioutas G, Kapetanakis S. Clinical anatomy and clinical significance of the cervical intervertebral foramen: a review. Folia Morphol 2016;75(2):143–8.

[18] Gkasdaris G, Tripsianis G, Kotopoulos K, Kapetanakis S. Clinical anatomy and significance of the thoracic intervertebral foramen: a cadaveric study and review of the literature. J Craniovert Junct Spine 2016;7(4):228–35. https://doi.org/10.4103/0974-8237.193266.

[19] Uchikado H, Nishimura Y, Hattori G, Ohara Y. Micro-anatomical structures of the lumbar intervertebral foramen for full-endoscopic spine surgery: review of the literature. J Spine Surg 2020;6(2):405.

[20] Vancamp T, Levy RM, Peña I, Pajuelo A. Relevant anatomy, morphology, and implantation techniques of the dorsal root ganglia at the lumbar levels. Neuromodulation Technol Neural Interf 2017;20(7):690–702.

[21] Cavazos DR, Higginbotham DO, Nham F, Court T, McCarty S, Sethi A, Vaidya R. Neuroforaminal stenosis in the lumbosacral spine: a scoping review of pathophysiology, clinical manifestations, diagnostic imaging, and treatment. Spartan Med Res J 2023;8(1):87848.

[22] Chapman KB, van Helmond N, Kallewaard JW, Vissers KC, Patel KV, Motivala S, Hagedorn JM, Deer TR, Dickerson DM. An anatomy-informed, novel technique for S1 dorsal root ganglion stimulation lead placement. Pain Med 2022;23(10):1750–6.

[23] Chapman KB, Groenen PS, Vissers KC, van Helmond N, Stanton-Hicks MD. The pathways and processes underlying spinal transmission of low back pain: observations from dorsal root ganglion stimulation treatment. Neuromodulation June 2021;24(4):610–21. https://doi.org/10.1111/ner.13150.

[24] Abbott. ProclaimTM DRG implantable pulse generator clinician's manual model 3664. 2018.

[25] Chapman KB, Groenen PS, et al. T12 dorsal root ganglion stimulation to treat chronic low back pain: a case series. Neuromodulation February 2020;23(2):203–12. https://doi.org/10.1111/ner.13047.

[26] Char S, Barman RA, Deer TR, Hagedorn JM. Dorsal root ganglion stimulation for chronic groin pain: a review. Neuromodulation 2022;25:965–9.

[27] Zuidema X, Breel J, Wille F. Paresthesia mapping: a practical workup for successful implantation of the dorsal root ganglion stimulator in refractory groin pain. Neuromodulation October 2014;17(7):665–9. https://doi.org/10.1111/ner.12113. ; discussion 669.

[28] Abraham ME, Potdar A, Ward M, Herschman Y, Mammis A. Risk factors associated with lead migration requiring revision in dorsal root ganglion stimulation. World Neurosurg 2019;128:e649–52.

[29] Liem L, Russo M, Huygen FJ, et al. One-year outcomes of spinal cord stimulation of the dorsal root ganglion in the treatment of chronic neuropathic pain. Neuromodulation Technol Neural Interf 2015;18(1):41–8.

[30] van Buyten JP, Linderoth B, Tan Y. The management of neuropathic pain with dorsal root ganglion stimulation. Curr Pain Headache Rep 2014;18(6):420.

[31] Kriek N, Groeneweg JG, Stronks DL, et al. Dorsal root ganglion stimulation in patients with failed back surgery syndrome: a prospective observational study. Pain Med 2021;22(3):481–90.

[32] Deer TR, Pope JE, Falowski S, et al. The neuromodulation appropriateness consensus committee on best practices for dorsal root ganglion stimulation. Neuromodulation Technol Neural Interf 2020;23(5):472–95.

Further reading

[1] Abd-Elsayed A, Stark CW, Topoluk N, Isaamullah M, Uzodinma P, Viswanath O, Dyara O. A brief review of complex regional pain syndrome and current management. Ann Med 2024;56(1). https://doi.org/10.1080/07853890.2024.2334398.

[2] Ahimsadasan N, Reddy V, Khan SMZ, et al. Neuroanatomy, dorsal root ganglion. In: StatPearls [Internet]. Treasure Island (FL): StatPearls Publishing; January 2025. Available from: https://www.ncbi.nlm.nih.gov/books/NBK532291/.

[3] Chapman KB, Mogilner AY, et al. Lead migration and fracture rate in dorsal root ganglion stimulation using anchoring and non-anchoring techniques: a multicenter pooled data analysis. Pain Pract November 2021;21(8):859–70. https://doi.org/10.1111/papr.13052.

[4] Deer TR, Pope JE, Lamer TJ, Grider JS, Provenzano D, Lubenow TR, FitzGerald JJ, Hunter C, Falowski S, Sayed D, Baranidharan G. The neuromodulation appropriateness consensus committee on best practices for dorsal root ganglion stimulation. Neuromodulation Technol Neural Interf 2019;22(1):1–35.

[5] Kato S, Smith JS, Driesman D, Shaffrey CI, Lenke LG, Lewis SJ, AO Spine Knowledge Forum Deformity. Post-operative bracing following adult spine deformity surgery: results from the AO Spine surveillance of post-operative management of patients with adult spine deformity. PLoS One April 16, 2024;19(4):e0297541. https://doi.org/10.1371/journal.pone.0297541.

[6] Meier K. Spinal cord stimulation: background and clinical application. Scand J Pain July 1, 2014;5(3):175–81. https://doi.org/10.1016/j.sjpain.2014.03.001.

[7] Peabody T, Black AC, Das JM. Anatomy, back, vertebral canal. In: StatPearls [Internet]. Treasure Island (FL): StatPearls Publishing; January 2025. Available from: https://www.ncbi.nlm.nih.gov/books/NBK557587/.

[8] Stelter B, Karri J, Marathe A, Abd-Elsayed A. Dorsal root ganglion stimulation for the treatment of non-complex regional pain syndrome related chronic pain syndromes: a systematic review. Neuromodulation June 2021;24(4):622–33. https://doi.org/10.1111/ner.13361.

[9] Chapter 4: The spinal nerves. In: Watson C, Paxinos G, Kayalioglu G, editors. The spinal cord: a Christopher and Dana Reeve Foundation text and atlas. Academic press; 2009. p. 37–56.

Chapter 15

Dorsal root ganglion stimulation

Kenneth B. Chapman[1, 2, 3], Christopher J. Mallard[4], Christopher A. Paul[4] and Ajax Yang[1, 2, 3]

[1]The Spine & Pain Institute of New York, New York, NY, United States; [2]Department of Anesthesiology, NYU Langone Medical Center, New York, NY, United States; [3]Department of Anesthesiology, The Zucker School of Medicine at Hofstra/Northwell, New York, NY, United States; [4]University of Kentucky, Department of Anesthesiology, Lexington, KY, United States

Introduction

Scope of procedure

Dorsal root ganglion stimulation (DRGS) is an advanced neuromodulation technique designed to treat chronic neuropathic pain conditions that are refractory to conventional therapies. DRGS is FDA-approved for the treatment of complex regional pain syndrome (CRPS) types I and II between the T10 through S2 vertebral levels [1]. Since its approval, DRGS' role has continued to evolve, showing effectiveness not only in treating persistent neuropathic pain syndromes but also in managing persistent spinal pain syndrome (PSPS) types I and II. DRGS is also potentially a treatment option for nociceptive conditions. DRGS provides precise dermatomal coverage, including anatomically challenging distal regions such as the foot, groin, and knee, making it a valuable tool for addressing focal neuropathic pain that may not be optimally managed with conventional neurostimulation.

This chapter aims to provide an evidence-based overview of DRGS and offer surgical guidance on a procedure that differs in many ways from its predecessor, spinal cord stimulation (SCS).

Brief historical perspective

DRGS was conceptualized to meet some of the shortcomings of SCS; namely, better distal dermatomal coverage, improving lead stability, reducing stimulation variability, and targeting pain more precisely. To stimulate the DRG, several modifications from the existing SCS systems were required. These changes included a smaller lead diameter, increased flexibility, reduced contact size, and a novel implantation technique. Furthermore, device programming needed to allow for finer adjustments, as DRGS requires a significantly lower dosing compared to traditional SCS.

DRGS was able to achieve these targets, and in 2016 demonstrated greater, more sustained relief than SCS in treating CRPS in the seminal ACCURATE study [1]. Given these advantages, DRGS was poised to become the gold standard neuromodulation technique for CRPS. Unfortunately, DRGS stumbled out of the gate, as the procedural complexity combined with the early potential complications of lead migration and fracture slowed adoption.

Brief procedure innovations in DRGS

Accessing the foramen from the epidural space requires a curved introducer sheath in addition to the 30% thinner four contact DRGS lead (0.9 vs. 1.25 mm). Placing the DRGS lead requires traversing the lateral recess and intervertebral foramen without direct visualization. Radiolucent obstacles and sensitive neural structures add to the technical challenge of lead placement.

The procedure was initially described with needle entry from the contralateral side and caudal to the target foramen. Since that time, several alternative techniques have been described. The introduction of an ipsilateral paramedian approach has been shown to reduce lead migration and fracture rates by minimizing fascial tension on the lead and without the leads crossing the midline, thereby improving overall lead positional stability [2,3].

A Modern Atlas for Implantable Devices of the Spine, Brain, and Nerve. https://doi.org/10.1016/B978-0-443-36528-7.00015-7

Additional alternative approaches for DRGS lead placement have been described, primarily introduced for cases with accessibility issues, particularly a history of laminectomy. The contralateral retrograde, or "transgrade" approach, accesses the rostral intervertebral space [4]. Should the lamina above and below the target foramen be compromised, an outside-in technique has also been described detailing a transforaminal approach [5]. And finally, several surgical techniques have also been described recently. These include placement through a laminotomy and endoscopic approaches, both of which will be described in this chapter [6–10].

At the time of this manuscript preparation, a new, more "kink" resistant introducer sheath has been released. A more durable lead currently remains in the development phase.

Brief most relevant advancements in DRGS

Advancements in DRGS have centered around energy delivery, with refinement of stimulation parameters and programming strategies that have optimized efficacy. Following this, the expanded application of this therapy has emerged, with results from back and leg pain with T12 and S1 placement [11–13], and its use for nociceptive, mechanical pain syndromes [14,15].

Since 2020, the following has been brought to light with DRGS:

Lowest energy usage and battery life

DRGS has efficacy at subthreshold, paresthesia-free levels. It is as efficacious at 4 Hz, cycled at up to 1 min "on" and 1 min "off". This reduces the charge delivered to neural tissue per second by more than 200 times less energy use per second than SCS [16,17]. This very low energy consumption directly contributes to IPG battery longevity, with other factors remaining similar, on the lifespan of the IPG's charge retaining carbon monofluoride/silver vanadium oxide cell is expected to exceed 10 years [18].

Mixed-type and nociceptive pain syndromes

The ability of DRGS to affect mixed-type pain syndromes cannot be made clearer than through the treatment of post total knee replacement pain. In over more than 50 years, SCS has produced little evidence in the literature for post-TKR pain, whereas the novel DRGS already has multiple case series demonstrating efficacy(refs). An ongoing study investigating the use of DRGS for nonsurgical osteoarthritis of the knee is currently underway [19].

Potential against infection

DRGS may carry a lower infection risk. Early European studies with extended staged trials, some up to 30 days before implant, have inflated the overall infection rate in the literature [20]. Real-world data showed only 1/249 patients undergoing device explant secondary to infection (0.4%). This is thought to be due to potentially earlier functional improvement or mechanisms related to the sympathetic nervous system [21].

Use in sympathetically mediated conditions

DRGS has demonstrated great improvements in sympathetically mediated conditions such as peripheral vascular disease and abdominopelvic pain, including postsurgical, visceral-type abdominal and pelvic pain, as well as chronic pelvic pain itself [22–25]. The potential for such relief in this challenging population warrants further investigation.

Use as 'a salvage' therapy

DRGS has emerged as a salvage therapy for patients who have become tolerant to conventional neurostimulation or lacked sufficient coverage to a particular anatomical area, often the hip, knee, ankle and foot. DRGS should be considered a first-line option for patients with CRPS who have SCS which has lost efficacy, and the therapy is available. A retrospective study using DRGS as a salvage therapy showed that out of 60 patients who lost efficacy to SCS trialed with DRGS, 93%, or 56/60 undergoing implant [26]. This group was followed for a mean of 34 months with maintained improvements in pain, function, and quality of life over that time. There are also multiple other examples of DRGS as a salvage therapy in the literature [27,28].

The potential resistance to habituation

DRGS may be less susceptible to habituation, one of the biggest challenges facing SCS. Levy et al. first noted a potential for decreased loss of efficacy (LOE) with DRGS in an ACCURATE study subanalysis, where DRGS maintained statistically significant pain relief over the 1 year study compared to SCS [29]. Another study comparing DRGS at L2 to SCS using BurstDR for the treatment of discogenic pain also showed similar results initially, with DRGS better maintaining improvements over the year [30]. And in the 249-patient pooled analysis studying complications, there were 10 explants over an average 27-month follow-up period, corresponding to an overall 2% rate per year [21].

Complications

Complications arose in the early days of DRGS adoption, with lead fracture and migration dominating early clinical DRGS dialog. Technique refinement was necessary, and it became evident that implanting DRGS leads presents a distinct set of challenges as compared to SCS. The sensitive nature of the DRG and nearby neural structures, combined with a thinner, more malleable lead, and a stiffer, curved introducer sheath, further compounds the challenges of lead placement.

In literature, DRGS has repeatedly shown a complication rate comparable to SCS in lead fracture, lead migration, and nerve insult [31–33]. However, real-world publications and experience with complications reflect the frustration of physician's faced with reoperative intervention to restore therapy. Below, we discuss these complications in more detail.

Lead and hardware related complications

Lead migration

Lead migration and lead fracture have been highlighted in the literature. In 2021, Chapman et al. published a pooled analysis of 249 implants (756 leads) with a mean follow-up of 27 months, demonstrating that anchoring leads reduced lead migration and fracture rates from 8.4% to 1.4% and 3.1%–1.9% per lead, respectively [21]. A follow-up paper documented long term migration rates with *anchored* DRGS leads to be less than 1% per lead [34]. This data and expert consensus suggest that anchoring of DRGS leads with a silastic anchor should be the standard of care to prevent lead migration.

Lead fracture

The hallmark of lead fracture is the reading of high lead impedances on the clinician programmer. A lead fracture may not always be visible on X-ray or fluoroscopy. Fractures are thought to be related to the transection of fascial planes with the DRGS lead, with the fascial plane locking a lead in place, and friction created, leading to fracture [3]. Lead fractures were not worsened with lead fixation, which was a concern, and rather were reduced slightly [21]. An ipsilateral approach was also developed to minimize the transection of these fascial planes and is recommended by experts to decrease the risk of fracture [2].

Neural injury

The DRG is susceptible to inflammatory and chemical stimuli. Moreover, its neurons are densely packed and highly excitable, which means even mild mechanical contact or compression such as: a herniated disc, surgical manipulation, or implant placement can result in significant neuropathic pain or sensory disturbances. This sensitivity underscores the importance of careful handling during clinical and surgical procedures involving the spine.

Procedural insult to neural tissue can present as a transient radiculopathy or neuritis, with most symptoms likely resolving over time. These risks can be minimized by using a controlled, gentle technique, preprocedural evaluation, MRI or CT scan, and through appropriate intraoperative monitoring of the patient's nervous system during lead implantation.

Relevant Anatomy

The DRG is a bundle of cell bodies of sensory afferent neurons situated within the intervertebral foramina of each of the 31 pairs of human spinal nerves. It is comprised not only of the cell bodies and axons, but also contains various supporting cells such as satellite glial cells, immune cells, and capillaries.

The DRG has unique factors that make it appealing as a therapeutic target. By stimulating the cell body of the neuron rather than the axon, one can decrease the hyperexcitability seen in chronic pain states. Additionally, there is little to no CSF overlying the majority of the DRG, allowing for lower energy requirements for therapeutic benefit. On the other hand, these hyperexcitable cells and a lack of CSF "cushioning" make the DRG particularly sensitive to physical or chemical stimuli, and render the DRG susceptible to insult from the introducer sheath.

Procedure

Indications and diagnosis (with ICD-10 codes)

On label

Complex Regional Pain Syndrome (CRPS I)—G90.50, G90.511, G90.512.

Causalgia or CRPS II—G57.70, G57.71, G57.72.

Causalgia is defined by the International Association for the Study of Pain (IASP) as a syndrome of sustained burning pain, allodynia, and hyperpathia after a traumatic nerve lesion, often combined with vasomotor and sudomotor dysfunction and later trophic changes.

Causalgia may encompass other postsurgical neuropathic pain syndromes, including but not limited to the following diagnoses if the criteria for causalgia are met (G57.70, G57.71, G57.72):

- Postsurgical Herniorrhaphy Pain—G58.8
- PostSurgical Neuropathy—G58.9
- Postjoint replacement pain (TKR, THR, TAR)- M25.569Chronic PostSurgical Joint Pain—M25.569

Off label

- PostSurgical Pain Syndromes Type I and II (Previously named Postlaminectomy syndrome and NonSurgical LBP)
- Osteoarthritis-related knee pain—M17.1
- Peripheral vascular disease—I73.9
- Chronic Pelvic Pain Syndrome—N94.89
- Diabetic Neuropathy—E11.40

Patient selection considerations

Selecting appropriate candidates for DRGS is crucial to achieving successful outcomes. While the ideal patients typically experience well-defined, localized neuropathic pain that corresponds to a specific dermatomal distribution, DRGS has shown efficacy in treating individuals with mixed-type pain and multi-dermatomal pain, such as back pain. The following factors should be carefully evaluated in patient selection:

Age

DRGS is primarily indicated for adults with chronic neuropathic pain that has been unresponsive to conservative management regardless of age. The ability to utilize technology and a cell phone is necessary to interact with the device.

Contraindications

Patients with active systemic or localized infections at the implantation site should not undergo DRGS until the infection is resolved.

Individuals with untreated coagulopathies or those on anticoagulation therapy without a proper bridging plan are at increased risk of procedural complications.

Severe psychiatric comorbidities, including uncontrolled anxiety, depression, or substance abuse, may interfere with postprocedure management and overall treatment success.

Anatomical limitations such as significant central and foraminal stenosis, extensive prior spinal surgeries, or existing hardware presence may hinder appropriate lead placement and reduce the efficacy of DRGS. Fluoroscopic visualization hindrance may increase inadvertent blunt trauma to the target DRG during lead installation.

Preoperative planning

Advanced imaging (MRI or CT scan) of the target spinal region should be reviewed preoperatively. If no MRI was performed, which is possible in the treatment of CRPS and other off-label indications is a possibility, an MRI of the target spinal region (lumbar or thoracic) should be performed. DRGS lead placement in the lumbar spine, where even in asymptomatic patients may contain severe central spinal stenosis, lateral recess stenosis, or severe foraminal stenosis, may provide an obstacle to placement or may be worsened by the addition of a lead or loops. This also allows for alternative lead placement approaches to be planned beforehand.

Targeted DRG for pain syndromes

The highest level of evidence for DRGS is for CRPS I and focal neuropathic pain related to nerve injury. Most dermatomal pain syndromes require placement at or adjacent to the level of nerve injury. This is consistent with the mechanism of action involved with the filtering of pain signals. However, as our understanding of the therapy grows, placement of leads at levels of convergence of nerve fibers can often provide coverage beyond the range of a single dermatome.

The following table can serve as a guideline for lead placement per condition/diagnosis and per body location . See Tables 15.1 and 15.2.

Maintenance concerns

- Optimizing patient education improves outcomes and reduces the need for office visits.
- Ongoing follow-up visits for device programming and optimization are essential to ensure sustained efficacy and to adjust stimulation parameters as needed.
- DRGS is an ultralow energy form of neuromodulation in which the IPG does not require recharging. Using low energy programming should maintain an IPG life of over 10 years [18].

TABLE 15.1 Level of lead placement per diagnosis.

Pain syndrome/diagnosis	Optimal lead combination(s)
Discogenic pain	Bilateral T12 or L2
Post-knee replacement syndrome	L 2,3, 4
Post-herpetic neuralgia	At level DRG, or above and below affected dermatome
Post-laminectomy syndrome	Bilateral T12 and S1
Post-thoracotomy syndrome	At the affected level(s)
Post-herniorrhaphy syndrome	L1 followed by T12 and L2
Pudendal neuralgia	L1 & S2
Sacroiliac joint pain/adjacent segment syndrome of the SI joint	T12 and S1

Adapted and modified from Chapman KB, et al. Best Practices for dorsal root ganglion stimulation for chronic pain: guidelines from the american society of pain and neuroscience. J Pain Res 2023;16:839–879.

TABLE 15.2 Level of lead placement per body region.

Area	Optimal lead combination(s)
Hand and elbow	C5/6/7/8
Hip joint	T12/L1, L4, and S1
Knee	L2, L3, and L4
Buttock/sacroiliac	T12, ±L1, and S1
Pelvic & genitalia	L1 & S2
Low back	Bilateral T12 or L2
Foot/ankle	L4/5/S1 (mechanical) or S1 alone (neuropathic)

These tables summarize commonly utilized dorsal root ganglion (DRG) lead placement levels according to specific diagnoses and broader body regions. The recommendations presented reflect a synthesis of published literature, clinical experience, and expert consensus, and are intended to serve as a practical reference to guide procedural planning. Variability in individual patient anatomy, pain distribution, and clinical response should be considered when applying these guidelines.
Adapted and modified from Chapman KB, et al. Best Practices for dorsal root ganglion stimulation for chronic pain: guidelines from the american society of pain and neuroscience. J Pain Res 2023;16:839–879.

- As the therapeutic window is narrow and the therapy is paresthesia-free, it is important to use the clinician programmer to assess if the patient is having worsening pain or has simply fallen out of the therapeutic window prior to considering other interventions.
- Remote programming is a consideration for patients who have accessibility issues and can be performed in areas with adequate internet access [35].

Training recommendations

ACGME fellowship and/or residency training specialty

- Following residency training, physicians performing DRGS implantation should undergo an interventional pain management fellowship. An ACGME-accredited or well-regarded fellowship program with high-procedural volume is most optimal to provide comprehensive hands-on exposure to neuromodulation therapies, including clinical decision-making process, procedural proficiency training, postimplantation care and potential complication management.

Suggested case volume for competence

- The FDA placed a requirement that physicians wishing to use the commercially available DRGS system complete a 2-day training program with the company. Adept skills with SCS are a prerequisite for physician eligibility. This training introduction for the DRGS procedures is intended to develop technical proficiency in lead placement, procedural safety, understanding device programming, and troubleshooting complications.

Proctoring recommendation

- The DRGS training course is performed under the supervision of experienced mentors to ensure proper technique and safety. The proctoring process should continue until the physician demonstrates consistent proficiency in procedural execution and postoperative care.

Case peer review

- Continuous professional development is maintained through case studies and training courses. Regular participation in case discussions and journal clubs allows for ongoing assessment of patient selection criteria, procedural effectiveness, and long-term outcomes. Neuromodulation societal and device manufacturer-sponsored quality assurance programs, and seminars should be integrated into one's practice to support continuous improvement and adherence to evolving neuromodulation guidelines.

Technique

Patient positioning

Prone positioning. Additional bolsters, pillows, and specific table frames would be at the discretion of the implanter. Caution should be used with excessive lumbar flexion.

Anesthesia considerations during DRGS placement

Anesthetic care of the patient undergoing DRGS is paramount to safety. Given the sensitive nature of the DRG and surrounding neural tissue combined with the stiffer curved bevel and anatomical challenges with placement, a method of monitoring the patient's neural status is imperative to limit neural insult.

Guidelines recommend performing a trial or implant with either an awake and responsive patient or neuromonitoring for those under general anesthesia. Options include:

Awake, responsive patient strategy

Maintaining an awake patient during DRGS placement provides the most direct neuromonitoring, as verbal feedback enables real-time detection of paresthesia or radicular symptoms. Short-acting benzodiazepines (e.g., midazolam) and opioids (e.g., fentanyl) are commonly used, with dexmedetomidine serving as an alternative that preserves responsiveness while providing analgesia and anxiolysis. Agents such as propofol or ketamine should be used sparingly, particularly before lead placement, to avoid suppressing neurological feedback. Once leads are fixated, deeper sedation may be administered as the risk of neural injury diminishes.

It is important to note that while moderate sedation is often used to enhance patient comfort, anesthetic depth must allow interaction with the operating physician. Inhaled or intravenous general anesthesia may be an appropriate or preferred anesthetic choice, but it should be combined with intraoperative neuromonitoring to compensate for the lack of patient verbal feedback.

Intraoperative neuromonitoring

Intraoperative neuromonitoring (IONM) has been increasingly recognized as a tool for enhancing safety in neuromodulation procedures in patients receiving general anesthesia. Real-time monitoring can help prevent neural injury. IONM consists of somatosensory evoked potentials (SSEP) and electromyography (EMG). Falowski et al. demonstrated IONM's effectiveness in ensuring accurate lead placement in asleep patients in a retrospective analysis of 304 lead placements [36]. Alerts from IONM led to corrective actions without causing severe complications, and no permanent adverse events were reported.

Operating room time estimate

Trial lead(s) placement approximately 20–60 min.

Permanent lead(s) and pulse generator implantation approximately 75–120 min.

Procedure

DRGS lead implantation differs significantly from SCS lead placement; approaches to lead placement are discussed here:

Contralateral approach

This traditional technique involves placing the lead at an oblique angle, contralateral to the target foramen, entering two levels below the target at the lateral pedicle border. While effective, this approach carries a risk of lead fracture due to friction as the lead traverses the paraspinal musculature and superficial fascia. This led to the development of an alternative ipsilateral paramedian approach.

Ipsilateral paramedian approach

The needle is inserted adjacent and parallel to the spinous process and avoids DRGS electrode(s) cross-angular trajectory of the DRGS electrode(s) through the paraspinal musculature and fascia. Key steps for optimized placement include aligning the rostral laminar border using cephalocaudal tilt, rotating the fluoroscope 5–10 degrees for optimal visualization, and advancing the needle to the periosteum before entering the ligamentum flavum. Guidewire placement is adjusted dynamically under fluoroscopic guidance to ensure precise foraminal entry. Once optimal lead placement is achieved, an "S" tension loop is created before it is anchored.

This implantation technique requires cutting down to the fascia and anchoring leads to the deep fascia, reducing the migration risk to approximately 1% per lead without increasing lead fracture rates. See Fig. 15.1.

Contralateral retrograde approach

Also known as the "transgrade" technique, this method allows for access from the interlaminar space cephalad to the target foramen. The Tuohy needle is directed to contact the lamina above the space on the lateral aspect and directed medially to the central interlaminar space. After loss of resistance, the introducer sheath and lead are advanced to the contralateral foramen. Use caution to avoid rotating the curved bevel toward the thecal sac. After the lead is advanced through the foramen, the S loop should be performed. See Fig. 15.2.

This approach is utilized by neuromodulators who use traditional SCS leads to perform transforaminal neurostimulation.

Outside-in approach

An outside-in, transforaminal approach has been described in the literature that was designed to limit contact with the DRG and associated structures. Contact is made first with the inferior articular process to assess depth and trajectory with a finder

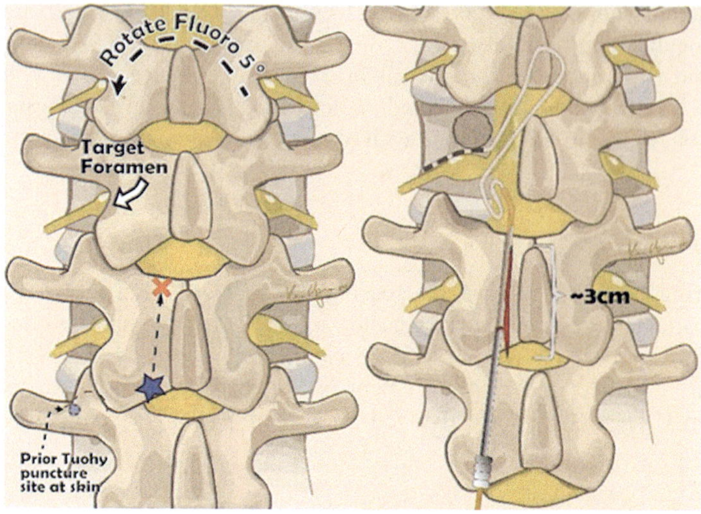

FIGURE 15.1 Anatomic landmarks for ipsilateral approach. The *blue* star (*) indicates needle puncture site. *Red* "X" indicates Tuohy needle contacting lamina. Lead advanced though foramen and ipsilateral "S" loop placed. For implant, incision can be made prior to lead placement, usually from infrapedicular line to infrapedicular line. *From Chapman KB, Spiegel MA, Dickerson DM, et al. A paramedian approach for dorsal root ganglion stimulation placement developed to limit lead migration and fracture. Pain Prac 2021;21(8):991–1000. https://doi.org/10.1111/papr.13063.*

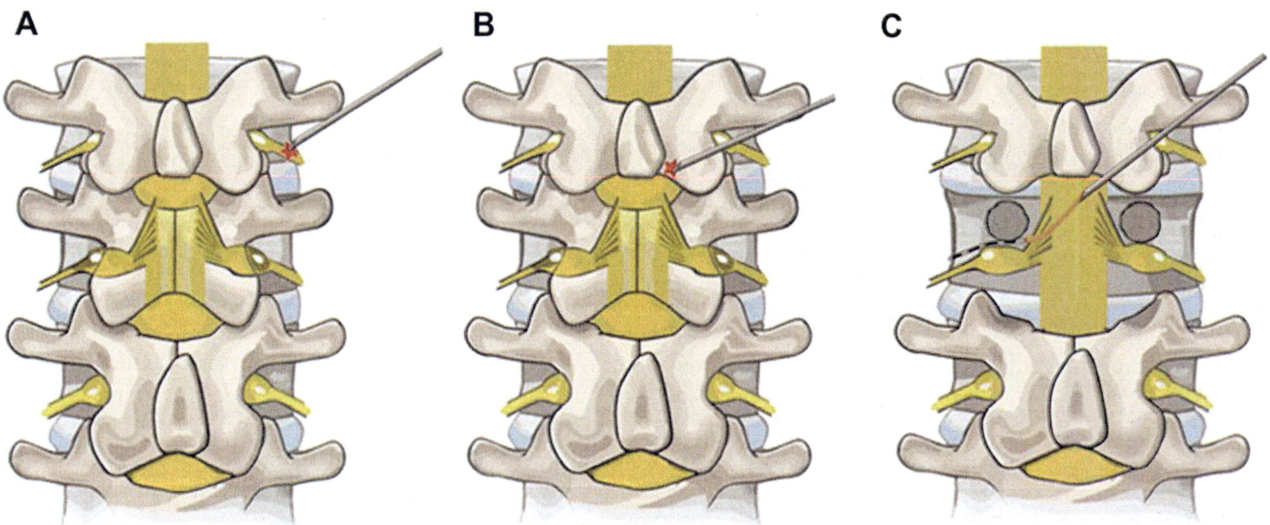

FIGURE 15.2 Schematic representation of transgrade DRG lead placement. (A) Depicts the initial position where the Tuohy needle enters the skin. (B) Depicts the Tuohy needle contacting the lamina prior to walking off and entering the epidural space. The *red cross* indicates graphic target for Tuohy needle. (C) Depicts the Touhy needle within the epidural space with the introducer sheath and lead positioned along the superior aspect of the contralateral foramen, one level below. *From Chapman KB, Ramsook RR, Groenen PS, Vissers KC, van Helmond N. Lumbar transgrade dorsal root ganglion stimulation lead placement in patients with post-surgical anatomical changes: a technical note. Pain Prac 2019;20(4):399–404. https://doi.org/10.1111/papr.12859.*

needle. After this, repeat with the Tuohy needle, and when contact is made with the lateral border, the Tuohy is walked off laterally and advanced several millimeters. The sheath is then advanced slightly, enough to direct the lead into the foramen. Tension loops can be made in the paravertebral space in a fashion similar to epidural "S" loops [5]. *See* Fig. 15.3.

Surgical approaches

Several surgical approaches to DRGS lead placement have been described in the literature using open, microsurgical, and endoscopic techniques. The reports describe these techniques as safe and effective, and although reported numbers have been small, there were no migrations or fractures noted in follow-ups at 1 year and longer.

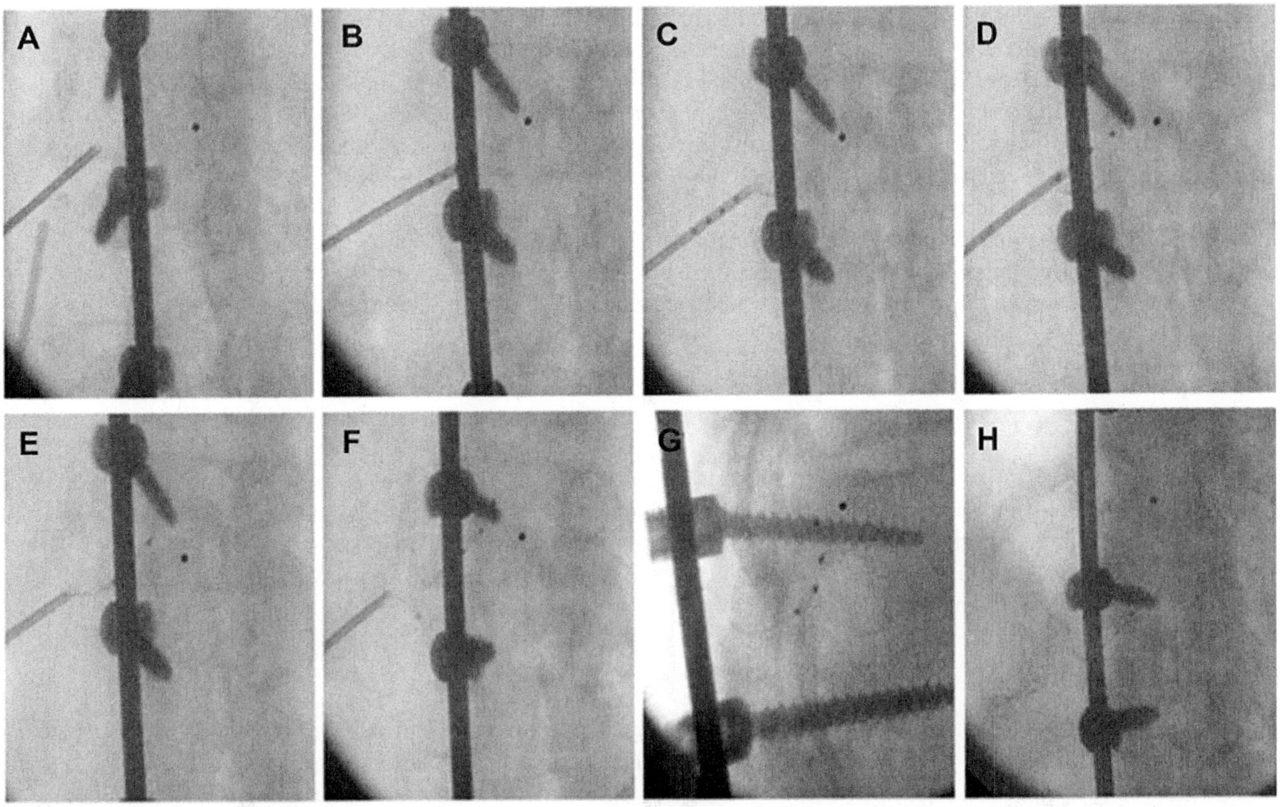

FIGURE 15.3 Outside in approach: (A) Far oblique view with Tuohy needle making contact with the SAP. (B) AP view with Tuohy needle contacting SAP. (C) Tuohy needle retracted slightly with introducer and lead loaded and directed ventrally to the foramen. (D) Lead advanced alone into. (E) Lead advanced and Tuohy retracted slightly. (F) Loops made in soft tissue by advancing the introducer slightly and advancing lead. Then rotating introducer caudally and repeating. (G and H) Final AP and lateral views of lead position. *From Chapman KB, Nagrani S, Patel KV., Yousef T, van Helmond N. Lumbar dorsal root ganglion stimulation lead placement using an outside-in technique in 4 patients with failed back surgery syndrome: a case series. A A Pract 2020;14(10):e01300. https://doi.org/10.1213/XAA.0000000000001300.*

Open techniques have been described with placement through a *laminectomy,* with lead fixation performed with a mini plate to the lamina below [6]. Microsurgical approaches with a *laminotomy*/foraminotomy from the level above have been reported on. In this minimally invasive surgical approach, lead stability is provided with a fibrin patch and fibrin glue after tension loop placement [8].

Intraoperative placement of DRGS leads during a lumbar decompression and fusion has been reported on in a case where decompression was indicated, but the patient also had coexisting CRPS of the knee. Leads were inserted under direct visualization in the foramen over the dorsal aspect of the DRG and were fixed using a braided resorbable suture anchored to the pedicle, followed by a strain relief loop [10].

Endoscopic placement of the DRGS leads has also been reported. The lateral endoscopic trajectory is a similar oblique entry to that used for an endoscopic transforaminal discectomy. This minimally invasive approach allows for lead placement without the need to access the spinal canal. This surgical placement mirrors the outside-in approach detailed above, although rather than paravertebral loops, the report placed a tension loop in the subcutaneous space, leaving concern for migration and or fracture. The report however, did not report any complications [9].

Lead explant considerations

Those suffering from a complication with DRGS were three times more likely to undergo revision surgery rather than device explant [33]. While a testament to the therapy, special consideration during DRGS revision surgery is required to prevent or limit a retained segment (broken piece of lead) and to navigate potential for adhesions and challenges when replacing leads. Neuromonitoring, as described above, should be applied to limit the potential for neural insult.

Lead fractures are often associated with tension points within fascia and muscular planes, and can be entrapped within this tissue. This is usually at or distal to the midline incision site. To reduce the risk of the lead breaking off deep during explant and causing a retained segment, we recommend a thorough dissection of the deep fascia where lead anchoring occurred, and loosening around the lead beyond the fascial anchor point. The lead should be removed with gentle traction. Using a Kelly clamp may apply a more evenly distributed tractional force at these deeper tension points. If there is a retained segment in the epidural space, a surgical consultation is recommended for removal.

When replacing leads during revision surgery, adhesions around the lead tract may form and be an obstacle to lead reimplantation. It is vital to have an awake or neuromonitored patient during lead removal and reimplantation to limit pain and neural insult during the procedure. In addition, there are several approaches described within this chapter that can be used as an alternative method should one face difficulty placing the lead with the initial technique.

Post-operative considerations

Recovery

Postoperative recovery following DRGS implantation is generally well-tolerated, with most patients discharged on the same day. Patients may experience mild to moderate discomfort at the implantation site, which is usually managed with oral analgesics. Close monitoring during the initial postprocedure period is recommended to assess complications such as infection or excessive pain at the surgical site. Patients should receive thorough postoperative instructions, including wound care, signs of infection, and activity limitations, to optimize recovery.

Efficacy estimates

Clinical studies have demonstrated that DRGS provides significant and sustained pain relief in well-selected patients. Reported pain reduction rates range from 50% to 80%, with improved functional outcomes and quality of life. Studies have shown that DRGS offers superior efficacy for CRPS and postsurgical neuropathic pain compared to traditional SCS. Additionally, long-term follow-ups indicate that many patients maintain therapeutic benefits beyond 12 months, with a reduction in opioid usage and improved patient-reported outcomes.

Bracing considerations

Routine bracing is not typically required. Patients should be advised to avoid excessive spinal flexion, extension, and rotational movements until adequate tissue healing has occurred.

Activity limitations

Patients should be instructed to limit strenuous physical activities, including heavy lifting, bending, and twisting, for the first 8 weeks after implantation. These precautions are meant to limit migration, as this typically occurs early in the postoperative period. Gradual reintroduction of activities is encouraged, with physical therapy as needed to facilitate functional recovery. Participation in sports with excessive truncal torque should be minimized if possible.

Maintenance considerations

While DRGS has been shown to be less prone to therapy tolerance and habituation, long-term success with DRGS requires ongoing surveillance. Routine follow-up visits are recommended to maintain a steady therapeutic window. For patients who live far away from the office, DRGS manufacturer remote programming technology enhances patient convenience by allowing real-time adjustments without the need for in-person visits. This secure, cloud-based system enables clinicians to fine-tune stimulation settings remotely and minimizes the need for frequent office appointments [35].

Pearls and Pitfalls

Preoperative

- Review MRI preoperatively to evaluate for central and foraminal stenosis. Severe central stenosis is of concern, and preparation should be made to avoid these levels.

- Planning for the level of lead placement should be performed preop, using the patient's pain condition and distribution as well as the evidence-based recommendations in this chapter.
- Patient education is pivotal to a good outcome and can prevent unnecessary office visits.

Intraoperative

- Plan lead placement with scout fluoroscopy imaging prior to initiation of case.
- Anesthetic considerations: either an awake, responsive patient or IONM with general anesthesia is required for neural monitoring to limit neural insult.
- Anchor placement after dissecting down to the deep fascia is the standard of care for cervical, thoracic, and lumbar lead implantation. Silastic anchor placement greatly reduces migrations and decreases lead fracture.

Postoperative

- Consider bringing trial patients in for a midtrial visit for reprogramming and therapy optimization.
- Use caution with postimplant programming in the recovery area, as fluid and blood near the lead site can alter the impedance and lead to overstimulation when these fluids dissipate.
- When a patient with a DRGS system presents with worsening pain complaints, ensure that the patient is in the therapeutic window with the programmer prior to consideration of procedures or medication changes.

Pitfalls

- Performing DRGS lead placement under deep sedation or general anesthesia without intraoperative neuromonitoring can increase the chance of neural insult.
- Lack of anchor placement will greatly increase the odds of a lead migration.

References

[1] Deer TR, Levy RM, Kramer J, et al. Dorsal root ganglion stimulation yielded higher treatment success rate for complex regional pain syndrome and causalgia at 3 and 12 months: a randomized comparative trial. J Pain 2017;158(4):669–81. https://doi.org/10.1097/j.pain.0000000000000814.

[2] Chapman KB, Spiegel MA, Dickerson DM, et al. A paramedian approach for dorsal root ganglion stimulation placement developed to limit lead migration and fracture. Pain Pract 2021;21(8):991–1000. https://doi.org/10.1111/papr.13063.

[3] Chapman KB, Patel KV, van Helmond N, Chien GCC. Dorsal root ganglion stimulation lead fracture within the superficial fascial layers in 4 cases. Practice 2020;14(11). https://doi.org/10.1213/XAA.0000000000001307.

[4] Chapman KB, Ramsook RR, Groenen PS, Vissers KC, van Helmond N. Lumbar transgrade dorsal root ganglion stimulation lead placement in patients with post-surgical anatomical changes: a technical note. Pain Pract 2019;20(4):399–404. https://doi.org/10.1111/papr.12859.

[5] Chapman KB, Nagrani S, Patel KV, Yousef T, van Helmond N. Lumbar dorsal root ganglion stimulation lead placement using an outside-in technique in 4 patients with failed back surgery syndrome: a case series. Practice 2020;14(10):e01300. https://doi.org/10.1213/XAA.0000000000001300.

[6] Mollica S, Awad M, Teddy PJ. Lead migration in neuromodulation. J Clin Neurosci 2021;90:32–5. https://doi.org/10.1016/j.jocn.2021.05.014.

[7] Bharthi R, Kusyk DM, Patterson M, Tomycz ND. Open surgical implantation of lumbosacral dorsal root ganglion stimulators for chronic pain: analysis of patient outcomes and operative technique. World Neurosurg 2024;18. https://doi.org/10.1016/J.WNEU.2024.09.112.

[8] Piedade GS, Cornelius JF, Chatzikalfas A, Vesper J, Slotty PJ. Open microsurgical dorsal root ganglion lead placement. Neuromodulation 2019;22(8):956–9. https://doi.org/10.1111/ner.12905.

[9] Thissen J, De Ridder D, Maciaczyk J, Bara GA. Endoscopic lateral approach for dorsal root ganglion burst stimulation: technical note and illustrative case series. Neuromodulation 2022;25(7):1033–9. https://doi.org/10.1016/j.neurom.2021.10.022.

[10] Schultheis BC, Willie C, Ross-Steinhagen NE, De Ridder D, Vancamp T, Weidle PA. Alternative dorsal root ganglion neuromodulation electrode implantation : a report of 2 cases with 3 different techniques. J. Neurol. Surg. 2021;4:1–6.

[11] Chapman KB, Groenen PS, Patel KV, Vissers KC, van Helmond N. T12 dorsal root ganglion stimulation to treat chronic low back pain: a case series. Neuromodulation 2020;23(2):203–12. https://doi.org/10.1111/ner.13047.

[12] Kallewaard JW, Edelbroek C, Terheggen M, Raza A, Geurts JW. A prospective study of dorsal root ganglion stimulation for non-operated discogenic low back pain. Neuromodulation 2020;23(2):196–202. https://doi.org/10.1111/ner.12937.

[13] Kallewaard JW, Nijhuis H, Huygen F, et al. Prospective cohort analysis of DRG stimulation for failed back surgery syndrome pain following lumbar discectomy. Pain Pract 2019;19(2):204–10. https://doi.org/10.1111/papr.12734.

[14] Chapman KB, Tupper C, Helmond N van, Yousef TA. Dorsal root ganglion stimulation for the treatment of joint pain with predominantly nociceptive characteristics: a case series. Pain Pract 2023;23(3):317–24. https://doi.org/10.1111/papr.13180. Epub 2022 Dec 8. PMID: 36334041.

[15] Chapman KB, Tupper C, Yousef T, van Helmond N. Dorsal root ganglion stimulation to treat chronic shoulder pain: a case report. Practice 2023;17(11). https://journals.lww.com/aacr/fulltext/2023/11000/dorsal_root_ganglion_stimulation_to_treat_chronic.6.aspx.

[16] Chapman KB, Tupper C, Yang AH, van Helmond N, Yousef T. Intermittent dorsal root ganglion stimulation is as efficacious as standard continuous dosing in treating chronic pain: results from a randomized controlled feasibility trial. Neuromodulation 2021;S1094–7159(21). https://doi.org/10.1016/j.neurom.2021.10.008. 06183-3.

[17] Chapman KB, Yousef TA, Vissers KC, van Helmond N, Stanton D, Hicks M. Very low frequencies maintain pain relief from dorsal root ganglion stimulation: an evaluation of dorsal root ganglion neurostimulation frequency tapering. Neuromodulation 2021;24(4):746–52. https://doi.org/10.1111/ner.13322.

[18] Chapman KB, Tupper C, Amireh A, van Helmond N, Yousef T. Impact of lowering frequency of dorsal root ganglion stimulation on implantable pulse generator consumption. Reg Anesth Pain Med 2022. https://doi.org/10.1136/rapm-2022-103644 (rapm-2022-103644).

[19] ClinicalTrials.gov. Dorsal root ganglion stimulation outcomes for the treatment of mechanical knee pain among patients with osteoarthritis of the surgical and non-surgical knee. 2022. https://clinicaltrials.gov/ct2/show/NCT05103527. [Accessed 10 April 2025].

[20] Moman RN, Peterson AA, Maher DP, et al. Infectious complications of dorsal root ganglion stimulation: a systematic review and pooled analysis of incidence. Neuromodulation 2021. https://doi.org/10.1111/ner.13473.

[21] Chapman KB, Mogilner AY, Yang AH, et al. Lead migration and fracture rate in dorsal root ganglion stimulation using anchoring and non-anchoring techniques: a multicenter pooled data analysis. Pain Pract 2021;21(8):859–70. https://doi.org/10.1111/papr.13052.

[22] Burns SL, Majdak P, Adler AR, et al. Dorsal root ganglion stimulation for patients with chronic pelvic pain: a retrospective review of patient experiences and long-term outcomes. Interv Pain Med 2024;3(1):100397. https://doi.org/10.1016/J.INPM.2024.100397.

[23] Hunter CW, Yang A. Dorsal root ganglion stimulation for chronic pelvic pain: a case series and technical report on a novel lead configuration. Neuromodulation 2019;22(1):87–95.

[24] Kloosterman JR, Yang A, van Helmond N, Chapman KB. Dorsal root ganglion stimulation to treat persistent abdominal pain after bypass surgery. Pain Med 2020;21(1):201–3. https://doi.org/10.1093/pm/pnz193.

[25] Ghorayeb JH, Chitneni A, Rupp A, Parkash A, Abd-Elsayed A. Dorsal root ganglion stimulation for the treatment of chronic pelvic pain: a systematic review. Pain Pract 2023;23(7):838–46. https://doi.org/10.1111/papr.13255.

[26] Chapman KB, Spiegel MA, van Helmond N, et al. Dorsal root ganglion stimulation as a salvage therapy following failed spinal cord stimulation. Neuromodulation 2022:1–9. https://doi.org/10.1016/j.neurom.2022.04.050.

[27] Yang A, Hunter CW. Dorsal root ganglion stimulation as a salvage treatment for complex regional pain syndrome refractory to dorsal column spinal cord stimulation: a case series. Neuromodulation 2017;20(7):703–7. https://doi.org/10.1111/ner.12622.

[28] Smith GL, Petersen EA, Paul C, Goree JH. Transgrade dorsal root ganglion stimulation as a salvage technique for three different anatomical barriers: A case series. Neuromodulation. 2020;2020. https://doi.org/10.1111/ner.13276.

[29] Levy RM, Mekhail N, Kramer J, et al. Therapy habituation at 12 Months: spinal cord stimulation versus dorsal root ganglion stimulation for complex regional pain syndrome type I and II. J Pain 2020;21(3–4):399–408. https://doi.org/10.1016/j.jpain.2019.08.005.

[30] Mons MR, Chapman KB, Terwiel C, Joosten EA, Kallewaard JW. Burst spinal cord stimulation as compared with L2 dorsal root ganglion stimulation in pain relief for nonoperated discogenic low back pain: analysis of two prospective studies. Neuromodulation 2024;27(1):172–7. https://doi.org/10.1016/J.NEUROM.2023.04.464.

[31] Horan M, Jacobsen AH, Scherer C, et al. Complications and effects of dorsal root ganglion stimulation in the treatment of chronic neuropathic pain: a nationwide cohort study in Denmark. Neuromodulation 2020;2020. https://doi.org/10.1111/ner.13171.

[32] Hines K, Swaminathan V, Thalheimer S, Kogan M, Wu C. Single-center retrospective analysis of device-related complications related to dorsal root ganglion stimulation for pain relief in 31 patients. Neuromodulation 2021:2021. https://doi.org/10.1111/ner.13498.

[33] Sivanesan E, Bicket MC, Cohen SP. Retrospective analysis of complications associated with dorsal root ganglion stimulation for pain relief in the FDA MAUDE database. Reg Anesth Pain Med 2019;44(1):100. https://doi.org/10.1136/RAPM-2018-000007.

[34] Chapman KB, Yousef T, Amireh A, Kallewaard JW, van Helmond N. Lead migration rate in dorsal root ganglion stimulation using lead anchoring techniques: a follow-up study. Pain Pract 2024;24(1):72–5. https://doi.org/10.1111/papr.13285.

[35] Deer TR, Esposito MF, Cornidez EG, Okaro U, Fahey ME, Chapman KB. Teleprogramming service provides safe and remote stimulation options for patients with DRG-S and SCS implants. J Pain Res 2021;14(October):3259–65. https://doi.org/10.2147/jpr.s332966.

[36] Falowski SM, Deer T, Tubic G, Mehta P. Multicenter retrospective analysis of dorsal root ganglion stimulator placement using intraoperative neuromonitoring in asleep patients during early periods of adoption. Neuromodulation 2020;2020. https://doi.org/10.1111/ner.13286.

Chapter 16

Sacral dorsal root ganglion stimulation

Trishul Kapoor[1], Andrew Dudas[2], Ammar Mahmoud[3] and Robert Heros[4]
[1]Department of Pain Management, Cleveland Clinic Foundation, Cleveland, OH, United States; [2]Mays & Schnapp Neuroscience and Spine, Memphis, TN, United States; [3]Alleviate Pain & Spine, Bangor, ME, United States; [4]Spinal Diagnostics, PC, Tualatin, OR, United States

Introduction

As of 2023, according to a National Health Survey conducted by the Centers for Disease Control and Prevention (CDC), it is estimated that nearly 24.3% of adults report chronic pain [1]. The presentation of chronic pain can be diverse, but some of the most common forms of chronic pain include mechanical and neuropathic low back pain, joint-related arthropathies, and chronic pelvic pain. The application of sacral nerve dorsal root ganglion stimulation (DRG-S) is primarily indicated for chronic pelvic pain syndromes and lower extremity complex regional pain syndrome (CRPS). In particular, DRG-S is a technique that is tailored toward treating neuropathic conditions with a sacral nerve distribution (i.e., lower back, buttocks, genitals, and thighs). The dorsal root ganglia (DRG) in the sacral foramina contain afferent nerve fibers from the S1, S2, S3 spinal nerves and cell bodies. These pseudo-unipolar type neurons project to the anterolateral spinal tracts and travel to cortical structures.

The utilization of DRG-S was first described in a case report published in 1998 to treat a patient with low back pain of discogenic etiology [2]. In this particular application, the author used conventional dorsal column spinal cord stimulation (SCS) leads to target the L2 DRG and achieved nearly 70% analgesic relief [2]. It was not until 2009 that a neurostimulation lead was developed to specifically target the DRG. The unique anatomy of and anatomic location of the DRG demanded certain lead characteristics to ensure safe and accurate stimulation. These included a smaller profile (diameter), greater flexibility, and a limited number of contacts (4 instead of 8) compared to a traditional dorsal column SCS lead. DRG-S was first approved by the European Union and Australia in 2011 after the publication of a multi-center study demonstrating the efficacy of this technique in patients with chronic neuropathic pain of the lower back and extremities [2]. Following this, numerous studies were published demonstrating therapeutic efficacy, improvement in quality of life, and increased functionality in patients treated with DRG-S [2–4]. In 2016, the US Food and Drug Administration (FDA) officially approved DRG-S for patients with CRPS of the groin and lower extremities [2–4].

DRG-S is unique in comparison to conventional SCS for several reasons. First, DRG-S utilizes a lower electrical current, but achieves a greater electrical efficiency and consumption without compromising therapeutic efficacy due to a focused DRG target [2]. This is made possible by the native anatomy of the spinal nerve root passing through the neural foramen; while there is CSF surrounding the DRG, it is significantly less so when compared to the dorsal column. The electrodes are therefore much closer to the target structure, allowing for lower energy requirements. In addition, DRG-S is generally thought to have more lead placement stability with positional changes. However, this is not always the case with lumbar dorsal root ganglion stimulation (DRG-L). As discussed in further detail later in this chapter, traditional DRG-S is performed via a minimally invasive approach and anchored with the formation of loops with the distal portion of the leads in the subcutaneous and subfascial layers. However, recent innovations have considerably improved DRG-S procedural efficiency and lead placement with smaller incisions, lead anchoring devices, and intraoperative navigation with fluoroscopy and 3D navigation.

DRG-S is also considerably evolving with technological advancements. The lead designs have been consistently refined to be smaller and remarkably flexible. Furthermore, the electrode contact configurations are uniquely designed to make maximal contact with the sacral DRG to improve focused target stimulation and minimize paresthesia. In addition, implantable pulse generators (IPGs) for DRG-S have significantly advanced to deliver customized programming of stimulation patterns based on the personalized needs of a patient. However, despite these advancements, there is a

A Modern Atlas for Implantable Devices of the Spine, Brain, and Nerve. https://doi.org/10.1016/B978-0-443-36528-7.00031-5

growing field of research with DRG-S focused on biofeedback integration, improved patient selection, target refinement, and treatment optimization.

Key points

- DRG-S is a specialized and selective application of neuromodulation therapy that is designed to target the sacral nerve dorsal root ganglia in an effort to treat CRPS and chronic pelvic pain syndromes.
- The DRG is the neuroforaminal dilatation of tissue that carries the axons of the primary afferent sensory neurons located as paired structures within the anterolateral epidural space at each spinal level (8 paired cervical 12 paired thoracic, five paired lumbar, and four paired sacral).
- DRG-S has current FDA approval for treating CRPS Type I and II of the lower extremities. CRPS Type 1 (ICD 10 code G90.5), formerly known as reflex sympathetic dystrophy (RSD), develops without definitive nerve injury. CRPS Type 2 (ICD 10 code G90.6), also known as causalgia, is typically the result of specific nerve damage following trauma or surgical injury.
- The Neuromodulation Appropriateness Consensus Committee (NACC) on the best practices for Dorsal Root Ganglion stimulation recommends that DRG-S only be considered in the treatment of pelvic pain using strict selection criteria. This includes a clear mechanism of injury be ascertained, post-surgical or trauma-related, and pain is categorized as being visceral or somatic. In this patient population, the decision to proceed with DRG-S should be multidisciplinary involving gynecology, urology, psychology and primary care.
- The ACCURATE trial published in 2017 is currently the only RCT evaluating efficacy of DRG-S. In this study, DRG-S showed greater efficacy in treating pain related to CRPS at 3 (81.2 vs. 55.7%) and 12 months (74.2 vs. 53%) as compared to DCS.

Relevant anatomy

The DRG is the neuroforaminal dilatation of the spinal nerve root carrying the axons of the primary afferent sensory neurons. Paired structures located within the anterolateral epidural space at each spinal level (8 paired cervical 12 paired thoracic, 5 paired lumbar, and 4 paired sacral), the DRG acts as a low pass filter for visceral and somatic stimuli originating from the periphery and traveling to the central nervous system. In addition, the DRG has T junctions which have been postulated to be the primary target for stimulation (Fig. 16.1) [5]. The location of the DRG within the neuroforamen varies based on the individual spinal level. The seminal anatomic study on the location of sacral DRGs was conducted by

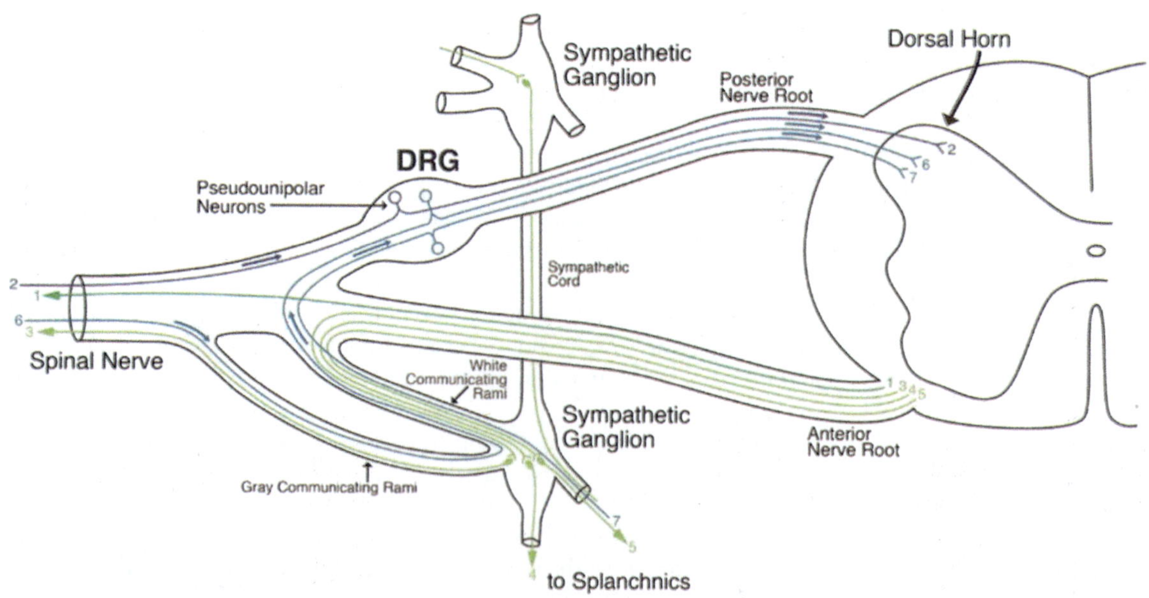

FIGURE 16.1 This figure demonstrates the anatomic framework of neuronal pathways within the DRG as it blocks, propagates, and filters peripheral nerve action potentials. a. Physical Medicine and Rehabilitation Clinics of North America, 2022-05-01, volume 33, issue 2, pages 359–378, copyright © 2022 Elsevier Inc.

Ebraheim and Lu in 1998 [6]. On examination of 20 cadavers, they found that the S1 DRG is intraforaminal in 55%–60% of patients and "intracanalar" in 40%–45% (medial to the medial border of the sacral pedicle) [6]. The S2 DRG was most commonly in the vertebral canal (ranging from 50%–85% of the time), and the S3 and S4 DRGs were always in the vertebral canal [6]. Therefore in the sacrum, the DRGs are actually more typically located within the vertebral canal itself and none are extraforaminal [5–8]. The sacrum tapers as it progresses inferiorly, making the inferior aspect of the sacrum (the apex) narrower than the superior aspect (the base) [7]. This size can vary from patient to patient and is typically larger in males than it is in females. The DRGs themselves also get smaller as one progresses inferiorly [7]. The sacrum is concave anteriorly which affects the angulation of the sacral foramina. The sacral foramen is triangular in shape at S1, becoming more ovoid as they progress inferiorly. Each level has an anterior (pelvic) and posterior (dorsal) foramen [8]. The foramina are typically angled from medial to lateral with the posterior foramen being more medial than the anterior foramen, therefore necessitating a more medial to lateral approach with needle entry for access. Each foramina varies slightly in anatomy as well. Of note, small segmental arteries and veins also exit through the foramina along with the sacral nerve root.

Procedure

While conventional dorsal column spinal cord stimulation (SCS) is commonly utilized for refractory trunk and limb pain, lack of precision with SCS limits its efficacy in treating focal pain in discrete anatomical regions. Dorsal root ganglion stimulation (DRG-S), in contrast, offers targeted dermatomal neuromodulation, which is a key factor in its proven superiority in treating focal pain conditions such as Complex Regional Pain Syndrome (CRPS) and causalgia [4]. Sacral DRG-S is considered for the management of refractory focal pain syndrome such as CRPS Type I and II of the lower extremities, painful diabetic neuropathy, phantom limb pain and refractory pelvic pain syndromes.

DRG-S has current FDA approval for treating CRPS Type I and II of the lower extremities. CRPS Type 1 (ICD 10 code G90.5), formerly known as reflex sympathetic dystrophy (RSD), develops without definitive nerve injury. CRPS Type 2 (ICD 10 code G90.6), also known as causalgia, is typically the result of specific nerve damage following trauma or surgical injury. CRPS is a clinical diagnosis of exclusion and is best diagnosed using the Budapest criteria which demonstrated a high sensitivity (0.99) and specificity (0.79) [9]. There are no established imaging or laboratory tests that are currently used to diagnose CRP. However, bone densitometry, electromyography (EMG), and quantitative sensory testing (QST) may be helpful [10]. The efficacy of DRG-S in treating CRPS, particularly CRPS affecting the lower extremities, was demonstrated by the ACCURATE study published in 2017 [4]. They found that 81.2% of patients (56/69) responded to DRGS versus 55.7% of patients (39/70) to SCS at 3-month follow-up. Long term, the proportion of subjects who achieved treatment success at 12 months in the DRG arm (74.2%; 49/66) also was greater than that in the SCS arm (53.0%; 35/66); these results demonstrated both noninferiority ($P < 0.0001$) and superiority ($P < 0.0004$) at the long-term follow-up. Sacral DRG-S, specifically at S1, has also been found to be a potential target in patients suffering from diabetic peripheral neuropathy [11]. Large randomized controlled clinical trials are needed to further explore and demonstrate the efficacy of DRG-S for DPN and other non-diabetic peripheral neuropathies.

Due to the complex neuroanatomy and innervation of the pelvic viscera, which receive innervation from both the lumbar and sacral plexuses, there is difficulty in providing consistent coverage of the affected area with SCS. Hence, out of all the diagnoses treated with SCS, CPP was found to have the highest explant rate [12]. Various lead placement locations and combination arrays have been proposed when targeting DRG for CPP [13–15]. The L1 and S2 lead array has reported the most success in ensuring coverage of the lower abdomen, groin, and pelvis [16,17]. The L1 DRG is a confluence for three lumbar plexus nerves commonly implicated including the ilioinguinal (L1-2), iliohypogastric (L1-2), and genitofemoral nerves (L1-2). This is in conjunction with S2 to interrupt primary afferent input from the sacral plexus including the pudendal nerve (S2–S4) and sacral splanchnic sympathetic plexus.

The evidence for DRG-S for pelvic pain is reported in one case series, three case reports, and one retrospective study, all of which have evaluated and established the efficacy of DRG-S implants in this patient population, with limitations present [13–20]. Hunter et al. reported with a case report of seven patients who underwent sacral DRG-S placement at S2, as well as L1, to cover the generalized dermatomal distribution involved in CPP [13]. This lead configuration of DRG-S is most widely accepted and is within on-label indications for placing leads between the T10-S2 levels. The DRG Focus paper also highlights other possible lead arrays that have been used to treat refractory CPP [13].

The Neuromodulation Appropriateness Consensus Committee (NACC) on the best practices for Dorsal Root Ganglion stimulation recommends that DRG-S only be considered in the treatment of pelvic pain using strict selection criteria [21]. They describe that a clear mechanism of injury be ascertained, post-surgical or trauma-related, and pain is categorized as being visceral or somatic. In this patient population, the decision to proceed with DRG-S should be multidisciplinary involving gynecology, urology, psychology and primary care. The use of DRG-S in the management of CPP is supported by level III evidence, suggesting the recommendations are based upon clinical experience-based opinions, descriptive studies, clinical observations, or reports of expert committees.

There are two case reports that discuss the utilization of sacral DRG-S in an off-label manner, both of which involved patients suffering from CPP. Zuidema et al. present a case report of utilizing DRG-S at S3 for a patient with chronic perineal pain after surgical resection of a Bartholin's cyst [22]. Santiago et al. discuss a case of a patient with refractory coccygodynia, who underwent bilateral S3 and S4 DRG-S implantation, with significant improvement of his underlying pain [23]. While placing leads in the S3 and S4 foramina allows for better coverage of perineal and coccygeal pain, the anatomic features of the sacral canal make placement of leads and the creation of strain relief loops technically difficult.

When selecting patients for DRG-S, there are general and anatomical considerations that need to be evaluated. Anatomical considerations can be assessed with MRI imaging to evaluate for spinal and neural foraminal stenosis at the index level and to ensure adequate foraminal patency to allow for safe device placement. General considerations for implantable therapies according to the NACC guidelines include [21]

- Appropriate psychological evaluation.
- No active substance abuse or ongoing addiction.
- Appropriate anticoagulant management that allows for safe placements of leads in the epidural space.
- Optimized medical comorbidities that may affect the outcome of the procedure.
- Appropriate patient education surrounding neuromodulation treatment with opportunities to ask questions and understand different treatment options.

The contraindications present for DRG-S overlap many of those for other SCS implantation procedures. Patient refusal, patient inability to understand and operate the device, active coagulopathy and infection, uncontrolled medical comorbidities, and an immunocompromised state all present general contraindications. When considering the utilization of sacral DRG-S in patients with CPP, a relative contraindication would be the presence of significant psychological comorbidity and a history of sexual abuse in a patient who has not undergone proper therapy or counseling.

There is no consensus regarding any age limitations or restrictions regarding the utilization of DRG-S. Similar to SCS, Most published studies on DRG-S involve adult patients (≥18 years of age). Extrapolating from the available SCS data, a retrospective study examining whether SCS outcomes correlate with age found that SCS outcomes are equivalent or better in patients 65 years of age or older [24]. There are limited studies regarding the utilization of neuromodulation in the pediatric population. In a literature review of a total of 183 children (ages 7–18 years old) with CRPS, SCS was reserved for severe cases of CRPS and the mean age of these patients was 11.6 years, with the youngest patient being 8 years old [25].

As spinal neuromodulation continues to expand to include newer targets and delivery techniques, such as DRG-S, there continues to be a notable paucity of guidelines to address standardization across training programs. The most recent Accreditation Council for Graduate Medical Education (ACGME) program requirements do not mandate case minimums for DRG-S neuromodulation. DRG-S certification is provided through industry-sponsored didactic and cadaver training. To complement fellowship training, several international and regional pain societies offered training curricula and courses for fellows and early practitioners. Notability, the American Society of Pain and Neuroscience (ASPN) has created the Pain Education and Knowledge (PEAK) Consensus Guidelines for Neuromodulation to provide a comprehensive perspective in establishing guidelines to allow for standardization across different fellowship and training programs [26].

Identifying the case volume required to obtain true proficiency is still debated and quite subjective. ASPN PEAK Consensus Committee recommends that trainees have at least 5 DRG-S trials and five permanent DRG-S implant procedures during training, amounting to about 1 a month [26]. While this is a relatively low number, it is realistically attainable across all fellowship and training programs. The PEAK Consensus Committee also recommends that all fellows receive foundational training in DRG-S, due to its growing evidence in treating CRPS and neuropathic pain. This includes additional engagement in society cadaver labs, company-sponsored labs, and lecture-based curricula during the academic year [26].

Peer-to-peer proctoring is typically recommended for DRG–S, both for post-graduate physicians and early attending physicians to gain experience and familiarity with DRG-S. Proctoring is typically accomplished by subject matter experts such as fellowship directors or qualified attending physicians. This is especially critical when it comes to sacral DRG-S, where the sacral anatomy may be more challenging to visualize and the creation of adequate strain relief loops can be more challenging.

Technique

When preparing for the DRG-S procedure, it is crucial to complete proper pre-procedural planning. Specifically, a proper radiological survey reviewing the cross-sectional MRI or CT imaging is important in evaluating the sacral foramina and needle trajectory. Once appropriate informed consent is obtained, the patient is positioned prone with a pillow placed underneath the lower abdomen to minimize lumbar spine lordosis and place the sacrum in counter-nutation to better visualize the sacral foramina. This positioning will allow for easier instrumentation and needle placement into the sacral foramina.

The DRG-S procedure is separated into two categories - trial and permanent implant. Anesthetic considerations vary depending on whether a DRG-S trial or permanent implant is being performed. A DRG-S trial is ideally performed under minimal anxiolysis or moderate sedation with local anesthetic subcutaneous infiltration. Whereas, a DRG-S permanent implant is performed under monitored anesthesia care (MAC). The operating room time estimate for a DRG-S trial is approximately 15–30 min. Whereas for a DRG-S permanent implant, the operating room time estimate is approximately 45–60 min.

Vendor support is crucial when planning for DRG-S trial and permanent implant. It is important to review the following features during pre-procedural planning with a vendor - number of DRG-S leads, length of DRG-S leads, epidural needle sizes and types, recharge-free IPG with a battery life up to 6.5 years, IPG software upgrades without IPG replacement, mobile device compatibility and communication for therapy selection, and MRI conditional labeling.

DRG-S trial

After the patient is brought to the operating room and a surgical time-out is completed, the patient is positioned in a prone position, as described previously, on the X-ray table. After the administration of preoperative antibiotics, the patient is prepped and draped in a standard sterile fashion. Subsequently, an antero-posterior (AP) fluoroscopic image is taken to visualize the sacral foramina. The S2 foramina should be readily visible in a standard AP view, but the S1 foramina may require cephalad angulation.

For the purpose of this chapter, the right S1 foramina will be targeted. If the right S1 foramen is targeted, a transforaminal epidural approach is taken with a needle entry target at the five o'clock position of the osseous perimeter of the foramen. If the left S1 foramen is targeted, a transforaminal epidural approach is taken with a needle entry target at the 7 o'clock position of the osseous perimeter of the foramen. Following this, local anesthetic is infiltrated in the skin and subcutaneous tissue overlying the site marked for needle entry. The straight introducer needle is subsequently percutaneously inserted in a caudal-oblique fashion along the anaesthetized tract until osseous contact is made at the five o'clock position of the S1 foraminal border. Next, the needle is advanced off the osseous edge into the foramen. The needle is advanced 1–1.5 cm in the trajectory of the foramen with the bevel at a 45 degrees degree facing the foraminal opening (Figs. 16.2 and 16.3).

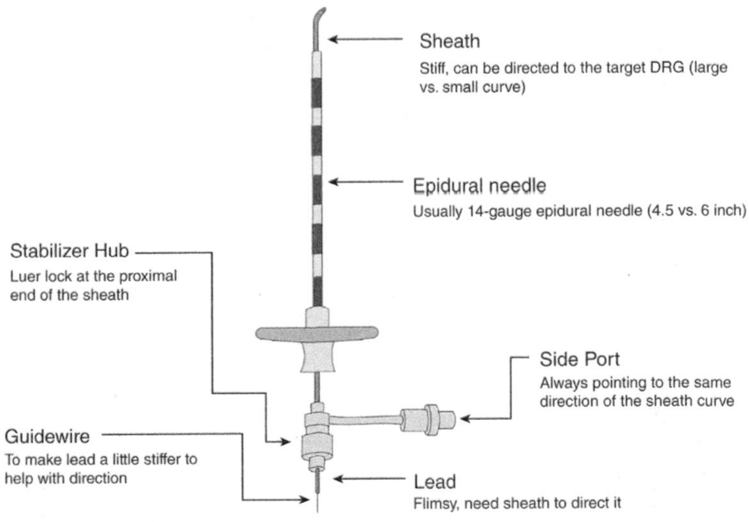

FIGURE 16.2 This figure demonstrates the equipment utilized in a DRG procedure. a. Neuromodulation Techniques for the Spine, Chapter 13, 109–119, copyright © 2024 Elsevier Inc.

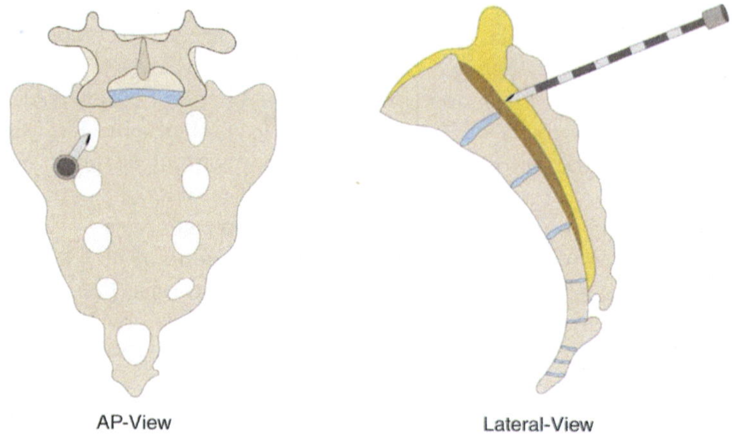

FIGURE 16.3 This figure demonstrates the correct placement of the epidural introducer needle in AP and lateral views. a. Neuromodulation techniques for the spine, Chapter 13, 109–119, copyright © 2024 Elsevier Inc.

Subsequently, the DRG large-curve introducer sheath is pre-loaded with the DRG lead. The DRG large-curve introducer should have at least 1 mm of the DRG lead tip exposed at the distal opening. The DRG introducer sheath and DRG lead is then locked into position. Next, the stylette is disengaged from the straight introducer and removed while maintaining the introducer needle position within the S1 foramen. The DRG introducer sheath pre-loaded with the DRG lead is inserted into the introducer needle. The sheath-lead combo is then advanced while maintaining the sheath injection port facing in caudal-oblique direction (projecting the S1 foraminal tract). The sheath-lead combo is advanced until the white marker on the sheath enters the straight introducer needle hub. This demarcates externalization of the DRG lead from the introducer needle cannula. The sheath-lead combo is carefully advanced under live fluoroscopic imaging in a lateral view until 1 DRG contact is positioned anterior to the ventral surface of the sacrum.

The sheath-lead combo is then unlocked and the sheath is carefully retracted into the introducer needle while maintaining the lead position as described previously. At this point, intraoperative testing should be performed to confirm optimal lead positioning. Next, the introducer needle is withdrawn slightly while being maintained within the epidural space and the bevel turned to face cephalad. The lead-sheath combo is relocked and then advanced to form the upper portion of the anchoring S-curve. Once the top portion of the curve is formed, the lead-sheath combo is unlocked and the sheath is carefully retracted into the introducer needle while maintaining the lead position. The bevel of the introducer needle is turned to face caudad and the relocked lead-sheath combo is advanced to form the lower portion of the anchoring S-curve (Fig. 16.4). Next, the lead-sheath combo is unlocked and the sheath is retracted carefully out of the introducer needle. Lastly, the introducer needle is removed while maintaining the lead position. The lead is then anchored at the level

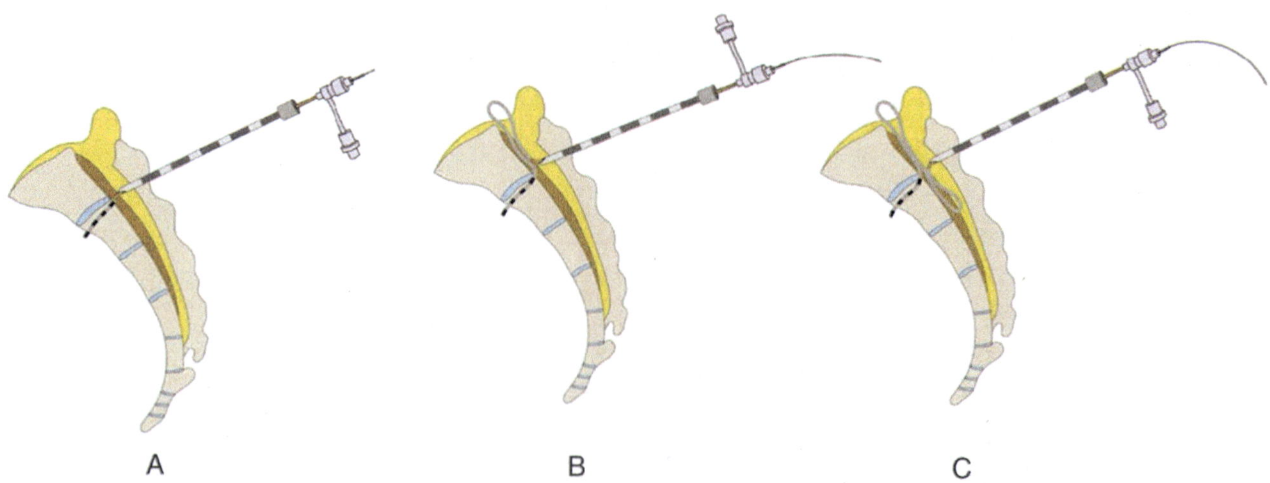

FIGURE 16.4 This figure demonstrates correct lead placement with superior and inferior loop creation at the S1 foramen. a. Neuromodulation techniques for the spine, Chapter 13, 109–119, copyright © 2024 Elsevier Inc.

of the skin with skin glue, adhesive dressing, or suture fixation. The percutaneous lead exit site is covered with a sterile dressing and the lead is connected to an external pulse generator (EXP). The EXP should be placed above the level of the iliac crest and on the side of patient preference.

DRG-S permanent implant

When completing a DRG-S permanent implant, all of the same steps as the DRG-S trial are performed along with a few additional steps. First, prior to placement of the introducer needle, a 1 cm vertical stab incision is made with a no. 15-blade or no. 11-blade. Alternatively, the incision can be extended to accommodate external subcutaneous anchoring devices. Second, a 4–5 cm horizontal incision is marked below the right or left iliac crest (based on patient preference) and local anesthetic is subcutaneously infiltrated over a broad area approximating the size of the IPG. Third, an incision is made and blunt dissection is carried out to create a subcutaneous pocket for the IPG without violating the gluteal fascia. Fourth, a subcutaneous tissue tunneler is used to create a tract from the lead insertion site to the IPG site. Fifth, the lead is passed through tunneling sheath and the sheath removed while avoiding lead traction (Fig. 16.5). Sixth, the lead is connected to the IPG and fixated. Lastly, the incisions are closed and re-approximated in a layered fashion with sutures and skin glue. Antibiotic cream is applied to incisions and the incisions are covered with sterile dressings.

Fluoroscopic images of correct lead placement and position are demonstrated in Fig. 16.6–16.8.

Post-operative considerations

Recovery time is typically minimal after both trial and implantation of DRG-S. Both trial and implantation procedures are routinely performed outpatient and, with very few exceptions, do not require hospital admission. Although general anesthesia is often used for implantation, both procedures can be done under local anesthesia with or without sedation. Some procedural discomfort is expected and can last for several days postoperatively. This can be treated with 5–7 days of postoperative opioids. However, this is generally neither necessary nor recommended.

An occlusive dressing is placed after implantation and should remain in place for at least 48 h postoperatively. It is common to have patients continue to wear the dressing until their initial postoperative visit 7–10 days following the procedure. At this time, the dressing is removed and incision assessed. If staples or nonabsorbable sutures have been left in place, these will also be removed at this time. Showering is allowed after 48 h postoperatively, but the patient should be counseled not to submerge in water for at least 2 weeks after the procedure or the wound is adequately healed [21,27,28]. The patient should also be educated on warning signs of poor wound healing, infection, or neurologic deficit so these can be identified early if present.

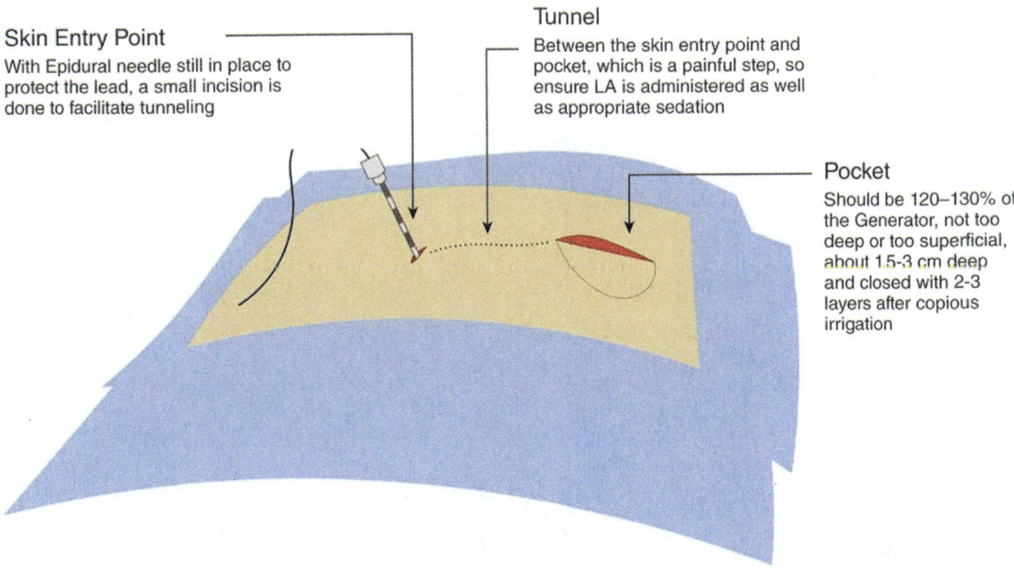

FIGURE 16.5 This figure demonstrates the ideal tunneling pathway of the lead to the IPG pocket site. a. Neuromodulation techniques for the spine, Chapter 13, 109–119, copyright © 2024 Elsevier Inc.

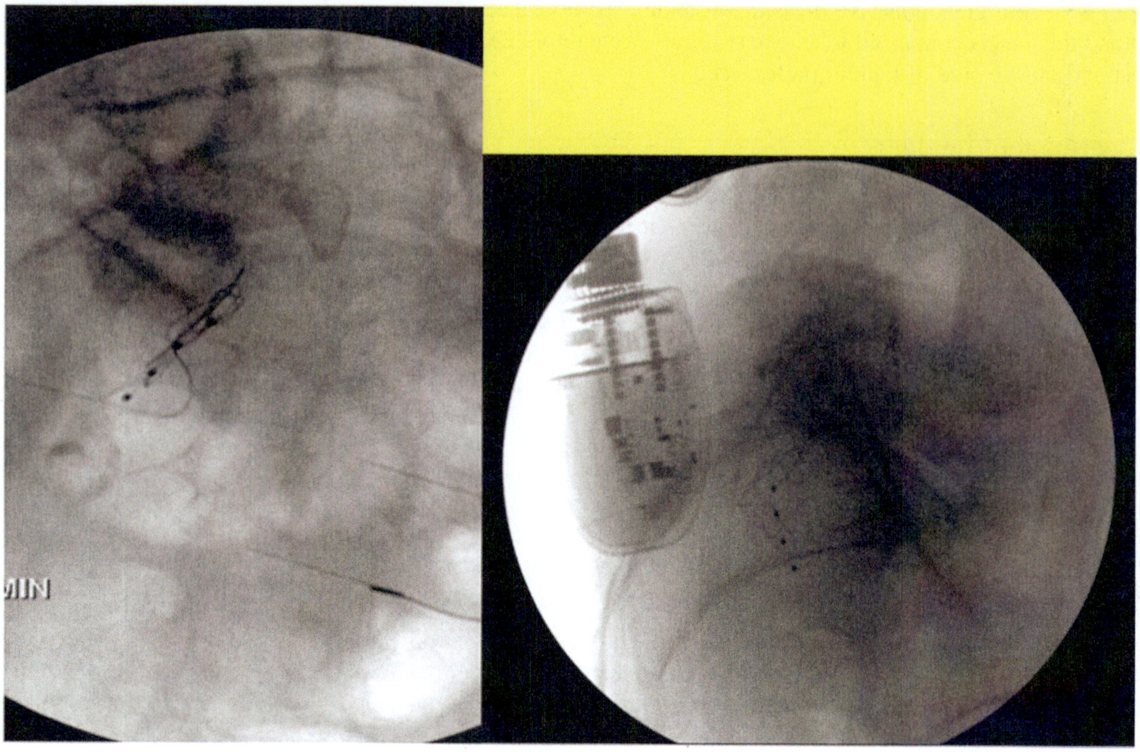

FIGURE 16.6 This figure demonstrates the ideal and correct placement of the S1 DRG lead and IPG in AP and lateral fluoroscopic views.

It is imperative to counsel the patient on specific activity limitations after implantation to limit risk of lead migration as well as aid in optimal incisional healing. This allows the leads more time to scar into the epidural space and limits lead migration risk [21]. Generally speaking, patients should be counseled to avoid large movements of bending and twisting that would risk incision dehiscence or lead migration. Limiting lifting to objects less than five pounds is recommended for 6–8 weeks following surgery and can be liberalized at that time under the guidance of the surgeon if no wound closure or

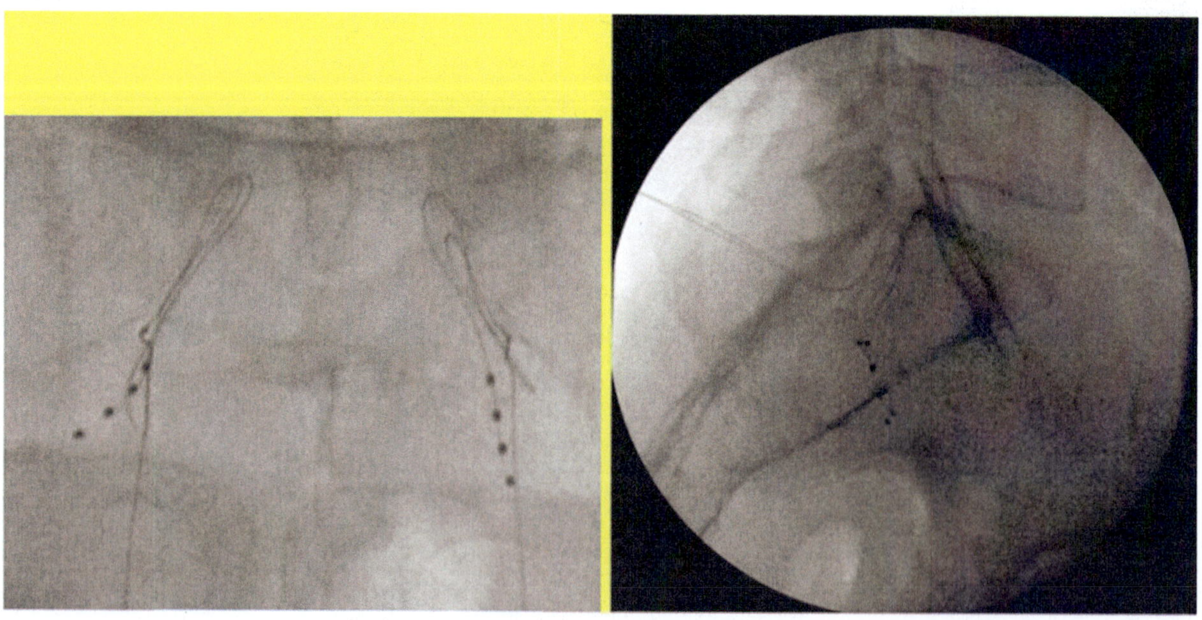

FIGURE 16.7 This figure demonstrates the ideal and correct placement of bilateral S1 DRG leads in AP and lateral fluoroscopic views.

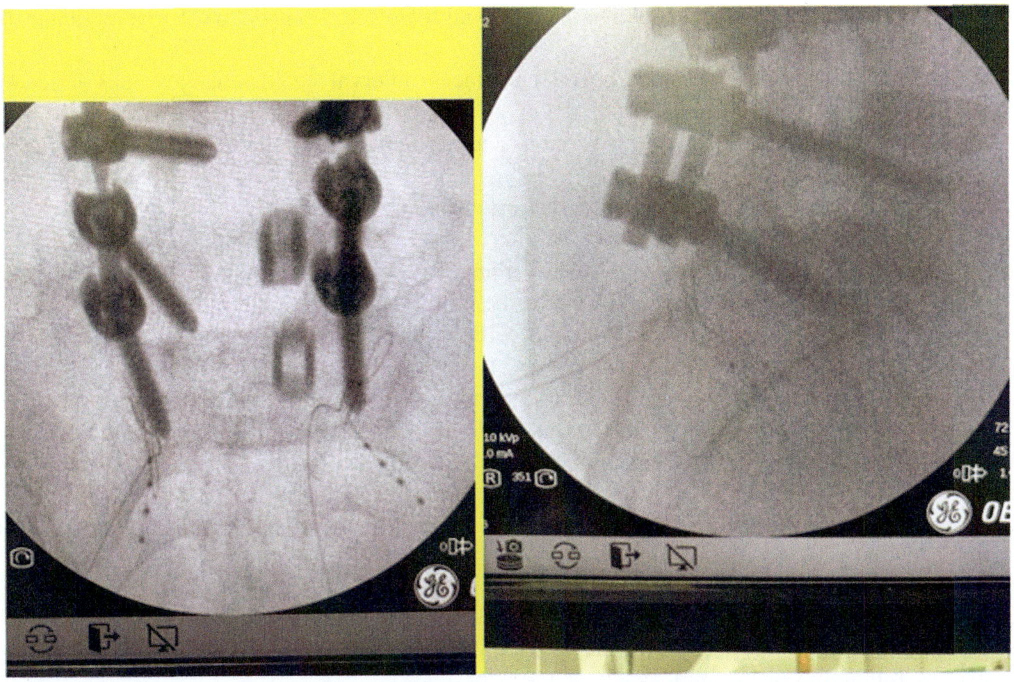

FIGURE 16.8 This figure demonstrates the ideal and correct placement of bilateral S1 DRG leads in AP and lateral fluoroscopic views in a patient with prior spinal fusion and instrumentation.

lead migration complications are suspected. Although no specific data exists to confirm their efficacy, abdominal binders are generally recommended for use up to 2 weeks following procedure to limit risk of seroma formation as well as aiding in appropriate wound healing and IPG discomfort [21]. Some providers will even employ an LSO brace postoperatively. This is not a requirement, but has been mentioned by the NACC as a consideration for reducing postoperative complications and has anecdotal evidence of efficacy.

Efficacy estimates for DRG-S depend on the location targeted and the data regarding efficacy is fluid as more procedures are performed and new target nerves and pathologies are addressed. While the only diagnoses currently approved for DRG-S in the United States are CRPS Type 1 and 2, many other pathologies have been treated and published in case studies. These include Failed Back Surgery Syndrome, post-herpetic neuralgia, Post-hernia pain, Pelvic Pain, phantom limb pain, and peripheral neuropathy [29]. The ACCURATE trial published in 2017 is currently the only RCT evaluating efficacy of DRG-S [4]. In this study, DRG-S showed greater efficacy in treating pain related to CRPS at 3 (81.2 vs. 55.7%) and 12 months (74.2 vs. 53%) as compared to DCS. A review published by Chapman et al. in 2023 evaluates efficacy rates published in case studies for other diagnoses listed above. Decrease in VAS scores is comparable in most of these case studies; however, the number of patients analyzed is still low and more research needs to be conducted.

Some patients have immediate relief following implantation of DRG-S; however, most patients will require some programming changes to reach optimal therapeutic effect. This involves close communication with the device representative as well as the patient care team to assess programming changes and their effects on pain relief. As the IPG software continues to improve, patients will continue to have more control over feedback as well as programming. It is important to have careful follow up with patients throughout the first year of therapy for multiple reasons. One reason is to monitor for therapeutic efficacy. Another reason is to monitor for device complications. Complications are discussed in another section; however, infections, lead migration, lead fracture, hardware damage can all occur within the first year after implantation and need to be monitored.

Pearls and pitfalls

A. Preoperative

- Personally review relevant spinal images such as lumbosacral X-rays and lumbar MRI images to assess spinal and procedural anatomy

- If MRI is contraindicated, a CT scan should be obtained and reviewed. Consider a CT myelogram if there is clinical concern for high-grade spinal stenosis
- Review pre-procedural laboratory tests, medical clearances, interval health changes, and anticoagulant hold if applicable.
- Counsel the patient regarding procedural expectations and encourage communication throughout the procedure during times of pain or discomfort.
- Communicate the anesthetic requirements with the anesthesiology team.

B. Intraoperative
- Use a flat-top table without a surgical base to allow for unobstructed cranial/caudal C-arm movements and imaging.
- Minimize lumbar lordosis by placing pillows under the umbilicus of the patient.
- Attempt to identify the dorsal sacral neural foramen without significant cephalic tilt if necessary, to make tension loop creation easier.
- Ensure purposeful tactile and verbal response during lead insertion and tension loop creation or consider general anesthesia with intraoperative EMG testing to confirm lead placement as well as detect iatrogenic nerve irritation.
- Anchor DRG-S leads to minimizing the risk of fracture and migration.
- Consider live fluoroscopy to observe for electrode migration while creating strain relief loops.
- The sheath should always be facing the same direction as the needle tip and should be retracted into the needle before turning the needle 180 degrees.
- Consider the placement of extra-spinal sacral tension relief loops as needed.

C. Postoperative
- Assess and document postoperative neurological examination.
- Facilitate early follow-up for wound check and consider postoperative X-ray imaging to assess post-implant placement.
- Consider abdominal binder use postoperatively to minimize the risk of pocket fluid collection and lead migration.

References

[1] Lucas JW, Sohi I. Chronic pain and high-impact chronic pain in U.S. adults, 2023. NCHS Data Brief, no 518. Hyattsville, MD: National Center for Health Statistics; 2024. https://doi.org/10.15620/cdc/169630.

[2] D'Souza RS, Kubrova E, Her YF, et al. Dorsal root ganglion stimulation for lower extremity neuropathic pain syndromes: an evidence-based literature review. Adv Ther 2022;39(10):4440–73. https://doi.org/10.1007/s12325-022-02244-9.

[3] Deer TR, Pope JE. Dorsal root ganglion stimulation approval by the Food and Drug Administration: advice on evolving the process. Expert Rev Neurother 2016;16(10):1123–5. https://doi.org/10.1080/14737175.2016.1206817.

[4] Deer TR, Levy RM, Kramer J, Poree L, Amirdelfan K, Grigsby E, Staats P, Burton AW, Burgher AH, Obray J, Scowcroft J, Golovac S, Kapural L, Paicius R, Kim C, Pope J, Yearwood T, Samuel S, McRoberts WP, Cassim H, Netherton M, Miller N, Schaufele M, Tavel E, Davis T, Davis K, Johnson L, Mekhail N. Dorsal root ganglion stimulation yielded higher treatment success rate for complex regional pain syndrome and causalgia at 3 and 12 months: a randomized comparative trial. Pain 2017;158(4):669–81. https://doi.org/10.1097/j.pain.0000000000000814.

[5] Van Buyten JP, Smet I, Liem L, Russo M, Huygen F. Stimulation of dorsal root ganglia for the management of complex regional pain syndrome: a prospective case series. Pain Pract 2015;15(3):208–16. https://doi.org/10.1111/papr.12170.

[6] Ebraheim NA, Lu J. Morphometric evaluation of the sacral dorsal root ganglia. A cadaveric study. Surg Radiol Anat 1998;20(2):105–8.

[7] Vialle E, Vialle LR, Contreras W, Jacob CJ. Anatomical study on the relationship between the dorsal root ganglion and the intervertebral disc in the lumbar spine. Rev Bras Ortop 2015;50(4):450–4. https://doi.org/10.1016/j.rboe.2015.06.013.

[8] Cramer GD, Ro C-S. The sacrum, sacroiliac joint, and coccyx. In: Clinical anatomy of the spine, spinal cord, and ANS; 2014. p. 312–39. https://doi.org/10.1016/b978-0-323-07954-9.00008-6.

[9] Harden NR, Bruehl S, Perez RSGM, Birklein F, Marinus J, Maihofner C, Lubenow T, Buvanendran A, Mackey S, Graciosa J, Mogilevski M, Ramsden C, Chont M, Vatine JJ. Validation of proposed diagnostic criteria (the "Budapest criteria") for complex regional pain syndrome. Pain 2010;150(2):268–74. https://doi.org/10.1016/j.pain.2010.04.030.

[10] Misidou C, Papagoras C. Complex regional pain syndrome: an update. Mediterr J Rheumatol 2019;30(1):16–25. https://doi.org/10.31138/mjr.30.1.16.

[11] Chapman KB, Van Roosendaal BW, Van Helmond N, Yousef TA. Unilateral dorsal root ganglion stimulation lead placement with resolution of bilateral lower extremity symptoms in diabetic peripheral neuropathy. Cureus 2020;12(9):e10735. https://doi.org/10.7759/cureus.10735.

[12] Hayek SM, Veizi E, Hanes M. Treatment-limiting complications of percutaneous spinal cord stimulator implants: a review of eight years of experience from an academic center database. Neuromodulation 2015;18:603–8.

[13] Dydyk AM, Gupta N. Chronic pelvic pain. In: StatPearls [internet]. Treasure Island (FL): StatPearls Publishing; 2025. https://www.ncbi.nlm.nih.gov/books/NBK554585/.

[14] Rowland DCL, Wright D, Moir L, FitzGerald JJ, Green AL. Successful treatment of pelvic girdle pain with dorsal root ganglion stimulation. Br J Neurosurg 2016;30(6):685–6. https://doi.org/10.1080/02688697.2016.1208810.

[15] Hunter CW, Yang A. Dorsal root ganglion stimulation for chronic pelvic pain: a case series and technical report on a novel lead configuration. Neuromodulation 2019;22(1):87–95. https://doi.org/10.1111/ner.12801.

[16] Patel KV. Dorsal root ganglion stimulation for chronic pelvic pain [39T]. Obstet Gynecol 2019;133:223S.

[17] Hunter CW, Sayed D, Lubenow T, Davis T, Carlson J, Rowe J, Justiz R, McJunkin T, Deer T, Mehta P, Falowski S, Kapural L, Pope J, Mekhail N. Drg FOCUS: a multicenter study evaluating dorsal root ganglion stimulation and predictors for trial success. Neuromodulation 2019;22(1):61–79. https://doi.org/10.1111/ner.12796.

[18] Giordano NL, Van helmond N, Chapman KB. Coccydynia treated with dorsal root ganglion stimulation. Case Rep Anesthesiol 2018;2018:1–4. https://doi.org/10.1155/2018/5832401.

[19] Hassanain M, Murphy P. Dorsal root ganglion stimulation for the treatment of bilateral intractable chronic testicular pain. Neuromodulation 2019;22(1):115–6. https://doi.org/10.1111/ner.12805.

[20] Burns SL, Majdak P, Adler AR, Jo C, Chiang MC, Yong RJ, Barreveld AM. Dorsal root ganglion stimulation for patients with chronic pelvic pain: a retrospective review of patient experiences and long-term outcomes. Interv Pain Med 2024;3(1):100397. https://doi.org/10.1016/j.inpm.2024.100397.

[21] Deer TR, Pope JE, Lamer TJ, Grider JS, Provenzano D, Lubenow TR, FitzGerald JJ, Hunter C, Falowski S, Sayed D, Baranidharan G, Patel NK, Davis T, Green A, Pajuelo A, Epstein LJ, Harned M, Liem L, Christo PJ, Chakravarthy K, Gilmore C, Huygen F, Lee E, Metha P, Nijhuis H, Patterson DG, Petersen E, Pilitsis JG, Rowe JJ, Rupert MP, Skaribas I, Sweet J, Verrills P, Wilson D, Levy RM, Mekhail N. The neuromodulation appropriateness consensus committee on best practices for dorsal root ganglion stimulation. Neuromodulation 2019;22(1):1–35. https://doi.org/10.1111/ner.12845.

[22] Zuidema X, Breel J, Wille F. S3 dorsal root ganglion/nerve root stimulation for refractory postsurgical perineal pain: technical aspects of anchorless sacral transforaminal lead placement. Case Rep Neurol Med 2016;2016:8926578. https://doi.org/10.1155/2016/8926578.

[23] Santiago N, Monaco BA, Santos PG, Jagid J, Cordeiro JG. Navigated dorsal root ganglion stimulation (DRGS) for the treatment of chronic refractory coccygodynia: a case report. Cureus 2023;15(7):e41663. https://doi.org/10.7759/cureus.41663.

[24] Bondoc M, Hancu M, DiMarzio M, Sheldon BL, Shao MM, Khazen O, Pilitsis JG. Age as an independent predictor of adult spinal cord stimulation pain outcomes. Stereotact Funct Neurosurg 2022;100(1):1–7. https://doi.org/10.1159/000517426.

[25] Mosquera-Moscoso J, Eldrige J, Encalada S, Mendonca LFP, Hallo-Carrasco A, Shan A, Rabatin A, Mina M, Prokop L, Hunt C. Interventional pain management of CRPS in the pediatric population: a literature review. Interv Pain Med 2024;3(4):100532. https://doi.org/10.1016/j.inpm.2024.100532.

[26] Pritzlaff SG, Goree JH, Hagedorn JM, Lee DW, Chapman KB, Christiansen S, Dudas A, Escobar A, Gilligan CJ, Guirguis M, Gulati A, Jameson J, Mallard CJ, Murphy MZ, Patel KV, Patel RG, Sheth SJ, Vanterpool S, Singh V, Smith G, Strand NH, Vu CM, Suvar T, Chakravarthy K, Kapural L, Leong MS, Lubenow TR, Abd-Elsayed A, Pope JE, Sayed D, Deer TR. Pain education and Knowledge (PEAK) consensus guidelines for neuromodulation: a proposal for standardization in fellowship and training programs. J Pain Res 2023;16:3101–17. https://doi.org/10.2147/JPR.S424589.

[27] Hagedorn JM, Misercola B, Comer A, Tari-Blake J, Hoffmann CM, Mehta P, Deer TR. The team approach to spinal cord and dorsal root ganglion stimulation: a guide for the advanced practice provider. Mayo Clin Proc Innov Qual Outcomes. 2021;5(3):663–9. https://doi.org/10.1016/j.mayocpiqo.2021.05.002.

[28] Deer TR, Stewart CD. Complications of spinal cord stimulation: identification, treatment, and prevention. Pain Med 2008;9(Suppl. 1):S93–101. https://doi.org/10.1111/j.1526-4637.2008.00444.x.

[29] Chapman KB, Sayed D, Lamer T, Hunter C, Weisbein J, Patel KV, Dickerson D, Hagedorn JM, Lee DW, Amirdelfan K, Deer T, Chakravarthy K. Best practices for dorsal root ganglion stimulation for chronic pain: guidelines from the American society of pain and neuroscience. J Pain Res 2023;16:839–79. https://doi.org/10.2147/JPR.S364370.

Chapter 17

Specific complications of dorsal root ganglion stimulation

Carlos E. Trigo[1], Kevin Ko[2], Jason D. Ross[3], Derron Keith Wilson[4] and Kiran V. Patel[5]
[1]*Alivio Pain Center, Carolina, PR, United States;* [2]*SamWell Pain Institute, Colonia, NJ, United States;* [3]*Department of Anesthesiology, Northwestern University, Feinberg School of Medicine, Chicago, IL, United States;* [4]*Goodman Campbell Brain & Spine, Carmel, IN, United States;* [5]*Lenox Hill Hospital, Barbara and Donald School of Medicine at Hofstra/Northwell, New Hyde Park, NY, United States*

Introduction

Dorsal Root Ganglion (DRG) stimulation is an advanced neuromodulation therapy for treating chronic, intractable neuropathic pain, particularly complex regional pain syndrome (CRPS), peripheral causalgia, and focal nerve-related pain syndromes [1,2]. By targeting the dorsal root ganglia—key sensory relay points—rather than the dorsal columns of the spinal cord, DRG stimulation can provide more focal and effective analgesia for certain pain phenotypes [2]. However, like any interventional procedure, DRG stimulation carries inherent risks, including potential neurological, biological, hardware-related, and intraprocedural complications that require careful consideration during pre-procedural planning, execution, and post-procedural management. The ACCURATE study, a large, prospective, multicenter, and randomized control trial that proved the effectiveness of DRG stimulation in comparison to dorsal column spinal cord stimulation (SCS) did not demonstrate a significant difference in serious adverse events (SAE) between these two groups. The rates of SAE were 10.5%(8/76) in the DRG arm and 14.5%(11/76) in the SCS arm [1]. The difference in rate between the two study arms did not prove to be statistically significant ($P = 0.62$), determining that the safety profile of DRG stimulation is comparable to SCS. In another study of >500 DRGs and >2000 SCS implants the safety event rate for DRG was 3.2% and 3.1% for SCS [3]. Determining that the safety profile for DRG stimulation is parallel to SCS.

Key points

- Identify Biological Complications related to DRG Stimulation
- Recognize Neurological Complications related to DRG Stimulation
- Understand Hardware-Related Complications related to DRG Stimulation
- Assess Surgical and Procedural Risk during DRG Stimulation

Biological complications

Infection

Infection is the most frequent safety event in neuromodulation accounting for one-third of all adverse events. The incidence rate of infection for DRG implants is 1.08%–1.3% [1,3].

Diagnosis and workup

Patients may present with localized erythema, swelling, tenderness, or drainage at the incision site. Systemic symptoms are more common in deep infections. Laboratory values such as complete blood count and elevation of inflammatory markers like C-reactive protein (CRP) and erythrocyte sedimentation rate (ESR) can indicate a state of infection or an

A Modern Atlas for Implantable Devices of the Spine, Brain, and Nerve. https://doi.org/10.1016/B978-0-443-36528-7.00013-3

inflammatory process. In addition, swab cultures from the wound or aspirated fluid are critical to guide antibiotic therapy. Ultrasound can be useful for assessing fluid collections in the superficial tissues and guiding needle aspiration. CT or MRI is useful when deep infections or hardware involvement is suspected; these modalities help delineate abscess formation or epidural collections.

Mitigation strategies

Preprocedural

Preoperative screening for staphylococcus aureus is often performed to detect colonization. Positive findings can lead to decolonization measures before DRG implantation.

Intraoperative prophylaxis

In addition, strict adherence to aseptic protocols during the entire procedure is essential. This includes full barrier precautions, proper skin antisepsis, minimization of operating room traffic and the use of intraoperative prophylactic antibiotics (Table 17.1).

Complication management

Patients with localized, superficial infections are typically managed with targeted antibiotic therapy based on culture results. Patients should be re-evaluated frequently to ensure resolution of symptoms. Repeat imaging or cultures may be indicated if the infection persists. Patients should also be instructed to send pictures of wounds to providers for progress monitoring. When the infection involves the IPG pocket, leads, or extends into the epidural space, explantation of the DRG system is required. This may involve debridement of the infected tissue and thorough irrigation of the infected site. After explantation, patients are managed with appropriate intravenous antibiotic therapy tailored to culture sensitivities.

Seroma

Seroma is a collection of clear, serous fluid that accumulates in a dead space created during the surgical procedure. Seromas are associated with several factors, including: tissue trauma, dead space creation, local inflammation, and post-implant trauma. Intraoperatively, the use of blunt dissection, aggressive tissue handling, or excessive cautery can disrupt lymphatic channels increasing the risk of seroma formation.

Diagnosis

Patients with a seroma typically present with visible swelling around the affected site. The swelling is often soft and fluctuant with minimal tenderness and usually lacks the redness, warmth, and systemic signs that might suggest an infection. Ultrasound imaging is a useful tool for confirming the diagnosis by demonstrating a well-circumscribed, fluid-filled cavity. If needed, aspiration of the fluid under image guidance can help rule out infection and differentiate a seroma from a hematoma or a cerebrospinal fluid leak.

Complication management

Small, asymptomatic seromas may resolve on their own with close observation and the application of a compression dressing. For larger or symptomatic seromas, needle aspiration under sterile conditions may be employed to remove the fluid. However, repeated aspirations can sometimes be necessary if the fluid reaccumulates. In cases where the seroma persists, enlarges, or shows signs of infection, surgical exploration may be required.

Prevention

Prevention strategies focus on minimizing tissue trauma and dead space during DRG implantation. The use of compression garments or abdominal binders may help reduce seroma formation.

Epidural hematomas

Diagnosis

Epidural hematomas are less common but more concerning due to their potential to compress neural structures. They occur within the epidural space and can lead to severe back pain, radiculopathy, and if not promptly addressed, irreversible neurological deficits. Patients with epidural hematomas may exhibit sudden onset of severe, localized back pain. There may be neurological deficits, including motor weakness, sensory disturbances, or bowel/bladder dysfunction. These symptoms typically arise within the first 72 h after implantation, although onset can be variable. MRI is the imaging

TABLE 17.1 This table depicts the recommended intraoperative prophylactic antibiotics.

Antibiotic	Standard IV dose	Weight-based dose	Timing prior to incision (min)	Redosing interval (based on CrCl)	Indications
Cefazolin	1 g (≤80 kg)	2 g (>80 kg)	Within 30–60	3–4 h (>50 mL/min)	First-line
		3 g(>120 kg)		8 h (20–50 mL/min)	
				16 h (<20 mL/min)	
Clindamycin	600 mg (≤80 kg)	900 mg (>80 kg)	Within 30–60	6 h (>50 mL/min)	β-lactam allergy
		1200 mg (>120 kg)		6 h (20–50 mL/min)	
				6 h (<20 mL/min)	
Vancomycin	1 g (≤80 kg)	2 g (>80 kg)	Within 120	8 h (>50 mL/min)	
		3 g (>120 kg)		16 h (20–50 mL/min)	Known MRSA colonization
				None (<20 mL/min)	

Modified from Bratzler et al. [4], Alexander et al. [5], and Bratzler et al. [6].

modality of choice for diagnosing epidural hematomas because of its superior soft-tissue resolution. CT may be employed when MRI is contraindicated.

Complication management

Epidural hematomas require immediate neurosurgical evaluation. Treatment typically involves urgent decompressive laminectomy and evacuation of the hematoma to relieve pressure on the spinal cord. Delays in surgical intervention may result in permanent neurological deficits.

Immunologic complications

The overall incidence rate of immunologic complications in patients undergoing DRG implantation is 0.18%–2.7% [1,3]. These reactions can range from mild local hypersensitivity to more pronounced inflammatory or granulomatous responses.

Diagnosis

A detailed history of allergic diseases or prior reactions to implants should be obtained. Physical examination should assess for signs of inflammation without purulence or systemic illness. Routine laboratory tests (e.g., CBC, inflammatory markers) may be nonspecific. Imaging studies such as ultrasound or MRI can help exclude fluid collections (e.g., seromas or hematomas) and may identify localized inflammatory masses. Skin patch testing can be useful to identify sensitivity to specific materials (e.g., silicone or metal components of DRG system). Providers can inquire about metal allergy testing with their device representatives (Fig. 17.1).

Complication management

Mild reactions may be managed with topical corticosteroids, oral antihistamines, or nonsteroidal anti-inflammatory drugs to reduce inflammation and alleviate symptoms. Occasionally, adjustments in stimulation parameters may help mitigate discomfort associated with a localized inflammatory response. For severe or persistent immunologic reactions that compromise device function or cause significant morbidity, removal of the offending device may be necessary.

(A) (B)

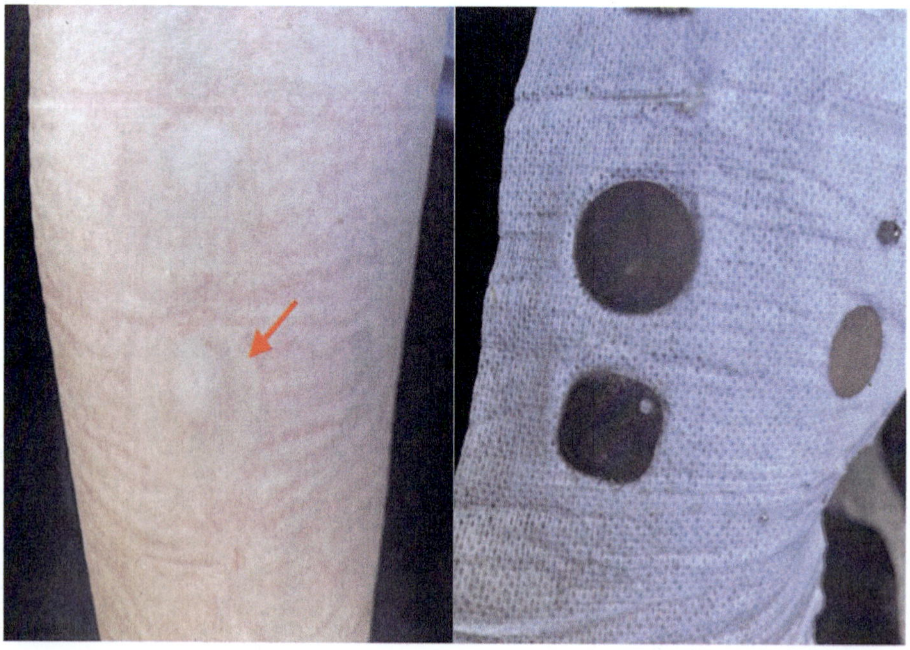

FIGURE 17.1 (A) Allergy test result showing a reaction (red arrow) to the, (B) IPG metal. *Photos courtesy by Carlos Trigo, MD.*

Neurological complications of dorsal root ganglion stimulation

Nerve injury

Nerve injury is a recognized complication of DRG stimulation procedures, typically caused by mechanical trauma from needles, leads, guidewires, or sheaths contacting or penetrating neural structures. Such injuries may result in sensory or motor deficits, including paresthesia, neuropathic pain, or muscle weakness. Often, these injuries are transient although long-term injury may rarely occur [7]. Proper pre-procedural planning and precise technique are critical to reducing the risk of nerve injury [8].

A detailed pre-procedural imaging review, particularly using MRI, is essential to evaluate patient anatomy and identify potential procedural risks. Key considerations include assessing the degree of neuroforaminal and central canal stenosis and identifying anatomical variations such as scoliosis, kyphosis, or the presence of implanted hardware. Severe or critical neuroforaminal stenosis is considered a contraindication for DRG stimulation due to the increased risk of nerve injury during lead placement [8]. Prior surgery at the target DRG level is another relative contraindication for DRG-S lead placement [8]. Intra-procedurally, the use of appropriate needle angles and entry points tailored to the patient's specific anatomy is crucial. Numerous techniques are documented. The most common are the contralateral and ipsilateral approaches. Continuous fluoroscopic guidance is recommended to maintain visualization and reduce the likelihood of neural trauma. Gentle handling of guidewires and sheaths is critical, avoiding abrupt movements or excessive force. Neuromonitoring or minimal sedation during the procedure can also provide valuable feedback and mitigate risks.

Although DRG stimulation is officially approved for use below the T10 spinal level (T10-S2), it has been reported that off-label lead placements at higher levels are performed in some clinical scenarios. These off-label procedures, however, may present additional risks and should be carefully evaluated on a case-by-case basis [9,10].

Complication management

Management of neural injury related to DRG is similar to the management of dorsal spinal cord stimulation (SCS). It requires prompt recognition and appropriate intervention to mitigate neurological deficits and optimize patient outcomes. Immediate cessation of stimulation and a detailed neurological assessment are essential first steps to evaluate the extent of the injury, including sensory or motor deficits, paresthesia, or neuropathic pain. Imaging studies, such as MRI or CT scan, may be warranted to confirm lead positioning, identify nerve impingement, or detect complications such as hematomas [11].

When improper lead placement or nerve compression is identified, lead repositioning or removal may be required. Surgical decompression may be necessary in rare cases involving significant hematoma formation or ongoing nerve impingement [8]. Conservative measures often involve pharmacological therapies, including the use of anti-inflammatory medications, steroids and neuropathic agents such as gabapentin or pregabalin, along with physical therapy to support recovery and reduce symptoms [11].

Neuromodulation adjustments may also help alleviate neural irritation while preserving the therapeutic benefits of stimulation. Reducing stimulation amplitudes or reprogramming lead configurations can mitigate discomfort associated with overstimulation. Close follow-up is essential to monitor neurological recovery and assess residual symptoms.

Dural puncture

Dural puncture is one of the most common compilations during the DRG-S trials and implants. It occurs when the needle or other instruments inadvertently breach the dura membrane, leading to cerebrospinal fluid (CSF) leakage [12]. The incidence rate of CSF leak during placement of DRG leads is 0.54%–2.7% [1,3].

Diagnosis

The clinical presentation typically includes post-dural puncture headache (PDPH), characterized by a positional headache that worsens when upright and improves when lying down. Other symptoms may include nausea, dizziness, tinnitus, visual changes and neck stiffness.

Prevention

Preventing dural puncture begins with meticulous attention to patient positioning, needle placement, and proper procedural techniques. Positioning aids, such as pillows or balloons, are utilized to reduce lumbar lordosis, facilitating a more straightforward needle trajectory. The contralateral oblique (CLO) fluoroscopic view enhances accuracy by providing a clear visualization of the interlaminar space, posterior epidural border, and needle trajectory, thereby reducing the risk of inadvertent dural puncture [13,14]. Studies have demonstrated that the CLO view offers superior needle tip visualization and more consistent identification of anatomical landmarks compared to the lateral view. For instance, research indicates that the needle tip location in the epidural space was most consistent at a CLO angle of 45 degrees, suggesting that this view should be considered the preferred method for gauging needle depth during interlaminar lumbar epidural access [15].

While the lateral fluoroscopic view can also be employed, it has limitations in accurately assessing needle depth relative to the epidural space. The CLO view addresses these limitations by providing better visualization of the needle tip and relevant anatomical structures, thereby enhancing the safety and efficiency of epidural access procedures [13,14].

Needle angles should be shallow, with a needle-to-skin angle of ≤30°. This technique minimizes the risk of dural puncture and increases the likelihood that the sheath and electrode remain in the dorsal aspect of the epidural space [12]. Special attention is required at the L5-S1 level due to its smaller epidural space and thinner ligamentum flavum [8].

If the event of an unintended dural puncture during a DRG-S trial or implant, consider the following intra-procedural steps to guide management:

1. **Assessing Whether to Abort the Procedure:** The decision to continue or abort the DRG trial/implant after a dural puncture depends on factors such as the severity of the puncture, patient symptoms, and the clinician's judgment. Currently, there is no consensus in the literature regarding the definitive course of action in such scenarios [8].
2. **Attempting Epidural Access on the Opposite Side:** If the initial approach results in a dural puncture, accessing the epidural space from the contralateral side may be considered. This strategy aims to bypass the compromised area and achieve successful lead placement. However, clinicians must weigh the risks of additional punctures against the potential benefits, as multiple attempts may increase the likelihood of further complications [8].
3. **Selecting an Alternative Vertebral Level:** Choosing a different vertebral level for epidural access is another viable option. This approach involves identifying a nearby level that provides safe access to the targeted neural structures while avoiding the site of the dural puncture. Careful imaging and anatomical considerations are essential to ensure effective and safe lead placement [8].

Complication management

Regarding the use of intraoperative epidural blood patches (EBP) to address dural punctures, the literature primarily supports their application in the postoperative setting for managing post-dural puncture headaches (PDPH). EBPs involve injecting autologous blood into the epidural space to seal the dural tear, with success rates ranging from 70% to 98% [16]. The optimal timing for EBP administration remains a topic of discussion; some studies suggest increased failure rates when performed within 24–96 h post-puncture [17]. Currently, there is a lack of substantial evidence supporting the routine use of intraoperative EBPs during DRG procedures. Therefore, their application should be considered on a case-by-case basis, guided by clinical judgment and patient-specific factors.

Management of dural puncture complications centers on the treatment of post-dural puncture headache (PDPH) and the diagnosis and management of cerebrospinal fluid (CSF) leaks. Initial conservative management includes hydration, bed rest, and the use of analgesics or caffeine-containing medications, which can help alleviate symptoms [18]. In cases of persistent or severe headache, an epidural blood patch (EBP) remains the gold standard intervention. The success rate of EBPs is high, and many patients experience rapid relief [19]. For patients with prolonged symptoms or suspected CSF leaks that do not respond to conservative measures, advanced imaging techniques, such as MRI with gadolinium contrast, may be used to localize the leak. Surgical intervention may rarely be necessary to repair the defect [20].

Conus medullaris irritation

Conus medullaris irritation is a rare but significant complication associated with neuromodulation. Conus irritation typically occurs when electrodes are placed in the lower thoracic or upper lumbar regions. The conus medullaris, the tapered terminal portion of the spinal cord, typically extends to the L1-L2 vertebral levels in adults. Given its anatomical proximity to DRG targets, improper lead placement or mechanical irritation may result in neurological symptoms, including radicular pain, motor deficits, and sensory disturbances. This has been documented in SCS placement but there is a paucity of data as it relates to DRG stimulators [21].

Prevention

Preventive measures for conus irritation start with careful pre-procedural imaging and anatomical evaluation. Identifying the precise location of the conus medullaris using MRI helps avoid inadvertent lead placement at inappropriate levels. Caution is especially warranted during off-label DRG lead placements above the T10 spinal level, as the risk of conus irritation may increase in these scenarios [8]. Additionally, using fluoroscopic guidance during lead placement ensures accurate targeting and minimizes excessive manipulation near the spinal cord structures [22].

Gentle handling of the sheath and lead, avoiding forceful advancement, and maintaining optimal insertion angles are essential intra-procedural techniques to prevent mechanical irritation. In patients with anatomical variations, such as low-lying conus medullaris or spinal deformities, alternative stimulation levels may be considered to reduce risks [7]. Furthermore, utilizing a contralateral approach at or above the conus medullaris has the potential to increase irritation due to the lead's trajectory and proximity to neural structures. In these cases, an ipsilateral approach or alternative lead positioning strategies should be considered to minimize the risk of conus-related complications.

Complication management

The management of conus medullaris irritation focuses on early recognition and intervention. Immediate reduction or cessation of stimulation is recommended if symptoms such as motor weakness, radicular pain, or unusual paresthesia develop. Re-evaluation of lead position through fluoroscopic imaging is essential to assess for potential misplacement or excessive lead tension. In some cases, repositioning or complete removal of the lead may be necessary to alleviate symptoms [21].

If conservative measures, including lead adjustment, are unsuccessful, short courses of corticosteroids may be prescribed to reduce inflammation and alleviate nerve irritation. Patients with persistent or severe neurological symptoms may benefit from consultation with neurology or spine specialists for further evaluation and management. Close follow-up is crucial to monitor symptom resolution and ensure the long-term safety and efficacy of neuromodulation therapy [11].

Anesthetic management for DRG placement and neuromonitoring

The American Society of Anesthesiologists emphasizes balancing patient comfort and safety during interventional pain procedures, recommending that patients remain responsive to minimize neural injury risks. Although sedation is commonly used, maintaining an appropriate anesthetic depth is critical to allow patient feedback. In cases requiring general anesthesia, intraoperative neuromonitoring (IONM) is recommended to enhance procedural safety [23].

Preoperative evaluation should consider patient-specific factors and procedural challenges, ensuring alignment between the anesthetic plan, patient tolerance, and implanter preferences. Discussions on patient positioning, pain management, and expected sensory feedback should occur beforehand to minimize intraoperative complications.

Given the sensitive nature of the DRG and the potential for neural injury, lead placement should be performed with the patient awake or under IONM when deep sedation or general anesthesia is required. Electrophysiologic monitoring, including somatosensory evoked potentials (SSEP) and electromyography (EMG), helps assess neural integrity and detect abnormalities early. Studies suggest that IONM may enhance safety, with two retrospective analyses reporting 16 IONM alerts across 182 DRG-S cases, resulting in only three transient postoperative paresthesia and no serious neurological complications [24]. While IONM is not yet universally adopted, it represents a valuable tool in optimizing DRG-S placement safety.

Hardware-related complications

Sheath kinking

Sheath kinking can occur during the placement of DRG leads. The specialized sheaths used for DRG stimulation must navigate tight neuroforaminal anatomies, which increases the risk of bending or folding [8]. Failure to recognize a kinked sheath may limit the ability to pass the lead into the foramen, prevent the formation of strain relief loops, or prevent the removal of the sheath once the lead and strain relief loops are in the proper position.

Prevention

Thus, proper technique is crucial for prevention. Clinicians must be thoroughly trained in the unique mechanical properties of the manufacturer's DRG delivery system, including how bend tolerances and coatings can influence handling. Prone positioning and appropriate table adjustments help maintain a more linear path to the targeted DRG, thereby decreasing the likelihood of undue angulation [25]. Advancing the sheath in small increments while continuously assessing resistance further minimizes the risk of mechanical stress that can lead to kinking [26].

Complication management

Immediate Recognition and Replacement: If the sheath kinks during insertion, further advancement should be stopped. In most cases, withdrawing the damaged or kinked sheath and replacing it with a new one is the most efficient intervention [27].

Lead migration

Lead migration is defined as the unintended displacement of the lead from its optimal position over the dorsal root ganglion. Even small shifts can alter paresthesia coverage and compromise pain relief [28]. Preventive measures primarily involve secure anchoring and the creation of high-quality strain relief loops in the epidural space. A recent multicenter pooled analysis reported that using anchoring techniques—whether with suture alone or a silastic anchor—significantly reduces migration and fracture rates in DRG systems (Figs. 17.2 and 17.3) [30] Incorporating a small loop of lead slack before anchoring accommodates typical spinal movements and reduces the tension that could pull the lead away from its target [31].

High-quality strain relief loops (thoracolumbar & sacral regions)

- In the thoracolumbar region, the first (superior) loop is intended to hug the medial border of the pedicle and create traction for the lead. The second (inferior) loop is intended to "bump up" the portion of the lead containing the electrodes, so it remains close to the pedicle (Fig. 17.4). Ensure that neither loop crosses midline, as this may increase the risk of spinal cord irritation (Fig. 17.6).
- In the sacral region, the first sacral loop should be rostral in the sacral epidural space, while the second sacral loop sits in the sacral foramen, effectively "locking" the lead in place (Fig. 17.5).

Patient education & activity modification

Patient education is essential; limiting vigorous activities during the early postoperative period may decrease mechanical stress on freshly implanted leads [32]. Limiting bending, twisting, and heavy lifting for about 4–6 weeks postoperatively often helps prevent lead migration [8]. Some clinicians also use abdominal binders to limit patient movements but also to remind patients to limit abrupt spinal movement.

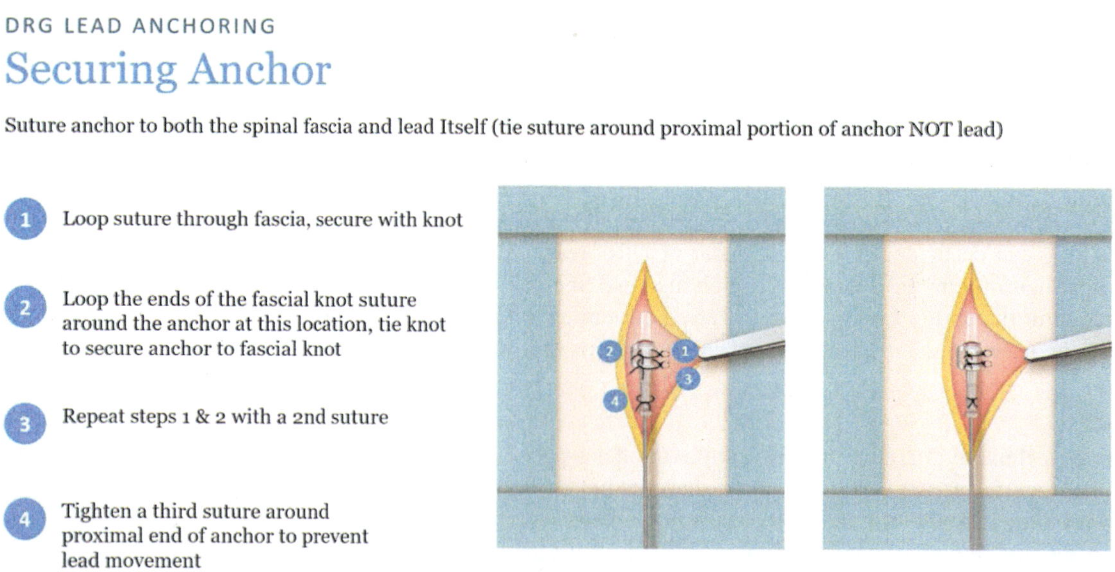

FIGURE 17.2 DRG lead anchoring technique to prevent lead migration and fracture [29]. Proper anchoring technique must ensure a secure connection between the anchor and the lead, as well as between the anchor and the thoracolumbar fascia. To properly secure the silastic anchors in place, 5 knots must be tied using a non-absorbable suture.

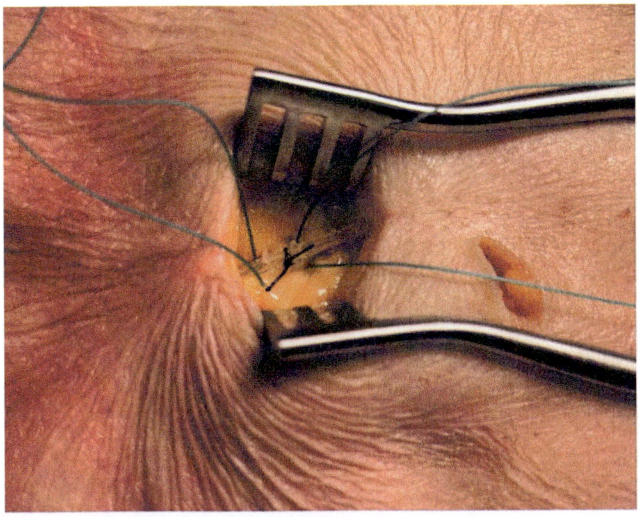

FIGURE 17.3 DRG lead anchoring technique to prevent lead migration and fracture. *Image courtesy of Carlos Trigo, MD.*

Management of suspected migration

When lead migration is suspected, imaging—often X-ray or fluoroscopy—can confirm displacement (Fig. 17.7) [33]. Surgical revision under fluoroscopic guidance may then be required to reposition or replace the lead. A revised anchoring strategy and properly placed strain relief loops can help prevent further migration [34].

Lead fracture

Lead fracture occurs when mechanical stress disrupts the conductor or insulating material [35]. DRG leads, thinner and more flexible than traditional SCS leads to accommodate the neural foramina, may be more susceptible to bending or shearing forces [36,37].

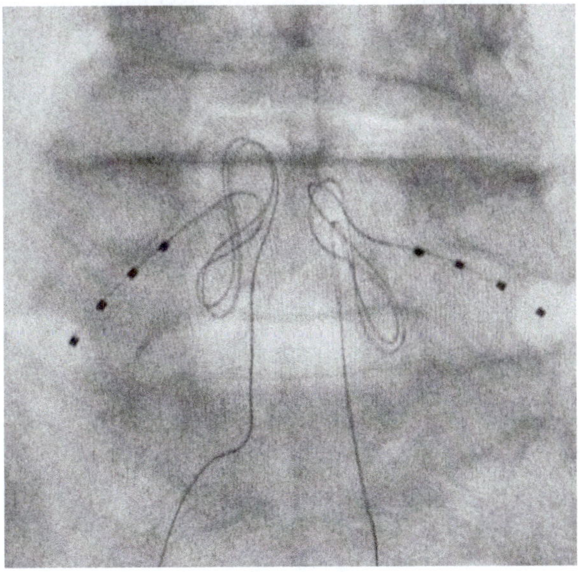

FIGURE 17.4 AP fluoroscopic view demonstrating bilateral L5 DRG leads with high quality loops. Note that the loops don't cross midline. Loops that cross the midline may irritate the spinal cord and cause discomfort. *Image courtesy of Kiran Patel, MD.*

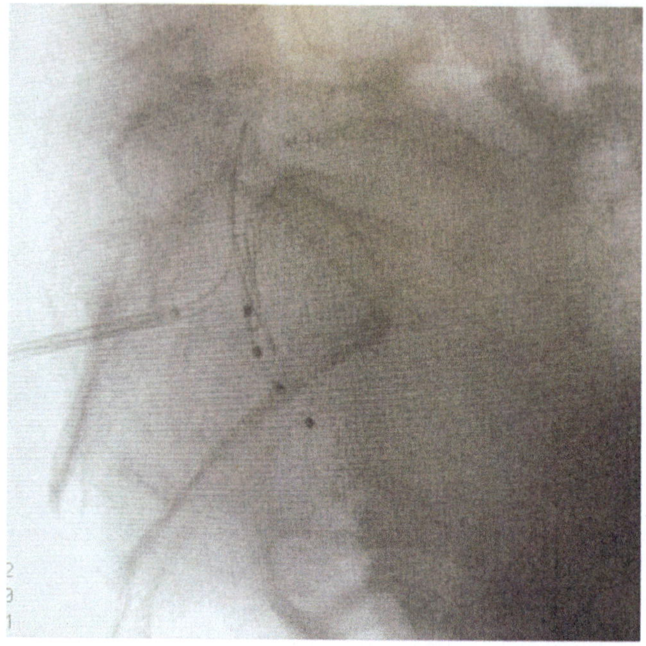

FIGURE 17.5 Lateral fluoroscopy view. S1 DRG lead with high-quality superior and inferior strain relief loops to minimize the risk of lead migration. The inferior sacral loop should not exceed the anterior border of the sacrum due to potentially irritating the sacral nerve root of the target DRG. *Image courtesy of Kiran Patel, MD.*

Preventive steps

1. **Gentle Handling**: Avoid excessive bending or torque during insertion, especially in anatomically challenging regions [36].
2. **Optimal Lead Routing & Anchoring**: Position the lead to minimize repeated flexion points and friction against bony structures or traversing fascial planes, which can lead to mechanical fatigue over time [30,37,38].
3. **Regular Device Interrogation**: Routine follow-up checks can detect partial fractures early by identifying changes in lead impedance or stimulation patterns [38].
4. **Technical Approaches**: Chapman and colleagues described a paramedian placement that may reduce torque and friction, thus potentially mitigating the risk of lead fracture [30].

When a fracture is suspected—signaled by abrupt changes in therapeutic effectiveness or device telemetry—imaging (X-ray or fluoroscopy) and electrical integrity testing can confirm the diagnosis (Fig. 17.8) [39]. Surgical revision is usually required to remove or replace the damaged lead, and optimizing lead path or anchoring technique may help prevent future recurrences.

Lead retention

Lead retention signifies significant difficulty in removing or exchanging a previously implanted lead. Over time, fibrous scar tissue may form around the lead—particularly where the DRG lead traverses the foramen—due to an inflammatory microenvironment near the dorsal root ganglion [40]. Excessive traction during removal should be avoided to limit the risk of complete fracture of the lead, especially in older DRG systems with more vulnerable "ball and tip" designs.

Complication management

- **Gentle Traction & Fluoroscopic Guidance**: This can sometimes free the lead if adhesions are not too extensive.

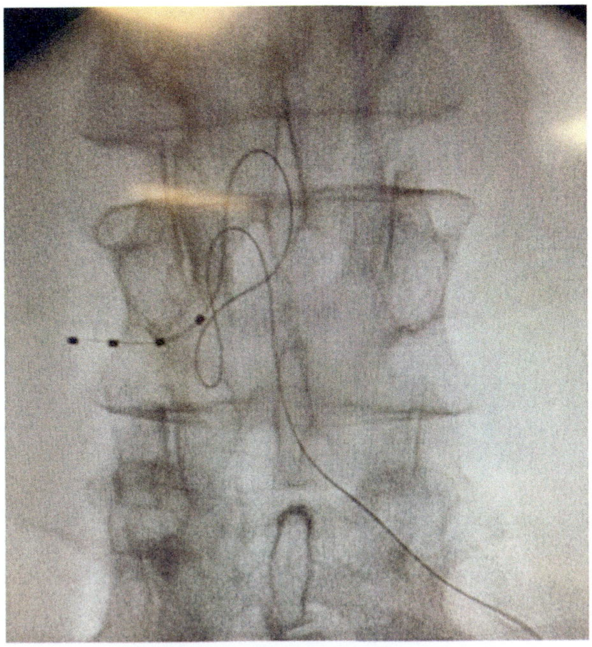

FIGURE 17.6 AP fluoroscopy view. Left L3 DRG with appropriate lead placement but the superior strain relief S-loop is crossing the midline. This can increase the risk of spinal cord irritation and patient discomfort. *Image courtesy of Carlos Trigo, MD.*

- **Surgical Intervention**: If traction efforts fail or if patient safety and spinal integrity become concerns, a neurosurgeon may perform a laminectomy or foraminotomy to dissect and remove the lead [40,41]. This approach is typically reserved for infection, uncontrolled pain, or the need to replace a nonfunctioning lead.
- **Partial Removal**: In rare cases, partial lead removal or leaving the lead in situ may be preferable if the risks of complete removal outweigh the potential benefits.
- **Avoiding Loops That Cross Themselves**: Minimizing leads crossing over during implantation may reduce fibrous anchor points, making future revision or explant less traumatic.

(A) (B)

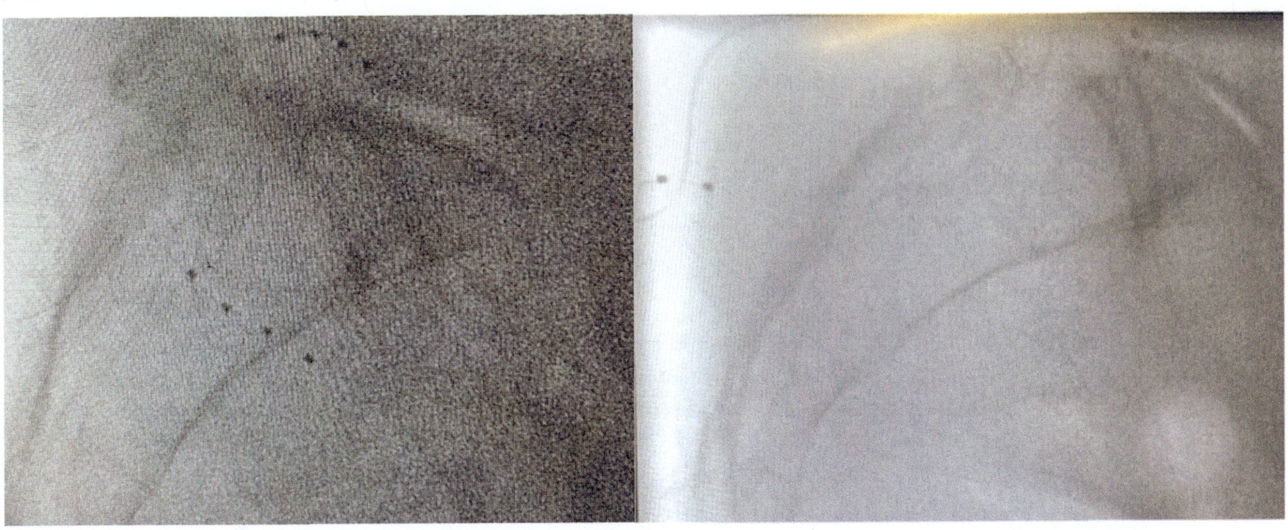

FIGURE 17.7 Lateral fluoroscopy view. (A) S1 and L5 DRG implant. (B) S1 DRG lead migration 6 months after DRG implant. Patient was complaining of reduction in pain relief. *Image courtesy of Carlos Trigo, MD.*

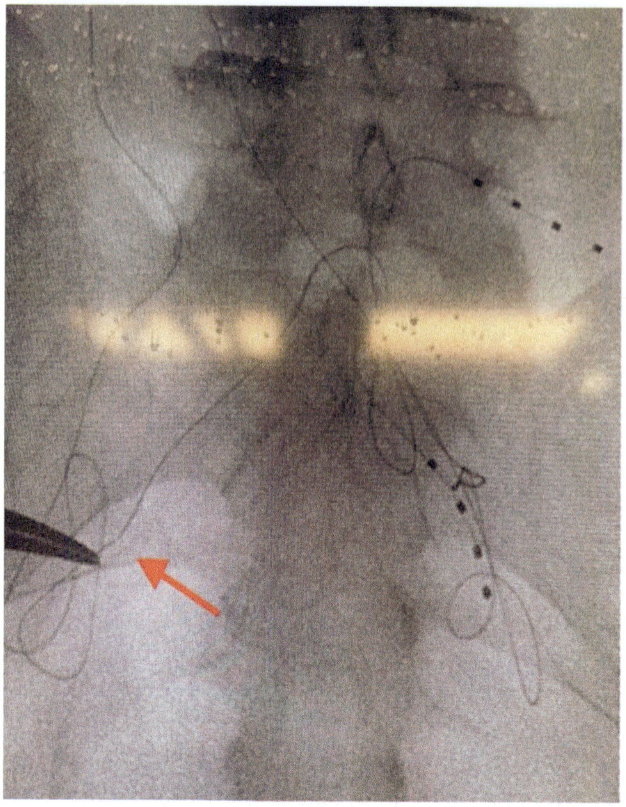

FIGURE 17.8 L5 lead fracture, the patient started complaining of worsening pain and reported a message on her remote that she was not able to increase the strength due to issue with the device. *Image courtesy of Carlos Trigo, MD.*

Technological innovation in hardware design

Manufacturers and researchers are continually refining DRG stimulation systems to reduce mechanical failures and simplify both implantation and revision [33,42,43]. New anchors feature ergonomic and radiopaque designs specifically tailored to DRG leads, such as low-profile anchors that minimize bulk and self-locking sleeves that reduce the need for complex suturing [44]. Improvements in lead materials aim to enhance durability and flexibility. Stronger, fatigue-resistant alloys reduce fractures caused by repetitive stress near the DRG [45]. Sheaths are also undergoing advancements, with kink-resistant constructions that use braided or coiled reinforcement to resist collapse when navigating tight pathways [26,46]. Emerging steerable sheaths further enhance precision and minimize torque, decreasing the risk of kinking or other mechanical complications [26].

Intra-procedural challenges

Lead keeps going anterior/ventral

Proper placement of DRG-S lead along the dorsal aspect of the target neuroforamen is crucial for successful stimulation of the DRG (Fig. 17.9). Ventral placement of DRG-S lead increases the risk of undesired motor stimulation (Fig. 17.10).

Needle angle and position

Ensure the needle angle is as shallow as possible and epidural access is obtained midline and in the superior aspect of the interlaminar space. If you are not satisfied with your needle placement, remove it and start again. Proper needle placement is key for the successful placement of DRG-S lead and reducing the risk of ventral lead deployment.

To determine the ideal needle entry point before skin puncture, place the Tuohy needle on the skin, obtain a CLO image, and adjust the entry site and needle angle to achieve the optimal trajectory toward the target interlaminar level (Figs. 17.11 and 17.12).

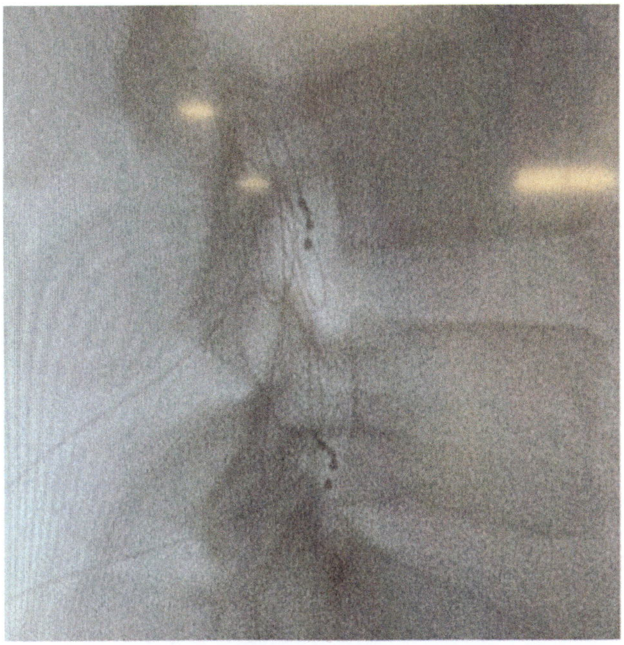

FIGURE 17.9 Lateral view. L3 and L4 DRG leads with electrodes placed within the dorsal aspect of the neuroforamen. *Image courtesy of Carlos Trigo, MD.*

Sheath advancement and navigation

As you advance the sheath through the neuroforamen, position the sheath side port dorsal [47]. Make this adjustment when the tip of the sheath is just under the pedicle to increase the likelihood of dorsal placement of DRG-S lead [47]. It is important to apply gentle force while advancing the sheath through the neuroforamen to not cause any neural damage to the DRG from direct trauma. Monitoring the awake patient and taking into consideration the feedback of changes in tolerance of procedural discomfort when placing the sheath and attempting lead deployment, provides useful feedback in technique. Similarly, change in neuromonitoring also provides similar feedback in technique when advancing the sheath and deploying the lead.

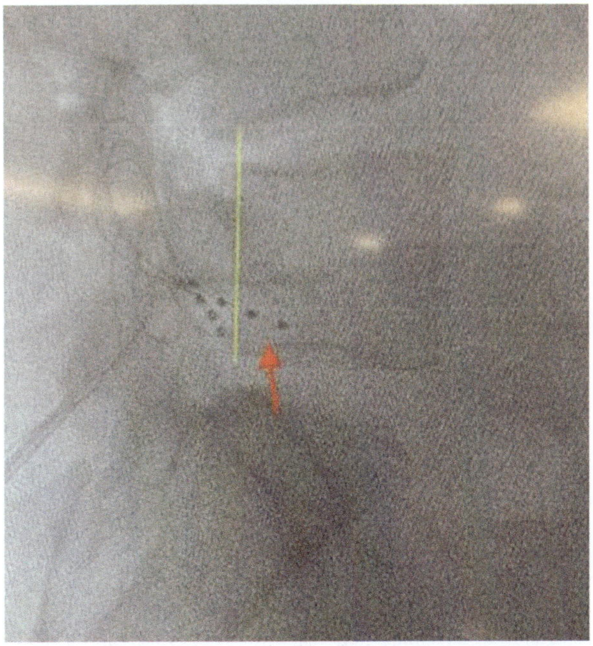

FIGURE 17.10 Lateral view. Red arrow shows L5 DRG lead breaching the posterior wall of the vertebral body which resulted in ventral placement of DRG electrodes within the neuroforamen, increasing the risk of motor stimulation at that level. The yellow line represents the posterior wall of the vertebral body, defining the boundary between dorsal and ventral DRG lead placement. *Image courtesy of Carlos Trigo, MD.*

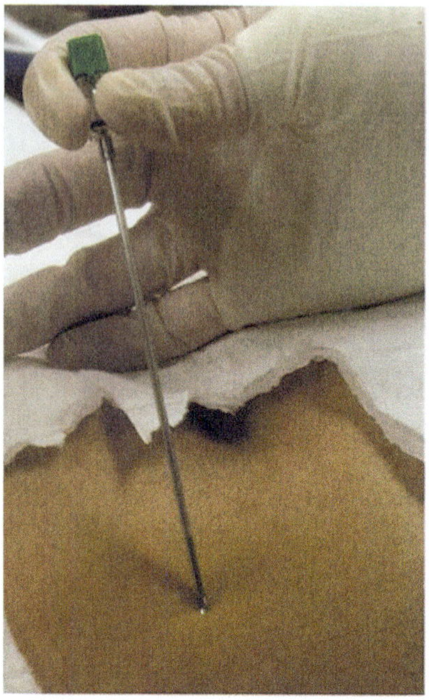

FIGURE 17.11 Presenting the needle on the patient's skin and obtaining a CLO image can help determine whether the selected entry point provides an optimal needle trajectory. *Image courtesy of Carlos Trigo, MD.*

Sheath/lead navigation on lateral fluoroscopy view

Attempt to guide sheath/lead on lateral view while advancing the lead through the neuroforamen. Make adjustments on sheath direction to ensure dorsal lead placement. Ensure you have a true lateral image before determining if the lead is dorsal or ventral.

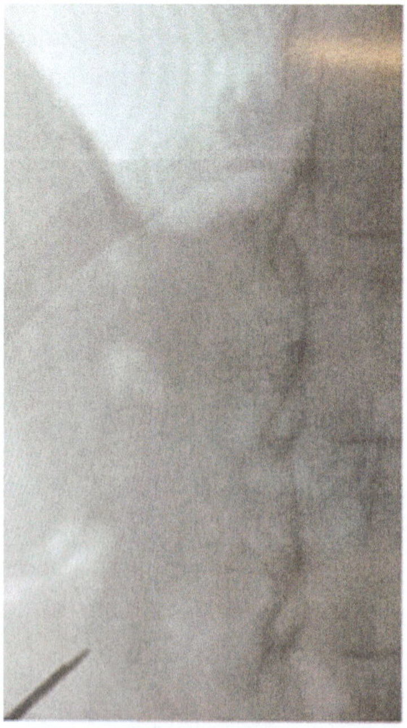

FIGURE 17.12 CLO image from Fig. 17.11 showing an optimal trajectory toward target interlaminar space prior to needle puncturing the skin. *Image courtesy of Carlos Trigo, MD.*

Challenges in accessing the target neuroforamen

Needle placement

Ensure proper needle placement: superior and midline within the interlaminar space being targeted. Ensure the needle angle is as flat as possible (this might be difficult for L4 and more difficult for the L5 level). You can also change from a contralateral approach on needle entry to an ipsilateral approach as another option if you continue with difficulty accessing the neuroforamen (Fig. 17.13) [7].

Guidewire

If unable to advance the lead through the neuroforamen, attempt to access the neuroforamen with gentle navigation of the guidewire, then remove it and replace it with the DRG-S lead [8]. Ensure the stylet is all the way in when introducing the lead. If you can't access the target neuroforamen after multiple attempts, choose a different level, above or below your original target. Choose the level that's closest to the dermatome you want to target.

Sheath kinking or shearing

If the sheath is kinked it will be difficult to navigate and access the target neuroforamen. If resistance is met while advancing the sheath and bowing is observed more force will ultimately kink the sheath. You can exchange the lead within the sheath for the guidewire to decrease the pliability of the sheath [8]. This rigidity generates greater lateral force, enabling the sheath to bypass most resistance from intraforaminal ligaments [8]. If you identify that the sheath has kinked, remove it and replace it with another one. Misalignment of the sheath and the needle during advancement or withdrawal of the sheath, can cause it to shear leading to difficulty advancing/withdrawing the lead and operating the sheath itself.

Needle dislodgement during sheath withdrawal

- Place a hand at the distal end of the introducer sheath, positioning the small finger just proximal to the needle hub to stabilize the needle while withdrawing the sheath into the needle [47] (Fig. 17.14). This technique facilitates lead deployment and the creation of the strain relief loops. Another technique is to place the distal end of the introducer sheath between the small and ring fingers, just proximal to the needle hub, to create counterforce and prevent needle dislodgment while withdrawing the sheath.
- Another option to prevent the needle from coming out of the epidural space is to have an assistant hold the needle while the sheath is being retracted.

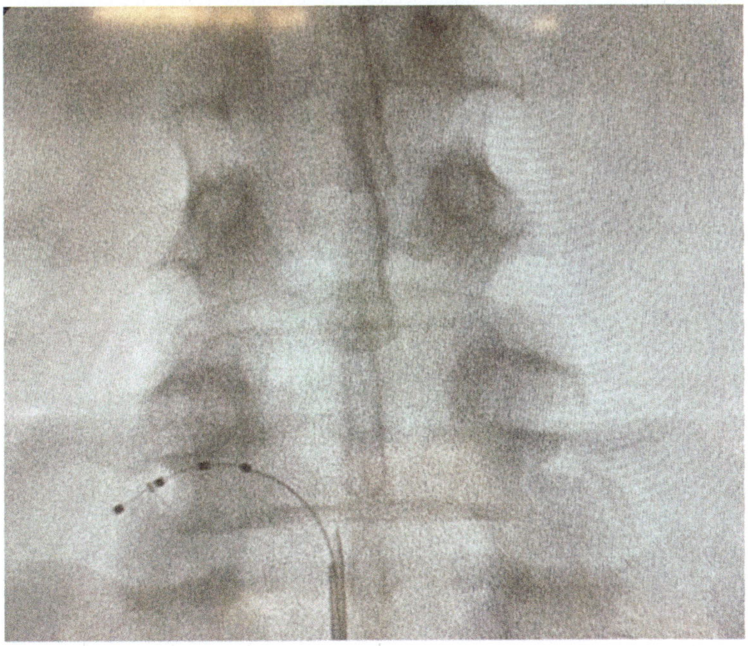

FIGURE 17.13 AP view. Ipsilateral technique for placement of left L5 DRG lead. *Image courtesy of Carlos Trigo, MD.*

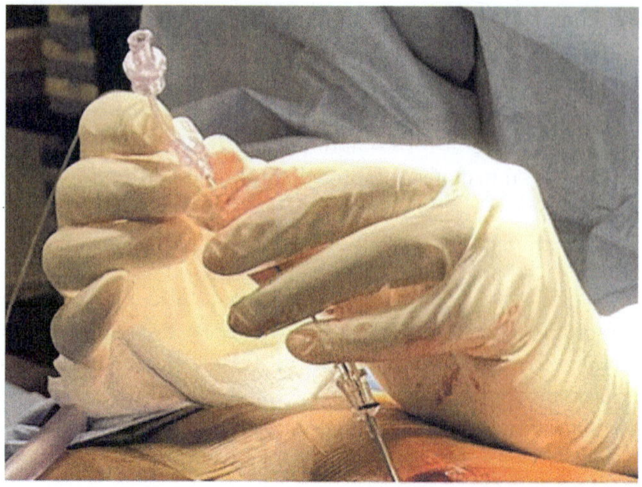

FIGURE 17.14 Hand positioning during sheath retraction, place the small finger just proximal to the needle hub as the sheath is being withdrawn to prevent the needle from coming out. The Tuohy needle and the sheath need to always move in the same direction to prevent shearing of the sheath or contributing to sheath kinking. *Image courtesy of Carlos Trigo, MD.*

- If the needle becomes dislodged, do not attempt to reintroduce it—except in sacral cases—as there is a high risk of dural puncture. This is because loss of resistance cannot be performed with the introducer sheath in place.

Pearls and pitfalls

- Gentle technique will prevent most complications related to DRG stimulation.
- The rate of safety events for DRG-S is comparable to SCS safety profile.
- Pre-procedural planning is essential to ensure patient safety and procedure success. Pre-procedural planning encompasses: imaging review and thorough review of the patient's comorbidities.
- Establish relationships with a multidisciplinary team to help you manage complications that are outside of the scope of practice of an interventional pain physician.

References

[1] Deer TR, Levy RM, Kramer J, et al. Dorsal root ganglion stimulation yielded higher treatment success rate for complex regional pain syndrome and causalgia at 3 and 12 months: a randomized comparative trial. Pain 2017;158(4):669–81. https://doi.org/10.1097/j.pain.0000000000000814.

[2] Pope JE, Deer TR, Kramer J. A systematic review: current practices and future directions of dorsal root ganglion stimulation. Expet Rev Med Dev 2019;16(10):883–91.

[3] Deer TR, Levy RM, Kramer J, Poree L, Amirdelfan K, Grigsby EJ, et al. Dorsal root ganglion stimulation safety and efficacy: a review of the literature. Neuromodulation 2021;24(5):837–46. https://doi.org/10.1016/j.neurom.2021.06.003.

[4] Bratzler DW, Houck PM. Antimicrobial prophylaxis for surgery: an advisory statement from the National Surgical Infection Prevention Project. Clin Infect Dis 2004;38:1706–15.

[5] Alexander JW, Solomkin JS, Edwards MJ. Updated recommendations for control of surgical site infections. Ann Surg 2011;253:1082–93.

[6] Bratzler DW, Dellinger EP, Olsen KM, et al. Clinical practice guidelines for antimicrobial prophylaxis in surgery. Am J Health Syst Pharm 2013;70:195–283.

[7] Chapman KB, Sayed D, Lamer T, Hunter C, Weisbein J, Patel KV, et al. Best practices for dorsal root ganglion stimulation for chronic pain: guidelines from the American Society of Pain and Neuroscience. J Pain Res 2023;16:839–79.

[8] Deer TR, Pope JE, Lamer TJ, Grider JS, Provenzano D, Lubenow TR, et al. The neuromodulation appropriateness consensus committee on best practices for dorsal root ganglion stimulation. Neuromodulation 2019;22(1):1–35.

[9] Graca MJ, Lubenow TR, Landphair WR, McCarthy RJ. Efficacy and safety of cervical and high-thoracic dorsal root ganglion stimulation therapy for complex regional pain syndrome of the upper extremities. Neuromodulation 2023;26(8):1781–7.

[10] Piedade GS, Vesper J, Chatzikalfas A, Slotty PJ. Cervical and high-thoracic dorsal root ganglion stimulation in chronic neuropathic pain. Neuromodulation 2019;22(8):951–5.

[11] Deer TR, Stewart CD. Complications of spinal cord stimulation: identification, treatment, and prevention. Pain Med 2008;9:S93–101.

[12] Vancamp T, Levy RM, Pena I, Pajuelo A. Relevant anatomy, morphology, and implantation techniques of the dorsal root ganglia at the lumbar levels. Neuromodulation 2017;20(7):690–702.

[13] Kim DH, Kwon HJ, Jeon B, Lee D, Shin JW, Choi SS. Comparison of the contralateral oblique view with the lateral view for mid-thoracic epidural access under fluoroscopic guidance: a randomized controlled trial. Reg Anesth Pain Med 2022. https://doi.org/10.1136/rapm-2021-103466.

[14] Kwon HJ, Kim CS, Kim J, Kim S, Shin JY, Choi SS, et al. Contralateral oblique view can prevent dural puncture in fluoroscopy-guided cervical epidural access: a prospective observational study. Reg Anesth Pain Med 2023;48(12):588–93.

[15] Gill JS, Nagda JV, Aner MM, Keel JC, Simopoulos TT. Contralateral oblique view is superior to the lateral view for lumbar epidural access. Pain Med 2016;17(5):839–50.

[16] Wong AK, Rasouli MR, Ng A, Wang D. Targeted epidural blood patches under fluoroscopic guidance for incidental durotomies related to spine surgeries: a case series. J Pain Res 2019;12:2825–33.

[17] Scavone BM. Timing of epidural blood patch: clearing up the confusion. Anaesthesia 2015;70(2):119–21.

[18] Patel R, Urits I, Orhurhu V, Orhurhu MS, Peck J, Ohuabunwa E, et al. A comprehensive update on the treatment and management of postdural puncture headache. Curr Pain Headache Rep 2020;24(6):24.

[19] Zetlaoui PJ, Buchheit T, Benhamou D. Epidural blood patch: a narrative review. Anaesth Crit Care Pain Med 2022;41(5):101138.

[20] Gandhi J, DiMatteo A, Joshi G, Smith NL, Khan SA. Cerebrospinal fluid leaks secondary to dural tears: a review of etiology, clinical evaluation, and management. Int J Neurosci 2021;131(7):689–95.

[21] Baranidharan G, Bretherton B, Black S. A case series of new radicular pain following the insertion of spinal cord stimulator. Br J Pain 2022;16(4):450–7.

[22] Sivanesan E, Bicket MC, Cohen SP. Retrospective analysis of complications associated with dorsal root ganglion stimulation for pain relief in the FDA MAUDE database. Reg Anesth Pain Med 2019;44(1):100–6.

[23] Lu L, Lau M, Akers L, Jones L, Selassie M, Burke M, et al. Intraoperative neurophysiological monitoring during lead placement for dorsal root ganglion stimulation: a literature review and case series. Neuromodulation 2024;27(1):160–71.

[24] Zhu AC, Tram J, Waterman R, Wallace M, Chakravarthy K. Recommendations for anesthetic management for intraoperative neuromodulation cases. Pain Manag 2022;12(4):557–67.

[25] Mackey S, Deer T, Pope J. A best-practice guide for dorsal root ganglion stimulation. Neurotherapeutics 2019;16(1):37–43.

[26] Eldabe S, Mounsey PJ, Madzinga G, et al. Dorsal root ganglion stimulation: a review of the literature and treatment recommendations. Pain Ther 2018;7(2):159–77.

[27] Verrills P, Sinclair C, Barnard A. A review of spinal cord stimulation systems for chronic pain. J Pain Res 2016;9:481–92.

[28] Hunter CW, Yang A, Davis T. The use of dorsal root ganglion stimulation in the treatment of chronic postoperative joint pain: initial report. Pain Pract 2016;16(5):300–6.

[29] Proclaim DRG neurostimulation clinician's manual. Plano, TX: Abbott; 2018.

[30] Chapman KB, Mogilner AY, Yang AH, et al. Lead migration and fracture rate in dorsal root ganglion stimulation using anchoring and non-anchoring techniques: a multicenter pooled data analysis. Pain Pract 2021;21(8):859–70. https://doi.org/10.1111/papr.13052.

[31] Deer TR, Pope JE, et al. The polyanalgesic consensus conference (PACC): recommendations for DRG stimulation. Pain Pract 2020;20(3):277–86.

[32] Pope JE, Falowski S, Provenzano D. Dorsal root ganglion stimulation for the treatment of focal neuropathic pain. Curr Pain Headache Rep 2021;25(8):1–8.

[33] Deer TR, Skaribas IM, Haider N, et al. Effectiveness of dorsal root ganglion stimulation for the treatment of complex regional pain syndrome compared with spinal cord stimulation. Pain Physician 2020;23(3):E251–78.

[34] Pope JE, Deer TR. A novel implanted epidural neuromodulation system for the treatment of chronic pain. Expet Rev Med Dev 2020;17(7):649–57.

[35] Baranidharan G, Athanassoglou V, Palmisani S. An overview of the mechanisms and use of spinal cord stimulation for pain management. Br J Pain 2021;15(2):122–9.

[36] Deer TR, Narouze S, Provenzano D, et al. The appropriate use of neurostimulation of the spinal cord and peripheral nervous system for the treatment of chronic pain and ischemic diseases: the Neuromodulation Appropriateness Consensus Committee. Neuromodulation 2014;17(6):515–50.

[37] Falowski S, Pope J. DRG stimulation: fundamentals and literature review. Front Pain Res 2021;2:7.

[38] Li S, Yu L, Sinha S, et al. Techniques and complications of dorsal root ganglion stimulation. Pain Manag 2020;10(5):311–22.

[39] Sommer C, Richter H, Rogausch JP, et al. Spinal cord stimulation and neuropathic pain: mechanisms of action and clinical application. Pain 2018;159(2):314–9.

[40] Levy RM, Mekhail N. Dorsal root ganglion stimulation in the treatment of chronic pain: a review and update on the clinical evidence. Neurosurgery 2021;88(5):877–89.

[41] Pangarkar S, Pham A. The role of dorsal root ganglion stimulation in the management of intractable pain: a critical analysis of the literature. Pain Med 2019;20(Suppl. 1):S35–42.

[42] Pope JE, Deer TR. Dorsal root ganglion stimulation: advancing the field of neuromodulation. Expet Rev Med Dev 2021;18(3):233–40.

[43] Yang A, Hunter CW. Dorsal root ganglion stimulation for chronic pain: a clinical review. Curr Pain Headache Rep 2017;21(3):12.

[44] Levy R, Deer T, Henderson J, et al. Neuromodulation for the treatment of chronic pain: review and update of the clinical evidence and recommendations for future trial designs. Neuromodulation 2021;24(1):68–78.

[45] Hunter CW. DRG stimulation and its effect on neuropathic pain: results from a prospective global registry. Reg Anesth Pain Med 2018;43(6):e129.

[46] Raza A, Morgan RJ, Pettifer R, et al. An overview of new spinal cord stimulators and technologies. Neuromodulation 2020;23(Suppl. 1):61–71.

[47] Abbott. Dorsal root ganglion stimulation: virtual certification [video]. Abbott; 2024. https://www.medworldlive.com.

Further reading

[1] Biancari F, Tiozzo V. Staples versus sutures for closing leg wounds after vein graft harvesting for coronary artery bypass surgery. Cochrane Database Syst Rev 2010;5:CD008057.

[2] Iavazzo C, Gkegkes ID, Vouloumanou EK, Mamais I, Peppas G, Falagas ME. Sutures versus staples for the management of surgical wounds: a meta-analysis of randomized controlled trials. Am Surg 2011;77:1206–21.

[3] Deer TR, Narouze S, Provenzano DA, et al. The neurostimulation appropriateness consensus committee (NACC): recommendations on bleeding and coagulation management in neurostimulation devices. Neuromodulation 2017;20(1):51–62. https://doi.org/10.1111/ner.12542.

[4] Dydyk AM, Tadi P. Spinal cord stimulator implant. In: StatPearls. Treasure Island (FL): StatPearls Publishing; 2025.

[5] Deer TR, Mekhail N, Provenzano D, et al. The appropriate use of neurostimulation: avoidance and treatment of complications of neurostimulation therapies for the treatment of chronic pain. Neuromodulation 2014;17(6):571–97.

[6] West T, Driver CN, D'Souza RS. Incidence of neuraxial and non-neuraxial hematoma complications from spinal cord stimulator surgery: systematic review and proportional meta-analysis. Neuromodulation 2023;26(7):1328–38.

[7] Deer TR, Provenzano DA, Hanes M, et al. The neurostimulation appropriateness consensus committee (NACC) recommendations for infection prevention and management. Neuromodulation 2017;20(1):31–50.

Section 5

Waveforms and frequencies

Introduction to section 5 waveforms and frequencies

Jeff Arle

The rapidly advancing field of neuromodulation is unlocking transformative possibilities for patients with chronic pain, neurological disorders, and other challenging conditions. In this textbook, we delve into the innovative procedures and techniques that are shaping the future of this dynamic field. This section, specifically, focuses on the exciting developments in wavelengths, high-frequency stimulation, closed-loop systems, and subperception waveforms, highlighting their current applications and potential future directions.

Neuromodulation techniques utilizing various wavelengths and frequencies are at the forefront of modern therapeutic strategies. The evolution from traditional low-frequency stimulation to high-frequency and burst stimulation has significantly improved patient outcomes. High-frequency stimulation, for instance, has demonstrated remarkable efficacy in reducing pain and improving quality of life without the tingling sensations typically associated with conventional spinal cord stimulation. This shift has opened new avenues for treating conditions that were previously challenging to manage with neuromodulation.

Closed-loop systems represent another leap forward in the field, offering personalized and adaptive treatment options. Unlike open-loop systems that deliver constant stimulation, closed-loop systems continuously monitor the body's response to therapy and adjust stimulation parameters in real time. This approach not only enhances therapeutic efficacy but also minimizes side effects, providing a more tailored and responsive treatment experience. The integration of feedback mechanisms from physiological signals such as electromyography (EMG) or local field potentials (LFP) marks a significant advancement in precision medicine.

Subperception stimulation, or the use of waveforms that do not elicit conscious sensations, is another revolutionary concept that has gained traction. By delivering stimulation below the threshold of patient perception, these methods aim to reduce discomfort and improve compliance while maintaining or even enhancing therapeutic benefits. The exploration of various waveform patterns and their impact on neuronal circuits is leading to the development of more sophisticated and effective neuromodulation therapies.

Looking forward, the future of neuromodulation is brimming with potential. The convergence of artificial intelligence, machine learning, and neuromodulation technologies promises to further refine and personalize treatments and speed up programming. Predictive algorithms could anticipate patient needs and adjust therapies accordingly, ushering in an era of truly individualized care. Additionally, ongoing research into novel materials and miniaturization of devices aims to make neuromodulation therapies less invasive and more accessible.

This section aims to provide a comprehensive understanding of these cutting-edge procedures, offering insights into their mechanisms, clinical applications, and future prospects. As we continue to explore the complexities of the human nervous system and harness technological advancements, the possibilities for improving patient outcomes through new neuromodulation waveforms and methodologies are vast and exciting.

Chapter 18

Burst waveforms

Harry Soar[1], Dirk De Ridder[2], Robin Mata[3] and Timothy Deer[4]
[1]*York and Scarborough Teaching Hospitals NHS Foundation Trust, Yorkshire, United Kingdom;* [2]*University of Otago, Dunedin, New Zealand;* [3]*University of Miami, Coral Gables, FL, United States;* [4]*The Spine and Nerve Centers of the Virginias and West Virginia University, Morgantown, WV, United States*

Introduction

Spinal cord stimulation (SCS) has long been a cornerstone in the management of chronic pain, particularly for patients refractory to conventional therapies. Traditional "tonic" or "paresthesia-based" SCS is characterized by electrical pulses at a consistent frequency and pulse width and has been used successfully for decades to treat patients with chronic and disabling, painful conditions.

Despite its widespread use, tonic SCS is associated with several limitations:

1) The induction of paresthesia, which, though therapeutic, can be uncomfortable or intolerable for some patients, particularly without a closed-loop mechanism.
2) The development of tolerance over time can diminish therapeutic efficacy, and a subset of patients experience suboptimal pain relief, thought to be due to reduced neural response.
3) Movement, especially in the cervical spine, can result in painful over or understimulation, due to changes in the distance between the stimulating electrode and the spinal column.

These limitations have led to the exploration of more physiologically nuanced stimulation patterns.

This chapter focuses on burst waveform stimulation, an innovative approach designed to address the shortcomings of traditional tonic SCS. Whereas tonic stimulation mimics tonic firing in the nervous system, burst stimulation mimics a second physiological firing pattern in the nervous system, called burst firing, which is the electrophysiological correlate of salience.

Burst stimulation delivers intermittent bursts of high-frequency pulses separated by quiescent periods, a pattern that closely approximates the physiological firing patterns of neural circuits. The most widely used burst waveform originally isolated and described by DeRidder (BurstDR, Abbott) is characterized in technical terms by a five-pulse train of monopolar spikes with internal frequency of 500 Hz, delivered at 40 Hz, with a 1 ms pulse width and 1 ms pulse interval, that utilizes a passive recharge pattern at the end of the pulses, recharging all pulses at once.

This chapter aims to provide surgical and pain medicine specialists with a detailed understanding of burst waveforms, including their neurophysiological mechanisms, clinical evidence and potential future applications.

Pain is a multidimensional experience, encompassing both the sensory-discriminative component (painfulness) and the affective-emotional component (suffering). The painfulness and suffering-evoking pathways are balanced by the pain-inhibitory pathway. If the descending pathway activity equals the pain-evoking activity, no pain ensues. If, however, the balance is negative, then pain ensues. Traditional tonic SCS primarily targets the lateral and descending pain pathways, modulating sensory-discriminative pain by inhibiting nociceptive signal transmission at the dorsal horn. In contrast, burst stimulation appears to engage both the lateral, medial and descending pain pathways, including the anterior cingulate cortex, which are integral to the affective and cognitive dimensions of pain. By activating medial pain pathways, burst stimulation simultaneously attenuates both the intensity of pain and its emotional burden, offering a more comprehensive and holistic therapeutic effect.

Multiple level-1 randomized placebo-controlled studies show that burst waveform SCS provides superior pain relief compared to tonic stimulation, as well as superior reduction in suffering encompassing patients with inadequate response

A Modern Atlas for Implantable Devices of the Spine, Brain, and Nerve. https://doi.org/10.1016/B978-0-443-36528-7.00034-0

to traditional SCS. Additionally, studies indicate a lower propensity for tolerance development, potentially extending the durability of therapeutic benefits. As the field of neuromodulation advances, burst waveforms represent a significant evolution in SCS technology. This chapter will delve into the neurophysiological underpinnings of burst stimulation, evaluate the clinical evidence supporting its use, and explore emerging research directions. By the conclusion of this chapter, pain specialists will gain a robust understanding of how burst waveforms have evolved the neuromodulation sector, offering a promising alternative for patients with complex chronic pain conditions.

Key points

- **Mimics Natural Neural Activity**: Burst waveforms replicate burst firing patterns, a universal phenomenon in both the central (CNS) and peripheral nervous systems (PNS), making them physiologically aligned with natural neural processes.
- **Comprehensive Pain Modulation**: Unlike traditional stimulation, burst waveforms engage the medial pathway alongside lateral and descending inhibitory pathways, addressing both the sensory (painfulness) and emotional (suffering) dimensions of pain.
- **Clinically Validated Efficacy**: The effectiveness of burst waveforms is supported by level-1 randomized placebo-controlled trials, placebo-controlled trials and a meta-analysis, providing robust evidence for their use in SCS.
- **Less is more**: Burst waveforms are most effective with lower energy supplied to the spinal cord. Utilizing lower amplitudes and intermittent use.
- **Power efficient**: The less is more principle of burst stimulation offers the added benefit of low power consumption, which enhances device longevity and patient convenience.

Waveform characteristics

When discussing SCS waveforms, it's important to understand their characteristics and associated mechanisms of action. The three parameters that describe most waveforms are frequency (Hz), pulse width (microseconds), and amplitude (V or mA) (Fig. 18.1).

What is a tonic waveform?

Key characteristics of traditional tonic waveform:

- **Continuous Stimulation:**
  - Tonic SCS delivers a constant, uninterrupted stream of electrical pulses, in which each individual pulse is charge-balanced.

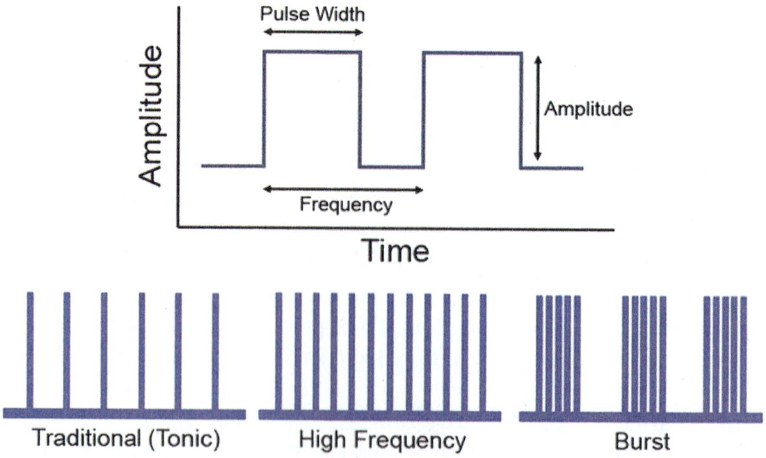

FIGURE 18.1 Artistic depiction illustrating the basic components of the stimulation waveform, including amplitude, frequency, and pulse width. Compared to traditional (tonic) stimulation, recent waveform innovations include high-frequency and burst stimulation. *Sheldon B, Staudt MD, Williams , Harland TA, & Pilitsis JG. Spinal cord stimulation programming: a crash course. Neurosurgical review 2021;44(2):709–720. https://doi.org/10.1007/s10143-020-01299-y.*

- **Parameters:**
  - **Frequency:** Typically ranges from 40 to 80 Hz.
  - **Pulse Width:** Usually varies between 200 and 500 μs (μs).
  - **Amplitude:** Adjusted to produce paresthesia that covers the patient's pain area.

Tonic conventional stimulation (TCS), also known as paresthesia-based or low-frequency SCS, was the only available stimulation paradigm from 1967 to 2006. This constant, low-frequency stimulation generates a tingling sensation (paresthesia). A drawback of TCS is that paresthesia can be very uncomfortable for patients. Furthermore, TCS's reported success rate is roughly 50% pain relief in approximately 50%–70% of patients, with diminishing effectiveness on long-term follow-up [1,2]. These limitations prompted research into other waveforms for more effective SCS therapy.

What is a burst waveform?

Instead of continuous electrical pulses, burst stimulation delivers bursts of multiple pulses followed by periods of rest. This pattern is designed to mimic the natural firing patterns of neurons.

Typical structure of a burst waveform:

- **Burst Structure:**
  - Five monophasic pulses lasting 1 ms.
- **Intra-Burst Frequency:**
  - Pulses within the burst are delivered at a frequency of 500 Hz.
- **Burst Delivery Rate:**
  - 40 such bursts are delivered per second.
- **Charge Balancing:**
  - The cumulative charge of the five monophasic pulses is balanced within 5 ms following the delivery of the entire burst (not after each individual pulse) (Fig. 18.2).

Burst stimulation was conceived as a novel stimulation design to mimic physiological burst firing. In the brain, burst firing is exhibited by certain neurons (e.g., thalamocortical neurons) and is considered a "wake-up call" as it exerts both a strong inhibitory and excitatory postsynaptic potential due to its nonlinear build-up and higher signal-to-noise ratio [3,4]. Burst firing within the central nervous system (CNS) has also been suggested to be involved in rerouting information, allowing parallel processing, and contributing to the synchronization of neural network activity [5,6].

How do these waveforms interact with the CNS? (Tonic vs. burst)

Based on the pain gate theory, tonic SCS alleviates pain in the spinal cord by stimulating dorsal column Aβ fibers, which creates paresthesias matching the painful area and activates inhibitory interneurons in the dorsal horn. In the brain, tonic SCS also modulates neuropathic pain through a supraspinal-spinal feedback loop and serotonergic descending fibers, also

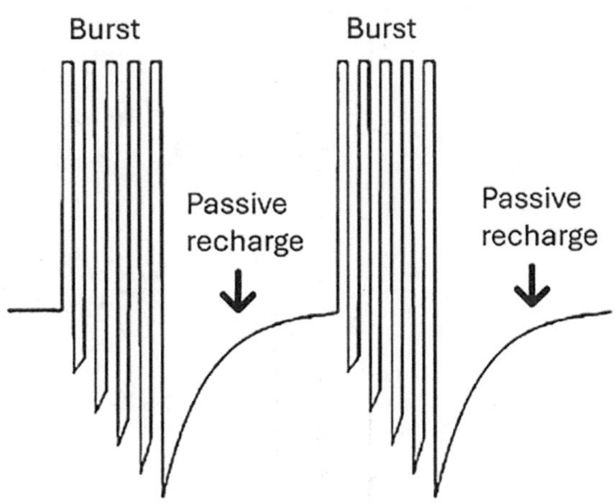

FIGURE 18.2 Burst stimulation waveform. *Image created by author Harry Soar.*

known as the descending pathway [7]. On functional magnetic resonance imaging (MRI) tonic SCS has been shown to *deactivate* the medial thalamus and its connections to the cingulate cortex and insula, also referred to as the medial pathway. Although immediate pain relief with tonic SCS most strongly correlated with reduced activity in the inferior olivary nucleus, cerebellum, and rostral anterior cingulate cortex, also referred to as the descending pathway.

Compared to tonic SCS, animal model studies suggest that burst waveforms are independent of GABAergic signaling in the spinal cord [8]. While not fully neurochemically understood, burst SCS has been shown to reduce inhibitory interneuron (wide dynamic range) firing within the dorsal horn of the spinal cord, with the exception of the gracile nucleus, which may explain pain relief without experiencing paresthesia. In the brain, burst SCS has been shown to enhance postsynaptic responses, boost synaptic connectivity via long-term potentiation, and more potently activate pain and emotional processing pathways compared to tonic SCS [9] (Figs. 18.3 and 18.4).

Mechanism of pain pathways

The traditional pain model

Traditionally, pain processing has been understood through three primary neural pathways: two ascending pathways (medial and lateral) and one descending pathway (Fig. 18.5). These pathways dynamically interact and are influenced by factors like context, expectations, and emotional state [10,11]

- **Lateral Pathway (Sensory/Discriminative):**
  - This pathway focuses on the "where" and "how intense" aspects of pain.
  - It's activated by various nerve fibers (Aβ, Aδ, and C fibers).
  - Information travels from the spinal cord to the thalamus (ventral posterolateral nuclei) and then to the somatosensory cortex and parietal areas [12,13].
- **Medial Pathway (Emotional/Motivational):**
  - This pathway deals with the "unpleasantness" or emotional response to pain.
  - It's primarily activated by C fibers.

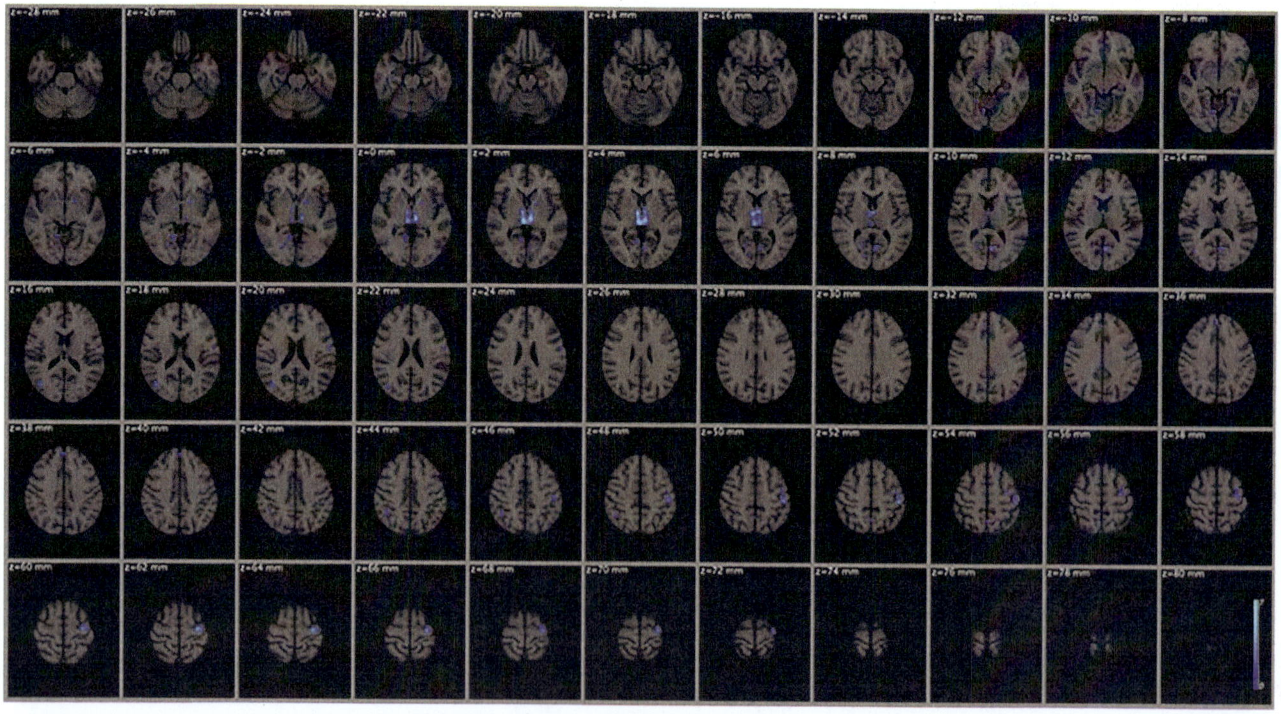

FIGURE 18.3 Group statistical map of functional alterations during short-term tonic SCS ($P < .05$ FWE corrected). Blue deactivation, z dorsoventral location according to MNI coordinates. *Moens M, Sunaert S, Mariën P, Brouns R, De Smedt A, Droogmans S, Van Schuerbeek P, Peeters R, Poelaert J, Nuttin, B. Spinal cord stimulation modulates cerebral function: an fMRI study. Neuroradiology, 2012;54(12):1399–1407.*

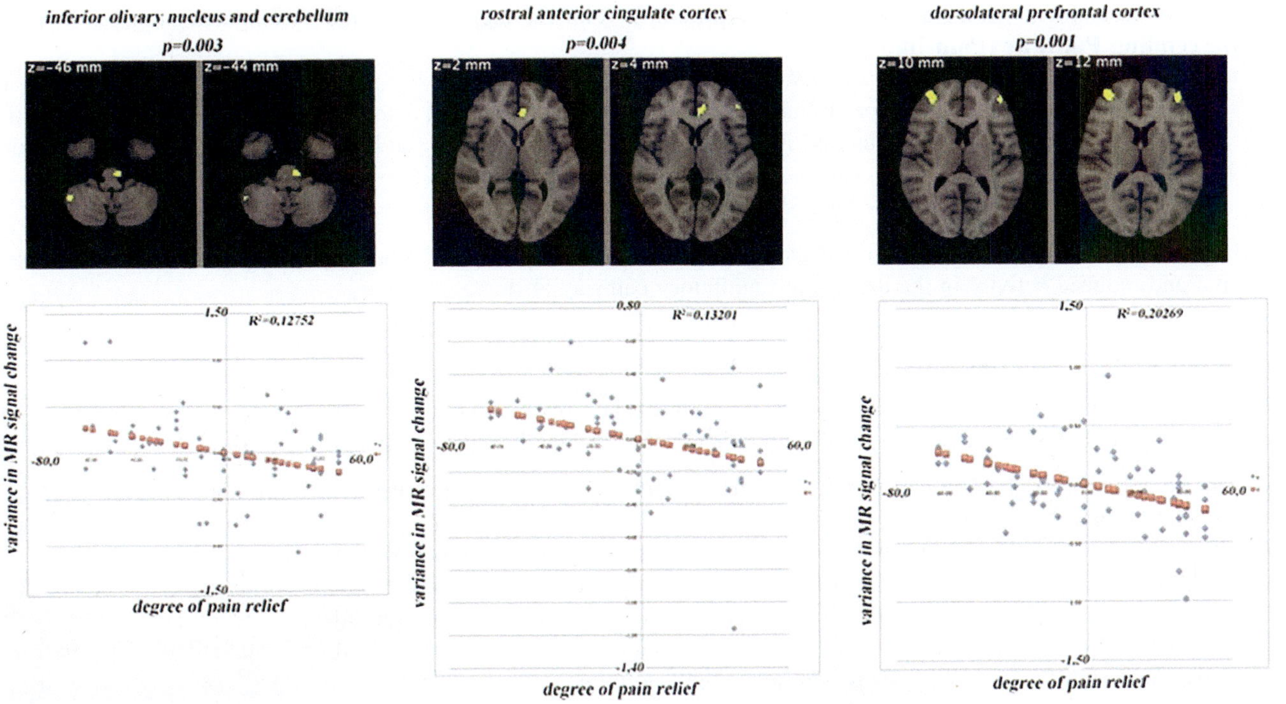

FIGURE 18.4 Correlation between degree of pain relief during short-term SCS and variance in MR signal change (percent change of MR signal in T2*-weighted BOLD images). This variance is mean-centered. z Dorsoventral location according to MNI coordinates. *Moens M, Sunaert S, Mariën P, Brouns R, De Smedt A, Droogmans S, Van Schuerbeek P, Peeters R, Poelaert J, Nuttin B. Spinal cord stimulation modulates cerebral function: an fMRI study. Neuroradiology, 2012;54(12):1399–1407.*

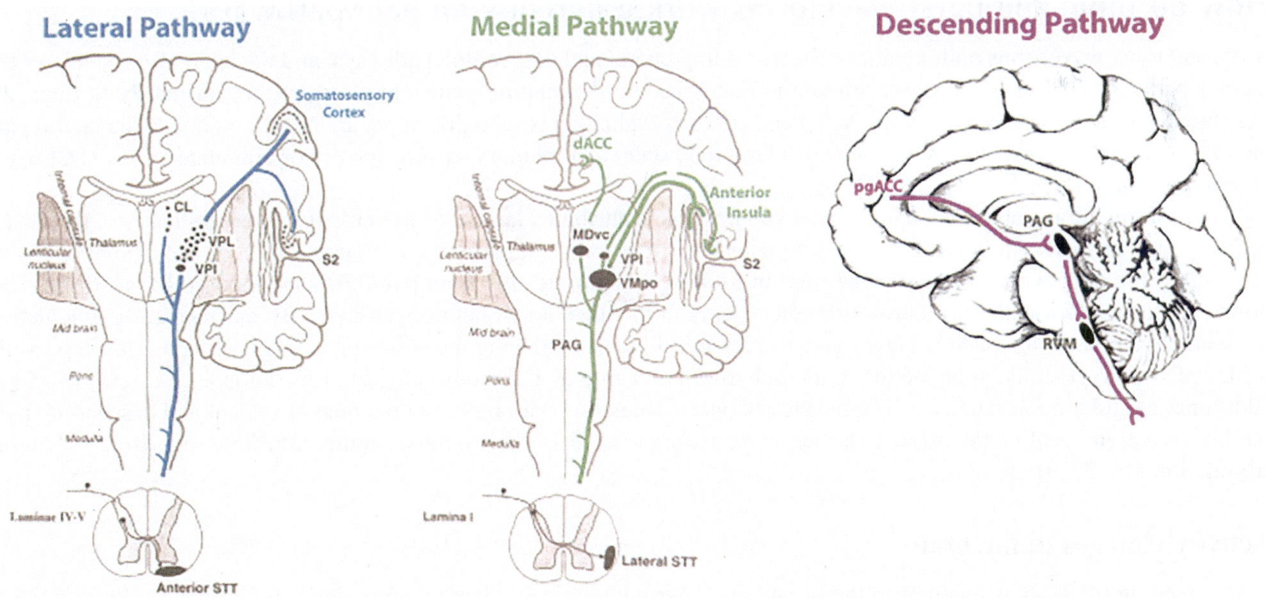

FIGURE 18.5 Ascending and descending pain pathways. Two ascending pain-supporting pathways have been described, and one pain-inhibitory descending pathway. The lateral ascending pathway processes the discriminatory components of pain, whereas the medial pathway processes the motivational, affective, and attentional components of pain. The pain-inhibitory pathway suppresses ongoing pain. *De Ridder D, Vanneste S. Burst and tonic spinal cord stimulation: Different and common brain mechanisms. Neuromodulation, 2016;19(1):47–59. https://doi.org/10.1111/ner.12368.*

    - It connects the thalamus (mediodorsal and ventral posterolateral nuclei) to the anterior cingulate cortex and insula.
- **Descending Pathway (Pain Inhibition):**
    - This pathway acts to reduce or modulate pain signals.
    - It originates in the dorsolateral prefrontal cortex and rostral and pregenual anterior cingulate cortex, connects to the reticular nucleus of the thalamus and further to the periaqueductal gray, and then projects to the somatosensory periphery.
    - In chronic pain, this pathway is often dysfunctional.

In chronic pain, there's often an imbalance, with increased activity in the ascending pathways (leading to more pain signals) and reduced activity in the descending inhibitory pathway [14].

Expanding the model: The triple network and chronic pain

While the traditional model is valuable, it doesn't fully explain the complexities of chronic pain. Recent research integrates the brain's "triple network model" to provide a more comprehensive understanding [15].

- The traditional model distinguishes between the "painfulness" (lateral pathway), "suffering" (medial pathway), and descending inhibitory pathways.
- The Triple Network Model expands on this by considering the interactions between three key brain networks:
    - **Default Mode Network (DMN):** Involved in self-representation and introspection. In chronic pain, the somatosensory cortex can become functionally connected to the DMN, making pain feel like an integral part of one's self.
    - **Salience Network (SN):** Responsible for detecting and responding to behaviorally relevant stimuli. This network overlaps with the medial pathway and hence the "suffering" aspect of pain.
    - **Central Executive Network (CEN):** Handles goal-oriented behavior and cognitive control. Disruptions in the CEN may explain the cognitive dysfunction often seen in chronic pain.
- This model helps explain a wider range of chronic pain symptoms, including cognitive and emotional issues, by highlighting the network interactions.
- The model also explains that pain can evolve into a chronic state as a method for the body to conserve energy.
- This framework distinguishes the experience of painfulness and suffering, and how context can change the experience of pain.

How do tonic and burst waveforms work differently on pain pathways?

Burst and tonic waveforms both modulate the ascending lateral and descending pathways, and the burst also modulates the medial pathway [16]. Both types of stimulation activate the descending pain inhibitory system, primarily through the pregenual anterior cingulate cortex (pgACC) and context-evaluating parahippocampal area. Both modulate the lateral pain pathways (somatosensory cortex) and a self-referential contextual memory system (posterior cingulate cortex (PCC) and parahippocampus).

Tonic stimulation's ability to achieve pain suppression is attributed largely to its activation predominantly of the lateral pathway and the descending [16,17]. It is yet unclear whether tonic stimulation has a direct effect on the medial pathway, or whether the improvement in suffering seen in tonic stimulation results from painfulness reduction. Burst stimulation, however, has a statistically more profound effect on both the medial and lateral pathways. By more potently modulating the medial pain pathway, burst achieves greater pain relief by also reducing the suffering element of pain. This is possibly achieved by direct modulation of the spinothalamic pathways, as indirectly suggested by animal research [18]. This additional modulation normalizes an imbalance between ascending pain input via the medial system and descending pain inhibitory activity and could explain the larger pain suppression effect by burst stimulation in comparison with tonic stimulation [19–22] (Fig. 18.6).

Activity changes in the brain

Understanding the activity changes in the brain that occur with tonic and burst stimulation requires a basic knowledge of key brain regions and brain wave frequencies. Several distinct brain regions play a role in mediating and relaying the effects of pain and SCS. The pregenual anterior cingulate cortex (pgACC) is a central component of the descending pain inhibitory system [23]. The parahippocampus, also part of the descending pain inhibitory pathway, links the default mode network to memory and is involved in contextual pain processing, appearing to act as a potential "control switch" between

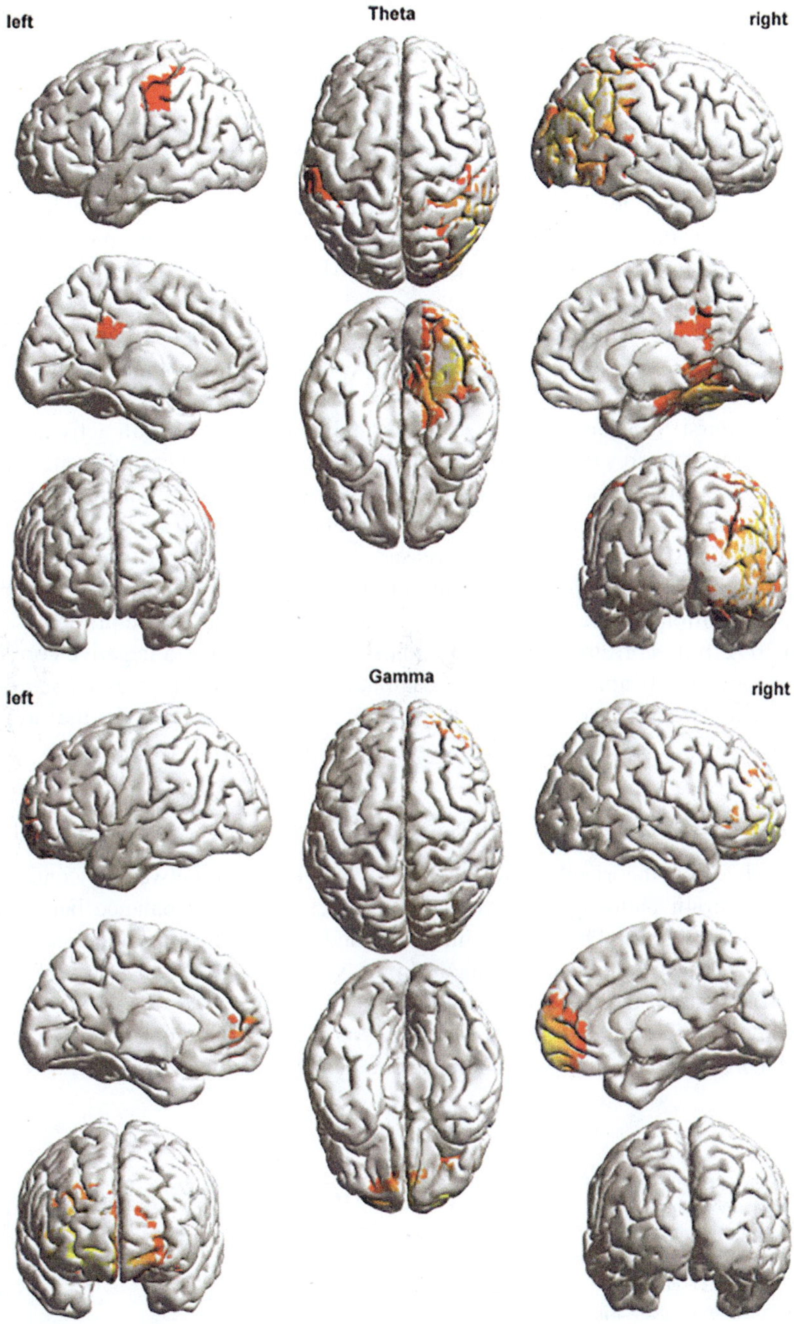

FIGURE 18.6 Conjunction analysis between tonic and burst stimulation corrected for baseline measures for the theta and the gamma frequency bands. Activation in tonic and burst stimulation goes in the same direction (yellow to red areas) for theta activity in the somatosensory cortex, posterior cingulate cortex, parahippocampal area, and inferior parietal area. For gamma activity, similar activation patterns are noted in the pregenual anterior cingulate cortex extending into the ventromedial prefrontal cortex bilaterally. *De Ridder, D., Vanneste, S. Burst and tonic spinal cord stimulation: Different and common brain mechanisms. Neuromodulation, 2016:19(1):47–59. https://doi.org/10.1111/ner.12368.*

pain pathways [24]. The posterior cingulate cortex (PCC) is another hub of the default mode network, which consists of a group of higher-order neurons that is the brain's "default state" when not focused on external stimuli and is implicated in self-referential pain processing (how an individual interprets their own pain as it relates to their identity). It strongly connects to the parahippocampus. The somatosensory cortex (SSC) is a main component of the lateral pain pathway, and the dorsal anterior cingulate cortex (dACC) and insula are the main hubs of the medial pain pathway.

Brain wave frequencies correlate with distinct mental states: delta waves (0.5–4 Hz) dominate during deep sleep, are related to autonomic and reward processing and physical restoration, while theta waves (4–8 Hz) are associated with memory processes, deep relaxation, drowsiness, and subconscious access, commonly seen in early sleep and meditation. Alpha waves (8–12 Hz) reflect a scanning mode in a relaxed, calm state, often experienced during daydreaming or meditation, and are linked to creativity and introspection. Conversely, beta waves (12–35 Hz) signify active thinking, alertness, and focused concentration, dominating during external attention, tasks, and problem-solving. Beta waves are related to a status quo, in which the brain makes sensory predictions without many prediction errors. Finally, gamma waves (30–80 Hz) represent the highest level of cognitive processing, peak mental performance, learning, and complex problem-solving [25].

Thalamocortical dysrhythmia, in which gamma is nested on theta waves by cross-frequency coupling, links the hypesthesia (theta) to painfulness (gamma), and has been posited to link pain to (contextual) memory processes (Fig. 18.7).

Compared to tonic SCS, burst SCS has been shown to normalize pathologic brain activity on electroencephalogram (EEG) in the medial and lateral pathways to a greater extent, as suggested by greater alpha activity in the dACC, SSC, and prefrontal cortex [16]. In a 2023 study, BurstDR SCS effects on brain activity were further analyzed [14]. Prior to SCS, γ activity in the SSC (main component of the lateral pathway) correlated with pain intensity. Following burst SCS, both θ (theta) and γ (gamma) oscillations in the SSC were decreased. In the dACC (part of the medial pain pathway), prior to stimulation, α (alpha) and β (beta) α and β activity correlate with pain catastrophizing. After burst SCS, a significant decrease in both α and β oscillations of the dACC was observed. In the pgACC (a central component of the descending pathway), prestimulation, θ activity correlated with pain intensity, and there was a negative correlation between θ and α. Following burst SCS, there are significant decreases in θ oscillations after stimulation and discontinuation of the negative correlation between θ and α. Overall, burst SCS reduces excessive brain activity in the areas associated with pain sensation (SSC), suffering (dACC), and pain suppression (pgACC) (Figs. 18.8–18.11).

Connectivity changes in the brain

Chronic pain has previously been theorized to be the result of imbalances between ascending (pain-provoking) and descending (pain-inhibitory) brain pathways. Pain reduction correlates with a balance between medial pain pathway activity and descending pain inhibition. Therefore, while tonic and burst SCS both modulate the lateral and descending pathways, burst SCS more strongly influences the medial pain system (dACC). In terms of brain activity, burst SCS effects more complete normalization compared to tonic SCS.

Further exploration of burst SCS suggests that its superiority is derived from its ability to alter both brain activity and connectivity. Functional connectivity with lagged phase coherence indicates how well two areas of the brain are

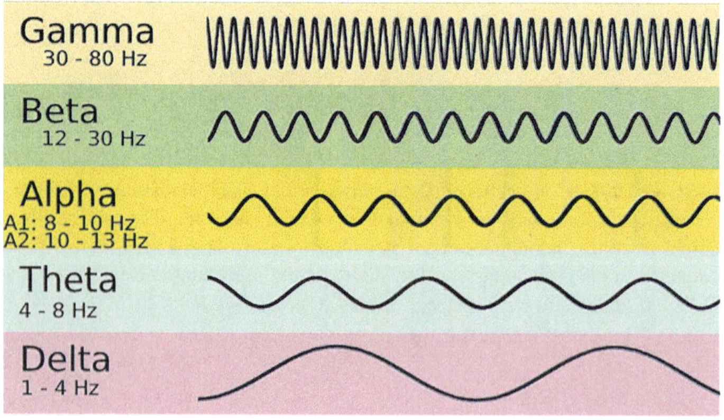
Gamma
30 - 80 Hz
Beta
12 - 30 Hz
Alpha
A1: 8 - 10 Hz
A2: 10 - 13 Hz
Theta
4 - 8 Hz
Delta
1 - 4 Hz

FIGURE 18.7 Conjunction analysis between tonic and burst stimulation corrected for baseline measures for the theta and the gamma frequency bands. Activation in tonic and burst stimulation goes in the same direction (yellow to red areas) for theta activity in the somatosensory cortex, posterior cingulate cortex, parahippocampal area, and inferior parietal area. Similar activation patterns are noted in the pregenual anterior cingulate cortex extending into the ventromedial prefrontal cortex bilaterally for gamma activity. *Attribution not legally required: Bondigoldwiki, CC0, via Wikimedia Commons.*

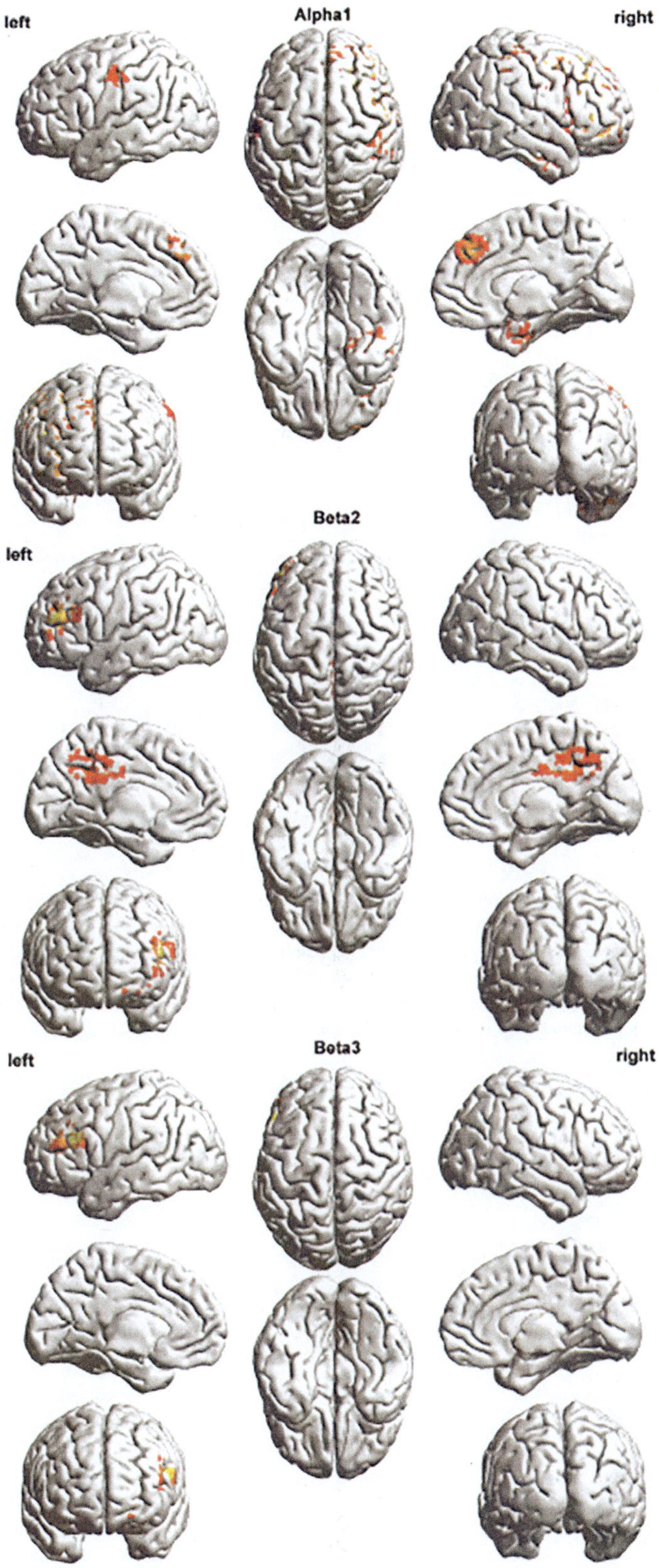

FIGURE 18.8 A comparison between tonic and burst stimulation on the source-localized EEG recording data revealed a significant ($P < .05$) increase in synchronized activity (yellow to red colored areas) in the left and right dorsal anterior cingulate cortex extending to the dorsomedial prefrontal cortex, as well as the primary somatosensory cortex for the alpha 1 frequency band and the left dorsal lateral prefrontal cortex (DLPFC) and posterior cingulate cortex for beta2 and DLPFC for beta3 frequency bands for burst stimulation in comparison with tonic stimulation. *De Ridder D, Vanneste S. Burst and tonic spinal cord stimulation: different and common brain mechanisms. Neuromodulation, 2016;19(1):47–59. https://doi.org/10.1111/ner.12368.*

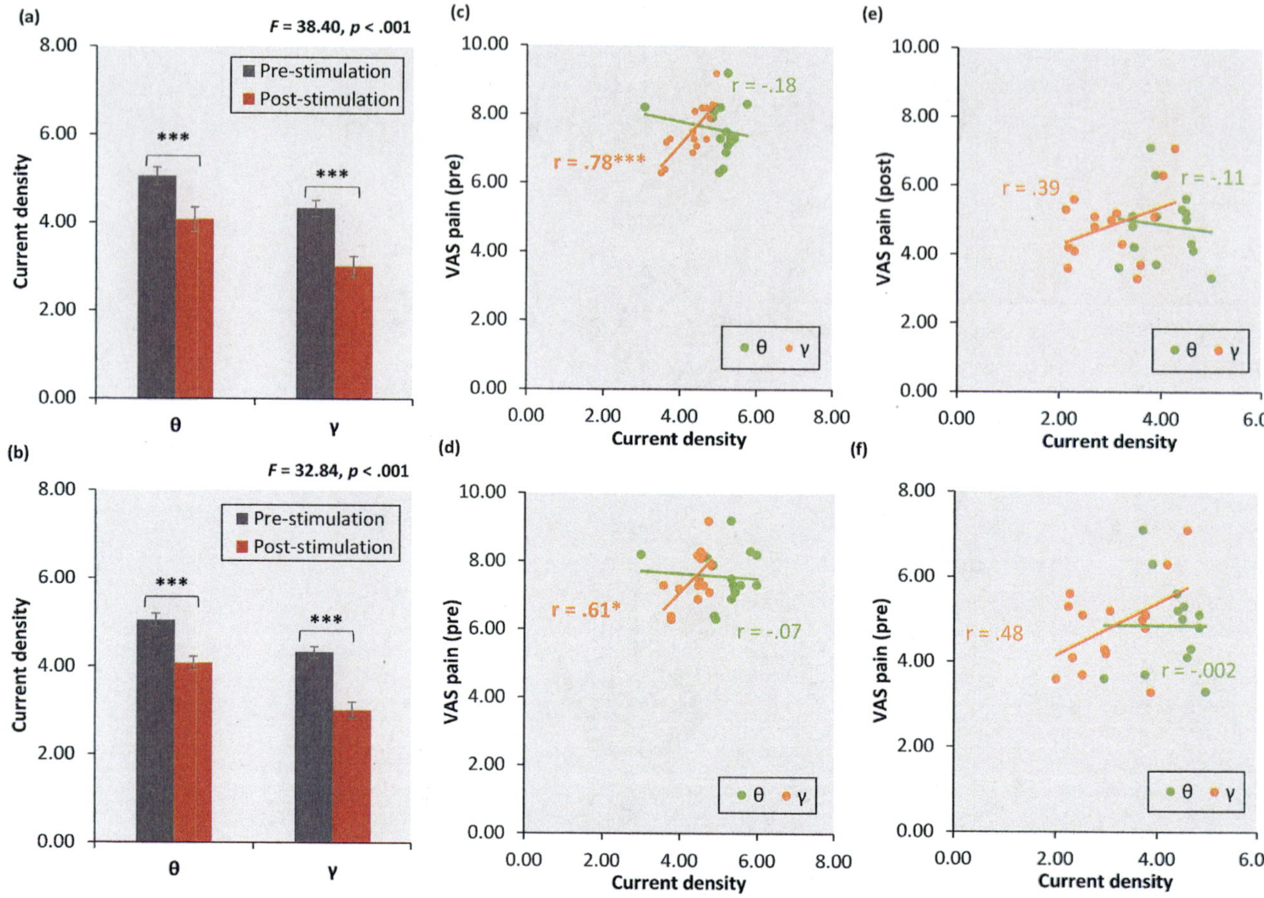

FIGURE 18.9 (a–b) A comparison between pre and postburstDR spinal cord identified a significant difference for both the θ and γ frequency band current density in the left and right SSC after stimulation in comparison to before stimulation. (c–d) Pre-stimulation, a significant positive correlation was found between the current density at γ for the left and right SSC and the pain intensity as measured by VAS. For the θ frequency band, no significant correlation was found between left and right SSC and the pain intensity. (e–f) Poststimulation, no significant correlation was obtained between current density for θ and γ frequency for left and right SSC and the pain intensity as measured by VAS. *Vanneste S, De Ridder D. BurstDR spinal cord stimulation rebalances pain input and pain suppression in the brain in chronic neuropathic pain. Brain stimulation, 2023;16(4):1186–1195. https://doi.org/10.1016/j.brs.2023.07.058.*

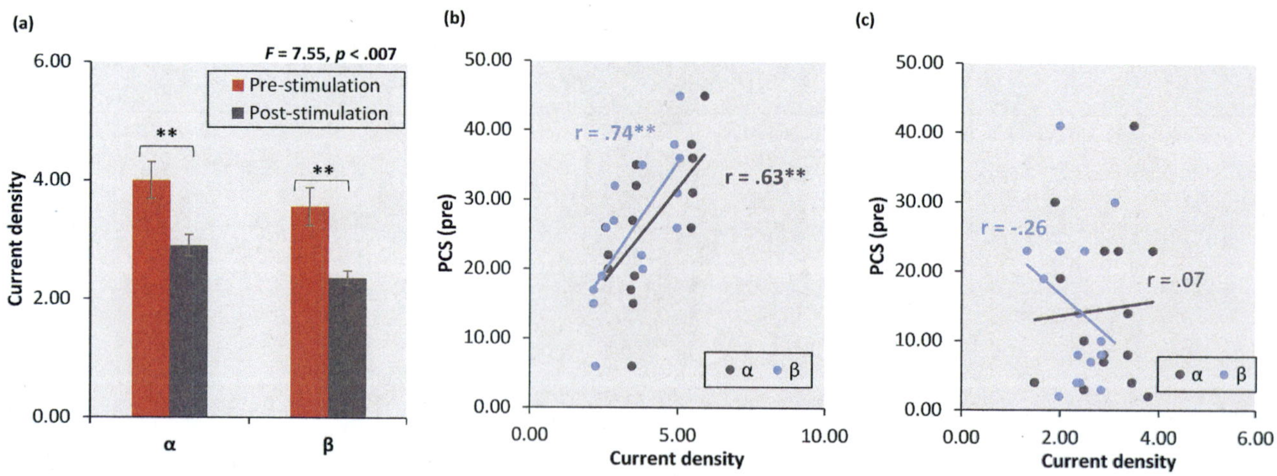

FIGURE 18.10 (a) A comparison between pre and postburstDR spinal cord stimulation identified a significant difference for both the α and β frequency band current density in the dACC after stimulation. (b–c) The current density for both the θ and α frequency bands for dACC correlates with the PCS prestimulation, but not after stimulation. *Vanneste S, De Ridder D. BurstDR spinal cord stimulation rebalances pain input and pain suppression in the brain in chronic neuropathic pain. Brain stimulation, 2023;16(4):1186–1195. https://doi.org/10.1016/j.brs.2023.07.058.*

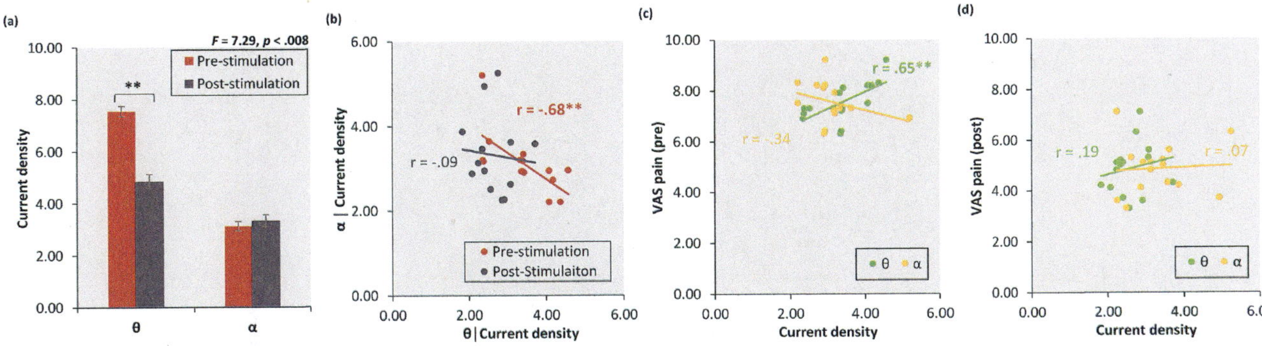

FIGURE 18.11 (a) A comparison between pre and postburstDR spinal cord stimulation identified a significant difference in current density for the θ frequency band in the pgACC after stimulation. No significant difference was found for the α-band. (b) A correlation was shown between the current density for the θ and α frequency band prestimulation, but not poststimulation. (c) An association was identified for the θ frequency band between the current density in pgACC and the pain intensity as measured by a VAS prestimulation. This association was not found for the α-band. (d) No association was shown for the θ and α frequency bands between the current density in pgACC and the pain intensity as measured by a VAS poststimulation. *Vanneste S. De Ridder D. BurstDR spinal cord stimulation rebalances pain input and pain suppression in the brain in chronic neuropathic pain. Brain stimulation, 2023;16(4):1186–1195. https://doi.org/10.1016/j.brs.2023.07.058.*

functionally connected by assessing how consistently their neural oscillations align over time, even if there is a slight delay between them. In pain, the communication (= functional connectivity) is decreased between the descending, lateral and medial pathways, resulting in a loss of balance between the three pain pathways. Burst SCS has been shown to increase connectivity between the pain pathways (pgACC and SSC, dACC and SSC, and pgACC and dACC), resulting in regained communication, permitting the normal balance to be restored. Effective connectivity, as measured by Granger Causality, indicates which brain region is driving the activity of another region rather than just correlating activity between them. Burst SCS has been shown to change information flow between the pgACC and the bilateral SSC, as well as the pgACC and the dACC and the bilateral SSC. In people without pain, the pain-inhibitory pgACC sends (inhibitory) information to the lateral and medial pathways, hypothetically resulting in their inhibition. In pain, however, the medial "salience" pathway sends (inhibitory) information to the pain-inhibiting pgACC, thereby suppressing its pain-inhibitory effect. BurstDR SCS reverts the effective connectivity to a normal directional signal transmission. Cross-frequency coupling (CFC) indicates the relationship between the frequency, amplitude, or phase of two different frequency bands in the brain. Burst frequency was shown to reduce θ-γ coupling in the SSC and α-β coupling in the dACC; in other words, it reduces the pathological thalamocortical dysrhythmia.

Overall, burst SCS has been shown to strengthen communication between pain processing pathways, with increased activity in the alpha frequency range, suggesting improved coordination of pain processing. It has also been shown to reduce the coupling of brain wave frequencies associated with pathological pain processing. Essentially, burst SCS does not merely block pain signals as occurs in tonic SCS; it actively reshapes brain network activity and connectivity to restore a more balanced and healthy state (Figs. 18.12–18.14).

Why not all burst stimulation designs are clinically the same

Beyond tonic and burst, other commercially available waveforms, such as high-frequency, high-dose, and clustered tonic, have emerged. When comparing waveforms, a clear distinction emerges between their mechanisms and the physiological responses they elicit. Traditional tonic stimulation delivers continuous, low-frequency pulses, relying on paresthesia induction for pain relief. This method generates predictable EMG responses, with stimulation artifact preceding muscle activation, and causes a reduction in SSEP signals [26].

In contrast, burst stimulation, particularly Abbott's BurstDR, introduces a pulsed approach with a quiescent phase, leading to unique neuromonitoring findings [27]. BurstDR stands out with its distal-to-proximal muscle recruitment, lower amplitude thresholds, and stimulation artifact following EMG responses. High-frequency stimulation, as exemplified by Nevro's HF10 and Medtronic's high-dose stimulation, diverges significantly by aiming for paresthesia-free pain relief [28]. HF10 elicits minimal neuromonitoring responses, while high-dose stimulation creates abdominal artifacts without lower extremity response, and neither reduces SSEP signals.

The critical difference between Abbott's BurstDR and Boston Scientific's clustered tonic (burst) stimulation lies in their pulse train dynamics and EMG response patterns. BurstDR utilizes a five-pulse train, in which the five monophasic

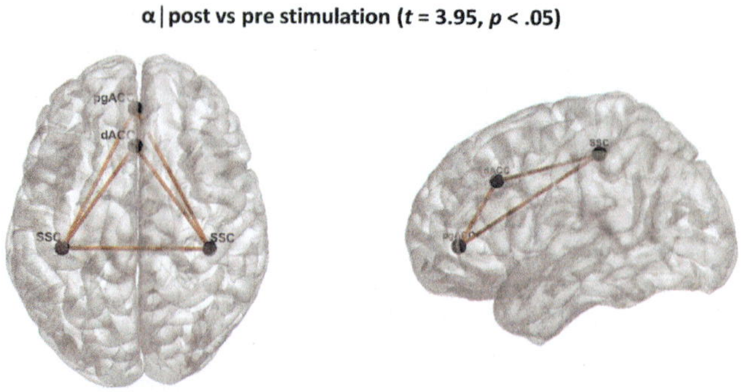

FIGURE 18.12 Functional connectivity posttreatment for α in comparison to pretreatment, revealing increased connectivity between the pgAAC and SSC, and the dACC and SSC, as well as pgACC and dACC. *Vanneste S, De Ridder D. BurstDR spinal cord stimulation rebalances pain input and pain suppression in the brain in chronic neuropathic pain. Brain stimulation, 2023;16(4):1186–1195. https://doi.org/10.1016/j.brs.2023.07.058.*

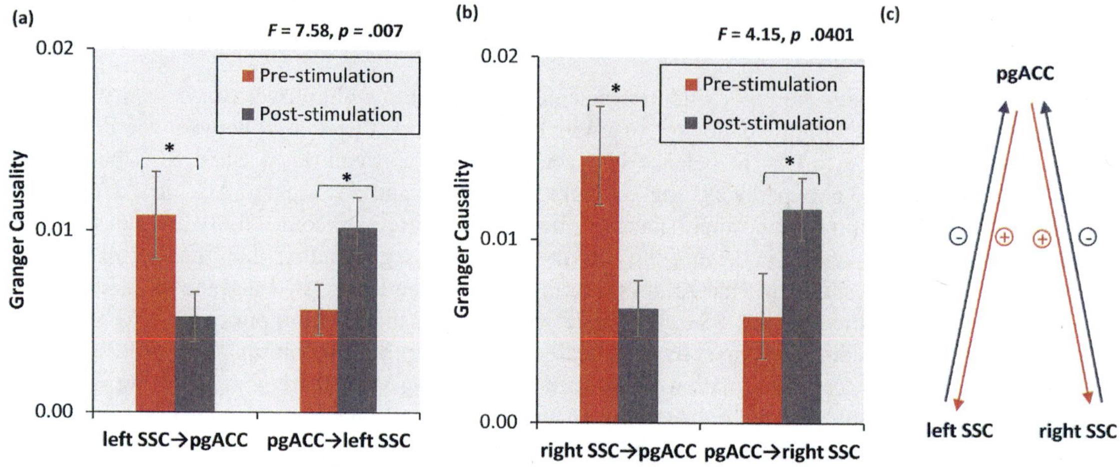

FIGURE 18.13 (a–b) A comparison between pre and post burstDR spinal cord stimulation for effective connectivity from left SSC → pgACC and pgACC → left SSC, as well as the right SSC → pgACC and pgACC → right SSC for the θ frequency band. This revealed for a significant reduction in effective connectivity for both the left SSC → pgACC and the right SSC → pgACC and increased effective connectivity for the pgACC → left SSC and right SSC → pgACC post-stimulation in comparison to pre-stimulation. (c) A summary figure of the results obtained for the θ frequency band [14].

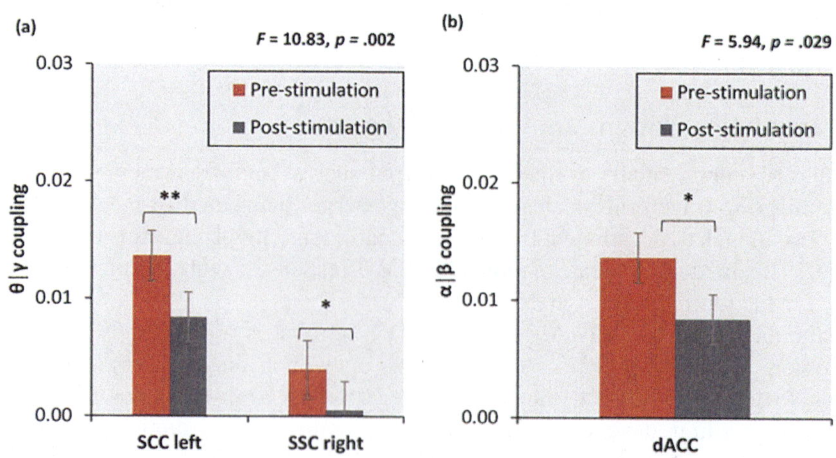

FIGURE 18.14 (a–b) A significant reduction for θ-γ coupling was identified for the left and right SSC and α-β coupling for dACC poststimulation in comparison to prestimulation. *Vanneste S, De Ridder D. BurstDR spinal cord stimulation rebalances pain input and pain suppression in the brain in chronic neuropathic pain. Brain stimulation, 2023;16(4):1186–1195. https://doi.org/10.1016/j.brs.2023.07.058.*

spikes are charge-balanced after the five pulses terminate, followed by a quiescent period, resulting in a single, large EMG spike and a hyperexcitable state for subsequent tonic stimulation, suggesting a deeper, more profound modulation of spinal pathways. Conversely, Boston Scientific's clustered tonic mimics traditional tonic stimulation by cycling four individually charge-balanced pulses with a rest phase, producing distinct EMG spikes that mirror each pulse. While both burst modalities reduce the amplitude required for EMG responses compared to standard tonic, they achieve this through different mechanisms. BurstDR's unique pattern appears to fundamentally alter neuronal excitability, while clustered tonic essentially delivers a more efficient version of tonic stimulation.

In essence, tonic stimulation provides a continuous paresthesia-based approach, while burst stimulation offers pulsed variations with distinct neuromodulatory effects. BurstDR's unique characteristics, such as reversed muscle recruitment and hyperexcitability, suggest a potentially more potent and efficient form of stimulation. In contrast, clustered tonic maintains the core principles of tonic stimulation but with enhanced energy efficiency. High-frequency and high-dose stimulation, by design, abandons paresthesia in favor of alternative pain relief mechanisms, resulting in vastly different neuromonitoring profiles. These waveform variations underscore the ongoing evolution of SCS technology, offering clinicians a range of options to tailor treatment to individual patient needs.

At the core of the complex interplay between stimulation parameters and the nervous system's response lies the thalamus, a key brain structure that acts as a relay station for sensory information. The thalamus operates in two primary firing modes: tonic and burst. Tonic firing provides a steady, detailed stream of information, while burst firing acts as a "wake-up call," enhancing the detection of subtle or sudden changes. The ability of the thalamus to switch between these firing modes based on input (cortical feedback and other inputs) underscores the dynamic nature of neural processing and the potential for SCS to modulate these processes differently [4]. Furthermore, research has shown that the dendrites of thalamic relay cells, independent of the cell bodies, also play an active role in signal amplification and integration, highlighting the intricate mechanisms through which neural signals are processed and transmitted [29].

Evidential controversies

BurstDR stimulation has been shown to be effective in multiple, multicenter randomized controlled trials, and its effects have been additionally confirmed through systematic review and pooled analysis of real-world evidence, as well as placebo-controlled trials and a meta-analysis [9,30,31].

The other form of burst stimulation, developed by Boston Scientific, has been tested in one placebo-controlled trial involving 50 participants. There was no benefit for the clustered tonic stimulation in comparison to the sham [21]. As the authors labeled the study a burst stimulation study, this results in a semantic confusion of what burst stimulation really is [32].

Clinical evidence

The adoption of burst waveforms in SCS has been underpinned by a growing body of clinical evidence demonstrating its efficacy, safety, and advantages over traditional tonic stimulation. This section reviews key studies and findings that have shaped the understanding and application of burst stimulation in clinical practice. The most widely researched and clinically utilized waveform is Abbott's BurstDR.

After decades of treating patients effectively with paresthesia-based SCS, in 2010, a landmark paper was published which heralded a paradigm shift in the world of neuromodulation. An experimental trial of 12 patients was conducted comparing tonic SCS to a novel "burst" waveform. Patients were operated under general anesthesia, based on anatomical lead placement. BurstDR stimulation demonstrated significantly greater efficacy in pain suppression compared to tonic stimulation, as measured by both the Visual Analog Scale (VAS) score and the McGill Short Form score. While paresthesia was reported in 92% of patients during tonic stimulation, it was present in only 17% of patients during burst stimulation [33].

In 2014, a prospective, randomized, double-blind, placebo-controlled study compared BurstDR with tonic SCS and placebo [31]. It involved 20 patients with persistent spinal pain syndrome type-2 (Failed Back Surgery Syndrome) who already had an SCS system implanted. Each participant received the three treatments in random order for 1 week: tonic stimulation, burst stimulation, and placebo stimulation. The primary outcome was pain intensity measured using a numerical rating scale (NRS). Results showed that burst stimulation produced the lowest mean NRS scores, indicating significantly better pain relief compared to both tonic stimulation and placebo. No significant differences in pain relief were observed between tonic stimulation and placebo. 80% of patients (16 out of 20) preferred burst stimulation over the other options.

A large randomized controlled trial was conducted in 2016. Named SUNBURST, this trial evaluated BurstDR SCS against traditional tonic SCS using a crossover design [22]. After a successful tonic SCS trial, 100 participants were randomized to receive one stimulation mode (either burst or tonic) for an initial 12 weeks, followed by the alternative mode for the subsequent 12 weeks. The primary endpoint evaluated the noninferiority of the within-subject difference in mean daily overall Visual Analog Scale (VAS) scores between tonic and burst stimulation. Following the crossover period, participants were allowed to choose their preferred stimulation mode and were monitored for a year to assess long-term outcomes. BurstDR stimulation was found to be noninferior to tonic stimulation ($P < .001$) and also demonstrated superiority ($P < .017$). A significant majority of participants (70.8%) preferred burst stimulation over tonic stimulation ($P < .001$). This preference remained consistent over the 1-year follow-up period, with 68.2% of participants favoring burst stimulation, 23.9% preferring tonic stimulation, and 8.0% expressing no preference. This pivotal study played a critical role in securing FDA approval for burst SCS therapy in October 2016.

A prospective, postmarket, single-arm study enrolled 269 participants across 22 sites in the United States, Canada, and Europe between 2016 and 2018. Its aim was to assess the long-term safety and effectiveness of SCS for chronic pain in the trunk and/or limbs using a burst SCS by following patients for 2 years [34]. The study had broad, real-world inclusion criteria. They included adults with chronic pain of the trunk and/or lower limbs of ≥6/10 on a numerical rating scale, who had been recommended for SCS by their physician. After a successful trial, subjects were implanted with an SCS system and were instructed to use whichever stimulation program they preferred: either tonic, burst, or a combination of waveforms. The group was followed up for 2 years, and at each study visit, ≥86% of participants reported using burst stimulation. Of these, ≥70% used it intermittently with a duty cycle of 30 s on and 90 s off. The majority of subjects preferred burst stimulation at all follow-up timepoints, ranging from 90.2% of subjects at 6 months to 85.0% at 24 months. Patient-reported pain relief was 60.3% (±27.6) at 6 months, 63.1% (±25.1) at 12 months, 61.7% (±26.2) at 18 months, and 60% (±24.1) at 24 months.

In 2019, a systematic review and pooled analysis of real-world evidence was published [9]. This review encompassed 15 studies, totaling 427 participants. The included studies utilized diverse prospective designs, such as crossover trials, single-arm cohorts, and a single randomized controlled trial, alongside retrospective case reports. At baseline, the weighted pooled mean pain rating was 76.7 (±27.4). Tonic SCS reduced this to 49.2 (±12.9), and burst SCS further decreased it to 36.7 (±11.6), representing a 12.5-point difference between the two SCS methods. Psychometric analyses of patient-reported outcomes indicated a preference for burst SCS, which was also reflected in 65% of subjects stating a preference for this modality.

In 2020, the first meta-analysis was performed, quantifying the difference between burstDR and tonic stimulation and demonstrating that burstDR was superior to tonic stimulation. It involved five studies, which is considered the minimum for a meta-analysis, but still showed superiority on painfulness, with a 1.64 VAS score difference [30].

Optimizing the dose—Less is more

Beyond the treatment's overall effectiveness, an interesting observation was made regarding the stimulation parameters used by patients receiving burst therapy. When using burst stimulation, participants preferred lower to higher amplitudes. This led to the hypothesis that lower burst amplitudes will correlate with lower pain scores, while higher amplitudes will be associated with higher pain scores. A secondary analysis of trial data revealed that, in contrast to tonic stimulation, when using burst stimulation, lower amplitudes are more effective in suppressing pain than high amplitudes [35].

A second way of reducing the amount of current that reaches the spinal cord is by intermittent stimulation, aka cycle mode stimulation. The practice of using intermittent periods of stimulation had been done with conventional SCS for years, alternating between periods of stimulation and nonstimulation. It was postulated that alternating between on and off periods of stimulation could provide sustained therapeutic effects while reducing the overall amount of current delivered to the spinal cord and decreasing the energy requirements of the device. After an initial small trial using 5 s on 10 s off that showed equally good outcome results as continuous stimulation, but a patient preference for intermittent stimulation, a second prospective, multicentre, feasibility trial was devised to evaluate the clinical efficacy of using a variety of "off" times [36]. 50 patients completed an SCS trial using intermittent dosing stimulation settings of 30 s on and 90 s off, with 38 (76%) receiving ≥50% pain relief. The 38 (76%) who had >50% pain relief received permanent implantation and underwent titration of their settings. They all began on a low dose (30 s on, 360 s off) for two to 3 days. If pain control matched or exceeded that achieved during the trial period, this setting was maintained. If not, the dose was incrementally increased by shortening the off time. Subjects progressed stepwise, decreasing the off time until they were satisfied or they had returned to the original settings during the trial period (30 s on and 90 s off). Ultimately, the patients' self-selected the lowest effective dose that replicated their trial-period pain relief [36]. 45.8% of the subjects that completed the 6-month follow-up visit used an off period of 360 s. These findings pointed toward the possibility of optimizing the dose of stimulation to achieve adequate pain relief, whilst also reducing the power consumption of these battery-driven devices. A low dose would mean low recharge burden, extended battery life and potentially reduced habituation and tolerance to stimulation.

The idea of using ultralow energy, intermittently cycled burst stimulation was validated by the analysis of large real-world data sets [37]. A retrospective data analysis compared programming and outcome data from two large burst SCS cohort studies. In one study, 100 patients had used burst in a 1:3 ratio (30 s on, 90 s off) for 6 months. In another study, 95 patients used burst in a 1:12 ratio (30-sec on, 360-sec off) for 6 months. Both groups demonstrated significant clinical improvements, with mean pain intensity decreasing by nearly 50% compared to baseline. Pain Catastrophizing Scale (PCS) scores also showed a significant reduction, and physical function improved notably. Importantly, no statistically significant differences were observed between the 1:3 and 1:12 groups.

Burst as a "rescue" waveform

Loss of efficacy (LOE) is a well-documented phenomenon with SCS therapy and remains the primary reason for device explantation. While recent advancements in neuromodulation have reduced the incidence of LOE, it continues to pose a significant clinical challenge. A retrospective study explored the idea that exchanging a previously used SCS waveform with a burst could reverse LOE [38]. The records of 307 patients who were receiving SCS therapy and transitioned from another waveform to burst therapy were reviewed. They made this transition to burst either through surgical replacement of an IPG or a software upgrade. Patients were further divided into two subgroups: those experiencing SCS failure (salvage group) and those satisfied with their current therapy but seeking greater pain relief (upgrade group). Both surgical revision and software upgrade resulted in statistically significant reductions in Numeric Rating Scale scores and improved percentage of pain relief. Subgroup analysis revealed that both the salvage and upgrade groups experienced a return of treatment effectiveness, regardless of the duration of prior therapy or the previous stimulation waveform.

Multisite burst stimulation

Many patients experience pain in two or more noncontiguous areas, complicating the programming of stimulation and limiting long-term efficacy. To address this, multiarea burst programming was developed, allowing stimulation to be delivered to multiple spinal cord areas simultaneously. A study investigated the location of burst stimulation on evoked electromyography (EMG) responses, aiming to optimize therapy for multisite pain [39].

Nine patients with chronic intractable back and/or leg pain who underwent permanent implantation of SCS leads. A Penta Paddle electrode was surgically placed via a laminectomy at the T8-T10 spinal levels. EMG recordings were obtained using subdermal electrodes in lower extremity muscle groups and the rectus abdominis muscles. The researchers compared evoked EMG responses across multiple trials of burst stimulation, varying the number of independent burst areas and stimulation parameters. When multisite burst stimulation was applied across up to four stimulation programs, the threshold for evoking a bilateral EMG response decreased, representing a 23% reduction in energy requirements compared to single-site stimulation. Stimulation across four electrode pairs resulted in more proximal muscle recruitment and more focal coverage of multiple pain areas compared to stimulation across two electrode pairs.

The study demonstrated that multisite burst stimulation offers several advantages over traditional single-site stimulation.

- Broader myotomal coverage: Multisite stimulation provided more extensive coverage of pain areas, addressing the challenge of noncontiguous pain distributions.
- Focal recruitment and differential control: It enabled precise recruitment of distal myotomes and differential control of noncontiguous pain areas.
- Reduced energy requirements: Multisite stimulation required lower energy thresholds, potentially improving the longevity of the device and patient comfort.

Expanding indication for burst

It was established early on through clinical studies that burst was often superior to tonic SCS for the traditional indications for which SCS has been historically used, such as persistent spinal pain syndrome type 2 (PSPS Type 2) or painful diabetic neuropathy (CRPS) [40]. Considering that burstDR mimics burst firing, which is a universal firing pattern found all over the nervous system, it was suggested that more indications and more targets could be studied by clinical trials.

Low back pain: The DISTINCT study enrolled 270 adults with chronic axial low back pain, who had not had prior lumbar spine surgery and whose condition was not surgically treatable [41]. Participants were required to have had a spinal MRI and/or CT scan within 12 months of screening to confirm the absence of surgically correctable pathology. Lumbar spondylosis accounted for 52.1% of diagnosis, 33.2% diagnosed with degenerative disc disease, and 38% with lumbar radiculopathy. Patients were randomized to either SCS with burst or conventional medical management (CMM), which included injections, radiofrequency denervation, physical therapy and medications. Patients had the option to crossover at 6 months. The primary outcome was the proportion of patients in each group who experienced ≥50% reduction in pain on NRS at 6 months. The SCS group had a significantly higher responder rate of 85.3% (87/102) compared to 6.2% (5/81) in the Conventional Medical Management (CMM) group. Of those in the SCS group who responded to treatment, 49% (43/87) achieved a substantial pain reduction of 80% or more.

Thoracic SCS for abdominal pain

Beyond back and leg pain, Burst has been explored for managing abdominal pain. Richter et al. (2020) and Segura et al. (2019) investigated the use of thoracic SCS with burst for chronic abdominal pain [42,43]. These studies suggest that burst delivered to this region may modulate visceral pain pathways, offering a potential treatment option for patients with chronic abdominal pain syndromes refractory to conventional therapies.

ONS stimulation for PSPS type 2

A patient with PSPS Type 2, following three lumbar discectomies, was successfully controlling her pain using transcutaneous electrical nerve stimulation (TENS) at the C2 level. However, the patient developed an allergic reaction to the skin-applied TENS electrodes, prompting a discussion of a new treatment strategy. A subcutaneous C2 electrode was subsequently inserted under local anesthesia and attached to an external pulse generator. With tonic stimulation, pain was reduced in her legs but not in the back, whereas with BurstDR stimulation, both legs and back improved dramatically. With placebo-stimulation, no improvement was seen [44].

C2 stimulation for movement disorders

The cervical spinal cord, particularly at the C2 level, has become a target of interest for neuromodulation in movement disorders due to its role in motor control, cognition, and autonomic function. Several studies have explored the efficacy of burst stimulation at C2 for various aspects of Parkinsons Disease and other movement disorders. One such study explored the effectiveness of two types of high cervical SCS in managing pain and Parkinson's disease (PD) [45]. Comparing tonic and burst stimulation modes. Tonic stimulation was applied to six PD patients with low back pain and failed back surgery syndrome, while burst was used in 12 PD patients primarily to address motor deficits. The stimulation was delivered via percutaneous quadripolar or octapolar electrodes. Clinical outcomes were measured using the Unified Parkinson's Disease Rating Scale (UPDRS), the Hoehn and Yahr (H&Y) scale, and a visual analog scale for pain. Results showed that burst was more effective and consistent than tonic in reducing pain. Burst also improved UPDRS score and H&Y scores, with motor benefits appearing quickly after stimulation onset. The study concluded that burst is more effective than tonic in alleviating pain and addressing specific motor and nonmotor deficits in PD patients for at least 1 year.

Conclusion

Burst stimulation represents a significant advancement in neuromodulation technology, offering a physiologically nuanced and clinically superior alternative to traditional tonic stimulation. By mimicking the natural burst firing patterns of the central and peripheral nervous systems, burst stimulation aligns more closely with the body's inherent neural processes, making it a universal and effective approach for pain management. This innovative waveform not only addresses the sensory-discriminative aspects of pain but also uniquely modulates the medial and lateral pain pathways, as well as the descending inhibitory pathways, providing a more comprehensive therapeutic effect. This dual modulation of both the intensity of pain and its emotional burden significantly improves painfulness, suffering, and overall quality of life for patients.

The clinical advantages of burst stimulation are well-supported by robust evidence, including level-1 randomized trials, placebo-controlled trials and meta-analyses. These studies consistently demonstrate that burst stimulation offers superior pain relief compared to tonic stimulation, particularly for patients who have experienced suboptimal results with traditional SCS. Furthermore, burst stimulation is associated with a lower propensity for tolerance development, ensuring sustained therapeutic benefits over time. Its ability to deliver effective pain relief with lower amplitudes and intermittent dosing not only enhances patient comfort but also improves device longevity and energy efficiency, reducing the need for frequent recharging and extending battery life.

Burst stimulation's unique mechanism of action, which involves rebalancing brain activity and connectivity, sets it apart from other SCS modalities. By normalizing pathological brain activity and strengthening communication among pain-processing pathways, burst stimulation actively reshapes neural networks to restore a healthier state. This approach goes beyond merely blocking pain signals, offering a more holistic and durable solution for chronic pain management.

The growing body of clinical evidence underscores the versatility and efficacy of burst stimulation across a wide range of conditions, from persistent spinal pain syndrome and painful diabetic neuropathy to chronic low back pain and abdominal pain. Its success in these diverse applications highlights its potential to expand the indications for SCS, providing hope for patients who have previously found little relief from conventional therapies.

In summary, burst stimulation represents a paradigm shift in neuromodulation, offering a more effective, efficient, and patient-friendly approach to chronic pain management. Its ability to address both the physical and emotional dimensions of pain, combined with its strong clinical validation, makes it a promising option for patients and clinicians alike. As the field of neuromodulation continues to evolve, burst stimulation represents a transformative innovation, paving the way for improved outcomes and enhanced quality of life for individuals suffering from chronic pain.

References

[1] Taylor RS, Desai MJ, Rigoard P, Taylor RJ. Predictors of pain relief following spinal cord stimulation in chronic back and leg pain and failed back surgery syndrome: a systematic review and meta-regression analysis. Pain Pract 2014;14(6):489–505. https://doi.org/10.1111/papr.12095.

[2] Heijmans L, Joosten EA. Mechanisms and mode of action of spinal cord stimulation in chronic neuropathic pain. PGM (Postgrad Med) 2020;132 (Suppl. 3):17–21. https://doi.org/10.1080/00325481.2020.1769393.

[3] Lisman JE. Bursts as a unit of neural information: making unreliable synapses reliable. Trends Neurosci 1997;20(1):38–43. https://doi.org/10.1016/S0166-2236(96)10070-9.

[4] Sherman SM. A wake-up call from the thalamus. Nat Neurosci 2001;4(4):344–6. https://doi.org/10.1038/85973.

[5] Cain SM, Snutch TP. T-type calcium channels in burst-firing, network synchrony, and epilepsy. Biochim Biophys Acta 2013;1828(7):1572–8. https://doi.org/10.1016/j.bbamem.2012.07.028.

[6] Izhikevich EM. Neural excitability, spiking and bursting. Int J Bifurcat Chaos 2000;10(6):1171–266. https://doi.org/10.1142/s0218127400000840.

[7] Joosten EA, Franken G. Spinal cord stimulation in chronic neuropathic pain: mechanisms of action, new locations, new paradigms. Pain 2020;161 (Suppl. 1):S104–13. https://doi.org/10.1097/j.pain.0000000000001854.

[8] Crosby ND, Weisshaar CL, Smith JR, Zeeman ME, Goodman-Keiser MD, Winkelstein BA. Burst and tonic spinal cord stimulation differentially activate GABAergic mechanisms to attenuate pain in a rat model of cervical radiculopathy. TBME 2015;62(6):1604–13. https://doi.org/10.1109/TBME.2015.2399374.

[9] Chakravarthy K, Malayil R, Kirketeig T, Deer T. Burst spinal cord stimulation: a systematic review and pooled analysis of real-world evidence and outcomes data. Pain Med 2019;20(Suppl. ment_1):S47–57. https://www.ncbi.nlm.nih.gov/pubmed/31152177.

[10] Bushnell MC, Ceko M, Low LA. Cognitive and emotional control of pain and its disruption in chronic pain. Nat Rev Neurosci 2013;14(7):502–11. https://doi.org/10.1038/nrn3516.

[11] Price DD. Psychological and neural mechanisms of the affective dimension of pain. Science 2000;288(5472):1769–72. https://doi.org/10.1126/science.288.5472.1769.

[12] Kong J, Loggia ML, Zyloney C, Tu P, LaViolette P, Gollub RL. Exploring the brain in pain: activations, deactivations and their relation. Pain 2010;148(2):257–67. https://doi.org/10.1016/j.pain.2009.11.008.

[13] Craig AD. How do you feel? interoception: the sense of the physiological condition of the body. Nat Rev Neurosci 2002;3(8):655–66. https://doi.org/10.1038/nrn894.

[14] Vanneste S, De Ridder D. BurstDR spinal cord stimulation rebalances pain input and pain suppression in the brain in chronic neuropathic pain. Brain Stimul 2023;16(4):1186–95. https://doi.org/10.1016/j.brs.2023.07.058.

[15] De Ridder D, Vanneste S, Smith M, Adhia D. Pain and the triple network model. Front Neurol 2022;13:757241. https://doi.org/10.3389/fneur.2022.757241.

[16] De Ridder D, Vanneste S. Burst and tonic spinal cord stimulation: different and common brain mechanisms. Neuromodulation 2016;19(1):47–59. https://doi.org/10.1111/ner.12368.

[17] Stančák A, Kozák J, Vrba I, et al. Functional magnetic resonance imaging of cerebral activation during spinal cord stimulation in failed back surgery syndrome patients. Eur J Pain 2008;12(2):137–48. https://doi.org/10.1016/j.ejpain.2007.03.003.

[18] Craig AD. Distribution of trigeminothalamic and spinothalamic lamina I terminations in the macaque monkey. J Comp Neurol 2004;477 (2):119–48. https://doi.org/10.1002/cne.20240.

[19] Van Havenbergh T, Vancamp T, Van Looy P, Vanneste S, De Ridder D. Spinal cord stimulation for the treatment of chronic back pain patients: 500-hz vs. 1000-hz burst stimulation. Neuromodulation 2015;18(1):9–12. https://doi.org/10.1111/ner.12252.

[20] De Ridder D, Plazier M, Kamerling N, Menovsky T, Vanneste S. Burst spinal cord stimulation for limb and back pain. World Neurosurg 2013;80 (5):642–9. https://doi.org/10.1016/j.wneu.2013.01.040.

[21] Hara S, Andresen H, Solheim O, et al. Effect of spinal cord burst stimulation vs placebo stimulation on disability in patients with chronic radicular pain after lumbar spine surgery: a randomized clinical trial. JAMA, J Am Med Assoc 2022;328(15):1506–14. https://doi.org/10.1001/jama.2022.18231.

[22] Deer T, Slavin KV, Amirdelfan K, et al. Success using neuromodulation with BURST (SUNBURST) study: results from a prospective, randomized controlled trial using a novel burst waveform. Neuromodulation 2018;21(1):56–66.

[23] Vanneste S, Alsalman O, De Ridder D. Top-down and bottom-up regulated auditory phantom perception. J Neurosci 2019;39(2):364–78. https://doi.org/10.1523/JNEUROSCI.0966-18.2018.

[24] Brandman T, Malach R, Simony E. The surprising role of the default mode network in naturalistic perception. Commun Biol 2021;4(1). https://doi.org/10.1038/s42003-020-01602-z. 79–79.

[25] Gawali BW, Abhang PA, Mehrotra SC. Technological basics of EEG recording and operation of apparatus. In: Introduction to EEG- and speech-based emotion recognition. United States: Elsevier Science & Technology; 2016. http://ebookcentral.proquest.com/lib/SITE_ID/reader.action?docID=4458824&ppg=30.

[26] Falowski SM. An observational case series of spinal cord stimulation waveforms visualized on intraoperative neuromonitoring. Neuromodulation 2019;22(2):219–28. https://doi.org/10.1111/ner.12781.

[27] Kirketeig T, Schultheis C, Zuidema X, Hunter CW, Deer T. Burst spinal cord stimulation: a clinical review. Pain Med 2019;20(Suppl. ment_1): S31–40. https://doi.org/10.1093/pm/pnz003.

[28] Russo M, Van Buyten J. 10-kHz High-Frequency SCS therapy: a clinical summary. Pain Med 2015;16(5):934–42. https://doi.org/10.1111/pme.12617.

[29] Crandall SR, Govindaiah G, Cox CL. Low-threshold Ca2+ current amplifies distal dendritic signaling in thalamic reticular neurons. J Neurosci 2010;30(46):15419–29. https://doi.org/10.1523/JNEUROSCI.3636-10.2010.

[30] Karri J, Orhurhu V, Wahezi S, Tang T, Deer T, Abd-Elsayed A. Comparison of spinal cord stimulation waveforms for treating chronic low back pain: systematic review and meta-analysis. Pain Physician 2020;23(5):451–60. https://doi.org/10.36076/ppj.2020/23/451.

[31] Schu S, Slotty PJ, Bara G, von Knop M, Edgar D, Vesper J. A prospective, randomised, double-blind, placebo-controlled study to examine the effectiveness of burst spinal cord stimulation patterns for the treatment of failed back surgery syndrome. Neuromodulation 2014;17(5):443–50. https://doi.org/10.1111/ner.12197.

[32] De Ridder D, Vancamp T, Falowski SM, Vanneste S. All bursts are equal, but some are more equal (to burst firing): burstDR stimulation versus boston burst stimulation. Expet Rev Med Dev 2020;17(4):289–95. https://doi.org/10.1080/17434440.2020.1736560.

[33] De Ridder D, Vanneste S, Plazier M, van der Loo E, Menovsky T. Burst spinal cord stimulation: toward paresthesia-free pain suppression. Neurosurgery 2010;66(5):986–90.

[34] Deer TR, Falowski SM, Moore GA, et al. Passive recharge burst spinal cord stimulation provides sustainable improvements in pain and psychosocial function: 2-year results from the TRIUMPH study. Spine 2022;47(7):548–56. https://doi.org/10.1097/BRS.0000000000004283.

[35] Leong SL, De Ridder D, Deer T, Vanneste S. Potential therapeutic effect of low amplitude burst spinal cord stimulation on pain. Neuromodulation 2021;24(3):574–80. https://doi.org/10.1111/ner.13090.

[36] Deer TR, Patterson DG, Baksh J, et al. Novel intermittent dosing burst paradigm in spinal cord stimulation. Neuromodulation 2021;24(3):566–73. https://doi.org/10.1111/ner.13143.

[37] Deer T, Wilson D, Schultz D, et al. Ultra-low energy cycled burst spinal cord stimulation yields robust outcomes in pain, function, and affective domains: a subanalysis from two prospective, multicenter, international clinical trials. Neuromodulation 2022;25(1):137–44. https://doi.org/10.1111/ner.13507.

[38] Hunter CW, Carlson J, Yang A, et al. BURST(able): a retrospective, multicenter study examining the impact of spinal cord stimulation with burst on pain and opioid consumption in the setting of salvage treatment and "upgrade". Pain Physician 2020;23(6):E643–58. https://doi.org/10.36076/ppj.2020.23.E643. https://www.ncbi.nlm.nih.gov/pubmed/33185383.

[39] Falowski SM, Benison AM, Nanivadekar AC. Regional coverage differences with single- and multi-area burst spinal cord stimulation for treatment of chronic pain. Neuromodulation 2023;26(7):1471–7. https://doi.org/10.1016/j.neurom.2023.01.015.

[40] de Vos CC, Bom MJ, Vanneste S, Lenders MWPM, de Ridder D. Burst spinal cord stimulation evaluated in patients with failed back surgery syndrome and painful diabetic neuropathy. Neuromodulation 2014;17(2):152–9. https://doi.org/10.1111/ner.12116.

[41] Yue JJ, Gilligan CJ, Falowski S, et al. Surgical treatment of refractory low back pain using implanted BurstDR spinal cord stimulation (SCS) in a cohort of patients without options for corrective surgery: findings and results from the DISTINCT study, a prospective randomized multi-center controlled trial. Spine J 2022;22(9):S120–1. https://doi.org/10.1016/j.spinee.2022.06.246.

[42] The efficacy of BurstDR spinal cord stimulation for chronic abdominal pain: a clinical series. . .

[43] Salvage therapy with burst spinal cord stimulation for chronic pancreatitis: a case report. . .

[44] De Ridder D, Plazier M, Menovsky T, Kamerling N, Vanneste S. C2 subcutaneous stimulation for failed back surgery syndrome: a case report. Neuromodulation 2013;16(6):610–3. https://doi.org/10.1111/j.1525-1403.2012.00518.x.

[45] Mazzone P, Viselli F, Ferraina S, et al. High cervical spinal cord stimulation: a one year follow-up study on motor and non-motor functions in Parkinson's disease. Brain Sci 2019;9(4):78. https://doi.org/10.3390/brainsci9040078.

Chapter 19

High-frequency stimulation

Leonardo Kapural
Carolinas Pain Institute and Best Opinion Doctorcom, Winston-Salem, NC, United States

Introduction

Over the past 40 years, spinal cord stimulation (SCS) has evolved from an experimental therapy into an evidence-based intervention for many refractory pain syndromes, including failed back surgery syndrome (FBSS), refractory, nonsurgical back pain, complex regional pain syndrome (CRPS), and painful diabetic peripheral neuropathy (DPN) [1–3]. On the horizon there are numerous new indications for SCS such as chronic abdominal pain, pelvic pain, movement disorders such as Parkinson's, and spinal cord injury [4–7].

Traditional low-frequency SCS relies on dorsal column stimulation producing paresthesias overlapping the area of chronic pain. Although effective for many patients, its therapeutic benefit is often limited to less than 40% of patients achieving more than 50% pain relief [1,2,8–12]. To address these shortcomings, several new waveforms and technological refinements have emerged, such as high-frequency 10 kHz therapy [7,12–15]. 10 kHz SCS delivers paresthesia-free stimulation that preferentially modulates dorsal horn wide-dynamic-range neurons, thereby eliminating the need for intraoperative paresthesia mapping [7,12].

a. Scope of Procedure

A large scale, randomized and prospective multicenter trial demonstrated that 10 kHz provided superior analgesia for both back and leg pain as compared with the control arm of conventional SCS in subjects with or without previous spine surgery [7]. In this study the authors note that standard 10 kHz lead placement was used, without trial-and-error paresthesia mapping:

For 10 kHz SCS therapy, the distal tip of one lead was placed at T8, whereas a second lead tip was placed atT9, both near anatomical midline. Lead position for 10 kHz therapy was based on extensive empirical observation that most patients respond to stimulation application near T9/T10, while allowing for patient variation by covering T8 toT11. Such standardized leads placement provided consistent clinical outcomes and long -term improvement in pain and functional capacity [7,12–15].

Petersen et al. in another large, multicenter RCT of 10 kHz SCS demonstrated profound pain relief, neurological improvement and improved health-related quality of life outcome measures sustained over 24 months in patients with painful diabetic peripheral neuropathy (PDN). Standard lead placement as described above of two 8-contact leads positioned midline in posterior epidural space between top of T9 and T11 vertebral bodies. The percentage of responders (greater than 50% pain relief of lower extremity PDN) in the permanent implant population was 90.1% at 24 months and 66% had improvement in neurological deficits (Figs. 19.1 and 19.2).

A third large RCT compared 10 kHz SCS with ongoing medical management in the treatment of chronic axial low back pain in the nonsurgical refractory back pain population (as determined by spinal surgical evaluation) demonstrated that 10 kHz SCS provides long-term improvement in pain disability, quality of life, and reduction in opioid use [16,17].

b. Brief Procedure Innovation

10 kHz SCS therapy involves percutaneous lead placement in the epidural space, very similar to traditional SCS. However, a combination of standardized anatomical midline lead placement and novel waveform with specific stimulation parameters results in paresthesia-free pain relief with 10 kHz SCS. In an initial multicenter, randomized controlled trial (SENZA-RCT) for approval by United States Food and Drug Administration (FDA), 10 kHz SCS provided superior, long-lasting back and leg pain relief, when compared with traditional, low-frequency SCS without the need for pain-

A Modern Atlas for Implantable Devices of the Spine, Brain, and Nerve. https://doi.org/10.1016/B978-0-443-36528-7.00060-1

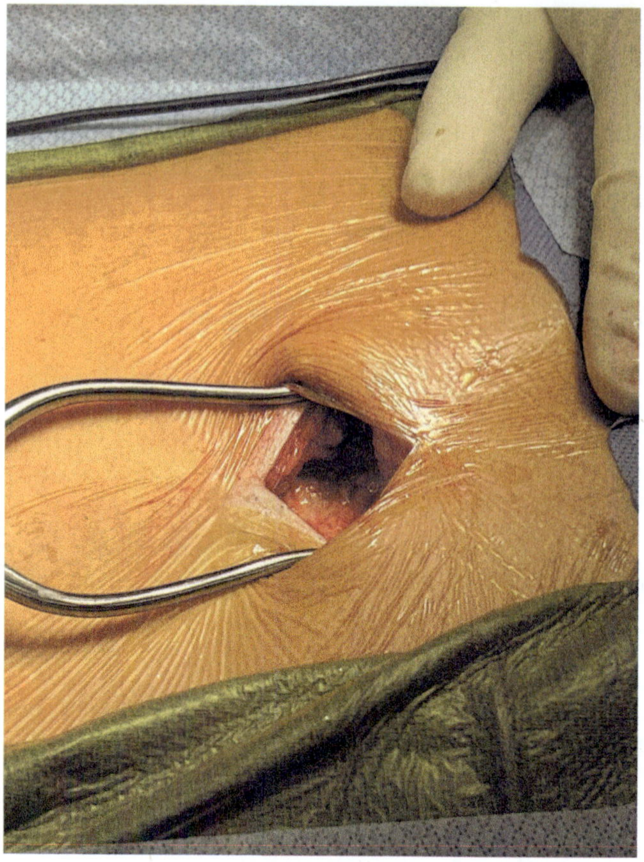

FIGURE 19.1 An initial vertical incision with clear view of interspinous fascia/ligament and extended same side pocket for the placement of anchors and leads (safety loop; see text above).

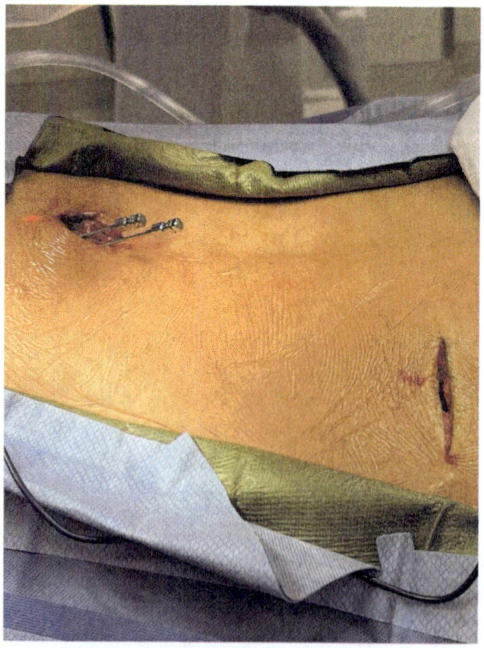

FIGURE 19.2 Same side placement of the two Tuohy epidural needles and already formed pocket for the SCS generator placement. Planning of the pocket location should take place in preoperative area (see text above).

paresthesia perception overlap. or postural changes related uncomfortable stimulation [7,12–17]. Therefore, trial and or lead placement is seamless and not complicated with unnecessary intraoperative programming of device. Additionally, difficulty of obtaining and maintaining paresthesia coverage of the low back, a well-known difficulty of conventional SCS, is obviated. 10 kHz SCS is not just paresthesia-based SCS with amplitude decreased to generally subthreshold as is seen with many low frequency paresthesia free SCS approaches. In fact, 10 kHz is completely paresthesia independent and does not activate the dorsal columns or produce evoked compound action potentials (ECAPs) at 10 kHz SCS therapeutic levels [18].

c. Brief Most Relevant Advancements

10 kHz SCS has expanded the therapeutic reach of SCS. Randomized prospective study evaluating patients with predominant axial low back pain demonstrated that 10 kHz SCS provides superior pain relief when compared with conventional medical management at 24 months [16,17]. In patients with diabetic peripheral neuropathy (DPN) 10 kHz SCS resulted in up to date the best improvements in pain and functional capacity [15] It has been suggested that 10 kHz SCS could provide long term improvements in pain disability, quality of life, and reduction in opioid use [12–17]. These findings emphasize the adaptability of 10 kHz, high-frequency stimulation (Figs. 19.3 and 19.4).

Key points

- **Paresthesia independent high-frequency spinal cord stimulation.**
- **Simple standardized anatomical lead placement without need for paresthesia mapping.**
- **Effective for axial and peripheral chronic pain.**
- **Algorithmic programming with extensive programming and outcomes data collection allows for AI guided programming.**
- **Multiple long term level 1 clinical trials.**
- **Device can also provide low frequency waveforms 2–1200 Hz.**

Relevant anatomy

a. Summary of Relevant Anatomy

The size of the spinal canal and spinal cord, the position of the cord within the canal, and the amount of cerebro-spinal fluid (CSF) vary at each vertebral level of the spine. When electrical current epidurally applied, travels through low

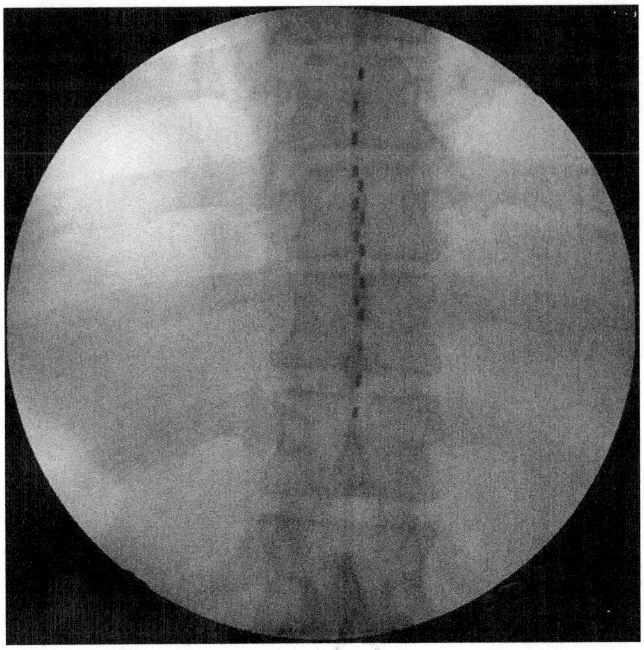

FIGURE 19.3 Anterior-posterior fluoroscopic view of most frequent final location of two Octrode leads when 10 kHz SCS is used. Midline location, leads staggered extending contacts from the top of T8 to the top of T11 vertebral bodies.

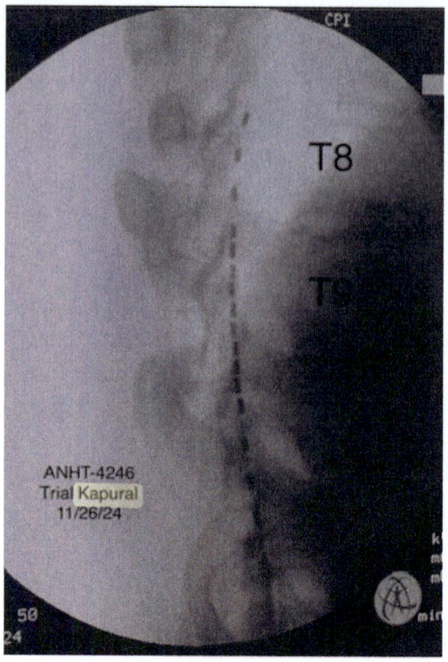

FIGURE 19.4 Obligatory lateral view after the placement of both leads to verify posterior epidural location.

and high impedance tissues. Thickness of CSF layer is frequently least at C6 disc level and largest at T6 [19]. Such anatomic variability can significantly change electrical current delivery to the targeted tissues. In addition, change in the patient's posture alters the amplitude of stimulation [20]. Cervical lead placement (Fig. 19.5) is frequently achieved by an entry to the posterior epidural space in the upper thoracic area and an effective stimulation of the upper extremities is provided through higher cervical stimulation. Frequent position of epidural leads is at the top of C2 and C3, respectively. An effective stimulation for visceral pain and thoracic neuropathic pain such as in postherpetic neuralgia (PHN) can be achieved by placing the leads tip to the mid-to-high thoracic region at T4 and T5, respectively,

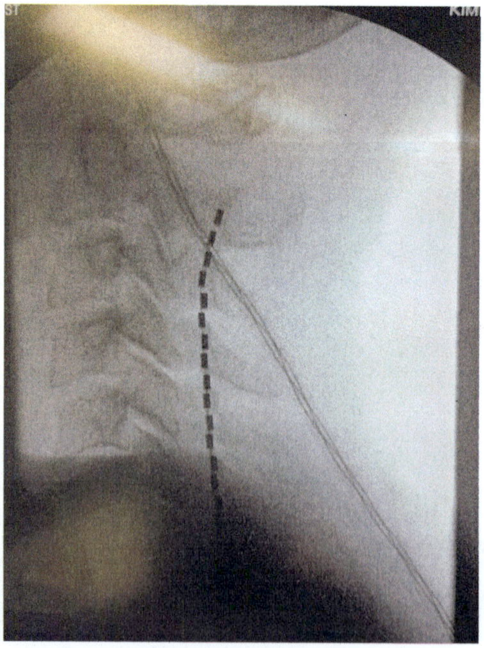

FIGURE 19.5 Most common placement of the cervical leads for 10 kHz SCS. Notice that the leads are staggered and placed on the top of C2 and C3 vertebral body. Posterior epidural placement of both leads is confirmed.

while pain in the lower extremities is commonly addressed by leads contacts positioned over T8 to T11. It is important to carefully asses fluoroscopic and anatomic spinal midline and to position leads accordingly [19].

Procedure

a. Indications
  a. On label:
    Painful diabetic neuropathy [15].
    Chronic pain of the trunk and limbs including FBSS [7,12].
    Refractory, nonsurgical back pain [16,17].
    Complex regional pain syndrome (CRPS) [21].
  b. Off label
  c. Chemotherapy-induced peripheral neuropathy [15,18].
    Chronic abdominal pain [4].
    Chronic pelvic pain [5].
b. Patient Selection Considerations
  a. Age
    No specific precautions regarding 10 kJz SCS regarding patient age except those listed below and general guidelines [22–24].
  b. Contraindications
    Like all implantable SCS systems, 10 kHz SCS contraindications include active infection, pregnancy, coagulopathy (unless properly corrected), failed trial, psychological issues preventing optimal therapy [22,23],
  c. Maintenance concerns
    Inability of patient to operate device and or communicating problems related to therapy sometimes presents later during the therapy maintenance phase and are for concern (e.g., dementia).
c. Training Recommendations
  a. ACGME Fellowship and or Residency Training Specialty
    As suggested and detailed in Neuromodulation Appropriateness Consensus Committee (NACC) PEAK (Pain Education and Knowledge) guidelines foundation residency training for implanters should be in Neurosurgery, Anesthesiology, Physiatry or Neurology. Neuromodulation procedural competence can be gained through ACGME Fellowship programs getting experience in hands-on trialing/implantation, fluoroscopic and ultrasound imaging, programming, and managing risks/complications [22–24].
  b. Suggested Case Volume for Competence
    There is no specific guidelines related to 10 kHz implantation, however one should follow already published Neuromodulation Appropriateness Consensus Committee (NACC) general guidelines applicable to all SCS device implantations regarding volume and type of appropriate training [22–24].
  c. Proctoring Recommendation
    As above, NACC guidelines provide such recommendations [22–24].

Technique

a. Patient positioning
  Permanent implantation of an SCS system should be performed in a sterile operating room environment. The patient is positioned prone (unless and only exceptionally required otherwise) with generous padding to correct lumbar lordosis (or cervical lordosis for cervical SCS implant).
b. Anesthesia considerations
  Choice of anesthesia for10 kHz implantation surgery is mainly decided by the anesthesia team. 10 kHz technology does not require intraoperative paresthesia mapping and therefore patient is not awakened during surgery. Monitored anesthesia care (MAC) is frequently utilized, however for some cases general anesthesia with endotracheal intubation is indicated (e.g., protection of airways in patients with gastroparesis etc).
c. Operating room time estimate
  40–60 min.
d. Relevant vendor support
  Globus/Nevro.

e. Procedure

A vertical incision site is marked under fluoroscopy starting at the level of the intervertebral disc caudal to the intended interlaminar insertion site, and extending caudally three to 5 centimeters to make enough space for as much horizontal and parallel to the skin Tuohy epidural needle placement. Such planning facilitates needle placement and minimizes possibility of any inadvertent access to an intrathecal space. The skin and subcutaneous tissue is anaesthetized with either 1% lidocaine containing 1:200,000 epinephrine or 50:50 combination with 0.5% bupivacaine. A vertical incision is made using a scalpel blade. Careful dissection should be assisted with electrocautery to achieve hemostasis, until the fascia overlying the spinous processes/supraspinous ligament is exposed. A retractor is helpful during the dissection and Tuohy needle placement. Epidural needles are inserted lateral to the palpable spinous processes at the shallow angle and directed toward the midline of targeted interlaminar space. Insertion site for both Tuohy needles should be at the cranial end of an incision in order to allow adequate space below for anchors positioning and suturing. Contact can be made with the lamina just caudad to the intended interlaminar space in order to gauge the depth. The needle is further advanced utilizing lateral or contralateral fluoroscopy, and a loss of resistance, or tip of lead tapping techniques until accessing an epidural space. The stimulator leads should access posterior epidural space under the lateral or contralateral fluoroscopy followed by careful advancement under continuous low-emission or intermittent AP fluoroscopy to reach the targeted vertebral level. Both needles should be placed ipsilaterally and if epidural space can be accessed at the same level, needles are closer and midline incision may be of the lesser size. Placement of the leads for 10 khz therapy is purely anatomical and for the most common indications are as follows: for the neck and upper extremity chronic pain and radiculopathy, one lead tip is typically placed on top of C2 and other top of C3 vertebral body, for back and chronic leg pain top of T8 and top of T9. Again, midline positioning is required.

Epidural needles are then gently removed leaving the leads in place while those are secured to the underlying fascia using anchoring device and nonabsorbable suture. A final fluoroscopy image confirms that there was no lead migration during the needle removal and anchoring of the leads. Documenting AP and lateral views is advised [13–18].

It is essential to discuss and to mark IPG location with the patient in a sitting position in preoperative area and before implantation to avoid postoperative discomfort and an overestimation of the generator site. The desired site is marked preoperatively before proceeding to the operating room [25,26].

To make generator pocket, 3–4-centimeter horizontal incision is made using a scalpel blade. Blunt dissection and electrocautery are used to create subcutaneous pocket no deeper than 2 cm below the skin to avoid any difficulties in charging the device. Consider enclosed sizer to assure that the pocket size will fit the IPG. After hemostasis is established, leads are tunneled from the midline incision to the pocket. The tunneling device is frequently bent and tip gently palpated on the skin to achieve proper superficial control of device and facilitate tunneling. Both leads are then fed through the tunneling device until located in the generator pocket. Any extra length of both leads will serve as a retention loop to reduce the risk of lead migration. It is important to clean distal leads contacts using wet and dry sponge, complete an impedance check, and lock the leads in place. Copious irrigation of both incisions is performed using antibiotic solution or saline before closure. Consider vancomycin powder or any commercial antibiotic impregnated mesh/bag The excess length of SCS lead is then looped behind the IPG as it is placed inside the pocket. Nonabsorbable suture is utilized to secure the IPG within the pocket. The wounds are closed in a layered fashion using a simple interrupted absorbable suture. The skin is closed using a running absorbable suture or staples [25–28].

Postoperative considerations

a. Recovery

Patient were told to slowly increase their activities after an implant spending that first week in bed rest and limited physical activities, followed by prolonged walking, jogging, during the weeks two and three, gradually increasing their activities during weeks three and four after implant. Delayed are intensive swimming, golf swings, and heavy weight lifting.

b. Bracing Considerations

Even a simple elastic brace is sufficient to warn the patient first weeks after the implant not to unconsciously make an excessive bending or other moves that would cause significant tension to freshly implanted leads and anchors.

c. Activity Limitations

Slow increase of basic activities first week after implantation is recommended, followed by walking, light jogging through week two. Exercises should be selected to those not engaging thoracic (or cervical) spine flexion through the first month after SCS implantation. Minimize lateral thoracic (or cervical) flexion with rotation (e.g., golf, joga) for at least 2 months.

d. Maintenance Considerations
Each patient is offered five different programs based on trial and current postimplant configuration. Reprogramming as needed, updates on IQ programs as needed

Pearls and pitfalls

a. Preoperative
Patient should have a proper screening for MSSA/MRSA and possible decolonization (IA). One way to do it is a nasal decontamination using 2% mupirocin twice a day for 5 days. It is important in diabetics to optimize their glucose control and assure that hemoglobin A1c is <8.0% within the 30 days before an implant. Precautions for trial are not as strict as some patient after successful trial are well motivated to control their food intake and their glucose level in order to have an uneventful implant and postoperative care. Similarly, we do recommend smoking cessation, preoperative chlorhexidine baths (night before an implant). General assessment of other risk factors such as chronic immunosuppression, those anticoagulated and on steroid therapy must be made much in advance [27,28].

b. Intraoperative
Intravenous antibiotic infusion timing is of great importance as the maximal peak concentration of various antibiotics in an epidural space varies between 30 and 90 min. In addition, dosing should be based on weight for the most used antibiotics.
Chlorohexidine skin preparation and incise drape (Ioban) should be used, as well as double gloves by all surgical personal accessing the sterile field. Also, the number of surgical personal and their movements in operating room should be minimized to those that are essential. Layered closure is and has been standard when it comes to all SCS implants [25–28].

c. Postoperative
Any type of occlusive dressing is placed over the wounds and kept for at least 48 h. Surgical wound needs to be monitored and any changes addressed promptly and, if any concerns, in follow-up.

References

[1] Mekhail NA. Narouze S, Kapural L, Mekhail MN, Deer T. Clinical applications of neurostimulation: forty years later. Pain Pract 2010;10:103–12. 302 2.

[2] Verrills P, Sinclair C, Barnard A. A review of spinal cord stimulation systems for chronic pain. J Pain Res 2016;9:481–92.

[3] Lo Bianco G, Al-Kaisy A, Natoli S, Abd-Elsayed A, Matis G, Papa A, Kapural L, Staats P. Neuromodulation in chronic pain management: addressing persistent doubts in spinal cord stimulation. J Anesth Analg Crit Care 2025;5(1):3.

[4] Kapural L, Gupta M, Paicius R, Strodtbeck W, Vorenkamp KE, Gilmore C, Gliner B, Rotte A, Subbaroyan J, Province-Azalde R. Treatment of chronic abdominal pain with 10-kHz spinal cord stimulation: safety and efficacy results from a 12-month prospective, multicenter, feasibility study. Clin Transl Gastroenterol 2020;11(2). e00133.

[5] Tate JL, Stauss T, Li S, Rotte A, Subbaroyan J. A prospective, multi-center, clinical trial of a 10-kHz spinal cord stimulation system in the treatment of chronic pelvic pain. Pain Pract January 2021;21(1):45–53.

[6] Zhang T, Jia Y, Wang N, Chai X, He Q, Cao T, Mu Q, Lan Q, Zhao J, Yang Y. Recent advances in potential mechanisms of epidural spinal cord stimulation for movement disorders. Exp Neurol October 2025;392:115330.

[7] Kapural L, Yu C, Doust MW, et al. Novel 10-kHz high-frequency therapy (HF10 therapy) is superior to traditional low-frequency spinal cord stimulation for the treatment of chronic back and leg pain: the SENZA-RCT randomized controlled trial. Anesthesiology 2015;123:851–60.

[8] North RB, Kidd DH, Farrokhi F, Piantadosi SA. Spinal cord stimulation versus repeated lumbosacral spine surgery for chronic pain: a randomized, controlled trial. Neurosurgery 2005;56:98–107. discussion 106–107.

[9] Kumar K, North R, Taylor R, et al. Spinal cord stimulation vs. conventional medical management: a prospective, randomized, controlled, multicenter study of patients with failed back surgery syndrome (PROCESS study). Neuromodulation 2005;8:213–8.

[10] Kriek N, Groeneweg JG, Stronks DL, de Ridder D, Huygen FJ. Preferred frequencies and waveforms for spinal cord stimulation in patients with complex regional pain syndrome: a multicentre, double-blind, randomized and placebo-controlled crossover trial. Eur J Pain 2017;21:507–19.

[11] Deer TR, Levy RM, Kramer J, et al. Dorsal root ganglion stimulation yielded higher treatment success rate for complex regional pain syndrome and causalgia at 3 and 12 months: a randomized comparative trial. Pain 2017;158:669–81.

[12] Kapural L, Yu C, Doust M, et al. Comparison of 10- kHz high-frequency and traditional low-frequency spinal cord stimulation for the treatment of chronic back and leg pain: 24-month results from a multi- center, randomized, controlled pivotal trial. Neurosurgery 2016;79(5):667–77.

[13] Al-Kaisy A, Palmisani S, Smith TE, et al. Long-term improvements in chronic axial low back pain patients without previous spinal surgery: a cohort analysis of 10-kHz high-frequency spinal cord stimulation over 36 months. Pain Med 2018;19:1219–26.

[14] Al-Kaisy A, Van Buyten JP, Smet I, et al. Sustained effectiveness of 10 kHz high-frequency spinal cord stimulation for patients with chronic, low back pain: 24-month results of a prospective multicenter study. Pain Med 2014;15(3):347–54.

[15] Petersen EA, Stauss TG, Scowcroft JA, Brooks ES, White JL, Sills SM, Amirdelfan K, Guirguis MN, Xu J, Yu C, Nairizi A, Patterson DG, Tsoulfas KC, Creamer MJ, Galan V, Bundschu RH, Paul CA, Mehta ND, Choi H, Sayed D, Lad SP, DiBenedetto DJ, Sethi KA, Goree JH, Bennett MT, Harrison NJ, Israel AF, Chang P, Wu PW, Gekht G, Argoff CE, Nasr CE, Taylor RS, Subbaroyan J, Gliner BE, Caraway DL, Mekhail NA. Effect of high-frequency (10-kHz) spinal cord stimulation in patients with painful diabetic neuropathy: a randomized clinical trial. JAMA Neurol June 1, 2021;78(6):687–98.

[16] Patel NP, Jameson J, Johnson C, Kloster D, Calodney A, Kosek P, Pilitsis J, Bendel M, Petersen E, Wu C, Cherry T, Lad S, Yu C, Sayed D, Goree J, Lyons MK, Sack A, Bruce D, Bharara M, Province-Azalde R, Caraway D, Kapural L. Durable responses at 24 months with high-frequency spinal cord stimulation for nonsurgical refractory back pain. J Neurosurg Spine 2023;40(2):229–39.

[17] Kapural L, Jameson J, Johnson C, Kloster D, Calodney A, Kosek P, Pilitsis J, Bendel M, Petersen E, Wu C, Cherry T, Lad SP, Yu C, Sayed D, Goree J, Lyons MK, Sack A, Bruce D, Rubenstein F, Province-Azalde R, Caraway D, Patel NP. Treatment of nonsurgical refractory back pain with high-frequency spinal cord stimulation at 10 kHz: 12-month results of a pragmatic, multicenter, randomized controlled trial. J Neurosurg Spine 2022;37(2):188–99.

[18] Carolis G, Paroli M, Tollapi L, Doust MW, Burgher AH, Yu C, Yang T, Morgan DM, Amirdelfan K, Kapural L, Sitzman BT, Bundschu R, Vallejo R, Benyamin RM, Yearwood TL, Gliner BE, Powell AA, Bradley K. Paresthesia-independence: an assessment of technical factors related to 10 kHz paresthesia-free spinal cord stimulation. Pain Physician May 2017;20(4):331–41.

[19] Rosenow J. Anatomy of the nervous system. In: Krames E, 303 Peckham H, Rezai A, editors. Textbook of Neuromodulation, vol 304; 2009. p. 95–108. 305 3.

[20] Grill WM. Principles of electric field generation for the stimulation of CNS. In: Krames E, Peckham H, Rezai A, editors. Textbook of Neuromodulation; 2009. p. 109–22.

[21] Sweeney J, Sheldon BL, Juneja A, Hadanny A, Foley J, Pilitsis JG, Sukul V. Efficacy of 10 kHz spinal cord stimulation in complex regional pain syndrome: a retrospective analysis. Clin Neurol Neurosurg May 2022;216:107220.

[22] Deer TR, Russo MA, Grider JS, Pope J, Rigoard P, Hagedorn JM, Naidu R, Patterson DG, Wilson D, Lubenow TR, Buvanendran A, Sheth SJ, Abdallah R, Knezevic NN, Schu S, Nijhuis H, Mehta P, Vallejo R, Shah JM, Harned ME, Jassal N, Gonzalez JM, Pittelkow TP, Patel S, Bojanic S, Chapman K, Strand N, Green AL, Pahapill P, Dario A, Piedimonte F, Levy RM. The neurostimulation appropriateness consensus committee (NACC): recommendations for surgical technique for spinal cord stimulation. Neuromodulation January 2022;25(1):1–34.

[23] Deer TR, Russo MA, Sayed D, Pope JE, Grider JS, Hagedorn JM, Falowski SM, Al-Kaisy A, Slavin KV, Li S, Poree LR, Eldabe S, Meier K, Lamer TJ, Pilitsis JG, De Andrés J, Perruchoud C, Carayannopoulos AG, Moeschler SM, Hadanny A, Lee E, Varshney VP, Desai MJ, Pahapill P, Osborn J, Bojanic S, Antony A, Piedimonte F, Hayek SM, Levy RM. The neurostimulation appropriateness consensus committee (NACC): recommendations for the mitigation of complications of neurostimulation. Neuromodulation August 2024;27(6):977–1007.

[24] Deer TR, Russo M, Grider JS, Sayed D, Lamer TJ, Dickerson DM, Hagedorn JM, Petersen EA, Fishman MA, FitzGerald J, Baranidharan G, De Ridder D, Chakravarthy KV, Al-Kaisy A, Hunter CW, Buchser E, Chapman K, Gilligan C, Hayek SM, Thomson S, Strand N, Jameson J, Simopoulos TT, Yang A, De Coster O, Cremaschi F, Christo PJ, Varshney V, Bojanic S, Levy RM. The neurostimulation appropriateness consensus committee (NACC): recommendations for spinal cord stimulation long-term outcome optimization and salvage therapy. Neuromodulation August 2024;27(6):951–76.

[25] Deer TR, Lamer TJ, Pope JE, et al. The Neurostimulation Appropriateness Consensus Committee (NACC) safety guidelines for the reduction of severe neurological injury. Neuromodulation 2017;20:13–30.

[26] Falowski S, Ali R, Sweet J, Mackel C, Kesarwani R, Arle J, Larkin MB, Pinckard-Dover HN, Stone L, Nerison C, Ben Haim S, Rosenow J, Viswanathan A, Petersen E, Lad N, Schwalb J, Raslan A. Technical and clinical overview: spinal cord stimulation. Neuromodulation September 25, 2025. S1094–7159(25)00691-9.

[27] Bendel MA, O'Brien T, Hoelzer BC, Deer TR, Pittelkow TP, Costandi S, Walega DR, Azer G, Hayek SM, Wang Z, Eldrige JS, Qu W, Rosenow JM, Falowski SM, Neuman SA, Moeschler SM, Wassef C, Kim C, Niazi T, Saifullah T, Yee B, Kim C, Oryhan CL, Warren DT, Lerman I, Mora R, Hanes M, Simopoulos T, Sharma S, Gilligan C, Grace W, Ade T, Mekhail NA, Hunter JP, Choi D, Choi DY. Spinal cord stimulator related infections: findings from a multicenter retrospective analysis of 2737 implants. Neuromodulation 2017;20(6):553–7.

[28] Falowski SM, Provenzano DA, Xia Y, Doth AH. Spinal cord stimulation infection rate and factors: Results from a United States payer database. Neuromodulation February 2019;22(2):179–89.

Chapter 20

Surround inhibition

Nitish Aggarwal[1], Roshan Santhosh[2], Ajay Antony[3], Sayed E. Wahezi[4], Ugur Yener[4] and James North[5]

[1]*Pain Management, TriState Pain Institute, Fort Mohave, AZ, United States;* [2]*Physical Medicine and Rehabilitation, Larkin Community Hospital, Miami, FL, United States;* [3]*Pain Management, The Orthopaedic Institute, Gainesville, FL, United States;* [4]*Montefiore Multidisciplinary Pain Program, Bronx, NY, United States;* [5]*Interventional Pain Management Department, The Center for Clinical Research, LLC, Winston–Salem, NC, United States*

Surround inhibition

Surround inhibition is a fundamental concept in neuroscience that plays a critical role in sensory processing, motor control, and neuromodulation systems. It refers to the neural mechanism by which the activation of a specific group of neurons suppresses the activity of neighboring neurons. This process enhances the contrast and sharpness of activated neural signals, allowing for more precise and efficient information processing. Surround inhibition is observed across various sensory systems, including vision, touch, and pain, as well as in motor systems, where it helps refine movement and coordination.

In sensory systems, surround inhibition is essential for distinguishing between stimuli and improving perceptual clarity. Initially discovered in the visual system, surround inhibition contributes to edge detection and the perception of contrast [1]. When light falls on the retina, photoreceptors in the center of a visual field are activated, while those in the surrounding area are inhibited [2]. This lateral inhibition, mediated by horizontal cells and amacrine cells in the retina, sharpens the boundaries between light and dark regions, enabling the brain to detect edges and contours more effectively. Similarly, in the somatosensory system, surround inhibition helps localize tactile stimuli by suppressing neural activity in adjacent areas, allowing for precise discrimination of touch [3].

In the motor system, surround inhibition is crucial for the execution of controlled and accurate movements. When a specific muscle group is activated to perform a movement, surrounding muscles are inhibited to prevent unwanted contractions [4]. This mechanism ensures that movements are smooth and coordinated. For instance, when reaching for an object, the brain activates the muscles responsible for the movement while simultaneously inhibiting antagonist muscles that could interfere with the action. Disruptions in surround inhibition have been linked to motor disorders such as dystonia, where excessive muscle contractions lead to involuntary movements and abnormal postures [5].

At the cellular level, surround inhibition is mediated by inhibitory interneurons that release neurotransmitters like gamma-aminobutyric acid (GABA) [6]. These interneurons, specifically the parvalbumin (PV)-positive interneurons, form synaptic connections with neighboring neurons, reducing their excitability and preventing the spread of neural activity [7]. The balance between excitation and inhibition is critical for maintaining neural circuit stability and function. Dysregulation of this balance can lead to neurological and psychiatric disorders, including chronic pain, epilepsy, schizophrenia, and autism spectrum disorders [8].

Surround inhibition in the pain sensory system is a neural mechanism that enhances the perception of localized pain by suppressing the activity of surrounding neurons. This process helps the brain accurately identify the precise location and intensity of a painful stimulus by sharpening the contrast between the activated area and its surroundings. When nociceptors are stimulated, the central nervous system employs inhibitory interneurons to dampen the signals from adjacent regions, ensuring that the pain is perceived as coming from a specific, well-defined area rather than a diffuse region [9]. This phenomenon is crucial for effective pain localization, severity, and response, allowing the body to focus its protective and healing mechanisms on the exact site of injury or damage. Defects in surround inhibition processing can lead to altered pain perception such as hyperalgesia or allodynia [10].

A Modern Atlas for Implantable Devices of the Spine, Brain, and Nerve. https://doi.org/10.1016/B978-0-443-36528-7.00002-9

Neuromodulation involves the regulation of neural activity through the release of neurotransmitters, neuropeptides, or other signaling molecules that can either enhance or dampen pain signals in ascending or descending spinothalamic pain pathways [11]. Therapeutic neuromodulation techniques, such as spinal cord stimulation or pharmacological interventions targeting neuromodulatory pathways, aim to restore balance in these systems, thereby improving pain localization and reducing pain intensity. The earliest form of spinal neuromodulation is a paresthesia-based mechanism which is explained by the suppression of ascending pain fibers by gate theory [12]. The balance between inputs from nociceptive and non-nociceptive Aβ mechanoreceptors is filtered by spinal inhibitory interneuron circuits (the 'gate'), which control the strength of the painful signals transmitted to higher brain centers [13]. Contemporary neurobiological and clinical studies have demonstrated that stimulation of this pathway alone is suboptimal to mitigate pain and that Wide Dynamic Range (WDR) neurons are the proxy for pain in animal models. This led to studies employing WDRs to surround receptive field inhibition to suppress [14]. Clinically, an important element of WDR suppression seems to be very specific activation of anatomical pain centers and thus seems to rely on accurate positioning of neurostimulation devices over spinal cord centers. Adherence to proper utilization of surround inhibition waveforms relies on the pain practitioner's ability to place active SCS electrodes directly over the spinal homuncular regions which correlate with the patient's pain complaints [15].

In summary, surround inhibition is a vital neural process that enhances the precision and efficiency of sensory, motor, and neuromodulation functions. By suppressing the activity of surrounding neurons, it sharpens neural signals, improves perceptual clarity, and enhances pain localization. Understanding the mechanisms and functions of surround inhibition provides valuable insights into the organization of neural circuits and thus this system can be targeted by neuromodulation techniques, such as Fast-Acting Sub-Perception Therapy.

Energy delivery to the surrounding dorsal column fibers: What cell lines are affected?

Spinal cord stimulation (SCS) as a therapeutic modality has been around for over 60 years, and to this date the pathways through which it mechanistically achieves pain relief are not completely understood [16]. Neurostimulation therapies rose in popularity after Melzack and Wall (1965) proposed a gate control theory of pain [12]. This foundational paradigm of neuromodulation suggests that stimulation of non-nociceptive large diameter A-beta fibers can inhibit ascending nociceptive signals carried by the A-delta and C-fibers at the level of the spinal dorsal horn. The initial clinical data supported this mechanism, as early SCS systems generated paresthesia over the desired coverage area, thought to stimulate large diameter afferents [17,18]. Early studies posited that as the dorsal column intraspinal structures were in closest proximity to a midline epidural electrode, the modulation of analgesic effects would be observed principally in these white matter tracts [19].

In reality, the changes observed in dorsal column stimulation are far more nuanced with multiple clinical trials demonstrating that SCS is far more effective at reducing chronic neuropathic pain when compared to acute nociceptive pain - findings not fully explained by the gate control theory [20]. Animal models have demonstrated that reduction in inhibitory signaling at the level of the dorsal horn can lead to hyperexcitability of wide dynamic range neurons thus modulating chronic neuropathic pain [21]. Invitro SCS studies in animal models have also demonstrated activation followed by inhibition of both excitatory glutaminergic as well as inhibitory GABA signaling in dorsal horn neurons [22]. Conversion of SCS non-responders to responders with the addition of intrathecal baclofen highlights the importance of GABA inhibitory signaling on ascending pain pathways [23,24].

Islet cells in the superficial dorsal horn are GABA-ergic neurons that are known to inhibit excitatory signals [21]. Studies in animal models have demonstrated that dorsal horn islet cell are often dysfunctional in chronic pain states, and loss of this rostral-caudal inhibition may be responsible for increased pain signaling [20]. Dorsal horn islet cells have been shown to be tonically firing neurons with relatively depolarized resting membrane potentials, making them particularly well suited to activation by SCS [20,25]. Recent work by Gmel et al. (2023) has demonstrated that SCS can also directly generate evoked compound action potentials (ECAPs) in post synaptic dorsal column pathway fibers which have traditionally been posited to carry non-nociceptive signals [26]. Numerous studies have demonstrated changes in cortical activity, particularly at the thalamus, cingulate cortex, and post central gyrus as demonstrated by fMRI [27]. As such, SCS can modulate pain signaling at the dorsal horn, ascending secondary interneurons both directly and indirectly. There are also proven supraspinal mechanisms involved.

Glial cells including oligodendrocytes, astrocytes, and microglia serve to modulate the response and function of central nervous system neurons and may play a role in the mechanism of action of SCS [15]. There are high concentrations of glial cells in the T8-T11 levels where SCS leads are often placed [28]. Oligodendrocytes have been shown to be upregulated in chronic neuropathic pain [28,29]. Vallejo and Kelley (2020) demonstrated that maximal oligodendrocyte activity is seen with stimulation with multiple waveforms when compared to traditional SCS. This compound waveform termed differential target multiplexed programming (DTMP) has been shown to increase glial cell gene expression and decrease pain when compared to conventional SCS in animal models [15,30].

Clinical data known: Time of onset to pain relief, % pain relief, and clinical trials

The use of FAST (Fast-Acting Sub-Perception Therapy) waveforms remains a relatively new addition to the SCS toolkit of paresthesia free therapies on the commercial market today. Metzger et al. (2021) conducted a prospective multicenter observational case-series of 41 patients with low back or lower extremity pain who were previously implanted with a permanent SCS system utilizing standard technique with up to 32 electrode leads placed between T7-T10 spinal levels. Patients were programmed to receive stimulation at 90 Hz with a pulse width of 210 ± 50 ms with a symmetric biphasic waveform [31]. This waveform was delivered via an SCS system with capabilities for multiple central points of stimulation, with the first phase characterized by a negative current introduced though cathodes and positive current introduced through anodes, with polarity being reversed in the second phase. Patients underwent paresthesia mapping at 90 Hz after which stimulation was reduced to 65% of the perception threshold. Pain was noted to decrease from 6.5/10 prior to initiation of therapy to 1.3/10 on average 11 min after initiation of therapy [31]. This is likely explained by the novel mechanism of surround inhibition achieved with FAST, which is in stark contrast to conventional SCS which takes hours to days to achieve peak efficacy [31]. This small cohort study did demonstrate durability of the NRS pain improvement at 3- and 6-month follow-up.

Another observational prospective, single center, 14 patient case-series by Matis et al. (2022) for patients with chronic mixed pain, half of whom were classified as having non-neuropathic pain per intake painDETECT questionnaire demonstrated durability FAST [32]. Oswestry Disability Index (ODI), pain scores (Numeric Rating Scale, NRS), and Quality-of-life (EQ-5D-5L) were collected. Baseline NRS was 8.3 ± 0.3 which remained reduced to 1.4 ± 0.3 ($P < 0.0001$) at 6 months post implant. There were also notable improvements in patient quality of life (53.1-point increase in EQ-5D-5L score at 6-month follow-up. In addition, mean ODI score was reduced by 48.9-points at 6-month follow-up, representing a change in patient disability from that of "crippling" (at baseline) to that of "minimal" disability at 6 month follow-up [33].

There is comparable efficacy of FAST demonstrated in a multi-center, observational consecutive case series of 167 patients with chronic pain from 13 European centers who utilized FAST-SCS [34]. Most patients (74%) suffered from persistent spine pain syndrome type 2% and 87% presented with low back and/or leg pain. Two-year follow up data (mean 1.6 years) demonstrated a decrease in overall pain (NRS) from 8.0 ± 1.2 to 2.9 ± 2.2 ($n = 167$, $P < .0001$). Encouragingly, 87% of patients reported greater than 50% pain relief and 55% of the cohort were "high responders" as defined by NRS <2/10 [34]. Oswestry Disability Index at final follow-up was noted to be decreased by 29.2 ± 21.5 points, and patients had a significant gain in quality of life (EQ-5D-5L) increased by 52.0 ± 26.9 points. This clinical data suggests that FAST SCS will be a valuable tool in the treatment of chronic pain.

References

[1] Blakemore C, Carpenter RH, Georgeson MA. Lateral inhibition between orientation detectors in the human visual system. Nature 1970;228 (5266):37–9. https://doi.org/10.1038/228037a0.

[2] Angelucci A, Levitt JB, Lund JS. Anatomical origins of the classical receptive field and modulatory surround field of single neurons in macaque visual cortical area V1. Prog Brain Res 2002;136:373–88. https://doi.org/10.1016/s0079-6123(02)36031-x.

[3] Abraira VE, Ginty DD. The sensory neurons of touch. Neuron 2013;79(4):618–39. https://doi.org/10.1016/j.neuron.2013.07.051.

[4] Beck S, Hallett M. Surround inhibition in the motor system. Exp Brain Res 2011;210(2):165–72. https://doi.org/10.1007/s00221-011-2610-6.

[5] Quartarone A, Hallett M. Emerging concepts in the physiological basis of dystonia. Mov Disord 2013;28(7):958–67. https://doi.org/10.1002/mds.25532.

[6] Buldyrev I, Taylor WR. Inhibitory mechanisms that generate centre and surround properties in ON and OFF brisk-sustained ganglion cells in the rabbit retina. J Physiol. 2013;591(1):303–25. https://doi.org/10.1113/jphysiol.2012.243113.

[7] Tremblay R, Lee S, Rudy B. GABAergic interneurons in the neocortex: From cellular properties to circuits. Neuron 2016;91(2):260–92. https://doi.org/10.1016/j.neuron.2016.06.033.

[8] Canitano R, Pallagrosi M. Autism spectrum disorders and schizophrenia spectrum disorders: Excitation/inhibition imbalance and developmental trajectories. Front Psychiatry 2017;8:69. https://doi.org/10.3389/fpsyt.2017.00069.

[9] Dubin AE, Patapoutian A. Nociceptors: The sensors of the pain pathway. J Clin Investig 2010;120(11):3760–72. https://doi.org/10.1172/JCI42843.

[10] Woolf CJ. Central sensitization: Implications for the diagnosis and treatment of pain. Pain 2011;152(3 Suppl. 1):S2–15. https://doi.org/10.1016/j.pain.2010.09.030.

[11] Nadim F, Bucher D. Neuromodulation of neurons and synapses. Curr Opin Neurobiol 2014;29:48–56. https://doi.org/10.1016/j.conb.2014.05.003.

[12] Melzack R, Wall PD. Pain mechanisms: A new theory. Science 1965;150(3699):971–9. https://doi.org/10.1126/science.150.3699.971.

[13] Metzger C, Hammond B, Ferro R, et al. Two-year outcomes using fast-acting sub-perception therapy for spinal cord stimulation: Results of a real-world multicenter study in the United States. Expert Rev Med Devices 2025;22(2):155–64. https://doi.org/10.1080/17434440.2025.2453554.

[14] Zhang TC, Janik JJ, Grill WM. Modeling effects of spinal cord stimulation on wide-dynamic range dorsal horn neurons: Influence of stimulation frequency and GABAergic inhibition. J Neurophysiol 2014;112(3):552–67. https://doi.org/10.1152/jn.00254.2014.

[15] Wahezi SE, Caparo MA, Malhotra R, Sundaram L, Batti K, Ejindu P, Veeramachaneni R, Anitescu M, Hunter CW, Naeimi T, Farah F, Kohan L. Current waveforms in spinal cord stimulation and their impact on the future of neuromodulation: A scoping review. Neuromodulation. Technol Neural Interface 2024;27:47–58. https://doi.org/10.1016/j.neurom.2023.11.002.

[16] Linderoth B, Foreman RD. Conventional and novel spinal stimulation algorithms: hypothetical mechanisms of action and comments on outcomes. Neuromodulation 2017;20(6):525–33. https://doi.org/10.1111/ner.12624.

[17] Barolat G, Massaro F, He J, Zeme S, Ketcik B. Mapping of sensory responses to epidural stimulation of the intraspinal neural structures in man. J Neurosurg 1993;78:233–9. https://doi.org/10.3171/jns.1993.78.2.0233.

[18] North RB, Roark GL. Spinal cord stimulation for chronic pain. Neurosurg Clin N Am 1995;6:145–55.

[19] Holsheimer J, Barolat G, Struijk JJ, He J. Significance of the spinal cord position in spinal cord stimulation. https://doi.org/10.1007/978-3-7091-9419-5_26; 1995.

[20] Jensen MP, Brownstone RM. Mechanisms of spinal cord stimulation for the treatment of pain: still in the dark after 50 years. Eur J Pain 2019;23:652–9. https://doi.org/10.1002/ejp.1336.

[21] Todd AJ. Neuronal circuitry for pain processing in the dorsal horn. Nat Rev Neurosci 2010;11:823–36. https://doi.org/10.1038/nrn2947.

[22] Fan W, Sullivan SJ, Sdrulla AD. Dorsal column and root stimulation at Aβ-fiber intensity activate superficial dorsal horn glutamatergic and GABAergic populations. Mol Pain 2022;18. https://doi.org/10.1177/17448069221079559.

[23] Chakravarthy K, Fishman MA, Zuidema X, Hunter CW, Levy R. Mechanism of action in burst spinal cord stimulation: Review and recent advances. Pain Med 2019;20:S13–22. https://doi.org/10.1093/pm/pnz073.

[24] Cui J-G, O'Connor WT, Ungerstedt U, Linderoth B, Meyerson BA. Spinal cord stimulation attenuates augmented dorsal horn release of excitatory amino acids in mononeuropathy via a GABAergic mechanism. Pain 1997;73:87–95. https://doi.org/10.1016/S0304-3959(97)00077-8.

[25] Zannou AL, Koochesfahani MB, Russo M, Bikson M. Dorsal horn dendrite polarization during Spinal Cord Stimulation (SCS) predicted using the quasi-uniform-mirror assumption. 2024. https://doi.org/10.1101/2024.01.17.575924.

[26] Gmel GE, Santos Escapa R, Benkohen TE, Mugan D, Parker JL, Palmisani S. Postsynaptic dorsal column pathway activation during spinal cord stimulation in patients with chronic pain. Front Neurosci 2023;17. https://doi.org/10.3389/fnins.2023.1297814.

[27] Sdrulla AD, Guan Y, Raja SN. Spinal cord stimulation: Clinical efficacy and potential mechanisms. Pain Pract 2018;18:1048–67. https://doi.org/10.1111/papr.12692.

[28] Vallejo R, Kelley C. Neuron-glial inflammasome enhanced reversal by DTM-SCS relative to high rate and low rate SCS in a neuropathic pain model. J Neurosurg 2020;132:1–124. https://doi.org/10.3171/2020.4.JNS.AANS2020abstracts.

[29] Gritsch S, Lu J, Thilemann S, Wörtge S, Möbius W, Bruttger J, Karram K, Ruhwedel T, Blanfeld M, Vardeh D, Waisman A, Nave K-A, Kuner R. Oligodendrocyte ablation triggers central pain independently of innate or adaptive immune responses in mice. Nat Commun 2014;5:5472. https://doi.org/10.1038/ncomms6472.

[30] Vallejo R, Kelley CA, Gupta A, Smith WJ, Vallejo A, Cedeño DL. Modulation of neuroglial interactions using differential target multiplexed spinal cord stimulation in an animal model of neuropathic pain. Mol Pain 2020;16. https://doi.org/10.1177/1744806920918057.

[31] Metzger CS, Hammond MB, Paz-Solis JF, Newton WJ, Thomson SJ, Pei Y, Jain R, Moffitt M, Annecchino L, Doan Q. A novel fast-acting sub-perception spinal cord stimulation therapy enables rapid onset of analgesia in patients with chronic pain. Expert Rev Med Devices 2021;18:299–306. https://doi.org/10.1080/17434440.2021.1890580.

[32] Matis G, Chen L, Jain R, Doan Q. Clinical utilization of fast-acting sub-perception therapy (FAST) in SCS-implanted patients for treatment of mixed pain. Interv Pain Med 2022;1:100165. https://doi.org/10.1016/j.inpm.2022.100165.

[33] Fairbank JCT, Pynsent PB. The oswestry disability Index. Spine 2000;25:2940–53. https://doi.org/10.1097/00007632-200011150-00017.

[34] Bayerl S, Paz-Solis J, Matis G, Rigoard P, Kallewaard JW, Canos-Verdecho MA, Vesper J, Llopis JE, Kyriakopoulos G, Gulve A, Raoul S, Papa A, Love-Jones S, Williams A. Two-year outcomes using fast-acting, sub-perception therapy for spinal cord stimulation: A European, real-world, multicenter experience. J Clin Med 2024;13. https://doi.org/10.3390/jcm13226999.

Chapter 21

Differential target multiplexed (DTM)

Ricardo Vallejo[2], Melissa Murphy[3], Matthew Chung[4] and Mark N. Malinowski[1]

[1]*Ohio Health Hospital System, Columbus, OH, United States;* [2]*CEO, CFLow Labs Inc., CMO, Capri-Medical Ltd, President Emeritus, MiVI, Madrid, Spain;* [3]*North Texas Orthopedics and Spine Center, Grapevine, TX, United States;* [4]*Department of Pain Medicine, Division of Critical Care Anesthesia and Pain Medicine, The University of Texas MD Anderson Cancer Center, Houston, TX, United States*

Introduction

Our understanding of the central nervous system (CNS) has been changed dramatically by the discovery that glial cells, once thought to be a mere supporting structure, sense and control electrical activity flowing through neural circuits. Neurons and glial cells are 2 cell types of the nervous system with close molecular and cellular. While neurons are specialized in conducting electrical signals, glial cells are nonconducting cells that provide nutrition, protection, and insulation to the neurons of the CNS. Glial cells represent 70% of the total cell population in the brain and spine. They are subdivided into two categories: microglia comprise 5%–10% of the glial population, and macroglia, which includes astrocytes and oligodendrocytes. Both cell populations are now known to play a fundamental role in the development and maintenance of neuropathic pain. Microglia cells are resident immune cells in the CNS. Under normal circumstances, microglia are in a resting state, but in response to pain, they migrate to the central terminals of afferent peripheral nerves in the dorsal horn and undergo proliferation and activation. This activation generates changes in the surface markers. Additionally, the activated microglia begin secreting a variety of signaling peptides such as cytokines, neurotrophic factors and chemokines. Among those cytokines, Interleukin 1-beta, Interleukin-6 and tumor necrosis alpha (TNK-alfa) lead to the activation of surrounding astrocytes. Astrocytes represent the majority of cells in the CNS. In a resting state, they play a fundamental role in the neuroglial homeostasis, regulating the extracellular ion concentration of K^+, Ca^{2+}, as well as the neurotransmitters concentration at the synaptic level, including deactivation of glutaminergic activity. The activation of astrocytes leads to the prolongation of the pain state. It is relevant to understand that one astrocyte can provide extensions to over 200 1000 synapsis while one oligodendrocyte may generate myelin to up to 100 axons. In vivo experiments have demonstrated that stimulation of oligodendrocytes may modulate axonal conduction velocity of action potentials through axons they myelinate [1].

Traditional approaches to electrical neuromodulation focus on modulating neural circuits based on the effects exerted on neuronal action potentials. As mentioned earlier, glial cells do not generate action potentials, and therefore, the recording electrodes commonly used to evaluate neuronal response to electrical signals are blind to the depolarizing effects exerted by electrical signals on these cells that represent the vast majority of cells in the spinal cord [2]. Since its inception in the 1960s, spinal cord stimulation (SCS) has been based on the gate control theory, focusing exclusively on a neuron-centric approach and ignoring the fundamental role of the neuroinflammatory process in the development of chronic pain [3].

In recent years, several highly effective stimulation paradigms that do not exert paresthesia prompted the question of what other mechanisms of action are engaged in the clinical benefits observed with those SCS modalities. Glial cells have a membrane potential and depolarize upon electrical stimulation. The depolarization of these cells is dependent on the electrical parameters of the stimulating signal. As an example, electrical stimulation of astrocytes induces the release of glutamate in a manner dependent on charge balancing. Astrocyte depolarization also modulates Ca^{2+} waves, which are the main form of communication of these cells.

Current molecular technologies allow us to evaluate how genes, proteins, and phosphoproteins are affected by injury and how different parameters (pulse charge, amplitude, pulse width, and frequency) have different effects in different cell populations. These studies have highlighted the modulation of neuroimmune regulation, inflammatory response, extracellular matrix and synaptic signaling as well as the transition from resting to activated states of glial cells when exposed

A Modern Atlas for Implantable Devices of the Spine, Brain, and Nerve. https://doi.org/10.1016/B978-0-443-36528-7.00035-2

to those parameters [3]. Considering that chronic pain is caused by unbalanced neuronal-glial interactions associated with glial-mediated activation of pathways that lead to central sensitization and maladaptive changes in neural plasticity, an SCS programming algorithm based on the multiplexing of electrical signals in order to differentially target neurons and glial cells was developed. The goal of this approach is the modulation of neuroglial interactions in the direction of the homeostatic balance found in normal neurotransmission. This differential target multiplexed programming (DTMP) approach has been compared with conventional low-rate SCS in both preclinical and clinical studies [4].

Glia cells role in chronic neuropathic pain

Microglia exist in the central nervous system (CNS) as a form of resident immune cells. Microglia are known to play a role in modulating pain perception throughout the pain pathway, and these cells represent key roles in the mediation of both acute and chronic pain processes. As previous research has suggested, they were known for their role in immune surveillance in brain homeostasis, but are now known to become activated by noxious stimuli such as direct injury of tissue, inflammation or subsequent neural damage.

As a result of these varied responses, microglia become activated and release cytokines, chemokines and other growth factors, all of which can influence the transmission and processing of pain in the spinal cord and the brain. The activation of microglia may also be known to mediate both peripheral and central sensitization and may play a role in amplification of pain signals, a role traditionally thought of exclusively for wide dynamic range neurons. Furthermore, microglia are thought to be involved in sustaining pain beyond the acute phase, and if these become maladaptive, they may perpetuate the pain signal disproportionately or in the absence of active tissue injury. Therefore, the role of microglia in the pain pathway and its understanding are critical for the development of treatments that focus on neural inflammation and processing of pain in the central nervous system.

Astrocytes are the most numerous cell population in the central nervous system. They are fundamental in the neuroglial interaction. It's important to emphasize their role at the synapse and along the axons. Interestingly, astrocytes membrane express cytokine and neurotransmitter receptors and become activated, among others, by glutamate and cytokines. The activation generates an inflow of Ca^{2+} into the cell and the activation of intracellular cascades like MAP kinases and mTOR that promote proinflammatory pathways [5]. At the synapse, astrocytes surround the synapse cleft and oversee the homeostasis of neurotransmitters like glutamate, GABA, Adenosine, and ions. Constant glutamate release at the clef leads to the disruption of astrocytic membrane glutamate receptors, generating an excess of the excitatory neurotransmitter and further generating sensitization of the postsynaptic neurons. Once activated, astrocytes will also start releasing pro- and antiinflammatory cytokines that eventually will facilitate pain chronification or resolution of the inflammatory process. Also relevant is the syphoning role of the astrocytes and the Ranvier nodes, where the removal of K^+ ions is essential to allow the axons to maintain depolarization of their membrane [6].

Furthermore, astrocytes are in charge of the synthesis of glutamate and GABA, as neurons are not capable of generating the main excitatory and inhibitory neurotransmitters.

Considering that one astrocyte may generate extensions that surround thousands of synapses, it is fundamental to understand the coordination of the CNS function.

Finally, it is important to mention the role of oligodendrocytes. Recent studies have highlighted the role of this cell population in chronic pain conditions. Oligodendrocytes provide the myelin sheaths to hundreds of adjacent axons, and electrical stimulation has been shown to modulate axonal conduction [7].

In vitro and *in vivo* studies have demonstrated the response of astrocytes to different forms of electrically applied pulses regarding charge balancing and intensities [8–10].

As mentioned in the introduction, in consideration of the role of the neuroglia interaction in the development of chronic pain, it is essential to consider all these cell populations when developing any programming paradigm. Differential Target Multiplex stimulation considers this foundation and the fact that different variables of the electrical signal (frequency, pulse width, intensity and charge balancing) generate different responses in different cell populations at the core of its formulation.

Differential targeted multiplexed stimulation

Differential targeted multiplexed stimulation (DTM) is known to be an emerging novel stimulation paradigm that is focused on specific microglial subpopulations. Specifically, simultaneous multi-frequency stimulation (multiplexing) is thought to selectively activate or potentially inhibit different aspects of the targeted glial function in a controlled manner such that these modulate either proinflammatory or neural protective pathways, simultaneously, through at least in part differential activation of gene translation of specific proteins.

Therefore, the ability to target specific populations of microglia both differentially and simultaneously, DTM stimulation allows for the potential to treat a wide range of conditions, including those specific to pain processing.

Differential targeted multiplexed (DTM) preclinical studies

To explore the role DTM has on glial cells, an animal model investigating the use of DTM programming for chronic neuropathic pain was explored [2]. Using a spared nerve injury model in 55 rats, comparison of DTM programming with conventional low rate (LR) [50 Hz, 150 µsec pulse width (PW)], and high rate (HR)[1200 Hz, 50 µs PW] programming was made by continuous stimulation for 48 h, and subsequently assessing mechanical and thermal hypersensitivity. Behavioral evaluations and RNA gene expression changes through sequencing revealed that while all treatment modalities reduced mechanical hypersensitivity, DTMP achieved greater improvement ($62.9 \pm 8.9\%$, $N = 9$) versus LR ($37.6 \pm 6.0\%$, $N = 10$) and HR ($38.3 \pm 5.5\%$, $N = 11$) and modulated gene expression effectively – restoring 48% (11/23) modules toward naïve expression patterns compared to 9% and 22% low and high rate programming, respectively. Weighted gene expression analysis further confirmed that DTM programming more closely approximated normal gene expression patterns compared to conventional stimulation observed in uninjured animals [2].

In a follow-up study to explore the impact of various SCS parameters (including DTM) for modulated gene expression, a randomized spared nerve injury model was implemented among rats [11]. Male rats were randomized to DTM, HR, LR or no stimulation for 48 h. Microglia-specific gene expression was assessed using Pearson correlations, revealing DTM restored 83% of resting microglial genes toward baseline levels, compared to 70% with a high rate, and 59% with a low rate. These findings support the hypothesis that SCS parameters significantly influence microglial activation, with DTM demonstrating the most robust effect in normalization of neuroinflammatory gene expression [11].

Preclinical studies that followed included proteomic and phosphoproteomic analysis, along with prior transcriptomics, demonstrating the ability of DTM to reverse changes in gene and protein expression levels induced by a neuropathic pain model.

Expression profiles of specific transcripts were assessed using RNA sequences to identify differences in gene expression correlated with pain states across various SCS therapies [4]. Pearson correlations and cell population analyses revealed that DTM programming produced strong and significant alignments with the expression levels observed in healthy animals across all examined cell-specific transcriptomes. In contrast, HR programming only showed a robust correlation for microglia-specific transcriptomes, while LR programming did not yield strong correlations with any cell type. These results provide evidence that differential target multiplexed programming selectively modulates cell-specific gene expression toward a healthy state, supporting its established role in regulating neuronal–glial interactions in a pain model [4].

Expanding the scope of molecular analysis, another study investigated the comparative effects of DTM and LR on the proteomic and phosphoproteomic profiles associated with the neuronal and inflammatory signaling of neuropathic pain, focusing on mitogen-activated protein kinases (MAPKs) and nuclear factor kappa-light-chain-enhancer of activated B cells (NFkB). In this study, rats in a spared nerve injury model were treated with DTM or LR, while control groups received no stimulation. A total of 7192 proteins were identified, with DTM significantly modulating 1451 proteins compared to those by low-rate stimulation of 705 proteins. Notably, DTM had a more pronounced impact on proteins involved in the MAPK and NFkB signaling pathways, including significant repression of complement pathway proteins that were elevated upon injury [12]. These results suggest that DTMP more effectively modulates neuroinflammatory processes, offering greater therapeutic potential for reversing the molecular changes associated with neuropathic pain and improving patient outcomes in chronic pain management [12].

Continuing the investigation into the molecular effects of SCS, Tilley et al. evaluated how various SCS paradigms – particularly DTM and low rate SCS – affect ion channels and related signaling pathways, in the dorsal spinal tissue of another spared nerve injury model, including rats [13]. The findings from this randomized study involving four arms (DTM, LR, No-SCS, and sham, each with a $N = 10$) identified and quantified 7200 proteins, of which DTM significantly modulated the expression of 1222 proteins compared to 705 by LR stimulation, indicating a greater impact on restoring ionic homeostasis. Notably, DTMP upregulated key components of potassium regulation, such as Na^+/K^+ ATPase subunits, altered the expression of calcium-regulating proteins like VDAC1/2/3 and PMCA isoforms to reduce neuronal excitability, and increased GABA and glycine receptor levels to promote chloride influx and hyperpolarization. These findings suggest that DTM more effectively reverses the injury-induced disruptions in ion transport pathways, thereby reducing pain perception. Overall, this study underscored the potential of DTMP as a superior modality for reestablishing ionic balance in the spinal cord [13].

Finally, an animal study investigated the impact of DTM upon the mTOR pathway using proteomic and phosphoproteomic analyses [5]. The mTOR has been identified as playing a central role in the regulation of inflammation, protein synthesis, cellular metabolism and its dysregulation is implicated in a range of pathological conditions, including chronic pain. mTOR influences neuro-glial interactions by modulating transcription factors and kinases such as MAPK and NFkB, which are critical for the production of inflammatory mediators. This makes the mTOR pathway an attractive therapeutic target for managing neuropathic pain, as modulating its activity could help restore cellular balance and reduce pain hypersensitivity. In a spared injury model, rats were randomized to no-SCS ($N = 10$), DTM ($N = 10$), low rate ($N = 10$) and an uninjured ($N = 10$) group. Following stimulation for the DTM and LR arm, over 7000 proteins were identified, with 1451 and 705 demonstrating changes in response to DTM and LR, respectively ($P < .05$). 192 mTOR-related proteins were identified, with 49 found to be significantly affected in the analyses. DTM modified the expression of 25 proteins, while LR affected 8. Further, DTM led to 66% reversal of phosphorylation changes compared to 58% by low rate. This differential modulation suggests that DTM may harness additional pathways for pain relief through targeted molecular actions rather than being limited to disrupting pain transmission [5].

Preclinical differential targeted multiplexed endurance

Amid growing interest in a recharge-free system that minimizes charge burden, Vallejo et al. examined pain relief using a reduced-energy differential target multiplexed (RE-DTM) stimulation setting. In a similar spared nerve injury model, rats were split into five groups: naive, no-SCS, DTM-RE1, DTM-RE2, and LR. Following SNI, the rats had 48 h of continuous stimulation, while the naive group underwent sham stimulation. Mechanical sensitivity was measured before SNI, before SCS, and after SCS. DTM-RE1 and DTM-RE2 both achieved superior improvements from their preinjury withdrawal threshold in comparison to the no-SCS and LR groups.

Spinal cord sections from the ipsilateral side of stimulation were subjected to RNA sequencing. Bioinformatic analyses demonstrated that DTM-RE provided reversal of expression of genes in neuroinflammation in significantly larger extent toward naïve expression compared to LR, shifting them toward a nonpainful state [6].

Evidence supporting DTM SCS

Multiple randomized controlled trials (RCTs) have shown the effectiveness of using differential target multiplexed (DTM) waveforms to deliver significant pain relief. The first groundbreaking study was the DTM RCT published by Dr. Fishman in 2021 [14]. This prospective, postmarket RCT compares DTM SCS with traditional SCS in treating chronic low back and leg pain. Patients were randomly assigned to these two groups and were followed for up to 12 months. The primary endpoint was the low back pain responder rate at 3 months. A total of 128 patients across 12 centers were enrolled in the study. 67 patients received DTM SCS, while 61 patients received traditional SCS. At the 3-month mark, the low back pain responder rate (defined as a reduction of ≥50%) was 80.1% in the DTM group and 51.2% in the traditional SCS group. The mean reduction in low back pain in the DTM group was 5.36 cm, compared to 3.37 cm in the traditional SCS group. These results were sustained at 6 and 12 months [14].

More recently, Gulve et al. published a UK cost-effectiveness analysis comparing DTM SCS, conventional SCS, and conservative medical management to treat chronic intractable low back pain over a 15-year follow-up period [15]. They found that DTM SCS was the most cost-effective option for payers with a cost-effectiveness ratio (ICER) of £6101 per QALY gained (incremental net benefit [INB] = £21,281), higher than conventional SCS (INB = £8551), and conventional medical management [15].

The second DTM RCT focused on chronic refractory axial low back pain not eligible for spine surgery (PSPS 1) [14]. This is a prospective, postmarket RCT across 20 centers in the U.S. Patients were randomized to either DTM SCS or conventional SCS and were followed up to 12 months. The primary endpoint was the responder rate at 3-month postimplant. An optional crossover was available at 6 months. Among 121 patients, the responder rate in the DTM SCS was 93.5% compared to the conventional SCS group (36.4%). The mean reduction in pain in the DTM SCS group was 6.52 cm compared to the conventional SCS group of 3.01 cm. The study also showed that DTM SCS provided significant leg pain reduction, improved overall quality of life and disability, better patient satisfaction, and global impression of change [16].

More recently, Kallaward JW et al., presented 24-month results of the first prospective, multicenter, multinational, randomized control trial comparing conventional medical management with DTM –SCS for patients with PSPS 1. Subjects were randomized in a 1:1 ratio to the test and control arms. The primary endpoint was the percentage of subjects reporting ≥50% reduction of VAS for chronic low back pain at 6 months. A superiority test compared the responder rate in both groups. Other reported outcomes include leg pain, functional disability, quality of life (QOL), patient satisfaction and global impression of change. A composite responder index was analyzed using CLBP, disability and QOL. Overall, DTM was superior with a responder rate of ≥80% with a >5.6 cm reduction (70% reduction) through the 24 months follow up. The CRI was 80% for DTM for DTM-SCS through the 24 months. An important consideration of the RCTs is the reproducibility of outcomes in selected patients with CLBP with or without previous surgery.

A third DTM study focused on using DTM to treat chronic, intractable upper limb pain. This prospective, open-label, single-arm study's primary endpoint was the percentage of responders to treatment 3 months after device activation [17]. 58 patients across 11 sites in the U.S. were enrolled. 47 patients were assessed at the primary endpoint. The responder rate was 92% at 3 months, and the result was consistent at 6 months (91%) and 12 months (86%). The VAS reduction at the primary endpoint was 81%. The study also shows significant improvement in disability and high patient satisfaction [17–19].

References

[1] Vallejo R, Tilley DM, Vogel L, Benyamin R. The role of glia and the immune system in the development and maintenance of neuropathic pain. Pain Pract 2010;10(3):167–84. https://doi.org/10.1111/j.1533-2500.2010.00367.x.

[2] Ruiz-Sauri A, Orduña-Valls JM, Blasco-Serra A, Tornero-Tornero C, Cedeño DL, Bejarano-Quisoboni D, Valverde-Navarro AA, Benyamin R, Vallejo R. Glia to neuron ratio in the posterior aspect of the human spinal cord at thoracic segments relevant to spinal cord stimulation. J Anat 2019;235(5):997–1006. https://doi.org/10.1111/joa.13061.

[3] Milligan ED, Watkins LR. Pathological and protective roles of glia in chronic pain. Nat Rev Neurosci 2009;10(1):23–36. https://doi.org/10.1038/nrn2533.

[4] Vallejo R, Cedeño D. The quest for neurobiological mechanisms of electrical stimulation of the spinal cord to reduce chronic neuropathic pain. Bioelectron Med 2020;2. https://doi.org/10.2217/bem-2020-0003.

[5] Cedeno DL, Tilley DM, Vetri F, Platt DC, Vallejo R. Proteomic and phosphoproteomic changes of MAPK-related inflammatory response in an animal model of neuropathic pain by differential target multiplexed SCS and low-rate SCS. J Pain Res 2022;15:895–907. https://doi.org/10.2147/JPR.S348738.

[6] Tilley DM, Cedeño DL, Vetri F, Platt DC, Vallejo R. Differential target multiplexed spinal cord stimulation programming modulates proteins involved in ion regulation in an animal model of neuropathic pain. Mol Pain 2022;18:17448069211060181. https://doi.org/10.1177/17448069211060181.

[7] Lee HU, Blasiak A, Agrawal DR, Loong DTB, Thakor NV, All AH, Ho JS, Yang IH. Subcellular electrical stimulation of neurons enhances the myelination of axons by oligodendrocytes. PLoS One 2017;12(7):e0179642. https://doi.org/10.1371/journal.pone.0179642.

[8] Guthrie PB, Knappenberger J, Segal M, Bennett MV, Charles AC, Kater SB. ATP released from astrocytes mediates glial calcium waves. J Neurosci 1999;19(2):520–8. https://doi.org/10.1523/JNEUROSCI.19-02-00520.1999.

[9] Agnesi F, Blaha CD, Lin J, Lee KH. Local glutamate release in the rat ventral lateral thalamus evoked by high-frequency stimulation. J Neural Eng 2010;7(2):26009. https://doi.org/10.1088/1741-2560/7/2/026009.

[10] Vallejo R, Gupta A, Kelley CA, Vallejo A, Rink J, Williams JM, Cass CL, Smith WJ, Benyamin R, Cedeño DL. Effects of phase polarity and charge balance spinal cord stimulation on behavior and gene expression in a rat model of neuropathic pain. Neuromodulation January 2020;23 (1):26–35. https://doi.org/10.1111/ner.12964.

[11] Vallejo R, Kelley CA, Gupta A, Smith WJ, Vallejo A, Cedeño DL. *Modulation of neuroglial interactions using differential target multiplexed spinal cord stimulation in an animal model of neuropathic pain. Mol Pain* 16, doi: 10.1177/1744806920918057.

[12] Smith WJ, Cedeño DL, Thomas SM, Kelley CA, Vetri F, Vallejo R. Modulation of microglial activation states by spinal cord stimulation in an animal model of neuropathic pain: comparing high rate, low rate, and differential target multiplexed programming. Mol Pain 2021;17:1744806921999013. https://doi.org/10.1177/1744806921999013.

[13] Cedeno DL, Smith WJ, Kelley CA, Vallejo R. Spinal cord stimulation using differential target multiplexed programming modulates neural cell-specific transcriptomes in an animal model of neuropathic pain. Mol Pain 2020;16:1744806920964360. https://doi.org/10.1177/1744806920964360.

[14] Tilley DM, Vallejo R, Vetri F, Platt DC, Cedeno DL. Activation of neuroinflammation via mTOR pathway is disparately regulated by differential target multiplexed and traditional low-rate spinal cord stimulation in a neuropathic pain model. J Pain Res 2022;15:2857–66. https://doi.org/10.2147/JPR.S378490.

[15] Vallejo R, Cedeno DL, Platt DC et al. *Differential target multiplexed SCS using reduced energy parameters in an animal model of neuropathic pain. NANS mid-year 2021 poster presentation. Orlando, Finland* (2021).

[16] Fishman M, Cordner H, Justiz R, Provenzano D, Merrell C, Shah B, Naranjo J, Kim P, Calodney A, Carlson J, Bundschu R, Sanapati M, Mangal V, Vallejo R. Twelve-Month results from multicenter, open-label, randomized controlled clinical trial comparing differential target multiplexed spinal cord stimulation and traditional spinal cord stimulation in subjects with chronic intractable back pain and leg pain. Pain Pract 2021;21(8):912–23.

[17] Gulve A, Mehta V, Provenzano DA, Eggington S, Scheffler S, Gasquet NC, Ricker CN. Differential target multiplexed spinal cord stimulation: A UK cost-effectiveness analysis. Neuromodulation 2024;27(5):908–15.

[18] White T, Justiz R, Almonte W, et al. 12-Month results from a randomized controlled trial comparing differential target multiplexed spinal cord stimulation and conventional spinal cord stimulation in subjects with chronic refractory axial low back pain not eligible for spine surgery. N Am Spine Soc J 2024:100528.

[19] White T, Justiz R, Fishman M, Schultz D, Calodney A, Cordner H, Almonte W, Millet Y, Wu K, Gekht G, Will A, Kim P, Bundschu R, Sirianni J, El-Naggar A, Gupta M, Park W, Cedeño DL, Vallejo R. Differential target multiplexed spinal cord stimulation for the treatment of chronic intractable upper limb pain: 12-month results from a prospective, Multicenter Study. Neuromodulation. 2024;24(24):S1094–7159.

Chapter 22

New waveform concepts for spinal cord stimulation

Vinicius Tieppo Francio[1], Lucas Bracero[2], Marco Lawandy[3], Daniel Pak[4], Marc Russo[5] and Mitsukuni Yoshida[1]

[1]*Division of Pain Medicine, Department of Anesthesiology, Washington University School of Medicine, St. Louis MO, United States;* [2]*The Spine and Nerve Centers of the Virginias, Charleston, WV, United States;* [3]*Department of Physical Medicine & Rehabilitation, Montefiore Medical Center, Bronx NY, United States;* [4]*Pain Medicine Division, University of Texas Health Science Center at Houston, Houston, TX, United States;* [5]*Hunter Pain Specialists, Broadmeadow, Australia*

Introduction and historical context of spinal cord stimulation waveforms

Spinal cord stimulation (SCS) has undergone a remarkable evolution since its inception, with advancements in waveform technology playing a pivotal role in enhancing clinical efficacy and expanding its application to novel indications. Initially developed as a tonic low-frequency stimulation modality, early SCS systems operated within the 40–100 Hz range, relying on paresthesia-based mechanisms to modulate pain perception. While effective for some patients, the reliance on paresthesia as a therapeutic endpoint introduced challenges, including sensory discomfort, variability in patient response, and complexities in optimal programming [1,2]. The evolution of SCS has been marked by groundbreaking technological advancements that extend beyond traditional paresthesia-based stimulation. Key developments include the introduction of novel waveforms, miniaturization of devices, enhanced stimulation programming capabilities, refined surgical techniques, and the advent of closed-loop stimulation. These innovations have not only broadened treatment options but have also improved efficacy by engaging distinct neurophysiological pathways and optimizing therapy based on patient-specific factors [2–4].

Recent advancements in SCS therapy have further leveraged artificial intelligence (AI) and biomarker-driven modulation to enhance precision and therapeutic effectiveness. AI-assisted programming has emerged as a valuable tool in optimizing parameter selection, reducing the trial-and-error approach, and improving long-term clinical outcomes. Additionally, the integration of objective biomarkers, such as electrophysiological and neurochemical signals, enables real-time adaptive modulation, facilitating a more personalized and responsive neuromodulation strategy. These advancements hold significant potential in addressing inherent variability in patient response and reducing the likelihood of treatment failures [4–6]. The continued evolution of SCS therapy is essential to meet the increasing complexity of chronic pain management and address the diverse needs of the patient population. In an era where the scientific foundation of interventional pain management is under constant scrutiny, advancing SCS technology remains a crucial endeavor in ensuring improved patient outcomes, sustained therapeutic efficacy, and broader acceptance within the medical community.

Fundamental parameters of spinal cord stimulation

The effectiveness of spinal cord stimulation (SCS) is determined by several key parameters, including frequency, pulse width, amplitude, pulse pairing, current/voltage, and impedance [7]. Table 22.1 summarize these concepts. In conventional tonic SCS, the primary adjustable parameters include electrode selection, stimulation frequency, pulse width, and amplitude [8]. Optimizing these parameters requires a sophisticated understanding of neurophysiological mechanisms and an individualized approach to patient care. The ability to fine-tune these variables allows clinicians to tailor therapy for

A Modern Atlas for Implantable Devices of the Spine, Brain, and Nerve. https://doi.org/10.1016/B978-0-443-36528-7.00047-9

TABLE 22.1 Summary of fundamental parameters and clinical implications.

Parameter	Definition	Clinical implication
Frequency	Number of electrical pulses delivered per second (Hz), influencing neural fiber activation.	Low-frequency SCS (40–100 Hz) activates A-beta fibers and dorsal horn inhibitory neurons; high-frequency SCS (>1 kHz) provides broader activation with potential paresthesia-free effects.
Pulse width	Duration of each electrical pulse (¬μs), affecting charge delivery and neural recruitment.	Shorter pulse widths activate larger fibers with reduced energy consumption; longer pulse widths recruit smaller fibers and expand paresthesia coverage.
Amplitude	Intensity of stimulation (V or mA), determining neural engagement and paresthesia strength.	Lower amplitudes engage superficial fibers for targeted pain relief; higher amplitudes increase paresthesia intensity but may cause discomfort or motor activation.
Pulse pairing	Delivery of multiple pulses in rapid succession to mimic physiological firing patterns.	Enhances analgesia by leveraging temporal summation; optimizes neural selectivity and reduces habituation.
Current and voltage	Current (mA) is the rate of charge flow; voltage (V) drives current through neural tissue.	Constant current (CC) adjusts voltage for stable activation, preferred for consistent effects; constant voltage (CV) maintains fixed voltage but allows variable current.
Impedance	Resistance to electrical flow in the SCS system, affecting efficiency and energy consumption.	High impedance requires greater voltage and may indicate poor electrode contact; low impedance suggests excessive current flow, risking overstimulation and battery depletion.
Duty cycle	Proportion of time that electrical stimulation is actively delivered to the spinal cord within a given stimulation period.	May influence both therapeutic efficacy and device longevity, since a higher duty cycle may enhance pain relief, yet it can also accelerate battery depletion and tolerance.

maximum analgesic benefit. A thorough understanding of the interrelationship among frequency, pulse width, amplitude, pulse pairing, current/voltage, and impedance is essential for refining SCS therapy. Through careful parameter adjustment, clinicians can achieve precise neuromodulation, enhance energy efficiency, and mitigate adverse effects, ultimately improving patient outcomes in the management of chronic pain. Figs. 22.1 and 22.2

Frequency

Frequency, measured in Hertz (Hz), denotes the number of electrical pulses delivered per second and plays a crucial role in determining the type and response of neural fibers to stimulation. Conventional SCS typically operates within the 40–100 Hz range, primarily activating A-beta fibers in the dorsal columns, which, in turn, engage inhibitory interneurons in the dorsal horn to modulate pain transmission. This approach is associated with a paresthesia-based mechanism and relatively low energy consumption [9–11]. Higher-frequency SCS (>1 kHz) results in broader neuronal recruitment, enhancing analgesic effects while also increasing the risk of unwanted sensory or motor activation [12]. Notably, 10 kHz SCS achieves pain relief without inducing paresthesia by directly modulating inhibitory interneurons in the dorsal horn without dorsal column activation [10,11,13].

Pulse width

Pulse width, measured in microseconds (μs), defines the duration of each electrical pulse and influences the charge delivered per amplitude. Shorter pulse widths preferentially activate large, fast-conducting A-beta fibers while minimizing off-target effects such as motor activation or discomfort. These shorter durations also improve spatial selectivity and optimize energy efficiency by reducing battery consumption [14]. In contrast, longer pulse widths (≥200 μs) enhance recruitment of smaller-diameter fibers, potentially expanding paresthesia coverage in a caudal direction due to the somatotopic organization of the dorsal columns [15]. However, longer pulse widths necessitate increased energy consumption, a factor mitigated by the advent of rechargeable implantable pulse generators (IPGs) [11].

Amplitude

Amplitude, expressed in volts (V) or milliamperes (mA), dictates the intensity of stimulation and the extent of neural recruitment. Lower amplitudes primarily engage superficial nerve fibers, offering targeted pain relief with minimal side effects. Conversely, higher amplitudes increase paresthesia intensity by recruiting deeper spinal structures but may inadvertently activate motor fibers, leading to discomfort or involuntary muscle contractions. Higher amplitude settings also elevate energy demands, potentially reducing battery longevity. Emerging evidence suggests that high-frequency and burst waveforms achieve effective analgesia at lower amplitudes compared to tonic SCS, thereby offsetting their inherently greater energy requirements [16–18].

Pulse pairing

Pulse pairing involves delivering multiple pulses in rapid succession, often structured into specific patterns designed to mimic physiological neuronal firing. This strategy is fundamental to advanced stimulation paradigms such as burst SCS, where high-frequency pulse trains (500–800 Hz) leverage temporal summation to enhance analgesic effects at lower amplitudes than tonic stimulation [19]. Optimizing pulse pairing parameters, including inter-pulse interval and burst

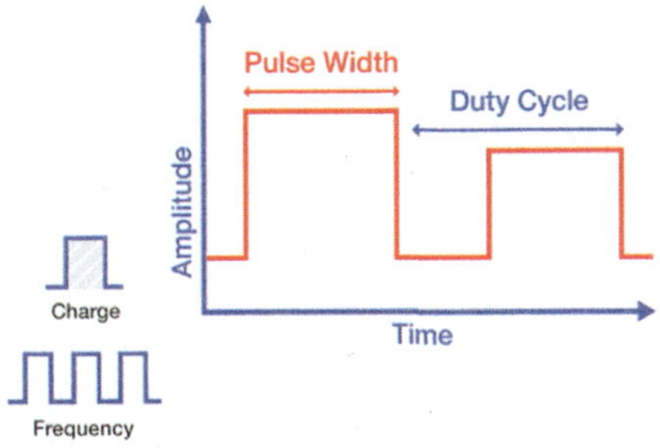

FIGURE 22.1 Key stimulation parameters in spinal cord stimulation. *Image created by Tieppo Francio, modified from Miller [9].*

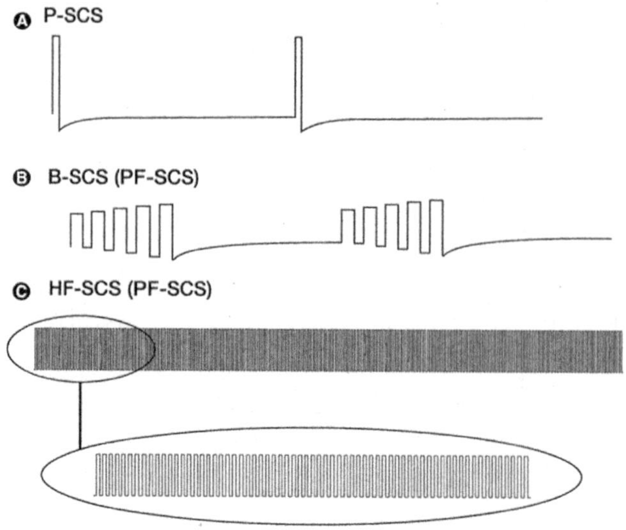

FIGURE 22.2 Stimulation patterns in paresthesia versus paresthesia-free spinal cord stimulation. (a) Traditional tonic stimulation, (b) Burst with an inter-burst stimulation; (c) High-frequency (10 kHz) stimulation without paresthesia. *Image from Miller [9], public domain CC BY.*

configuration, may improve neural selectivity and mitigate tolerance or habituation to therapy. Additionally, pulse pairing has been shown to modulate distinct cortical and subcortical pain-processing centers, differentiating its mechanism from conventional SCS [16,19].

Current and voltage

Current (mA) represents the rate of electrical charge flow, while voltage (V) reflects the driving force propelling this current through neural tissue. Clinically, SCS systems operate using either constant current (CC) or constant voltage (CV) paradigms. CC stimulation maintains a stable current by dynamically adjusting voltage in response to impedance fluctuations, ensuring consistent neural activation. This approach has been associated with improved patient preference and enhanced pain relief during the trial phase [20]]. In contrast, CV stimulation delivers a fixed voltage, leading to variable current levels in response to impedance changes, which may result in inconsistent neural recruitment [9]. While CC stimulation is generally favored for its reliability, the optimal modality remains an area of ongoing investigation.

Impedance

Impedance, defined by Ohm's law as the ratio of voltage to current, governs the resistance encountered by electrical flow within the SCS system. High impedance necessitates greater voltage to maintain effective stimulation, potentially compromising therapy efficiency and increasing energy consumption. Conversely, low impedance facilitates energy-efficient stimulation but may indicate excessive current flow, raising concerns about overstimulation and accelerated battery depletion. Real-time impedance monitoring during lead placement aids in optimizing electrode positioning within the epidural space. Excessively high impedance often suggests posterior lead placement within epidural fat, while excessively low impedance may indicate proximity to the spinal cord, increasing the risk of overstimulation [21,22]. The advent of MRI-conditional SCS systems has introduced an additional layer of complexity, as some devices require impedance within a predefined range to maintain MRI compatibility. Recent innovations in lead insulation have led to the development of impedance-independent MRI-conditional systems, which preserve compatibility irrespective of impedance fluctuations [23]. Ongoing impedance surveillance remains essential for maintaining lead integrity, assessing therapy effectiveness, and preemptively identifying potential device malfunctions, such as lead fractures, migration, or epidural fibrosis.

Duty cycle

Duty cycle refers to the proportion of time that electrical stimulation is actively delivered to the spinal cord within a given stimulation period. Expressed as a percentage, it reflects the ratio of time when current is actively being delivered to the total cycle duration, including "on and off" intervals. This is a critical parameter that may influences both therapeutic efficacy and device longevity, since a higher duty cycle may enhance pain relief by sustaining neuromodulatory effects, particularly in patients with high-frequency or burst stimulation paradigms, yet it can also accelerate battery depletion and increase the risk of stimulation-induced tolerance [9,24–26].

Open-loop spinal cord stimulation waveforms

Dorsal column SCS delivers epidural analgesia by modulating pain transmission at the spinal cord level. This technique primarily activates large-diameter Aβ fibers in the dorsal column, which subsequently engage inhibitory interneurons in the dorsal horn. This interaction suppresses nociceptive signaling via wide dynamic range (WDR) neurons, effectively reducing pain perception [27–29]. The foundational mechanism of SCS is based on the gate control theory, first proposed by Melzack and Wall, which posits that stimulation of non-nociceptive afferents can inhibit nociceptive transmission at the spinal cord level [29–32]. More recent research has identified additional mechanisms, including the modulation of inhibitory neurotransmitters such as gamma-aminobutyric acid (GABA) and the activation of supraspinal pathways, further refining the understanding of SCS-induced analgesia [28,32,33].

Traditional spinal cord stimulation

Traditional open-loop SCS operates with fixed stimulation parameters that do not dynamically adjust to physiological variations. While widely used, this system lacks adaptability to changes in spinal cord-electrode distance caused by movement, potentially leading to inconsistent pain relief [27]. Consequently, postural changes such as spine flexion-extension or sitting-standing can alter the stimulation intensity. With fixed output stimulation, patients may experience discomfort from overstimulation due to these positional shifts. To mitigate discomfort, patients often underdose their therapy, ultimately reducing overall efficacy and potentially leading to SCS explant [34–37]. Moreover, open-loop therapies typically may necessitate frequent clinical appointments for parameter adjustments, where patients are often lost to follow up and do not optimize the therapy. In contrast, closed-loop SCS utilizes real-time evoked compound action potential (ECAP)-based feedback to continuously modulate stimulation intensity. This adaptive approach maintains stable neural recruitment, optimizing therapeutic efficacy while reducing the need for frequent manual reprogramming [28,32,33,38,39]. By automatically adjusting stimulation parameters in response to neural activity, closed-loop SCS may enhance pain relief and minimizes variability in patient outcomes, representing a significant advancement in neuromodulatory therapy [27,28,32,33,38,39]. The ability to record ECAPs in real time provides an objective measure of neural engagement, allowing clinicians to fine-tune stimulation parameters for individualized therapy optimization [27,28].

Modern waveform paradigms

The technological evolution of SCS has led to multiple waveform paradigms, each designed to optimize pain relief while minimizing adverse effects. Tonic SCS operates at frequencies between 40 and 100 Hz, continuously activating Aβ fibers and relying on paresthesia to achieve analgesia in accordance with the gate control theory [31,32,40,41]. High-frequency (10 kHz) SCS provides paresthesia-free analgesia by modulating pain signaling at the dorsal horn without directly engaging WDR neurons. Additionally, intermittent pulse dosing (15%–25% duty cycle) can be used to reduce energy consumption and mitigate neural adaptation [28,32,33]. BurstDR SCS delivers bursts of five pulses at an intraburst frequency of 500 Hz and an interburst frequency of 40 Hz. By engaging both sensory and affective pain processing pathways, BurstDR SCS mimics medial and lateral thalamic firing patterns to enhance analgesia and cortical modulation [31,41–45]. A variant, MicroBurst 360, employs ultra-short pulses and low duty cycles to optimize energy efficiency while maintaining sub-perception modulation. Differential Target Multiplexed (DTM) SCS targets neuroglial interactions by delivering multiplexed waveforms with variable frequency, pulse width, and voltage. This enhances pain relief by modulating both neuronal and glial activity [2,5,28,31,46,47]. Additionally, Inceptiv technology integrates AdaptivStim, which dynamically adjusts stimulation based on real-time posture sensing and can be combined with DTM if desired. Fast-Acting Sub-perception Therapy (FAST) SCS leverages surround inhibition principles to selectively activate inhibitory interneurons and WDR neurons, using a proprietary algorithm to minimize central excitatory responses and provide rapid analgesic effects [2,32,46]. These advancements in waveform technology continue to refine the clinical application of SCS, offering more personalized and effective strategies for managing chronic pain. Table 22.2 summarizes key features of open loop SCS waveforms and Table 22.3 summarizes key level I landmark studies in neuromodulation.

TABLE 22.2 Open-loop spinal cord stimulation waveforms key features.

Feature	Low frequency	High-frequency (10) kHz	BurstDR	DTM	FAST
Mechanism of action	Activates Aβ fibers, inhibits WDR neurons	Paresthesia-free modulation of dorsal horn activity	Mimics burst firing, targets sensory and affective pathways	Targets neurons and glial cells for pain modulation	Uses low frequency sub perception stimulation to activate inhibitory interneurons
Paresthesia	Dependent	Independent	Variable	Independent	Independent

TABLE 22.3 Key level I landmark studies in spinal cord stimulation.

Waveform	Study name and year	Study design	Patient population and indication	Objective	Key findings
Tonic low-frequency	[48,49] (EVIDENCE trial)	Multicenter crossover Randomized clinical trial	Neuropathic radicular leg pain and back pain after failed back surgery	Comparison of tonic SCS versus re-operation	SCS was more successful and effective than reoperation for failed back surgery syndrome
10 kHz high frequency	[50] (SENZA trial)	Multicenter Prospective Randomized clinical trial	Chronic back and leg pain, failed back surgery syndrome	Comparison of 10 kHz SCS versus tonic SCS	HF10 SCS was superior in providing back and leg pain relief compared to tonic SCS. HF10 provided 84.5% response for back pain and 83.1% response for leg pain while tonic SCS provided 43.8% response for back pain and 55.5% response for leg pain.
BurstDR SCS	[42] (SUNBURST trial)	Prospective, Crossover Randomized clinical trial	Chronic pain syndromes including failed back surgery syndrome	Comparison of BurstDR versus tonic SCS effectiveness in pain relief and patient preference	Burst SCS resulted in significantly greater pain relief and was preferred by 70.8% of patients over tonic SCS. Burst SCS provided superior outcomes in both sensory and affective pain modulation.
DTM SCS	[46]	Prospective Randomized clinical trial	Chronic low back pain and leg pain.	Comparison of DTM SCS to tonic SCS	DTM SCS had a greater low back pain responder rate than tonic SCS, 80.1% versus 51.2%, respectively. Mean pain reduction was greater with DTM SCS than tonic SCS, 5.36 versus 3.37 cm, respectively.
Closed-loop SCS ECAP	[27] (EVOKE)	Multicenter Double-blind Randomized clinical trial	Chronic trunk and limb pain	Open-loop SCS versus closed-loop SCS	Closed-loop SCS maintains optimal and stable activation of the spinal cord. Closed-loop SCS uses feedback from the spinal cord to adjust stimulation while open-loop SCS does not. Closed-loop ECAP-controlled SCS modulates the stimulation delivered in real time.
Open versus **closed loop**	[39] (ECHO-MAC) [21]	Multicenter prospective Single-blind randomized clinical tria	Chronic back pain and leg pain	Open-loop SCS versus closed-loop SCS	97.6% of participants had a reduction in sensation in the closed-looped SCS group versus the open-loop SCS group. 88.1% of participants preferred closed-loop over open-loop SCS.

Closed-loop and biomarker based spinal cord stimulation waveforms

Evoked compound action potentials (ECAPs)

The emergence of electrophysiological biomarkers, particularly evoked compound action potentials (ECAPs), has significantly advanced the field of neuromodulation by introducing an objective and dynamic method for optimizing therapy. ECAPs quantify the electrophysiological responses elicited within dorsal column fibers upon electrical stimulation, reflecting the aggregated action potentials of numerous nerve fibers activated by each stimulation pulse [28]. By precisely measuring the neural recruitment of Aβ-fibers within the dorsal columns, ECAPs offer immediate and quantifiable feedback, thereby elucidating the direct relationship between applied spinal stimulation and resultant neural activation. Extensive research has validated the utility of ECAP recordings across various experimental models, including rodents, sheep, and humans, underscoring their reliability and potential as objective biomarkers for optimizing SCS parameters [6,51–53]. Compared to traditional open-loop programming approaches, ECAP-based titration has demonstrated enhanced stability and consistency in the recruitment of dorsal column fibers. Furthermore, the integration of ECAP measurements into automated feedback systems has facilitated the evolution of closed-loop spinal cord stimulation. These advanced systems dynamically adjust stimulation parameters in real time, ensuring consistent and optimal neural engagement. This adaptive approach aims to enhance therapeutic outcomes, extend therapy longevity, and improve patient comfort and overall experience [54].

The epidural space represents a dynamic physiological environment, subject to continual fluctuations arising from spinal movements and alterations in cerebrospinal fluid dynamics, thereby influencing the relationship between epidural leads, energy delivery, and their neural targets [33,55,56]. Traditional spinal cord stimulation (SCS) systems, utilizing fixed-output (open-loop) paradigms, fail to accommodate these inherent physiological variances. This shortcoming frequently results in suboptimal neural activation, manifesting as under- or overstimulation, increased necessity for frequent device reprogramming, and potential habituation leading to diminished therapeutic efficacy. Although subperception waveforms have partially addressed these limitations, they do not fully resolve the fundamental challenge of achieving stable, consistent, and therapeutically effective neural recruitment [34–37]. The introduction of ECAP-guided closed-loop SCS represents a significant advancement by enabling continuous sensing and adaptive modulation of stimulation parameters to maintain optimal neural activation [6,33,57]. Neural activation in dorsal column neuromodulation encompasses the spinal cord's physiological responses to targeted electrical stimulation, specifically affecting dorsal column fibers, inhibitory interneurons, microglial activity, and elements within the medial and lateral thalamic pain pathways. Consistent and stable neural activation is imperative for achieving durable analgesic outcomes in epidural pain management. ECAPs serve as direct and objective biomarkers of neural activation and are integral to closed-loop SCS, facilitating precise therapy optimization [6]. The magnitude of the ECAP signal correlates directly with the extent of dorsal column neural activation: larger ECAP signals suggest excessive neural recruitment, smaller signals indicate insufficient therapeutic activation, and optimal ECAP amplitudes reflect ideal neural dosing. By defining a targeted ECAP amplitude, closed-loop systems dynamically monitor and adjust stimulation output in real-time, responding appropriately to physiological changes and ensuring consistent therapeutic neural activation [33,57].

Therapeutic dosing

Therapeutic dosing in closed-loop SCS can be quantitatively assessed using the therapy dose ratio, defined as the current ECAP amplitude divided by the established ECAP threshold. This ratio facilitates the creation of dose-response curves, or objective neural activation plots. Empirical evidence identifies a dose ratio between 1.3 and 1.4 as optimal for pain relief, minimizing the necessity for frequent device reprogramming. Deviations from this therapeutic range suggest either suboptimal or excessive dosing, necessitating programming refinements or reevaluation of patient candidacy [33,58]. Real-world evidence further indicates variability in mean therapeutic dose ratios based upon pain etiology and spinal implant location. Specifically, cervical electrode placements have demonstrated steeper activation curves and heightened neural sensitivity. Studies have demonstrated that adherence to a neural dosing regimen, characterized by a neural dose accuracy of approximately 2.8 μV and a targeted dose ratio of 1.4, results in substantial clinical improvements, achieving maximal analgesic outcomes. This underscores the critical role of closed-loop ECAP monitoring in establishing evidence-based neural dosing, enabling optimized clinical efficacy, adherence monitoring, and comprehensive management of patients undergoing SCS therapy [33,57,58].

Closed-loop spinal cord stimulation systems

Closed-loop SCS represents a substantial advancement within the field of neuromodulation. As of 2024, two commercially available closed-loop SCS systems are prominent: the Saluda Evoke and Medtronic Inceptiv. Both systems utilize ECAP to optimize therapeutic efficacy, though each employs distinct methodologies for implementing closed-loop control. Given their novelty, randomized controlled trials directly comparing distinctive closed-loop SCS systems remain lacking. However, insights have emerged from the ECHO-MAC study, which assessed patient experiences concerning overstimulation using ECAP-based closed-loop versus conventional open-loop SCS systems. This study revealed that 97.6% of patients reported decreased sensations of overstimulation with closed-loop stimulation. Furthermore, a substantial majority (88.1%) expressed a preference for closed-loop SCS over the traditional open-loop system, with only 11.9% favoring the latter [39].

The Saluda Evoke system was the first closed-loop SCA platform commercially introduced in the United States, engineered specifically to modulate stimulation dynamically in real-time utilizing ECAP feedback. Subsequently, Medtronic introduced the Inceptiv system as the second commercially available closed-loop SCS technology. The Medtronic closed-loop platform integrates seamlessly with their preexisting waveform ecosystem, including compatibility with subperception DTM therapy. This advanced system employs positional sensors, specifically accelerometers, to detect changes in patient posture, along with intermittent ECAP measurements, facilitating adaptive adjustments in stimulation. These capabilities aim to mitigate overstimulation and under stimulation during positional shifts by limiting stimulation intensity according to predetermined ECAP thresholds. Employing a proprietary closed-loop algorithm, the Medtronic Inceptiv system continuously monitors neural responses at a frequency of 50 measurements per second, totaling 3000 measurements per minute. The stimulation intensity automatically increases upon detection of decreased neural responses and decreases correspondingly when neural activity is elevated. However, as outlined by the manufacturer, ECAP sensing signals may not always be measurable in every clinical scenario [59] https://www.medtronic.com/content/dam/medtronic-wide/public/united-states/products/neurological/inceptiv-hcp-brochure.pdf.

In contrast, Saluda's EVOKE closed-loop SCS technology continuously auto-adjusts energy delivery on a pulse-by-pulse basis, achieving adjustments over four million times per day. These real-time modifications are guided by measurable electrically ECAPs and positional changes, thereby sustaining consistent neural activation within a precisely defined therapeutic window. Should the amplitude of stimulation deviate from the targeted therapeutic range, the system instantly adapts within milliseconds to maintain optimal energy delivery [33]. By continuously monitoring dorsal column neural activation, this closed-loop system enhances therapeutic precision by eliminating risks associated with overstimulation or under-stimulation, both at rest and during positional transitions. Consequently, it ensures a stable and durable therapeutic dose response and maintains dorsal column activation consistently within the ECAP-defined therapeutic parameters. The clinical efficacy of Saluda's closed-loop SCS technology was initially demonstrated through the AVALON and EVOKE studies. Notably, the EVOKE trial was groundbreaking as the first randomized, double-blinded, pivotal neuromodulation study to objectively measure spinal cord activation. This study provided robust level I clinical evidence supporting the superiority of closed-loop SCS over traditional open-loop approaches [27,60]. Follow-up data extending to 36 months further validated these findings, confirming sustained and clinically meaningful improvements in pain reduction, functional capacity, and quality-of-life indices [38,54,61]. These represents a significant advancement in neuromodulation technology, delivering biomarker-driven therapy that dynamically adapts to physiological variations. This capability to maintain uniform neural activation markedly reduces the risk of therapeutic habituation, lowers explantation rates, and optimizes the long-term effectiveness and sustainability of SCS therapy.

Cutting-edge developments

In addition to advancements in closed-loop SCS, several innovative technologies have recently emerged aiming to deliver personalized and durable neuromodulation outcomes. These cutting-edge developments incorporate artificial intelligence (AI)-driven programming, remote monitoring capabilities, and novel waveform strategies to optimize analgesia while concurrently reducing patient and clinician burdens.

Artificial intelligence (AI) integrated systems

In 2024, Nevro introduced the HFX AdaptivAI platform powered by HFXiQ, marking the first commercially available AI-enabled SCS system in the United States. This platform utilizes a proprietary algorithm informed by extensive data analytics, compiling over 500 daily data points across 187 variables, and aggregating more than 100 million data points from over 100,000 patients collected across a decade, supported by Level I clinical evidence. This sophisticated system seamlessly integrates AI-driven learning with real-time patient-reported outcome measures, enabling automatic, remote adjustment or recommendation of therapy settings. Moreover, the inclusion of bipole interlacing technology allows optimization of stimulation patterns directly informed by patient feedback captured via a manufacturer-provided mobile application, while cloud-based analytics continually refine individualized treatment recommendations [62] https://nevro.com/English/us/providers/Product-HFX-AdaptivAI/default.aspx.

Automated patient programming

In 2025, Saluda Evoke Automated Algorithm (EVA) received approval from the U.S. Food and Drug Administration (FDA). EVA employs a proprietary, biomarker-driven approach using ECAP assessments to objectively and autonomously optimize neural activation. By analyzing multi-point ECAP sensing across a tripolar lead configuration comprising 12 contacts that span four vertebral segments, EVA accurately determines individualized neural response patterns. This advanced automation minimizes programming variability, thereby enhancing consistency across clinical practices while empowering patients to actively participate in personalized therapy adjustments [63] https://www.prnewswire.com/news-releases/saluda-medical-receives-fda-approval-for-first-automated-programming-platform-in-scs-302359124.html.

Remote monitoring systems

The Biotronik Prospera SCS system introduces another distinct approach, prioritizing remote monitoring and proactive therapy management. Utilizing automated, daily remote monitoring, this system evaluates therapy adherence, system integrity, and patient-reported outcome data by capturing over 200 data points daily. Such comprehensive remote data collection allows clinicians to efficiently monitor patient progress and therapy optimization remotely, significantly reducing the necessity for frequent in-person clinical visits. This also features a proprietary multiphase stimulation approach termed Resonance, incorporating an advanced BioARC (Biotronik Advanced Return Current) charge-balancing mechanism. This system differs significantly from traditional single-phase stimulation methods, which necessitate periodic interruptions for passive charge balancing to prevent electrode and tissue injury. Instead, this employs sequential micro-pulse rotations across multiple electrodes, achieving dynamic, real-time charge balancing. The rapid rotation of micro-pulses, typically applied through tripolar or quadripolar electrode arrays, facilitates both temporal and spatial summation, potentially enhancing dorsal column fiber activation across multiple vertebral levels in a continuous stimulation pattern, thereby broadening therapeutic coverage and improving longevity of relief [64].

While these technologies represent significant innovations, head-to-head comparative studies remain lacking due to their novelty. Nonetheless, the advancements in remote monitoring, closed-loop neuromodulation, biomarker-guided interventions, and AI-driven therapy mark a transformative evolution within the field. These technological strides promise highly personalized, responsive, and sustained analgesic outcomes, substantially alleviating burdens on healthcare providers and patients alike. Consequently, they may contribute to enhanced therapy monitoring, improved patient adherence, and reduced rates of habituation and explantation.

Novel neural targets

High-density (HD) SCS represents a modification of traditional tonic stimulation designed to deliver a higher charge per second by increasing frequency and pulse width, without elevating amplitude beyond patient tolerance. This approach has been used to enhance dorsal column engagement in patients with limited response to conventional low-frequency SCS. Prior to the development of DTM SCS, *Medtronic* utilized an HD waveform characterized by high-frequency and subperception or low-perception amplitude settings. *Biotronik* later introduced a novel iteration of HD stimulation using a cascading bipolar configuration, in which active stimulation bipoles dynamically shift along the lead array to create a traveling stimulation field across the dorsal column. This design aims to broaden spatial recruitment, reduce neural habituation, and maintain therapeutic efficacy with minimal or no paresthesia [64]. These advancements reflect a broader trend in neuromodulation toward personalized, sub-perception therapies that optimize stimulation parameters and spatial targeting to improve patient outcomes.

Dorsal horn dendrite stimulation

The dorsal horn dendrite stimulation waveform was developed by one of the authors (MR) to selectively and preferentially target dendrites located along the lateral aspect of the dorsal horn, using a midline electrode placement in a paresthesia-free manner. Originally conceived as a theoretical counterpoint to dorsal column axonal stimulation, the waveform was subsequently translated into clinical practice as a salvage approach for patients with implanted neuromodulation systems who were refractory to conventional therapies. Encouraging clinical outcomes prompted an investigator-initiated trial, with 12-month results now published [65]. The waveform employs a gapped bipole configuration (cathode–off–anode) centered at the T9–T10 intervertebral disc space. Stimulation parameters include a frequency of 100 Hz, pulse width of 1000 μsec, and amplitude titrated in stages: 80% of the paresthesia perception threshold (PT) for the first month, followed by 60% and 40% in subsequent months, with patients ultimately selecting their preferred setting among these options. The chosen parameters are physiologically grounded, as dorsal horn dendrites are optimally responsive only at frequencies exceeding 75 Hz and pulse widths greater than 900 μsec? In the Russo et al. study, the 52-week responder rate—defined as ≥50% pain relief—was 66%, while the high responder rate (≥80% relief) reached 56%. The average reduction in pain intensity, measured by the visual analog scale (VAS), was 44 mm. Furthermore, 87% of participants achieved the minimum clinically important difference (MCID) in quality of life, as measured by the EQ-5D-5L index. Treatment satisfaction was reported by 83% of subjects, and 91% rated their global improvement as "much improved" or better on the Clinical Global Impression of Change (CGIC) scale. No serious study-related adverse events were observed [65]. Importantly, this novel waveform was released as open-source and remains unpatented. It is fully programmable across all currently available neuromodulation platforms, offering clinicians an additional tool to deliver personalized, precision-based care in spinal cord stimulation.

Pearls and pitfalls with novel spinal cord stimulation waveforms

Key considerations

As clinicians consider integrating SCS into their practice and the appropriate waveform to utilize, it is essential to evaluate several key factors to ensure optimal outcomes. These considerations include a thorough assessment of the patient's specific pain characteristics, an understanding of the underlying mechanisms of each waveform, and an evaluation of the available clinical evidence supporting their efficacy. Additionally, practical aspects such as energy consumption, device longevity, and the potential for remote programming should be considered to meet the individual needs of patients and enhance overall treatment effectiveness. As previously detailed, conventional paresthesia-based SCS paradigms have been used to treat various pain syndromes refractory to conventional medical management with significant improvements in pain, quality of life, and function. Non-responder rates, however, have been found to be particularly high in patients with predominantly axial low back pain, with up to 50% failing to achieve sustained 50% relief or more [66,67]. Furthermore, difficulty with tolerating paresthesia stimulation and/or undesirable paresthesias in other anatomical areas can make it a poor choice for many patients. Paresthesia-free approaches may therefore present a compelling alternative. Burst, high frequency, differential targeted multiplexed stimulation waveforms have demonstrated pain relief that is equivalent or superior to conventional tonic SCS and may offer a solution as a salvage therapy for those who have failed traditional stimulation [65]. Paresthesia-free waveforms are often preferred for neck and arm pain where cervical lead placement is required, as dynamic neck movement can cause variability in paresthesias. Paresthesia-free waveforms have also been found to be effective for other clinical indications, including painful diabetic neuropathy and nonsurgical refractory back pain [34,50]. By maintaining neural activation and spinal cord activation within a therapeutic window, closed-loop SCS can also avoid the pitfalls of traditional and high frequency stimulation paradigms, including under and overstimulation [34].

Optimizing device longevity

Higher energy demands and decreased device longevity can be seen with high frequency waveforms. Optimizing stimulation parameters such as utilizing pulse dosing or cycled stimulation paradigms can reduce this. Closed-loop SCS can additionally reduce unnecessary energy use to maintain consistent spinal cord activation as previously discussed. Other efforts have been made to utilize the lowest-effective stimulation dose to reduce recharge burden and extend battery life. Keeping patients within the therapeutic window and avoiding overstimulation may also help to combat the loss of SCS therapy and habituation over time, which can be achieved through closed-loop SCS and next-generation post-implant care strategies, including AI-driven personalization. SCS platforms that utilize AI algorithms, which can adjust stimulation parameters based on patient-specific inputs, and remote daily monitoring can allow patients to optimize their therapy without having to be seen for in-person device interrogations and reprogramming. This improves therapy accessibility for patients living in remote areas where frequent clinic visits for device optimization are not feasible.

Future directions

SCS continues to evolve with the aforementioned advancements in waveforms. However, the exact mechanism of action for each respective waveform and its efficacy compared to other novel waveforms remains unclear and requires additional investigation [31]. The emergence of wearable smart health devices has also generated interest within the neuromodulation community due to the ability to monitor daily physiological and biochemical changes. Efforts to integrate these technologies with SCS platforms remain ongoing. With advancements in clinical indications, hardware innovations, and the adoption of newer waveforms, SCS continues to be a vital tool for pain interventionists. Therefore, it is essential for practitioners to stay informed on the latest developments and adapt to the evolving needs of their patients.

References

[1] Viswanath O, Urits I, Bouley E, Peck JM, Thompson W, Kaye AD. Evolving spinal cord stimulation technologies and clinical implications in chronic pain management. Curr Pain Headache Rep 2019;23(6):39. https://doi.org/10.1007/s11916-019-0778-9.

[2] Malinowski MN, Chopra PR, Tieppo Francio V, Budwany R, Deer TR. A narrative review and future considerations of spinal cord stimulation, dorsal root ganglion stimulation and peripheral nerve stimulation. Curr Opin Anaesthesiol 2021;34(6):774–80. https://doi.org/10.1097/ACO.0000000000001072.

[3] Strand N, Tieppo Francio V, Murphy M, Turkiewicz M, El Helou A, Maita M, Covington S, Singh N, Wie C. Advances in pain medicine: A review of new technologies. Curr Pain Headache Rep 2022;26(8):605–16. https://doi.org/10.1007/s11916-022-01062-6.

[4] Ho JS, Poon C, North R, Grubb W, Lempka S, Bikson M. A visual and narrative timeline review of spinal cord stimulation technology and US food and drug administration milestones. Neuromodulation 2024;27(6):1020–5. https://doi.org/10.1016/j.neurom.2024.05.006.

[5] Chitneni A, Jain E, Sahni S, Mavrocordatos P, Abd-Elsayed A. Spinal cord stimulation waveforms for the treatment of chronic pain. Curr Pain Headache Rep 2024;28(7):595–605. https://doi.org/10.1007/s11916-024-01247-1.

[6] Muller L, Pope J, Verrills P, Petersen E, Kallewaard JW, Gould I, Karantonis DM. First evidence of a biomarker-based dose-response relationship in chronic pain using physiological closed-loop spinal cord stimulation. Reg Anesth Pain Med 2024. https://doi.org/10.1136/rapm-2024-105346.

[7] Deer TR, Jain S, Hunter C, Chakravarthy K. Neurostimulation for intractable chronic pain. Brain Sci 2019;9(2):23. https://doi.org/10.3390/brainsci9020023.

[8] Gordon AT, Zou SP, Kim Y, Gharibo C. Challenges to setting spinal cord stimulator parameters during intraoperative testing: Factors affecting coverage of low back and leg pain. Neuromodulation 2007;10(2):133–41. https://doi.org/10.1111/j.1525-1403.2007.00101.x.

[9] Miller JP, Eldabe S, Buchser E, Johanek LM, Guan Y, Linderoth B. Parameters of spinal cord stimulation and their role in electrical charge delivery: A review. Neuromodulation June 2016;19(4):373–84. https://doi.org/10.1111/ner.12438.

[10] Petersen EA. Spinal cord stimulation in painful diabetic neuropathy: An overview. Diabetes Res Clin Pract 2023;206(Suppl. 1):110760. https://doi.org/10.1016/j.diabres.2023.110760.

[11] Hatheway J, Yang M, Fishman M, Verdolin M, McJunkin T, Rosen S, Slee S, Kibler A, Amirdelfan K. Defining the boundaries of patient perception in spinal cord stimulation programming. Neuromodulation 2024;27(1):108–17. https://doi.org/10.1016/j.neurom.2023.08.011.

[12] Gmel GE, Santos Escapa R, Parker JL, Mugan D, Al-Kaisy A, Palmisani S. The effect of spinal cord stimulation frequency on the neural response and perceived sensation in patients with chronic pain. Front Neurosci 21, 2021;15:625835. https://doi.org/10.3389/fnins.2021.625835.

[13] Lee KY, Bae C, Lee D, Kagan Z, Bradley K, Chung JM, La JH. Low-intensity, kilohertz frequency spinal cord stimulation differently affects excitatory and inhibitory neurons in the rodent superficial dorsal horn. Neuroscience 2020;428:132–9. https://doi.org/10.1016/j.neuroscience.2019.12.031.

[14] Grill Jr WM, Mortimer JT. The effect of stimulus pulse duration on selectivity of neural stimulation. IEEE Trans Biomed Eng 1996;43(2):161–6. https://doi.org/10.1109/10.481985.

[15] Yearwood TL, Hershey B, Bradley K, Lee D. Pulse width programming in spinal cord stimulation: A clinical study. Pain Physician 2010;13(4):321–35.

[16] Chakravarthy K, Malayil R, Kirketeig T, Deer T. Burst spinal cord stimulation: A systematic review and pooled analysis of real-world evidence and outcomes data. Pain Med 2019;20(Suppl. 1):S47–57. https://doi.org/10.1093/pm/pnz046.

[17] Leong SL, De Ridder D, Deer T, Vanneste S. Potential therapeutic effect of low amplitude burst spinal cord stimulation on pain. Neuromodulation 2021;24(3):574–80. https://doi.org/10.1111/ner.13090.

[18] El-Naggar AO, Reis CL, Hatheway JA, Schmidt TE, Pico TC, Sanapati MR, Abd-Elsayed A, Patel AS, Calodney A, Johanek L, Tan Y, McCammon S. Using lower amplitudes to maintain effective high dose spinal cord stimulation therapy (SCS dosing pilot study). Neuromodulation 2021;24(3):532–9. https://doi.org/10.1111/ner.13258.

[19] Patil AS, Levasseur B, Gupta M. Neuromodulation and habituation: A literature review and conceptional analysis of sustaining therapeutic efficacy and mitigating habituation. Biomedicines 2024;12(5):930. https://doi.org/10.3390/biomedicines12050930.

[20] Washburn S, Catlin R, Bethel K, Canlas B. Patient-perceived differences between constant current and constant voltage spinal cord stimulation systems. Neuromodulation 2014;17(1):28–35. https://doi.org/10.1111/ner.12085.

[21] Alò K, Varga C, Krames E, Prager J, Holsheimer J, Manola L, Bradley K. Factors affecting impedance of percutaneous leads in spinal cord stimulation. Neuromodulation 2006;9(2):128–35. https://doi.org/10.1111/j.1525-1403.2006.00050.x.

[22] Jotwani R, Abd-Elsayed A, Villegas K, Shakil A, Gulati A, Sayed D, Lam C, Mehta N. Failure of SCS MR-conditional modes due to high impedance: A review of literature and case series. Pain Ther 2021;10(1):729–37. https://doi.org/10.1007/s40122-020-00219-8.

[23] Mullins CF, Harris S, Pang D. A retrospective review of elevated lead impedances in impedance-dependent magnetic resonance-conditional spinal cord stimulation devices. Pain Pract 2024;24(2):270–7. https://doi.org/10.1111/papr.13301.

[24] North RB, Brigham DD, Khalessi A, Calkins SK, Piantadosi S, Campbell DS, Daly MJ, Dey PB, Barolat G, Taylor R. Spinal cord stimulator adjustment to maximize implanted battery longevity: A randomized, controlled trial using a computerized, patient-interactive programmer. Neuromodulation 2004;7(1):13–25. https://doi.org/10.1111/j.1525-1403.2004.04002.x.

[25] Linderoth B, Foreman RD. Conventional and novel spinal stimulation algorithms: Hypothetical mechanisms of action and comments on outcomes. Neuromodulation 2017;20(6):525–33. https://doi.org/10.1111/ner.12624.

[26] Sheldon B, Staudt MD, Williams L, et al. Spinal cord stimulation programming: A crash course. Neurosurg Rev 2021;44:709–20.

[27] Levy R, Deer TR, Poree L, et al. Multicenter, randomized, double-blind study protocol using human spinal cord recording comparing safety, efficacy, and neurophysiological responses between patients being treated with evoked compound action potential-controlled closed-loop spinal cord stimulation or open-loop spinal cord stimulation (the Evoke study). Neuromodulation 2019;22(3):317–26. https://doi.org/10.1111/ner.12932.

[28] Vallejo R, Chakravarthy K, Will A, Trutnau K, Dinsmoor D. A new direction for closed-loop spinal cord stimulation: Combining contemporary therapy paradigms with evoked compound action potential sensing. J Pain Res 2021;14:3909–18. https://doi.org/10.2147/JPR.S344568.

[29] Sharma M, Bhaskar V, Yang L, et al. Novel evoked synaptic activity potentials (ESAPs) elicited by spinal cord stimulation. eNeuro 2023;10(5). https://doi.org/10.1523/ENEURO.0429-22.2023.

[30] Melzack R, Wall PD. Pain mechanisms: A new theory. Science 1965;150(3699):971–9. https://doi.org/10.1126/science.150.3699.971.

[31] Lam CM, Latif U, Sack A, et al. Advances in spinal cord stimulation. Bioengineering (Basel) 2023;10(2):185. https://doi.org/10.3390/bioengineering10020185.

[32] Wahezi SE, Caparo MA, Malhotra R, et al. Current waveforms in spinal cord stimulation and their impact on the future of neuromodulation: A scoping review. Neuromodulation 2024;27(1):47–58. https://doi.org/10.1016/j.neurom.2023.11.002.

[33] Pope JE, Antony A, Petersen EA, et al. Identifying SCS trial responders immediately after postoperative programming with ECAP dose-controlled closed-loop therapy. Pain Ther 2024;13(5):1173–85. https://doi.org/10.1007/s40122-024-00631-4.

[34] Wang VC, Bounkousohn V, Fields K, Bernstein C, Paicius RM, Gilligan C. Explantation rates of high frequency spinal cord stimulation in two outpatient clinics. Neuromodulation 2021;24(3):507–11.

[35] Van Buyten JP, Wille F, Smet I, Wensing C, Breel J, Karst E, Devos M, Poggel-Kramer K, Vesper J. Therapy-related explants after spinal cord stimulation: Results of an international retrospective chart review study. Neuromodulation 2017;20(7):642–9.

[36] Pope JE, Deer TR, Falowski S, Provenzano D, Hanes M, Hayek SM, Amrani J, Carlson J, Skaribas I, Parchuri K, McRoberts WP, Bolash R, Haider N, Hamza M, Amirdelfan K, Graham S, Hunter C, Lee E, Li S, Yang M, Campos L, Costandi S, Levy R, Mekhail N. Multicenter retrospective study of neurostimulation with exit of therapy by explant. Neuromodulation 2017;20(6):543–52.

[37] Dupre DA, Tomycz N, Whiting D, Oh M. Spinal cord stimulator explantation: motives for removal of surgically placed paddle systems. Pain Pract 2018;18(4):500–4.

[38] Mekhail NA, Levy RM, Deer TR, et al. ECAP-controlled closed-loop versus open-loop SCS for the treatment of chronic pain: 36-Month results of the EVOKE blinded randomized clinical trial. Reg Anesth Pain Med 2024;49(5):346–54. https://doi.org/10.1136/rapm-2023-104751.

[39] Will A, Fishman M, Schultz D, et al. Improvements in therapy experience with evoked compound action potential controlled, closed-loop spinal cord stimulation-primary outcome of the ECHO-MAC randomized clinical trial. J Pain 2024;25(11):104646. https://doi.org/10.1016/j.jpain.2024.104646.

[40] Ranjan M, Kumar P, Konrad P, Rezai AR. Finding optimal neuromodulation for chronic pain: waves, bursts, and beyond. Neurol India 2020;68 (Suppl. ment):S218–23. https://doi.org/10.4103/0028-3886.302465.

[41] Rigoard P, Ounajim A, Moens M, et al. Should we oppose or combine waveforms for spinal cord stimulation in PSPS-T2 patients? A prospective randomized crossover trial (multiwave study). J Pain 2023;24(12):2319–39. https://doi.org/10.1016/j.jpain.2023.07.015.

[42] Deer T, Slavin KV, Amirdelfan K, et al. Success using neuromodulation with BURST (SUNBURST) study: results from a prospective, randomized controlled trial using a novel burst waveform. Neuromodulation 2018;21(1):56–66. https://doi.org/10.1111/ner.12698.

[43] Kirketeig T, Schultheis C, Zuidema X, Hunter CW, Deer T. Burst spinal cord stimulation: A clinical review. Pain Med 2019;20(Suppl. 1):S31–40. https://doi.org/10.1093/pm/pnz003.

[44] Dinsmoor DA, Usoro JO, Barka ND, Billstrom TM, Litvak LM, Poree LR. Using evoked compound action potentials to quantify differential neural activation with burst and conventional, 40 Hz spinal cord stimulation in ovines. Pain Rep 2022;7(6):e1047. https://doi.org/10.1097/PR9.0000000000001047.

[45] De Ridder D, Plazier M, Kamerling N, Menovsky T, Vanneste S. Burst spinal cord stimulation for limb and back pain. World Neurosurg 2013;80(5):642–649.e1. https://doi.org/10.1016/j.wneu.2013.01.040.

[46] Fishman M, Cordner H, Justiz R, et al. Twelve-Month results from multicenter, open-label, randomized controlled clinical trial comparing differential target multiplexed spinal cord stimulation and traditional spinal cord stimulation in subjects with chronic intractable back pain and leg pain. Pain Pract 2021;21(8):912–23. https://doi.org/10.1111/papr.13066.

[47] Metzger CS, Hammond MB, Paz-Solis JF, et al. A novel fast-acting sub-perception spinal cord stimulation therapy enables rapid onset of analgesia in patients with chronic pain. Expert Rev Med Devices 2021;18(3):299–306. https://doi.org/10.1080/17434440.2021.1890580.

[48] North RB, Kidd DH, Farrokhi F, Piantadosi SA. Spinal cord stimulation versus repeated lumbosacral spine surgery for chronic pain: A randomized, controlled trial. Neurosurgery 2005;56(1):98–107. https://doi.org/10.1227/01.neu.0000144839.65524.e0.

[49] North RB, Kumar K, Wallace MS, et al. Spinal cord stimulation versus re-operation in patients with failed back surgery syndrome: An international multicenter randomized controlled trial (EVIDENCE study). Neuromodulation 2011;14(4):330–6. https://doi.org/10.1111/j.1525-1403.2011.00371.x.

[50] Kapural L, Yu C, Doust MW, et al. Novel 10-kHz high-frequency therapy (HF10 therapy) is superior to traditional low-frequency spinal cord stimulation for the treatment of chronic back and leg pain: The SENZA-RCT randomized controlled trial. Anesthesiology 2015;123(4):851–60. https://doi.org/10.1097/ALN.0000000000000774.

[51] Dietz BE, Mugan D, Vuong QC, Obara I. Electrically evoked compound action potentials in spinal cord stimulation: Implications for preclinical research models. Neuromodulation 2022;25(1):64–74.

[52] Parker JL, Karantonis DM, Single PS, Obradovic M, Laird J, Gorman RB, Ladd LA, Cousins MJ. Electrically evoked compound action potentials recorded from the sheep spinal cord. Neuromodulation 2013;16(4):295–303.

[53] Parker JL, Karantonis DM, Single PS, Obradovic M, Cousins MJ. Compound action potentials recorded in the human spinal cord during neurostimulation for pain relief. Pain 2012;153(3):593–601. https://doi.org/10.1016/j.pain.2011.11.023.

[54] Mekhail N, Levy RM, Deer TR, Kapural L, Li S, Amirdelfan K, Hunter CW, Rosen SM, Costandi SJ, Falowski SM, Burgher AH, Pope JE, Gilmore CA, Qureshi FA, Staats PS, Scowcroft J, Carlson J, Kim CK, Yang MI, Stauss T, Poree L, Evoke SG. Long-term safety and efficacy of closed-loop spinal cord stimulation to treat chronic back and leg pain (Evoke): A double-blind, randomised, controlled trial. Lancet Neurol 2020;19(2):123–34.

[55] Cullis K, Isaac J. Epidural endeavour and the pressure principle. Anaesthesia 2007;62(11):1187–8. https://doi.org/10.1111/j.1365-2044.2007.05331.x.

[56] Taccola G, Kissane R, Culaclii S, Apicella R, Liu W, Gad P, Ichiyama RM, Chakrabarty S, Edgerton VR. Dynamic electrical stimulation enhances the recruitment of spinal interneurons by corticospinal input. Exp Neurol 2024;371:114589. https://doi.org/10.1016/j.expneurol.2023.114589.

[57] Levy RM, Mekhail NA, Kapural L, Gilmore CA, Petersen EA, Goree JH, Pope JE, Costandi SJ, Kallewaard JW, Thomson S, Gilligan C, AlFarra T, Broachwala MY, Chopra H, Hunter CW, Rosen SM, Amirdelfan K, Falowski SM, Li S, Scowcroft J, Lad SP, Sayed D, Antony A, Deer TR, Hayek SM, Guirguis MN, Boeding RB, Calodney AK, Bruel B, Buchanan P, Soliday N, Duarte RV, Leitner A, Staats PS. Maximal analgesic effect attained by the use of objective neurophysiological measurements with closed-loop spinal cord stimulation. Neuromodulation 2024;27(8):1393–405. https://doi.org/10.1016/j.neurom.2024.07.003.

[58] Gmel GE, Santos Escapa R, Benkohen TE, Mugan D, Parker JL, Palmisani S. Postsynaptic dorsal column pathway activation during spinal cord stimulation in patients with chronic pain. Front Neurosci 2023;17:1297814. https://doi.org/10.3389/fnins.2023.1297814.

[59] Medtronic. Inceptiv™ spinal cord stimulator. 2024. https://www.medtronic.com/content/dam/medtronic-wide/public/united-states/products/neurological/inceptiv-hcp-brochure.pdf.

[60] Russo M, Cousins MJ, Brooker C, Taylor N, Boesel T, Sullivan R, Poree L, Shariati NH, Hanson E, Parker J. Effective relief of pain and associated symptoms with closed-loop spinal cord stimulation system: Preliminary results of the avalon study. Neuromodulation 2018;21(1):38–47. https://doi.org/10.1111/ner.12684.

[61] Mekhail N, Levy RM, Deer TR, Kapural L, Li S, Amirdelfan K, Hunter CW, Rosen SM, Costandi SJ, Falowski SM, Burgher AH, Pope JE, Gilmore CA, Qureshi FA, Staats PS, Scowcroft J, McJunkin T, Carlson J, Kim CK, Yang MI, Stauss T, Pilitsis J, Poree L, Evoke SG, Brounstein D, Gilbert S, Gmel GE, Gorman R, Gould I, Hanson E, Karantonis DM, Khurram A, Leitner A, Mugan D, Obradovic M, Ouyang Z, Parker J, Single P, Soliday N. Durability of clinical and quality-of-life outcomes of closed-loop spinal cord stimulation for chronic back and leg pain: A secondary analysis of the Evoke randomized clinical trial. JAMA Neurol 2022;79(3):251–60. https://doi.org/10.1001/jamaneurol.2021.4998.

[62] Nevro. Product HFX AdaptivAI. 2025. https://www.nevro.com/providers/product-hfx-adaptivai/.

[63] PR Newswire. Saluda Medical Receives FDA Approval for First Automated Programming Platform in SCS. 2025. https://www.prnewswire.com/news-releases/saluda-medical-receives-fda-approval-for-first-automated-programming-platform-in-scs-302359124.html.

[64] Naidu RK, Kapural L, Li S, Tourje C, Rutledge J, Dickerson D, Lubenow TR. A review of the Prospera spinal cord stimulation system with multiphase stimulation and proactive care. Curr Pain Headache Rep 2025;29(1):25.

[65] Russo MA, Volschenk W, Bailey D, Santarelli DM, Holliday E, Barker D, Dizon J, Graham B. Twelve-month clinical trial results of a novel, dorsal horn dendrite stimulation waveform for chronic neuropathic low back pain. Neuromodulation 2025;28(2):263–73. https://doi.org/10.1016/j.neurom.2024.09.007.

[66] Koeze TH, Williams AC, Reiman S. Spinal cord stimulation and the relief of chronic pain. Neurol Neurosurg Psychiatry 1987;50(11):1424–9. https://doi.org/10.1136/jnnp.50.11.1424.

[67] Karri J, Orhurhu V, Wahezi S, Tang T, Deer T, Abd-Elsayed A. Comparison of spinal cord stimulation waveforms for treating chronic low back pain: systematic review and meta-analysis. Pain Phys 2020;23(5):451–60.

Further reading

[1] Pope JE, Deer TR, Sayed D, Antony AB, Bhandal HS, Calodney AK, Chakravarthy K, Costandi S, Diep J, Durbhakula S, Fishman MA, Gilligan C, Goree JH, Guirguis M, Hagedorn JM, Hunter CW, Kallewaard JW, Kapural L, Lam CM, Li S, Mayrsohn B, Nijhuis H, Nikolic S, Petersen EA, Poree LR, Puri SK, Reece DE, Rosen SM, Russo MA, Shah JM, Staats PS, Verrills P, Vu CM, Levy RM, Mekhail N. The American society of pain and neuroscience (ASPN) guidelines and consensus on the definition, current evidence, clinical use and future applications for physiologic closed-loop controlled neuromodulation in chronic pain: A neuron Group project. J Pain Res 2025;18:531–51. https://doi.org/10.2147/JPR.S475527.

Section 6

Closed loop systems

Introduction to section 6 closed loop systems

Neuromodulation is undergoing a period of remarkable progress, especially in the realm of closed-loop spinal cord stimulation (SCS) and peripheral nervous system (PNS) therapies. These technologies, once considered theoretical, are now being integrated into everyday clinical practice, offering new possibilities for treating complex neurologic and pain conditions. This section, *Closed-Loop SCS Systems*, brings together a thorough and thoughtful examination of these developments, shaped by the diverse expertise of several contributing authors whose work bridges clinical care, research, and technological innovation.

The opening chapter on *EVOKE* closed-loop system provides a detailed walkthrough of this foundational modality, charting its clinical origins, the rationale behind its design, and the key technological advances that define its use today. From diagnostic frameworks and patient selection to operative technique and postoperative management, the chapter offers practical insights grounded in real-world application. It's an invaluable starting point for anyone looking to understand not just the "how," but the "why" of closed-loop SCS.

The next chapter on *Inceptiv* closed loop promises to build on this base, exploring another approach to closed-loop neuromodulation with emerging applications.

The section comes to an end with an in-depth analysis of closed-loop stimulation in the peripheral nervous system, which extends the discussion beyond the central nervous system to encompass biosensing-driven adaptive neurostimulation in the periphery. By synthesizing the current applications in deep brain, spinal cord, cochlear, vagas, and sacral nerve stimulation with ongoing research into the future possibilities, this chapter offers critical perspectives on the optimization of the stimulation parameters through real-time feedback mechanisms.

What stands out across all the three chapters is a shared commitment to precision, innovation, and patient-centered care. The content reflects a multidisciplinary understanding where physiology, engineering, and clinical practice intersect, and it's this interplay that makes the section especially valuable for trainees, practicing clinicians, and researchers alike.

For those working in or entering the field, I hope this collection not only serves as a practical resource, but also inspires continued curiosity. Closed-loop neuromodulation is still in its early stages, and the work documented here represents both where we are and where we might go next.

The comprehensive insights presented in this section are the result of the dedicated efforts of several esteemed experts in the fields of neuromodulation, neurophysiology, and pain management. I am genuinely grateful for the opportunity to read and reflect on their insights while putting this foreword together. Their collective input makes this section a rich and relevant resource for anyone looking to better understand the direction neuromodulation is heading in.

Nagy A Mekhail, MD, PhD

Carl E. Wasmuth Endowed Chair

Director of the Evidence-Based Pain Medicine Research

Department of Pain Management

Cleveland Clinic, Cleveland, OH

Chapter 23

Physiologic closed loop controlled spinal cord stimulation

Trishul Kapoor[1], Chau Vu[2], Chheany Ung[3], Timothy Deer[4] and Jason E. Pope[5]

[1]Department of Pain Management, Cleveland Clinic Foundation, Cleveland, OH, United States; [2]Interventional Pain Specialist, Evolve Restorative Center, Santa Rosa, CA, United States; [3]Virginia Interventional Pain and Spine Centers, Virginia Tech Carilion School of Medicine, INJX Group Purchasing Organization, Roanoke, VA, United States; [4]The Spine and Nerve Center of the Virginias, Anesthesiology and Pain Medicine, WVU School of Medicine, American Society of Pain and Neuroscience, Charleston, WV, United States; [5]Evolve Restorative Center, American Society of Pain and Neuroscience, Santa Rosa, CA, United States

Introduction

It is estimated that approximately 34,000 patients undergo spinal cord stimulation (SCS) implant surgeries every year to treat chronic pain [1]. SCS is a subcategory of neuromodulation. Neuromodulation is a field of therapy in which the delivery of electrical, chemical, or mechanical stimuli to nerve targets results in the alteration of neuronal signal processing. The primary purpose of neuromodulation is analgesic therapy. In addition to SCS, there are many types of neuromodulation including deep brain stimulation (DBS), transcranial magnetic stimulation (TMS), transcranial direct current stimulation (tDCS), transcranial ultrasound stimulation (TUS), vagus nerve stimulation (VNS), sacral nerve stimulation (SNS), motor cortex stimulation (MCS, and peripheral nerve stimulation (PNS). This chapter is focused on SCS and, more specifically, a form of SCS called closed-loop stimulation.

After appropriate diagnostic evaluation, as discussed later in this chapter, SCS is achieved through implantation of small-profile percutaneous leads in the epidural space overlying the dorsal columns of the spinal cord. The leads are connected to an implantable pulse generator (IPG) that is surgically placed subcutaneously in the lower back, or upper buttock region, above or below the level of the posterior iliac crest. SCS is first completed as a trial with an external pulse generator (EPG) and, depending on the results of the trial, a permanent implant is surgically placed. The mechanism of SCS is focused around modulation of pain pathways in the spinal gray matter through Aβ sensory fibers within the dorsal column of the spinal cord [2]. The preferential stimulation targets are favored by proximity to the stimulating electrodes [2]. In addition, SCS stimulation preferentially activates larger-diameter axonal profile and nerve axons [2].

The first known SCS implant in a human being was placed by Dr. Norman Shealy in 1967 [3]. Following this, the first commercially available SCS system was released by Medtronic in 1968. [3] In 1975, the first percutaneous lead was developed and this was further advanced to contain multiple electrode contacts by 1981. In 2004, the first rechargeable SCS system was commercially released. In 2013, the U.S. Food and Drug Administration (FDA) approved the first MRI-compatible SCS system. Following this, the FDA approved the first wireless SCS system in 2014. After 2014, there were several landmark FDA approvals in terms of SCS programming modalities - high frequency SCS (2015), burst SCS (2016), differential target multiplexed SCS (2020), and closed-loop SCS (2022).

Closed-loop SCS (CL-SCS) is a novel neuromodulation modality that, in real-time, measures the response of the spinal cord to stimulation and adjusts the stimulation output with every pulse to maximally optimize analgesic therapy using a precise neural dose that is within a patient's measured therapeutic window. The first CL-SCS system to be FDA-approved and introduced commercially was the Evoke system by Saluda Medical. This represents a significant procedural innovation from traditional SCS for several reasons. Unlike traditional SCS, CL-SCS allows for precise biomarker-based neural dosing of stimulation to provide dynamic analgesic relief through the continual measurement of evoked compound

A Modern Atlas for Implantable Devices of the Spine, Brain, and Nerve. https://doi.org/10.1016/B978-0-443-36528-7.00011-X

action potentials (ECAPs). Traditional SCS is also referred to as fixed-output SCS because there is a fixed dosing of stimulation (i.e., pulse duration, current amplitude, and frequency) without any real-time adjustments based on physiologic feedback. This is particularly important because postural and physiological functions (i.e., postural changes, respiratory variability, pulse variation, medication changes, CSF/hydration levels) can dramatically alter the distance between the epidural SCS electrode contacts and the target fibers of the spinal cord [2]. The utilization of ECAPs in CL-SCS has markedly advanced the field of neuromodulation by providing patients with improved and, more importantly, sustained analgesic relief through patient-centered customization. There is a growing field of research with CL-SCS focused on development of advanced stimulation algorithms, interpretation of neural signals, and delivery mechanisms of stimulation [4].

Key points

- Closed-loop SCS (CL-SCS) is a novel neuromodulation modality that measures the response of the spinal cord to stimulation and, in real-time, adjusts the stimulation output with every pulse to maximally optimize analgesic therapy within a patient's measured therapeutic window. The first CL-SCS system to be FDA-approved and introduced commercially was the Evoke system by Saluda Medical.
- Unlike traditional SCS, CL-SCS allows for precision neural dosing of stimulation to provide dynamic analgesic relief through the continual measurement of evoked compound action potentials (ECAPs).
- The therapy aims for precise neural activation at a patient-specific neural dose target, thus improving functional outcomes and quality of life. Capturing and responding to this neurophysiological biomarker offers the potential for long-term efficacy by preventing habituation and tolerance, with insights that can guide treatment and diagnose pain issues.
- The gray matter structures of the spinal cord are the primary target of SCS. The closest structures to the epidural layer are the dorsal columns (primary target for SCS which carry sensory information associated with touch and proprioception), dorsal horns (entry zone of sensory information associated with pain processing), and laminae of Rexed (multiple layers of spinal cord gray matter containing interneurons).
- Closed-loop SCS shares the same indications as traditional fixed-output spinal cord stimulation and is considered on-label for chronic intractable pain of the trunk and/or limbs.
- Patients must pass a psychological screening assessment to determine if they are an appropriate candidate for this therapy prior to the trial. If deemed an appropriate candidate for a trial, ensuring realistic goals for trial and implant as well as optimizing a patient's psychological health is of utmost importance, especially in chronic pain patients.
- The FDA has recently approved the first automated programming paradigm (EVA; Evoke Virtual Assistant) with the Evoke Closed-Loop SCS System. Specifically, EVA utilizes objective neural biomarker-based measurements to optimize programming more efficiently compared to that performed independently by a human programmer. Suboptimal stimulation levels could be addressed by CL-SCS.

Relevant anatomy

Although there are numerous anatomic structures that are important to consider when pursuing SCS trial or permanent implant, the following structures are crucial to understand: spinal canal, interlaminar window, intervertebral ligamentous complex, ligamentum flavum, spinal meninges, and the spinal cord (Fig. 23.1) (Fig. 23.2). The spinal canal is an osseous cavity that is bordered by the intervertebral disc (anterior), vertebral body (anterior), pedicles (lateral), and laminae (posterior). The spinal canal, also known as the vertebral canal, is the widest in the cervical region to accommodate the largest dimension of the spinal cord. The spinal canal subsequently narrows in the inferior regions. The spinal canal extends from the foramen magnum of the skull to the sacral hiatus. The spinal canal forms an osseous cavity to protect numerous critical structures such as the spinal cord, spinal nerve roots, spinal meninges, blood vessels, and adipose tissue. The spinal canal is prone to pathologic narrowing secondary to zygapophyseal joint hypertrophy, intervertebral disc herniation, and ligamentum flavum thickening.

The interlaminar window is formed by the laminae of two adjacent vertebral bodies. The interlaminar window is widest in the lumbar region and narrows significantly in dimension in the thoracic and cervical regions. The interlaminar window is prone to pathologic narrowing secondary to osteophytes secondary to osteoarthritic changes and degenerative intervertebral disc disease.

The intervertebral ligamentous complex is a series of ligaments that stabilize the vertebral column. The most superficial ligament along the tips of the spinous processes is the supraspinous ligament and it extends from the C7 vertebra to the L4 vertebra. This ligament becomes significantly thicker and broader in dimension as it extends into the lumbar

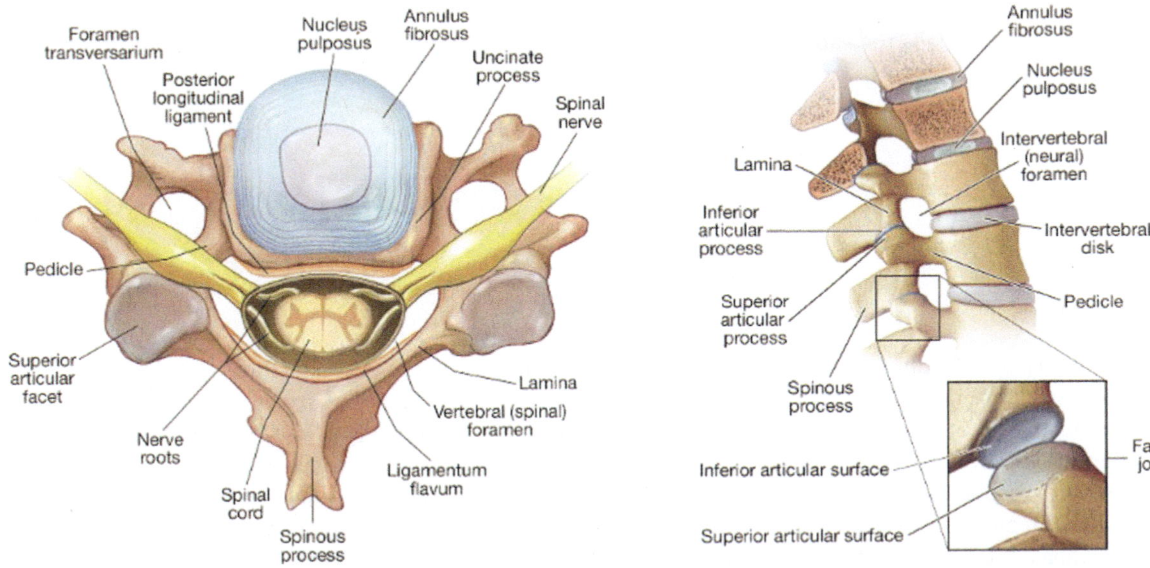

FIGURE 23.1 This image demonstrates the cross sectional anatomy of the vertebral column and spinal canal components. *a. Hines RL, Jones SB: Stoelting's Anesthesia and Co-Existing Disease, ed 14, 2022, Elsevier.*

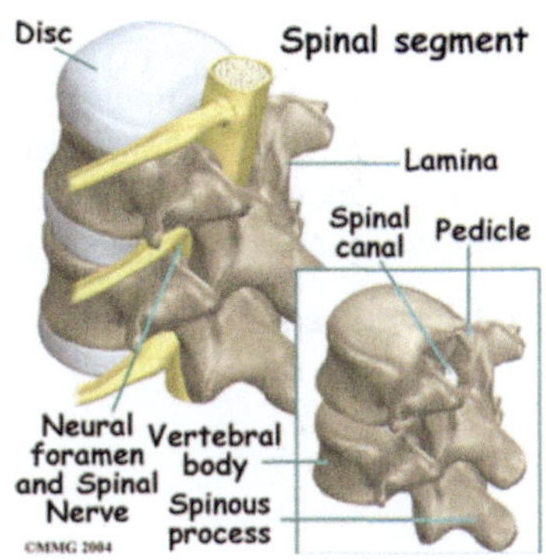

FIGURE 23.2 This image demonstrates the cross sectional anatomy of the vertebral column and spinal canal components. *a. Hines RL, Jones SB: Stoelting's Anesthesia and Co-Existing Disease, ed 14, 2022, Elsevier.*

spine. Deep to the supraspinous ligament, the interspinous ligament extends between adjacent spinous processes. This ligament is an extension of the supraspinous ligament through a network of collagenous fibers. The interspinous ligament extends into the ligamentum flavum.

The ligamentum flavum is a ligamentous structure found within the spinal canal abutting the vertebral laminae extending from the C2 to S2 laminae. This dense structure is largely composed of elastin fibers. The ligamentum flavum is the thinnest in the cervical region and the thickest in the lower thoracic and lumbar regions. The potential anatomic space between the ligamentum flavum and the spinal meninges is the epidural space. The epidural space contains fat, veins, and connective tissue.

The spinal meninges encompasses the spinal cord circumferentially and is composed of three components (superficial to deep) - the dura mater, arachnoid mater, and the pia mater. The dura mater is the toughest layer of the spinal meninges and spans from the foramen magnum to S2. This structure forms the dural sac and attaches to the coccyx by forming the filum terminale. Deep to the dura mater, the arachnoid mater is a thin membrane separated by the dura mater through a film of lymph fluid and forms a potential space known as the subdural space. The pia mater is deep to the arachnoid mater and encompasses the spinal cord to be contiguous with the epineurium. There are lateral extensions of the pia mater called denticulate ligaments that attach to the dura mater throughout the course of the spinal cord. The potential space between the pia mater and the arachnoid mater is called the subarachnoid space which contains cerebrospinal fluid (CSF), arteries, veins, and arachnoid trabecule.

TABLE 23.1 This table details the various levels of the spinal cord associated with SCS therapeutic targets.

Anatomic level of spinal cord	Correlating SCS target
C2 to C4	Lower half of the face, neck, shoulder, and upper extremities
T5 to T6	Abdomen
T7 to T9	Upper and lower back
T10 to L1	Lower extremities and pelvis

The spinal cord extends from the brainstem to L1-L2 level to form the conus medullaris. Inferior to the conus medullaris, the spinal cord forms the cauda equina. The spinal cord is formed by an outer layer of axonal nerve fibers called the white matter and an inner layer of neuronal cell bodies called the gray matter. The gray matter structures of the spinal cord are the primary target of SCS. The closest structures to the epidural layer are the dorsal columns (primary target for SCS which carry sensory information associated with touch and proprioception), dorsal horns (entry zone of sensory information associated with pain processing), and laminae of Rexed (multiple layers of spinal cord gray matter containing interneurons). The following anatomic levels of the spinal cord have been associated with correlating SCS targets (Table 23.1).

Procedure

Indications

Closed-loop SCS shares the same indications as traditional fixed output spinal cord stimulation and is considered on-label for chronic intractable pain of the trunk and/or limbs [5]. This definition encompasses a wide range of neuropathic pain conditions, many of which remain on-label as long as they involve the trunk or limbs.

Below is a list of selected pain conditions for which closed loop SCS therapy could be utilized for on-label use:

- Post-laminectomy pain syndrome or Failed back surgery syndrome
- Complex regional pain syndrome (CRPS) Type I and II
- Diabetic peripheral neuropathy
- Radicular pain
- Chemotherapy-induced peripheral neuropathy
- Pelvic pain
- Abdominal pain
- Post-herpetic neuralgia
- Chronic refractory angina
- Peripheral arterial disease/Limb ischemia
- Raynaud's syndrome
- Phantom limb pain
- Pain associated with multiple sclerosis
- Spinal cord injury-related pain
- Chest wall pain syndromes
  - Post-thoracotomy pain syndrome
  - Post-mastectomy pain syndrome

Although there are a limited number of case reports, off-label indications include:

- Chronic intractable headache
- Chronic intractable facial pain/Atypical facial pain
- Post-herpetic neuralgia of the face

Patient selection considerations

Spinal cord stimulation can be effective for a variety of neuropathic conditions, but success can largely hinge on careful patient selection. The following factors should be taken into consideration before proceeding [6,7]:

Cognitive and behavioral considerations

- Ability to comprehend therapy and provide informed consent
- Patient has realistic goals and expectations for pain relief and functional improvement
- Ability to recharge or operate the device
- Ability to attend follow up or reprogramming visits

Age considerations

- While there is no definitive age limit, considerations in pediatric and geriatric patient populations include:
  - The ability to manage the device independently (or if unable to, help is available)
  - Comorbidities that could increase surgical or anesthesia risk
  - Potential anatomic/developmental concerns in younger patients

Medical considerations

- Smoking increases risk of infection
- Ability to safely hold anticoagulation for trial or permanent procedure
- Ability to safely tolerate anesthesia for trial (if used) or permanent procedure
- Patients with cardiac pacemakers/defibrillators can often safely have SCS therapy, but NACC guidelines recommend verification and cardiologist clearance prior to proceeding
- Caution in pregnancy including radiation and anesthesia risks
- Patients who may need for serial MRIs (i.e., cancer, multiple sclerosis, etc.)
  - It is essential to ensure MRI conditionality of the device aligns with the patients' imaging needs
- Comorbidities associated with increased medical/anesthesia risk
- Previous spine surgeries where epidural space is violated

Contraindications

- Active infection or sepsis
- Critical central stenosis in areas of planned lead entry or placement
- Neurologic deficits or spine instability that is at risk of progression. Consider surgical evaluation before proceeding
- Coagulopathy
  - Patient cannot discontinue or bridge anticoagulation for trial or permanent implant
  - Thrombocytopenia with platelet count <50,000
- Inadequately controlled psychiatric disorders
- Cognitive impairment without acceptable caregiver
- Living situation that poses safety risk

Maintenance concerns

Maintenance concerns for closed looped SCS is similar to fixed output SCS [6,7]

- Need for recharging of the impulse generator
- Need for Impulse generator replacement
  - Saluda's EVOKE SCS impulse generator has an approximate battery life of 10 years [5].
- Need for replacement of ancillary items such as charging device or belt
- Need for follow up/reprogramming
  - The EVOKE closed loop SCS trial showed that once initial relief achieved, need for reprogramming is < 1 time per year on average [2].
- Risk of lead migration or lead fracture
- Concern for infection or dehiscence

Training and proctoring recommendations

There is no standardized requirement within ACGME-accredited fellowship training to perform spinal cord stimulation. PEAK consensus guidelines do recommend a total of 10 neuromodulation procedures during fellowship which can include five trials and five permanent implants to establish proficiency [8]. For established physicians/new implanters, the NACC guidelines recommend implanters should be trained in interventional pain management or spinal surgical intervention at a credentialed high volume center and perform a minimum of 10 cases as the primary implanter under supervision [6].

Both NACC and PEAK guidelines suggest that implanters be able to properly select patients, understand contraindications, and be able to identify and manage complications related to SCS therapy [6,8]. While closed-loop SCS is procedurally similar to traditional fixed-output SCS, differences in technology and the availability of real-time metrics, such as neural activation and maximal analgesic effect (MAE), provide deeper insight into patient needs and enable more personalized treatment decisions [9]. Additionally, the advent of automated programming for closed loop SCS provides more efficient and optimized programming [10]. Adapting to these differences in programming, workflow, and patient management scenarios may require time and additional learning.

- The following is a suggested approach for new adopters of CL-SCS:
  - Initially focus on standard, well-established SCS indications before tackling complex, non-traditional cases
  - Gradually expand to more challenging cases as experience with the therapy grows
  - Consider peer review discussions or case debriefs to refine programming, patient selection strategies, treatment algorithms, and workflow.

Technique

Pre-procedural planning is crucial when preparing for the CL-SCS procedure. First, a proper radiological survey is essential to complete. This involves reviewing the cross-sectional MRI or CT imaging in order to evaluate the epidural space, interlaminar window, and epidural needle trajectory. Next, after appropriate informed consent is obtained, the patient is positioned prone with a pillow placed underneath the lower abdomen. This minimizes lumbar spine lordosis and maximizes lumbar flexion in order to better visualize the target interlaminar window. In addition, this positioning will allow for easier instrumentation and needle placement into the target interlaminar window.

The CL-SCS procedure consists of two specific and sequential techniques - trial and permanent implant procedure. Depending on whether a closed loop trial or permanent implant is being performed, anesthetic consideration can vary. A CL-SCS trial is ideally performed under minimal anxiolysis or moderate sedation with local anesthetic subcutaneous infiltration. Whereas, a CL-SCS permanent implant procedure is performed under monitored anesthesia care (MAC). The operating room time estimate for a CL-SCS trial is approximately 15–30 min. Whereas for a CL-SCS permanent implant procedure, the operating room time estimate is approximately 45–60 min.

Vendor support is crucial when planning for a CL-SCS trial and permanent implant procedure. It is important to review the following features during pre-procedural planning with a vendor - number of closed loop-specific SCS leads, length of closed loop-specific SCS leads, epidural needle sizes and types, rechargeable IPG with a battery life up to 10 years, IPG software upgrades without IPG replacement, mobile device compatibility and communication for therapy selection, automated programming, and 1.5T full-body MRI compatibility labeling.

Closed loop SCS trial

After the patient is brought to the operating room and a surgical time-out is completed, the patient is positioned in a prone position, as described previously, on the X-ray table. After the administration of preoperative antibiotics, the patient is prepped and draped in a standard sterile fashion. Subsequently, an antero-posterior (AP) fluoroscopic image is taken to visualize the target low thoracic (T10-T12) or upper lumbar (L1-L2) interlaminar space. However, it is important to obtain a true AP image of the target level. This is achieved by adjusting the fluoroscopy to align the endplates of the vertebral bodies to create a square border of each vertebral body. This in turn allows for optimal visualization of the lamina and interlaminar space.

For the purpose of this chapter, the T10-T11 interlaminar space will be targeted. Prior to beginning the procedure, appropriate preoperative antibiotics should be administered. Next, using fluoroscopic guidance, the skin should be marked at the midpoint of the medial border of the pedicle of the vertebra one level below. Subsequently, a spinal needle can be utilized to create a local anesthetic infiltration tract from the skin into the subcutaneous tissues. In this particular example, the spinal needle can be advanced at a 45 degrees angle from the medial border of the T12 pedicle to the upper edge of the T11 lamina abutting the spinous process (Fig. 23.3). The spinal needle is removed and an epidural introducer needle

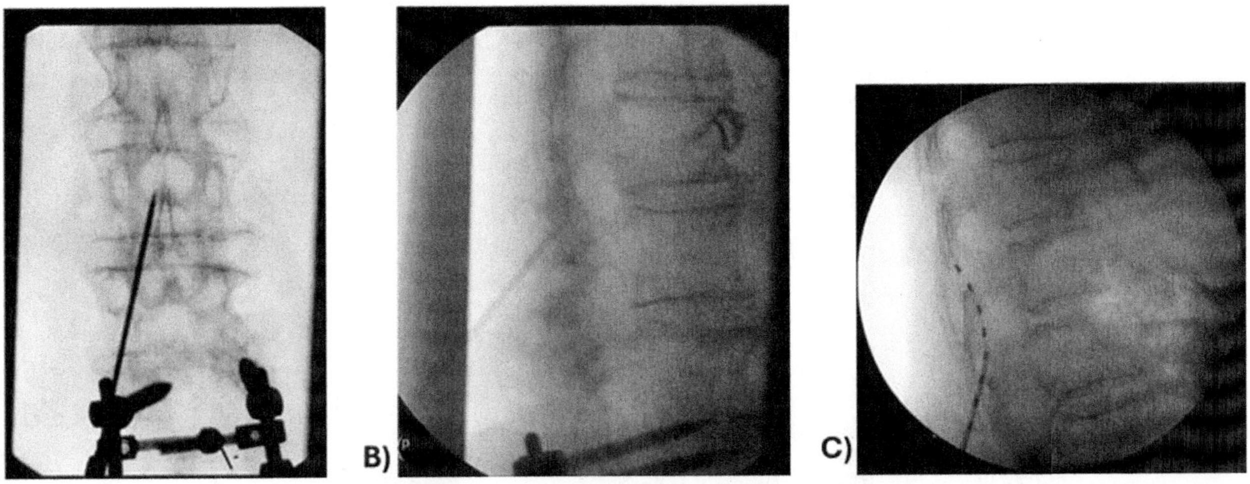

FIGURE 23.3 A) AP image of 14 gauge Tuohy needle placement on approach to the interlaminar space. Note the paramedian approach of the needle. This and a shallow needle angle to the skin (less than 45°) will help to improve lead steering in the epidural space. B) and C) Lateral images of 14 gauge Tuohy needle placement during loss of resistance (LOR). Lateral image may help guide with depth of needle placement during the LOR. Note the needle bevel is facing "up" (i.e., posterior) at this point, which may help aid guiding the lead to remain posterior in the epidural space. *a. Permission obtained from Saluda Medical.*

(EIN), with the bevel facing up, is advanced in an identical trajectory to make osseous contact with the upper edge of the T11 lamina. The EIN is then stepped off the T11 laminar edge. The stylet is removed from the EIN and a loss-of-resistance syringe with air and saline is attached at the hub. The EIN is advanced slowly while paying close attention to tactile feedback until there is a loss of resistance and the epidural space is entered.

Next, a percutaneous closed loop SCS lead preloaded with a curved stylet is inserted into the EIN needle slowly. The SCS lead is advanced, under live AP and lateral fluoroscopy, utilizing the torque stylet hub and positioned according to the patient's needs at the appropriate level and laterality. If another percutaneous closed loop SCS lead needs to be placed, the previous steps can be completed in an identical fashion from the contralateral side. Once the SCS lead is at an appropriate position, a screen cable connector is attached to the distal externalized portion of the SCS lead and intra-operative testing is completed to capture an ECAP while confirming optimal SCS lead positioning (Fig. 23.4). Next, the screen cable connectors are disconnected and the EIN is removed along with the percutaneous SCS lead stylet. It is crucial to ensure the percutaneous SCS lead position is maintained while withdrawing the EIN and stylet.

The percutaneous SCS lead is then anchored at the level of the skin with skin glue, adhesive dressing, or suture fixation. The percutaneous lead exit site is covered with a sterile dressing and the lead is connected to an external pulse generator (EXP). The EXP should be placed above the level of the iliac crest and on the side of patient preference.

Closed loop permanent implant procedure

When completing a CL-SCS permanent implant procedure, all of the steps described in the closed loop SCS trial are performed along with a few additional steps (Fig. 23.4). First, prior to placement of the EIN, a 4–5 cm vertical midline incision is made with a no. 15-blade. Electrocautery is utilized to separate subcutaneous tissues until the tips of the spinous processes are encountered. The EIN can then be placed in a paramedian approach under direct visualization and live fluoroscopy as previously described. Second, upon removal of the EIN, the SCS lead is secured subcutaneously with a lead anchor device (Fig. 23.5). Third, a 4–5 cm horizontal incision is marked below the right or left iliac crest (based on patient preference) and local anesthetic is subcutaneously infiltrated over a broad area approximating the size of the IPG. Next, an incision is made and blunt dissection is carried out to create a subcutaneous pocket for the IPG without violating the gluteal fascia. Subsequently, a subcutaneous tissue tunneler is used to create a tract from the lead insertion site to the IPG site (Fig. 23.6). The lead is passed through tunneling sheath and the sheath removed while avoiding lead traction. Next, the lead is connected to the IPG and fixated with a torque wrench (Fig. 23.7). Lastly, the incisions are closed and re-approximated in a layered fashion with sutures and skin glue. Antibiotic cream is applied to incisions and the incisions are covered with sterile dressings (Fig. 23.8).

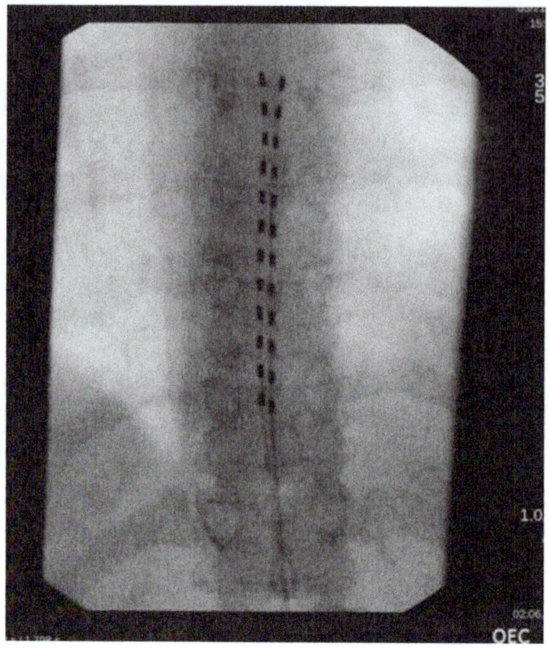

FIGURE 23.4 AP image of lead placement for closed-loop system implantation. General lead placement is T7 due to the 12-contact lead that typically spans between 3-4 vertebral segments in most adults. A suggestion for lead placement is to leave a "leads width" of gap between the leads as this helps prevent shunting of energy from one lead to the other, via touching contacts, and thus potentially improving IPG battery life. *a. Permission obtained from Saluda Medical.*

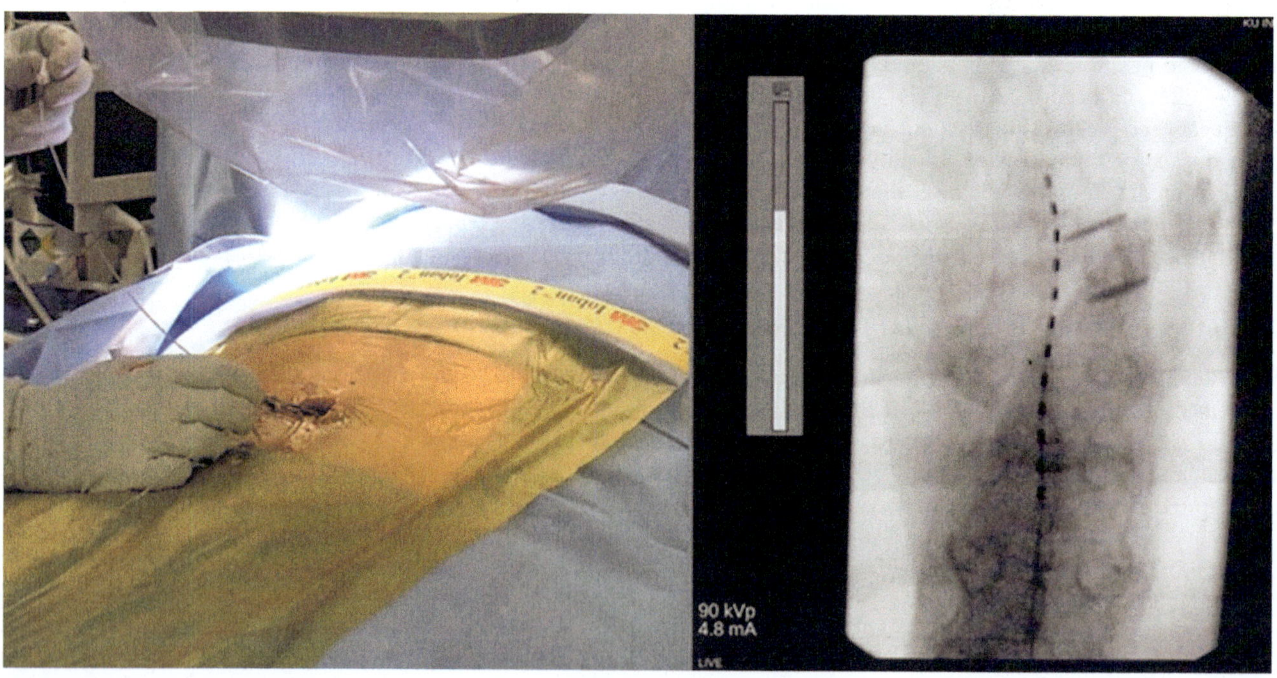

FIGURE 23.5 This figure demonstrates advancement of the lead in a permanent implant case. Vertical midline incision is done prior to needle placement. *a. Permission obtained from Saluda Medical.*

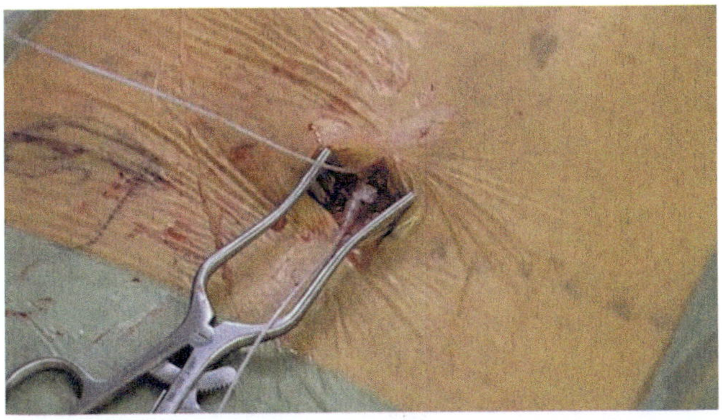

FIGURE 23.6 This image demonstrates proper anchoring technique in a permanent implant case. It is important to bury the nose of the anchor in the paraspinal fascia while suturing the anchor to the paraspinal muscle in order to minimize lead migration risk. This is an example of an active anchor that has a mechanical hold on the lead. *a. Permission obtained from Saluda Medical.*

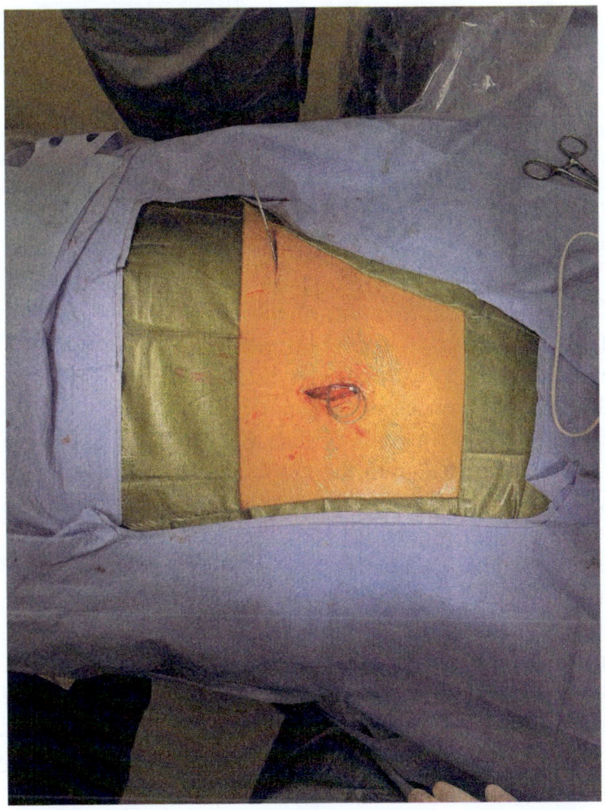

FIGURE 23.7 This figure demonstrates the midline incision overlying the thoracic spine for epidural lead placement and tunneling of leads to subcutaneous IPG site above the gluteal fascia. *a. Practical Management of Pain, Chapter 71, 957-962, Copyright © 2023 Elsevier.*

Post-operative considerations

The majority of patients follow up within 10–14 days following surgical implantation. Patients are given postoperative instructions and limitations similar to what is given after their trial. This includes sedentary instructions such as no bending, lifting or twisting as well as to keep the incisions clean and dry. In addition, patients are advised to monitor for signs of infection locally and systemically. A lumbar brace is often recommended to help aid in reminding patients of these limitations as the most common complication is lead migration. Any degree of lead migration can directly affect

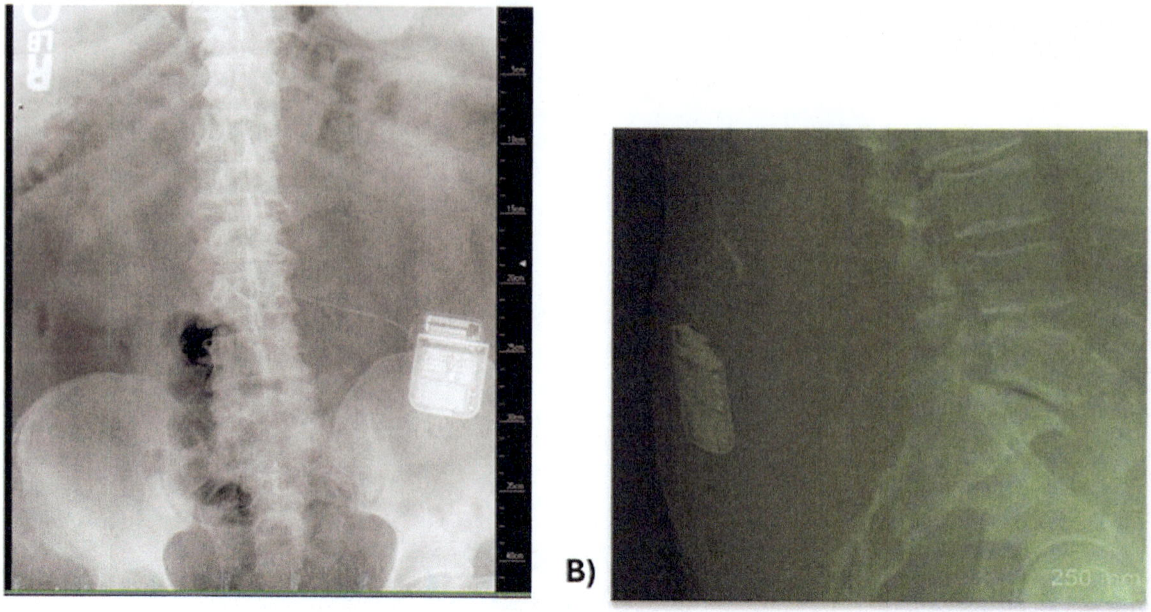

A) B)

FIGURE 23.8 A) AP image of the IPG pocket and battery implantation site. Note the strain relief loop of excess lead can be seen behind the battery. This is a good practice to potentially help prevent lead migration by providing a loop of excess lead to pull rather than pulling the anchor site. B) Lateral image of IPG pocket and battery implantation site. Note the strain relief loop above the battery in this example. Always take note of the orientation of your battery in the pocket as the charging coil is only on one side. It is important to have the correct orientation and implant depth in order to prevent charging issues. *a. Permission obtained from Saluda Medical.*

the programming of the CL-SCS system. Programming of the CL-SCS system is often delayed until the first post-operative visit to allow the patient to recover from post-surgical pain. Furthermore, the patient may have difficulty providing accurate information and recalling instructions while recovering from the sedative effects of anesthesia. Lastly, delayed programming also reduces the risk of surgical site infections associated with repeated exposure of the incision while attempting to recharge the IPG. In general, activities are limited for up to 4–6 weeks to decrease the risk of lead migration and to allow the leads to scar into the epidural space. The recommendations are proposed by The Neurostimulation Appropriateness Consensus Committee (NACC) based on a review of peer-reviewed evidence-based literature [11].

If a patient's analgesic efficacy from the CL-SCS system is not as effective as the trial, several scenarios must be considered to determine the causality. Lead migration is the most common "complication" of SCS therapy (88.5%) resulting in loss of analgesic or therapeutic efficacy [12]. In this circumstance, there should be a low threshold in obtaining spine X-ray imaging to assess for lead position. This is a crucial step as the CL-SCS system programming is entirely based on the location of the leads. If the electrode contacts are not programmed relative to the correct anatomic lead position within the epidural space, there may be significant loss of degree and duration of therapeutic relief. Following a diagnostic radiology survey (i.e., X-ray imaging), interrogation of the Cl-SCS system should be performed to evaluate whether the leads have shifted independently or relative to each other. Another complication to be aware of is a lead fracture. This complication is identified through interrogation of the CL-SCS system. If a lead fracture is present, high impedances will be present and this can significantly affect CL-SCS system programming. Assuming the patient does present with any new complaints of pain since the Cl-SCS trial procedure, they should be continually educated on the expectations of the CL-SCS therapy throughout the procedural and surgical pathway (i.e., prior to the CL-SCS trial and after CL-SCS surgical implantation). If patient expectations are not met at any point after the CL-SCS surgical implant, performing a "stim holiday" may be beneficial. A "stim holiday" is achieved by having the patient turn off their CL-SCS system for a duration of time. This step may serve as a reminder to patients with regards to the degree of therapeutic relief they obtained with CL-SCS therapy and could potentially reset patient expectations. Lastly, encouraging and assuring frequent communication between the CL-SCS vendor representative, patient, and clinical provider is crucial in optimizing therapy.

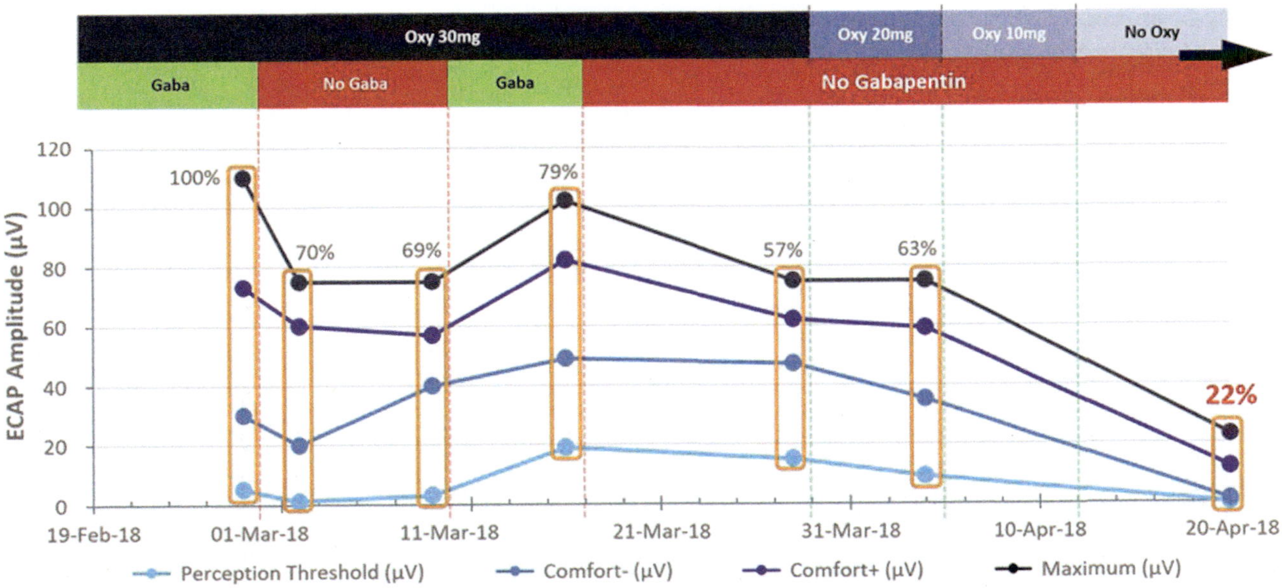

FIGURE 23.9 This figure demonstrates medication dose status, data collection points, ECAP amplitude measured at different activation levels, and comparisons to the TW at baseline (as a % at each time point). In this example, patient's therapeutic window and SCS dose decreased after titration off of Gabapentin and opiates. a. *Permission obtained from Saluda Medical.*

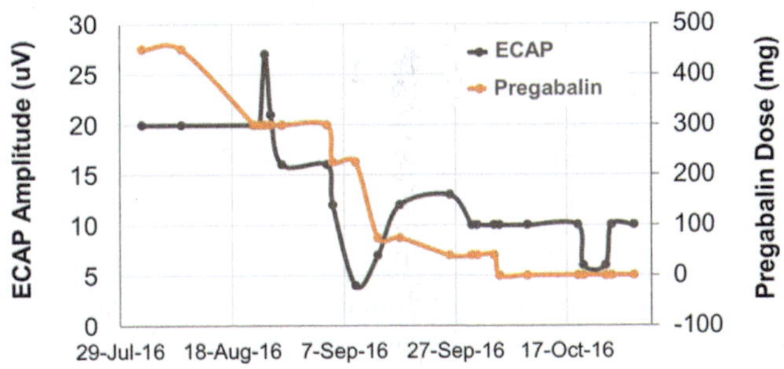

FIGURE 23.10 This figure demonstrates (preferred) ECAP amplitude (µV) decreased as the dose of pregabalin (mg) decreased over several weeks. a. *Permission obtained from Saluda Medical.*

Postoperatively, programming in CL-SCS systems is markedly different from open-loop tonic stimulation programming. In open-loop spinal cord stimulation (OL-SCS), a fixed-output of energy is delivered, regardless of the distance of the electrodes to the cord. This translates to constant energy being delivered to provide pain relief that can produce variable feelings of intensity of stimulation. Stimulation is adjusted based upon a patient's preferred level of stimulation; or sometimes to prevent uncomfortable stimulation. This can vary based upon their body posture, medications, or physiology (i.e., heartbeat, breathing) that could lead to either over or under-stimulation resulting in inconsistent and suboptimal pain control. In contrast, closed-loop stimulation is based on interpreting an objective neural biomarker, known as an ECAP and adjusting stimulation parameters millions of times per day. This allows for individualized programming unique to each patient's measured therapeutic window while minimizing side effects, such as uncomfortable stimulation or suboptimal/subtherapeutic stimulation. These real-time ECAP measurements are used to detect changes in neural activity, allowing for adaptive modulation of stimulation output in real-time on a pulse-to-pulse basis. This ensures consistent pain control, reducing the need for manual adjustments and reprogramming visits. The therapy aims for precise neural activation at a patient-specific neural dose target, thus improving functional outcomes and quality of life. Capturing and responding to this neurophysiological feedback offers the potential for long-term efficacy by preventing habituation and tolerance, with insights that can guide treatment and diagnose pain issues. The technology is advancing rapidly, potentially leading to more personalized and precise neuromodulation therapies in the future.

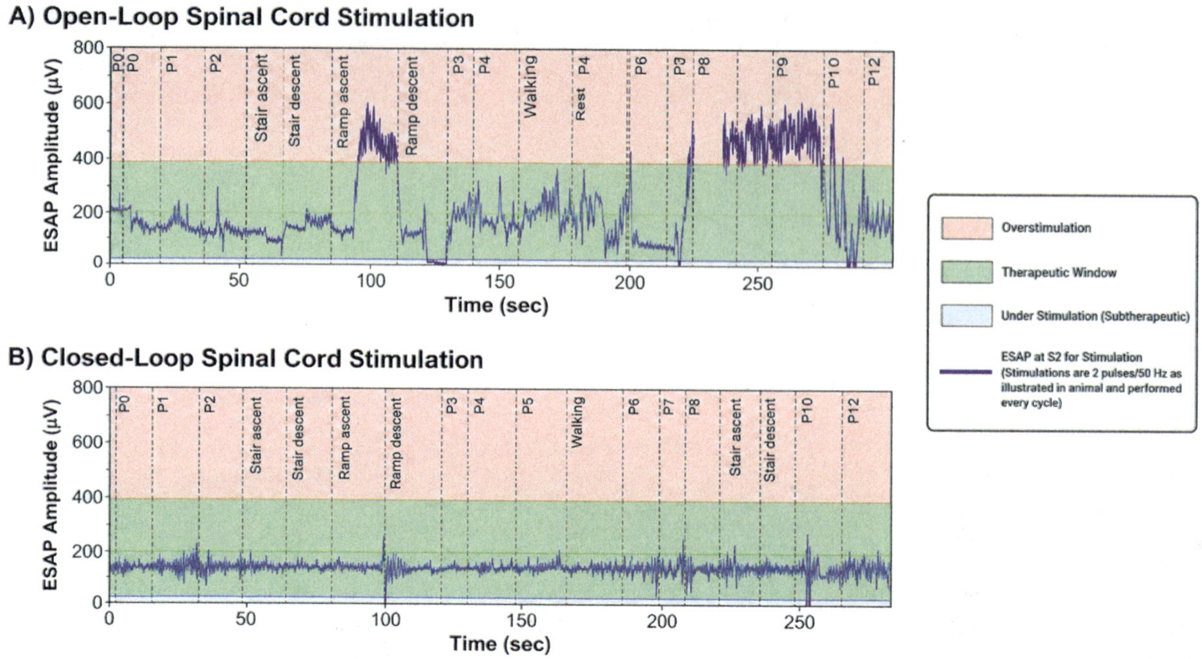

FIGURE 23.11 Above are examples of A) open-loop stimulation and B) closed-loop stimulation over various postures and physiological changes. Notice in open-loop stimulation in figure A) that there is tremendous variability in dorsal column neural activation due to changes in posture, physiology, even heartbeat and respiration. Some of these activations can fall into subtherapeutic (under-stimulation) or supratherapeutic (over-stimulation) as a result of the variability in the distance between the cord and the electrodes. Patients will experience this as inconsistent stimulation sensation, some of which may be uncomfortable or unwanted. In figure B), with closed-loop stimulation, the system is modulating the output of the device on every single pulse thus preventing subtherapeutic or supratherapeutic stimulation. It is this consistency in neural activation which results in more long-term durable therapeutic benefit as demonstrated in the EVOKE 36-Month double-blinded RCT. *a. Permission obtained from Saluda Medical.*

The primary goal of any chronic pain therapy is to provide pain relief and functional improvement. However, of equal importance as the primary goal, the secondary goal is to ultimately reduce medication usage. Neural activation changes can be seen while titrating medications and this can ultimately affect the spinal cord's response to stimulation therapy. Diagnostic evaluation of medication titration and its effect on the spinal cord's sensitivity to stimulation is a phenomenon that is only seen with closed-loop stimulation (Figs. 23.9 and 23.10). Until recently, postoperative programming could be relatively time consuming as measurements needed to be taken in various clinical situations and scenarios to determine the variability in stimulation and response. This upfront investment has shown to decrease the number of interim reprogramming visits as well as patient daily stimulation adjustments [9]. In addition, recent innovations have greatly decreased this time burden of optimizing patient programming post implant. The FDA has recently approved the first automated programming paradigm (APP) with the Evoke Closed-Loop SCS System. Specifically, the APP utilizes objective neural biomarker-based measurements to optimize programming more efficiently compared to that performed independently by a human programmer. Across all devices, roughly 22% of devices are explanted due to loss of efficacy at 2 years following surgical implantation [13–16]. There are numerous reasons that could account for this, but one overlooked issue is patient manipulation of therapy. Some patients continually adjust their stimulation parameters as a result of too much or too little stimulation. Suboptimal stimulation levels could be addressed by CL-SCS (Fig. 23.11).

Pearls and pitfalls

Spinal cord stimulation is an indispensable treatment option in providing pain relief for chronic pain patients. Because of this, as well as the recent significant advances within the neuromodulation space, utilization rates have skyrocketed over the past 10 years. That being said, it is important to follow best practices to avoid any preventative complications that may arise utilizing this therapy.

From a preoperative perspective, patient selection is key. A patient must have a primary clinical diagnosis and symptoms that support the use of this therapy; generally a pain that is neuropathic in nature. Obtaining updated diagnostic

TABLE 23.2 This table lists a few high-yield recommendations from the 2024 NACC guidelines.

High-yield recommendations from the 2024 NACC guidelines
Proper technique and training: Ensuring that practitioners are adequately trained in neuromodulation techniques and the appropriate use of equipment to reduce procedural errors and complications. Standardized surgical procedures must be adopted to minimize risks. This includes meticulous planning of electrode placement, ensuring proper lead positioning, and securing leads to prevent migration. Exercise caution to avoid nerve damage during implantation. Employ techniques that reduce the risk of nerve injury and monitor for neurological deficits during and after the procedure.
Monitoring and follow-up: Continuous monitoring during the procedure and regular follow-ups to detect complications early, including infection, lead migration, and device malfunctions.
Infection prevention: Strict adherence to aseptic techniques to minimize the risk of infections and ensure appropriate use of antibiotics when indicated. Strict infection control protocols must be implemented during and after surgery. This encompasses the use of prophylactic antibiotics, maintaining sterile environments, and monitoring for signs of infection postoperatively.
Patient education: Educating patients on potential risks, proper care, and the need for adherence to follow-up appointments to ensure early detection of complications.
Management of complications: Prompt recognition and management of complications such as device malfunction, lead displacement, infections, and pain. Specific interventions include device revisions, antibiotics for infections, and physical therapy or reprogramming in cases of discomfort.
Multidisciplinary approach: Collaboration among neurologists, pain specialists, surgeons, and other healthcare professionals to provide comprehensive care and mitigate risks.
Bleeding and coagulation management: Assess and manage coagulation status to prevent bleeding complications. This includes evaluating patients' bleeding risks and adjusting anticoagulant therapy as necessary.
Long-term outcome optimization: Regularly monitor patients to assess device function and therapeutic efficacy. Be prepared to adjust stimulation parameters or consider salvage therapies if optimal outcomes are not achieved.

studies, including X-ray imaging and MRIs of the lumbar and thoracic spine, can help support the clinical diagnosis and assist in planning for the patient's upcoming trial. Prior surgical consultation and support is recommended especially if any prior instrumentation and/or pathology is present at the levels of lead placement. Patients must pass a psychological screening assessment to determine if they are an appropriate candidate for this therapy prior to the trial. If deemed an appropriate candidate for a trial, ensuring realistic goals for trial and implant as well as optimizing a patient's psychological health is of utmost importance, especially in chronic pain patients. Lastly, anticoagulants should be held in the appropriate time frame per the recommended guidelines at the discretion of the prescribing provider. Furthermore, perioperative glucose control should be optimized in diabetic patients to help minimize risk of surgical site infection. Lastly, smoking cessation is highly recommended [17,18].

From a technical standpoint, patients should be marked for the IPG site in a level, seated position. A flat plane should be located on the patient's flank/gluteal region above or below the beltline depending on patient preference. Generally, the upper outer quadrant of the flank can be a good site for battery implantation. Care should be taken to mark the level of the lowest rib as well as the lowest point where the buttocks contact the bed. Typically, IPG placement should avoid any bony prominences, be on the opposite side of where the patient lays to sleep and opposite to any side with shoulder issues. Furthermore, the 2024 NACC guidelines should be routinely referenced. These guidelines are focused on mitigating complications related to neuromodulation, focusing on ensuring patient safety and optimizing treatment outcomes [11]. These guidelines emphasize a proactive approach to avoid, detect, and manage complications, ensuring that neuromodulation remains a safe and effective therapeutic option for patients. Specific high-yield recommendations from the 2024 NACC guidelines are referenced in Table 23.2 [11].

From a post-operative standpoint, recommendations for physical activity restrictions and phasic activity progression are detailed in Table 23.3 [11,19]. It is crucial that patients are provided with specific instructions and visual examples of allowable activity in various phases of post-operative recovery following surgical implantation. Most patients have little clarity on terms such as mild, moderate, or strenuous activity. Hence, a visual aid with specific day-by-day or week-by-week examples of physical activity recommendations can drastically improve post-operative recovery and therapeutic efficacy of the CL-SCS system.

TABLE 23.3 This table details recommendations for physical activity restrictions and phasic activity progression following surgical implantation of a CL-SCS system.

Post-operative physical activity recommendations
Immediate Post-Operative Phase (0–7 Days After Surgical Implantation)
1. Educate patient and family on safe bed mobility and transfers
2. Encourage diaphragmatic breathing-based training
3. Initiate a walking program
4. Avoid positions requiring flexion of the spine greater than 50° for at least 14 weeks
5. Avoid combined movements of the spine in flexion for at least 14 weeks
6. Avoid straight leg hip flexion greater than 45° for at least 14 weeks
7. Avoid combined hip flexion and spinal flexion for at least 14 weeks
Protective Phase (1–4 Weeks After Surgical Implantation)
1. Initiate an aerobic activity and home exercise program
2. Implement proper lifting guidelines: **a.** Maintain a symmetric upright posture **b.** Keep object close to the body **c.** Keep the weight of the object low **d.** Lift symmetrically using both hands **e.** Lift without jerking and maintaining a moderate speed
Controlled Motion Phase (5–16 Weeks After Surgical Implantation)
1. Ensure proper contraction and muscle firing patterns of cervico-thoracic and lumbo-pelvic stabilizer muscles during functional mobility exercises
2. Continue to improve coordination, strength, and endurance of cervical and lumbar muscles
3. Continue to increase aerobic tolerance through general strength and conditioning exercises (up to 30–60 min for at least 5 or more days per week)
4. At 16 weeks following surgical implantation, return to baseline function and normal activities with baseline range of motion in spine, upper extremities, and lower extremities
5. Establish functional independence in activities of daily living and self-care routine
6. Develop and maintain independent home exercise program and cardiovascular endurance training program

References

[1] Vakkala M, Järvimäki V, Kautiainen H, Haanpää M, Alahuhta S. Incidence and predictive factors of spinal cord stimulation treatment after lumbar spine surgery. J Pain Res 2017;10:2405–11. https://doi.org/10.2147/JPR.S143633.

[2] Mekhail N, Levy RM, Deer TR, et al. Durability of clinical and quality-of-life outcomes of closed-loop spinal cord stimulation for chronic back and leg pain: A secondary analysis of the Evoke randomized clinical trial [published correction appears in JAMA neurol. JAMA Neurol 2022;79 (4):420. https://doi.org/10.1001/jamaneurol.2022.0022.

[3] Nahm FS. From the torpedo fish to the spinal cord stimulator. Korean J Pain 2020;33(2). https://doi.org/10.3344/kjp.2020.33.2.97. 97-98.

[4] Lam CM, Latif U, Sack A, et al. Advances in spinal cord stimulation. Bioengineering (Basel) 2023;10(2):185. https://doi.org/10.3390/bioengineering10020185.

[5] Saluda Medical. Evoke® SCS system user manual. Rev. 4.01. Saluda Medical 2022. https://www.accessdata.fda.gov/cdrh_docs/pdf19/P190002C.pdf. [Accessed 23 February 2025].

[6] Deer TR, Mekhail N, Provenzano D, et al. The appropriate use of neurostimulation of the spinal cord and peripheral nervous system for the treatment of chronic pain and ischemic diseases: The Neuromodulation Appropriateness Consensus Committee. Neuromodulation 2014;17 (6):515–50. https://doi.org/10.1111/ner.12208.

[7] Deer TR, Mekhail N, Petersen E, et al. The appropriate use of neurostimulation: stimulation of the intracranial and extracranial space and head for chronic pain. Neuromodulation Appropriateness Consensus Committee. Neuromodulation 2014;17(6):551–70. https://doi.org/10.1111/ner.12215.

[8] Pritzlaff SG, Goree JH, Hagedorn JM, et al. Pain education and knowledge (PEAK) consensus guidelines for neuromodulation: A proposal for standardization in fellowship and training programs. J Pain Res 2023;16:3101–17. https://doi.org/10.2147/JPR.S424589.

[9] Mekhail NA, Levy RM, Deer TR, et al. ECAP-controlled closed-loop versus open-loop SCS for the treatment of chronic pain: 36-month results of the EVOKE blinded randomized clinical trial. Reg Anesth Pain Med 2024;49(5):346–54. https://doi.org/10.1136/rapm-2023-104751.

[10] Antony A, Pope J, Goree J, Smith G, Petersen E, Sayed D, Lam C, Gilmore C, Kapural L. Novel automated platform to upgrade SCS programming experience from subjective to objective - results from a prospective, dose-controlled closed-loop clinical study. In: Presented at: 2025 north American neuromodulation conference; 2025.

[11] Tekmyster G, Jonely H, Lee DW, et al. Physical therapy considerations and recommendations for patients following spinal cord stimulator implant surgery. Neuromodulation 2023;26:260–9. https://doi.org/10.1111/ner.13391.

[12] Dombovy-Johnson ML, D'Souza RS, Ha CT, Hagedorn JM. Incidence and risk factors for spinal cord stimulator lead migration with or without loss of efficacy: a retrospective review of 91 consecutive thoracic lead implants. Neuromodulation Technol Neural Interface 2022;25(5):731–7. https://doi.org/10.1111/ner.13487.

[13] Pope JE, Deer TR, Falowski S, et al. Multicenter retrospective Study of neurostimulation with exit of therapy by explant. Neuromodulation 2017;20(6):543–52. https://doi.org/10.1111/ner.12634.

[14] Van Buyten JP, Wille F, Smet I, et al. Therapy-related explants after spinal cord stimulation: Results of an international retrospective chart review study. Neuromodulation 2017;20(7):642–9. https://doi.org/10.1111/ner.12642.

[15] Al-Kaisy A, Royds J, Al-Kaisy O, et al. Explant rates of electrical neuromodulation devices in 1177 patients in a single center over an 11-year period. Reg Anesth Pain Med 2020;45(11):883–90. https://doi.org/10.1136/rapm-2020-101681.

[16] Wang VC, Bounkousohn V, Fields K, Bernstein C, Paicius RM, Gilligan C. Explantation rates of high frequency spinal cord stimulation in two outpatient clinics [published correction appears in neuromodulation. Neuromodulation 2021;24(8):1503. https://doi.org/10.1111/ner.13544. .

[17] Mekhail N, Costandi S, Mehanny DS, Armanyous S, Saied O, Taco-Vasquez E, Saweris Y. The impact of tobacco smoking on spinal cord stimulation effectiveness in complex regional pain syndrome patients. Neuromodulation 2020;23(1):133–9. https://doi.org/10.1111/ner.13058.

[18] Mekhail N, Azer G, Saweris Y, Mehanny DS, Costandi S, Mao G. The impact of tobacco cigarette smoking on spinal cord stimulation effectiveness in chronic spine-related pain patients. Reg Anesth Pain Med 2018;43(7):768–75. https://doi.org/10.1097/AAP.0000000000000870.

[19] Deer TR, Russo M, Grider JS, et al. The neurostimulation appropriateness consensus committee (NACC)®: recommendations for the mitigation of complications of neurostimulation. Neuromodulation 2024;24:S1094–7159. https://doi.org/10.1016/j.neurom.2024.04.004.

Chapter 24

Closed loop: Spinal cord stimulation

Michael Fishman[1], Melissa Murphy[2], Thomas Salazar[3], Harman Chopra[3] and Nomen Azeem[4]
[1]Brixton Biosciences Cambridge, Cambridge, MA, United States; [2]North Texas Orthopedics and Spine Center, Grapevine, TX, United States; [3]Colorado Rehabiliation and Occupational Medicine, Denver, CO, United States; [4]Florida Spine & Pain Specialists, Tampa, FL, United States

Introduction

Spinal cord stimulation (SCS) or neurostimulation has proven effective in managing various pain syndromes, including persistent spinal pain syndrome, complex regional pain syndrome, and neuropathic pain. However, despite the advances in stimulation patterns and frequencies, loss of efficacy remains one of the most leading causes for lead explant. This is partly because, until recently, SCS systems have relied on fixed-output, open-loop stimulation. This system, although initially effective, can be unsustainable without the use of objective physiologic feedback on target engagement or therapy delivery. The advent of closed-loop technology has bridged this gap and brings several potential advantages for patients who may experience overstimulation or subtherapeutic stimulation through traditional Open Loop SCS systems.

When nerves are repolarized during electrical stimulation, there is a measurable response corresponding to their magnitude of activation. During this process, it also produces an Evoked Compound Action Potential or ECAP, the amplitude of which provides an objective measurement of neural activation. In fixed-output SCS, the absence of this feedback results in a constant current with fixed parameters, aka "fixed-output". However, the use of real-time ECAP measurement in a closed-loop SCS system allows the automatic adjustment of stimulation intensity (current amplitude or charge) of each electrical pulse, thereby administering therapy that maintains precise and consistent neural activation. ECAP-controlled closed-loop SCS has overcome the limitations of fixed-output SCS by measuring spinal cord activation and accurately administering therapeutic doses, even in the face of dynamic physiologic processes that impact SCS therapy delivery [1–3].

ECAPs are generated when a stimulus pulse activates a group of neurons, leading to a synchronization of action potentials. The ECAP waveform consists of a positive P1 peak, a negative N1 trough, and a second positive P2 peak. The N1 component represents the direct activation of axons, while the P1 component reflects the subsequent postsynaptic response. Changes in the latency or shape of waveform provides information about the timing and degree of neural activation within the dorsal columns. A suboptimal amplitude alerts the system to increase stimulation intensity, while an abnormally high amplitude leads to a reduction in stimulation to prevent overstimulation. Alterations in the latency of the N1 trough signals changes in neural conduction, necessitating real-time adjustments to pulse width or frequency for optimal therapy [4,5].

By the continuous monitoring and analysis of ECAPS, specifically the N1 and P1 waveforms, closed-loop systems provide the dynamic ability to adjust the stimulation parameters in real-time. ECAPs respond to changes in the patient's physiology, such as postural movements or variations in tissue impedance, seen with complex movements such as walking, running, biking or even subtle changes in CSF fluid properties during simple functions such as coughing, sneezing or bending over resulting in changes within the spinal canal diameter and fluid shifts [6–9].

Key points

- Closed Loop SCS Systems are designed to adjust stimulation and dosing in real-time
- Closed Loop SCS is possible in parasthesia-free systems such as the Inceptive System.
- Closed Loop SCS may drastically increase patient satisfaction and treatment durability

A Modern Atlas for Implantable Devices of the Spine, Brain, and Nerve. https://doi.org/10.1016/B978-0-443-36528-7.00039-X

- Closed Loop SCS can further improve a long-standing data supported treatment for neuropathic and sympathetically mediated conditions.

Existing closed loop systems

As defined by the US Food and Drug Administration (FDA), a physiologic closed-loop controlled (PCLC) device is "a system consisting of sensors, actuators, and control algorithms that adjusts or maintains a physiologic variable through automatic adjustments to delivery or removal of energy or article (e.g., drugs, or liquid or gas regulated as a medical device) using feedback from a physiologic-measuring sensor(s)" [10]. Simply put, a PCLC device measures a physiologic variable in a patient, enters the input into a predetermined algorithm, and adjusts a separate response variable accordingly. It must have the ability to process data and respond as necessary to meet predetermined parameters.

PCLC systems have been successfully utilized in other specialties for decades, with early examples including pacemakers, ventilators, hemodialysis, and anesthesia delivery. These devices have all evolved as the technology has become more refined. Initially, for example, pacemakers were crude systems which did not involve a closed loop system at all; they now are complex PCLC devices which are able to treat a variety of wide-range of arrhythmias [11]. More specifically, with bradycardia, when the heart rate drops below a set, defined value, the pacemaker can sense that change and respond by delivering an appropriate amount of electrical stimulation to speed the heart rate up to a predetermined range.

With diabetes being one of the most common chronic diseases worldwide, there also has been significant progress in developing an efficient system to improve glycemic control. These implantable devices, sometimes referred to as the "artificial pancreas," continuously record blood glucose levels and automatically respond by adjusting insulin delivery per a set formula to avoid the peaks and valleys that can frequently lead to complications in diabetics [12].

Within the central nervous system, cochlear implants and deep brain stimulators are historically the most well-utilized PCLC devices. Cochlear implants can sense sound and in response electrically stimulate the auditory nerve to treat deafness. Though the first devices were successful in managing hearing loss, initial cochlear implants in the 1960s were open-loop systems requiring frequent fine-tuning [13,14]. More modern devices can measure evoked compound action potentials (ECAPs) and adjust their input accordingly, similar to how PCLC systems in spinal cord stimulators record ECAPs and respond based on a programmed algorithm [15].

Unmet need for open loop neurostimulators

The field of neuromodulation is fundamentally based on the theory that neural interfaces allow clinicians to programmatically influence biological effects. Over the years, the programming of spinal cord stimulation therapy has evolved to include a variety of proprietary and non-proprietary frequency-pulse width combinations. However, the development of novel programming modalities is only useful if those pulses can be effectively and reliably delivered to the neural tissue they are intended to modulate.

Herein lies a fundamental challenge of neuromodulation of the dorsal columns of the spinal cord—the cord is a moving target in a living organism.

Macro-movements of the body can substantially influence the activation threshold for the cord as the thickness of the dorsal cerebrospinal fluid (dCSF) layer changes with posture. Initial technology to change stimulation intensity with respect to changes in posture relied on a three-axis accelerometer to adapt stimulation intensity to patient body position (Medtronic AdaptiveStim). This was evaluated in the 2010 RestoreSensor study, which prospectively compared the use of adaptive stimulation versus standard stimulation in a randomized crossover study. The study demonstrated efficacy of neurostimulation in both groups, with a trend toward improved pain relief and improved convenience with adaptive stimulation [16]. Programming of adaptive stimulation is performed in clinic, where the comfort threshold parameters for each posture are set. The three-axis accelerometer and adaptive stimulation functions also allow the device to track the amount of time spent in each position, which can be useful in understanding the impact of therapy on patient macro-movement activities.

Micromotion also impacts the transmission of electrical activity across the thecal sac and its contents to the spinal cord. The cardiac and pulmonary cycles also induce micro-oscillations in the dCSF, which influences the distance between the electrodes and intended neural tissue targets. An accelerometer-based system cannot account for this physiological variability. Using accelerometry and dCSF thickness as a surrogate for cord activation is essentially using an imprecise mechanical measurement to estimate a neurophysiological response. Finite Element Models (FEM) are theoretical models that use the relative impedance of tissues to estimate the extent and breadth of electrical field activity with respect to the spinal cord [17,18]. FEMs fail as they cannot possibly account for the variability of the moving, breathing, living human being as they are static. In order to dynamically understand the impact of neurostimulation in real time, a direct measurement of spinal cord activation is required [19].

ECAPs are a well-characterized neurophysiological signal that represent a measure of spinal cord activation in response to a calibrated impulse, called a "ping pulse" [20,21]. Advancements in neural interface technology have now transformed the spinal cord stimulator electrode from being a unidirectional therapy delivery conduit to a bidirectional therapy delivery and response monitoring interface. Sensing activation of the cord is typically performed by delivering a 50Hz "ping" pulse from a proximal contact and then sensing the cord response between a pair of distal electrodes, in an either adjacent (narrow-spaced) or skipped (wide-spaced) configuration [22]. Isolating the electrical activity at the level of the cord under these circumstances relies on sophisticated artifact suppression algorithms that account for not only the macro-motion of the organism and its physiologic micro-motion, but also for the concurrent stimulation artifact and the residual stimulation artifact.

Inceptiv specific closed-loop algorithm

One challenge of measuring ECAPs is to create a high-fidelity filtering system to filter out artifacts and detect true ECAPs—the distance between the electrodes and neural target ia mediated by the CSF thickness in between [23]. A template correlation method calculates ECAPs by correlating the measured ECAP with an artificial ECAP signal.

This may over or under-estimate ECAPs in a conventional paresthesia-based closed-loop system [24]. Another method is called the high-pass filter, which can maintain a high neural response-to-artifact output [24].

The closed-loop algorithm in inceptiv can be used with paresthesia-based therapy and subperception therapy. During paresthesia-based therapy, the closed loop algorithm works closely to maintain the sensed ECAP amplitude between the upper and lower limits. For subperception therapy, stimulation intensity is programmed near or below perception, such as differential target multiplexed (DTM) SCS. In the DTM SCS programming, there are low-frequency and high-frequency components. The low-frequency component is used to detect ECAPs through a special processing mechanism. Then, the detected ECAP is used to control both the low-frequency and high-frequency waveforms in a pulse-to-pulse fashion [25].

Inceptiv closed-loop SCS studies

The Electrically Evoked Compound Action Potentials Human Observation Medtronic Algorithm Comparion Study (ECHO-MAC) study was performed in 2021. It tested clinical performance of the closed loop algorithm in a randomized setting. At the end of the commercial SCS trial, 42 subjects were connected to an investigational device in clinic. Subjects were randomized and crossed over to open-loop SCS and closed-loop SCS. Devices were programmed with a 50 Hz near the perception threshold. The subjects were asked to perform activities such as bending, coughing, or laughing that normally elicit overstimulation discomfort and rate their discomfort level with closed-loop on and closed-loop off while being blinded on the programming setting. The study showed 97.6% of subjects preferred closed-loop on instead of open-loop [5].

The Programming Optimization for Spinal Evoked Compound Action Potentials (PROSE) study conducted in 2022 was used to develop a workflow using closed-loop with Differential Target Multiplexed waveforms (DTM). At the end of a commercial SCS trial, subjects were connected to an external investigational hardware. 39 out of 42 patients had a measurable ECAP. On average, it took about 9 min (range 2–38 min) to program DTM with closed-loop [26].

In Australia, there is an ongoing prospective, multi-center, single arm study evaluating patients with implanted closed-loop device up to 24 months. The objective of this study is to evaluate the performance of flexible, ECAP-based, closed-loop feature in a representative population of pain patients. The study design includes in-clinic, randomized, crossover to test closed-loop performance at 1 month, 3 months, 12 months. At these time points, for patients with a clear ECAP, they were randomized to test closed loop versus open loop. They were instructed to perform activities that may cause over stimulation and were asked to rate the discomfort level from 0 to 4. This was retested again after cross over [27].

The primary objective of this study was to demonstrate reduction in overstimulation by performing in-clinic randomized, crossover testing with the closed loop versus open loop at the 1 month visit for the first 28 subjects. The secondary objective was to determine the responder rate (measured as 50% reduction in VAS) in this single arm study at 3 months for a minimum of 45 subjects with low back-leg pain [27].

The study showed 9 out of 10 subjects reported overstimulation reduction with closed-loop on through 12 months and they prefer closed-loop over open-loop stimulation.

ECAPs were detected in 93%–94% of subjects through the 12 months visit. 82% of subjects reported $\geq$50% reduction in low back pain. The mean reduction in pain was 67% at 12 months. The overall composite success includes overall low back/leg pain reduction, improved quality of life, improved physical function, improved mood, and improved sleep. 87% of patients reported improvement in at least 3 domans. The study shows consistent performance of closed-loop feature through 12 months and 9 out of 10 patients prefer the closed-loop feature to engage in daily activities [27].

Inceptiv versus Evoke

Despite the initial success seen in SCS trial procedures and early stages in the implant period, loss of efficacy remains as the most common reason for explant in long-term patients. The reasons for this have largely been speculative, but the recent deployment of ECAP-based measurements may provide the bridge to this roadblock, and early studies have already demonstrated its value and contribution to the therapeutic ability of SCS technology. In the US, two major medical device companies currently offer CL-SCS (see Table 24.1).

Inceptive future considerations

Applying closed loop stimulation principles using ECAPs to contemporary therapy paradigms that are independent of paresthesia has been accomplished [5]. In the case of subthreshold stimulation paradigms, the goal of ECAPs closed loop is the same as in tonic therapy—to minimize variability in delivery of therapy to the spinal cord to maintain consistent therapy delivery. It is now imperative that there is an effort to collect long term data using the Inceptive system with a

TABLE 24.1 Comparison of inceptive closed loop system and Evoke closed loop system [9,23,28–33].

Category	Medtronic Inceptiv (closed-loop SCS)	Saluda Evoke (closed- loop SCS)
Closed-loop method	ECAP-sensing amplitude control; automatically adjusts to maintain therapy during activity. Senses approximately 50 times per second.	ECAP-controlled closed loop; automatically adjusts current of the next pulse to hold target ECAP amplitude.
Closed-loop adjustment cadence	Samples and adjusts ~50 times per second during movement.	Updates pulse-to-pulse based on ECAP reading (every pulse in real time).
Programmable frequency range	Published by waveform rather than one universal spec; e.g., DTM programs span ~50–1200 Hz. Exact Inceptiv master range not publicly listed.	10–1400 Hz.
Pulse width range	Not publicly listed for Inceptiv; varies by program.	20–1000 μs.
Max output (current)	Not publicly listed.	0–50 mA.
Lead types supported	Vectris SureScan percutaneous leads and Specify SureScan paddle (surgical) leads.	CAP12 percutaneous leads (12-contact).
Example lead specs	Percutaneous: Vectris 1 × 8 contacts, 3.0 mm contact length, 1.5–4.0 mm spacing, lengths 60–90 cm. Paddle: Specify 2 × 8 (7.6 mm wide, 1.9 mm thick) or specify 5-6-5 (10 mm wide, 2.0 diameter ~1.32 mm mm thick).	Percutaneous: CAP12, 12- contact, 3 mm contact length, 4 mm spacing, lengths 60 or 90 cm
IPG thickness/ dimensions	Thickness ~6 mm (marketed as Medtronic's thinnest SCS). Other dimensions not publicly posted.	68 × 48 × 12 mm; thickness 12 mm; ~50 g; 33 cc volume.
Ports/channel configuration	Dual-port IPG; supports two leads (percutaneous or paddle) with up to 16 contacts.	Supports CAP12 lead with 12 contacts.
Battery & recharge	Rechargeable; adaptive recharging profile; battery longevity varies by program parameters. 8–10+ years	Rechargeable; typical recharge every few days to weekly depending on program; battery longevity 8–10+ years.
Waveform families	Supports tonic, burst, high-frequency (up to 1200 Hz in some programs), DTM, and ECAP-based closed loop.	Primarily tonic stimulation in ECAP-controlled closed loop.
MRI labeling	Full-body 1.5T and 3T MRI access under specified conditions.	MRI conditions vary by model and region; not

focus on SCS explant rates. Currently, the Inceptive closed loop system cannot be utilized during the SCS trial period, future iterations of the inceptive system should be incorporated into the trial period. Near-infrared reflectometry (NIR) technology is a technology being developed for use in closed loop neurostimulation. NIR uses light reflected off the spinal cord to measure the distance between the stimulating electrode and its neural target in real-time [34]. Closed loop SCS is the future and that is evidenced by further advancements to develop more nuanced systems such as the NIR technology.

References

[1] Parker JL, Karantonis DM, Single PS, Obradovic M, Cousins MJ. Compound action potentials recorded in the human spinal cord during neurostimulation for pain relief. Pain 2012;153(3):593–601. https://doi.org/10.1016/j.pain.2011.11.023.

[2] Parker JL, Karantonis DM, Single PS, Obradovic M, Laird J, Gorman RB, Ladd LA, Cousins MJ. Electrically evoked compound action potentials recorded from the sheep spinal cord. Neuromodulation 2013;16(4):295–303. https://doi.org/10.1111/ner.12053.

[3] Parker J, Karantonis D, Single P. Hypothesis for the mechanism of action of ECAP-controlled closed-loop systems for spinal cord stimulation. Healthc Technol Lett 2020;7(3):76–80. https://doi.org/10.1049/htl.2020.0021.

[4] Dietz BE, Mugan D, Vuong QC, Obara I. Electrically evoked compound action potentials in spinal cord stimulation: implications for preclinical research models. Neuromodulation 2022;25(1):64–74. https://doi.org/10.1111/ner.13322.

[5] Will A, Fishman M, Schultz D, et al. Improvements in therapy experience with evoked compound action potential controlled, closed-loop spinal cord stimulation – primary outcome of the ECHO-MAC randomized clinical trial. J Pain 2024;25:104646.

[6] Single PS, Scott JB, Mugan D. Measures of dosage for spinal-cord electrical stimulation: review and proposal. IEEE Trans Neural Syst Rehabil Eng 2023;31:4653–60. https://doi.org/10.1109/TNSRE.2023.3115470.

[7] Versantvoort EM, Dietz BE, Mugan D, Vuong QC, Luli S, Obara I. Evoked compound action potential (ECAP)-controlled closed-loop spinal cord stimulation in an experimental model of neuropathic pain in rats. Bioelectron Med 2024;10(1):2. https://doi.org/10.1186/s42234-023-00028-0.

[8] Pilitsis JG, Chakravarthy KV, Will AJ, et al. The evoked compound action potential as a predictor for perception in chronic pain patients: tools for automatic spinal cord stimulator programming and control. Front Neurosci 2021;15:673998. https://doi.org/10.3389/fnins.2021.673998.

[9] Su PP, Arle J, Poree L. Closing the loop and raising the bar: automated control systems in neuromodulation. Pain Pract 2024;24(1):177–85. https://doi.org/10.1111/papr.13290.

[10] United States Food and Drug Administration (FDA), Health and Human Services. In: Technical considerations for medical devices with physiologic closed-loop control technology; guidance for industry and food and drug administration staff; 2023. https://www.fda.gov/regulatory-information/search-fda-guidance-documents.

[11] Mulpuru SK, Madhavan M, McLeod CJ, Cha YM, Friedman PA. Cardiac pacemakers: function, troubleshooting, and management: Part 1 of a 2-part series. J Am Coll Cardiol 2017;69(2):189–210. https://doi.org/10.1016/j.jacc.2016.09.979.

[12] Hovorka R. Closed-loop insulin delivery: from bench to clinical practice. Nat Rev Endocrinol 2011;7:385–95. https://doi.org/10.1038/nrendo.2011.32.

[13] Mudry A, Mills M. The early history of the cochlear implant: a retrospective. JAMA Otolaryngol Head Neck Surg 2013;139(5):446–53. https://doi.org/10.1001/jamaoto.2013.293.

[14] Mc Laughlin M, Lu T, Dimitrijevic A, Zeng F-G. Towards a closed-loop cochlear implant system: application of embedded monitoring of peripheral and central neural activity. IEEE Trans Neural Syst Rehabil Eng 2012;20(4):443–54. https://doi.org/10.1109/TNSRE.2012.2186982.

[15] Van Dijk B, Botros AM, Battmer R-D, Begall K, Dillier N, Hey M, Lai WK, Lenarz T, Laszig R, Morsnowski A, Müller-Deile J, Psarros C, Shallop J, Weber B, Wesarg T, Zarowski A, Offeciers E. Clinical results of AutoNRT, a completely automatic ECAP recording system for cochlear implants. Ear Hear 2007;28(4):558–70. https://doi.org/10.1097/AUD.0b013e31806dc.

[16] Schultz D, Schultz DM, Webster L, Kosek P, Dar U, Tan Y, Sun M. Randomized trial sensor-driven position-adaptive spinal cord stimulation for chronic pain. Pain Physician 2012;15:1–12.

[17] Holsheimer J. Computer modelling of spinal cord stimulation and its contribution to therapeutic efficacy. Spinal Cord 1998;36(8):531–40. https://doi.org/10.1038/sj.sc.3100717.

[18] Holsheimer J, Barolat G. Spinal geometry and paresthesia coverage in spinal cord stimulation. Neuromodulation 1998;1(3):129–36. https://doi.org/10.1111/j.1525-1403.1998.tb00006.x.

[19] Dinsmoor DA, Usoro JO, Barka ND, Billstrom TM, Litvak LM, Poree LR. Using evoked compound action potentials to quantify differential neural activation with burst and conventional, 40 Hz spinal cord stimulation in ovines. Pain Reports 2022;7(6):E1047. https://doi.org/10.1097/PR9.0000000000001047.

[20] Pilitsis J, Chakravarthy K, Hageman K, Litvak L, Dinsmoor D. The spinal evoked compound action potential as a predictor for perception. Neuromodulation 2011;25(5):S54.

[21] Poree L, Pope JE, Levy RM, Kapural L, Deer TR, Gorman RB, Obradovic M, Khurram A, Parker JL. In: Long-term robustness of evoked compound action potentials (ECAPs) as a physiological monitoring tool; 2011.

[22] Fishman M, Wolf J, Will A, Dinsmoor D, Skerker A. The effect of electrode selection on optimal spinal evoked compound action potential sensing. Neuromodulation 2021;25(5):S55.

[23] Chakravarthy K, Bink H, Dinsmoor D. Sensing evoked compound action potentials from the spinal cord: novel preclinical and clinical considerations for the pain management researcher and clinician. J Pain Res December 4, 2020;13:3269–79. https://doi.org/10.2147/JPR.S289098.

[24] Chakravarthy K, FitzGerald J, Will A, Trutnau K, Corey R, Dinsmoor D, Litvak L. A clinical feasibility study of spinal evoked compound action potential estimation methods. Neuromodulation 2022;25(1):75–84. https://doi.org/10.1111/ner.13510.

[25] Vallejo R, Chakravarthy K, Will A, Trutnau K, Dinsmoor D. A new direction for closed-loop spinal cord stimulation: combining contemporary therapy paradigms with evoked compound action potential sensing. J Pain Res 2021;14:3909–18. https://doi.org/10.2147/JPR.S344568.

[26] Will A, Franke A, Schultz D, et al. Early experience with closed-loop SCS during in-clinic testing. Neuromodulation 2023;26(4):S92.

[27] Charkravarthy K, Mohabbati V, et al. 12-month outcomes with a flexible closed loop spinal cord stimulation system. In: North American Neuromodulation Society (NANS) Meeting. January 30-Feburary 1; 2025.

[28] Sharan A, Mohabbati V, Sullivan R, et al. Closed-loop SCS therapy outcomes at 3-months with waveforms optimized per patient preference. In: American Society of Regional Anesthesia and Pain Medicine (ASRA); November 10-11; 2023.

[29] Leitner A, Hanson E, Soliday N, et al. Real world clinical utility of neurophysiological measurement utilizing closed-loop spinal cord stimulation in a chronic pain population: the ECAP study protocol. J Pain Res 2023;16:2497–507. https://doi.org/10.2147/JPR.S411927.

[30] Poree L, Foster A, Staats PS. Device profile of the Evoke physiologic closed-loop spinal cord stimulation system for the treatment of chronic intractable pain: overview of its safety and efficacy. Expet Rev Med Dev 2023;20(11):885–98. https://doi.org/10.1080/17434440.2023.2255520.

[31] London D, Mogilner A. Spinal cord stimulation: new waveforms and technology. Neurosurg Clin 2022;33(3):287–95. https://doi.org/10.1016/j.nec.2022.02.006.

[32] Mekhail N, Levy RM, Deer TR, et al. Long-term safety and efficacy of closed-loop spinal cord stimulation to treat chronic back and leg pain (Evoke): a double-blind, randomised, controlled trial. Lancet Neurol 2020;19(2):123–34. https://doi.org/10.1016/S1474-4422(19)30414-4.

[33] Mekhail N, Levy RM, Deer TR, et al. Durability of clinical and quality-of-life outcomes of closed-loop spinal cord stimulation for chronic back and leg pain: a secondary analysis of the Evoke randomized clinical trial. JAMA Neurol 2022;79(3):251–60. https://doi.org/10.1001/jamaneurol.2021.4998.

[34] Wolf EW. Dynamic detection of spinal cord position during postural changes using near-infrared reflectometry. Neuromodulation 2015;18(6):448–59. https://doi.org/10.1111/NER.12319.

Chapter 25

Biosensing and closed-loop stimulation in the peripheral nervous system

Jeffery Kramer[1, 2, 3], Hemant Kalia[4], Ramana Naidu[5], Aydin Babakhani[6, 7] and Timothy Deer[8]

[1]*Volta Research, Minneapolis, MN, United States;* [2]*University of Illinois, Chicago, IL, United States;* [3]*Nervonik, Los Angeles, CA, United States;* [4]*Center for Research & Innovation in Spine & Pain, Rochester, NY, United States;* [5]*MarinHealth Spine Institute, Larkspur, CA, United States;* [6]*Nervonik, Los Angeles, CA, United States;* [7]*UCLA, Los Angeles, CA, United States;* [8]*The Spine and Nerve Centers of the Virginias, Charleston, WV, United States*

Biosensing and closed-loop therapy

- Electrical biosensing detects signals generated in excitable cell tissues to help improve and automate therapy.
- Signals include local field potentials (LFP) evoked compound action potentials (ECAP), and compound muscle action potentials (CMAP).
- Closed-loop therapies are already in use for brain and spinal cord stimulation.
- Uses in peripheral nerve stimulation are commercially limited but show great promise.

Introduction

The human body produces electrical biosignals that are related to voltage potentials being generated due to excitable cell membrane function. Examples of these biosignals include electrocardiographic, electromyographic and electroencephalographic potentials from the heart, skeletal muscles and brain, respectively. In particular, electrical biosignals from the nervous system have garnered interest not only due to diagnostic information that may be decoded from the signals but also for their use as a means to control electrical stimulation-based therapies [1].

Beyond the source of the electrical biosignal (e.g., the heart, spinal cord, and peripheral nerves), there are also other ways to describe these measured voltage potentials. In some cases, biosignals are recorded passively without provocation. An example of this is local field potentials, which can be recorded from discrete regions of the brain [2] and other regions of the CNS and PNS. In this way, focal activity within a specified region of the nervous system can be obtained and related to a clinical symptom or outcome of interest. Some examples of this include the ability to measure local brain activity, which, when analyzed in the frequency domain, has rhythms tuned to beta-band patterns [2]. This biosignal has been shown to be related to motor symptoms in Parkinson's disease [3]. Still another contemporary example is utilized in brain-computer interfacing to read brain signals and then decode them for augmentative and assistive communication or motor function.

Another class of biosignal is evoked rather than passively recorded. An example of this is an evoked compound action potential (ECAP). In this case, an electrical field is utilized to excite neural tissue, which in turn generates synchronized action potential ensembles. This coordinated and summated activation can be recorded and filtered to yield a signal that is related to the stimulation used to evoke it as well as other characteristics such as changes in distance from the stimulating electrode and neural tissue, dynamic physiologic properties of the neural element(s) of interest or physiologic results of stimulation that may be downstream from the neural tissue being targeted.

Common types of evoked potentials are recorded from both neural and muscle tissues (Fig. 25.1). ECAPs recorded from neural tissues are small and typically require: 1) recording electrodes to be close to the tissue generating the voltage potentials, 2) large amplification, and 3) selective filtering of recording artifacts (stimulation, movement, etc.). Neurally

A Modern Atlas for Implantable Devices of the Spine, Brain, and Nerve. https://doi.org/10.1016/B978-0-443-36528-7.00008-X

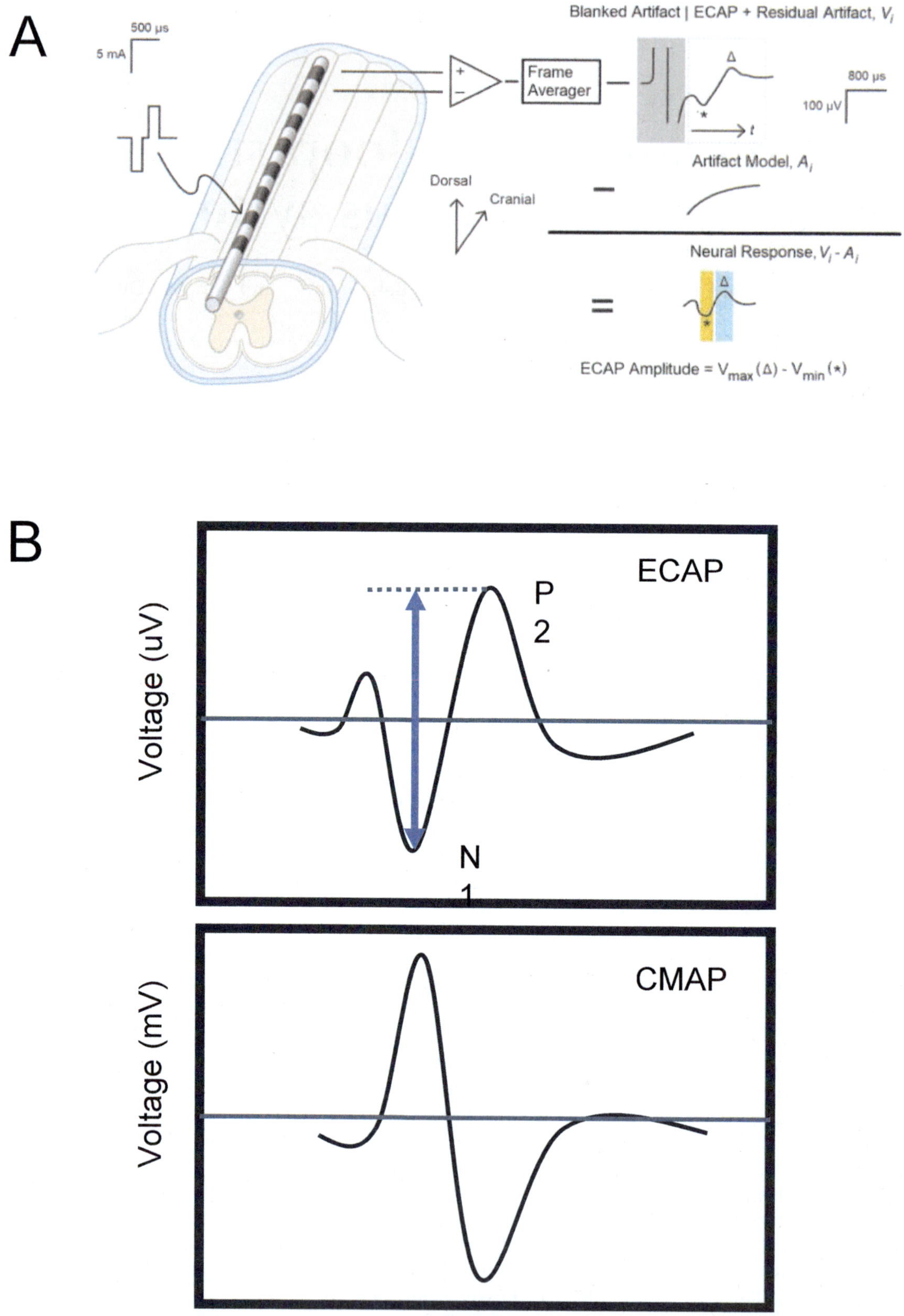

FIGURE 25.1 Evoked compound action potential (ECAP) and compound muscle action potential (CMAP) signatures and recording methods from the epidural space. Panel a depicts an epidural lead stimulating the dorsal surface of the spinal cord and recording evoked potentials from the same lead [4]. Panel B shows the relevant ECAP and CMAP waveforms and, in the case of an ECAP, the relevant markers utilized for measurement and use in closed-loop therapy control algorithms.

based ECAPs are fast-moving because the conduction of neural tissue propagates quickly. As such, both the location of the stimulating and recording components are critical to ensure efficient and appropriate signal detection. Compound muscle action potential (CMAP) recordings are generally larger since the mass of muscle being activated is much larger than the volume of neural tissue generating coordinated action potentials. Also, CMAPs that are being activated by neural stimulation also have the advantage of being slightly delayed relative to ECAP signals, thus allowing one to separate this signal from other potential artifact sources.

Aside from the recording techniques, it is important to understand the biosignal being measured and what information it is encoding. This will help determine the utility as a diagnostic or, in some cases, as a basis for therapy control. The latter of these examples is the basis for closed-loop stimulation therapy. In this case, the biosignal is being used to help control a therapy output, thus resulting in a better means by which to deliver electricity. In some cases, a biosignal that is related to a symptom can be used, while in other cases, a signal that conveys physical distance or proximity can be used to physiologically control stimulation. In both examples, the recorded biosignal is conveying an important piece of information that provides guidance on how, when and/or where stimulation should be provided.

Closed-loop neurostimulation – CNS examples

Deep Brain Stimulation. Biosensing and closed-loop neurostimulation in the treatment of symptoms such as tremor and dyskinesia with deep-brain stimulation (DBS) has been well documented [5]. The basis for this approach involves detecting a synchronized brain signal typically recorded from the subthalamic nucleus (STN), a common brain target for stimulation therapy. The brain signal from the STN is a collection of extracellular signals that amalgamate into multiple field potentials being recorded at once. Analysis of these signals demonstrates that in the frequency domain, these field potentials in patients suffering from Parkinson's Disease (PD) show a peak in the beta band (13–25 Hz) [2]. This signal has been shown to be related to symptoms in PD, thereby providing a potential means to relate stimulation therapy to a symptom-linked biomarker [3]. The approach also utilizes the ability of stimulation to modulate both the beta signal and symptoms concurrently, thereby hoping to optimize the appropriate therapy dose at any given time. This closed-loop approach aims to provide consistent therapy while multiple factors may shift neurologic functioning (and symptoms), including pharmacotherapy and the natural instability of neurologic function due to underlying neuropathology.

Similar to anatomic region, evoked potentials have also been studied in the STN with DBS. The observation of evoked resonant responses to stimulation provides another dimension to the ability to sense field potentials in the brain [6]. Although it is unclear how these resonant biosignals might reflect brain network dysfunction or be utilized therapeutically, it provides another basis by which to inform and, perhaps, enhance therapy delivery in the treatment of movement disorders.

Spinal Cord Stimulation. Using a similar approach, epidural neural sensing from the spinal cord of chronic pain patients utilizing spinal cord stimulators has yielded an interesting approach to enhance analgesic therapy. By measuring an ECAP biosignal, observations can be made about the relative amount of electrical dose that is reaching the spinal cord, thereby gauging therapy delivery consistency and efficiency [7]. The ECAP is evoked by stimulating contact pairs on one side of an epidural lead placed over the dorsal surface of the spinal cord and then recording some rostral or caudal distance away via sensing contact pairs on the same epidural lead array. Figure 25.1 depicts the measurement configuration and waveform of a spinal ECAP, and denotes the marker points that help determine the relative amplitude of the ECAP biosignal. The amplitude is an index of the volume of neural tissue activated and a direct measurement of the received electrical dose. Multiple factors can influence the ECAP amplitude, including the distance of the lead from the neural tissue as well as pharmacological influences from analgesic drugs. While it is known that epidural lead positions relative to the spinal cord vary widely based upon spinal segment and gravitational effect from body position (e.g., upright vs. supine), what was not as well appreciated was how widely the received dose can vary with even small amounts of movement or inherent physiologic rhythms (respiratory and cardiac cycles). In this way, the epidural ECAP is not a symptom-related biosignal, which differs from the previously mentioned LFP signal in the STN. Rather, the ECAP is a dose-meter of sorts which allows a more consistent therapy delivery over time, as well as potentially automating various programming functions [7].

The closed-loop therapy embodiment utilizes the ECAP signal to automatically adjust the pulse amplitudes to enable more or less electrical dose delivery. A feedback loop enables a control policy to utilize the objective dose measured and then corrects the stimulation output if needed. A smaller ECAP indicates that a lower dose was received than needed, so pulse amplitude is increased. Similarly, if the ECAP is too large relative to the programmed maximal set point, then the pulse amplitude is lowered to reduce the total dose delivered.

Biosensing signals from the peripheral nervous system

Although biosensing is an integral part of various peripheral-nerve neuromodulation therapies, sensing in PNS for pain has yet to see commercial applications. Peripheral nerve ECAPS are used routinely in preclinical pain research to identify the fiber types (Aβ,Aα, Aδ, or C fibers) stimulated based on ECAP morphology and latency [e.g., Ref. [8]]. Relationships have been found between ECAPS and cognitive elements of stimulation [4], thus providing a means to understand electrical dosing in a way that is translational to human subjects [9,10]. Biosensing of ECAP and CMAP signals is utilized clinically to diagnose neurological damage as part of nerve conduction studies in patients suffering from carpal tunnel syndrome, inflammatory neuropathies, and other diseases [11].

Cuff-style electrodes that encompass the peripheral nerve have been used for neural recordings in VNS applications [12]. But, as percutaneous, circumferential leads are increasingly utilized for PNS applications, it is desirable to use this type of lead for biosensing as well. Recording ECAPS from peripheral electrodes with cylindrical leads, however, can be challenging. The ability to record ECAPS, particularly at relatively low stimulation levels (such as those used with leads close to peripheral nerves), generally requires a close proximity to neural tissue, with the ECAP signal dropping approximately with the square of the distance [13]. In addition, since the volume of neural tissues is much lower in peripheral nerves relative to the spinal cord, for example, the resultant ECAP can be small. Depending on the application, it may be possible to utilize signal analysis techniques such as averaging (repeated measurement of ECAP signal) to partially overcome the decrease in the ECAP signal strength. Signals below a microvolt have been recorded through cylindrical leads utilizing averaging technique [4], demonstrating this potential measurement enhancement approach.

Commercial uses

Cochlear Implants. Several sensing modalities are routinely utilized in cochlear implants. Cochlear implant prosthesis is one of the most successful peripheral neuromodulation devices, designed to treat hearing loss by bypassing the normal hearing mechanism and directly stimulating the auditory nerve. These devices are often implanted at a very young age (e.g., 6 months). For these recipients, clinicians are greatly challenged with obtaining proper stimulation levels based on behavioral feedback and thus utilize ECAPs to assist in the programming of these devices. One common practice is to set the maximum stimulation level of each electrode to its ECAP threshold. Although this practice has been challenged as the correlation between comfortable levels in adults and ECAP thresholds is low [14], it is used routinely for initial pediatric fitting. Performance with ECAP-informed maps is generally comparable to performance with clinically generated maps [15]. Typically, ECAPS growth curves are measured for a set of stimulation electrodes, with another nearby intracochlear electrode utilized as the recording electrode. Monopolar configuration is used for both stimulation and recording, with the same or separate recording and stimulation grounds depending on the device. Because such a monopolar configuration results in a very large artifact, specialized techniques, such as masker-probe [16] and alternating polarity, have been developed to reduce the artifact to an acceptable level.

Vagus Nerve Stimulation. Implantable vagus nerve stimulation utilizing biosensing is used in the treatment of drug-resistant epilepsy. Cardiac changes (increases in HR) are recorded from the ECG signal and utilized for controlling stimulation output. The intent is to detect preictal events in order to drive stimulation at opportunistic windows to increase antiseizure therapy effectiveness [12].

Sacral Nerve. While not implemented into a commercial therapy yet, compound muscle potentials have been recorded from human sacral leads. These potentials are large (up to 1 mV) and have distinct morphological features. The CMAP thresholds appear to be tightly correlated with therapeutic levels utilized for stimulation, suggesting that they may be useful for appropriate dosing of the therapy [17,18]. In addition, the morphology of the signal is thought to relate to the quality of the therapy.

Future PNS application

Peripheral nerve stimulation (PNS) is poised to revolutionize pain management through advanced biosensing and closed-loop control mechanisms. Current research focuses on integrating evoked compound action potentials (ECAPs) and compound muscle action potentials (CMAPs) as biomarkers for personalized therapy modulation. Another potential option could be to simply develop a closed biosensing loop based on nerve conduction studies (NCS), which is a very widely used application in electromyographic studies. All these signals offer real-time insights into nerve activation, ensuring precise dosing and minimizing side effects.

Future PNS systems will likely incorporate machine learning algorithms to optimize stimulation parameters based on patient-specific neural and behavioral responses. Additionally, advancements in percutaneous and implantable electrodes will improve long-term stability and signal fidelity, allowing for more effective closed-loop therapies. By dynamically adjusting stimulation based on biosensed signals, future PNS applications could provide reliable lead placement based upon objective biosignals and consistent electrical dosing, thereby producing optimal pain relief while minimizing side effects and the need for manual recalibration. The latter of these points, system function automation and ease of use, are already being realized in the SCS and DBS therapy spaces and could significantly ease the burden on physicians and patients.

Application of closed-loop approaches in peripheral nerve stimulation will probably follow a redefined construct. As there is less chance of medium (cerebrospinal fluid) variability in signal transmission as compared to SCS, the goal of closed-loop stimulation in PNS will primarily be to remain within the identified therapeutic index of the dose-response curve. The goal of closed-loop PNS will be to achieve personalized, precise and predictable improvements in pain, function and quality of life.

Moreover, integrating PNS with wearable biosensors may enable remote monitoring, paving the way for adaptive neuromodulation strategies tailored to individual needs. These innovations hold promises for transforming chronic pain management, enhancing both efficacy and patient experience.

Pearls and pitfalls

- Contemporary adaptive and closed-loop neuromodulation therapy features utilize advanced biosensing to help optimize stimulation therapies.
- When to stimulate, how much to stimulate, and where to stimulate are automation goals. Better clinical outcomes are presented as one positive feature while also increasing ease of use for programming and reducing side effects.
- Optimization can be fully automatic or an assistive aid to the patient and clinician.
- Closed-loop therapies are still relatively new, and clinical utility is still being understood; not all patients may be good candidates for this therapy feature.
- Applications in peripheral nerve stimulation are being investigated for multiple possible therapy enhancements.

References

[1] Pope JE, Deer TR, Sayed D, et al. The American society of pain and neuroscience (ASPN) guidelines and consensus on the definition, current evidence, clinical use and future applications for physiologic closed-loop controlled neuromodulation in chronic pain: A neuron group project. J Pain Res 2025;18:531–51.

[2] van Wijk BCM, de Bie RMA, Beudel M. A systematic review of local field potential physiomarkers in Parkinson's disease: From clinical correlations to adaptive deep brain stimulation algorithms. J Neurol 2023;270(2):1162–77.

[3] Morelli N, Summers RLS. Association of subthalamic beta frequency sub-bands to symptom severity in patients with Parkinson's disease: A systematic review. Parkinsonism Relat Disord 2023;110:105364.

[4] Pilitsis JG, Chakravarthy KV, Will AJ, et al. The evoked compound action potential as a predictor for perception in chronic pain patients: Tools for automatic spinal cord stimulator programming and control. Front Neurosci 2021;15:673998.

[5] Cuschieri A, Borg N, Zammit C. Closed loop deep brain stimulation: A systematic scoping review. Clin Neurol Neurosurg 2022;223:107516.

[6] Hageman K, Stypulkowski P, Stanslaski S. Characterization of subthalamic nucleus deep brain stimulation evoked resonant neural activity in a large animal model: A pilot study. Brain Res 2025;1846:149233.

[7] Poree L, Foster A, Staats PS. Device profile of the evoke physiologic closed-loop spinal cord stimulation system for the treatment of chronic intractable pain: Overview of its safety and efficacy. Expert Rev Med Devices 2023;20(11):885–98.

[8] Castoro MA, Yoo PB, Hincapie JG, et al. Excitation properties of the right cervical vagus nerve in adult dogs. Exp Neurol 2011;227(1):62–8.

[9] Cedeno DL, Vallejo R, Kelley CA, et al. Spinal evoked compound action potentials in rats with clinically relevant stimulation modalities. Neuromodulation 2023;26(1):68–77.

[10] Dietz BE, Mugan D, Vuong QC, Obara I. Electrically evoked compound action potentials in spinal cord stimulation: Implications for preclinical research models. Neuromodulation 2022;25(1):64–74.

[11] Mallik A, Weir AI. Nerve conduction studies: Essentials and pitfalls in practice. J Neurol Neurosurg Psychiatry 2005;76(Suppl. 2):ii23–31.

[12] Mertens A, Raedt R, Gadeyne S, et al. Recent advances in devices for vagus nerve stimulation. Expert Rev Med Devices 2018;15(8):527–39.

[13] Parker JL, Shariati NH, Karantonis DM. Electrically evoked compound action potential recording in peripheral nerves. Bioelectron Med 2018;1(1):71–83.

[14] de Vos JJ, Biesheuvel JD, Briaire JJ, et al. Use of electrically evoked compound action potentials for cochlear implant fitting: A systematic review. Ear Hear 2018;39(3):401–11.

[15] Craddock L, Cooper H, van de Heyning P, et al. Comparison between NRT-based MAPs and behaviourally measured MAPs at different stimulation rates–a multicentre investigation. Cochlear Implants Int 2003;4(4):161–70.
[16] Miller CA, Abbas PJ, Brown CJ. An improved method of reducing stimulus artifact in the electrically evoked whole-nerve potential. Ear Hear 2000;21(4):280–90.
[17] Goudelocke C, Jungbauer Nikolas LM, Bittner KC, et al. Sensing in sacral neuromodulation: A feasibility study in subjects with urinary incontinence and retention. Neuromodulation 2024;27(2):392–8.
[18] Powell C, Goudelocke C, Ruiz H, et al. 255 - beyond sensory: SNM lead sensing consistently measures patient-specific sacral evoked responses. Continence 2024;12:101597.

Section 7

Remote care and monitoring

Introduction to section 7 remote care and monitoring

Chronic pain remains a pervasive and debilitating condition affecting millions worldwide. For patients whose pain is refractory to conventional pharmacologic and interventional therapies, spinal cord stimulation (SCS) has emerged as a powerful neuromodulation strategy. Over the past decades, SCS devices have evolved in sophistication, offering multiple waveforms, closed-loop capabilities, and more precise targeting of neural substrates. However, despite these advances, the long-term success of SCS does not rest solely on the implant hardware—it depends critically on ongoing patient follow-up, parameter optimization, adherence, and early detection of complications or device issues. In this context, remote monitoring and remote care are poised to transform the practice of neuromodulation by shifting a portion of care from clinic visits into the patient's home environment, providing new insights to maintain successful therapy and to intervene more quickly and prudently.

Remote patient monitoring (RPM) refers broadly to the use of digital technologies to collect and transmit physiologic, device, usage, or patient-reported data from a patient's setting (home or community) to clinicians, enabling timely oversight and intervention. In the realm of SCS, remote monitoring may encompass stimulation usage metrics; enhanced diagnostics, such as lead impedance or electrical delivery integrity; battery status; patient activity levels; or patient-reported outcomes such as patient satisfaction, subjective pain scores, function, sleep quality, and activity logs. ASPN (American Society of Pain and Neuroscience) expert consensus guidelines for remote SCS device management have recently emphasized a tripartite classification of remote metrics: (1) device-related (e.g., usage logs, lead performance), (2) physiologic or disease-related (e.g., activity, biometrics), and (3) patient-reported outcomes (e.g., pain, quality of life).

Remote care more broadly encompasses not only monitoring, but also interactive management: remote programming of stimulation parameters, teleconsultations, automated alerts and decision support, and patient coaching. During the COVID-19 pandemic, several centers reported successful remote reprogramming of SCS settings when in-person access was constrained, demonstrating proof-of-concept for this model. Moreover, commercial platforms now offer physician dashboards and patient mobile apps to facilitate continuous engagement and dynamic therapy adjustments outside the clinic environment.

This paradigm brings multiple potential advantages. It may increase the responsiveness of care, allowing clinicians to detect and remediate suboptimal performance or adverse signals before patients even notice symptoms; reduce the burden of clinic visits, especially for patients in remote or underserved areas; and allow for a patient-centric and scalable data collection of validated measures, creating a never-achieved device chain of custody and management hygiene that enables a more scalable, cost-effective, and unbiased maintenance of neuromodulation therapy as compared to historical strategies.

Remote monitoring and care deployment are not without challenges. Developing technology that has been dramatized in movies like Skynet in Terminator or Big Brother in 1984 is not just for conspiracy theorists. Technical hurdles (secure data transmission, interoperability, latency, and actionable trigger pulls), clinical and regulatory concerns (patient safety, audits, liability, privacy and compliance, and HIPAA), and integration into practice and workflow development, as well as defining best practices and benchmarks, are just a few of the variables that need to be addressed.

Furthermore, integration with closed-loop control systems introduces added complexity. As physiological feedback loops (e.g., biomarkers of neural response) become incorporated into next-generation SCS controllers, robust frameworks for control design, risk management, and clinical validation will be needed. This section explores the next generation of clinician and patient engagement as it pertains to remote monitoring and care.

Chapter 26

Remote care and monitoring

Christopher Andriano[1], Ramana Naidu[2] and Johnathan Goree[3]

[1]Georgia Pain Care, Atlanta, GA, United States; [2]MarinHealth Spine Institute, Larkspur, CA, United States; [3]University of Arkansas for Medical Sciences, Little Rock, AR, United States

Introduction

Implantable neuromodulation devices have emerged as an effective adjunct therapy for managing chronic pain and improving quality of life in appropriately selected patients [1,2]. These systems typically use electrical stimulation to modulate neural activity in the central or peripheral nervous system. Common modalities include spinal cord stimulation (SCS), dorsal root ganglion stimulation, peripheral nerve stimulation, and brain stimulation.

The initial success of neuromodulation therapy depends on multiple factors including appropriate patient selection, underlying comorbidities, device choice, surgical technique, provider expertise, and postoperative care [3]. Once the device is implanted, the durability of the therapy may hinge on ongoing device management and patient follow-up. Explantation of neuromodulation systems carries substantial clinical and financial consequences, often leading to increased healthcare utilization through additional procedures and follow-up visits [4,5]. Among the leading causes of device explant is a loss of therapeutic efficacy, which can be addressed through proactive monitoring and timely programming adjustments [6].

Traditionally, adjustments to neuromodulation devices such as parameter changes, troubleshooting, or coverage optimization have required in-person clinic visits, often coordinated with industry representatives. These visits can be reactive, prompted by patient reports of diminished pain relief, unwanted stimulation, or technical difficulties with device operation. Delays in care can be consequential, as most patients experience a return to baseline pain levels within 24 h of therapy disruption [7]. Additional challenges such as posture-related fluctuations in paresthesia or variability in stimulation effectiveness may evolve daily and remain unaddressed between clinic visits. Moreover, a subset of patients may not recognize that their therapy is suboptimal, further contributing to inadequate pain control and dissatisfaction.

The logistical burden of in-person programming, including mobility limitations, transportation challenges, and dependence on caregivers, can reduce patient engagement with therapy or result in loss to follow-up - both of which may compromise long-term outcomes. These access challenges are particularly pronounced in patients with advanced neurological disease, rural residency, or limited caregiver support [7].

As the complexity of neuromodulation therapies grows and patient expectations continue to evolve, the need for care models that are responsive, scalable, and patient-centered has become increasingly evident. The addition of remote monitoring represents a natural progression in neuromodulation care, helping to close gaps between regions with varying levels of medical resources and device support. Remote monitoring, a component of remote patient management (RPM), refers to the ongoing collection and secure transmission of device and patient data from outside the clinical setting to enable timely, informed adjustments to therapy and support continuous patient engagement.

The growing emphasis on virtual care has been reinforced by recent regulatory and reimbursement changes. The Centers for Medicare & Medicaid Services (CMS) introduced new billing codes for remote therapeutic monitoring (RTM) in 2022, allowing clinicians to be reimbursed for the interpretation of remotely collected physiologic and therapeutic data. These policy updates, combined with increasing expectations from both patients and payers for connected care models, have accelerated the adoption of remote management in neuromodulation.

A Modern Atlas for Implantable Devices of the Spine, Brain, and Nerve. https://doi.org/10.1016/B978-0-443-36528-7.00058-3

Clinical rationale for remote monitoring

Remote monitoring has been utilized in cardiac rhythm management for over 2 decades, with robust evidence supporting its clinical and operational benefits in patients with cardiovascular implantable electronic devices (CIED). The key milestones in this evolution are summarized in Table 26.1. These systems enable automated, daily transmission of device and physiological data to the care team, guided by pre-specified clinical and device-related alerts. Early detection of arrhythmias, lead malfunctions, or programming issues through remote surveillance allows for timely interventions that might otherwise be delayed until a scheduled in-clinic evaluation. This capability has been linked to reductions in inappropriate and unnecessary shocks, optimization of device parameters that prolong system longevity, and significant improvements in patient satisfaction and engagement [8]. Moreover, extensive registry and trial results indicate these systems boost survival rates and lower healthcare use, reducing emergency visits and hospital admissions through proactive care.

Due to technical advances in neuromodulation, SCS systems are beginning to incorporate remote monitoring features in ways that parallel the early evolution of remote management of CIED. These capabilities hold the potential to accelerate problem identification, intervention, and prompt resolution, ultimately improving both patient care and system efficiency. Expert consensus highlights key goals of SCS device management, referenced in Table 26.2, as well as core objectives for remote monitoring in SCS. Among these is the ability to track patient response to therapy and ensure stimulation parameters remain optimized over time. Continuous device oversight can also help maximize system longevity, promptly detect and address hardware or programming issues, and identify patients who may require additional support in operating or managing their device. In some cases, remote surveillance may uncover other health concerns, enabling timely referral to the appropriate provider [7].

From the patient's perspective, these capabilities aim to preserve quality of life by ensuring consistent pain control, minimizing therapy interruptions, and simplifying device management. For providers and health systems, they create opportunities to reduce unnecessary in-person visits, lessen the time and financial burden on patients and caregivers, and enhance operational efficiency. Additional advantages include streamlined communication between clinicians and industry representatives, improved allocation of time for programming visits, and more robust longitudinal documentation of therapy performance. Collectively, these elements may facilitate a more proactive and data-driven model of neuromodulation care, paralleling the paradigm established in remote cardiac rhythm management.

Remote monitoring in SCS mirrors many of the established benefits seen in cardiac remote care, particularly in leveraging continuous device oversight to detect problems early, optimize therapy delivery, and improve efficiency. While CIED monitoring is well-established, SCS remote monitoring is still in the early stages, with expanding capabilities and increasing clinical adoption as technology, connectivity, and data analytics continue to mature.

Remote monitoring modalities and data types

Remote management of neuromodulation systems incorporates multiple data inputs categorized as objective device-based data, physiologic metrics, and patient-reported outcomes. These data streams are reviewed by healthcare providers and industry representatives to optimize therapeutic efficacy and support timely intervention. Automated notifications may alert the care team when any parameter falls outside a predefined acceptable range, prompting assessment and corrective action. The overall framework of remote monitoring is illustrated in Fig. 26.1.

Objective device-based data

Implantable pulse generators (IPGs) and external programmer (EPG) accessories generate a continuous stream of objective diagnostic data including stimulation program parameters (stimulation electrode configuration, amplitude, pulse width, frequency), stimulation usage (such as percentage time on/off and programs used), battery usage (battery voltage, recharging trends), and lead status (impedance, position of implanted leads). These metrics help assess adherence to prescribed therapy, verify device integrity, and detect signs of hardware or programming issues [7].

Some systems also record physiologic or electrophysiologic signals that provide insight into neural and autonomic responses. Evoked compound action potentials (ECAPs) can be used to confirm neural recruitment and maintain stimulation within an optimal therapeutic range, while emerging on-device sensing technologies capture cardiac metrics such as heart rate and heart rate variability as potential biomarkers of pain modulation and overall wellbeing [12,13].

Across platforms, data are securely transmitted via Bluetooth or radiofrequency signals from the implant to patient controllers automatically, which relay the information to encrypted cloud platforms for review and long-term analysis.

TABLE 26.1 Evolution of remote monitoring in healthcare.

Early remote monitoring in cardiac rhythm management (CRM)	• Concept of remote management of CIEDs first introduced in the 1970s. • Initial trans-telephonic monitoring (TTM) captured only basic information such as rate, rhythm, and battery status. • By the 1990s, advancements in TTM enabled interrogation of implantable cardioverter-defibrillators (ICDs) through a telephone headset, allowing review of pacing parameters, tachycardia detection criteria and therapy logs. • Wand-based radiofrequency (RF) systems further enabled data transfer from the patient's CIED to a home transceiver, which relayed information via phone lines or cellular networks to secure servers accessible by clinicians. • These systems were time consuming and cumbersome, still requiring patient effort and scheduled sessions.
Shift to automatic continuous monitoring	• From the mid-2000s, manufacturers began embedding automatic data transmission in pacemakers and ICDs • Remote monitoring transitioned from concept to gold standard due to continuous automated data transfer which reduced clinic visits roughly 50%, while maintaining safety and improved early detection of device problems and arrhythmias.
Expansion across healthcare	• Widespread adoption of remote monitoring across multiple medical specialties, including endocrinology, cardiology, weight management, and chronic disease care. • Digital health technologies enabled passive, continuous collection and transmission of physiologic and therapeutic data through connected sensors, wearables, and mobile applications.
From CRM to neuromodulation	• Recognizing the benefits of automatic alerts and reduced clinic visits in CRM, neuromodulation companies explored applying the same principles to spinal cord stimulation. • Remote monitoring and remote programming of neuromodulation devices began to emerge around 2020, culminating in systems capable of monitoring and adjusting therapy parameters without requiring patients to travel to clinic

CIEDs, Cardiac implantable electronic devices; *ICD*, implantable cardioverter defibrillators; *TTM*, trans-telephonic transmissions; *VF*, ventricular fibrillation; *VT*, ventricular tachycardia; Refs. [8–10].

TABLE 26.2 Key goals of SCS device management.

• Monitor patient response to SCS therapy • Maximize device longevity • Identify and quickly resolve any SCS device issues • Identify patients who need assistance in managing their device • Identify other health issues so that the patient is appropriately referred for management • Optimize patient's quality of life • Optimize device function • Optimize neurostimulation parameters • Optimize physiologic function • Document SCS function and patient symptoms over time • Improve ease of use • Decrease time and financial burden for patients and/or caregivers • Increase efficiencies for the healthcare practice • Streamline device representative programming time management • Improve patient and clinician satisfaction

Adapted from Ref. [11].

The completeness and granularity of transmitted data vary by manufacturer and depend on the device's telemetry architecture, sensor configuration, and daily transmission frequency.

Physiologic or disease related data

External devices such as smartwatches, activity trackers, or smartphone-linked sensors can capture physiologic metrics including step count, heart rate, sleep quality, and general mobility. These measures complement stimulation and patient-reported data by providing an objective view of functional status and daily activity levels. Expert consensus classifies such information as measurable physiologic data relevant to remote therapeutic monitoring [7]. These physiologic inputs are beginning to be incorporated into neuromodulation systems, where they can guide algorithm-driven programming adjustments and enhance real-time therapy personalization.

Despite their potential, external wearables are often limited by patient compliance, variability across manufacturers, and inconsistencies in data capture. Integrating physiologic sensing directly into implanted neuromodulation systems may address these challenges by enabling continuous, passive data collection. Newer platforms are exploring the use of embedded sensors such as accelerometers within implantable pulse generators to monitor posture and movement in real time, providing additional objective data for therapy optimization.

Recent research has also explored the feasibility of using spinal cord stimulation (SCS) electrodes to record cardiac activity. In a 2024 feasibility study, SCS leads reliably detected R-peaks and derived heart rate and heart rate variability (HRV) across multiple postures [13]. This capability introduces the potential for longitudinal cardiac monitoring directly through the implanted system, offering opportunities to investigate the relationships between physiologic markers, pain modulation, autonomic function, and overall wellbeing. Although the clinical utility of these biomarkers in guiding neuromodulation therapy remains under investigation, their integration represents a promising step toward objective, data-driven assessment of chronic pain [7,13].

Theoretically, clinically relevant physiologic parameters that may be incorporated into future neuromodulation systems include exercise duration, gait characteristics, posture-related changes such as time spent standing or lying, walking steadiness as an indicator of fall risk, sleep quality, and temperature. Integration of these metrics into remote monitoring platforms could enable a more comprehensive assessment of patient function and physiologic status [7].

Patient-reported outcomes

Patient-reported outcomes (PROs) are collected directly from the patient or caregiver to provide insight into health status and functional capacity. Using validated questionnaires, PROs translate a patient's subjective experience into quantifiable data across domains such as pain intensity, functional ability, mood, sleep quality, and overall quality of life [7].

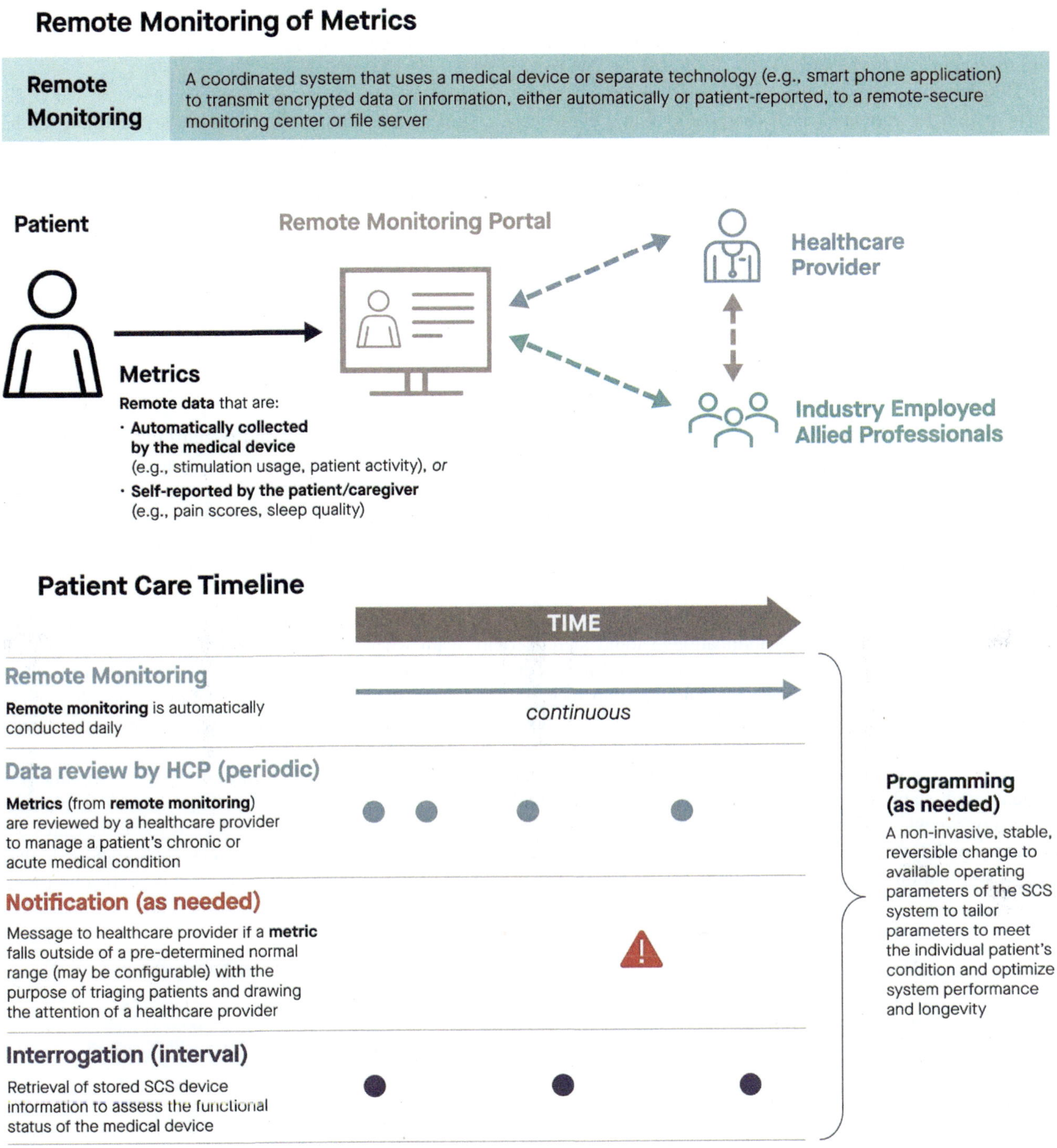

FIGURE 26.1 Overview of remote monitoring workflow and care team interaction in neuromodulation management. *Adapted from Ref. [7].*

Examples of PRO data relevant to neuromodulation include pain intensity score (i.e., numerical rating scale), location and distribution of pain areas, activity and sleep patterns, activities of daily living (ADL) performance, mood, medication use, patient satisfaction, and progress toward individualized treatment goals.

Neuromodulation platforms increasingly incorporate PRO collection through secure web portals and mobile applications. These tools enable longitudinal, HIPAA-compliant tracking of patient responses during both the trial and chronic phases of therapy. In a large real-world study of 13,331 patients undergoing spinal cord stimulation (SCS) trials, use of a mobile tracking application significantly enhanced patient engagement, with more than 60% of participants completing daily assessments. App users achieved a 91% trial success rate compared to 85% among non-users, suggesting that structured, real-time digital engagement may enhance trial outcomes and support more informed evaluation of SCS use and therapeutic effectiveness [14].

Despite these encouraging findings, the utility of PROs remains dependent on consistent engagement and active participation by patients and/or caregivers. While evidence for clinical use remains limited, standardized longitudinal tracking of PROs may help identify declining therapeutic response earlier and support more personalized, data-driven management of chronic pain. Incorporating clinically relevant variables, such as the number of days per week with controlled versus uncontrolled pain, could further refine clinical decision-making and facilitate timely interventions.

Follow-up paradigms in remote neuromodulation management

Expert consensus from Staats et al. [7] provides the most comprehensive recommendations to date for best practices in spinal cord stimulation (SCS) device follow-up, particularly regarding remote monitoring. These recommendations are intended as guiding principles rather than prescriptive standards, as follow-up must be tailored to each patient's unique clinical circumstances and response to therapy. In practice, approaches to SCS follow-up vary considerably among providers.

The frequency of monitoring is determined by a combination of clinical, technical, and patient-related factors. Key considerations include the frequency and severity of pain symptoms, therapeutic response, the presence of device-related issues (with the lead and/or generator), and patient circumstances such as distance from the treating center, comorbid medical conditions, and the availability of caregiver or social support. More frequent assessments are typically warranted during the initial stages of therapy, including the SCS trial and early postoperative period following implantation. Fig. 26.2 provides a conceptual framework demonstrating how these factors influence individualized monitoring schedules in SCS management.

The optimal paradigm combines continuous monitoring of device and physiologic data with periodic review of patient-reported outcomes. Automated notifications should alert the care team when any parameter falls outside a predefined acceptable range, prompting timely assessment and intervention. Clinically meaningful notifications may include device parameters such as low battery status, abnormal impedance in active contacts, or reduced stimulation usage, physiologic indicators such as decreased activity levels, and patient-reported findings including increased pain intensity or reduced satisfaction, each of which may signal the need for review by the clinical team.

The frequency of metric review depends on both clinical relevance and the expected rate of change over time. For patients with stable therapy more than 1 year after implantation, parameters warranting more frequent review, typically every few weeks to months, include activity level, step count, pain intensity, and medication use, as these measures can fluctuate rapidly and provide early insight into therapeutic response. Intermediate frequency measures such as battery status, stimulation usage, and lead impedance generally vary more gradually and should be reviewed periodically. Lower

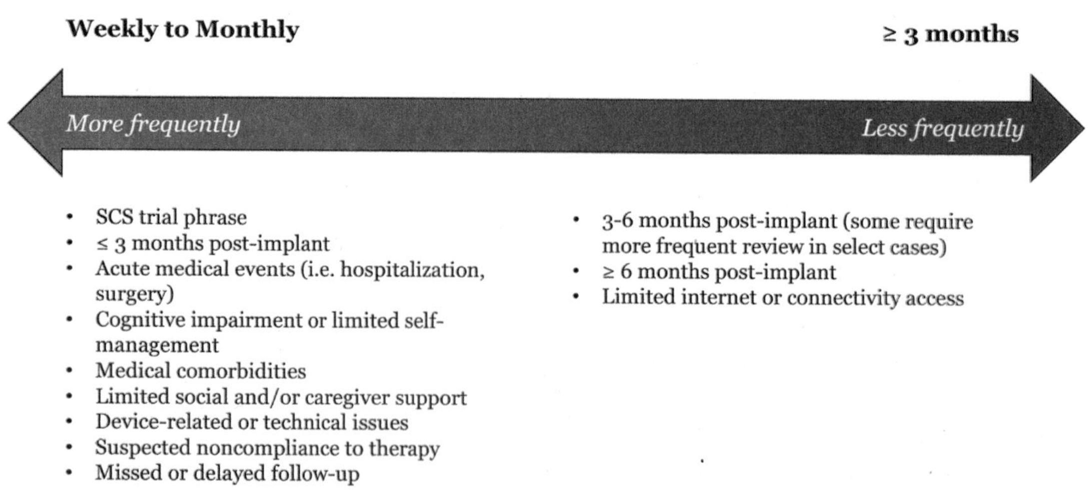

FIGURE 26.2 Framework for determining frequency of remote monitoring review in patients with spinal cord stimulation Monitoring frequency should be individualized according to therapy phase, patient stability, and clinical context. The framework illustrates typical ranges from more frequent review during early or complex clinical scenarios to less frequent review in stable patients. *Adapted from Ref. [7].*

frequency parameters including stimulation program settings, charging duration and intervals, activities of daily living, sleep quality, mood, pain distribution, patient satisfaction and goals, and quality of life surveys evolve over longer timescales and can be evaluated quarterly or at longer intervals to ensure accurate trend assessment.

While these recommendations provide a practical framework, real-world data and prospective studies are still needed to validate optimal follow-up intervals and alert thresholds in remote SCS management.

Current landscape of remote monitoring in spinal cord stimulation

Remote monitoring in neuromodulation remains in the early stages of clinical adoption, with ongoing development and varying degrees of integration among major device manufacturers. As technology advances and the clinical value of connected care becomes increasingly recognized, most systems are expected to incorporate some form of remote monitoring functionality. These innovations help to evolve traditional spinal cord stimulation care models by enabling more proactive management of therapy use, facilitating early identification and resolution of device-related issues, and enhancing the overall patient and clinician experience, potentially leading to improved therapeutic outcomes.

Substantial heterogeneity exists among currently available systems regarding the types of data collected, the frequency and automation of transmission, and the extent of clinician interaction. Nonetheless, remote monitoring and programming are increasingly being incorporated into next-generation neuromodulation platforms. A comparative summary of most currently available systems and their associated features is presented in Table 26.3.

Reimbursement considerations

Reimbursement for remote monitoring of neuromodulation systems remains an evolving component of digital health policy. While payment models for device implantation and in-person programming are well established, standardized coverage for remote monitoring and data review continues to vary among payers and regions [24,25]. Current reimbursement pathways are generally adapted from broader telehealth and remote monitoring codes rather than being specific to neuromodulation services [26,27].

Remote patient management should be applied when clinically relevant decisions or therapeutic adjustments are anticipated. The recommended frequency of follow-up is summarized in Fig. 26.2. When monitoring is required more frequently than monthly, an in-person evaluation is advised to assess for other contributing factors or device-related issues.

As remote management becomes more integrated into neuromodulation platforms, reimbursement policies are expected to evolve to reflect the associated clinical workload, infrastructure needs, and incentivize the potential benefits for patient care. Clinicians and institutions should routinely review current regulatory and payer guidance to ensure documentation aligns with medical necessity and accepted professional standards.

Barriers and limitations

Technical and operational limitations

Implementation of remote neuromodulation management faces several technical and operational challenges, including connectivity limitations, variable technological literacy among stakeholders, and the additional effort required to integrate these systems into clinical workflows.

Reliable internet connectivity is essential for remote monitoring, yet access remains inconsistent across the United States. Approximately one in seven households lacks reliable broadband service, with rural and low-income populations disproportionately affected [28]. These disparities limit the feasibility of real-time data transmission in certain populations. Potential solutions include expansion of state and federal broadband infrastructure programs, provision of subsidies or rebates for connectivity services, and integration of cellular-based systems such as 4G or 5G-enabled transmitters. For example, Biotronik's use of 5G Health Cloud architecture illustrates how manufacturers may enhance connectivity for patients without reliable Wi-Fi access.

Limited familiarity with digital technologies among patients, caregivers, and healthcare providers can further hinder adoption. Older adults who represent a large proportion of the neuromodulation population often exhibit lower technology readiness levels and may require additional support to effectively engage with remote platforms [29]. In such cases, patients may depend on direct assistance from healthcare providers or industry representatives to facilitate device setup and data transmission. Time and reimbursement constraints may limit provider capacity for ongoing education, emphasizing the importance of industry involvement and intuitive, user-friendly system design.

Interoperability also remains a significant barrier. Proprietary software and fragmented data streams between implantable devices, electronic medical records, and monitoring dashboards can increase workflow complexity, delay data

TABLE 26.3 Manufacturers with remote monitoring and programming.

Company	Remote monitoring			Remote programming	Additional notes
	Objective device-based data	*Physiologic data*	*Patient reported outcomes*		
Abbott	**Partial** Remote system checks and parameter settings; sessions initiated by the patient.	**Partial** Data obtained through PROs.	**Yes** Patient-reported outcome survey and education through NeuroSphere Digital health app.	**Yes** NeuroSphere virtual clinic enables remote programming via secure video sessions.	
Biotronik	**Yes** Daily automatic uploads from IPG via bluetooth and 5G to Biotronik health cloud. Data includes: active status, charging, therapy usage, program adjustments and amplitude shifts.	**No**	**Yes** Validated questionnaires, routine outcome and patient progress reports through Biotronik patient app	**Yes** Embrace one remote programming via portal	Automatic data transmission to the health cloud enables proactive review and follow-up by the Embrace care team when predefined triggers are detected. These triggers may include therapy compliance parameters (such as low device usage or stimulation within the therapeutic window), technical performance metrics (including charging behavior), and system integrity indicators (such as out-of-range active electrode impedance).
Boston Scientific	**Partial** Weekly cloud-based data uploads, primarily supporting ongoing therapy development.	**No**	**Yes** Patient-report pain and quality of life surveys through mySCS app.	**No**	
Medtronic	**No/Partial** Inceptiv neurostimulator allows for automated closed-loop programming based on evoked compound action potentials.	**No**	**Yes** Patients report pain level, and a Promis-29 survey through the CareGuidePro^{TM} app.	**No**	Inceptiv allows for automated programming via a closed loop system that may limit need for in-person program adjustments.
Nevro/ Globus medical	**Partial** Data uploads to NevroCloud. Aggregate data utilized by the research and development team to further improve program algorithms. May provide alerts to the Nevro care team.	**Partial** Sleep and activity data collected through wearables or patient-reported outcomes.	**Yes** Patient-report pain relief and quality of life assessments through the HFX app.	**No**	Proprietary algorithms analyze longitudinal data to support adaptive therapy.
Saluda medical	**Partial** Automated closed-loop programming based on evoked compound action potentials.	**No**	**No**	**No**	Automated programming via a closed loop system may limit need for in-person program adjustments.

Based on data from published literature and manufacturer-provided information (Abbott [15,16], Deer [17], BIOTRONIK [18], Boston Scientific [19], Hale [20], Nevro Corp [21], Saluda Medical [22], Naidu [23]); As of March 2026.

review, and contribute to clinician fatigue. Streamlined reporting systems and third-party data integration platforms may help mitigate this burden. Despite these challenges, recent surveys indicate that both clinicians and patients hold generally favorable perceptions of remote monitoring and programming as components of neuromodulation care [30,31].

Patient engagement and reporting challenges

Consistent patient engagement with patient-reported outcomes (PROs) remains a challenge in remote neuromodulation management. Some individuals may have difficulty using digital platforms due to limited health or technological literacy, cognitive or psychological barriers, or restricted internet access. Reduced participation can limit the accuracy of symptom tracking and diminish the potential effectiveness of therapy optimization.

Education on the importance of PRO submission and its role in guiding therapy adjustments may help to improve adherence. Strategies can include simplifying user interfaces and involving caregivers when appropriate to assist with data entry. Incentivizing participation, such as through fewer in-person visits or providing visual feedback on patient progress, may further support compliance [7].

Limitations in objective and physiologic metrics

A limitation in remote neuromodulation monitoring is the absence of validated physiologic biomarkers that reliably reflect pain intensity or therapeutic response. While patient-reported outcomes provide valuable subjective insights, they are inherently limited by compliance, recall bias, and cognitive or psychological factors that may affect accuracy. Developing objective and physiologic measures, captured through wearable or implantable sensors, represents a critical step toward complementing subjective reporting with more quantifiable indicators of clinical status.

Recent research highlights the feasibility of wearable devices in capturing physiologic parameters such as heart rate, heart rate variability, activity level, and mobility metrics. These data have shown correlations with pain severity and functional improvement, suggesting potential utility as adjunctive indicators of therapy response [32–34]. While encouraging, these approaches remain constrained by device variability, inconsistent adherence, and the lack of standardized analytic frameworks. Further research is required to determine how these physiologic signals can be translated into actionable therapeutic insights and integrated within existing clinical pathways.

Ethical and regulatory dimensions of remote neuromodulation

The expansion of remote neuromodulation introduces complex ethical and regulatory considerations related to patient privacy and cybersecurity risks. These systems transmit sensitive health data that must be protected in accordance with federal and state privacy regulations, including the Health Insurance Portability and Accountability Act (HIPAA) and the Health Information Technology for Economic and Clinical Health (HITECH) Act [35].

Healthcare providers should be prepared to educate patients on privacy and cybersecurity risks when discussing remote spinal cord stimulation (SCS) management during the informed consent process. However, many clinicians are unfamiliar with data privacy and cybersecurity risks in regard to implanted medical devices [36]. Improving clinician awareness and establishing standardized counseling practices are essential to ensure patients fully understand both the benefits and potential risks of remote device management.

Manufacturers and healthcare institutions share responsibility for protecting data integrity and responding promptly to cybersecurity threats. Recommended safeguards include end-to-end encryption, multi-factor authentication, and restricted access controls. The U.S. Food and Drug Administration (FDA) requires manufacturers to report cybersecurity vulnerabilities and encourages clinicians and patients to submit suspected issues through its MedWatch program [7]. Sustaining ethical standards in remote neuromodulation will depend on continued vigilance, transparent reporting, and shared accountability among clinicians, patients, and industry partners.

Future directions in remote neuromodulation

Future development of remote neuromodulation will likely focus on advancing data integration, automation, and clinical decision support. As device connectivity, sensing capabilities, and computational power evolve, these systems may transition from reactive monitoring to predictive and adaptive management models.

Closed-loop stimulation, guided by physiologic feedback such as evoked compound action potentials (ECAPs), represents one of the most promising areas of innovation. ECAP-guided systems can quantify spinal cord activation in real time and automatically adjust stimulation parameters to maintain consistent neural recruitment despite physiologic or positional changes [12,37,38]. Future research should focus on defining optimal response thresholds and evaluating the long-term clinical impact of adaptive stimulation.

Artificial intelligence (AI) and machine learning algorithms may further enhance these platforms by identifying complex relationships across objective and physiologic metrics from implantable devices, wearable sensors, and patient-reported data. Predictive modeling could enable early detection of declining efficacy, overstimulation, or device malfunction, allowing individualized therapy adjustments before clinical deterioration occurs.

Continued research is needed to establish the clinical value, usability, and cost-effectiveness of these technologies for patients, caregivers, healthcare providers, and payers. Key outcome measures for future investigation may include loss of SCS efficacy, opioid utilization, functional outcomes, healthcare resource use, patient satisfaction, stimulation usage patterns (on/off time, therapeutic window, overstimulation, understimulation), explant and virtual explant rates, sleep quality, clinical event detection, and pain intensity [7]. As evidence accumulates, emerging standards may parallel those established in cardiac rhythm management, where remote monitoring has progressed from a supplemental feature to an integral component of long-term care.

Conclusions

Remote management in neuromodulation represents a shift toward more continuous, data-informed, and patient-centered care. Beyond improving access and operational efficiency, these technologies have the potential to transform how clinicians understand and optimize therapy response over time. The path forward will rely on validating objective and physiologic biomarkers, integrating advanced data analytics, and establishing evidence-based frameworks that demonstrate clinical and economic value.

As connectivity, automation, and interdisciplinary collaboration advance, remote monitoring may evolve from an adjunct feature to a standard of care in neuromodulation, much as it has in cardiology. Its success will rely not only on technological innovation but also on thoughtful implementation that upholds patient trust, ensures regulatory compliance, and adapts to evolving governmental and payer policies.

Key points

- Remote management in neuromodulation reflects a gradual transition toward more continuous and data-informed care, aimed at improving follow-up efficiency and therapy optimization.
- Current remote monitoring systems collect a combination of device-based data, physiologic measures, and patient-reported outcomes to support clinical decision-making, though evidence for their long-term impact remains limited.
- Implementation continues to face practical barriers including inconsistent connectivity depending on manufacture, variable technology literacy among patients and providers, and the additional effort and costs required to integrate these systems into existing clinical workflows.
- Ethical and regulatory considerations surrounding data privacy, cybersecurity, and informed consent are central to responsible adoption. Ongoing provider education, manufacturer safeguards, and transparent governance are essential to maintain patient trust.
- Future development will depend on validating physiologic and objective biomarkers, improving integration of device and clinical data, and aligning technological advances with evolving regulatory and reimbursement frameworks.

References

[1] Sdrulla AD, Guan Y, Raja SN. Spinal cord stimulation: clinical efficacy and potential mechanisms. Pain Pract 2018;18(8):1048–67. https://doi.org/10.1111/papr.12692.

[2] Zheng Y, Liu CW, Hui Chan DX, Kai Ong DW, Xin Ker JR, Ng WH, Wan KR. Neurostimulation for chronic pain: a systematic review of high-quality randomized controlled trials with long-term follow-up. Neuromodulation 2023;26(7):1276–94. https://doi.org/10.1016/j.neurom.2023.05.003.

[3] Yoo Y, Roh H, Moon JY, Choi EJ, Nahm FS, Lee PB. Predictive factors of successful spinal cord stimulation in patients with chronic pain: a retrospective cohort study. Brain Sci 2025;15(6):614. https://doi.org/10.3390/brainsci15060614.

[4] Han JL, Murphy KR, Qasim M, Yang S, Parente B, Xie J, Promila P, Lad SP. Explantation rates and healthcare resource utilization in spinal cord stimulation. Neuromodulation 2017;20(4):331–9. https://doi.org/10.1111/ner.12567.

[5] Dougherty MC, Woodroffe RW, Wilson S, Gillies GT, Howard MA, Carnahan RM. Risk factors and survival analysis of spinal cord stimulator explantation. Neuromodulation 2021;24(1):61–7. https://doi.org/10.1111/ner.13173.

[6] Hagedorn JM, Lam CM, D'Souza RS, Sayed D, Bendel MA, Ha CT, Romero J, Hall M, Freeman E, Richardson BF, Hoelzer BC. Explantation of 10 kHz spinal cord stimulation devices: a retrospective review of 744 patients followed for at least 12 months. Neuromodulation 2021;24 (3):499–506. https://doi.org/10.1111/ner.13359.

[7] Staats PS, Deer TR, Hunter C, Li S, Dickerson D, Petersen E, Kapural L, Shravani D, Gilligan C, Slavin KV, Pope JE, Kasra A, Poree L, Naidu R, Levy RM. Remote management of spinal cord stimulation devices for chronic pain: expert recommendations on best practices for proper utilization and future considerations. Neuromodulation 2023;26(7):P1295–308. https://doi.org/10.1016/j.neurom.2023.07.003.

[8] Slotwiner D, Varma N, Akar JG, Annas G, Beardsall M, Fogel RI, Galizio NO, Glotzer TV, Leahy RA, Love CJ, McLean RC, Mittal S, Morichelli L, Patton KK, Raitt MH, Pietro Ricci R, Rickard J, Schoenfeld MH, Serwer GA, Shea J. HRS Expert Consensus Statement on remote interrogation and monitoring for cardiovascular implantable electronic devices. Heart Rhythm 2015;12(7):e69–100. https://doi.org/10.1016/j.hrthm.2015.05.008.

[9] Varma N, Braunschweig F, Burri H, Gerhard H, Linz D, Michowitz Y, Ricci RP, Nielsen JC. Remote monitoring of cardiac implantable electronic devices and disease management. Europace 2023;25(9). https://doi.org/10.1093/europace/euad233.

[10] Tan VH, See Tow HX, Fong KY, Wang Y, Yeo C, Ching CK, Lim TW. Remote monitoring of cardiac implantable electronic devices using smart device interface versus radiofrequency-based interface: a systematic review. J Arrhythmia 2024;40(3):596–604. https://doi.org/10.1002/joa3.13054.

[11] Staats PS, et al. Expert consensus on the role of remote management in spinal cord stimulation. Pain Pract 2023.

[12] Mekhail N, Levy RM, Deer TR, Kapural L, Li S, Amirdelfan K, Hunter CW, Rosen SM, Costandi SJ, Falowski SM, Burgher AH, Pope JE, Gilmore CA, Qureshi FA, Staats PS, Scowcroft J, Carlson J, Kim CK, Yang MI, Stauss T. Long-term safety and efficacy of closed-loop spinal cord stimulation to treat chronic back and leg pain (Evoke): a double-blind, randomised, controlled trial. Lancet Neurol 2020;19(2):123–34. https://doi.org/10.1016/S1474-4422(19)30414-4.

[13] Brinda AK, Goudman L, Moens M, Hincapie J, Dinsmoor DA, Litvak LM, Straka M. Cardiac sensing at a spinal cord stimulation lead: a promising on-device potential biomarker for pain and wellbeing. Front Physiol 2024;15. https://doi.org/10.3389/fphys.2024.1342983.

[14] Lee JM, Woon R, Ramsum M, Halperin DS, Jain R. User engagement and assessment of treatment effectiveness in patients using a novel digital mHealth App during spinal cord stimulation screening trials. JMIR Human Fact 2022;9(1). https://doi.org/10.2196/35134.

[15] Abbott. NeuroSphere™ Digital Care. Abbott Neuromodulation. https://www.neuromodulation.abbott/us/en/healthcare-professionals/hcp-chronic-pain/neurosphere-digital-care.html. [Accessed 30 March 2026].

[16] Abbott. Abbott introduces NeuroSphere™ Virtual Clinic, first-of-its-kind remote neuromodulation patient care technology in the U.S. Abbott MediaRoom. March 8, 2021. https://abbott.mediaroom.com/2021-03-08-Abbott-Introduces-NeuroSphere-TM-Virtual-Clinic-First-of-its-Kind-Remote-Neuromodulation-Patient-Care-Technology-in-the-U-S. [Accessed 30 March 2026].

[17] Deer TR, Esposito MF, Cornidez EG, Okaro U, Fahey ME, Chapman KB. Teleprogramming service provides safe and remote stimulation options for patients with DRG-S and SCS implants. J Pain Res Published online October 2021:3259–65. https://doi.org/10.2147/jpr.s332966.

[18] BIOTRONIK. Prospera™ spinal cord stimulation (SCS) system with Embrace One™. BIOTRONIK Neuro. https://www.biotronik.com/en-us/professionals/prospera-scs. [Accessed 30 March 2026].

[19] Boston Scientific. WaveWriter Alpha™ spinal cord stimulation system. https://www.bostonscientific.com/en-US/medical-specialties/pain-management/wavewriter-alpha-scs.html. [Accessed 30 March 2026].

[20] Hale C. Medtronic debuts virtual spinal cord stimulation treatment guide. Fierce Biotech. May 5, 2021. https://www.fiercebiotech.com/medtech/medtronic-debuts-virtual-spinal-cord-stimulation-treatment-guide. [Accessed 30 March 2026].

[21] Nevro Corp. HFX AdaptivAI™ spinal cord stimulation platform. Nevro. https://www.nevro.com/providers/product-hfx-adaptivai/. [Accessed 30 March 2026].

[22] Saluda Medical. Saluda Medical receives FDA approval for first automated programming platform in spinal cord stimulation (SCS). January 23, 2025. https://www.saludamedical.com/press-releases/saluda-medical-receives-fda-approval-for-first-automated-programming-platform-in-scs/. [Accessed 30 March 2026].

[23] Naidu RK, Kapural L, Li S, Tourjé C, Rutledge J, Dickerson D, Lubenow TR. A review of the prospera spinal cord stimulation system with multiphase stimulation and proactive care. Curr Pain Headache Rep 2025;29(1). https://doi.org/10.1007/s11916-024-01318-3.

[24] Romaniuk M, Mahdi G, Singh R, Haglin J, Brown NJ, Gottfried O. Recent trends in Medicare utilization and reimbursement for spinal cord stimulators: 2000–2019. World Neurosurg 2022;166:e664–71. https://doi.org/10.1016/j.wneu.2022.07.075.

[25] Manchikanti L, Pampati V, Vangala BP, Soin A, Sanapati MR, Thota S, Hirsch JA. Spinal cord stimulation trends of utilization and expenditures in fee-for-service (FFS) Medicare population from 2009 to 2018. Pain Phys 2021;5:293–308. https://doi.org/10.36076/ppj.2021.24.293.

[26] Telehealth and remote patient monitoring: billing for remote patient monitoring; 2025. https://telehealth.hhs.gov/providers/best-practice-guides/telehealth-and-remote-patient-monitoring/billing-remote-patient.

[27] Ra OH, Sou BS, Streid J, Davis D, Pablo J, King R, Lurie JM, Vu K, Oh DJ, Robinson CL, Yong RJ, Lee KWK, Issa M. Reviewing the advances in remote therapeutic and physiological monitoring and applicability for chronic pain management. J Pain Res 2025;18:3757–64. https://doi.org/10.2147/jpr.s530553.

[28] Curtis ME, Clingan SE, Guo H, Zhu Y, Mooney LJ, Hser Y. Disparities in digital access among American rural and urban households and implications for telemedicine-based services. J Rural Health 2021;38(3). https://doi.org/10.1111/jrh.12614.

[29] Liu L, Stroulia E, Nikolaidis I, Miguel-Cruz A, Rios Rincon A. Smart homes and home health monitoring technologies for older adults: a systematic review. Int J Med Inf 2016;91:44–59. https://doi.org/10.1016/j.ijmedinf.2016.04.007.

[30] Haddad TC, Maita KC, Avila FR, Torres-Guzman RA, Coffey JD, Christopherson LA, Leuenberger AM, Bell SJ, Pahl DF, Garcia JP, Manka L, Forte AJ, Maniaci MJ. Patient satisfaction with a multi-site, multi-regional remote patient monitoring program for acute and chronic condition management: a survey-based descriptive analysis. J Med Internet Res 2023;25. https://doi.org/10.2196/44528.

[31] Bouabida K, Malas K, Talbot A, Desrosiers M-È, Lavoie F, Lebouché B, Taghizadeh N, Normandin L, Vialaron C, Fortin O, Lessard D, Pomey M-P. Healthcare professional perspectives on the use of remote patient-monitoring platforms during the COVID-19 pandemic: a cross-sectional study. J Personalized Med 2022;12(4):529. https://doi.org/10.3390/jpm12040529.

[32] Goudman L, Brouns R, Linderoth B, Moens M. Effects of spinal cord stimulation on heart rate variability in patients with Failed Back Surgery Syndrome. PLoS One 2019;14(7):e0219076. https://doi.org/10.1371/journal.pone.0219076.

[33] Hamm-Faber T, Arnts I, Dylan G, van F, Dongen R van, Engels Y, Kris. Feasibility of collecting objective data and exploring patient's experiences on physical activity in persistent spinal pain syndrome type 2 patients receiving spinal cord stimulation: a mixed feasibility study. Pain Pract 2025;25(3):e70013. https://doi.org/10.1111/papr.70013.

[34] Patterson DG, Wilson D, Fishman MA, Moore G, Skaribas I, Heros R, Dehghan S, Ross E, Kyani A. Objective wearable measures correlate with self-reported chronic pain levels in people with spinal cord stimulation systems. npj Digit Med 2023;6:146. https://doi.org/10.1038/s41746-023-00892-x.

[35] Zhong T, William HM, Jin MY, Abd-Elsayed A. A review of remote monitoring in neuromodulation for chronic pain management. Curr Pain Headache Rep 2024;28(12):1225–33. https://doi.org/10.1007/s11916-024-01302-x.

[36] Martin E, Petersen E, Shah J. Evaluating physician knowledge of data privacy and cybersecurity risks in neuromodulation: an online cross-sectional survey. J Pain Res 2025;18:3101–6. https://doi.org/10.2147/jpr.s506509.

[37] Poree L, Foster A, Staats PS. Device profile of the Evoke physiologic closed-loop spinal cord stimulation system for the treatment of chronic intractable pain: overview of its safety and efficacy. Expet Rev Med Dev 2023;20(11):885–98. https://doi.org/10.1080/17434440.2023.2255520.

[38] Mekhail NA, Levy RM, Deer TR, Kapural L, Li S, Amirdelfan K, Hunter CW, Rosen SM, Costandi SJ, Falowski SM, Burgher AH, Pope JE, Gilmore CA, Qureshi FA, Staats PS, Scowcroft J, McJunkin T, Kim CK, Yang MI, Stauss T. Neurophysiological outcomes that sustained clinically significant improvements over 3 years of physiologic ECAP-controlled closed-loop spinal cord stimulation for the treatment of chronic pain. Reg Anesth Pain Med 2024;50(6):rapm–105370. https://doi.org/10.1136/rapm-2024-105370.

Section 8

Remote programming

Introduction to section 8 remote programming

Author: Denis G. Patterson, DO

When I graduated from my Interventional Pain Fellowship at Emory University in 2007, neuromodulation of the nervous system had not yet advanced significantly. At that time, all devices relied on tonic stimulation, and the primary discussion centered around whether constant current or constant voltage was the best approach to power the system. In essence, there was little to debate—most decisions came down to vendor relationships or which company offered the "brighter, shinier device." Patient outcomes were modest, with 50% of patients experiencing only 50% pain relief. Concerns about the long-term viability of these devices were also prevalent, as they suffered from issues such as nonspecific stimulation (paresthesia outside of the targeted pain area) and instability due to postural changes.

Over the past decade, however, significant advancements have been made in neuromodulation therapy. These include innovations such as novel waveforms—particularly paresthesia-free stimulation with high-frequency and passive recharge burst stimulation—along with improvements in energy delivery through closed-loop stimulation. Additionally, new systems have been developed to access previously unexplored targets, like dorsal root ganglion stimulation, and peripheral nerve stimulation equipment has seen substantial improvements. The integration of smart devices to interface with neuromodulation systems, along with the development of primary cell generators and Bluetooth-enabled upgradability (eliminating the need for surgical revisions to access technological upgrades), has further enhanced the therapeutic options available. As a result, patient outcomes have significantly improved, with many now experiencing up to 80% sustained pain relief, while issues related to tolerance and device longevity have been minimized.

The onset of the COVID-19 pandemic in March 2020 introduced unprecedented challenges worldwide. With social distancing and reduced in-person interactions, physicians faced the task of continuing to care for patients despite the inability to meet face-to-face. During this period, the need to maintain the functionality of neuromodulation devices became critical. This necessity led to a groundbreaking innovation in the field—remote programming. While remote programming had long been used in cardiology to optimize pacemakers and defibrillators, it was only through collaboration between the cardiac and neuromodulation fields that this technology was adapted to meet the needs of patients during a global pandemic.

This section of the book will explore the current state of remote programming, discussing its benefits—such as enhanced convenience, improved access to care, and the potential for early intervention—along with an explanation of how it works (involving the patient device, secure connection, and remote programming interface). Additionally, safety considerations such as patient oversight and cybersecurity will be addressed. The future of neuromodulation is bright, offering exciting prospects not only for patients but also for clinicians dedicated to helping those with chronic pain. I am grateful to practice pain management during this transformative period, as it allows me to witness firsthand the incredible innovations shaping our field.

Chapter 27

Remote programming

Marcin Karcz[1], Lucas Bracero[1], Anuj Shah[2], Warren Mackie-Jenkins[3] and Timothy Deer[1]
[1]The Spine and Nerve Centers of the Virginias, Charleston, WV, United States; [2]Department of Anesthesiology, Division of Pain Management, New York Presbyterian Hospital/Weill Cornell Medicine, New York, NY, United States; [3]Interventional Pain Medicine, NOVA Orthopedic and Spine, Center for Advanced Orthopedics, Woodbridge, VA, United States

Introduction

Scope of remote programming

Neuromodulation, integral in the treatment of chronic pain and movement disorders, involves placement of implantable therapies such as deep brain stimulation (DBS), spinal cord stimulation (SCS), dorsal root ganglion stimulation (DRG), and peripheral nerve stimulation (PNS). Despite advancements in technology, optimization of these devices to effectively treat symptoms involves making changes to programming parameters to meet changes in physiology, pathology of symptoms, or electrode movement [1]. Traditionally, these changes have taken place though an in-person encounter in the clinician's office, which requires coordination between the clinician, a representative from the implantable device manufacturer, and the patient [2]. The challenges associated with this often place a burden on the patient that limits access to care and optimization of therapy [3]. Remote programming offers the ability to monitor and adjust implantable therapies without the need for the patient to make an in-person visit to the clinician's office [3]. Remote programming through digital platforms affords patients the ability to access care for their implanted device while decreasing the burden that multiple in-person visits to their clinician's office creates, which in turn can improve patient outcomes [3].

Brief historical perspective

Conventional programming of neuromodulation systems historically required direct physical contact and interaction with the patient's implanted device using an external programmer. During the COVID-19 pandemic, telemedicine services, which have been available and used since the late 1990s, were expanded to continue to provide patient care despite the challenges of the pandemic; however, an FDA-approved digital platform for reprogramming neuromodulation devices was lacking [2]. Remote programming of spinal cord stimulation was first studied in China during the COVID-19 pandemic, which demonstrated high patient uptake [4]. Similar technology had been available for monitoring cardiovascular implantable electronic devices (CIEDs) for decades, with a body of literature supporting its use [4]. The first digital platform for remote care and reprogramming was developed and launched in 2021 with the introduction of Abbott's NeuroSphere Virtual Clinic (Abbott, Austin, Texas) [5]. Consensus guidelines for remote management of spinal cord stimulation were established in 2023 [5].

Brief explanation of innovation and advancements in remote programming

Innovation around remote programming has come with the confluence of new technologies in neuromodulation hardware and waveforms and the associated plethora of data available through advancements in data aggregation, wireless technology and user-friendly platforms [6]. The concept of remote therapeutic monitoring (RTM) in spinal cord stimulation, currently available only through Biotronik's system (BIOTRONIK SE and Co KG, Berlin, Germany), allows the clinician and manufacturer's representative real-time and secure access to a patient's therapeutic utilization and performance data and is a billable service if coding requirements are met [6]. Interpretation of this data can permit prompt resolution of a

A Modern Atlas for Implantable Devices of the Spine, Brain, and Nerve. https://doi.org/10.1016/B978-0-443-36528-7.00016-9

device-related issue through expert-directed remote programming without the need for the patient to schedule an in-person visit [7,8].

Key points

- Remote programming allows clinicians to fine-tune implantable neuromodulation devices without requiring an in-person visit, improving access to care.
- The development of wireless platforms has resulted in the ability of the clinician to access, interpret, and provide prompt solutions to commonly encountered issues in neuromodulation.
- Development of remote programming platforms has advanced with the expansion of telemedicine services since the COVID-19 pandemic.
- The ability to track device performance, utilization, and therapy delivery has provided clinicians with a multitude of data points that can improve the ability to optimize device settings in an individualized manner.
- Innovation around wireless technology, data transmission, and remote therapeutic monitoring (RTM) may further enhance the capabilities of remote programming, modernizing the management of implantable neuromodulation devices.
- Remote device programming and management can be subject to technical limitations (for example, need for cellular network connectivity or Wi-Fi access), as well as the potential for lack of familiarity with the technology amongst both patients and clinicians, which could lead to suboptimal use of the technology.

Overview of remote programming

Spinal Cord Stimulation (SCS) has evolved significantly since its introduction in the 1960s, with advances in waveform technology, lead configurations, and programming capabilities enhancing patient outcomes [9]. Traditional SCS devices rely on in-person adjustments, requiring patients to visit clinics for programming changes. However, as telemedicine and digital health innovations have advanced, remote programming has emerged as a viable alternative, allowing clinicians to fine-tune therapy in real time without necessitating travel or in-person consultations [10].

Remote programming represents a paradigm shift in neuromodulation, allowing clinicians to make parameter adjustments from a distance via secure cloud-based platforms. This capability has gained traction due to its ability to improve access to care, enhance patient convenience, and reduce healthcare system burdens. Platforms such as Abbott's NeuroSphere Virtual Clinic and BIOTRONIK's Embrace One provide real-time clinician-patient interaction, enabling secure remote SCS adjustments [8].

Benefits of remote programming

Remote programming addresses systemic gaps in traditional SCS management. Rural patients, who previously traveled an average of 120 miles per clinic visit, now access specialist care via encrypted video consultations [8]. This improved accessibility has significant implications for treatment adherence and long-term outcomes, particularly for patients in underserved areas. Han et al. [9] noted that qualified SCS implantation and programming centers are primarily located in major cities, leading to long journeys and high costs for patients in rural locations. This inconvenience contributes to poor medical compliance and impedes therapeutic effects. Real-time optimization improves therapeutic precision: clinicians modify parameters based on patient-reported pain scores or activity levels. This dynamic approach to therapy management allows for more frequent, fine-tuned adjustments that can better accommodate the fluctuating nature of chronic pain conditions [10].

Additionally, remote systems reduce healthcare costs annually per patient through minimized travel and missed workdays [2]. This cost-effectiveness extends beyond direct medical expenses, encompassing broader socioeconomic benefits such as improved productivity and reduced caregiver burden. Han et al. [2] emphasized that remote programming is more efficient and economic, widely recognized among participants as beneficial.

In addition to remote programing of SCS device, the addition of digital biomarkers, such as gait patterns and heart rate variability derived from wearable devices, enables personalized therapy adjustments, enhancing long-term outcomes [11]. These objective measures provide clinicians with a more comprehensive view of patient status, allowing for data-driven decision-making in therapy management.

High-speed wireless networks (4G/5G) enhance the reliability of remote programming sessions by ensuring minimal latency and robust connectivity [2]. Furthermore, artificial intelligence (AI) and machine learning algorithms are emerging as adjunctive tools for predictive modeling, refining stimulation parameters based on historical patient data and physiological biomarkers [8]. The Prospera SCS system, utilizing proactive care via remote monitoring and multiphase stimulation, exemplifies the next generation of automated neuromodulation adjustments [10].

Challenges and limitations

Despite its promise, remote programming faces several challenges. Not all patients are comfortable with technology, and digital literacy may be a barrier. Additionally, cybersecurity concerns and regulatory restrictions vary by region, potentially hindering adoption. While most software platforms comply with HIPAA and other privacy regulations, maintaining robust security against data breaches remains a critical priority. Moreover, remote programming may not fully replace in-person evaluations in cases requiring lead repositioning, device troubleshooting, or complex therapy modifications [8].

In addition, technical and regulatory hurdles persist. Intermittent connectivity disrupts 4.8% of remote sessions, particularly in regions with limited 5G infrastructure [12]. This highlights the need for robust, reliable telecommunication networks to ensure consistent care delivery. Hardware issues, such as lead migration or battery failure, necessitate in-person intervention in 22% of cases, underscoring the need for hybrid care models [8]. These technical challenges emphasize the importance of ongoing research and development in SCS hardware to improve reliability and reduce the frequency of in-person interventions. In addition, regulatory variability further complicates adoption; while the FDA approved Abbott's NeuroSphere for remote use in 2021, European approvals remain fragmented [13]. This regulatory landscape necessitates a coordinated effort among healthcare systems, device manufacturers, and regulatory bodies to establish standardized protocols for remote SCS management.

Clinical applications and patient outcomes

Remote programming has demonstrated significant clinical utility across diverse patient populations, particularly among individuals with restricted mobility, rural residency, or complex pain phenotypes requiring frequent recalibration. A study by Deer et al. [13] confirmed that remote programming achieved clinical outcomes equivalent to in-person programming, with 100% of surveyed clinicians successfully addressing patient needs and 93.8% of patients preferring remote adjustments due to logistical convenience and efficiency.

Han et al. [2] investigated remote programming efficacy in China during the COVID-19 pandemic, reporting that 81% of patients experienced clinically significant benefits. The study highlighted the economic and functional advantages of teleprogramming, such as reduced healthcare costs and improved patient satisfaction. Staats et al. [8] emphasized the role of remote programming in early intervention strategies, mitigating therapy abandonment and device explanation rates through proactive monitoring and timely parameter adjustments.

The Prospera SCS (Biotronik) system has further expanded the scope of remote programming by integrating proactive care mechanisms, allowing for continuous device monitoring and automated therapy optimization. Clinical trials, such as BENEFIT-02 and BENEFIT-03, have demonstrated that multiphase stimulation improves patient outcomes by minimizing therapy gaps and reducing the risk of overstimulation [10]. Additionally, the integration of remote programming with wearable biometric devices provides a more comprehensive understanding of patient physiology, enabling precise and responsive therapy adjustments.

As remote programming becomes more refined, the potential for hybrid models of care emerges. A combination of remote and in-person interventions may provide the optimal balance between accessibility and direct clinical oversight. Hybrid approaches allow for real-time adjustments while ensuring that patients who require hands-on care can receive it promptly. Such an approach could further expand the adoption of remote programming, addressing hesitations from clinicians and regulatory bodies while maintaining patient safety.

Implementation framework and best practices

The successful deployment of remote programming requires a structured approach encompassing clinician, training, patient education, cybersecurity protocols, and regulatory compliance. Staats et al. [8] outline best practices for integrating remote programming into clinical workflows. Clinician competency and training are essential, requiring targeted education on device-specific programming methodologies, troubleshooting algorithms, and remote patient engagement techniques. Standardized certification programs bolster clinician proficiency and ensure adherence to best practices.

Patient selection is another critical consideration, as not all individuals are optimal candidates for remote programming. Ideal candidates possess stable psychiatric profiles, technological literacy, and reliable internet connectivity. Structured patient education on device functionality, remote platform navigation, and symptom tracking is vital for optimizing therapeutic outcomes. Comprehensive patient support resources, including instructional videos, mobile applications, and dedicated technical support teams, are critical for ensuring long-term adherence and satisfaction [8].

Cybersecurity and data protection remain paramount concerns. Robust encryption protocols, HIPAA-compliant communication platforms, and multi-tier authentication frameworks must safeguard patient confidentiality. Continuous collaboration with medical device manufacturers is necessary to fortify data security and provide real-time technical support [8].

An integral component of effective remote programming is the integration of biometric and behavioral analytics. Incorporating wearable biosensors and patient-reported outcome measures into remote programming platforms facilitates personalized therapy refinement. Quantifiable metrics, such as activity level, sleep patterns, and pain severity, can inform algorithmic parameter adjustments, enhancing treatment precision [10].

Challenges and limitations

Despite its transformative potential, remote programming faces several challenges, including disparities in digital infrastructure, reimbursement ambiguities, and limitations in addressing complex device complications. Regulatory and payer policies governing remote neuromodulation services exhibit considerable variability, posing barriers to widespread implementation [13]. Additionally, while remote programming suffices for routine parameter optimization, cases requiring lead repositioning or hardware revision necessitate in-person intervention.

Psychosocial factors also merit consideration, as some patients perceive remote care as impersonal, potentially impacting adherence and overall treatment engagement. Integrating virtual patient counseling, digital support groups, and hybrid telehealth models can mitigate these concerns, fostering a more comprehensive remote care experience. As remote programming expands, addressing disparities in access to broadband internet and digital literacy will be crucial for ensuring equitable healthcare delivery.

Future trajectory and innovations

Several emerging innovations are poised to further enhance remote programming. AI-assisted programming adjustments based on real-time patient feedback will enable autonomous therapy optimizations, reducing the need for clinician intervention. Integration with wearable devices and biometrics will allow for more personalized therapy, dynamically adjusting parameters in response to physiological changes. Improved internet and 5G connectivity will expand access to remote programming, making it more widely available to patients in remote locations [10]. Overcoming regulatory and reimbursement hurdles will be critical in ensuring broader adoption and equitable access to this transformative approach in neuromodulation. The evolution of remote programming is inextricably linked to advancements in AI-driven decision support, expanded telehealth reimbursement models, and enhanced interoperability across digital health platforms. Machine learning-based optimization algorithms promise to automate stimulation adjustments in response to real-time patient data, further refining therapeutic precision [8].

Additionally, legislative initiatives aimed at expanding reimbursement for remote neuromodulation services will be critical in ensuring equitable access to care. Emerging research is also investigating biofeedback-integrated programming, where physiological signals such as heart rate variability and muscle tension dynamically inform stimulation modifications. Such an approach has the potential to revolutionize neuromodulation by making therapy more responsive to patient-specific neurophysiological patterns [10]. Remote programming for spinal cord stimulators represents a vanguard advancement in neuromodulation, redefining paradigms of accessibility, efficiency, and therapeutic personalization. As digital health technologies evolve, integrating AI, biometric analytics, and telehealth infrastructure will further enhance the scope and efficacy of remote programming.

Spinal cord stimulator remote programming technique

Remote programming of spinal cord stimulators represents a paradigm shift in pain management, offering unprecedented flexibility and convenience for both patients and clinicians. Remote programming leverages wireless communication technologies to enable adjustments to stimulation parameters from a remote location, thereby circumventing the geographical and logistical constraints of traditional programming. Moreover, remote programming facilitates more frequent and personalized optimization of therapy, leading to improved pain relief and overall quality of life. The ability to fine-tune stimulation parameters remotely empowers clinicians and manufacturer representatives to proactively manage patient care, intervening promptly to address any issues or concerns that may arise.

Remote programming can be initiated in several ways. Remote monitoring plays a vital role in remote programming initiation. Currently different SCS manufacturers allow for different degrees of remote monitoring. As of 2023, one SCS manufacturer had the capability of remotely monitoring SCS device-related data on a daily basis [8].

Daily device-related data collection and transmission allows manufacturer representatives and/or healthcare providers to access and review this data via the manufacturer's device platform on an as needed basis or when prompted by the patient or device itself. Parameters can be set and individualized for each patient to trigger alerts for review from the patient's healthcare team. The other form of remote monitoring involves self-reported data. This is data that is input by the patient or caregiver and includes metrics such as pain scores, sleep duration/quality, and functional assessments [8]. Remotely monitored data whether automatically collected from the device or self-reported by the patient/caregiver can be viewed remotely via manufacturer portals and can then prompt reprogramming.

Different metrics have been proposed that may be clinically relevant to remote monitoring in order to better facilitate recognition of when reprogramming may be necessary to optimize a patient's therapy and promote better outcomes. Lastly, remote reprogramming can be requested at the patient's request at any time via the patient interface.

Remote programming typically has three main components: patient interface, communication infrastructure, and clinician interface [2,8]. The patient interface is carefully designed to be user-friendly and intuitive, typically comprising a handheld programmer or a dedicated smartphone application that serves as the patient's primary means of interaction with the SCS system [13].

The patient must first connect their controller to their IPG via Bluetooth/RF, then they are able to connect to the communication infrastructure and initiate a video session with the clinician. This must be done through a secure wireless network, such as cellular or internet connectivity, incorporating robust encryption protocols to protect patient data and maintain confidentiality. The communication network enables seamless and secure data transmission between the patient's device and the clinician's remote programming station.

A secure server infrastructure, meticulously maintained within a HIPAA-compliant data center, forms the backbone of the remote programming system, providing not only essential data storage and management capabilities, but also orchestrating secure communication pathways between the patient's device and the clinician's workstation. The final component is the clinician interface, which provides healthcare professionals (manufacturer representative and/or clinician) with the ability to participate in a video session with the patient and a comprehensive suite of tools for monitoring patient progress, adjusting stimulation parameters, and managing overall therapy. The healthcare professional has the ability to access the patient's device through a secure, cloud-based platform, permitting modifications to stimulation parameters, such as pulse width, amplitude, frequency, and electrode configuration all while also allowing a video session to occur to monitor the patient while making adjustments to the device parameters [2,13].

Manufacturer representatives and clinicians must be vigilant in monitoring for signs of overstimulation or adverse effects, such as paresthesia, motor weakness, or changes in bowel or bladder function, and be prepared to remotely adjust parameters or instruct patients to temporarily suspend stimulation.

Remote monitoring and reprogramming will likely not replace in-person reprogramming but these two modalities of monitoring/reprogramming can and should be used in conjunction with one another. Remote monitoring and reprogramming can allow for data collection and troubleshooting of issues as well as identification of device related issues that may warrant in-person visits. If issues persist despite remote reprogramming this should prompt an in person follow up for further evaluation [8].

Spinal cord stimulation remote programming: Navigating the pearls and pitfalls

Traditional methods of SCS programming often require in-person visits to specialized clinics, which can be burdensome for patients, particularly those in rural areas or with mobility limitations. Studies have shown that patients prefer remote monitoring over in-office visits/monitoring [2,13]. This innovative approach allows for real-time adjustments to stimulation parameters, optimizing pain relief and minimizing side effects without requiring in-office visits. Clinicians and/or manufacturer representatives can remotely modify stimulation amplitude, pulse width, frequency, and electrode configuration, tailoring the therapy to individual patient needs and fluctuations in pain levels. This capability is particularly valuable in managing dynamic pain conditions, where symptoms may vary throughout the day or in response to specific activities.

Furthermore, remote monitoring functionalities can provide clinicians and device manufacturers with valuable insights into patient usage patterns, adherence to therapy, and overall treatment response, facilitating data-driven decision-making and proactive intervention [13]. The ability to remotely interrogate device impedance, battery status, and lead integrity streamlines troubleshooting and reduces the need for unnecessary office visits while also allowing for early detection of any potential device-related issue and the ability to schedule prompt intervention. Thus, overall, enhancing patient convenience and reducing healthcare costs [13].

The implementation of remote spinal cord stimulation programming, however, is not without its challenges, necessitating careful consideration of potential pitfalls. A primary concern revolves around cybersecurity. Unauthorized access to the data or implanted pulse generator could lead to inappropriate stimulation or device malfunction as well as the breach of confidential patient information [13]. Robust encryption protocols and authentication mechanisms are essential to safeguard patient data and prevent malicious attacks. Ensuring reliable connectivity is crucial, as intermittent or lost connections during programming sessions can lead to incomplete parameter adjustments or device errors. The need and availability of a strong and reliable cellular network or Wi-Fi connection is a possible constraint for some patients in certain areas and/or demographics. Another major consideration regarding this modality of programming is the complexity of interfaces and the multitude of available parameters can be daunting for both patients and clinicians. This could lead to suboptimal utilization as well as programming choices [13].

Comprehensive training programs and user-friendly software interfaces are vital to promote effective and safe utilization of remote programming capabilities for both patients as well as the manufacturer representatives and clinicians performing the reprogramming. Remote monitoring for a majority of the SCS manufacturers currently relies heavily, if not completely, on patient-reported metrics such as pain scores, sleep duration/quality, and functional assessments. Thus the success of remote monitoring and its utility in initiating remote or in-person reprogramming currently relies on the patient's ability to participate with data entry and continued active participation over time.

References

[1] Aspher telematics. J Publ Health 1997;5(3):298–9. https://doi.org/10.1007/bf02956344.

[2] Han Y, Lu Y, Wang D, Ran M, Ren Q, Xie D, Aziz TZ, Li L, Wang JJ. The use of remote programming for spinal cord stimulation for patients with chronic pain during the COVID-19 outbreak in China. Neuromodulation 2021;24(3):441–7. https://doi.org/10.1111/ner.13382.

[3] Wilkoff BL, Auricchio A, Brugada J, et al. HRS/EHRA expert consensus on the monitoring of cardiovascular implantable electronic devices (CIEDs): Description of techniques, indications, personnel, frequency and ethical considerations. Heart Rhythm 2008;5(6):907–25. https://doi.org/10.1016/j.hrthm.2008.04.013.

[4] Slotwiner D, Varma N, Akar JG, et al. HRS Expert Consensus Statement on remote interrogation and monitoring for cardiovascular implantable electronic devices. Heart Rhythm 2015;12(7):e69–100. https://doi.org/10.1016/j.hrthm.2015.05.008.

[5] Silburn P, DeBates S, Tomlinson T, et al. Rapid development of a NeuroSphere™ virtual clinic (Abbott, Austin, Texas). In: Consensus guidelines for remote management of spinal cord stimulation were established; 2023.

[6] Silburn P, DeBates S, Tomlinson T, et al. Rapid development of an integrated remote programming platform for neuromodulation systems through the biodesign process. Sci Rep 2022;12(1). https://doi.org/10.1038/s41598-022-06098-7.

[7] Abbott Introduces NeuroSphereTM Virtual Clinic, *First-of-its-Kind Remote Neuromodulation Patient-Care Technology in the U.S.. Abbott MediaRoom.* https://abbott.mediaroom.com/2021-03-08-Abbott-Introduces-NeuroSphere-TM-Virtual-Clinic-First-of-its-Kind-Remote-Neuromodulation-Patient-Care-Technology-in-the-U-S.

[8] Staats P, Deer TR, Hunter C, Li S, Dickerson D, Petersen E, Kapural L, Durbhakula S, Gilligan C, Slavin KV, Pope J, Amirdelfan K, Poree L, Naidu R, Levy RM. Remote management of spinal cord stimulation devices for chronic pain: Expert recommendations on best practices for proper utilization and future considerations. Neuromodulation 2023;26(7):1295–308. https://doi.org/10.1016/j.neurom.2023.07.003.

[9] Ali R, Schwalb JM. History and future of spinal cord stimulation. Neurosurgery 2024;94(1):20–8. https://doi.org/10.1227/neu.0000000000002654.

[10] Naidu RK, Kapural L, Li S, Tourjé C, Rutledge J, Dickerson D, Lubenow TR. A review of the Prospera spinal cord stimulation system with multiphase stimulation and proactive care. Curr Pain Headache Rep 2025;29(1):25. https://doi.org/10.1007/s11916-024-01318-3.

[11] Pathak YJ, Greenleaf W, Verhagen Metman L, Kubben P, Sarma S, Pepin B, Lautner D, DeBates S, Benison AM, Balasingh B, Ross E. Digital health integration with neuromodulation therapies: The future of patient-centric innovation in neuromodulation. Front Digit Health 2021;3:618959. https://doi.org/10.3389/fdgth.2021.618959.

[12] Lu Y, Xie D, Zhang X, Dong S, Zhang H, Yu B, Wang G, Wang JJ, Li L. Management of intractable pain in patients with implanted spinal cord stimulation devices during the COVID-19 pandemic using a remote and wireless programming system. Front Neurosci 2020;14:594696. https://doi.org/10.3389/fnins.2020.594696.

[13] Deer TR, Esposito MF, Cornidez EG, Okaro U, Fahey ME, Chapman KB. Teleprogramming service provides safe and remote stimulation options for patients with DRG-S and SCS implants. J Pain Res 2021;14:3259–65. https://doi.org/10.2147/JPR.S332966.

Section 9

Peripheral nerve stimulation

Introduction to section 9 peripheral nerve stimulation

Seven years of implanting peripheral nerve stimulators has changed my understanding of chronic pain. Historically, pain medicine has struggled with tachyphylaxis. Oral analgesics work well initially, and then later analgesia requires dose escalation or medication rotation. Intrathecal medications likewise can work well initially, but over time require dose escalations or medication rotations. Spinal cord stimulation historically generally follows a similar pattern, with excellent results initially followed by reprogramming sessions and troubleshooting after 2–3 years. The body adjusts to electricity in the same way it adjusts to medication exposure over time.

When I started implanting peripheral nerve stimulators, I expected to see the same pattern, but was surprised to see the opposite pattern emerge. When the device is on the correct target and the patient perceives the paresthesia in the correct area, then the use of the device generally decreases over time, sometimes with resolution of pain. With SCS systems, I explanted them due to loss of efficacy. With PNS systems, I explant them due to lack of use when the original pain has resolved and remains resolved for 18 months. That stated, I do have patients who move towards early resolution of pain within months of stimulation, and I also have patients with daily use of 7-year-old peripheral nerve stimulators. What is the difference between these two patient groups? Why do some patients move towards resolution of pain, and some patients need ongoing treatment with peripheral nerve stimulators? I suspect it is related to anatomic differences and nerve entrapment.

When a non-neuronal structure in the body is injured, peripheral nociceptors detect this tissue damage and send nociceptive action potentials to the spinal cord only for a few days until healing occurs. When the tissue damage is directly to a nerve, however, the nerve may fire ectopically for weeks to months, strengthening the nociceptive pathway over time and possibly inducing swelling in the nerve. This nerve enlargement into tight anatomic tunnels may help maintain the neuropathic pain.

The key aspect of the peripheral nerve stimulator implantation is to find this lesion if it exists. If a patient responds well to a diagnostic nerve block with very short-term (hours) analgesia, then this could be a more injured nerve with possible entrapment. The patient may need more imaging or workup, and the nerve may need to be decompressed for optimal PNS outcome. On the other hand, if the patient has resolution of pain from the nerve block and has persistent analgesic benefit that lasts days to weeks, then that suggests the nerve is less injured and less likely to be significantly entrapped, and PNS should provide longer-term analgesia.

The ensuing chapters detail the best current evidence in peripheral nerve stimulator implant techniques along with their potential complications. Further research into the mechanism of action, patient selection, and optimizing long-term efficacy will be essential in continuing PNS's role in chronic pain management.

Einar Ottestad, MD, FIPP, CIPS, Clinical Professor

Associate Division Chief of Acute Pain Medicine

Medical Director, Acute Pain Service, and the Stanford Comprehensive Interdisciplinary Pain Program

Stanford University School of Medicine

Department of Anesthesiology, Perioperative, and Pain Medicine

Chapter 28

The upper extremity peripheral nerve stimulation

Mansoor M. Aman, David M. Gallacher, Lawson Smith, Tyler Burns and David M. Dickerson
Endeavor Health, Evanston, IL, United States

Key points

- Peripheral nerve stimulation (PNS) should be considered for focal pain along one to two dermatomes with predominant neuropathic clinical features
- Both temporary and permanent stimulation can provide durable relief
- When using ultrasound guidance for lead placement, an in-plane technique is recommended to optimize safety
- Best practice guidelines on anticoagulation medications and infection prevention should be followed
- Lead implantation should avoid crossing a joint such as the shoulder or elbow.

Introduction

In 1967, Wall and Sweet described the successful use of peripheral nerve stimulation (PNS) for the treatment of cutaneous, sensory or nerve root pain in eight patients. During stimulation, pain thresholds were improved for all eight patients, and in half the patients they observed relief of pain for more than 30 min after stimulation was used for only 2 min [1]. This phenomenon has been described as targeted neuroplasticity. Applying an external current may induce and maintain a long-term effect on the nervous system through long term potentiation or depression such that symptom improved is observed after cessation of stimulation [2]. Over the last 50 years, PNS has been successfully used for the treatment of chronic headache, chronic joint pain, post stroke pain, post operative pain, complex regional pain syndrome, post amputation pain, mechanical low back pain, and a multitude of neuropathic chronic pain conditions of peripheral origin [3–10].

PNS is best utilized for the treatment of focal pain along one to two dermatomes but can be used in proximity to nerve roots to target a larger area of pain. Initial limitations to adoption were bulky lead design that required open surgical placement, external pulse generators (EPG) that were not portable, limited magnetic resonance imaging (MRI) compatibility, and a narrow therapeutic window due to the available stimulation paradigms. In the last decade, numerous systems have been introduced that are thoughtfully designed for use in the periphery and offer MRI conditional labeling. Open invasive placement has largely transitioned to percutaneous electrode deployment using ultrasound or fluoroscopic guidance. Depending on the system, the lead communicates with an external pulse generator, with or without an implantable pulse generator at the end of the lead. Microelectrodes (0.3 mm diameter) and conventional peripheral electrodes (1.2–1.35 mm) can deliver monopolar and bipolar stimulation. In a monopolar stimulation system, a cathode (negative electrode) creates the field of stimulation while the anode (positive electrode) is at the external pulse generator. A monopolar stimulation system offers the advantage of larger field of stimulation, and when placed remote to a nerve can allow for lower thresholds for efficacy while mitigating unwanted stimulation. In bipolar systems a more focal, dense field of stimulation is created from cathode to anode located adjacent to the nerve. Multiple programing options are available for both types of system that can provide low frequency stimulation (10–30 Hz) to create comfortable contractions or high frequency stimulation (>90 Hz) that results in paresthesia overlying the area of pain without the presence of muscular contractions. There have been reports of using a combination of motor and sensory stimulation allowing for both afferent and efferent pathway capture resulting in a more significant pain relief when compared to either modality alone [11]. For

A Modern Atlas for Implantable Devices of the Spine, Brain, and Nerve. https://doi.org/10.1016/B978-0-443-36528-7.00030-3

example, in a patient with two leads implanted for shoulder stimulation, one lead may be placed along the axillary nerve and another along the suprascapular nerve. The axillary lead may utilize low frequency motor stimulation with instructions to use for 12 h a day, while the suprascapular lead will operate at high frequency setting providing a comfortable paresthesia continuously. The duration of each stimulation session varies based upon manufacturer labeling, patient tolerance to stimulation, and the need to rest the skin from adhesive required for the EPG.

In this chapter, we describe the relevant anatomy, pre procedure, intraoperative and post operative considerations when using PNS for upper extremity pain.

Anatomy

Understanding the relevant anatomy and targets is essential for effectively applying peripheral nerve stimulation (PNS). Although the utility for PNS is expanding, this section provides an overview of common targets in the upper extremity and anatomical considerations.

Brachial plexus nerve roots, trunks, cords

The brachial plexus comprises a complex network of nerves formed by the anterior rami of the C5 through T1 spinal nerves [12]. This structure provides both motor and sensory innervation to the upper limbs. It is organized into five roots, three trunks, six divisions, three cords, and five primary terminal branches [13] that can be targeted with PNS. The primary approaches to targeting the brachial plexus nerve roots include:

- *Interscalene Approach:* This approach targets the brachial plexus at the level of the roots and upper trunks as they pass between the anterior and middle scalene muscles. When in a supine position, the patient will turn their head away from the side being stimulated. With ultrasound guidance, the interscalene groove can be located, and the electrode can be positioned adjacent to the nerve root. Accessing between the posterior border of the levator scapulae muscle and posterior border of the trapezius muscle (posterior approach) allows for the lead to "tunnel" toward the interscalene target providing stability for placement.
- *Supraclavicular Approach:* This approach targets the brachial plexus superior to the clavicle and lateral to the sternocleidomastoid muscle (SCM). In a supine position, the patient's head is turned contralaterally. Ultrasound guidance allows visualization of the plexus above the clavicle bone, facilitating electrode placement near the target site. A similar approach to the interscalene approach can be used via the trapezius and levator scapulae muscle window.
- *Infraclavicular Approach:* This technique targets the cords of the brachial plexus located below the clavicle. When the patient is in a supine position with their arm abducted, ultrasound guidance aids in identifying the axillary artery, around which the three cords of the brachial plexus are arranged. The cords are named according to their position relative to the artery. The electrode can be placed on the targeted cord based on the patient's symptoms. The pectoral muscles are traversed which provides stability but requires awareness of the thoracoacromial artery, a branch of the axillary artery.

Suprascapular nerve

The suprascapular nerve originates from the upper trunk of the brachial plexus through the C5 and C6 nerve roots, and occasionally has contributors from C4. It traverses the suprascapular notch beneath the transverse scapular ligament after running deep to the omohyoid muscle. This nerve supplies the supraspinatus and infraspinatus muscles, which are part of the rotator cuff and assist with shoulder abduction and external rotation. Additionally, the suprascapular nerve conveys sensation to the acromioclavicular (AC) joint and the glenohumeral (GH) joint, making it an important target for managing chronic shoulder pain.

Axillary nerve

The axillary nerve arises from the posterior cord of the brachial plexus via the C5 and C6 nerve roots. It passes through the quadrilateral space, formed by the surgical neck of the humerus, long head of the triceps brachii, teres major, and teres minor. The axillary nerve innervates the deltoid muscle, which is critical for shoulder abduction, and the teres minor, which facilitates external rotation [14]. The nerve also provides sensory input over the deltoid region, making it a suitable target for managing chronic shoulder pain or proximal humeral fracture related nerve injury.

Radial nerve

The radial nerve forms from the posterior cord of the brachial plexus through the C5 to T1 nerve roots. It spirals around the humerus via the radial groove, innervating the triceps brachii muscle. The nerve continues distally, wrapping anteriorly around the lateral epicondyle of the humerus, where it divides into deep motor and superficial sensory branches. The motor portion provides extensor activation of the elbow and forearm, while the sensory portion innervates the posterior arm, forearm, and dorsal hand.

Median nerve

The median nerve receives contributions from the medial and lateral cords of the brachial plexus via the C5 through T1 nerve roots. It runs along the medial aspect of the arm, crosses the elbow anteriorly through the cubital fossa, and moves distally through the forearm between the flexor digitorum superficialis (FDS) and flexor digitorum profundus (FDP). PNS targeting the median nerve is used for conditions such as carpal tunnel syndrome, neuropathic pain [15], and complex regional pain syndrome (CRPS) [3].

Ulnar nerve

The ulnar nerve arises from the medial cord of the brachial plexus via the C8 and T1 nerve roots. It travels along the medial aspect of the arm, passes posterior to the medial epicondyle of the humerus, and enters the forearm. In the forearm, it courses between the two heads of the flexor carpi ulnaris (FCU) muscle and provides innervation to the hypothenar muscles, interossei, adductor pollicis, and medial two lumbricals. The ulnar nerve can be a target for PNS in conditions such as ulnar neuropathy or cubital tunnel syndrome.

Procedure

Diagnosis and indications

Peripheral nerve stimulation (PNS) of the upper extremity (UE) can be utilized as treatment for a myriad of pain syndromes. The United States Food and Drug Administration (FDA) has approved PNS devices for chronic intractable pain of peripheral nerve origin including nerve injuries or entrapment syndromes, as well as postoperative and post-traumatic neuropathic pain including complex regional pain syndromes (CRPS) Type 1 and 2. PNS may also be utilized for diabetic peripheral neuropathy, hemiplegic shoulder pain, phantom limb pain, and post stroke pain. A summary of the diagnosis with each subsequent ICD-10 code is included in Table 28.1.

Patient selection considerations

Appropriate patient selection, pre-operative evaluation, surgical technique, and follow up is key to any success with PNS. PNS therapy should be considered in any patient who has pain that is focal to a distinct nerve distribution, >6 months of duration, and has failed conservative therapy (physical therapy, pharmacologic therapy, and, when indicated, injection-based therapy) (1,2). For patients undergoing surgery of the upper extremity, there is a growing body of randomized controlled trial evidence for reduced opioid consumption and reduction of pain in acute, post-surgical pain compared to sham treatment.

PNS is not without risk as placing an electrode within close proximity to a nerve can result in negative sequelae, i. e.,: direct trauma, nerve compression, bleeding, infection [16,17]. The physician performing PNS and their advanced practice providers should individualize the risk for each patient, especially those seen as high risk such as: patients undergoing cancer treatment, immunocompromised status, chronic infections, or with an anticoagulation requirement. PNS is stratified in the low to intermediate risk category by the American Society of Regional Anesthesiologists and Pain Physicians (ASRA) guidelines, and is commonly performed in compressible areas of the body [16,18]. Therefore the risk of bleeding is small for most patients. The risk of bleeding increases if the peripheral nerve target is next a large vascular structure or when an anticoagulant is unable to be adequately held. Appropriate image guidance during implantation mitigates this risk. Using tined leads or fascial anchors reduce migration and potential lead fracture.

TABLE 28.1 Common conditions and associated ICD-10 codes treated with upper extremity peripheral nerve stimulation.

Condition	ICD-10 code	Description
Phantom limb pain (upper extremity)	G54.7	Phantom limb syndrome with pain
Median nerve neuropathy	G56.00	Carpal tunnel syndrome, unspecified upper limb
	G56.01	Carpal tunnel syndrome, right upper limb
	G56.02	Carpal tunnel syndrome, left upper limb
	G56.10	Other lesions of median nerve, unspecified upper limb
	G56.11	Other lesions of median nerve, right upper limb
	G56.12	Other lesions of median nerve, left upper limb
Median nerve entrapment	G56.00-G56.02	Carpal tunnel syndrome (wrist entrapment)
	G56.10-G56.12	Pronator teres syndrome (elbow entrapment)
Ulnar neuropathy	G56.20	Lesion of ulnar nerve, unspecified upper limb
	G56.21	Lesion of ulnar nerve, right upper limb
	G56.22	Lesion of ulnar nerve, left upper limb
Cubital tunnel syndrome (ulnar nerve entrapment at elbow)	G56.30	Lesion of ulnar nerve at elbow, unspecified upper limb
	G56.31	Lesion of ulnar nerve at elbow, right upper limb
	G56.32	Lesion of ulnar nerve at elbow, left upper limb
Radial nerve neuropathy	G56.30	Lesion of radial nerve, unspecified upper limb
	G56.31	Lesion of radial nerve, right upper limb
	G56.32	Lesion of radial nerve, left upper limb
Radial nerve entrapment syndromes	G56.3X	Includes Saturday night palsy, radial tunnel syndrome, wrist drop
Brachial plexopathy	G54.0	Brachial plexus disorders
Traumatic brachial plexopathy	S14.3XXA	Injury of brachial plexus, initial encounter
	S14.3XXD	Injury of brachial plexus, subsequent encounter
	S14.3XXS	Injury of brachial plexus, sequela
Inflammatory brachial plexopathy	G54.0	Includes Parsonage-Turner syndrome (neuralgic amyotrophy)
	M79.2	Neuralgia and neuritis, unspecified
Radiation-induced brachial plexopathy	G54.0	Brachial plexus disorders (due to radiation)
Postoperative brachial plexopathy	G54.0	Brachial plexus disorders (post-surgical)
	T81.89XA	Other complications of procedures, initial encounter
Diabetic peripheral neuropathy (type 2)	E11.40	Type 2 diabetes mellitus with diabetic neuropathy, unspecified
	E11.42	Type 2 diabetes mellitus with diabetic polyneuropathy
Diabetic peripheral neuropathy (type 1)	E10.40	Type 1 diabetes mellitus with diabetic neuropathy, unspecified
	E10.42	Type 1 diabetes mellitus with diabetic polyneuropathy
Other specific types of diabetes with neuropathy	E08.42	Diabetes due to underlying condition with diabetic polyneuropathy
	E09.42	Drug- or chemically-induced diabetes mellitus with diabetic polyneuropathy
	E13.42	Other specified diabetes mellitus with diabetic polyneuropathy
Hemiplegic shoulder pain	M25.519	Pain in unspecified shoulder
	M25.511	Pain in right shoulder
	M25.512	Pain in left shoulder

Training recommendations

A number of medical specialties utilize PNS therapy. Physicians wishing to utilize PNS therapy must have the necessary clinical acumen and skill for appropriate patient selection, surgical technique, knowledge of anatomy under fluoroscopy and ultrasound, and appropriate management of maintaining the therapy after implant as well as any complication. American Council of Graduate Medical Education (ACGME) accredited pain medicine fellowship programs and neurosurgical training programs provide training in PNS, but with varying levels of breadth of exposure [19–22]. Several professional societies including American Society of Pain and Neuroscience (ASPN) and the North American Neuromodulation Society (NANS) that have created specific training curriculum for specialists involved in PNS therapy [21,22]. Additionally, device manufacturers commonly provide hands-on training and proctorships to ensure physicians are safely and effectively utilizing their devices as intended.

Technique

Most PNS systems can be implanted in awake patients with local anesthesia or with conscious sedation in an outpatient setting. Ultrasound guided placement is recommended whenever possible, particularly when targeting nerves that are near large vessels. In plane and out of plane techniques are described in the literature and both require the operator to be proficient in principles of ultrasonography including relevant anatomy, angle of incidence, attenuation, velocity of propagation, and frequency. A fluoroscopic guided placement may be performed when targeting nerves that reside in a predictable location along an osseous target. Case times will vary depending on the type of system being used, experience with imaging, anatomic considerations and challenges and procedural/surgical proficiency. It is recommended to conduct intraoperative sensory or motor paresthesia mapping prior to lead deployment and securement to ensure adequate coverage and avoid unwanted stimulation. Relevant neural target technique is described in Table 28.2.

Post operative considerations

Recovery

Patients should be advised there will be soreness at the site where the introducer needle was placed and at the site of the lead and pulse generator when applicable. Patients should be cautioned to monitor for signs of infection such as swelling, erythema, drainage, and excessive pain. The dressing should be left in place and not changed until advised by the physician. If the dressing becomes soiled or begins to come off secondary to movement or sweating, the patient should notify the physician regarding care and how to proceed. The patient should avoid submerging the site in water for the duration of the trial and for the first weeks after an implant, utilizing sponge bath when appropriate. Percutaneous systems should never be submerged in water.

Efficacy

Studies have shown efficacy ranging from 60% to 75% pain relief with permanent PNS [17]. With percutaneous 60-day PNS treatment, 71% of patients had a least 50% pain relief at end of treatment [23].

Bracing considerations

This is dependent on the location of the nerve treated. Bracing should be considered for trials and implants as it may help prevent excessive movement of the body region. This will help prevent potential migration of the lead which would decrease effectiveness of the therapy. Bracing of the thoracic and lumbar spine can be considered for axial procedures to help reduce flexion, extension, rotation of the spine, bracing of the upper extremity can help to reduce reaching overhead in the setting of a suprascapular nerve or brachial plexus placement. Within 4–6 weeks healing will take place which should prevent further movement of the lead via scar tissue formation.

Activity limitations

Similarly, to traditional SCS, limitations following a trial or implant should be followed including limited bending, twisting, heavy lifting, or climbing. These limitations are to help prevent migration of the leads and loss of effective therapy. Once the lead has scarred into place, patients may resume all regular activities.

TABLE 28.2 Summary of upper extemity neural targets and associated procedural approaches.

Nerve	Imaging	Patient position	Approach
Suprascapular	US or fluoroscopic	Sitting (+/− beach chair) or prone with pillows underneath the chest	Ultrasound-transducer in a coronal oblique orientation over the posterior shoulder, parallel to the lateral third of the scapular spine. Tilt anterior to identify the floor of the supraspinous fossa deep to the trapezius and supraspinatus muscles. Insert the needle in-plane and medial to lateral direction until tip contacts the bone.
Axillary	US or fluoroscopic	Sitting or prone	Ultrasound-transducer in a sagittal orientation over the posterior aspect of the upper arm midway between the acromion and the axillary fold. Slide proximal to distal until the neck of the humerus is visualized, adjust tilt until posterior circumflex humoral artery is visualized between terries minor, deltoid and triceps, superficial to the bone. Needle can be inserted in-plane or out of plane.
Radial (above the elbow)	Ultrasound	Supine	Position the transducer in a transverse orientation 3–4 cm proximal to the lateral epicondyle. Scan with moderate pressure, adjusting the tilt to identify the nerve between the brachioradialis and brachialis, superficial to the humerus. Insert the needle in plane.
Median (above the elbow)	Ultrasound	Supine	Position the transducer in a transverse orientation on the antecubital fossa just proximal to the elbow crease. Identify the brachial artery, the median nerve is next to it on the medial side and appears hyperechoic. It is located between the brachialis and pronator teres. The needle is inserted in plane.
Ulnar (above the elbow)	Ultrasound	Supine or prone	Position the transducer in a transverse orientation proximal to the medial epicondyle and move posterior to identify the ulnar nerve on the triceps muscle. The needle is inserted in plane.

Maintenance considerations

Most available therapies have an external battery that requires a wearable device to have the battery within range of the PNS lead. Patient should remain in close contact with the company representative and treating physician's clinical team to ensure adequate programing of the device and to ensure appropriate stimulation coverage.

Pearls and pitfalls

Preoperative

Patients should have a neuropathic diagnosis amenable to PNS treatment, an understanding of the PNS treatments possible risks, benefits and alternatives, and a commitment to the ongoing management of the device and their overall health care. Preoperative discussion identifies a patient's preparedness for PNS treatment as well as other determinants of health that may impede optimal response to treatment. Before pursuing PNS, non-neuropathic pain complaints and diagnoses should be inventoried to help patients recognize that comprehensive care for those issues may be needed separately from PNS treatment. Lastly, selecting the optimal PNS treatment approach employs shared decision making that marries patient preference for implant site and wearable components with MRI conditionality and anatomical considerations. The preop area is ideal for confirming pulse generator and lead placement sites but these discussions and planning ideally begin well before the day of surgery.

Intraoperative

Patient positioning, adequate surgical cut down depth, ideal lead path to optimal target site, intraoperative testing when applicable, anchoring, or tined lead selection and a multilayer wound closure seek to reduce patient discomfort, lead migration, infection or other patient injury or dissatisfaction. A wide surgical prep area and a comfortably positioned, secured patient are key determinants of a smooth procedure and are challenging to readdress after the beginning of the procedure.

Postoperative

Timely follow up and continued patient support after device implantation is paramount. Tracking outcomes and ensuring clinic access for patients living with PNS devices post implant are critical to sustained patient response and mitigating negative outcomes.

References

[1] Wall PD, Sweet WH. Temporary abolition of pain in man. Science 1967;155(3758):108–9.
[2] Asp AJ, et al. Targeted neuroplasticity in spatiotemporally patterned invasive neuromodulation therapies for improving clinical outcomes. Front Neuroinf 2023;17.
[3] Chmiela MA, et al. Direct peripheral nerve stimulation for the treatment of complex regional pain syndrome: a 30-year review. Neuromodulation 2021;24(6):971–82.
[4] de Leon-Casasola OA. Spinal cord and peripheral nerve stimulation techniques for neuropathic pain. J Pain Symptom Manag 2009;38(2 Suppl. 1): S28–38.
[5] Deer T, et al. Prospective, multicenter, randomized, double-blinded, partial crossover study to assess the safety and efficacy of the novel neuromodulation system in the treatment of patients with chronic pain of peripheral nerve origin. Neuromodulation 2016;19(1):91–100.
[6] Gilmore C, et al. Percutaneous peripheral nerve stimulation for the treatment of chronic neuropathic postamputation pain: a multicenter, randomized, placebo-controlled trial. Reg Anesth Pain Med 2019;44(6):637–45.
[7] Gilmore CA, et al. Percutaneous peripheral nerve stimulation for chronic low back pain: prospective case series with 1 year of sustained relief following short-term implant. Pain Pract 2020;20(3):310–20.
[8] Jasper JF, Hayek SM. Implanted occipital nerve stimulators. Pain Physician 2008;11(2):187–200.
[9] Goree JH, et al. Randomized placebo-controlled trial of 60-day percutaneous peripheral nerve stimulation treatment indicates relief of persistent postoperative pain, and improved function after knee replacement. Neuromodulation 2024;27(5):847–61.
[10] Aman MM, et al. Retrospective evaluation of bipolar peripheral nerve stimulation for nociceptive and neuropathic pain: a pilot study. J Pain Res 2024;17:2929–36.
[11] Gutierrez GJ, et al. A single-center retrospective chart review of percutaneous PNS for treatment of chronic shoulder pain. Interv Pain Med 2024;3 (3):100419.
[12] Leinberry CF, Wehbé MA. Brachial plexus anatomy. Hand Clin 2004;20(1):1–5.
[13] Silver S, et al. Peripheral nerve entrapment and injury in the upper extremity. Am Fam Physician 2021;103(5):275–85.
[14] Leechavengvongs S, et al. Surgical anatomy of the axillary nerve branches to the deltoid muscle. Clin Anat 2015;28(1):118–22.
[15] Kaye AD, et al. Peripheral nerve stimulation: a review of techniques and clinical efficacy. Pain Ther 2021;10(2):961–72.
[16] Strand N, et al. Evidence-based clinical guidelines from the American society of pain and neuroscience for the use of implantable peripheral nerve stimulation in the treatment of chronic pain. J Pain Res 2022;15:2483–504.
[17] Xu J, et al. Peripheral nerve stimulation in pain management: a systematic review. Pain Physician 2021;24(2):E131–e152.
[18] Narouze S, et al. Interventional spine and pain procedures in patients on antiplatelet and anticoagulant medications (second edition): guidelines from the American Society of Regional Anesthesia and Pain Medicine, the European Society of Regional Anaesthesia and Pain Therapy, the American Academy of Pain Medicine, the International Neuromodulation Society, the North American Neuromodulation Society, and the World Institute of Pain. Reg Anesth Pain Med 2018;43(3):225–62.
[19] Kalia H, et al. Educational curriculum for peripheral nerve stimulation developed by the North American neuromodulation society. Neuromodulation 2023;26(3):483–9.
[20] Henderson JM, et al. NANS training requirements for spinal cord stimulation devices: selection, implantation, and follow-up. Neuromodulation 2009;12(3):171–4.
[21] Abd-Elsayed A, et al. Development of an educational curriculum for spinal cord stimulation. Neuromodulation 2020;23(5):555–61.
[22] Pritzlaff SG, et al. Pain education and knowledge (PEAK) consensus guidelines for neuromodulation: a proposal for standardization in fellowship and training programs. J Pain Res 2023;16:3101–17.
[23] Huntoon MA, et al. A retrospective review of real-world outcomes following 60-day peripheral nerve stimulation for the treatment of chronic pain. Pain Physician 2023;26(3):273–81.

Chapter 29

Peripheral nerve stimulation of the trunk and abdomen

Nasir Khatri[1], Evan Peskin[1] and Mayank Gupta[2]
[1]*Insight Health Systems, Flint, MI, United States;* [2]*Kansas Pain Management, Overland Park, KS, United States*

Introduction

Peripheral nerve stimulation (PNS) of the trunk and abdomen is a neuromodulation technique that involves the implantation of electrodes near peripheral nerves to modulate pain signals [1]. Unlike spinal cord stimulation (SCS), which targets the central nervous system, PNS directly influences specific peripheral nerves, offering a targeted approach for patients with focal pain syndromes. This technique has gained traction in the management of chronic, refractory pain conditions such as post-surgical pain, post-herpetic neuralgia, and abdominal wall pain caused by entrapped or irritated cutaneous nerves. With growing evidence supporting its efficacy, PNS is now an integral component of the interventional pain management landscape [1].

The concept of neuromodulation for pain relief dates back to the early 20th century, when researchers first recognized the potential of electrical stimulation to alter pain perception. However, it was not until the 1960s, following Melzack and Wall's Gate Control Theory of Pain, that clinical applications of neuromodulation began to take shape [2]. Spinal cord stimulation emerged as the primary method of neuromodulation, but as the understanding of pain pathways evolved, attention shifted toward peripheral nerve stimulation as a viable alternative, especially for focal neuropathic pain conditions [3]. In the 1990s, early PNS systems were developed, initially involving cumbersome implantable pulse generators. However, a significant limitation existed. Targeting individual nerves with fluoroscopy only was quite difficult, often resulting in field stimulation with nonoptimal long-term relief. Over the past 2 decades, technological advancements have refined electrode design, programming capabilities, and implant techniques, making PNS a more accessible and effective treatment option [1,4].

PNS has evolved significantly from its early iterations. Initially, percutaneous lead placement was challenging due to anatomical constraints and limitations in imaging guidance. Today, fluoroscopic and ultrasound-guided techniques have enhanced precision in lead placement, minimizing complications and improving patient outcomes. Innovations such as wireless technology, rechargeable battery systems, and smaller electrode arrays have further improved the feasibility of PNS [5]. These advancements have expanded the indications for PNS beyond traditional pain syndromes to include post-amputation pain, intercostal neuralgia, and even functional disorders such as abdominal wall spasticity. The introduction of wearable and externalized neuromodulation systems has also provided a non-permanent option for patients who may not require long-term implantation. As machine learning and artificial intelligence become integrated into device programming, PNS therapy will continue to offer personalized, adaptive treatment strategies, enhancing both safety and efficacy [1].

Key points

- Peripheral nerve stimulation (PNS) provides targeted relief for focal neuropathic pain syndromes of the trunk and abdomen, including post-surgical pain, post-herpetic neuralgia, and intercostal neuralgia.
- Advancements in imaging, lead design, and device technology have made PNS more precise, minimally invasive, and accessible for both trial and permanent implantation.

A Modern Atlas for Implantable Devices of the Spine, Brain, and Nerve. https://doi.org/10.1016/B978-0-443-36528-7.00050-9

- Appropriate patient selection—including diagnostic nerve blocks and exclusion of contraindications—is critical to ensuring therapeutic success with PNS.
- Intraoperative testing, accurate electrode placement, and gentle nerve handling are essential for effective stimulation and minimizing complications.
- Long-term success depends on patient education, routine device follow-up, and early recognition of issues such as lead migration or infection.

Relevant anatomy

Innervation of the abdomen and trunk

The anterolateral abdominal wall receives innervation primarily from the anterior rami of the T7–L1 spinal nerves, which supply both the musculature and overlying skin.

External abdominal oblique: Innervated by the anterior rami of T7–T12 spinal nerves.

Internal abdominal oblique: Innervated by the anterior rami of T7–T12 spinal nerves.

Transversus abdominis: Innervated by the anterior rami of T7–L1 spinal nerves.

Quadratus lumborum: Innervated by the anterior rami of T12–L1 spinal nerves.

Rectus abdominis: Innervated by the anterior rami of T7–T12 spinal nerves.

Pyramidalis: Innervated by the anterior ramus of T12 spinal nerve via the subcostal or iliohypogastric nerves [4].

The thoracoabdominal nerves (T7–T11) provide segmental innervation to the abdominal wall, while the lateral cutaneous branches from T7–T9 supply sensation to the hypochondriac regions. The subcostal nerve (T12) contributes to the innervation of the lower external oblique and its overlying skin. Additionally, the iliohypogastric and ilioinguinal nerves (L1) innervate the inguinal and hypogastric regions, with the ilioinguinal nerve also supplying the mons pubis and anterior scrotal/labial areas [6].

Procedure—TAP and intercostal

Diagnoses

Chronic abdominal pain syndromes associated with neuropathic etiologies are frequently underdiagnosed and undertreated. Some of the most relevant trunk and abdominal conditions amenable to PNS include complex regional pain syndrome (CRPS) of the trunk (ICD-10: G90.59) [7], mononeuropathy of the abdominal wall (ICD-10: G58.9) [8], postherpetic neuralgia (ICD-10: B02.2, B02.22, B02.23, B02.29) [9], anterior cutaneous nerve entrapment syndrome (ICD-10: G58.8) [10], and intercostal neuralgia (ICD-10: G58.0) [11]. These conditions often manifest with persistent pain that is unresponsive to conventional treatments, making them prime candidates for neuromodulation strategies such as PNS.

Indications

Peripheral nerve stimulation is FDA-approved for chronic intractable neuropathic pain of the trunk and limbs [12]. This category, considered on-label usage, includes conditions such as complex regional pain syndromes and intercostal neuralgia. These diagnoses are characterized by neuropathic pain mechanisms, including aberrant nerve firing, peripheral sensitization, and central amplification of pain signals. Patients with these conditions typically exhibit positive responses to neuromodulation due to the direct influence of peripheral stimulation on pathologic nerve activity.

Off-label applications of PNS, while not officially approved, have gained traction in clinical practice due to emerging evidence supporting their effectiveness. These indications include non-neuropathic pain syndromes, such as chronic post-surgical pain that does not conform to traditional neuropathic mechanisms, as well as field stimulation, where PNS is applied without targeting a specific named nerve. For example, anterior cutaneous nerve entrapment syndrome is sometimes treated using PNS despite its classification as a localized nerve entrapment rather than a classic neuropathic pain disorder [10]. Similarly, post-surgical abdominal pain syndromes that lack definitive nerve pathology but respond to PNS suggest an emerging role for field stimulation techniques, where broad coverage of an affected area provides analgesia via indirect neural modulation. This concept is most applicable to Transversus Abdominis Plane targeting nerves that come from the thoracolumbar spinal nerves (T6 to L1) with consideration for peripheral stimulation altering pain transmission within the dorsal horn, leading to decreased visceral hyperalgesia and attenuation of centralized pain sensitization.

Patient selection considerations

Candidates for PNS treatment typically range in age from 18 and older with patients identified as suitable candidates if they have clear indications for its use and no contraindications. While peripheral nerve stimulation is commonly used in adults, its application in the pediatric population is less frequently reported and remains an area of active review. Pediatric patients require careful evaluation, taking into account their developmental stage, anatomy, and psychological readiness, as well as special consideration of the anatomical and physiological differences between children and adults [13].

There are several absolute and relative contraindications to peripheral nerve stimulation for the trunk and abdomen. Among the absolute contraindications are active infection, patients with uncontrolled bleeding disorders, allergy to any stimulator component, patient refusal, and pregnancy. Relative contraindications include cognitive impairment or psychiatric disorders that may prevent patients from optimally managing their devices, as well as anticoagulant use whose continuation increases risk of bleeding and discontinuation increases risk of thromboembolic or ischemic events [14].

Once a patient has been selected and undergone peripheral nerve stimulation implantation, ongoing considerations must be addressed to ensure long-term success and the avoidance of complications. Regular follow-up visits are necessary to monitor the device. Patients should be educated on the appropriate use and adjustment of their devices, as settings may require modified over time to maintain efficacy. A significant concern for the long-term success of the therapy is lead migration, where the leads may shift from their initial position. Patients should be educated on signs such as reduced pain relief or altered sensations that may indicate lead displacement. Infection prevention is another key aspect of maintenance, as infections can lead to complications including the need for device removal. Additionally, psychosocial factors play an essential role in the effectiveness of PNS therapy [15]. Adherence to follow-up care, device management, and adjustment protocols can be influenced by a patient's mental health, support system, and understanding of the long-term commitment required. Clinicians should ensure that patients are supported in their journey with PNS therapy and offer support when needed to improve outcomes and adherence to treatment protocols [16].

Training recommendations

The administration of peripheral nerve stimulation for pain management requires advanced training that encompasses a combination of anatomical knowledge and hands-on procedural experience. In the United States, the Accreditation Council for Graduate Medical Education (ACGME) offers fellowship and residency training programs that provide the foundation necessary for physicians to gain expertise in the use of interventional pain management techniques, including neuromodulation. Most commonly, the training to perform these advanced procedures occurs during an ACGME-accredited pain medicine fellowship, which generally follows a clinical residency in anesthesiology or physical. Fellowship training in pain medicine typically includes both didactic education and supervised clinical exposure to a broad array of pain interventions, including education regarding neuroanatomy, pain pathophysiology, and procedural techniques. For practitioners who are already in independent practice, structured educational didactics from professional societies or industry events are recommended to foster familiarity and understanding of the procedure. Organizations like the American Society of Regional Anesthesia and Pain Medicine (ASRA), the North American Neuromodulation Society (NANS), and the International Neuromodulation Society (INS), among several others at the state and national level, frequently offer structured didactic courses, hands-on workshops, and cadaver labs that provide practical training in PNS techniques that allow independent practitioners to gain experience under the guidance of experienced faculty.

Suggested case volume, proctoring, and peer review

Achieving competence in the use of peripheral nerve stimulation for the trunk and abdomen requires exposure to sufficient number of cases to ensure that the practitioner can perform the procedure confidently and address complications or difficulties. As with other advanced interventional pain techniques, volume is a necessary component of mastering the procedure. There are no specific cutoffs or numerical requirements broadly recommended, but practitioners should aim to develop the necessary skills including technical approach, appropriate patient selection, familiarity with device selection, lead placement, intraoperative adjustments, post-operative care, and potential complications. Given the diversity of nerve targets and nuance of neuromodulation, consideration for proctoring, or supervision of a less experienced clinician by an expert, can ensure patient safety and the proper execution of the technique with real-time feedback. It has been recommended that at least 5 to 10 applicable proctored cases be performed before completing complex interventional procedures independently to mitigate risks, optimize patient outcomes, and facilitate appropriate training. Peer review, or the review of individual cases by colleagues who have expertise in the field, provide an opportunity to discuss facets such as patient selection, technique, outcomes, and complications. The peer review process should be conducted regularly during the beginning of a practitioner's use of PNS to provide a structured mechanism for continuous feedback and ensure adherence to best practices. Peer reviews are particularly valuable when complications arise, as they allow the practitioner to gain insight into how similar cases are managed by peers. Through this collaborative process, practitioners can refine their technique and improve their overall outcomes.

Technique

Patient positioning

Proper patient positioning is essential for accurate lead placement and optimal stimulation coverage. For PNS procedures involving the trunk and abdomen, the patient position may vary widely depending on anatomical location of the target nerve. Prone positioning is commonly used for posterior approaches targeting the dorsal rami, intercostal nerves. Supine positioning is commonly used for iliohypogastric and ilioinguinal nerves as well as traditional TAP approaches. The lateral position may be preferred for certain abdominal wall pain cases where an oblique approach is needed or in unilateral patient presentations. Adequate padding is necessary to prevent pressure injuries [1] (Fig. 29.1).

Anesthesia considerations

Anesthesia planning is critical for procedural success, particularly when intraoperative testing is required. In most cases, PNS lead placement is performed under local anesthesia with or without anxiolysis/minimal sedation to allow for patient feedback during intraoperative testing to confirm the stimulation pattern. Sedation should be titrated carefully to avoid oversedation, which can diminish the patient's ability to provide accurate sensory feedback. In rare cases where deeper anesthesia is necessary, such as in pediatric patients, electrophysiologic mapping may be used as an alternative to patient-reported responses [1].

Operating room time estimates

The duration of PNS procedures varies depending on whether a trial or permanent system is being implanted. A trial procedure typically takes 15–30 min intraoperatively, as it involves percutaneous lead placement under fluoroscopic or ultrasound guidance without implantation of pulse generator. The permanent implantation requires additional surgical time, generally lasting up to 60 min, to accommodate lead tunneling and placement of the IPG. The location of the IPG site may also change intraoperative time, as certain locations may require patient repositioning or more extensive tunneling for appropriate access [1].

Relevant vendor support

Advancements in PNS technology have led to a variety of system configurations that clinicians may consider. Currently available options include temporary external systems, implantable systems with a wearable external component, and fully implantable systems. Trial procedures for the permanent PNS systems allow for evaluation of symptomatic control before proceeding to permanent implantation, providing valuable insight into patient response. Vendor support during procedures often proves essential for all system configurations with regards to device programming and troubleshooting, proper approach, lead placement, and function of the device [1].

Procedure and imaging

The procedural steps for PNS implantation involve appropriate planning to provide optimate results and avoid complications. All procedures should start sterile preparation of the surgical field and accepted sterile physician precautions. Imaging with ultrasound or fluoroscopic imaging is used to identify the target nerve or corresponding surround anatomical structures [1]. Fluoroscopy is more commonly used for abdominal nerve targets with osseous structures used as anatomical landmarks, such as intercostal nerves being targeted along the path of the ribs. Ultrasound is more commonly used for abdominal nerve targets with soft tissue used as anatomical landmarks, such as the fascial plane between the transversus abdominis and internal oblique muscles for a TAP approach [4].

A percutaneous introducer needle is inserted under visualization, followed by the passage of a trial or permanent lead along the nerve pathway. Once the lead is placed, intraoperative testing is often performed to confirm appropriate

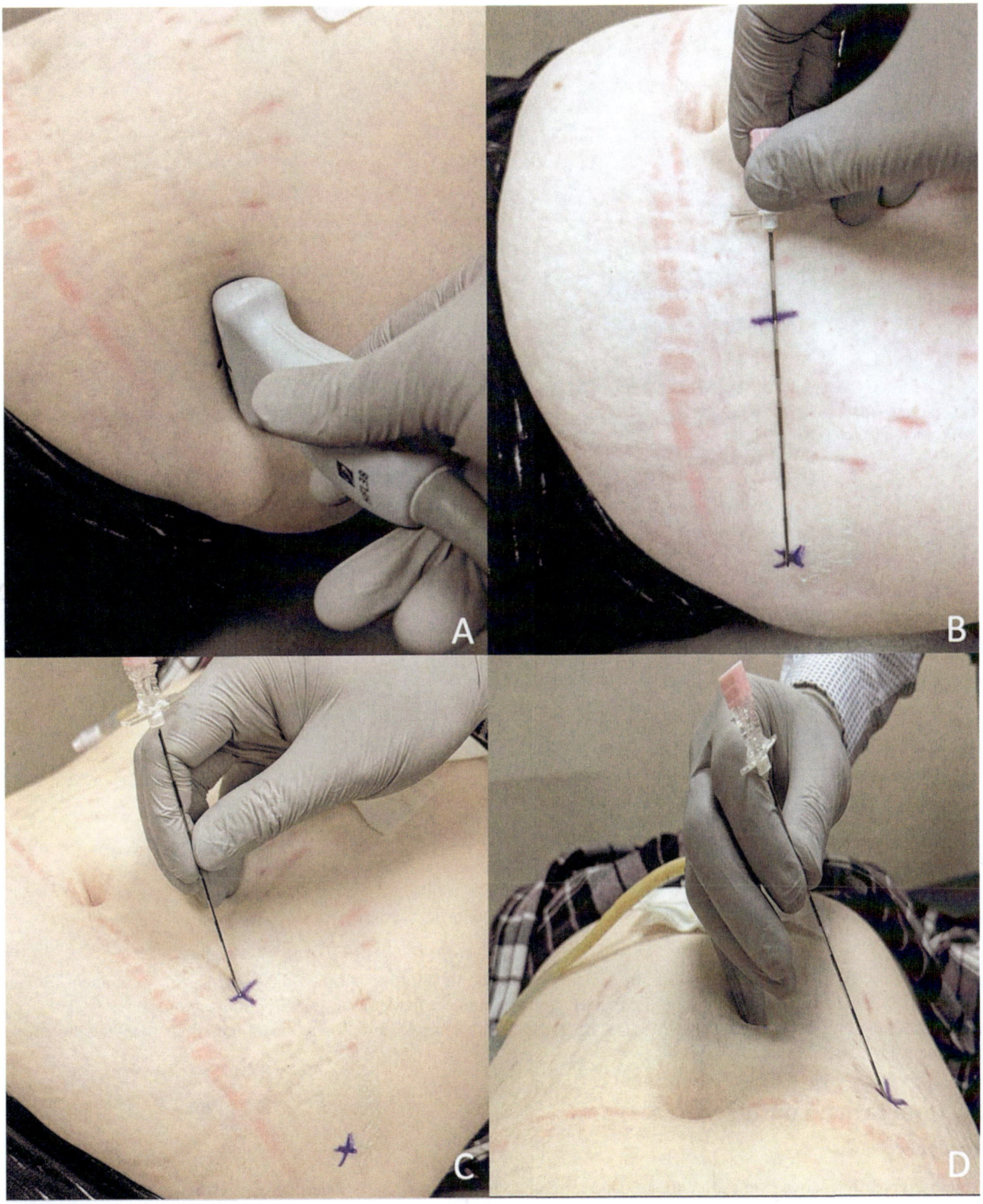

FIGURE 29.1 Example of a patient positioning and scanning with an ultrasound probe to evaluate underlying anatomy as described in figure (A). Patient marking to determine the starting access point and the final proposed lead trajectory (B). The needle is placed from a medial to lateral fashion from the demarked starting point (C) with the proposed angling to parallel the fascial plane once reached (D) [1].

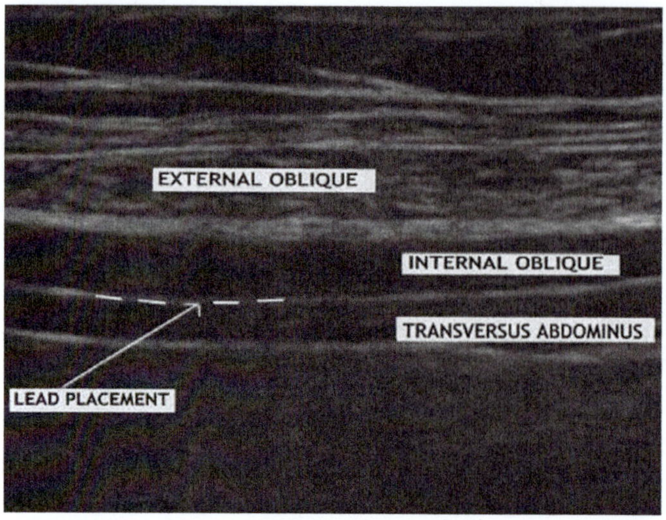

FIGURE 29.2 Cross-sectional ultrasound view of a percutaneous stimulator laying between the internal oblique and transversus abdonimus muscle in a TAP plane approach [17].

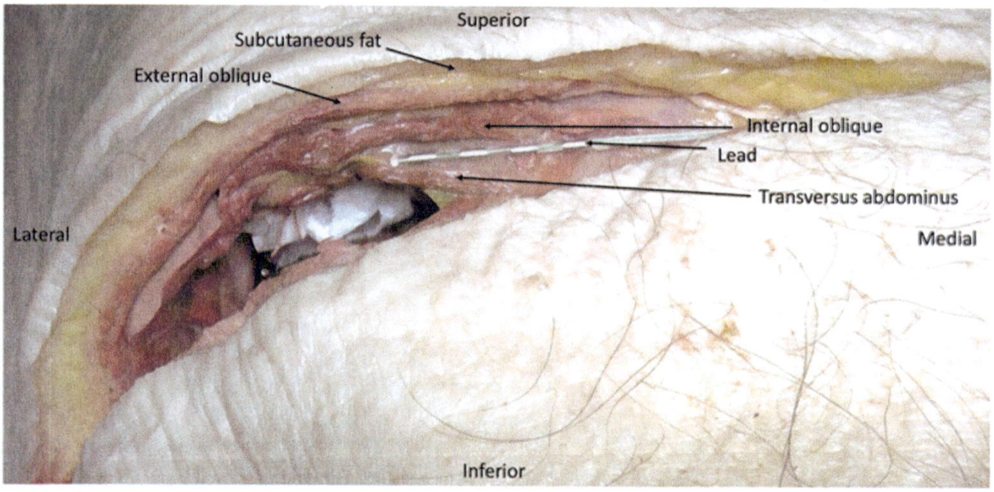

FIGURE 29.3 Cadaveric photo of a percutaneous PNS lead laying in the TAP plane with fascial and muscle layers labeled [1].

paresthesia coverage. If necessary, lead adjustments are made to improve stimulation patterns. For permanent implantation of applicable systems, lead tunneling is performed to connect the leads to the IPG in a subcutaneous pocket. Post-procedure imaging, such as live fluoroscopy or X-ray confirmatory views, may be obtained to demonstrate proper placement [1] (Figs. 29.2 and 29.3).

Post operative considerations

Recovery

Patients typically recover well after thoracoabdominal PNS implantation. For permanent systems, discharge is usually same-day or after short observation, depending on the patient's comorbidities and procedural complexity. Early recovery focuses on managing activity levels to minimize lead migration and support tissue integration. Gradual return to daily activities is encouraged over 1–2 weeks, with specific precautions to avoid twisting or strain on the abdominal wall [1]. Routine follow-up within the first 1–2 weeks post-procedure is critical to assess healing, detect infections early, and verify device function [18].

Efficacy estimates

Although long-term randomized data are limited, initial evidence supports the clinical benefit of thoracoabdominal PNS for chronic abdominal pain (CAP). In the study by Lam et al., PNS using a transversus abdominis plane (TAP) approach was shown to be a viable alternative in patients refractory to conventional therapies [1]. Additional case series, such as by Eden et al., have reported substantial reductions in pain intensity and opioid use with multicontact PNS systems placed in the TAP [19]. Similarly, Paicius et al. demonstrated improved quality of life and functional outcomes in chronic abdominal pain patients treated with peripheral nerve field stimulation [20]. These findings reinforce PNS as a promising therapy, especially in patients with focal or segmental neuropathic pain.

Bracing considerations

While not universally required, light abdominal bracing may be considered during the first 1–2 weeks post-implantation for patients at higher risk of lead migration—such as those with a thin abdominal wall, increased activity levels, or prior lead displacement. Soft bracing can help limit excessive motion and support lead stability during early healing. The decision to use bracing should be individualized based on anatomy, surgical technique, and provider preference [17].

Activity limitations

Postoperatively, patients should avoid bending, twisting, or heavy lifting for at least 2 weeks to reduce the risk of lead migration or dislodgement [17,21]. Walking and light activity are encouraged early on, but core or abdominal workouts, contact sports, and significant physical exertion should be delayed until healing is complete and stimulation settings are stable. Providers should emphasize the importance of these restrictions to preserve therapeutic efficacy and avoid unnecessary re-interventions [21].

Maintenance considerations

Ongoing maintenance of PNS therapy requires a structured follow-up regimen. Patients should be seen periodically to monitor stimulation efficacy, check for lead migration, manage hardware issues, and assess skin integrity [18]. Education is critical—patients must be trained on proper use of remote programming devices, battery recharging (if applicable), and signs of complications such as infection, stimulation loss, or unusual paresthesias [18,22].

Psychosocial factors significantly influence long-term outcomes. Psychological readiness, adherence to care protocols, and a strong support system are positively associated with therapeutic success [15]. For patients with evolving pain or inadequate coverage, periodic reprogramming of the device may be necessary. Encouraging realistic expectations and open communication improves satisfaction and reduces premature explantation or dissatisfaction with therapy [22].

Pearls and pitfalls

Preoperative considerations

Pearls

- **Proper Patient Selection:** Identify candidates with chronic neuropathic pain that is refractory to conservative treatments such as multiple medications and nerve blocks [23].
- **Diagnostic Nerve Blocks:** A successful local anesthetic block of the targeted peripheral nerve can predict responsiveness to PNS [24].
- **Imaging for Target Identification:** High-resolution ultrasound or fluoroscopy enhances precision in electrode placement and avoids vascular or organ injury [25].

Pitfalls

- **Misdiagnosis of Pain Source:** Incorrect identification of the target nerve may result in ineffective stimulation and suboptimal pain relief [26].
- **Contraindications:** Absolute contraindications to the placement of a peripheral nerve stimulator include allergy to any stimulator component or patient refusal. Relative contraindications include coagulopathy and local infection near the access site [14].

- **Infection Risk Underestimation:** Poor sterile technique during trial or implantation increases the risk of infection, potentially leading to device removal [27].
- **Unrealistic Patient Expectations:** Patients must understand that PNS may not eliminate pain entirely but rather modulate it for improved quality of life [28].

Intraoperative considerations

Pearls

- **Precise Electrode Placement:** Use ultrasound guidance or fluoroscopy to ensure accurate lead positioning along the targeted peripheral nerve [16].
- **Avoiding Nerve Trauma:** Gentle handling of nerve structures reduces the risk of neuritis, paresthesia, or worsening pain [16].
- **Intraoperative Testing:** Confirm appropriate nerve activation and patient response before finalizing implantation [29].

Pitfalls

- **Lead Migration:** Poor anchoring or excessive lead tension can lead to displacement and ineffective stimulation [21].
- **Inadvertent Organ or Vessel Injury:** Misplaced leads near visceral structures or blood vessels may cause unintended complications [30].
- **Inappropriate Stimulation Settings:** Suboptimal programming may lead to discomfort, paresthesia, or failure to relieve pain [31].

Postoperative considerations

Pearls

- **Gradual Activity Resumption:** Patients should follow post-op restrictions to minimize lead displacement while allowing tissue healing [17].
- **Regular Device Monitoring:** Scheduled follow-ups ensure optimal programming adjustments and device integrity [18].
- **Patient Education on Device Use:** Clear instructions on external controllers, battery management, and lifestyle modifications enhance long-term success [18].
- **Early Detection of Infection or Complications:** Close monitoring of the surgical site prevents delayed diagnosis of infections or device failure [18].

Pitfalls

- Clinically, common device-related complications include migration of the stimulator lead, lead fracture, and device malfunction. Other complications that are common with similar invasive procedures include infection, bleeding, surgical site pain, and nerve injury [26].

Scope-related considerations

Pearls

- For PNS in the transversus abdominis plane. The results indicate significant pain relief and reduced reliance on opioids. This study presents a case series of patients with chronic abdominal wall pain treated with multicontact PNS in the transversus abdominis plane. The results indicate significant pain relief and reduced reliance on opioids [19].
- This article discusses three cases where peripheral nerve field stimulation provided significant pain relief in patients with chronic abdominal pain, leading to decreased opioid use and improved quality of life [20].

Pitfalls

- This case report highlights how anatomical variations in nerve distribution can influence the effectiveness of PNS, emphasizing the need for individualized treatment planning [32].

- This case report illustrates that while PNFS can provide significant pain relief, it may offer only partial coverage in complex cases, underscoring the importance of comprehensive patient assessment [31].
- This study reviews cases where chronic abdominal pain was multifactorial, suggesting that PNS should be part of a multidisciplinary approach to address various pain sources [30].

References

[1] Lam CM, Keim SA, Sayed D, et al. Novel implantation technique for thoracoabdominal peripheral nerve stimulation via a transversus abdominal plane approach for treatment of chronic abdominal pain. J Pain Res 2024;17:981–7. https://doi.org/10.2147/JPR.S451955.

[2] Melzack R, Wall PD. Pain mechanisms: a new theory. Science 1965;150(3699):971–9. https://doi.org/10.1126/science.150.3699.971.

[3] Wie C, Ghanavatian S, Pew S, et al. Interventional treatment modalities for chronic abdominal and pelvic visceral pain. Curr Pain Headache Rep 2022;26(9):683–91. https://doi.org/10.1007/s11916-022-01072-4.

[4] Rozen WM, Tran TM, Ashton MW, et al. Refining the course of the thoracolumbar nerves: a new understanding of the innervation of the anterior abdominal wall. Clin Anat 2008;21(4):325–33. https://doi.org/10.1002/ca.20621.

[5] Nizamuddin SL, Koury KM, Lau ME, Watt LD, Gulur P. Use of targeted transversus abdominus plane blocks in pediatric patients with anterior cutaneous nerve entrapment syndrome. Pain Phys 2014;17(5):E623–7.

[6] Nayak R, Banik RK. Current innovations in peripheral nerve stimulation. Pain Res Treat 2018;2018:9091216. https://doi.org/10.1155/2018/9091216.

[7] Pilania C, Morvadiya D, Sheenam N, Agrawal H, Gonnade NM. Management of chronic truncal wall Type-I complex regional pain syndrome in a patient with uncontrolled diabetes mellitus: case report. Indian J Phys Med Rehab 2023;33(2):95–8. https://doi.org/10.4103/ijpmr_17_23.

[8] Fazekas D, Doroshenko M, Horn DB. Intercostal neuralgia. In: StatPearls. Treasure Island (FL): StatPearls Publishing; 2025.

[9] Chrona E, Kostopanagiotou G, Damigos D, Batistaki C. Anterior cutaneous nerve entrapment syndrome: management challenges. J Pain Res 2017;10:145–56. https://doi.org/10.2147/JPR.S99337.

[10] Gallacher DM, Gastelum P, Park SA. Intercostal neuralgia successfully managed with peripheral nerve stimulation. Cureus 2024;16(10):e71964. https://doi.org/10.7759/cureus.71964.

[11] Implantable peripheral nerve stimulation devices as a treatment for pain.*Blue cross blue shield of Tennessee medical policy manual*. Available from: https://www.bcbst.com/mpmanual/Implantable_Peripheral_Nerve_Stimulation_Devices_as_a_Treatment_for_Pain.htm.

[12] Sheen S, Riazuddin I, Javed S. Suprascapular nerve peripheral nerve stimulation for pediatric cancer pain: a case series. Pain Manag 2024;14(5–6):247–50. https://doi.org/10.1080/17581869.2024.2376523.

[13] Trent AR, Chopra P, Jain A. Peripheral nerve stimulator. In: StatPearls. Treasure Island (FL): StatPearls Publishing; 2025.

[14] Novak C, Anastakis DJ, Beaton D, Mackinnon SE, Katz J. Biomedical and psychosocial factors associated with disability after peripheral nerve injury. J Bone Joint Surg Am 2011;93(10):929–36. https://doi.org/10.2106/JBJS.J.00110.

[15] Kaye AD, Ridgell S, Alpaugh ES, et al. Peripheral nerve stimulation: a review of techniques and clinical efficacy. Pain Ther 2021;10(2):961–72. https://doi.org/10.1007/s40122-021-00298-1.

[16] Hoffmann CM, D'Souza RS, Hagedorn JM. An advanced practice provider guide to peripheral nerve stimulation. J Pain Res 2022;15:2283–91. https://doi.org/10.2147/JPR.S370037.

[17] Kasoff WS, Bina RW. Placement and anchoring of trigeminal neurostimulation electrodes: technical report. Stereotact Funct Neurosurg 2019;97(5–6):285–92. https://doi.org/10.1159/000503731.

[18] Eden C, Kang RS, Patel AA, Gulati A. Case series of multicontact peripheral nerve stimulation in the transversus abdominis plane for chronic abdominal wall pain. Neuromodulation 2024;27(5):862–5. https://doi.org/10.1016/j.neurom.2024.02.006.

[19] Paicius RM, Bernstein CA, Lempert-Cohen C. Peripheral nerve field stimulation in chronic abdominal pain. Pain Phys 2006;9(3):261–6.

[20] Kaye AD, Plaisance TR, Smith SA, et al. Peripheral nerve stimulation in postoperative analgesia: a narrative review. Curr Pain Headache Rep 2024;28(7):691–8. https://doi.org/10.1007/s11916-024-01257-z.

[21] Gupta M, Goodson R. Transverse abdominal plane neurostimulation for chronic abdominal pain: a novel technique. Pain Phys 2014;17(5):E619–22.

[22] Hoffmann CM, Butler CS, Pingree MJ, et al. Is response to a pre-implant diagnostic peripheral nerve block associated with efficacy after peripheral nerve stimulation implantation? A ten-year enterprise-wide analysis. Neuromodulation 2024;27(5):873–80. https://doi.org/10.1016/j.neurom.2023.10.003.

[23] Han D, Xu L, Xu J. Clinical application of ultrasound-guided electrode placement and detection of nerve action potential. J Neurol Surg Cent Eur Neurosurg 2024;85(6):594–601. https://doi.org/10.1055/a-1842-4343.

[24] Eldabe S, Buchser E, Duarte RV. Complications of spinal cord stimulation and peripheral nerve stimulation techniques: a review of the literature. Pain Med 2016;17:325–36. https://doi.org/10.1093/pm/pnv025.

[25] Ki YM, Park HJ, Yi SH, Sim WS, Lee JY. Latent infection after spinal cord stimulation device implantation for complex regional pain syndrome: a case report. Medicine (Baltim) 2023;102(19):e33750. https://doi.org/10.1097/MD.0000000000033750.

[26] Jayathilake NJ, Phan TT, Kim J, et al. Modulating neuroplasticity for chronic pain relief: noninvasive neuromodulation as a promising approach. Exp Mol Med 2025;57:501–14. https://doi.org/10.1038/s12276-025-01409-0.

[27] Zelenski NA, et al. Intraoperative neuromonitoring for peripheral nerve surgery. J Hand Surg Am 2023;48(4):396–401.

[28] Strand N, D'Souza RS, Hagedorn JM, et al. Evidence-based clinical guidelines from the American Society of Pain and Neuroscience for the use of implantable peripheral nerve stimulation in the treatment of chronic pain. J Pain Res 2022;15:2483–504. https://doi.org/10.2147/JPR.S362204.

[29] Helm S, Shirsat N, Calodney A, et al. Peripheral nerve stimulation for chronic pain: a systematic review of effectiveness and safety. Pain Ther 2021;10:985–1002. https://doi.org/10.1007/s40122-021-00306-4.

[30] Amorizzo E, De Sanctis F, Baldeschi GC, Ricci F, Varrassi G. Peripheral nerve stimulation (PNS): a valid and definitive therapeutical option for a case of anterior cutaneous nerve entrapment syndrome (ACNES). Agri 2024;36(2):126–8. https://doi.org/10.14744/agri.2023.07673.

[31] Zhou L, Chou H, Holder E. Abdominal wall Type-I complex regional pain syndrome treated effectively with peripheral nerve field stimulation: a case report. J Surg Case Rep 2017;2017(1):rjw222. https://doi.org/10.1093/jscr/rjw222.

[32] Gullapalli PA, Javed S. Multidisciplinary chronic pain management strategies in patients with Ehlers-Danlos syndromes. Pain Manag 2023;13(1):5–14. https://doi.org/10.2217/pmt-2022-005.

Chapter 30

Peripheral nerve stimulation of the lower extremity

Colin M. Buday[4], Daniyal Bashir[5], Donovan Wilcox[3], Justin McCarthy[3], Shashank Vodapally[6], Amit Gulati[7], Sayed E. Wahezi[2], Ugur Yener[2], Dustin Reynolds[1], Michael Cannone[8] and Timothy Deer[4, 9]

[1]*Ortho Alliance, Columbus, OH, United States;* [2]*Montefiore Multidisciplinary Pain Program, Bronx, NY, United States;* [3]*Mary Free Bed Rehabilitation Hospital, Grand Rapids, MI, United States;* [4]*The Spine and Nerve Centers of the Virginias and West Virginia University, Morgantown, WV, United States;* [5]*Trinity Health West Michigan, Muskegon, MI, United States;* [6]*Trinity Health Medical Group - Hauenstein Neurosciences, PM&R and Pain Management, Grand Rapids, MI, United States;* [7]*Chronic Pain, Memorial Sloan Kettering Cancer Center, New York, NY, United States;* [8]*Rocky Vista University, Montana College of Osteopathic Medicine, Billings, MT, United States;* [9]*Anesthesiology and Pain Medicine, WVU School of Medicine; American Society of Pain and Neuroscience, Charleston, WV, United States*

Historical perspective

Curiosity regarding the potential modulation of neurophysiology can be traced back to ancient Mesopotamia. The therapeutic use of "electroceuticals" to the nervous system for medicinal purposes was introduced during the first century CE, when Scribonius Largus, physician to Roman Emperor Claudius, observed the electric discharges from knifefish (genus *Gymnotiformes*) could relieve pain from podagra [1]. This serendipitous discovery laid the groundwork for electrotherapeutic approaches to headaches and other ailments. Modern understanding of peripheral nerve stimulation (PNS) emerged in the 20th century following the introduction of Melzack and Wall's 1965 groundbreaking paper on "gate control" theory of pain [2,3]. It proposed, stimulation of large-diameter, low threshold, non-nociceptive Aβ fibers results in the excitation of inhibitory dorsal horn interneurons that are involved in the processing and transmission of nociceptive information from the Aδ and C nerve fibers, thus inhibiting pain signal transmission from the spinal cord to higher centers in the central nervous system (CNS).

In simpler terms this theory posits a gating mechanism in the spinal cord that relies on the relative ratio of firing between small (nociceptive) and large (sensory) diameter neurons. Increased firing of the larger diameter neurons act to "close" the gate, thereby reducing transmission of painful stimuli to the brain. Conversely, firing of small diameter neurons would "open" the gate.

In 1990, renewed enthusiasm for PNS emerged after Weiner and Reed were the first to percutaneously place a lead in the vicinity of the greater occipital nerve to treat occipital neuralgia [4]. This has spearheaded growth in technology, percutaneous approach and improved understanding of indications. As of current multiple options are available for percutaneous placement of leads which are stimulated with an external or hybrid system with internal pulse generator powered by an external power source.

Nerve targets and patient considerations

Peripheral nerve stimulation is indicated for a variety of chronic pain conditions, particularly when the pain is localized to a specific dermatomal and/or cutaneous sensory distribution, and is refractory to conventional treatments. PNS may offer greater efficacy in cases with well-defined neuronal targets.

The lower extremities offer multiple nerve targets that are well-suited for percutaneous PNS lead implantation [5]. Ideal candidates for PNS typically experience chronic, severe pain that significantly impairs daily functioning and quality of life. These patients often fail to respond adequately to standard medical or interventional therapies. Additionally, patients with painful diabetic neuropathy (PDN) with relatively focal neuropathic pain may be good candidates for PNS [5–7].

A Modern Atlas for Implantable Devices of the Spine, Brain, and Nerve. https://doi.org/10.1016/B978-0-443-36528-7.00022-4

Common lower extremity nerve targets include, but are not limited to:

- Sciatic nerve
- Femoral nerve
- Lateral femoral cutaneous nerve
- Genicular nerves
- Saphenous nerve
- Common peroneal nerve
- Tibial nerve

Mechanisms of energy modulation

Although the precise mechanisms by which peripheral nerve stimulation (PNS) produces analgesia remain under investigation, current evidence supports a multifactorial model involving both peripheral and central nervous system modulation. Peripheral mechanisms include alterations in nociceptor excitability, local inflammatory responses, and afferent signal interference. Centrally, PNS has been shown to influence spinal cord dorsal horn activity, brainstem pain modulatory centers, and even cortical plasticity, contributing to both immediate and sustained pain relief.

A foundational understanding of electrophysiology is essential for the effective clinical application of PNS. Two key principles—rheobase and chronaxie—form the basis for how electrical currents interact with neural tissue [8–10] :

- **Rheobase** is defined as the minimum current intensity needed to elicit a response from a nerve fiber when using a long-duration stimulus. It reflects the excitability of a nerve and serves as a threshold measurement.
- **Chronaxie** is the shortest duration of an electrical pulse required to activate a nerve fiber using a current that is twice the rheobase. It is a time-dependent parameter that helps characterize the responsiveness of different types of nerve fibers.

These concepts are clinically important because different types of nerve fibers—categorized by size, degree of myelination, and function—have unique rheobase and chronaxie values. For example:

- **Aα fibers** (large, myelinated motor fibers) have a low rheobase and short chronaxie, making them easier to stimulate with brief pulses.
- **Aδ fibers** (small, myelinated nociceptive fibers) require slightly higher intensity and longer durations comparative to Aα fibers
- **C fibers** (unmyelinated, slow-conducting fibers associated with dull pain) have the highest thresholds, with a high rheobase and long chronaxie, making them more difficult to stimulate directly.

Nerve fiber type	Rheobase	Chronaxie	Required stimulation intensity
Aα fibers	Low	Short	Low intensity, brief pulses
Aδ fibers	Moderate	Moderate	Moderate intensity, longer pulses
C fibers	High	Long	High intensity, prolonged pulses

Understanding these relationships allows for targeted stimulation strategies, where device parameters such as pulse width, amplitude, and frequency can be fine-tuned to preferentially activate specific nerve populations while avoiding unwanted activation (e.g., motor contraction or discomfort). For example, shorter pulse durations and lower amplitudes may preferentially activate large-diameter sensory fibers without triggering nociceptive or motor fibers. This knowledge is essential for selecting appropriate stimulation settings during programming and follow-up of PNS devices, maximizing both efficacy and patient comfort.

Mechanisms of energy modulation: stimulation of motor versus sensory fibers

Two primary methods of peripheral nerve stimulation (PNS) have demonstrated efficacy in managing various pain conditions, each targeting different neural components and using distinct stimulation parameters [11].

Method one focuses on sensory nerves and utilizes high-frequency stimulation between ~100 Hz with *Nalu proprietary technology >500 Hz* to activate large-diameter afferent fibers [12]. This approach has shown efficacy in treating both neuropathic and non-neuropathic pain, including [13–15].

Method two targets motor (efferent) fibers using a lower frequency ~12 Hz with stimulation intensities sufficient to induce comfortable, visible muscle contractions in the area innervated by the nerve of interest. This technique has been associated with sustained relief in musculoskeletal pain conditions such as:

Both techniques deliver stimulation via open-coiled leads placed percutaneously near the target nerve. Adjusting the stimulation parameters allows for selective activation of different fiber types. Specifically:

- High-frequency stimulation ~100–500 Hz preferentially activates large-diameter sensory afferents—including tactile and muscle afferents—while avoiding motor efferents and nociceptive fibers.
- Low-frequency stimulation ~12 Hz, when applied at appropriate intensities, can activate mixed nerves by engaging muscle efferents along with large-diameter cutaneous and muscle afferents, while still avoiding nociceptive afferents [16].

Characteristic	A fibers	C fibers
Myelination	Myelinated	Unmyelinated
Conduction velocity	5–120 m/s	<2 m/s
Diameter	1–22 μm	0.2–1.5 μm
Function	Aβ: Touch & proprioception Aδ: Fast pain & temperature Aα: Motor functions	Slow pain, temperature, itch, affective tactile sensations
Response to stimuli	Rapid, sharp sensations (mechanical & thermal stimuli); Aδ detects fast-rising noxious heat & punctate mechanical stimuli	Slow, dull, diffuse pain (mechanical, thermal, and chemical stimuli); mediates warmth & pleasant touch

Image guidance: ultrasound versus fluoroscopy

Effective peripheral nerve stimulation (PNS) requires a detailed understanding of peripheral nerve pathways and their corresponding dermatomal and myotomal distributions. Optimal clinical outcomes are achieved by targeting a specified nerve, with precise lead placement in close proximity to the nerve structure. Image-guided techniques—primarily high-resolution ultrasound and fluoroscopy—are essential to ensure accurate lead localization. Intraoperative nerve mapping, using patient feedback during stimulation, can further refine lead positioning and enhance treatment efficacy [17,18].

Ultrasound has become the preferred technique for most PNS procedures due to its ability to provide real-time, high-resolution visualization of adjacent soft tissue structures, including vasculature, tendons, ligaments, and other nerves. Much of its use in PNS evolved from established techniques originally developed for perioperative pain management. Ultrasound enables direct visualization of the nerve and surrounding anatomy, improving accuracy and minimizing complications.

Fluoroscopy, while less commonly used for soft tissue imaging, can be advantageous in specific clinical scenarios—such as in patients with difficult anatomy, when bony structures obscure ultrasound visualization, or in those with challenging body habitus. Moreover, certain peripheral nerves that follow predictable paths over bony landmarks—such as the greater occipital, suprascapular, axillary, intercostal, cluneal, and genicular nerves—may be effectively targeted using fluoroscopic guidance alone.

Currently, no large-scale studies directly compare ultrasound-versus fluoroscopy-guided PNS placement. However, the American Society of Pain and Neuroscience (ASPN) recommends the use of ultrasound whenever feasible, as it facilitates precise lead placement and enhances procedural safety [17].

Intraoperative preparation and procedure

In the perioperative period care should be taken to ensure optimal patient positioning. This will serve to maximize visualization of the nerve of interest. Strict aseptic technique is essential during peripheral PNS. Preoperative preparation includes skin antisepsis with chlorhexidine-alcohol, limited hair removal, and prophylactic IV antibiotics (e.g., cefazolin) administered 30–60 min prior to the procedure. Full sterile barrier precautions—sterile gown, gloves, drapes, and mask—must be used, and the procedure should be performed in a controlled environment such as an operating or procedure room. Ultrasound probes require sterile covers and sterile gel. Leads and equipment must be handled only with sterile instruments and care taken to avoid contamination. After implantation, ensure hemostasis, close incisions with sterile technique, and apply sterile dressings. Postoperative care includes maintaining a clean, dry site and monitoring for signs of infection.

Percutaneous lead trial placement: A PNS lead can be implanted as a short-term trial or as a much longer-term treatment, and when warranted, the patient may be advanced to receive implantation of a permanent PNS system.

The skin will be anaesthetized with local anesthetic. This is followed by a 3–5 mm entry incision to allow for smooth insertion of a Tuohy needle into the subcutaneous space overlying the target nerve. A guidewire is then introduced into the Tuohy needle which will be advanced while simultaneously using ultrasound/fluoroscopy guidance to track trajectory. With the target nerve localized, withdraw the Tuohy needle, place the plastic cannula through guidewire and advance. Remove the guidewire then advance the electrode lead via the remaining cannula then connect lead to generator. The device will then be interrogated for amplitude, frequency, and pulse width. Typical trial periods consist of 2–14 days. During this time the patient should be instructed to refrain from strenuous activity and to avoid submerging in water.

Percutaneous Placement: After a trial is determined successful placement of a permanent stimulator is then considered. The lead(s) will be placed in a similar fashion to that described above. For permanent placement additional plastic anchors and non-absorbable suture are used to ensure stabilization of the leads in the fascia [18]. A strain relief loop is also created at the incision to prevent lead migration and kinking. Finally, a subcutaneous pocket is created for the implantable pulse generator. The pocket is then irrigated with antibiotic irrigation or powder then completed with layered closure.

Tibial nerve

In patients with PDN, the tibial nerve is a promising target for peripheral nerve stimulation (PNS). Due to the length-dependent nature of PDN, the plantar surface of the foot is frequently affected in cases of distal symmetric polyneuropathy. Symptoms typically begin in the toes and feet and gradually ascend in a proximal direction [19,20].

Anatomical course, landmarks, and ideal placement

Anatomically, the tibial nerve originates from the L4, L5, S1, and S2 (S3) nerve roots. These fibers arise from the medial portion of the sciatic nerve and travel distally through the posterior compartment of the lower extremity. In the distal third of the thigh, just above the popliteal fossa, the sciatic nerve bifurcates into the tibial and common peroneal nerves. The tibial nerve then continues posterior to the knee, descending toward the soleus muscle. At this level, it is referred to as the posterior tibial nerve, which then passes beneath the flexor retinaculum and divides into three terminal branches: medial plantar nerve (MPN), lateral plantar nerve (LPN) and medial calcaneal nerve (MCN).

Peripheral nerves in the lower extremity—particularly the tibial and common peroneal nerves are vulnerable to entrapment at anatomical sites such as the tarsal tunnel and fibular head, respectively. When planning PNS placement, it is essential to position leads proximal to any suspected site of entrapment, lesion, or injury. Electrodiagnostic studies can assist in identifying optimal lead placement and improving clinical outcomes.

1. **Femoral Branch of the Genitofemoral Nerve**
   - Anatomical course, landmarks, and ideal placement :
     - **i.** The genitofemoral nerve (GFN) originates from the ventral rami of L1 and L2 and arises from the upper lumbar plexus. After penetrating the Psoas muscle anteriorly at around the L3 and L4 level, the nerve courses medially over the psoas muscle at which point it separates into the genital and femoral branch just above the inguinal ligament [21].
     - **ii.** The femoral branch (more caudal and lateral branch) travels alongside and just lateral to the external iliac artery. It then travels superficially through the fascia lata of the thigh before entering the femoral sheath just behind the inguinal ligament. The femoral branch of the GFN can be found just lateral to the femoral artery where it arborizes to give off sensory branches that provide sensation over the anteromedial thigh [22]. Ideal placement when targeting the femoral branch is to place the electrode array next to the nerve in a caudal to cephalad direction overlying the fascia lata and lateral to the femoral artery. Testing stimulation can help confirm optimal placement as well [23].
     - **iii. Actual Ultrasound image**
       1. At the level of the inguinal crease in both men and women, the femoral branch can be found just superficial and lateral to the femoral artery.
     - **iv. Ultrasound illustration**
     - **v.** 1. https://link.springer.com/article/10.1007/s00330-023-10148-7

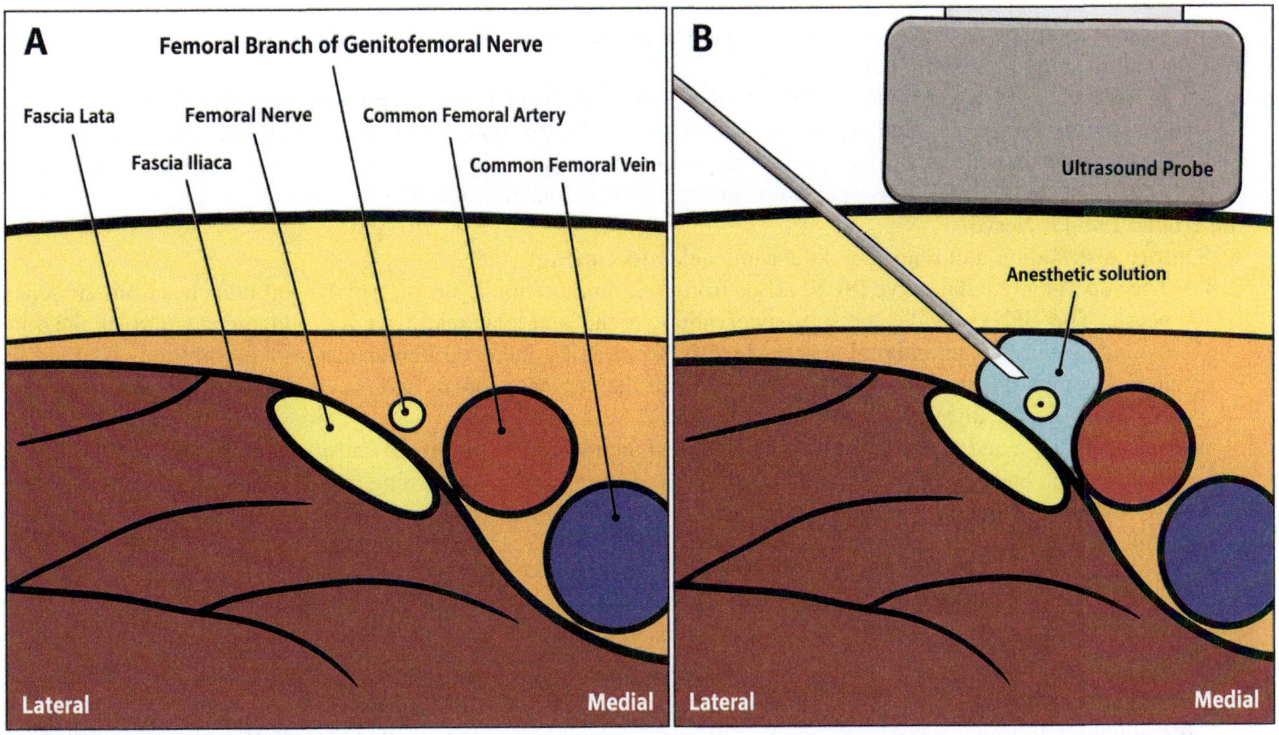

- Clinical indications: groin pain, post-hernia repair pain:
  - **i.** Patients with burning/stabbing pain in the inguinal region may have entrapment of the GFN, which can be confirmed from patient history, physical exam and utilization of diagnostic blocks proximal to the area of suspected entrapment. Sensory overlap with the bordering iliohypogastric nerve (IHN) and ilioinguinal nerves (IIN) can exist in this patient population as well, so careful consideration and ruling these other commonly entrapped nerves is a crucial step.
  - **ii.** Some common causes for entrapment of the GFN include psoas/retroperitoneal hematoma or abscess, post post abdominal surgery nerve injury (c-sections, appendectomy, inguinal hernia surgeries, groin surgeries, and pelvic surgeries) [23].

2. Lateral Femoral Cutaneous Nerve (LFCN)

- Anatomy and relevance to meralgia paresthetica:
  - **i.** The lateral femoral cutaneous nerve (LFCN) is a purely sensory nerve that arises from the lumbar plexus and provides sensation to the anterolateral aspect of the thigh. Specifically, it originates from the dorsal divisions of the L2 and L3 spinal nerve roots. It takes form within the psoas major muscle and emerges from its lateral border. The LFCN then travels obliquely downward and laterally across the iliacus muscle, deep to the iliac fascia. At this point, it most commonly runs medially to the anterior superior iliac spine (ASIS), and exits the pelvis typically under the inguinal ligament. It has been described to pass through the inguinal ligament as well as through the sartorius muscle. In the thigh, the LFCN divides into anterior and posterior branches:
    - **1.** Anterior Branch: The anterior branch travels down the anterolateral thigh, providing sensation to the skin over the anterior and lateral thigh. This branch courses more superficially and is more prone to compression.
    - **2.** Posterior Branch: The posterior branch supplies the skin over the greater trochanter and lateral thigh.
  - **ii.** Meralgia paresthetica is a condition caused by compression or entrapment of the LFCN, most often at the inguinal ligament. This compression leads to numbness and or pain in the anterolateral thigh. Common risk factors include tight clothing, obesity, pregnancy, prolonged standing, and trauma. Diagnosis is clinical, but can be confirmed with sensory nerve conduction studies. It is prudent to rule out other diagnoses, including

lumbar radiculopathy and space-occupying lesions. If conservative treatment fails, PNS is a reasonable treatment option, particularly for patients experiencing pain as opposed to dysesthesia.

- PNS techniques for lateral thigh pain
  - i. As with many PNS procedures, a trial phase is commonly used. In the trial, a temporary electrode is placed near the LFCN under ultrasound or fluoroscopic guidance. The most common target location is medial to the ASIS, just distal to the inguinal ligament. If the patient experiences significant relief, a permanent electrode lead is implanted, as well as a pulse generator in the lower abdomen or thigh.

3. Superficial Fibular Nerve
   - Sensory distribution and relevance to chronic ankle/foot pain [24,25].
     - i. The superficial fibular nerve (SFN) arises from the common fibular nerve, which itself branches from the sciatic nerve. The SFN provides sensory innervation to the anterolateral lower leg and the dorsum of the foot, excluding the first interdigital space which is supplied by the deep fibular nerve. The SFN travels along the lateral compartment of the leg, coursing between the peroneus longus and brevis muscles before emerging superficially in the distal third of the leg.
     - ii. Chronic ankle and foot pain related to SFN dysfunction can occur due to various etiologies including trauma, entrapment, and neuropathic conditions. Patients may present with burning pain, paresthesia, or hypersensitivity over the dorsum of the foot and lateral shin. Provocative maneuvers, such as Tinel's sign at the nerve's emergence site, may help localize the pathology.
   - Lead placement for neuromodulation [26,27].
     - i. Peripheral nerve stimulation (PNS) of the SFN is an emerging option for patients with refractory neuropathic pain in the lower leg and foot. Ultrasound guidance is used to target the nerve at its emergence from the deep fascia in the lower third of the leg, just proximal to the lateral malleolus. The lead should be placed parallel to the nerve in a proximal-to-distal direction, ensuring optimal contact and stimulation coverage. Pre-placement stimulation testing is recommended to verify sensory coverage in the affected area. Proper positioning is crucial to avoid stimulation of adjacent structures, such as the deep fibular nerve or sural nerve, which could lead to unwanted motor effects or incomplete pain relief.

Anatomical approach to PNS in the lower extremities

Proximal nerves (pelvis & upper thigh)

1. **Femoral Nerve & Saphenous Nerve (Knee Pain)**
   - Distinction between femoral proper versus saphenous branch
   - The femoral nerve originates from the lumbar plexus at levels L2 through L4 and provides both motor and cutaneous innervation to the anterior thigh and knee [28]. Just proximal to the adductor canal, the femoral nerve gives rise to the saphenous branch, which is purely sensory and comprises nerve fibers from L3 and L4. This branch provides sensation to the medial, anteromedial, and posteromedial lower leg, ankle, and foot [29]. Distally, the saphenous nerve divides into the infrapatellar branch—innervating the skin below the patella and anterior inferior knee capsule—and the sartorial branch, which extends to the medial leg and foot [30].
   - Pathologies treated: knee osteoarthritis, post-surgical pain
   - Knee osteoarthritis is one of the most common causes of knee pain, significantly impacting patients' quality of life as the condition progresses [31]. Peripheral nerve stimulation (PNS) is a viable treatment modality that involves placing one or multiple leads along the affected nerve, producing electrical impulses that can substantially reduce pain [31–33]. Studies have shown that post-surgical patients who undergo PNS experience pain relief exceeding 50% in many cases [34–37]. When stimulating a single nerve, dual electrodes can enhance impulse strength and efficacy to provide greater relief.
   - PNS approaches: proximal versus distal saphenous targeting
   - The optimal placement of electrodes and leads depends on the origin of the patient's pain. Proximal targeting within the adductor canal is preferred to minimize lead migration or erosion, while distal targeting may involve the infrapatellar saphenous (IFS) nerve or the sartorial saphenous (SS) nerve [38,39].
   - Include Genicular discussions (branch distributions/targets)
   - The genicular nerves play a significant role in knee pain modulation. The superior medial genicular nerve (SMGN) and inferior medial genicular nerve (IMGN) originate from the tibial nerve, whereas the superior lateral genicular nerve (SLGN) and inferior lateral genicular nerve (ILGN) arise from the common fibular nerve [40,41]. Each

branch provides sensory innervation to its respective knee joint region, with targeted stimulation of the SLGN especially showing effectiveness in alleviating post-operative knee pain [42–44].

Sciatic & its branches (thigh & popliteal region)

1. **Sciatic Nerve**
   - Anatomical course and segmentation
   - The sciatic nerve, the largest in the human body, arises from the ventral rami of L4 through S3. It descends through the gluteal region via the greater sciatic foramen, passing beneath the piriformis muscle before continuing down the posterior thigh and terminating in the popliteal fossa [45,46]. At this point, it bifurcates into its two terminal branches: the common fibular nerve (L4-S2) and the tibial nerve (L4-S3) [45].
   - Pathologies: post-surgical pain (hip, knee, amputation), sciatic neuralgia
   - The sciatic nerve provides extensive motor innervation to the posterior thigh and lower leg while also contributing to sensory innervation in these regions [47]. In a longitudinal study done by Gilmore, Ilfeld et al. investigating stimulation therapy for amputees with residual limb pain (RLP) or phantom limb pain (PLP), patients receiving nerve stimulation reported significantly greater pain relief compared to a placebo group [11]. In the same study, it was reported patients were also able to discontinue opioid and non-opioid pain medications. A study by Ilfeld, Ball et al. demonstrated that patients who underwent total knee arthroplasty (TKA) and received sciatic nerve stimulation experienced mild postoperative pain, with nearly 60% achieving opioid cessation within 1 week, and faster functional recovery [36].
   - Lead placement strategies
   - Ultrasound guidance, along with key anatomical landmarks such as the greater trochanter, ischial tuberosity, femur, and popliteal artery, is essential for accurate lead placement [48]. Stimulation testing should be performed by gradually increasing proximity to the nerve until desired paresthesia is achieved, with a primary concern being potential lead migration over time. There are many approaches to lead placement that can become dependent on various individual patient factors but there are two more common approaches. The first is a distal approach where the leads are positioned at the popliteal fossa, using the popliteal artery and veins as landmarks to track the tibial and common fibular nerves proximally. The second is a sub-gluteal approach working distally, which in lower extremity amputee patients is preferred [49].
2. **Common Fibular (Peroneal) Nerve & Fibular Neuralgia**
   - Anatomical course at the fibular head
   - The common fibular nerve, a branch of the sciatic nerve, contains fibers from L4 to S2. It courses posterolateral through the popliteal fossa, passing behind the long head of the biceps femoris before wrapping around the fibular neck, where it divides into its superficial and deep branches [45,50].
   - Common indications: post-knee surgery pain, entrapment neuropathy
     - The common fibular nerve entrapment at the fibular head is one of the most common neuropathies of the lower extremity and results in sensory deficits (e.g., numbness along the anterolateral leg and dorsum of the foot) and motor impairment such as foot drop.
   - PNS placement considerations
     - Some key concerns for PNS placement include avoiding lead placement across large joints to prevent migration and minimizing interference from the external stimulator in daily activities [23]. A compiled set of case studies by Huntoon and Burgher suggests that the optimal electrode positioning for the common peroneal nerve is 6–12 cm proximal to the popliteal crease, with the electrode anchored in the superficial fascia of the biceps femoris muscle [48]. There is also flexibility in placement to allow for distal stimulation of either branch of the common fibular nerve While stimulation near the fibular head can help modulate the pain, care must be taken to avoid excessive motor activation.

Distal nerves (leg, ankle & foot)

1. **Tibial Nerve (Thigh Level)**
   - Anatomical considerations for stimulation at the thigh
   - The tibial nerve, composed of fibers from the ventral rami of L4 through S3, branches from the sciatic nerve and courses through the popliteal fossa, between the heads of the gastrocnemius where it shifts medially, passing posterior to the medial malleolus [48,51]. Since the tibial nerve provides both motor and sensory innervation to the

posterior leg and foot, precise lead placement and stimulation parameters are crucial. Providing percutaneous stimulation within the thigh level

- Sciatic division: tibial versus peroneal fibers (posterior and lateralization at popliteal fossa)
  - The popliteal fossa serves as the primary landmark where the sciatic nerve bifurcates into the tibial and common fibular nerves. Techniques such as ultrasound assist in accurately localizing the bifurcation site as the sciatic nerve provides extensive variability on where this occurs and moving proximal to the popliteal crease by about 6–12 cm will generally provide the location [52–54]. The tibial nerve parallels the popliteal vessels deep and posterior to the knee, while the peroneal fibers run along the lateral edge of the fossa alongside the biceps femoris muscle [52].

Procedural techniques & considerations

1. **Imaging & Guidance Strategies**
   - Ultrasound versus fluoroscopy
   - For PNS systems to be effective requires that the electrodes are precisely placed and in proximity to the nerve(s) being stimulated. Ultrasound is a highly effective technique and provides direct visualization with its real time assessment of the leads and ability to precisely scan for soft tissue and neurovascular structures [49,55]. Fluoroscopy can be used as well or in conjunction with ultrasound but is the preferred modality when needing to visualize bony structures or nerves that have predictable courses over bony prominences.
   - Mapping nerve courses and lead placement strategies
     - There is a list of factors to consider for lead placement strategy including size of the lead, distance needed from target nerve to start approach, course of placement to be in parallel or cross the nerve, and more [49]. Prior to a procedure nerve mapping occurs to guide the physician for the procedure and gives insight to the nerve's path for the best initial incision and approach. Ultrasound or fluoroscopic guidance can be particularly helpful in mapping and with permanent marker, a physician can demarcate the path on the patient [56,57].

Future directions & emerging technologies

As we continue to revolutionize peripheral nerve stimulation, advanced technology should improve the outcomes for treating our pain patients with these systems. Our hope is similar to spinal cord stimulator systems. Peripheral nerve systems should read and react to painful stimuli being conducted along a peripheral nerve and deliver electrical fields to mitigate the pain response. As access to technology grows, modular and internalized systems may be preferential for treating a wider range of pain syndromes. Promising innovations for wireless stimulation options offer numerous benefits, such as the ability to customize lead lengths to fit specific nerve targets and eliminating the need for future surgeries related to battery replacement or implantation complications [58]. Certain populations of patients may benefit from specialized devices designed to target specific pain populations, such as diabetic neuropathy. This is already established in spinal cord stimulation [59,60]. The technology may advance to target damaged peripheral nerves with specialized electrical fields for healing and pain relief. The potential future options for advancement in this space are endless.

References

[1] Francis J, Dingley J. Electroanaesthesia–from torpedo fish to TENS. Anaesthesia 2015;70(1):93–103. https://doi.org/10.1111/anae.12887.

[2] Deer TR, Eldabe S, Falowski SM, Huntoon MA, Staats PS, Cassar IR, Crosby ND, Boggs JW. Peripherally induced reconditioning of the central nervous system: a proposed mechanistic theory for sustained relief of chronic pain with percutaneous peripheral nerve stimulation. J Pain Res 2021;14:721–36. https://doi.org/10.2147/JPR.S297091.

[3] Melzack R, Wall PD. Pain mechanisms: a new theory. Science 1965;150(3699):971–9. https://doi.org/10.1126/science.150.3699.971.

[4] Weiner RL, Reed KL. Peripheral neurostimulation for control of intractable occipital neuralgia. Neuromodulation 1999;2(3):217–21. https://doi.org/10.1046/j.1525-1403.1999.00217.x.

[5] Deer T, Pope J, Benyamin R, et al. Prospective, multicenter, randomized, double-blinded, partial crossover study to assess the safety and efficacy of the novel neuromodulation system in the treatment of patients with chronic pain of peripheral nerve origin. Neuromodulation 2016;19(1):91–100. https://doi.org/10.1111/ner.12381.

[6] Sayed D, Deer TR, Hagedorn JM, Sayed A, D'Souza RS, Lam CM, Khatri N, Hussaini Z, Pritzlaff SG, Abdullah NM, Tieppo Francio V, Falowski SM, Ibrahim YM, Malinowski MN, Budwany RR, Strand NH, Sochacki KM, Shah A, Dunn TM, Nasseri M, Lee DW, Kapural L, Bedder MD, Petersen EA, Amirdelfan K, Schatman ME, Grider JS. A systematic guideline by the ASPN workgroup on the evidence, education, and treatment algorithm for painful diabetic neuropathy: SWEET. J Pain Res 2024;17:1461–501. https://doi.org/10.2147/JPR.S451006.

[7] Chmiela MA, Hendrickson M, Hale J, et al. Direct peripheral nerve stimulation for the treatment of complex regional pain syndrome: a 30-year review. Neuromodulation 2021;24(6):971–82. https://doi.org/10.1111/ner.13295.

[8] Tsui BC. The effects of general anaesthesia on nerve-motor response characteristics (rheobase and chronaxie) to peripheral nerve stimulation. Anaesthesia 2014;69(4):374–9. https://doi.org/10.1111/anae.12540.

[9] Holsheimer J, Dijkstra EA, Demeulemeester H, Nuttin B. Chron-axie calculated from current-duration and voltage-duration data. J Neurosci Methods 2000;97:45–50.

[10] Goroszeniuk T, Pang D. Peripheral neuromodulation: a review. Curr Pain Headache Rep 2014;18:412. https://doi.org/10.1007/s11916-014-0412-9.

[11] Gilmore CA, Ilfeld BM, Rosenow JM, et al. Percutaneous 60-day peripheral nerve stimulation implant provides sustained relief of chronic pain following amputation: 12-month follow-up of a randomized, double-blind, placebo-controlled trial. Reg Anesth Pain Med 2020;45:44–51. https://doi.org/10.1136/rapm-2019-10093740.

[12] Hatheway J, Hersel A, Song J, et al. Clinical study of a micro-implantable pulse generator for the treatment of peripheral neuropathic pain: 3-month and 6-month results from the COMFORT-randomised controlled trial. Reg Anesth Pain Med 2024. https://doi.org/10.1136/rapm-2023-105264.

[13] Rauck RL, Kapural L, Cohen SP, et al. Peripheral nerve stimulation for the treatment of postamputation pain–a case report. Pain Pract 2012;12:649–55. https://doi.org/10.1111/j.1533-2500.2012.00552.x54.

[14] Rauck RL, Cohen SP, Gilmore CA, et al. Treatment of post-amputation pain with peripheral nerve stimulation. Neuromodulation 2013;17:188–97. https://doi.org/10.1111/ner.1210255.

[15] Gilmore CA, Ilfeld BM, Rosenow J, et al. Percutaneous peripheral nerve stimulation for the treatment of chronic neuropathic postamputation pain: a multicenter, randomized, placebo-controlled trial. Reg Anesth Pain Med 2019;44:637–45. https://doi.org/10.1136/rapm-2018-10010956.

[16] Rosenow JM, Gilmore C, Ilfeld BM, et al. One year follow-up of a randomized, double-blind, placebo-controlled trial of percutaneous peripheral nerve stimulation for chronic neuropathic pain following amputation. Neurosurgery 2019;66. https://doi.org/10.1093/neuros/nyz310_144.

[17] Strand N, D'Souza RS, Hagedorn JM, Pritzlaff S, Sayed D, Azeem N, Abd-Elsayed A, Escobar A, Huntoon MA, Lam CM, Deer TR. Evidence-based clinical guidelines from the American Society of Pain and Neuroscience for the use of implantable peripheral nerve stimulation in the treatment of chronic pain. J Pain Res 2022;15:2483–504. https://doi.org/10.2147/JPR.S362204.

[18] Gilmore CA, Kapural L, McGee MJ, et al. Percutaneous peripheral nerve stimulation for chronic low back pain: prospective case series with 1 year of sustained relief following short-term implant. Pain Pract 2020;20:310–20. https://doi.org/10.1111/papr.12856.

[19] Sayed, Dawood, others. In: Minimally invasive surgical procedures for pain. New York: Oxford Academic; 2024. https://doi.org/10.1093/med/9780197616734.001.0001.

[20] Dellon AL. Treatment of symptomatic diabetic neuropathy by surgical decompression of multiple peripheral nerves. Plast Reconstr Surg 1992;89(4):689–97.

[21] Garrett A, Black AC, Launico MV, et al. Anatomy, bony pelvis and lower limb: superficial peroneal nerve (superficial fibular nerve). In: StatPearls. Treasure Island (FL): StatPearls Publishing; 2025. https://www.ncbi.nlm.nih.gov/books/NBK534793/.

[22] Lezak B, Massel DH, Varacallo MA. Peroneal nerve injury. In: StatPearls. Treasure Island (FL): StatPearls Publishing; 2025. https://www.ncbi.nlm.nih.gov/books/NBK549859/.

[23] Hanyu-Deutmeyer A, Pritzlaff SG. Peripheral nerve stimulation for the 21st century: sural, superficial peroneal, and tibial nerves. Pain Med 2020;21:S64–7. https://doi.org/10.1093/pm/pnaa202.

[24] Muto CM, Pedana N, Scarpelli S, Galardo R, Guida G, Schiavone V. Inguinal neurectomy for nerve entrapment after open/laparoscopic hernia repair using retroperitoneal endoscopic approach. Surg Endosc 2005;19(7):974–6. https://doi.org/10.1007/s00464-004-2007-8.

[25] Rab M, Ebmer And J, Dellon AL. Anatomic variability of the ilioinguinal and genitofemoral nerve: implications for the treatment of groin pain. Plast Reconstr Surg 2001;108(6):1618–23. https://doi.org/10.1097/00006534-200111000-00029.

[26] Del Ray MLP. Chapter 18: genitofemoral nerve. In: Peripheral nerve stimulation: a comprehensive guide. Philadelphia , PA: Elsevier; 2023. p. 122–7.

[27] Rho RH, Lamer TJ, Fulmer JT. Treatment of genitofemoral neuralgia after laparoscopic inguinal herniorrhaphy with fluoroscopically guided tack injection. Pain Med 2001;2(3):230–3. https://doi.org/10.1046/j.1526-4637.2001.01032.x.

[28] Awad IT, Duggan EM. Posterior lumbar plexus block: anatomy, approaches, and techniques. Reg Anesth Pain Med 2005;30:143–9.

[29] Marsland D, Dray A, Little NJ, Solan MC. The saphenous nerve in foot and ankle surgery: its variable anatomy and relevance. Foot Ankle Surg 2013;19(2):76–9. https://doi.org/10.1016/j.fas.2012.10.007.

[30] Trescot AM, Brown MN, Karl HW. Infrapatellar saphenous neuralgia—diagnosis and treatment. Pain Phys 2013;16(3):E315–24.

[31] Kelly TD, Pazzol ML, Rahimi Darabad R. Peripheral nerve stimulation in chronic knee pain: a case series. Cureus 2023;15(12):e50127. https://doi.org/10.7759/cureus.50127.

[32] Amirianfar E, Rosales R, Logan A, Doshi TL, Reynolds J, Price C. Peripheral nerve stimulation for chronic knee pain following total knee arthroplasty: a systematic review. Pain Manag 2023;13(11):667–76. https://doi.org/10.2217/pmt-2023-0057.

[33] Lin CP, Chang KV, Wu WT, Özçakar L. Ultrasound-guided peripheral nerve stimulation for knee pain: a mini-review of the neuroanatomy and the evidence from clinical studies. Pain Med 2020;21(Suppl. 1):S56–63. https://doi.org/10.1093/pm/pnz318.

[34] Ilfeld BM, Grant SA, Gilmore CA, et al. Neurostimulation for postsurgical analgesia: a novel system enabling ultrasound-guided percutaneous peripheral nerve stimulation. Pain Pract 2017;17:892–901. https://doi.org/10.1111/papr.12539.

[35] Ilfeld BM, Said ET, Finneran JJ, et al. Ultrasound-guided percutaneous peripheral nerve stimulation: neuromodulation of the femoral nerve for postoperative analgesia following ambulatory anterior cruciate ligament reconstruction: a proof-of-concept study. Neuromodulation 2019;22:621–9. https://doi.org/10.1111/ner.12851.

[36] Ilfeld BM, Ball ST, Gabriel RA, et al. A feasibility study of percutaneous peripheral nerve stimulation for the treatment of postoperative pain following total knee arthroplasty. Neuromodulation 2019;22:653–60. https://doi.org/10.1111/ner.12790.

[37] Früh A, Sargut TA, Hussein A, et al. Peripheral nerve stimulation for the treatment of chronic knee pain. Sci Rep 2023;13(1):15543. https://doi.org/10.1038/s41598-023-42608-x.

[38] Rayegani SM, Eliaspour D, Bahrami MH, Baghbani M. Comparing distal and proximal techniques of saphenous nerve conduction study in healthy subjects. Electromyogr Clin Neurophysiol 2005;45(2):67–70.

[39] Li Q, Aierken A, Qin J, et al. Targeting the infrapatellar branch of the saphenous nerve for pain relief in patients with acute or chronic knee pain: a systematic review of randomized controlled trials and cohort studies. Orthop Surg 2025;17. https://doi.org/10.1111/os.14349.

[40] Cho JS, Grisham A, Wang A, et al. Focused anatomic review: ultrasound-guided peripheral nerve stimulation of the saphenous, lateral femoral cutaneous, and genicular nerves. Pain Med 2025;28:pnaf007. https://doi.org/10.1093/pm/pnaf007.

[41] Kim JH, Shustorovich A, Arel AT, et al. Genicular nerve anatomy and its implication for new procedural approaches for knee joint denervation: a cadaveric study. Pain Med 2022;23(1):144–51. https://doi.org/10.1093/pm/pnab238.

[42] Tran J, Peng PWH, Lam K, et al. Anatomical study of the innervation of the anterior knee joint capsule: implication for image-guided intervention. Reg Anesth Pain Med 2018;43(4):407–14. https://doi.org/10.1097/AAP.0000000000000778.

[43] Chitneni A, Berger AA, Orhurhu V, et al. Peripheral nerve stimulation of the saphenous and superior lateral genicular nerves for chronic pain after knee surgery. Orthop Rev 2021;13(2):24435. https://doi.org/10.52965/001c.24435.

[44] Busch C, Smith O, Weaver T, et al. Peripheral nerve stimulation for lower extremity pain. Biomedicines 2022;10(7):1666. https://doi.org/10.3390/biomedicines10071666.

[45] Standring S. Gray's anatomy: the anatomical basis of clinical practice. 39th ed. London: Churchill Livingstone; 2005. p. 1364–458.

[46] Cho JS, Grisham A, Wang A, et al. Focused anatomic review: ultrasound-guided peripheral nerve stimulation of the sciatic, posterior tibial, and obturator nerves. Pain Med 2025;26(3):166–9. https://doi.org/10.1093/pm/pnae12.

[47] Atoni AD, Oyinbo CA, Francis DAU, Tabowei UL. Anatomic variation of the sciatic nerve: a study on the prevalence, and bifurcation loci in relation to the piriformis and popliteal fossa. Acta Med Acad 2022;51(1):52–8. https://doi.org/10.5644/ama2006-124.370.

[48] Huntoon MA, Huntoon EA, Obray JB, Lamer TJ. Feasibility of ultrasound-guided percutaneous placement of peripheral nerve stimulation electrodes in a cadaver model: part one, lower extremity. Reg Anesth Pain Med 2008;33(6):551–7. https://doi.org/10.1016/j.rapm.2008.04.007.

[49] di Benedetto P, Casati A, Bertini L, Fanelli G, Chelly JE. Postoperative analgesia with continuous sciatic nerve block after foot surgery: a prospective, randomized comparison between the popliteal and subgluteal approaches. Anesth Analg 2002;94(4). https://doi.org/10.1097/00000539-200204000-00041.

[50] Kim GY, Ryou CH, Kim KH, Kim D, Rhyu IJ, Kim DH. Branching patterns and anatomical course of the common fibular nerve. Ann Rehabil Med 2019;43(6):700–6. https://doi.org/10.5535/arm.2019.43.6.700.

[51] Warehime JM, Gaskins JT, Gupta AS, et al. Proximity of percutaneous tibial nerve stimulation needle insertion to surrounding anatomic structures: a cadaveric study. Am J Obstet Gynecol 2023;229(4):430.e1–6. https://doi.org/10.1016/j.ajog.2023.06.048.

[52] Vloka JD, Hadzić A, April E, Thys DM. The division of the sciatic nerve in the popliteal fossa: anatomical implications for popliteal nerve blockade. Anesth Analg 2001;92(1):215–7. https://doi.org/10.1097/00000539-200101000-00041.

[53] Shrestha U, Lama MS, Shrestha SB. Ultrasonographic assessment of the distance of sciatic nerve bifurcation from the popliteal crease and its depth from skin in volunteers. Kathmandu Univ Med J 2020;18(70):176–80.

[54] McCartney CJ, Brauner I, Chan VW. Ultrasound guidance for a lateral approach to the sciatic nerve in the popliteal fossa. Anaesthesia 2004;59(10):1023–5. https://doi.org/10.1111/j.1365-2044.2004.03872.x.

[55] Skaribas I, Aló K. Ultrasound imaging and occipital nerve stimulation. Neuromodulation 2010;13(2):126–30. https://doi.org/10.1111/j.1525-1403.2009.00254.x.

[56] Singh H, Gargya A, Lin T, Gulati A. Sciatic, femoral, and lateral femoral cutaneous nerve ultrasound-guided percutaneous peripheral nerve stimulation. Pain Med 2020;21(Suppl. 1):S47–50. https://doi.org/10.1093/pm/pnaa040.

[57] Gofeld M, Bristow SJ, Chiu S, Kliot M. Preoperative ultrasound-guided mapping of peripheral nerves. J Neurosurg 2013;119(3):709–13. https://doi.org/10.3171/2013.5.JNS122243.

[58] Perryman LT. Wireless novel nanotechnology in neuromodulation of chronic pain: a safe minimally invasive, effective treatment option. Biomed J Sci Tech Res 2018;2:4.

[59] Pieber K, Herceg M, Paternostro-Sluga T. Electrotherapy for the treatment of painful diabetic peripheral neuropathy: a review. J Rehabil Med 2010;42(4):289–95. https://doi.org/10.2340/16501977-0554.

[60] Petersen EA, Stauss TG, Scowcroft JA, Brooks ES, White JL, Sills SM, Amirdelfan K, Guirguis MN, Xu J, Yu C, Nairizi A, Patterson DG, Tsoulfas KC, Creamer MJ, Galan V, Bundschu RH, Paul CA, Mehta ND, Choi H, Sayed D, Mekhail NA. Effect of high-frequency (10-kHz) spinal cord stimulation in patients with painful diabetic neuropathy: a randomized clinical trial. JAMA Neurol 2021;78(6):687–98. https://doi.org/10.1001/jamaneurol.2021.0538.

Chapter 31

60-Day peripheral nerve stimulation

Benjamin Gill[1], Harman Chopra[2], Ali Valimahomed[3], Vinny Francio[4] and Denise Lester[5]

[1]Nevada Advanced Pain Specialists, Reno, NV, United States; [2]Department of Physical Medicine & Rehabilitation, Johns Hopkins University, Baltimore, MD, United States; [3]Advanced Orthopedics and Sports Medicine Institute-Harvard Medical School, Freehold, NJ, United States; [4]Division of Pain Medicine, Department of Anesthesiology, Washington University School of Medicine in St. Louis, Barnes-Jewish Hospital, Center for Advanced Medicine, St. Louis, MO, United States; [5]Department of Physical Medicine & Rehabilitation, Richmond VA Medical Center, Virginia Commonwealth University, Richmond, VA, United States

Introduction

Temporary peripheral nerve stimulation (PNS) is a neuromodulatory technique used to manage chronic pain by electrically stimulating specific peripheral nerves. PNS was first tested in 1967 with direct nerve stimulation to alleviate neuropathic pain, though early results were limited by short-lived effects and surgical challenges [1–3]. Despite initial interest, PNS research stagnated for decades as spinal cord stimulation (SCS) gained prominence due to technological advancements and broader applications [4]. Interest in PNS resurged in 1999 when Weiner and Reed demonstrated its efficacy in occipital neuralgia. Recent advancements, including ultrasound-guided placement and improved lead designs, have enhanced PNS accessibility and safety, reducing complications like lead migration and infection [5–8])

The introduction of a 60-day temporary PNS system represents a significant procedural innovation, allowing for prolonged neuromodulation without permanent implantation. The currently available system uses a helically coiled monopolar lead that encourages fibrotic ingrowth, decreasing lead displacement and infection rates [9–11]. Emerging evidence suggests that even short-term stimulation can modulate peripheral and central sensitization, potentially leading to lasting pain relief by reversing maladaptive neuroplastic changes [12]. Studies have demonstrated its efficacy in treating various pain conditions, including chronic back, shoulder, knee, and postamputation pain, with many patients experiencing sustained benefits after lead removal [13–16]. These advancements have shifted the paradigm of PNS, offering a minimally invasive alternative to permanent implants while maintaining long-term therapeutic effects [17–19].

Key points

- Mechanism and Indications: 60-day PNS alleviates chronic pain by electrically modulating peripheral nerves and disrupting maladaptive pain signaling.
- Key Innovations: The introduction of ultrasound-guided PNS lead placement and a helically coiled monopolar lead reduced migration, infection risks, and the need for permanent implants. Leads are intended to be placed remotely (e.g., ~1 cm) from target nerves to increase selective activation of target fibers.
- Clinical Advancements: 60-day PNS treatment has shown long-term pain relief even after lead removal, supporting its use for chronic pain conditions like back, neck, shoulder, knee, and postamputation pain.
- Paradigm Shift: 60-day PNS offers a viable alternative to permanent implants for a variety of pathologies.

Procedure: General information

Indications: Patients aged 18 or older for symptomatic relief of chronic intractable pain, postsurgical pain, and post-traumatic acute pain. Indications for 60-day PNS have distinct advantages over SCS, as 60-day PNS may offer better utility for well-defined targets, such as nociceptive pain of the knee, shoulder, and zygapophyseal joints. Currently, the

A Modern Atlas for Implantable Devices of the Spine, Brain, and Nerve. https://doi.org/10.1016/B978-0-443-36528-7.00040-6

FIGURE 31.1 Example system used for 60-day PNS.

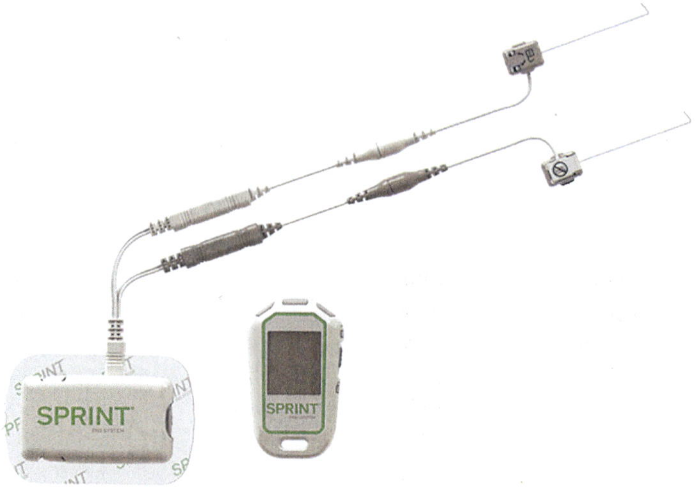

temporary PNS system has a 510K approval for placement for up to 60 days in painful conditions (Fig. 31.1, Table 31.1) [20].

Specific nerves are targeted depending on the painful condition (Table 31.2).

Although there are reports in literature of PNS being deployed for facial pain, per the 60-day PNS 510K submission, it is not currently cleared to be placed in the region innervated by the craniofacial nerves.

Patient Selection Considerations: Thorough preoperative evaluation optimizes success for PNS candidates. As the procedure calls for placing leads in proximity to nerves, there is a risk for direct nerve injury, nerve compression, bleeding, or infection. Optimization of bleeding disorders, chronic anticoagulation, diabetes mellitus, and infection risk is a priority [4]. PNS trial and implant is a low- to intermediate-risk procedure as classified by the American Society of Regional Anesthesiologists [21]. Diagnostic blocks have utility for localization of isolated nerves, but in some cases of complex chronic pain syndromes, identifying single culprits may be difficult, particularly in the distal extremities [22]. Patients with longstanding chronic pain syndromes, such as phantom limb pain or complex regional pain syndrome, may not exhibit a robust clinical response to nerve blocks but may still be a good candidate for PNS [23].

Contraindications: Standard contraindications include infection or active malignancy at the insertion site [24]. Additional concerns include: (1) lead placement (a) over the heart or across the thoracic volume; (b) in the front or side of the neck; (c) on the top of the head; (d) in patients with a deep brain stimulator system; (e) in patients with an active cardiac implant; (f) in patients with any implantable neurostimulator whose stimulus current pathway may overlap with that of the 60-day device; (2) patients who require MRIs during the treatment timeframe; (3) patients who have epilepsy if the leads are intended for the head or neck; (4) patients who have a tape or adhesive allergy [7].

Maintenance Considerations:

- Patient selection should consider compliance with proper use and care of the device, including hours of use and bandage care.
- Lead exit sites are to remain clean and dry.
- Showering is allowed, but avoidance of submerging during the 60-day implant period (swimming/bathing) is mandatory.

TABLE 31.1 General approved indications for 60-day PNS.

Chronic intractable pain	Postsurgical pain	Posttraumatic pain
G89.4: Chronic pain syndrome	**G89.18**: Other acute postprocedural pain	**G89.11**: Acute pain due to trauma
G89.29: Other chronic pain	**G89.28**: Other chronic postprocedural pain	**G89.21**: Chronic pain due to trauma

TABLE 31.2 Example 60-day PNS nerve targets and associated pain syndromes.

Upper extremity	
Suprascapular	Shoulder pain (e.g., rotator cuff injury, adhesive capsulitis, degenerative osteoarthritis), postsurgical shoulder pain, chronic shoulder impingement
Axillary	Shoulder pain (e.g., degenerative osteoarthritis, dislocation-related), posttraumatic shoulder neuropathy, quadrilateral space syndrome
Radial	Radial tunnel syndrome, postsurgical wrist/hand pain, forearm neuropathic pain
Median	Carpal tunnel syndrome, postcarpal tunnel release pain, forearm/wrist neuropathic pain
Ulnar	Cubital tunnel syndrome, ulnar neuropathy at elbow/wrist, posttraumatic forearm pain
Brachial plexus (at interscalene interval)	Brachial plexopathy (e.g., traumatic, postsurgical), complex regional pain syndrome (CRPS) Type I/II, hemiplegic shoulder pain (poststroke)
Lower extremity	
Sciatic	Sciatica, piriformis syndrome, postsurgical leg pain, lower extremity phantom limb pain
Femoral	Femoral neuropathy, anterior thigh pain (e.g., posthip surgery), meralgia paresthetica-like symptoms
Obturator	Obturator neuropathy, groin/thigh pain (e.g., posthernia repair), hip adductor pain
Lateral femoral cutaneous	Meralgia paresthetica, lateral thigh neuropathic pain
Saphenous	Medial knee/leg pain (e.g., postknee surgery), saphenous neuralgia
Posterior femoral cutaneous	Posterior thigh/buttock pain, posttraumatic neuropathy
Common peroneal	Peroneal neuropathy, footdrop-related pain, lateral leg pain
Tibial	Tarsal tunnel syndrome, posterior ankle/foot pain, postsurgical foot pain, phantom limb pain
Sural	Lateral ankle/foot pain, sural neuralgia, posttraumatic neuropathy
Superficial peroneal	Anterior/lateral leg pain, peroneal neuropathy, postankle surgery pain
Genicular nerves (knee)	Knee osteoarthritis pain, postknee replacement pain, chronic knee pain
Trunk/Pelvis	
Genitofemoral	Groin pain (e.g., postinguinal hernia repair), genitofemoral neuralgia
Ilioinguinal	Inguinal neuralgia, posthernia surgery pain, lower abdominal pain
Iliohypogastric	Lower abdominal/flank pain, postsurgical neuropathy (e.g., cesarean section)
Pudendal	Pudendal neuralgia, pelvic floor pain, posttraumatic perineal pain
Cluneal	Gluteal pain, cluneal nerve entrapment, chronic low back pain
Medial branch (cervical, thoracic, lumbar)	Chronic neck pain, thoracic pain, low back pain (facet joint-mediated), posttraumatic spine pain
Occipital nerves	Occipital neuralgia, migraine

- Patients are encouraged to increase and decrease the intensity of stimulation to maintain comfortable coverage of their area of pain.
- Robust vendor support is essential for optimizing neuromodulation therapy outcomes. Vendors should offer comprehensive training and online resources that provide step-by-step procedural guidance, best practices, and safety protocols.
- Vendors should collaborate with clinical researchers through postmarket surveillance, multicenter studies, and ongoing feedback to refine device design and surgical techniques.

Training Recommendations: To ensure proper technique and reduce complications, standardized training is recommended as part of an accredited pain fellowship program. This includes formal didactic training on treatment indications, contraindications, patient selection, initial diagnosis, procedural training, operative considerations, and follow-up. In clinical practice, exposure through conference-led cadaver courses or industry-sponsored surgical skills labs. There is no absolute number as the benchmark for proficiency, and depending on provider skills and learning abilities, 5–10 procedures may be required before providers feel comfortable with independent placement. There have been concerns regarding the lack of standardization amongst ACGME-accredited programs; a 1-year fellowship may not provide sufficient procedure volume and exposure [25]. For safe and effective clinical practice, competency and skill with ultrasound and fluoroscopic guidance are a requirement. Initial cases should ideally be performed under the supervision of an experienced proctor to reduce complications and enhance procedural efficiency.

General Procedural Technique Considerations [26,27]:

1) 60-day PNS placement is typically performed with local anesthesia, avoiding excessive blockade that could hinder intraoperative assessment. The patient must be sufficiently alert for real-time feedback on neural targeting.
2) Procedure may use fluoroscopic or ultrasound guidance with sterile technique and standard supplies.
3) Identify the target region for stimulation and perform sterile prep and drape.
4) Identify the target region with fluoroscopy or ultrasound as appropriate.
5) Inject numbing agents into the skin and avoid deep injections that would blunt stimulator testing nerve responses.
6) Assemble the stimulating probe and percutaneous sheath and insert them into the target region using image assistance.
7) At a location 1–2 cm away from the target, begin to test stimulation.
8) Consider multiple views of imaging to confirm needle tip location.
9) Optimal lead placement can be confirmed with (a) comfortable sensations overlapping the region of pain, (b) palpation of muscle contractions, (c) electromyographic responses, (d) visualization of needle movement, (e) patient-reported sensations, and (f) occasionally turning motor stimulation on and off can assist confirmation of subtle responses.
10) Remove the stimulating probe, maintaining the sleeve in place.
11) Insert the lead and lead introducer into the sleeve, rotating the interlocking hub.
12) Test the lead by connecting to the pulse generator and reconfirm stimulating activities.
13) Apply pressure over the exit site and withdraw the lead introducer and sleeve, leaving only the lead within the tissue.
14) Grasp the lead as it exits the skin and apply a single drop of adhesive at the exit site.
15) Return the lead connector to the lead, allowing a nickel ring-sized strain relief loop between exit site and connector.
16) Apply bandaging.

Examples of common 60-day PNS targets

Occipital nerves

Diagnoses: Occipital Neuralgia M54.2; Cervicogenic Headache G44.86; Migraine Headache G43.0.

Indications: Occipital nerve stimulation at C2 articular pillar to stimulate the third occipital nerve (TON), greater occipital nerve (GON), and/or C3 medial branch nerve.

Technique: Position, target, fluoroscopic approach, etc.

Position: Prone with neck in flexion; a seated or lateral decubitus position may be necessary, especially for patients with spasticity, dystonia, or joint contractures.

Target: 0.5–1 cm from the occipital nerve at the lateral border of C2 lamina. Locations near the inferior border of the inferior articular process of C2 (just superior to the C2/C3 joint line) may facilitate stimulation of GON and TON.

Fluoroscopy Approach: In the antero-posterior (AP) view, insert stimulating probes two levels caudad to the C2-3 facet joint at the C4-5 vertebral segment, well below the hairline to facilitate bandaging; the insertion site and angle should ensure at least 4 cm of lead length under the skin; the lateral view should show the needle juxtaposed to the C2 lamina.

Ultrasound Approach: Linear probe at the midline of the C2 vertebra with a shallow trajectory, inserting medially at the midline of the C2 vertebra, traveling laterally until medial to the C2-3 facet joint. Needle passes between the fascial planes of the trapezius, semispinalis, and inferior oblique muscles.

Confirmation: Comfortable sensations should cover the region of pain. The lead may be redirected locally around the C2 lamina (e.g., cephalad or caudad) to optimize stimulation.

Programming: (sensory) Continuous 60-day sensory stimulation at 100 Hz, 24 h per day, ensuring coverage of the pain region.

Pearls and Pitfalls:

1) Ensure at least 3–4 cm of lead under the skin.
2) Entering below the hairline and clipping hair may be required to facilitate bandaging.
3) The vertebral artery may have an aberrant anatomy from C2 to C6; therefore, imaging of the vertebral artery preprocedurally is recommended (Figs. 31.2–31.5).

Cervical medial branch nerves

Diagnoses: Cervical Facet Syndrome M53.82, Chronic Neck Pain M54.2, Cervical Post-Laminectomy Syndrome M96.1.

Indications: Chronic neck pain primarily attributed to cervical facet joint degeneration or chronic neck pain refractory to additional pain management options.

Technique: Position, target, approach, etc.

Position: Prone with neck in flexion; a seated or lateral decubitus position may be necessary, especially for patients with spasticity, dystonia, or joint contractures.

Target: 0.5–1 cm posterior to the medial branch, where it lies inferior to the facet joint.

Approach: In AP view, insert the introducer one to two vertebral levels caudal to the target level, advancing the needle until it is 1 cm from the lateral portion of the intended vertebra; the insertion site and angle should ensure at least 3–4 cm of lead length under the skin; the lateral view should show the needle posterior to the respective lamina.

Confirmation: Selective activation of cervical musculature, multifidus, and semispinalis may be confirmed with needle movement, patient report, and/or ultrasound evidence.

Programming: (motor) 12 Hz use for 6 h per day during the first week and then 12 h per day in subsequent weeks.

Pearls and Pitfalls:

1) Be aware of postsurgical changes in anatomy (i.e., postlaminectomy situations require awareness of needle depth given loss of bone and may require stimulation at surgically naive levels for intact neuromuscular structures.
2) Although the lateral pillars provide a bony backstop, the medial laminae have large intervertebral gaps that could cause unintended intraspinal entry of the introducer.
3) The vertebral artery may have an aberrant anatomy from C2 to C6; therefore, imaging of the vertebral artery preprocedurally is recommended (Figs. 31.6–31.9).

Brachial plexus interscalene stimulation

Diagnoses: Chronic Upper Extremity Pain M79.62, Complex Regional Pain Syndrome G90.5, Brachial Plexus Injury S14.3, Post-Operative Shoulder Pain G89.18.

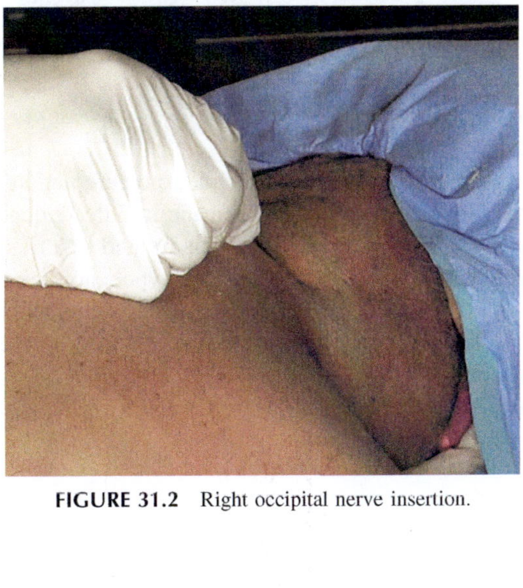

FIGURE 31.2 Right occipital nerve insertion.

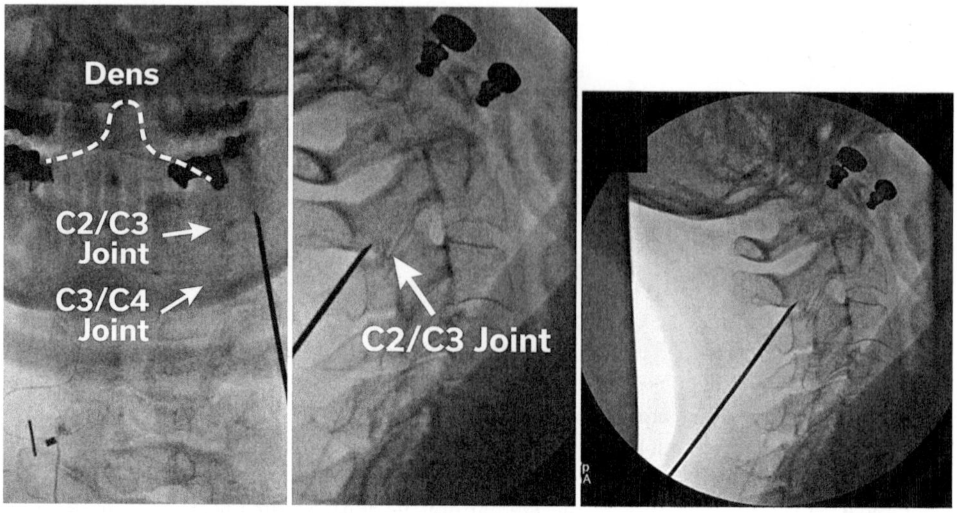

FIGURE 31.3 Occipital nerve placement with fluoroscopic guidance.

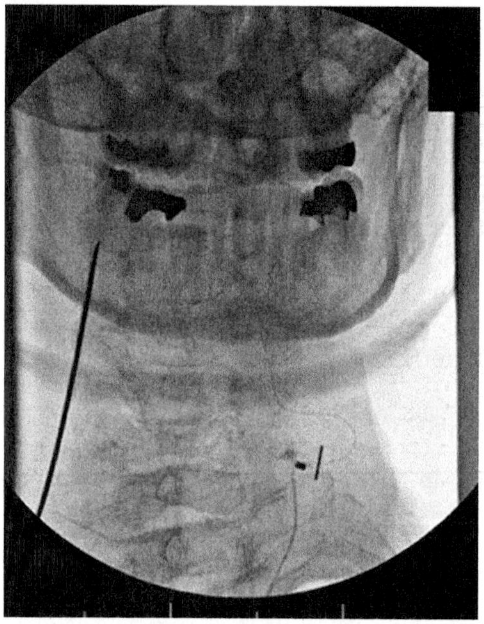

FIGURE 31.4 Fluoroscopic visualization of anatomical targets for left occipital nerve placement.

Indications: Chronic neuropathic upper extremity pain.

Technique: Position, target, etc.

Position: Patient positioned either supine or in a seated/reclined posture and slight contralateral neck flexion.

Target: 1 cm above, below, or next to the brachial plexus at the middle scalene muscle.

Approach: A linear probe is placed at the clavicle. The probe is rotated to a transverse view and advanced superiorly until the C5-7 brachial plexus roots are visualized in three stacked hypoechoic circles. Insertion follows a posterior-to-anterior path in plane with the ultrasound probe, targeting approximately 1 cm near the desired nerve, ensuring at least 4 cm of lead length under the skin. The lead is typically placed slightly anterior to the middle scalene muscle but posterior to the brachial plexus and anterior scalene.

Confirmation: Comfortable sensations reported in the shoulder and/or arm.

Programming: 100 Hz (sensory) use for 24 h per day.

Pearls and Pitfalls:

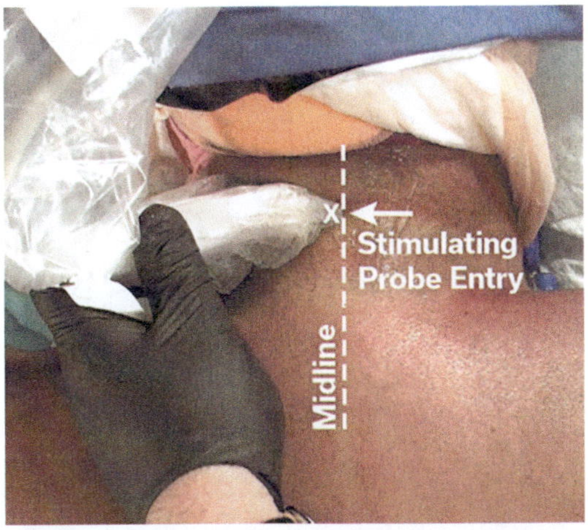

FIGURE 31.5 Left occipital nerve with inserted needle under ultrasound.

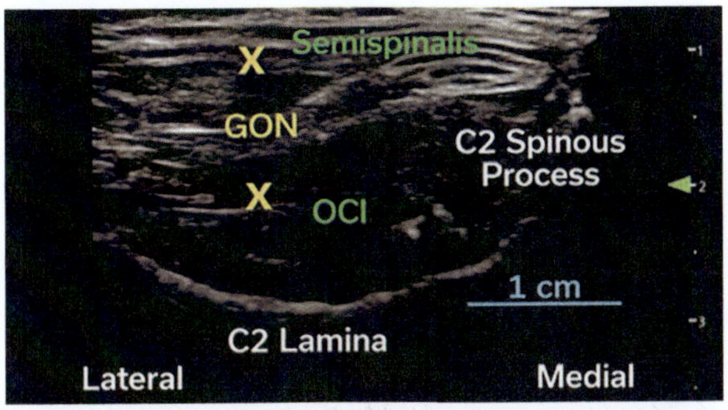

FIGURE 31.6 Cervical medial branch nerve insertion with ultrasound guidance.

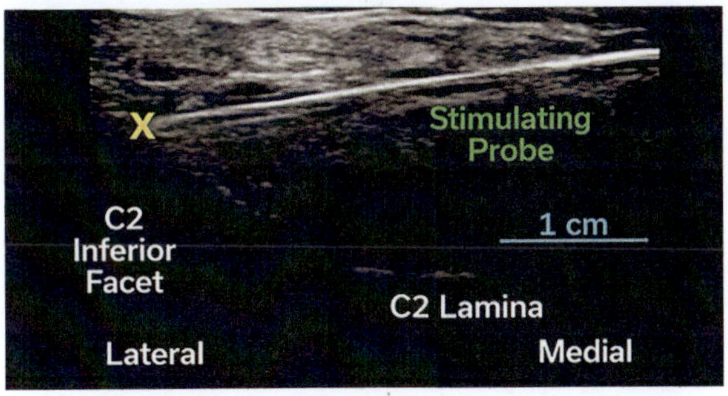

FIGURE 31.7 Cervical medial branch nerve insertion.

1) The electrode should be positioned with its long side facing the nerve, avoiding advancement beyond the brachial plexus to prevent contact with neurovascular structures, including the phrenic and vagus nerves.
2) Cervical nerve roots lie cephalad to the roots of the brachial plexus.
3) Do not advance anteriorly beyond the brachial plexus, which may place the needle tip in proximity to off-target neurovascular bundles (such as the phrenic and vagus nerves) (Figs. 31.10 and 31.11).

Brachial plexus infraclavicular stimulation

Diagnoses: Chronic Upper Extremity Pain M79.62, Complex Regional Pain Syndrome G90.5, Brachial Plexus Injury S14.3, Post-Operative Shoulder Pain G89.18.

Indications: Chronic neuropathic upper extremity pain.

Technique: Position, target, approach, etc.

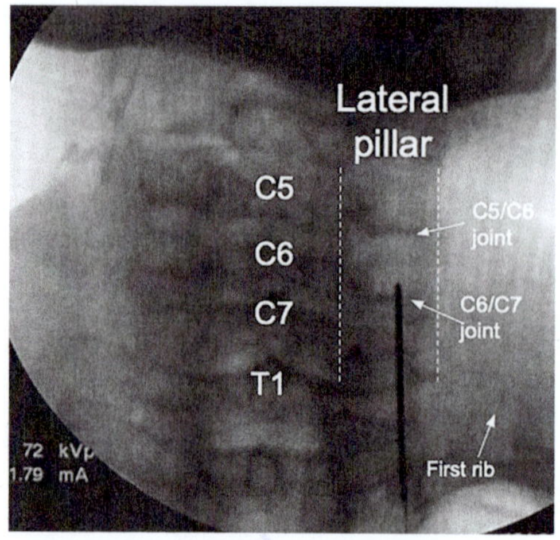

FIGURE 31.8 Right cervical medial branch insertion under fluoroscopic guidance.

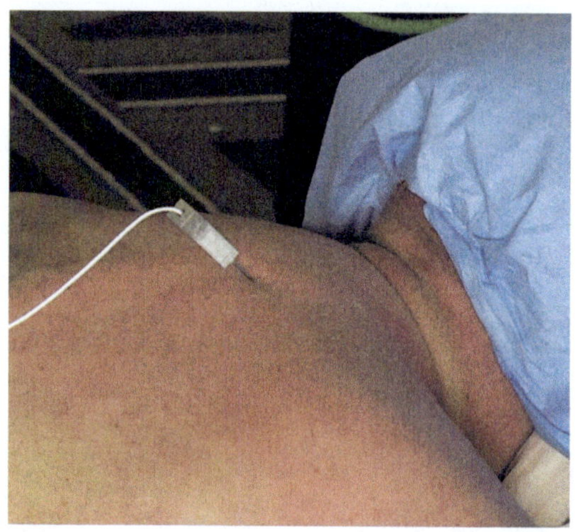

FIGURE 31.9 Right cervical medial branch insertion.

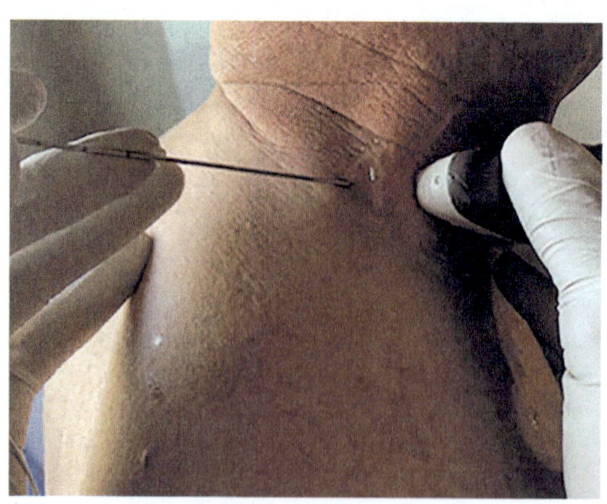

FIGURE 31.10 Right brachial plexus interscalene insertion with ultrasound guidance.

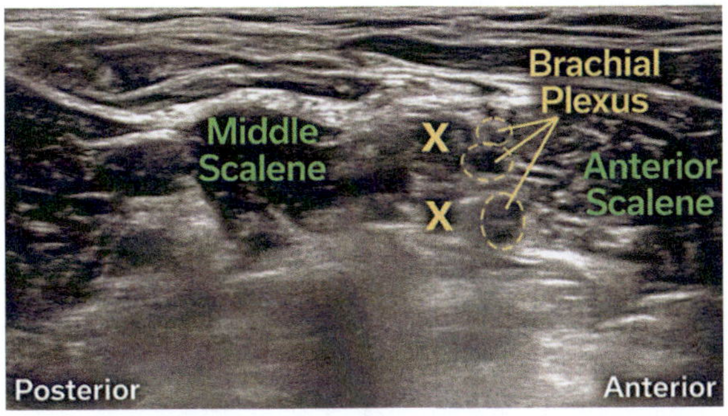

FIGURE 31.11 Anatomical landmarks for PNS insertion targeting the brachial plexus with the infraclavicular approach.

Position: Supine or in a seated/reclined posture with slight contralateral neck flexion.

Target: Superficial, or among the cords of the brachial plexus. Lead may be positioned in or under the pectoralis muscle.

Approach: A linear probe is placed beneath the clavicle, identifying the humeral head, and then advanced medially to identify the brachial plexus and neurovascular bundles. Insertion follows a medial-to-lateral path in plane with the ultrasound probe, targeting approximately 1 cm near the desired nerve, ensuring at least 4 cm of lead length under the skin.

Confirmation: Comfortable sensations reported in the shoulder and/or arm.

Programming: 100 Hz (sensory) use for 24 h per day.

Pearls and Pitfalls:

1) The trajectory should remain shallow, as the lung pleura is deep to the brachial plexus.
2) The use of color Doppler may help differentiate between nerve fascicles and branches of the axillary artery.
3) Other approaches to the brachial plexus at the interscalene or supraclavicular locations may be alternatives (Figs. 31.12 and 31.13).

Suprascapular nerve stimulation

Diagnoses: Chronic Upper Extremity Pain M79.62, Complex Regional Pain Syndrome G90.5, Brachial Plexus Injury S14.3, Post-Operative Shoulder Pain G89.18, Primary Osteoarthritis Shoulder M19.011.

Indications: Chronic upper extremity pain.

Technique: Position, target, approach, etc.

Position: Prone (fluoroscopy-guided) or seated (ultrasound-guided).

Target: 0.5–1 cm from the suprascapular nerve as it enters the groove at the suprascapular notch.

Ultrasound Approach: A linear probe is placed over the spine of the scapula at the outer 1/3. Scan cephalad parallel to the scapular spine to identify the suprascapular notch, the nerve, and vessels. The needle is inserted in-plane with a

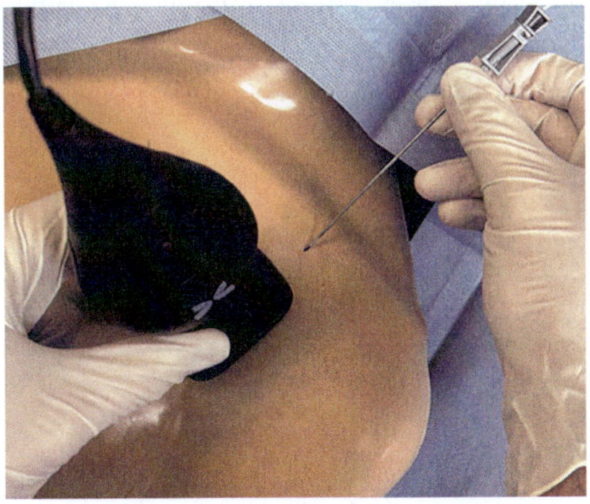

FIGURE 31.12 Insertion for infraclavicular brachial plexus stimulation.

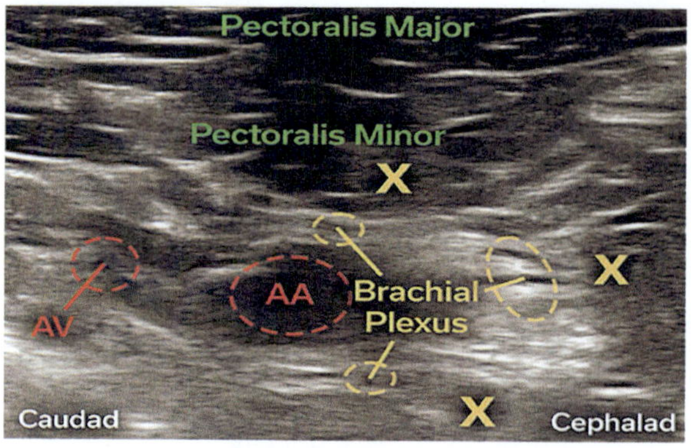

FIGURE 31.13 Anatomical landmarks for PNS insertion targeting the brachial plexus.

medial-to-lateral trajectory. The electrode is ideally beneath the superior transverse ligament in the suprascapular notch, just lateral to the neurovascular bundle, targeting approximately 1 cm near the desired nerve, ensuring at least 4 cm of lead length under the skin.

Fluoroscopy Approach: Using the AP view, identify the spinoglenoid fossa. Insert the needle over the medial scapula with a trajectory toward the fossa, ensuring placement using the scapula as a bony stop to reduce pleural injury risk.

Confirmation: Comfortable sensations reported in the shoulder and/or arm.

Programming: 100 Hz (sensory) use for 24 h per day.

Pearls and Pitfalls.

1) The trajectory should remain shallow as the lung pleura is deep to the suprascapular notch.
2) The use of color Doppler may help identify and avoid the suprascapular artery.
3) Maintaining the needle over the scapula reduces the risk of pneumothorax (Figs. 31.14–31.16).

Axillary nerve stimulation

Diagnoses: Chronic Upper Extremity Pain M79.62, Complex Regional Pain Syndrome G90.5, Brachial Plexus Injury S14.3, Post-Operative Shoulder Pain G89.18, Primary Osteoarthritis Shoulder M19.011.

Indications: Chronic upper extremity pain; adding a bimodal component (motor and sensory) to sensory-only stimulation.

Technique: Position, target, approach, etc.

Position: Seated position (ultrasound guided).

Target: Middle of the deltoid muscle at the inferior border of the humeral head swelling.

Ultrasound Approach: At 3 finger widths or 6 cm below the acromion, a neurovascular bundle can be located via ultrasound as the inferior location of the deltoid muscle. A linear probe is placed vertically over the humerus where the head meets the humeral shaft. After scanning for vessels to avoid, the linear probe is rotated 90 degrees, and the needle is inserted in-plane to reach the target, ensuring that at least 4 cm of trajectory is under the skin.

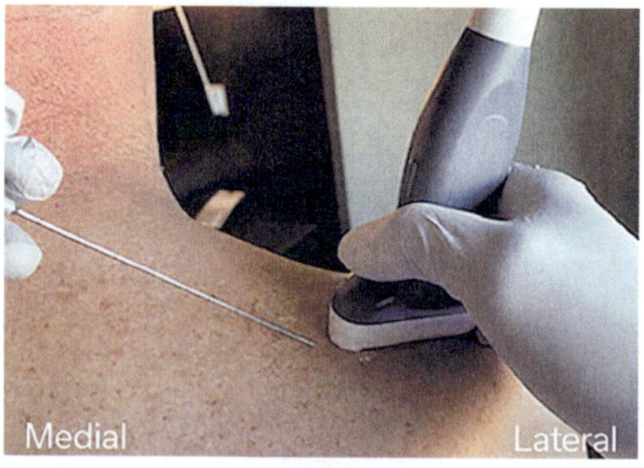

FIGURE 31.14 Right suprascapular nerve insertion under ultrasound.

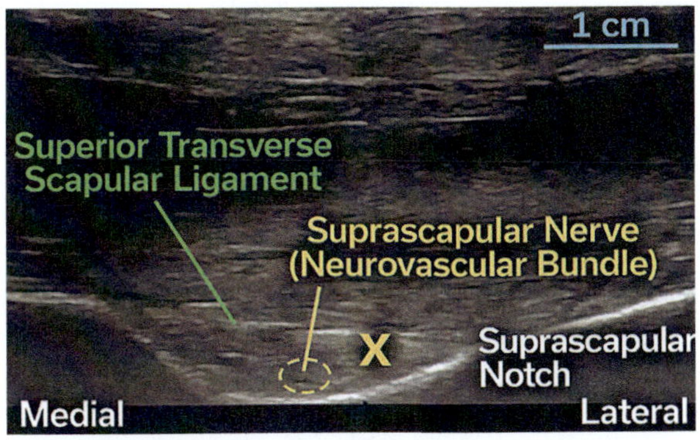

FIGURE 31.15 Anatomical landmarks for PNS insertion targeting suprascapular nerve.

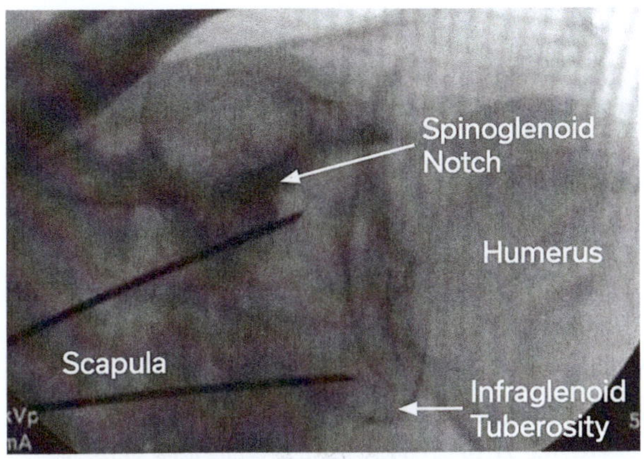

FIGURE 31.16 Right suprascapular and axillary nerve targets under fluoroscopy.

Confirmation: Comfortable sensations reported in the shoulder and/or arm.
Programming: 12 Hz (motor) use for 6 h per day, first week, then 12 h a day for 7 weeks.
Pearls and Pitfalls:

1) The use of color Doppler may help identify and avoid the circumflex artery.
2) Depending upon body habitus, a perpendicular approach may need adjustment to an angle that ensures lead length secured beneath the skin.
3) This nerve has been used for bimodal stimulation of the shoulder.
4) The axillary nerve may also be targeted with sensory or motor stimulation under ultrasound guidance at the quadrangular space (Figs. 31.16–31.18).

Lumbar medial branch of the dorsal ramus stimulation

Diagnoses: Chronic Axial Low Back Pain M54.5, Lumbar Spondylosis Without Myelopathy or Radiculopathy M47.816.
Indications: Chronic low back pain.
Technique: Position, target, approach, etc.
Position: Prone position.

Target: The patient's pain is mapped by identifying each lumbar segment with imaging and palpating that segment while asking the patient if the back pain has been severe in that area in the prior 2 weeks. Then, the vertebral segment most painful in the middle of the affected segments is chosen as the medial branch target for the implant. 1 cm distal to the medial branch, where it lies inferior and medial to the facet joint. The needle is advanced until the electrode is 1 cm from the lamina, approx. 4–6 cm deep. A preferred approach is introducing the needle at a 45-degree angle from a more cephalad vertebra, ending at the target vertebrae. A 45-degree entry angle is suggested and can be achieved by determining the depth of muscle overlying the target using ultrasound and starting the skin entry that number of centimeters away on the skin above the target.

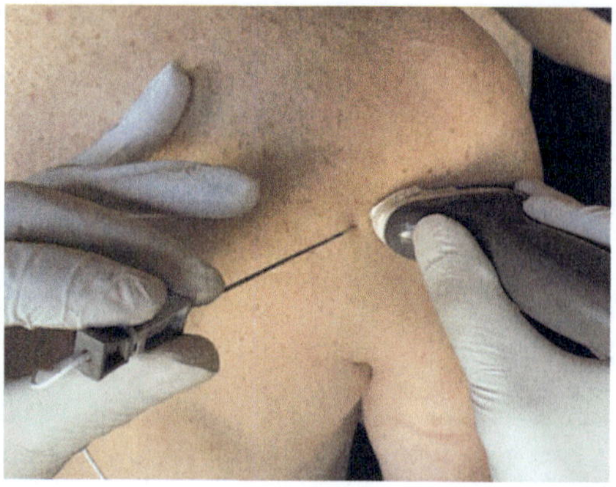

FIGURE 31.17 Right shoulder insertion with ultrasound guidance.

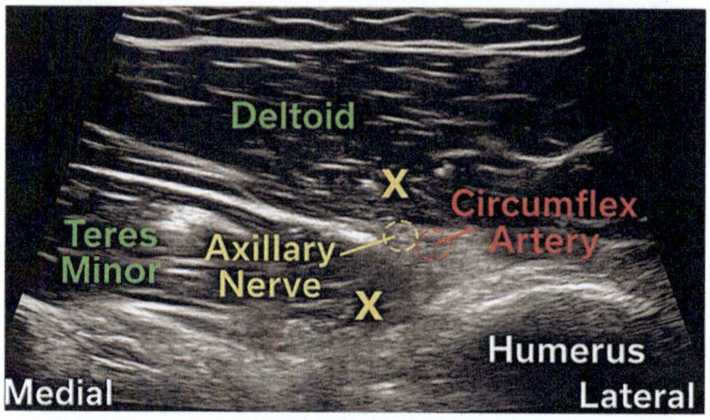

FIGURE 31.18 Axillary nerve targeting using ultrasound.

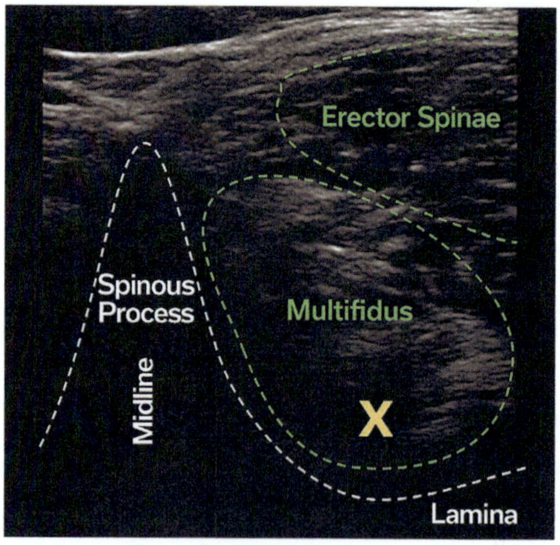

FIGURE 31.19 Lumbar medial branch nerve targeting under ultrasound.

Confirmation: Comfortable sensations reported in the low back, as well as ultrasound confirmation of multifidi contractions if used.

Programming: 12 Hz (motor) use for 6 h per day, first week, then 12 h a day for 7 weeks.

Pearls and Pitfalls:

1) A lateral view of the needle trajectory is helpful if using airplane approach to ensure depth, especially if there's a prior laminectomy.

2) Occasionally, additional multifidi vertebral levels will be scanned for contractions if not seen at the level of treatment.
3) Additionally, medial branches in the thoracic and cervical levels are also options for axial spine pain outside the lumbar region (Figs. 31.19 and 31.20).

Superior cluneal nerve stimulation

Diagnoses: Chronic Axial Low Back Pain M54.5, Superior Cluneal Neuralgia M79.2.

Indications: Chronic low back pain associated with superior cluneal nerve distribution.

Technique: Position, target, approach, etc.

Position: Prone.

Target: 0.5–1 cm from the superior cluneal nerves at the superior border of the ilium. The transverse approach to the iliac crest may allow several superior cluneal nerve branches. The target lies between the medial and middle thirds of the iliac crest and then travels medially or laterally along the ilium to optimize electrode location. An alternative approach would walk from the medial crest to the lateral ending at the target.

Confirmation: Comfortable sensations reported in the low back over the superior cluneal location.

Programming: 100 Hz (sensory) use for 24 h per day.

Pearls and Pitfalls:

1) Avoid walking off the iliac crest, which could lead to entering the peritoneal cavity.

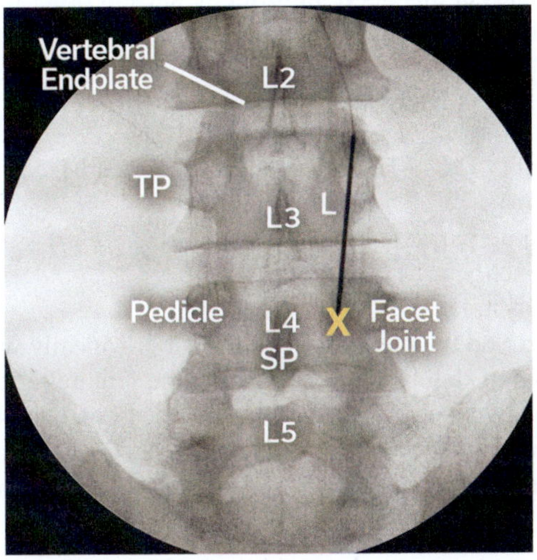

FIGURE 31.20 Right lumbar medial branch nerve insertion under fluoroscopy .

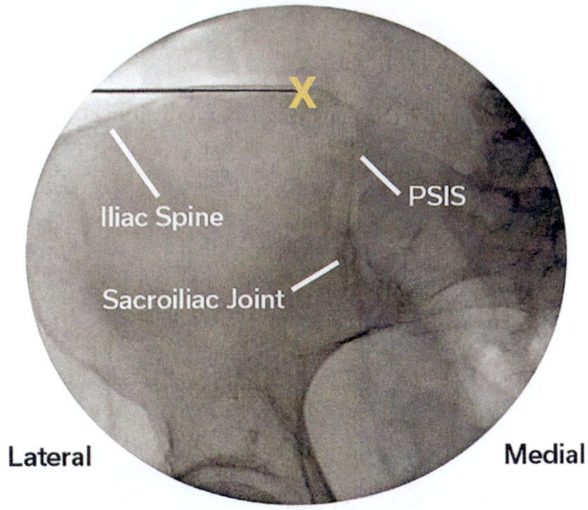

FIGURE 31.21 Anatomical landmarks for PNS insertion targeting the left superior cluneal nerves.

2) Alternatively, ultrasound may be used to place the lead, but the nerve is often difficult to identify (Fig. 31.21).

Femoral nerve stimulation

Diagnoses: Neuropathic Lower Extremity Pain M79.2, Chronic Knee Pain M25.5, Complex Regional Pain Lower Limb G90.52, Femoral Neuropathy G57.2, Chronic Amputation Phantom Pain G54.6, Post-Operative Amputation Pain T87.89.

Indications: Lower extremity chronic pain; acute postoperative pain.

Technique: Position, target, approach, etc.

Position: Supine.

Target: Superficial to the femoral nerve between the fascia lata and the fascia iliaca. The insertion is 1–2 cm distal to the inguinal crease with a lateral to medial trajectory nearly parallel to the skin to lie superficial to the nerve prior to its branching.

Confirmation: Comfortable sensations were reported in the leg over the intended locations.

Programming: 100 Hz (sensory) use for 24 h per day.

Pearls and Pitfalls:

1) Identify and mark the location where undergarments rest on the skin to ensure the lead exit site does not interfere with clothing.
2) The nerve is large and can lead to painful paresthesia or motor involvement if stimulation is too close to the nerve. It is recommended to start stimulating at approximately 1.5 cm distal to the nerve.
3) It may be beneficial to place two leads at this nerve in different sites in order to obtain better control and comfortable tonic stimulation of the nerve without receiving unintentional pain or motor stimulation (Figs. 31.20 and 31.21).

Saphenous nerve stimulation

Diagnosis: Neuropathic Lower Extremity Pain M79.2, Chronic Knee Pain M25.5, Complex Regional Pain Lower Limb G90.52.

Indications: Lower extremity chronic pain.

Technique: Position, target, approach, etc.

Position: Supine with hip externally rotated.

Target: Deep to the sartorius muscle on the medial side of the thigh—ideally with the full electrode within the fascial plane. At mid-thigh between the vastus medialis and the sartorius, the femoral artery is identified by scanning medially. The needle is inserted in the in-plane view using a shallow trajectory at 1 cm distal to the divergence of the femoral artery and saphenous nerve in a lateral to medial approach.

Confirmation: Comfortable sensations were reported in the leg over the intended locations.

Programming: 100 Hz (sensory) use for 24 h per day.

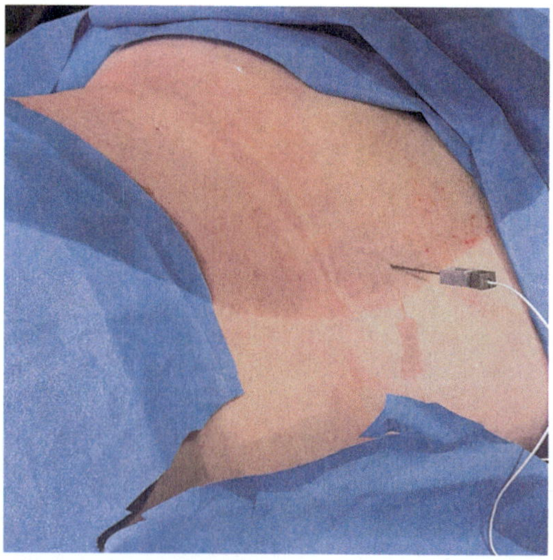

FIGURE 31.22 Right saphenous nerve ultrasound insertion.

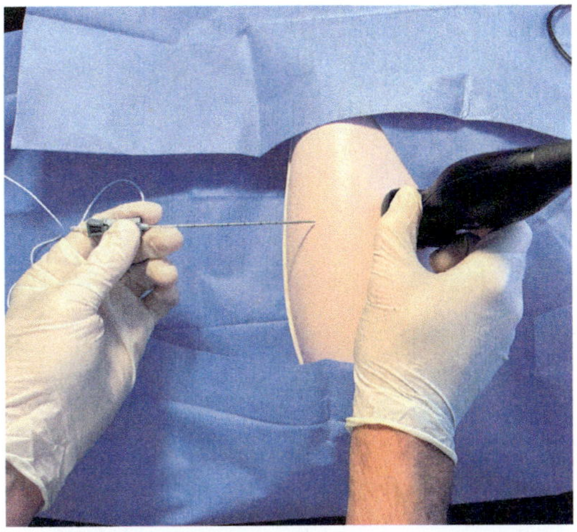

FIGURE 31.23 Anatomical landmarks for PNS insertion targeting the right saphenous nerve.

Pearls and Pitfalls:

1) Targeting the nerve above the joint line will most likely capture the infrapatellar branch of the saphenous nerve, providing analgesia to the anterior knee.
2) Ensure at least 4 cm of lead is beneath the skin (Figs. 31.21–31.24).

Sciatic nerve stimulation

Diagnosis: Neuropathic Lower Extremity Pain M79.2, Chronic Knee Pain M25.5, Complex Regional Pain Lower Limb G90.52, Femoral Neuropathy G57.2, Chronic Amputation Phantom Pain G54.6, Post-Operative Amputation Pain T87.89.

Indications: Lower extremity chronic pain.

Technique: Position, target, approach, etc.

Position: Prone or lateral decubitus with affected side up.

Target:

Popliteal: Target is 0.5–1 cm superficial to the nerve, although it could be placed deep, lateral, or medial to the nerve for better response. The needle is inserted superiorly in the popliteal fossa in-plane with the ultrasound probe, traveling laterally to medially, using scanning to identify the nerve while avoiding the vascular structures.

Subgluteal: Target is 0.5–2 cm from the sciatic nerve above or below the gluteal crease. Using a curvilinear low-frequency probe, identify the sciatic nerve at the gluteal crease and enter the skin laterally to medially, ending at the target using in-plane guidance.

Trans-gluteal: The target is 0.5–2 cm away from the sciatic nerve as it travels deep into the gluteus maximus muscle. It is often identified midway between the bony greater trochanter and ischial tuberosity on ultrasound scanning. Using a curvilinear low-frequency probe, identify the sciatic nerve at the target and enter the skin laterally to medially, ending at the target using an in-plane view.

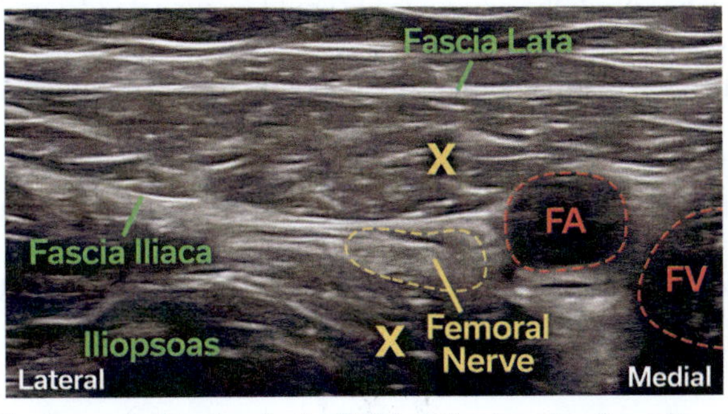

FIGURE 31.24 Anatomical landmarks for PNS insertion targeting the right saphenous nerve.

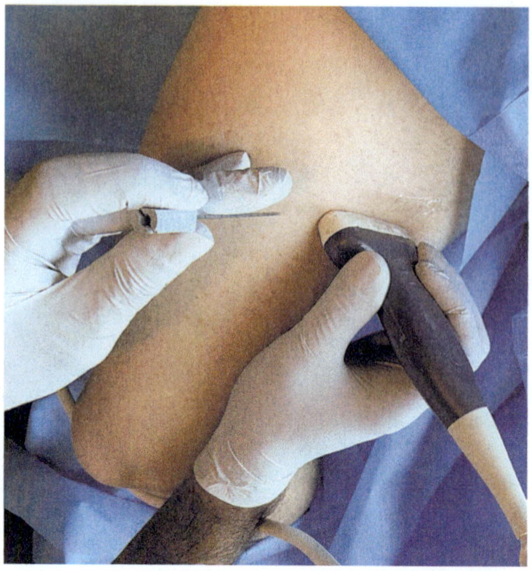

FIGURE 31.25 Right popliteal sciatic nerve ultrasound insertion.

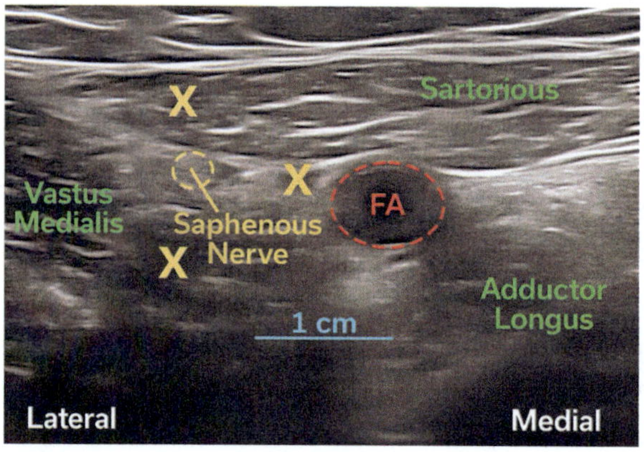

FIGURE 31.26 Anatomical landmarks for PNS insertion targeting the right popliteal sciatic nerve.

Confirmation: Comfortable sensations were reported in the leg over the intended locations.
Programming: 100 Hz (sensory) use for 24 h per day.
Pearls and Pitfalls:

1) Nerve is best targeted superior to the joint line, as lead placement in the joint line can result in lead migration and fracture.
2) Medial to lateral placement of the lead should be avoided, as the exiting lead site may become irritated or the lead displaced when the thighs rub together.
3) If a cephalad-to-caudad approach is used, the exiting lead should be tunneled laterally to avoid irritation of the exiting lead site while in a seated position.
4) Medial placement for the popliteal may preferentially treat the tibial nerve, and lateral may treat the common peroneal nerve.
5) The subgluteal location may lie in connective tissue near the biceps femoris.
6) If the subgluteal is difficult to locate, begin tracing the sciatic nerve from a more distal location to arrive at the subgluteal.
7) The transgluteal approach is deep and may require the lead to pass over the nerve rather than pointing to the side of the nerve (Figs. 31.25–31.32).

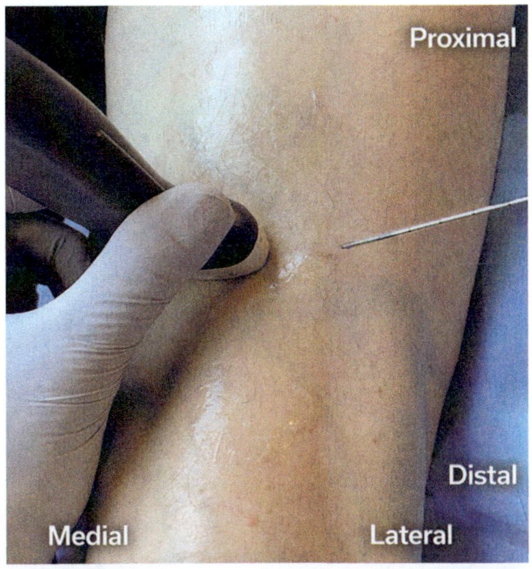

FIGURE 31.27 Right saphenous nerve insertion with ultrasound.

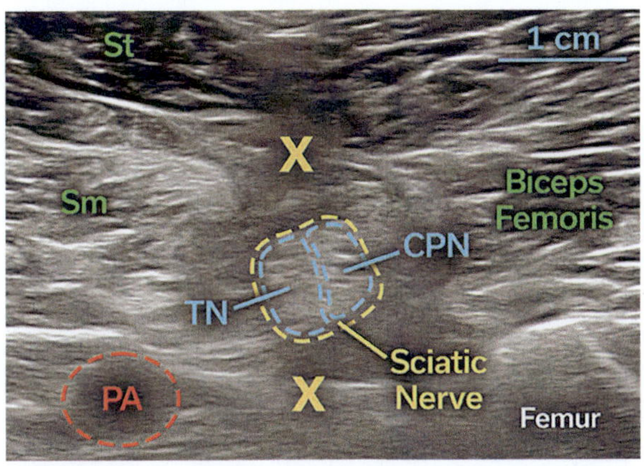

FIGURE 31.28 Anatomical landmarks for PNS insertion targeting the sciatic nerve with a transgluteal approach.

Complications

Most complications noted in commercial use are minor. Skin irritation, infection, minor bleeding, nerve injury, or lead migration have been reported (Table 31.3). Lead fractures resulting in remnants during explantation are reported as 2%–3%.

Preventive strategies

- Adherence to sterile technique following all applicable infection control procedures per the specific institution's guidelines.
- Avoid traversing joint capsules, as this breaches the capsule's barrier to infection. Avoid nerve targets in close proximity to orthopedic hardware, which can increase infection risk; do not place any components of the device (i.e., connector box or mounting cable) on top of the microlead connector.
- Ensure regular bandage changes by the patient or clinical staff and observe for signs of infection.
- Do not submerge any components of the device in water, alcohol, or other fluids, as this could lead to electrical shock and/or increased infection risk.
- Avoid simultaneous connection of the system and high-frequency surgical equipment (electrocautery), as this may result in burns at the site of the electrode tip and/or the mounting pad.

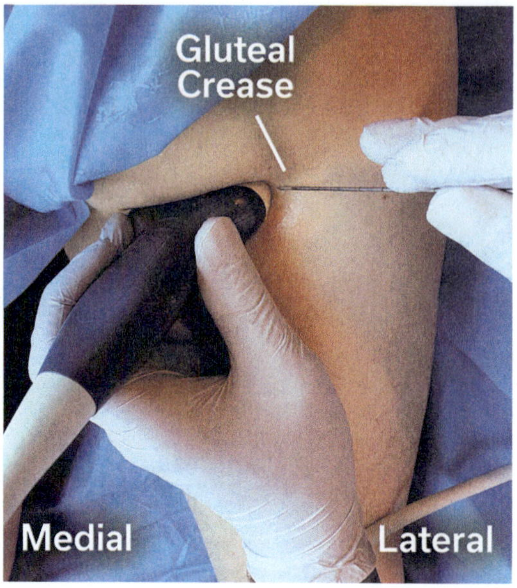

FIGURE 31.29 Right transgluteal sciatic nerve insertion.

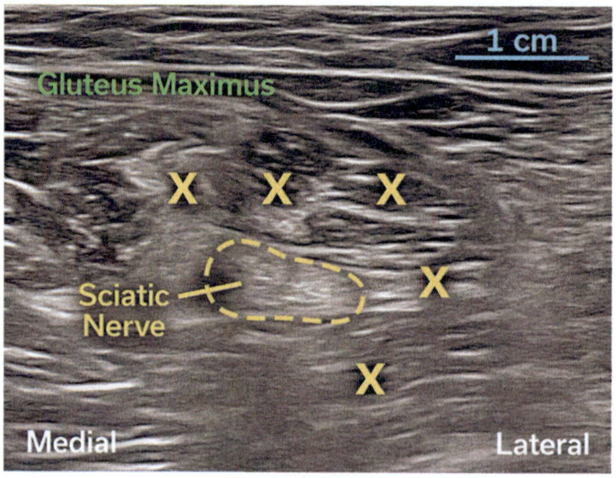

FIGURE 31.30 Subgluteal sciatic nerve target landmarks under ultrasound.

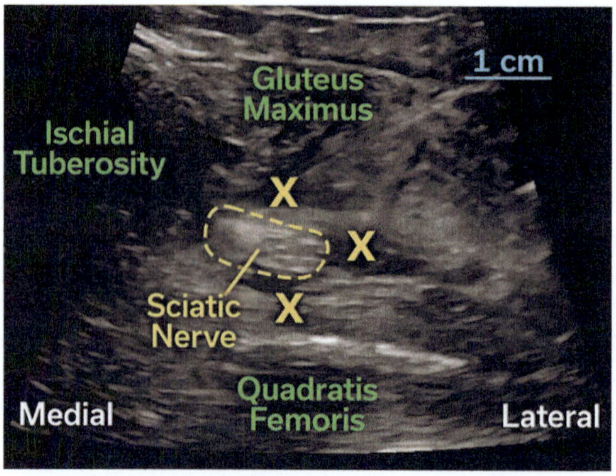

FIGURE 31.31 Subgluteal sciatic nerve insertion with ultrasound.

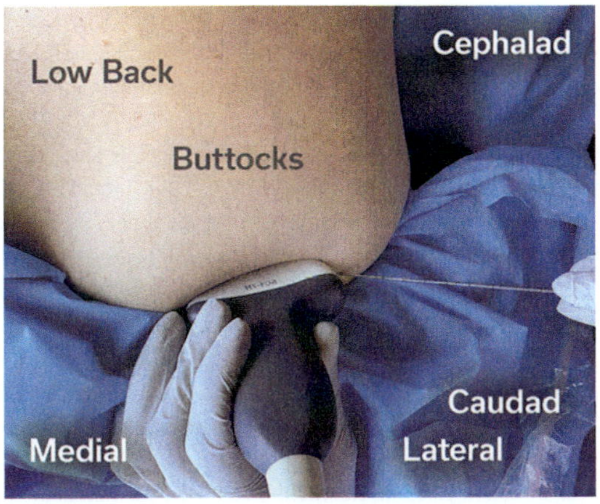

FIGURE 31.32 Setup for sciatic nerve targeting in the gluteal region.

TABLE 31.3 Reported complications of 60-day PNS in commercial use.

	Number of patients	Number of events	Percentage of patients (%)
Overall	*369*	*435*	*6*
Skin irritation	160	163	2.6
Confirmed	7	7	0.11
Suspected	70	73	1.1
Painful or uncomfortable stimulation	70	73	1.1
Change in sensation/location of stimulation	35	38	0.6
Pain in the lead exit site	18	20	0.3
Swelling	11	11	0.2
All other	48	50	0.8

Huntoon et al. Pain physician: May/June 2023 26:273–28

- Remove leads within the 60-day window and use a slow, controlled hand-over-hand technique to remove the lead at the 60-day completion of treatment.
- If lead is difficult to remove, consider applying a few milliliters of local anesthetic near the lead tip via a 25-gauge needle and then reattempting gentle removal.

When to Remove the Device: Criteria for discontinuation of therapy include completion of 60-day treatment, concern for infection, lead fracture or migration with poor efficacy, and preparation for an MRI scan. Specifically, regarding MRI compatibility, all MRI procedures, no matter the anatomic site, are contraindicated at this time for patients with a 60-day PNS system. Exposure can cause tissue heating and injury or unwanted stimulation. Pull out the lead and remove all other system components from the patient before an MRI examination is performed. In the case of a lead fracture beneath the skin resulting in a retained lead remnant, an MRI examination is safe to perform under the conditions described in the MR conditionality labeling. Specifically, a person with a retained lead remnant may be safely scanned anywhere in the body at 1.5T or 3.0T under specific conditions [28]. As always, consultation with the device manufacturer's manual is essential.

References

[1] Melzack R, Wall PD. Pain mechanisms: a new theory. Science. 1965;150(699):971–9.

[2] Wall PD, Sweet WH. Temporary abolition of pain in man. Science 1967;155(3758):108–9. https://doi.org/10.1126/science.155.3758.108.

[3] Deer TR, Levy RM, Verrills P, Mackey S, Abejon D. Perspective: peripheral nerve stimulation and peripheral nerve field stimulation birds of a different feather. Pain Med 2015;16(3):411–2. https://doi.org/10.1111/pme.12662.

[4] Strand N, D'Souza RS, Hagedorn JM, et al. Evidence-based clinical guidelines from the American Society of Pain and Neuroscience for the use of implantable peripheral nerve stimulation in the treatment of chronic pain. J Pain Res 2022;15:2483–504. https://doi.org/10.2147/JPR.S362204.

[5] Weiner RL, Reed KL. Peripheral neurostimulation for control of intractable occipital neuralgia. Neuromodulation 1999;2(3):217–21. https://doi.org/10.1046/j.1525-1403.1999.00217.x.

[6] Huntoon M, Huntoon E, Obray J, Lamer T. Feasibility of ultrasound-guided percutaneous placement of peripheral nerve stimulation electrodes in a cadaver model: Part One, lower extremity. Reg Anesth Pain Med 2008;33(6):551–7. https://doi.org/10.1016/j.rapm.2008.04.007.

[7] Huntoon MA, Burgher AH. Ultrasound-guided permanent implantation of peripheral nerve stimulation (PNS) system for neuropathic pain of the extremities: original cases and outcomes. Pain Med 2009;10(8):1369–77. https://doi.org/10.1111/j.1526-4637.2009.00745.x.

[8] Burgher AH, Huntoon MA, Turley TW, Doust MW, Stearns LJ. Subcutaneous peripheral nerve stimulation with inter-lead stimulation for axial neck and low back pain: case series and review of the literature. Neuromodul Technol Neural Inter 2012;15(2):100–7. https://doi.org/10.1111/j.1525-1403.2011.00388.x.

[9] Corriveau M, Lake W, Hanna A. Nerve stimulation for pain. Neurosurg Clin 2019;30(2):257–64. https://doi.org/10.1016/j.nec.2018.12.008.

[10] Singh V. A comparison of various peripheral nerve stimulators available currently on the market. ASRA News 2022;47(4). https://doi.org/10.52211/asra110122.045.

[11] Ilfeld BM, Gabriel RA, Saulino MF, et al. Infection rates of electrical leads used for percutaneous neurostimulation of the peripheral nervous system. Pain Pract 2017;17(6):753–62. https://doi.org/10.1111/papr.12523.

[12] Deer TR, Eldabe S, Falowski SM, et al. Peripherally induced reconditioning of the central nervous system: a proposed mechanistic theory for sustained relief of chronic pain with percutaneous peripheral nerve stimulation. J Pain Res 2021;14:721–36. https://doi.org/10.2147/JPR.S297091.

[13] Gilmore CA, Desai MJ, Hopkins TJ, et al. Treatment of chronic axial back pain with 60-day percutaneous medial branch PNS: Primary end point results from a prospective, multicenter study. Pain Pract 2021;21(8):877–89. https://doi.org/10.1111/papr.13055.

[14] Wilson RD, Harris MA, Gunzler DD, Bennett ME, Chae J. Percutaneous peripheral nerve stimulation for chronic pain in subacromial impingement syndrome: a case series. Neuromodul Technol Neural Interface 2014;17(8):771–6. https://doi.org/10.1111/ner.12152.

[15] Ilfeld BM, Ball ST, Gabriel RA, et al. A feasibility study of percutaneous peripheral nerve stimulation for the treatment of postoperative pain following total knee arthroplasty. Neuromodul J Int Neuromodul Soc 2019;22(5):653–60. https://doi.org/10.1111/ner.12790.

[16] Gilmore CA, Ilfeld BM, Rosenow JM, et al. Percutaneous 60-day peripheral nerve stimulation implant provides sustained relief of chronic pain following amputation: 12-month follow-up of a randomized, double-blind, placebo-controlled trial. Reg Anesth Pain Med 2020;45(1):44–51. https://doi.org/10.1136/rapm-2019-100937.

[17] Pingree MJ, Hurdle MF, Spinner DA, Valimahomed A, Crosby ND, Boggs JW. Real-world evidence of sustained improvement following 60-day peripheral nerve stimulation treatment for pain: a cross-sectional follow-up survey. Pain Manag 2022;12(5):611–21. https://doi.org/10.2217/pmt-2022-0005.

[18] Huntoon M. A retrospective review of real-world outcomes following 60-day peripheral nerve stimulation for the treatment of chronic pain. Pain Phys J 2023;26(3):273–81. https://doi.org/10.36076/ppj.2023.26.273.

[19] Naidu R, Li S, Desai MJ, Sheth S, Crosby ND, Boggs JW. 60-Day PNS treatment may improve identification of delayed responders and delayed non-responders to neurostimulation for pain relief. J Pain Res 2022;15:733–43. https://doi.org/10.2147/JPR.S349101.

[20] U.S. Food and Drug Administration. 510(k) premarket notification: SPRINT peripheral nerve stimulation system, K223306. Rockville, MD: U.S. Food and Drug Administration; 2023. https://www.accessdata.fda.gov/cdrh_docs/pdf22/K223306.pdf.

[21] Narouze S, Benzon HT, Provenzano D, Buvanendran A, de Andres J, Deer T, Rauck R, Huntoon MA. Interventional spine and pain procedures in patients on antiplatelet and anticoagulant medications (2nd ed.). Reg Anesth Pain Med 2018;43:225–62. Guidelines From the American Society of Regional Anesthesia and Pain Medicine, the European Society of Regional Anaesthesia and Pain Therapy, the American Academy of Pain Medicine, the International Neuromodulation Society, the North American Neuromodulation Society, and the World Institute of Pain.

[22] Hoffmann CM, Butler CS, Pingree MJ, Moeschler, et al. Is response to a pre-implant diagnostic peripheral nerve block associated with efficacy after peripheral nerve stimulation implantation? A ten-year enterprise-wide analysis. Neuromodulation 2024;27:873–80.

[23] Abd-Elsayed A, Keith MK, Cao NN, Fiala KJ, Martens JM. Temporary peripheral nerve stimulation as treatment for chronic pain. Pain Ther 2023;12:1415–26.

[24] Wahezi SE, Emerick TD, Caparó M, Choi H, et al. The current state of training in pain medicine fellowships: an Association of Pain Program Directors (APPD) survey of program directors. Pain Pract 2024;24:895–903.

[25] Singh V, Sandhu D, Xiang N. Techniques for peripheral nerve stimulator implantation of the upper extremity. Pain Med August 1, 2020;21(Suppl. 1):S27–31. https://doi.org/10.1093/pm/pnaa185.

[26] Kaye AD, Ridgell S, Alpaugh ES, Mouhaffel A, Kaye AJ, Cornett EM, Chami AA, Shah R, Dixon BM, Viswanath O, Urits I, Edinoff AN, Urman RD. Peripheral nerve stimulation: a review of techniques and clinical efficacy. Pain Ther December 2021;10(2):961–72. https://doi.org/10.1007/s40122-021-00298-1.

[27] Zhu AC, Tram J, Waterman R, Wallace M, Chakravarthy K. Recommendations for anesthetic management for intraoperative neuromodulation cases. Pain Manag May 2022;12(4):557–67. https://doi.org/10.2217/pmt-2020-0109.

[28] Orhurhu V, Hussain N, Karri J, Mariano ER, Abd-Elsayed A. Perioperative and anesthetic considerations for the management of neuromodulation systems. Reg Anesth Pain Med June 2023;48(6):327–36. https://doi.org/10.1136/rapm-2022-103660.

Chapter 32

Permanent peripheral nerve stimulation: Implant techniques and clinical applications

Robert Moghim[1], Ioannis Skaribas[2], Alaa Abd-Elsayed[3], Dustin Reynolds[4] and Chad Gorman[5]

[1]*Interventional Spine and Pain, Denver, CO, United States;* [2]*Expert Pain PA, Houston, TX, United States;* [3]*Department of Anesthesiology, University of Wisconsin School of Medicine and Public Health, Madison, WI, United States;* [4]*Ortho Alliance, Columbus, OH, United States;* [5]*Partner at Physician Partners of America, Tampa, FL, United States*

Introduction

The term "permanent" Peripheral Nerve Stimulation (PNS) implant refers to the surgical implantation of a peripheral neuro-stimulating system. Historically, the first implantable peripheral nerve stimulation systems used radiofrequency receivers powered by an external transmitter to deliver stimulation through neuro-stimulating electrodes or paddles surgically placed close to or in direct contact with the peripheral nerves (Einar Ottestad, August 20th, 2020).

Since the modern introduction of neuromodulation in 1967 and over the past 60 years, PNS hardware advancements in conjunction with fluoroscopy and ultrasound guidance have facilitated the percutaneous placement of electrodes and their connection to Internal Pulse Generators. These advancements have allowed for surgical implantation of devices that function independently from the limitations of earlier externally operated systems (Einar Ottestad, August 20th, 2020).

Until this last decade, implantable PNS systems utilized conventional components designed for spinal cord stimulation. Depending on the nerve target the energy requirements of the implantable IPG differed significantly. The growth of Interventional Pain Medicine, combined with the demand for long-term pain management solutions, has driven innovation, leading to the current renaissance in PNS technology and applications.

Currently there are multiple FDA-approved PNS devices, each tailored for specific indications. The individual components of these systems differ significantly indicative of the significant innovation that has occurred; some use temporary micro leads, coils, and external pulse generators or high frequency-electromagnetic coupling via an external transmitter requiring practically very little or no surgical placement. Other systems utilize more traditional electrodes comparable to the ones used for SCS that connect to implantable IPGs or micro-IPGs making traditional surgical implantation necessary.

Overall, the primary purpose of a PNS surgical implant remains consistent, and that is to position a PNS element close to specific nerves, secure it through anchoring, and connect it to an implantable IPG that operates internally (using either primary cells or rechargeable IPGs) or is powered externally in the case of a micro-IPG. The surgical implantation of PNS systems must always occur in a sterile environment, with imaging capabilities, anesthesia, and full surgical and resuscitative support available.

A Modern Atlas for Implantable Devices of the Spine, Brain, and Nerve. https://doi.org/10.1016/B978-0-443-36528-7.00038-8

Summary of relevant anatomy

Nerve	Innervation	Function	Associated pain distribution	Relevant anatomical landmarks
Greater occipital nerve	C2	Sensory	Posterior scalp up to the vertex	Emerges between the obliquus capitis inferior and semispinalis capitis muscles
Lesser occipital nerve	C2–C3	Sensory	Lateral scalp behind the ear	Runs along the posterior border of the sternocleidomastoid
Suprascapular nerve	C5–C6	Mixed	Shoulder region	Passes under the transverse scapular ligament through the suprascapular notch
Axillary nerve	C5–C6	Mixed	Lateral shoulder and upper arm	Wraps around the surgical neck of the humerus through the quadrangular space
Radial nerve	C5–T1	Mixed	Posterior arm, forearm, and hand	Runs in the radial groove of the humerus, vulnerable at the midshaft
Median nerve	C5–T1	Mixed	Anterior forearm and lateral palm	Travels through the carpal tunnel under the flexor retinaculum
Ulnar nerve	C8–T1	Mixed	Medial hand, including the little finger	Passes through the cubital tunnel at the elbow and Guyon's canal at the wrist
Intercostal nerves	T1–T11	Mixed	Thoracic wall and upper abdominal region	Run in the intercostal spaces under the rib grooves
Ilioinguinal nerve	L1	Mixed	Lower abdominal wall and upper medial thigh	Emerges through the superficial inguinal ring
Iliohypogastric nerve	L1	Mixed	Lower abdominal wall above the inguinal ligament	Runs superior to the inguinal canal near the ASIS
Genitofemoral nerve	L1–L2	Mixed	Anterior thigh and genital region	Emerges through the psoas major and travels along the external iliac artery
Lateral femoral cutaneous nerve	L2–L3	Sensory	Lateral thigh	Passes under the inguinal ligament near the ASIS
Femoral nerve	L2–L4	Mixed	Anterior thigh and medial leg	Passes through the femoral triangle lateral to the femoral artery
Obturator nerve	L2–L4	Mixed	Medial thigh	Travels through the obturator foramen
Sciatic nerve	L4–S3	Mixed	Lower back, buttocks, posterior thigh and leg	Emerges below the piriformis muscle and runs down the posterior thigh
Tibial nerve	L4–S3	Mixed	Posterior leg and sole of the foot	Passes through the tarsal tunnel behind the medial malleolus
Common peroneal nerve	L4–S2	Mixed	Lateral and anterior aspects of the leg and foot	Wraps around the fibular head
Sural nerve	S1–S2	Sensory	Posterolateral aspect of the leg and lateral foot	Runs with the small saphenous vein, posterior to the lateral malleolus
Saphenous nerve	L3–L4	Sensory	Medial aspect of the leg and foot	Runs with the great saphenous vein along the medial leg
Superior cluneal nerves	L1–L3	Sensory	Upper buttocks	Pierce the thoracolumbar fascia near the iliac crest
Middle cluneal nerves	S1–S3	Sensory	Medial buttocks	Emerge from the dorsal sacral foramina
Inferior cluneal nerves	S2–S3	Sensory	Lower buttocks	Branch from the posterior femoral cutaneous nerve
Pudendal nerve	S2–S4	Mixed	Perineum, genitalia, and anus	Passes through Alcock's canal (pudendal canal) in the ischioanal fossa

Procedure

Peripheral nerve stimulation (PNS) is an innovative neuromodulation therapy that delivers targeted electrical impulses to peripheral nerves to modulate pain signals. This minimally invasive approach is designed for patients with chronic, refractory pain who have not found relief through conventional treatments. A comprehensive understanding of the diagnostic criteria, appropriate ICD-10 coding, clear identification of on-label versus off-label indications, and thoughtful patient selection, especially with regard to age, are essential for optimizing clinical outcomes.

Diagnosis (with ICD 10 codes)

Here is an expanded academic list of diagnoses commonly associated with peripheral nerve stimulation (PNS), their ICD-10 codes, and a brief discussion of some of the more common diagnosis and their relevance in clinical practice. These diagnoses represent conditions that often lead to chronic neuropathic pain, which may be refractory to conventional treatments and thus require neuromodulation strategies such as PNS.

https://icd.who.int/browse10/2019/en

It is important to note that countless diagnoses can be treated with PNS, including nerve conditions and chronic pain conditions.

Mononeuritis- ICD-10: G58.9

The general ICD-10 code for mononeuritis is G58.9—*Mononeuritis, unspecified*. More specific codes exist based on the nerve affected (e.g., G56.41 for mononeuritis of the right upper limb). Mononeuritis refers to inflammation or damage to a single peripheral nerve, often caused by trauma, infection, autoimmune disorders, or vascular conditions such as diabetes. It typically presents with localized pain, weakness, numbness, or tingling along the affected nerve's distribution.

Trigeminal neuralgia—ICD-10: G50.0

Characterized by sudden, severe facial pain due to irritation of the trigeminal nerve, this condition is one of the classic neuropathic pain disorders.

Carpal tunnel syndrome—ICD-10: G56.0

This diagnosis applies to patients with median nerve compression at the wrist, presenting with numbness, tingling, or pain in the hand and fingers.

Unspecified peripheral neuropathy—ICD-10: G62.9

This is used when a patient presents with symptoms of peripheral neuropathy without a clearly defined etiology, often leading to chronic pain.

Polyneuropathy in diseases classified elsewhere—ICD-10: G63.2

This code is applicable when a patient has a polyneuropathy associated with another systemic disease, which can contribute to chronic pain syndromes.

Radiculopathy, lumbar region—ICD-10: M54.16

This diagnosis involves nerve root compression in the lumbar spine that can cause radiating leg pain, frequently leading patients to explore interventional pain management options.

Cervicalgia (neck pain)—ICD-10: M54.2

This condition describes pain in the cervical spine, which may be due to various underlying pathologies, including nerve impingement, often considered in the context of neuromodulation.

Occipital neuralgia- ICD-10 G52.81

Occipital neuralgia is a type of headache characterized by sharp, shooting pain in the distribution of the greater or lesser occipital nerves, typically at the back of the head and upper neck. It is often caused by nerve irritation or compression from muscle tension, trauma, or inflammation.

Low back pain, unspecified—ICD-10: M54.5

A broad category covering chronic low back pain, this code is often used when specific etiologies have not been identified, but pain persists despite conservative management.

Indications

The clinical applications of PNS can be divided into on-label and off-label indications. Understanding these categories is key to both regulatory compliance and appropriate patient care.

On-label indications

PNS comprises therapeutic applications that have received regulatory approval based on substantial clinical evidence and rigorous scientific validation. PNS is FDA-approved for chronic intractable pain, postsurgical pain, post-traumatic pain, and post-amputation pain. One of the most prominent and clinically significant on-label uses of PNS is its role in the management of chronic, intractable neuropathic pain, particularly in cases where patients have demonstrated resistance to traditional medical therapies.

For example, patients with well-documented post-surgical pain often experience enduring discomfort even after comprehensive treatment interventions have been instituted. PNS is a targeted approach in these scenarios, enabling healthcare providers to precisely stimulate the specific nociceptive pathways involved in the pain experience. Furthermore, individuals enduring chronic pain associated with nerve injury—who have systematically exhausted all conventional therapeutic modalities, including pharmacotherapy, physical rehabilitation, and less invasive interventional techniques—are recognized as optimal candidates for on-label PNS. This strategic utilization of PNS reflects its potential to significantly enhance patient outcomes and provide a viable alternative in managing complex pain syndromes, underpinning the need for its broader acceptance and integration into clinical practice.

The use of ICD-10 codes, such as G89.29, helps underscore the chronic and refractory nature of the pain, supporting the clinical rationale for PNS. This code, alongside others that specify nerve-related conditions, is critical in ensuring that the treatment indication is well-documented and that insurance providers recognize the therapeutic need.

Off-label indications

Off-label indications refer to using PNS for conditions beyond those for which it was initially approved. As research and clinical experience with PNS evolve, physicians are increasingly exploring its application in managing a broader spectrum of pain disorders. For instance, off-label use has been reported in conditions such as chronic migraine, where traditional pharmacologic treatments have failed. In such cases, targeting occipital or cervical nerves with PNS may reduce the frequency and severity of migraine attacks.

Another notable off-label indication is the treatment of complex regional pain syndrome (CRPS), a condition characterized by severe, disproportionate pain following injury. Although CRPS has not been a primary focus during initial FDA approval processes for PNS, emerging evidence suggests that neuromodulation can offer significant relief in carefully selected cases.

Phantom limb pain is yet another off-label area where PNS is being investigated, with early studies indicating potential benefits in reducing pain perception in amputees.

Off-label use requires that clinicians weigh the potential benefits against the risks on a case-by-case basis. Detailed patient counseling and thorough documentation of the decision-making process are essential to ensure informed consent and appropriate management of patient expectations. When used off-label, PNS should be viewed as an extension of its approved applications, guided by the latest clinical research and individual patient factors.

Patient selection considerations: Age

Age is a significant factor in selecting candidates for peripheral nerve stimulation. While PNS can be effective across a broad age range, the patient's age influences several aspects of the procedure and its long-term outcomes.

In younger patients, the advantages include generally robust healing capacities and longer potential durations of benefit from the device. However, these patients may also be more active, which can raise concerns about the longevity of the implanted device and the potential for repeated interventions over time. Younger individuals may also have higher expectations regarding improvements in function and quality of life, necessitating comprehensive pre-procedural counseling to ensure realistic goals. Moreover, the need for device maintenance, programming adjustments, or eventual replacements should be discussed in long-term management planning.

In older patients, several unique factors must be considered. Aging is often accompanied by comorbidities—such as diabetes, cardiovascular disease, or osteoporosis—that can affect both the safety and the efficacy of PNS. Age-related nerve conduction and tissue integrity changes may alter the response to electrical stimulation. Furthermore, older adults might face practical challenges in managing an implanted device, such as reduced manual dexterity or cognitive decline, which could impact their ability to operate the system effectively. A thorough assessment of the overall health status, including cardiovascular and metabolic risk factors, is critical to ensure that the benefits of PNS outweigh any potential risks.

A multidisciplinary evaluation—including input from pain specialists, geriatricians, and, when needed, neurosurgeons—can help tailor the intervention to the individual patient. Rather than using age as an exclusionary criterion, clinicians should consider it one element within a broader context of overall functional status and treatment goals. This balanced approach ensures that younger and older patients have access to PNS when it is likely to improve their quality of life.

Conclusion

Peripheral nerve stimulation offers a promising alternative for managing chronic neuropathic pain by directly modulating peripheral nerve activity. Establishing an accurate diagnosis—supported by appropriate ICD-10 coding—is essential for identifying suitable candidates. Distinguishing between on-label and off-label indications helps clinicians navigate regulatory requirements while addressing unmet clinical needs. Finally, carefully evaluating patient selection criteria, especially age-related factors, is crucial in optimizing outcomes and ensuring that the therapy is safe and effective. Through a comprehensive and individualized approach, PNS can significantly enhance pain management and improve the quality of life for patients with chronic pain.

Contraindications

Identifying appropriate candidates for PNS implantation is paramount to ensure optimal outcomes and minimize potential risks. Contraindications to permanent PNS implantation include:

- Coagulopathy- Patients with bleeding disorders or those on anticoagulant therapy may face heightened risks of bleeding during implantation. While many PNS targets are superficial and considered low risk for bleeding, exceptions may be made based on individual assessments.
- Active Infections- The presence of systemic or localized infections can increase the risk of postoperative complications, including device-related infections.
- Unoptimized Behavioral or Mental Health Conditions- Significant psychological disorders, if not adequately managed, can adversely affect postoperative outcomes and patient compliance.
- Failed Diagnostic Trial- An unsuccessful trial stimulation, where effective pain relief is not achieved, suggests that permanent implantation may not be beneficial. This approach aligns with the standard practice of conducting a trial phase before permanent implantation to assess the potential effectiveness of the therapy.
- Complete Sensory Loss- Patients lacking sensory perception in the target area may not experience the intended benefits of PNS therapy.
- Requirement for Periodic MRI Scans- Some PNS devices may not be compatible with magnetic resonance imaging (MRI). Patients requiring regular MRI evaluations may face limitations due to potential device interference.

A thorough preoperative evaluation is essential to identify these contraindications and ensure patient safety.

Maintenance concerns

The longevity and functionality of PNS devices are contingent upon diligent maintenance and patient adherence to prescribed guidelines. Key considerations include:

- Device Integrity: Regular assessments are crucial to detect any hardware malfunctions or lead migrations that could compromise therapeutic efficacy.
- Infection Surveillance: Continuous monitoring for signs of infection at the implantation site is vital. Prompt intervention is necessary to prevent systemic involvement.
- Battery Management: Patients should be educated on the expected lifespan of the device's battery and the need for timely replacements to maintain uninterrupted therapy.
- Activity Modification: Advising patients to avoid activities that may exert undue stress on the implanted device can prevent mechanical complications.

A collaborative approach involving regular follow-ups with the healthcare team ensures the device's optimal performance and addresses any emerging issues promptly.

Training recommendations and case peer review

Proficiency in PNS implantation and management necessitates specialized training and adherence to established guidelines. The following recommendations aim to standardize and enhance the competency of practitioners:

- ACGME Fellowship and Residency Training Specialty: The Accreditation Council for Graduate Medical Education (ACGME) underscores the importance of incorporating neuromodulation techniques, including PNS, into pain medicine fellowship programs. A structured curriculum ensures that trainees acquire the requisite knowledge and skills for effective PNS therapy.
- Suggested Case Volume for Competence: To achieve clinical proficiency, it is recommended that trainees perform a minimum of three PNS implantation procedures, encompassing both temporary and permanent systems, during their training period. This hands-on experience is crucial for developing technical expertise and clinical judgment. This recommendation aligns with the Pain Education and Knowledge (PEAK) Consensus Guidelines published by the American Society of Pain and Neuroscience (ASPN) [1].
- Proctoring Recommendation: Novice practitioners should engage in proctored procedures under the mentorship of experienced clinicians. This supervised approach facilitates the transition from theoretical knowledge to practical application, ensuring adherence to best practices and patient safety [1].
- Case Peer Review: Implementing regular peer review sessions fosters a culture of continuous improvement. Through critical appraisal of clinical cases, practitioners can share insights, address challenges, and uphold high standards of care in PNS therapy [1].

By integrating these training recommendations, healthcare institutions can cultivate a workforce adept in the nuances of PNS implantation and management, ultimately enhancing patient outcomes.

Technique

Patient positioning

Patient positioning is a crucial aspect of the permanent PNS implantation procedure. It ensures both access to the target nerve and comfort for the patient. The type of positioning depends on the nerve targeted for stimulation, the surgical approach, and the comfort required during the procedure. Patient positioning should accommodate the use of ultrasound or fluoroscopy for the procedure as needed.

Positioning for common nerve targets

Sciatic nerve stimulation

- For targeting the sciatic nerve, the patient is typically placed in the lateral decubitus position. This position allows for easier access to the lower back, sacral, and gluteal regions, where the stimulator lead can be positioned. The upper leg may be slightly flexed at the hip and knee to reduce tension on the nerve, ensuring that the surgical team can visualize and manipulate the nerve with minimal interference.
- The lower leg is usually supported with padding to prevent any pressure points or injury.

Femoral nerve stimulation

- The patient is positioned in the supine position with the hip and knee flexed. The femoral area is exposed, allowing the surgical team to access the inguinal ligament for lead placement.
- The flexion of the hip and knee provides better exposure of the femoral nerve while minimizing tension in the region [2].

Upper limb nerve stimulation

- For brachial plexus or radial nerve stimulations, the patient can be positioned in a semi-reclining or lateral decubitus position. The arm is positioned to provide access to the shoulder or elbow regions, with soft supports placed under the joints to prevent injury during the procedure.

General principles for positioning

Regardless of the specific nerve targeted, certain principles apply universally to positioning:

- Stability: The patient should be secured to avoid accidental movements that may disrupt the surgical procedure. A stable position also ensures proper access to the surgical site.
- Comfort: The patient should be positioned to avoid unnecessary muscle strain. Padding, particularly in areas of high pressure, is essential to reduce discomfort during the procedure.
- Exposure: Proper exposure of the nerve or area of stimulation is necessary for accurate placement of the stimulator lead.

Anesthesia considerations

Permanent peripheral nerve stimulator (PNS) implantation is often performed with monitored anesthesia care (conscious sedation) combined with local anesthetic infiltration, rather than general anesthesia, to allow patient feedback during lead placement. Under sedation (e.g., with propofol and short-acting opioids), the patient can communicate sensations during test stimulation, helping optimize lead positioning. In contrast, general anesthesia is usually avoided because an unconscious patient cannot report paresthesias, and intraoperative neuromonitoring would be needed to confirm nerve activation. Local anesthetics (such as lidocaine or bupivacaine) are used at the incision sites for comfort, but care is taken to avoid injecting near the target nerve to prevent blocking nerve conduction during testing. Overall, a sedation-based technique with agents like propofol and fentanyl, supplemented by local anesthetic, provides adequate analgesia while preserving the ability to perform intraoperative nerve testing and reduces the hemodynamic risks associated with general anesthesia. Preoperative antibiotics are routinely given to minimize infection risk, typically started just before surgery and discontinued within 24 h post-op. If general anesthesia is utilized, prior device trial results, fluoroscopy, and/or ultrasound may guide optimal lead placement.

Operating room time estimate

PNS implantation procedures generally last around 1–2 h from start to finish. Registry data indicate an average procedure duration of approximately 88 min for PNS, which is slightly shorter than spinal cord stimulator implants (~98 min) and much shorter than intrathecal pump placements (~112 min). The time required for permanent PNS implantation can vary based on the complexity of the case, patient-specific factors, and the surgeon's experience.

Time breakdown

The timeline can be broken down into several phases. Initial patient positioning and sterile preparation (e.g., prone or supine depending on the nerve target) typically take 10–15 min. The lead placement phase often requires 30–60 min, as the clinician carefully advances the electrode near the nerve under imaging guidance and performs test stimulation to confirm optimal placement. Once satisfactory lead position is achieved, the implantation of the pulse generator (IPG) or receiver and the creation of a subcutaneous pocket for it may add another 20–30 min. Finally, closure of incisions and dressing takes about 10–15 min in total.

In summary, most of the intraoperative time is spent on precise lead localization and testing, whereas positioning, IPG pocket creation, and wound closure comprise a smaller portion of the operative duration. Complex cases with multiple leads or challenging anatomy can extend beyond these estimates, but in most cases the entire permanent PNS implantation is efficiently completed in well under 2 hours.

Relevant vendor support

Vendor support is a crucial component in successfully implementing permanent PNS devices. Bioventus, Nalu Medical, SPR, and Curonix are major companies that provide these systems. Other companies with innovative PNS devices entering the market include: Nervonik and Neuspera. These vendors supply not only the devices but also a variety of services that enhance the surgical process. Physician team coordinates device procurement, implantation, and patient follow-up visits with vendor representatives.

Vendor contributions

- Technical Support:

Device manufacturer representatives play a vital role in the PNS implantation process. These vendor representatives (often neurostimulation specialists) are typically present in the operating room to provide technical support and guidance on the specific equipment. Intraoperatively, the representative assists the surgical team with device setup and programming—for example, using a programming console to test different stimulation settings (waveform, amplitude, pulse width, etc.) once the lead is in place.

- Educational Resources:

Vendors offer comprehensive training for the surgical team and other clinical staff. This training ensures that everyone involved in the procedure understands the proper use of the devices and how to address potential challenges.

- Software and Programming Support:

The representative often performs or guides the initial programming of the implanted generator post-procedure and ensures the patient knows how to use the controller. Some companies offer software platforms that allow real-time monitoring and adjustments of the stimulator during the surgery. Surgeons can use this software to ensure the stimulator is correctly calibrated for optimal patient outcomes.

- Post-Implantation Follow-up:

Vendor representatives provide ongoing support such as software updates, technical troubleshooting, and education on device features. This collaborative involvement of industry experts helps optimize the PNS therapy, both at the time of implantation and throughout the maintenance period, and is an established part of modern neuromodulation practice.

Procedure

The permanent PNS implantation procedure involves several key steps. The surgeon and surgical team must perform each step with precision to ensure the correct placement and function of the stimulator.

Step-by-step process

- Preoperative Evaluation:

Patients undergo a thorough evaluation to confirm that they are appropriate candidates for a permanent PNS implant. This includes a review of their chronic pain condition and confirmation that the target pain is peripheral nerve mediated. Often a positive response to a diagnostic peripheral nerve block or a trial stimulation is obtained before proceeding to permanent implantation. Psychological screening is recommended to ensure the patient has reasonable expectations and no unmanaged mental health issues that could impact outcomes. Preoperative planning also involves choosing the stimulator system and lead type and obtaining any necessary imaging of the anatomical region. Prophylactic IV antibiotics are administered prior to incision as recommended to reduce infection risk.

- Positioning, Incision and Lead Placement:

On the day of surgery, the patient is positioned to best expose the area of the target nerve (e.g., prone for dorsal lower extremity nerves or lateral decubitus for brachial plexus). The procedure is typically done under local anesthesia with conscious sedation, so the patient is lightly sedated but able to respond. Monitors are applied, and sedation is started (e.g., with propofol infusion and analgesics) while maintaining spontaneous breathing. The skin over the surgical field is prepped and draped in sterile fashion. The physician identifies the target peripheral nerve using imaging—usually high-frequency ultrasound for superficial nerves, or fluoroscopy if needed for deeper structures [2]. A needle or introducer is advanced toward the vicinity of the nerve without penetrating or damaging it. Through the needle, a test stimulation probe may be inserted to deliver electrical pulses, at this point the awake patient can report if they feel tingling in the distribution of their pain, confirming the correct target. The lead is deployed (for example, tines on the lead are expanded to anchor into tissue) and test stimulation is performed again via the implanted lead to verify proper function before moving on. To prevent migration, the leads are anchored at the site of insertion once their final position has been achieved. This is typically done via suture fixation to the fascia (Strand, 2022). Throughout this step, minimal sedation ensures the patient can provide feedback, and ultrasound or fluoroscopy is used to visualize the lead relative to the nerve.

- Pulse Generator Placement:

If the PNS system includes an implantable pulse generator (IPG) or receiver, the next step is to create a pocket for that component. A second incision is made in a convenient location (such as the lateral gluteal area or lower abdomen for lower-extremity nerves, or the infraclavicular area for upper-extremity nerves), typically about 5–10 cm away from the lead entry point.

The pulse generator is inserted, and the leads are tunneled subcutaneously to connect to the generator. This is typically done at an angle to increase lead slack and minimize tension on leads. The leads are to be anchored again at the pulse generator pocket.

- Intraoperative Testing:

At this stage, the surgical team (often with the vendor's assistance) programs initial stimulation settings. With the patient still awake, they may fine-tune the electrode configurations and amplitude to confirm that stimulation from the implanted system yields the intended sensations and pain coverage. Any adjustments to lead position can still be made, if necessary, prior to securing the leads. The IPG and receiver element is then placed in the pocket and all incisions are ready to be closed.

- Closure:

The incisions (lead entry site and IPG pocket site) are irrigated and then closed in layers using sutures or staples in the usual sterile fashion. The external components of the system (programmer or antenna) are positioned to test the device one more time before final dressings. Sterile dressings are applied to all wounds. The patient then emerged from sedation. In the recovery area, the stimulator is typically turned on to ensure it is providing pain relief and to check that the patient tolerates the sensations. Initial device programming may be adjusted at this time. The patient is given instructions on keeping the incisions clean and how to operate any external device controllers. The incision is closed with sutures or staples, and a sterile dressing is applied.

Appropriate intraoperative imaging

High-quality imaging is essential for accurate lead placement during PNS implantation [2]. Ultrasound is commonly used because it allows direct visualization of the peripheral nerve, surrounding anatomy, and the advancing needle or lead in real time. Using ultrasound, the operator can see the nerve and ensure the lead is placed a few millimeters away from it (usually the lead is positioned about 0.5–3.0 cm from the nerve, rather than directly on it, to avoid trauma while still achieving stimulation). Ultrasound guidance provides a dynamic view, enabling fine adjustments to the lead position and confirmation of adequate distance between the electrode and nerve throughout the procedure. Fluoroscopy is another imaging modality employed, particularly for deeper nerves or when an anatomical landmark approach is preferred. Fluoroscopy offers a continuous X-ray view and is often used in a manner analogous to traditional spinal cord stimulator placement or nerve blocks, relying on bony landmarks to guide the lead near the nerve's location. There are currently no large studies definitively favoring ultrasound versus fluoroscopy for PNS lead placement, and in practice the choice depends on the nerve targeted and the clinician's expertise. In some cases, both modalities may be utilized—for example, ultrasound to get the needle near the nerve, and a fluoroscopic snapshot to document lead position relative to skeletal landmarks. After the lead is deployed, imaging can be used to confirm that the electrode has remained in the intended location (ultrasound can show the lead and nerve alignment, while fluoroscopy can verify the lead hasn't migrated on X-ray). Overall, the use of intraoperative imaging (ultrasound, fluoroscopy, or both) improves the precision of lead placement and increases the likelihood that the stimulator will effectively cover the target nerve once activated.

Postoperative considerations

1. Recovery: After permanent PNS implantation, patients typically recover quickly and can often be discharged the same day, especially if only sedation (not general anesthesia) was used. Typically, healing and soft tissue recovery takes between 2 and 6 weeks depending on depth and location of lead placement. Special consideration should be taken for patients that have risk factors for poor healing. Patients who have diabetes, smoke, peripheral artery disease, auto immune disease or immunocompromised can take longer to heal. The patient's surgical sites are relatively small (often a centimeter or two for lead entry and a few centimeters for the IPG pocket), so postoperative pain is usually modest and managed with a short course of analgesics if needed. For the first week, patients should expect procedural pain and soreness in the incision area as well as the path of the lead placement. Prophylactic antibiotics are routinely prescribed. Patients are counseled on wound care and signs of infection to watch for, as infection is a notable risk with any implanted device (reported infection rates for neuromodulators range from ~4% to 10%). They are instructed to keep incisions clean and dry, and a follow-up is scheduled (typically 1–2 weeks post-op) for wound check and suture

removal if necessary. In addition to infection, practitioners watch for any signs of skin erosion over the hardware, electrode migration, or hardware malfunctions (e.g., lead fracture or battery failure) (Hoffmann, 2022). Most such complications are uncommon, but if they occur, they may necessitate interventions ranging from reprogramming to surgical revision or device removal.

2. Efficacy estimate: The overall efficacy can vary depending on anatomy and which nerve is being stimulated. Typically, over time a loss of efficacy happens in 20%–25% of pts who receive a permanent peripheral nerve stimulator. This may require reprogramming of the leads, revision or removal of the PNS system.
3. Bracing Considerations: Typically bracing is unnecessary after a permanent peripheral nerve implant. Most PNS leads have tines that help with securing leads and minimizing risk of migration. Some physicians prefer bracing to limit range of motion after lead placement. A lumbar support orthosis may be placed after placement of cluneal nerve or medial branch placement. Another example would be the wrist. For radial or ulnar nerve stimulation, a physician may consider short arm wrist brace to prevent excessive wrist flexion extension or supination during the healing process. Do not wear a brace without a clean bandage covering the incision.

d. Activity limitations: Patients who are post op permanent PNS are typically given a list of do's and don'ts after surgery. Activity should be limited in the initial postoperative period to prevent lead displacement. Because lead migration is the most common hardware-related complication of neurostimulators, patients are advised to avoid excessive bending, twisting, or stretching involving the region where the lead is implanted for at least a few weeks. Sudden movements or heavy lifting could dislodge the lead before fibrous healing secures it in place. If the lead traverses a highly mobile joint, the surgical team often provided extra slack in the lead and anchored it to tissue to mitigate tension, but the patient may still be asked to use caution or even wear a soft brace to restrict motion in that area during early healing. By about 6–8 weeks post-implant, tissue fibrosis tends to stabilize the lead, and patients can progressively resume normal activities with their physician's guidance.

e. Maintenance: Device maintenance is another important long-term consideration. Patients are educated on how to care for and operate their specific PNS system. For devices with an internal battery (IPG), the patient learns how to recharge the battery (usually via a transcutaneous charging pad) and is reminded to do so at the recommended interval (which might be every few days to weekly, depending on usage). Fully implantable IPGs typically last for several years before the battery is depleted; at that point, a minor surgery is needed to replace the generator. Newer PNS systems minimize this issue by using either rechargeable batteries or external power sources. Some systems, for example, have no implanted battery at all—the implanted lead is powered by an external transmitter patch worn on the skin, which the patient must keep in place and periodically replace or recharge. In such cases, the patient is instructed on the daily use of the external unit (positioning it over the lead's receiver and turning the stimulation on/off with a controller). Regular follow-ups with the clinic allow the team to address any maintenance issues, update software, and ensure the patient is comfortable with managing the device. Over the long term, successful PNS implantation can lead to sustained pain relief, improved function, and reduced reliance on pain medications, but it requires diligent post-operative care, patient education, and support from the healthcare team and device vendor to achieve the best outcomes.

Pearls and pitfalls

Preoperative

Prior to a permanent peripheral nerve stimulation (PNS) implant, it is essential to provide a detailed explanation of the procedure and all associated risks, with particular emphasis on the most significant risks, including nerve injury, infection, migration, and lead fracture. The informed consent must be detailed, accurate, and discussed with the patient immediately before the procedure.

The importance of an accurate psychological assessment cannot be overstated. Depending on the targeted nerve, appropriate imaging should be considered and completed before implantation. Since PNS devices are either non-MRI compatible or MRI conditional, the need for an MRI of the specific targeted or other anatomical areas must be addressed in advance, with the specifications and limitations of each system disclosed to the patient.

When choosing a system, hardware specifications, as well as the patient's anatomy (body habitus, height, weight, and specific nerve target), need to be considered. The adequacy of PNS electrode length should be determined in advance. Smaller implantable pulse generators (IPGs) are considered less likely to cause pocket pain. It is also important to assess patients' allergies or sensitivity to adhesives when using wearables that must be secured to the patient's skin. During the trial period, it is prudent to wear the adhesive material for a couple of days to ensure the absence of reactions to the material.

A thorough evaluation of the patient's pre-operative comorbidities is essential. Most surgical PNS implants occur under local only or Monitored Anesthesia Care (MAC). General Endotracheal Anesthesia (GETA) or Total Intravenous Sedation (TIVA) may be alternative ways to provide anesthesia. Significant comorbidities, particularly those involving the patient's pulmonary and cardiovascular systems, need to be addressed, and appropriate coordination of care with the anesthesia team should take place before the implant.

Anticoagulation issues often present challenges. Strict ASRA and ASPN anticoagulation guidelines must be followed, and appropriate clearances should be obtained in writing before the procedure. Some practitioners find it helpful for patients to use Hibiclens soap the day before and the morning of the procedure to minimize the risk of infection.

Intraoperative

If General Endotracheal Anesthesia (GETA) is utilized, one must consider the appropriateness of using neuromonitoring (EMG and/or SSEP) for both the safety and accuracy of PNS placement. A sterile surgical environment with fluoroscopy and/or ultrasound availability is mandatory. During the procedure, imaging is performed and recorded.

The use of pre-incision long-acting local anesthetics will provide adequate postoperative pain relief that lasts. Additionally, using local anesthetics mixed with epinephrine will optimize surgical exposure and minimize bleeding. Intravenous antibiotics should be administered before the incision, and antibiotic irrigation can be used during the surgical procedure.

Patient positioning is crucial to optimize fluoroscopic or ultrasound imaging and to expose the nerve target adequately. Any pressure points must be well-padded. When tunelers are used to connect PNS electrodes to the implantable pulse generator (IPG), the surgeon must be acutely aware of all anatomical areas being traversed to avoid any injury. Once the electrodes are connected to the IPG, the PNS system must be checked intraoperatively for function.

Anchoring is essential for all surgically implantable PNS electrodes to prevent migration. Given the anatomical nature of the PNS implant, bulky anchors present a challenge and often cannot be used. Anchoring sutures can be employed instead; however, the risk of electrode disruption or fracture is a possibility, depending on the type of electrode used, and must be considered. Tined electrodes available with some PNS products adequately address the risk of migration but present their own challenges, such as the inability to revise or correct placement once the electrode is in position.

The use of telemetry for most systems allows for intraoperative verification of system integrity and function. When implanting an IPG or Mini-IPG, the area of implantation is important. The distance from the skin must be appropriate to allow connectivity to an external power source. For implantable IPGs, the possibility of skin erosion when too close to the dermis must be considered. Additionally, proximity to osseous areas or joints can lead to pain or unwanted mobility, resulting in disconnection from the external source, loss of efficacy, and patient dissatisfaction.

Before completing the permanent PNS implantation, final fluoroscopic images should be obtained, recorded, and retained for documentation.

Postoperative

In the immediate postoperative period, it is important to ensure the functional status of the system and the patient's response to PNS therapy. After the patient has adequately recovered from anesthesia, the system should be tested in the postoperative area.

Oral antibiotic coverage following a PNS surgical implant has been a topic of debate; however, most practitioners will cover the patient for 7–10 days. Anticoagulants should be initiated after the procedure, following established anticoagulation guidelines. Appropriate postoperative pain management should be considered by providing the patient with up to 5 days of postoperative pain medications of choice.

Clear postoperative care instructions should be given to the patient, emphasizing the importance of keeping the surgical site clean and dry while monitoring for signs of infection (such as redness, swelling, or discharge). Before discharge, the patient should have a scheduled follow-up appointment for post-implant evaluation, during which the effectiveness of the PNS device will be monitored, and necessary adjustments can be made (Figs. 32.1–32.6).

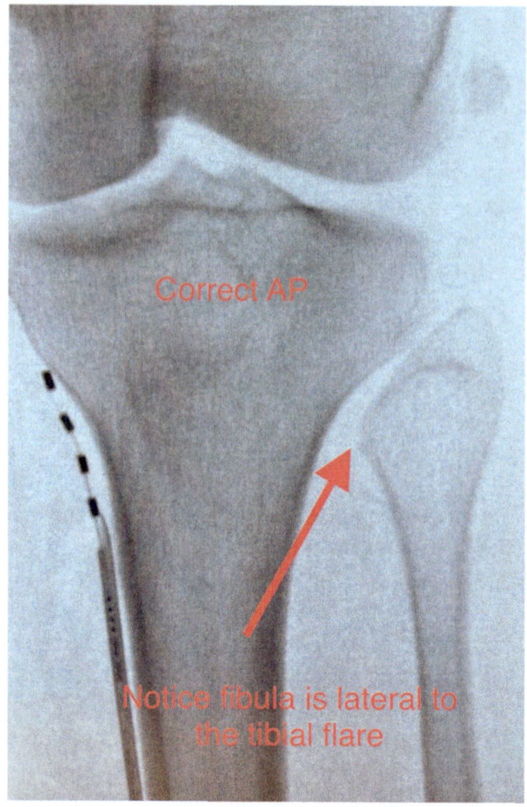

FIGURE 32.1 Infrapatellar saphenous nerve (AP view)- Courtesy of Dr. Robert Moghim.

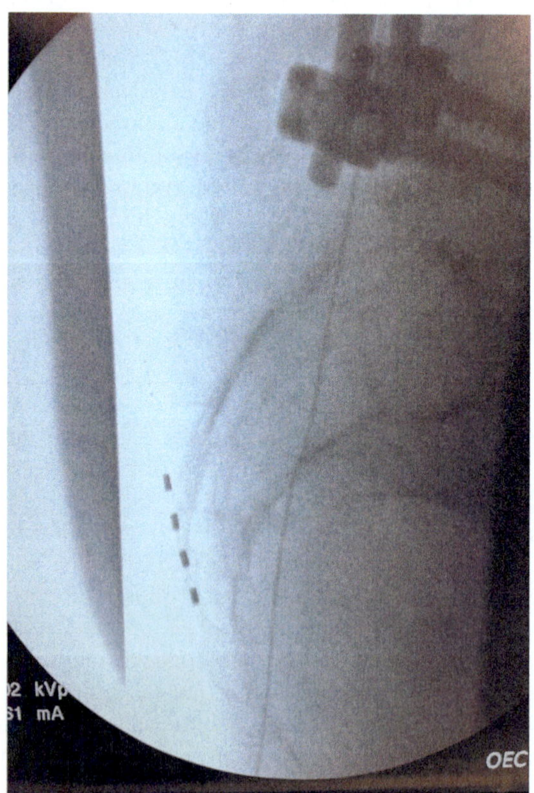

FIGURE 32.2 Middle cluneal nerve (lateral)- Courtesy of Dr. Robert Moghim.

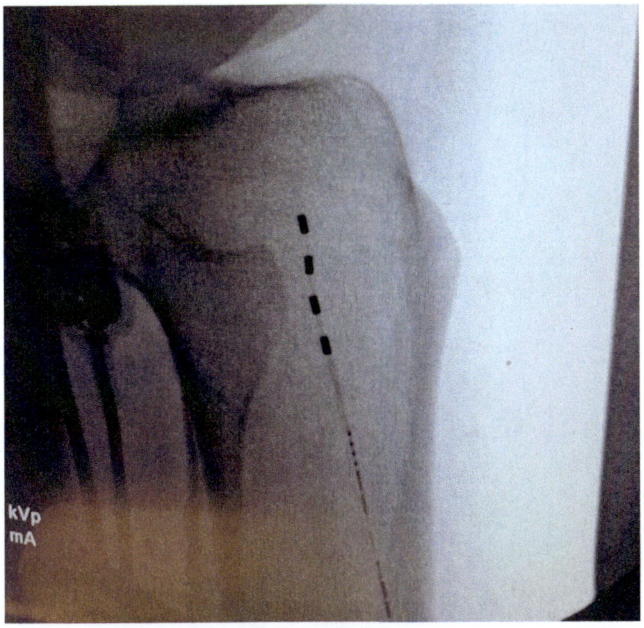

FIGURE 32.3 Infrapatellar saphenous nerve (lateral view)- Courtesy of Dr. Robert Moghim.

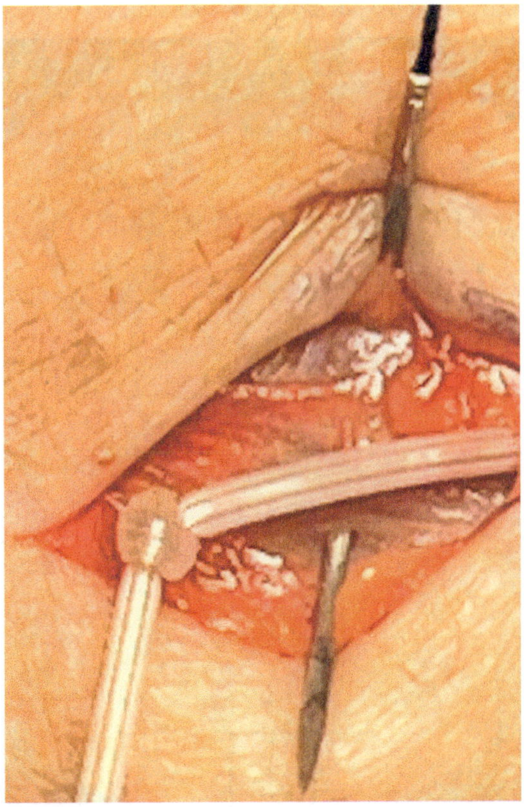

FIGURE 32.4 Lead anchoring- Courtesy of Dr. Robert Moghim.

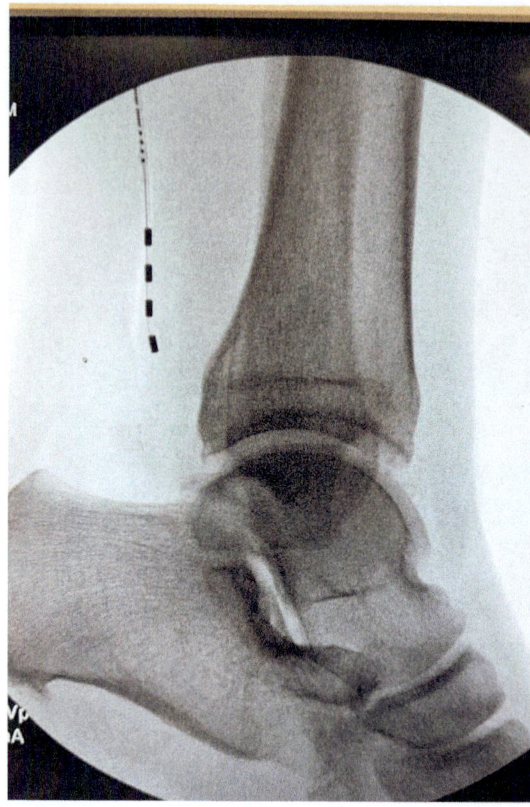

FIGURE 32.5 Posterior tibial nerve (lateral view)- Courtesy of Dr. Robert Moghim.

Figure 5Posterior Tibial Nerve (Lateral view)- Courtesy of Dr. Robert Moghim

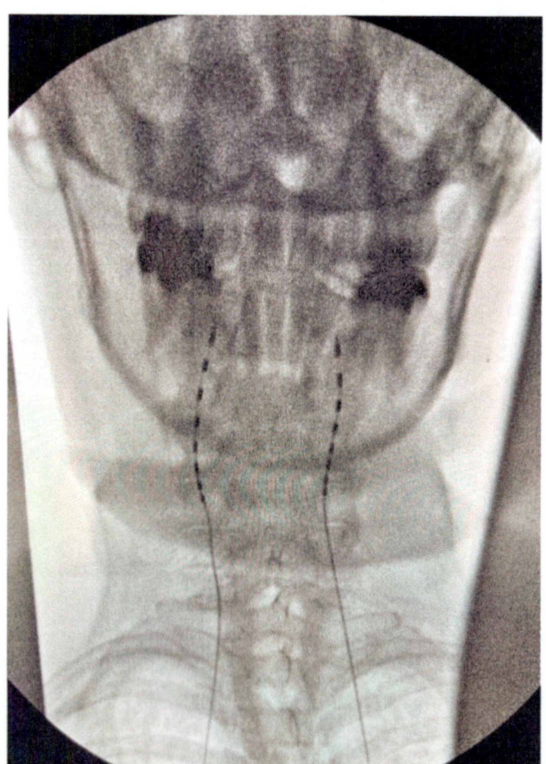

FIGURE 32.6 Occipital nerve (AP view)- Courtesy of Dr. Dustin Reynolds.

References

[1] Deer TR, Abejon D, Barolat G. Stimulation of the peripheral nervous system. In: Deer TR, editor. Atlas of implantable therapies for pain management. Springer; 2011. p. 71–8. https://doi.org/10.1007/978-0-387-88567-4.

[2] Kaye AD, Ridgell S, Alpaugh ES, Mouhaffel A, Kaye AJ, Cornett EM, Chami AA, Shah R, Dixon BM, Viswanath O, Urits I, Edinoff AN, Urman RD. Peripheral nerve stimulation: a review of techniques and clinical efficacy. Pain Ther 2021;10(2):961–72. https://doi.org/10.1007/s40122-021-00298-1.

Further reading

[1] Furman MB, Berkwits L, Cohen I, Goodman BS, Kirschner JS, Lee TS, Lin PS, editors. Atlas of image-guided spinal procedures. 2nd ed. Elsevier; 2017. p. 1–107.

[2] Huntoon MA. Ultrasound-guided peripheral nerve stimulation. In: Narouze SN, editor. Atlas of ultrasound-guided procedures in interventional pain management. 2nd ed. Springer; 2018. p. 311–6. https://doi.org/10.1007/978-1-4939-7754-3.

[3] Nalu Medical. Peripheral nerve stimulator. Retrieved March 2, 2025, from https://nalumed.com/patients/peripheral-nerve-stimulator/.

[4] Nervonik. Nervonik completes first-in-human clinical trial of nerve stimulation technology for chronic pain treatment. Biospace; 2024. Retrieved March 2, 2025, from, https://www.biospace.com/press-releases/nervonik-completes-first-in-human-clinical-trial-of-nerve-stimulation-technology-for-chronic-pain-treatment.

[5] Neuspera Medical. Neuspera Medical announces FDA clearance of its system for peripheral nerve stimulation. Neuspera; 2023. Retrieved March 2, 2025, from, https://neuspera.com/neuspera-medical-announces-fda-clearance-of-its-system-for-peripheral-nerve-stimulation/.

[6] Hayek, et al. Curonix LLC Announces Commercial Availability of the Freedom Peripheral Nerve Stimulation (PNS) System as the Only Full-Body PNS Therapy Available in the United States for Craniofacial Pain. Hayek SM, Haider N, Viswanathan A, Desai M, Rosenberg J, Vanquathem NE. A Prospective, Randomized, Controlled Clinical Trial of High-Frequency Electromagnetic Coupling Powered Permanent Peripheral Nerve Stimulator for the Treatment of Chronic Craniofacial Pain. Pain Physician. 2025 Sep;28(5):417-429. PMID: 40986904.. https://www.globenewswire.com/news-release/2026/01/16/3220297/0/en/Curonix-LLC-Announces-Commercial-Availability-of-the-Freedom-Peripheral-Nerve-Stimulator-PNS-System-as-the-Only-Full-Body-PNS-Therapy-Available-in-the-United-States-for-Craniofacia.html.

[7] Curonix LLC. FDA 510(k) K233162 Premarket Notification (https://www.accessdata.fda.gov/cdrh_docs/pdf23/K233162.pdf). https://www.accessdata.fda.gov/cdrh_docs/pdf23/K233162.pdf.

[8] Abd-Elsayed A, Moghim R. Abd-Elsayed A, Moghim R. Efficacy of peripheral nerve stimulation with a high frequency electromagnetic coupled (HF-EMC) powered implanted receiver in treating different pain targets/neuralgias. J Pain Res. 2023;16:589-596.. https://pmc.ncbi.nlm.nih.gov/articles/PMC9969801/.

Chapter 33

Complications of peripheral nerve stimulation

Jonathan Silverman[1], Brandon Gish[2], Sushanth Boda[3], Christine Haddad[4] and Hemant Kalia[5]

[1]Orthopedic Associates of SW Ohio, Dayton, OH, United States; [2]Lexington Clinic, Lexington, KY, United States; [3]Southern Pain and Spine, Newnan, GA, United States; [4]Innovative Pain and Wellness, Phoenix, AZ, United States; [5]Center for Research & Innovation in Spine & Pain, Rochester, NY, United States

Introduction

Peripheral nerve stimulation (PNS) has evolved significantly as a therapeutic approach for managing chronic pain, leveraging advancements in technology and understanding of neural anatomy. Initially developed from techniques similar to spinal cord stimulation (SCS), PNS has faced unique challenges due to the dynamic nature of peripheral nerves. Early systems, often repurposed from SCS hardware, encountered high rates of complications such as lead migration and skin erosion. However, recent innovations have led to the development of specialized leads and systems designed specifically for PNS, significantly reducing these complications. Despite these improvements, PNS still poses challenges, including hardware-related issues like lead migration and fracture, as well as biological complications such as infections and neurological injuries. This chapter delves into the complexities and advancements in PNS, exploring both the hardware-related and biological complications that arise from its use, and discusses strategies for mitigating these risks to optimize patient outcomes.

Hardware-related complications

Lead migration/fracture

Electricity has been utilized since antiquity to relieve pain and improve function [1], primarily by way of transcutaneous delivery. To help patients with pain from nerve targets inaccessible to transcutaneous stimulation, open surgical techniques were developed [2–6]. Concerns over surgical morbidity led Weiner and colleagues to introduce the concept of percutaneous PNS [7]. Although the conceptual framework for PNS is not all that different from dorsal column SCS, the anatomy and dynamics surrounding the nerve targets differ considerably.

SCS gained widespread use prior to PNS, as did manufacturer interest in the development of suitable hardware. Utilizing repurposed SCS leads and pulse generators, early PNS efforts were associated with alarmingly high rates of lead migration, skin erosion, fibrosis and nerve injury [7,8]. Compared to the epidural space, SCS leads are poorly suited to the more dynamic locations required by peripheral nerve stimulator systems [9]. Lead migration and fracture were estimated to be as high as 13% in one retrospective analysis of PNS systems utilizing SCS hardware, with 2.1% requiring surgical revision [10]. Another retrospective analysis of early PNS implants found that over 13 years, 20 of 72 patients implanted with a PNS system ultimately required the system to be removed, with the most common reasons for explant being lead migration (23.6%), infection and lead erosion (each 6.9%) [11].

As interest in PNS grew, so too did industry investment, resulting in the production of leads intended specifically for use in the periphery. The most utilized risk mitigation strategy employed by current PNS systems is the use of flexible tines (Fig. 33.1) to encourage scar tissue ingrowth and reduce migration. All but one of the currently available US Food and Drug Administration (FDA)-approved PNS systems utilizes this strategy. When combined with coiling and anchoring to the fascia of the proximal lead, one system's tines reduce migration risk to less than 1% [12]. Even more impressively, a

A Modern Atlas for Implantable Devices of the Spine, Brain, and Nerve. https://doi.org/10.1016/B978-0-443-36528-7.00010-8

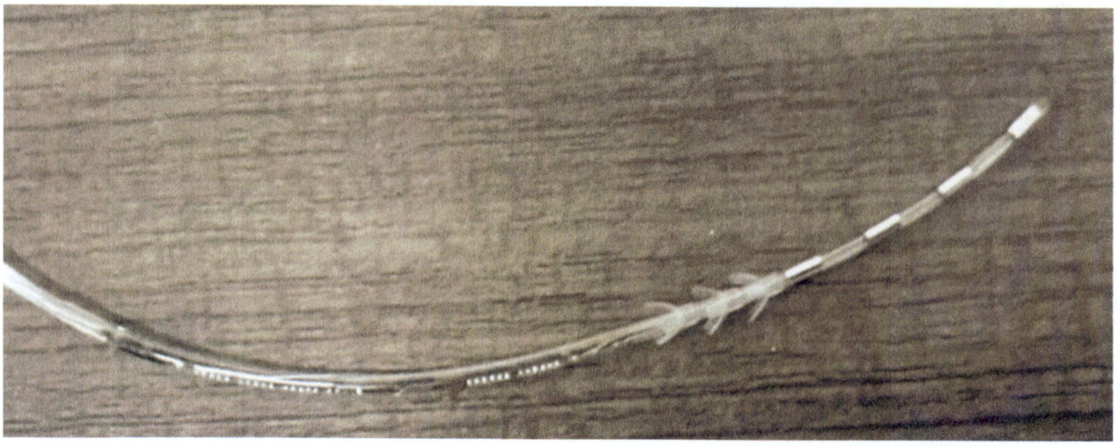

FIGURE 33.1 Tined PNS leads are intended to reduce migration risk. *Photo taken from patient demonstration device.*

5-year follow-up of 126 participants from another device's investigational device exemption (IDE) study revealed zero lead migrations [13], despite its placement across a highly mobile segment of the lumbar spine. Of the current commercially available systems, only one lacks a built-in migration mitigation system. Of the 46 patients implanted as part of the COMFORT RCT utilizing this device, 13 lead- and/or IPG-migration events were reported at 24 months, all requiring revision [14–16].

Despite the overwhelmingly positive outlook regarding the use of tined PNS leads, one case report [17] notes that scarring has the potential to limit the reversibility of the procedure. The authors opine that it may also increase tissue impedance over time, resulting in a gradual loss of therapeutic efficacy [18,19]. Despite the risk, adherence of current systems seems to remain less than that seen with early cuff and paddle leads that required surgical dissection for implantation.

Another strategy, utilized by the manufacturer of a temporary microcoiled peripheral nerve stimulator lead (Fig. 33.2), features a retroverted distal segment that resists posteriorly directed forces, thereby reducing migration. In addition to this barb, the lead is designed to uncoil under traction [20], allowing several centimeters of movement at the proximal lead before the distance between the conductive segment and its nerve target changes.

During removal, complete release of the lead's coiled structure eases removal but also significantly increases the risk of lead fracture. In one retrospective study of 80 patients [21] who underwent scheduled device removal after the prescribed 60-day dwell time, retained lead fragments occurred in 6.25% of patients. Other published data suggest a rate of

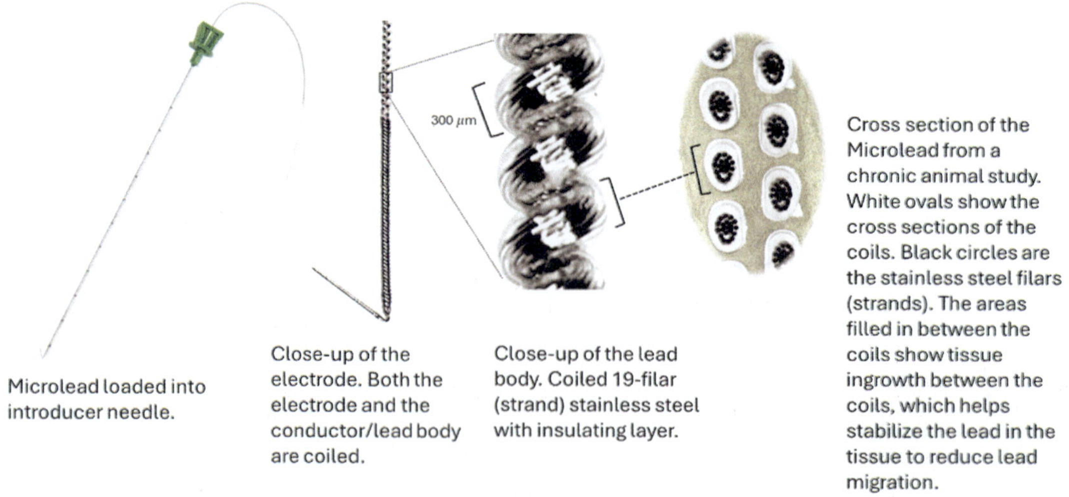

FIGURE 33.2 Coiled peripheral nerve stimulator lead demonstrating tissue ingrowth. *Image is used with the express permission of SPR Therapeutics, Inc.*

retained lead fragments as high as 21% [22–25]. A recent analysis utilizing a revised lead design found a reduction in retained lead fragments from 19.1% with version 1.0 to 3.1% with version 2.0 [26].

Although uncommon compared with lead migration, lead fracture can also occur with permanent PNS systems. This complication is more likely when the leads traverse a mobile joint [27] or while attempting to reverse the implantation process. Five-year data of the restorative neuromodulation device that is implanted across a highly mobile segment of the lumbar spine revealed six instances of lead fracture requiring revision [13]. Apart from this device, which is implanted in the same manner in all patients, the risk of fracture can be reduced by thorough preoperative planning, ensuring close proximity of the lead's contacts and generator, thereby reducing mobility of the system. Careful diagnosis, thoughtful pairing of patient and device, accurate lead placement and close postimplant follow-up with the clinical and device teams are all necessary to optimize patient outcomes and reduce the likelihood that device removal will be required.

Battery failure

Currently, only one available PNS system utilizes hardware reminiscent of a traditional SCS system—i.e., leads hard-wired to a fully implanted pulse generator (IPG). This system, used exclusively to stimulate the L2 medial branch of the dorsal ramus, takes advantage of the same anatomy used successfully by SCS systems to implant a full-size (29.6 cc) programmable pulse generator [28]. In their 5-year data, no device required replacement due to battery depletion—a fact the authors attribute to the low energy levels required to run the system [13].

The remaining approved PNS systems each utilize external power sources, which are either directly connected to a transcutaneous lead or communicate wirelessly through the skin with an implanted receiver. By miniaturizing or foregoing implanted batteries altogether, complication rates can be reduced [29–31]. With these systems, recharging and battery replacement are not necessary in the traditional sense. External power generators (Fig. 33.3) must be worn for activation of the system, which some patients may find burdensome, but the surgical risk of implantation/replacement, erosion, migration and IPG site pain is nonexistent. Charging is no longer a therapy-limiting burden requiring precise alignment of external chargers with internally implanted systems. Instead, patients are provided two generators, one to actively power the system and provide pain relief while the other charges, ready to be utilized when necessary.

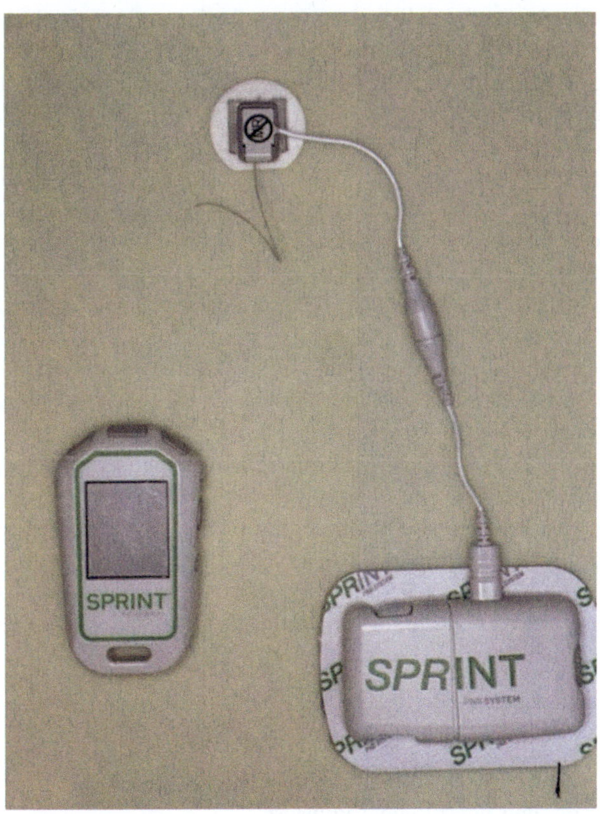

FIGURE 33.3 External power supply unit for the SPRINT PNS system. *Photos taken of patient demonstration units.*

Connection issues

Purpose-built PNS systems required developers to devise a safe and reliable method of delivering energy from a power generator to a remotely implanted electrode. The solution, as demonstrated in contemporary PNS systems, was many. Of the five PNS systems approved by the FDA for the management of chronic pain, two feature a direct connection between the lead and a surgically implanted pulse generator. The temporary PNS system utilizes a direct connection between a transcutaneous lead and an external pulse generator (Fig. 33.2 and 33.3). Three systems deliver energy percutaneously via externally worn components to receivers implanted near the peripheral nerve target. At the time of this writing, there are no published data regarding the prevalence of receiver complications or failure.

The micro IPG utilized by one previously discussed PNS system lacks a battery but contains a receiver to which the system's external battery, referred to as a therapy disc, transmits a radio frequency signal [32]. Radio frequency waves are susceptible to attenuation by the water present in human tissues, predisposing to connection failures if the distance between the signal generator and implanted receiver is too great or their alignment is imprecise. The manufacturer of this system mitigates this limitation by requiring superficial, subcutaneous placement of their micro IPG [32]. While this, in turn, increases the risk of IPG site discomfort or erosion, no instances of pocket pain or skin breakdown were reported at 6 months in the pivotal COMFORT RCT [14] and only one device required explanation due to an unspecified "wound complication" in the 24-month follow-up period [,14–16].

To circumvent the flaws of this energy delivery system, one manufacturer developed "electrical field conduction" technology, which relies on a tissue's water content to create a receptive field capable of producing a consistent connection over a greater range of depth and component alignment [33]. Similarly, high-frequency electromagnetic coupling is used by a third system [34] to deliver energy percutaneously to a copper receiver implanted in the lumen of the electrode array. The energy is transmitted from the receiver to an application-specific integrated circuit (ASIC) microchip (Fig. 33.1) integrated into the lead just proximal to the contacts. Provided that the external antenna is roughly parallel with the implanted lead, this technology extends the depth of effective communication to a maximum of 6 cm [35], dramatically increasing the catalog of available nerve targets.

Other considerations: IPGs, wearability

Following the development of reliable energy delivery systems, further refinement in the field of PNS has come in the form of hardware- and implant-related risk mitigation strategies, many of which were discussed previously.

In studies of various implanted devices, up to 31% of patients report pain at the site of their implanted pulse generator. Fortunately, few find the discomfort to be functionally limiting [36]. Erosion of the generator can also be problematic, particularly when larger generators are placed near common peripheral nerve stimulator targets, where the available soft tissues are not as robust as those at sites traditionally utilized for placement of SCS batteries (flank, buttock and abdomen). In part due to its use of similar anatomy as SCS, these theoretical pitfalls did not limit therapy for any of the 126 patients whose 5-year data were available in the study of restorative neuromodulation [13], the only PNS system which features a full-sized implanted pulse generator.

For all other systems, although IPG site pain and migration are not concerns, wearability of external device components can be a significant barrier to device utilization. Most systems utilize adhesives to affix their external components to the skin, although one manufacturer recently introduced a belt that can be used in certain applications to hold the therapy disc over the micro IPG of patients with an adhesive allergy. Reliance on adhesives limits the number of places over which the external device can be worn, increases the risk of skin irritation even in the absence of a recognized allergy, prevents use during strenuous activity and can complicate a patient's ability to don or adjust the device without assistance. Alternatively, application-specific belts, bands and braces (collectively referred to as "wearables") can be utilized. One system, which relies exclusively on this strategy, utilizes a system of specialized wearable components to hold a flexible fabric antenna parallel to the implanted lead. The antenna is connected by a wire to the external pulse generator, which is placed in a pocket or clipped to the wearable itself and allows easy access for programming adjustments. Owing to the full-length receiver and high-frequency electromagnetic coupling, the patient has the freedom to choose how they prefer to wear their device.

Biological complications

Peripheral nerve stimulators are generally well tolerated with low complication rates. Biological complications include infections, pocket pain, skin erosion, and neurological injuries.

Wound infection

Surgical site infection is one of the most common biological complications affecting PNS. Wound infection is one of the most common biological complications aguing peripheral nerve stimulation. Studies have estimated the infection rate of PNS systems to be around 2.5%–5% [37], although infection rates have been described as high as 10%–15% at certain institutions [37,38]. SSIs are classified as superficial, which often respond to medical management, or deep, which require source control including device removal and surgical debridement and, often, hospitalization. Wound infections can be superficial and treated with medical management or deep, requiring surgical debridement and hospitalizations.

Given the limited evidence on risk factors and prevention of PNS infection [39], most recommendations are extrapolated from data on spinal cord stimulators and other surgical procedures [40–42]. A retrospective study of 195 neuromodulation cases demonstrated increased SSI in patients with diabetes mellitus, elevated hemoglobin A1c and perioperative hyperglycemia [43]. Additionally, surgical factors such as increased operative time are associated with higher odds of infection [44]. The Neuromodulation Appropriateness Concensus Committee (NACC) guidelines for infection control and prevention include screening for Methicillin sensitive and resistant staphylococcus aureus (MSSA/MRSA) decolonization if positive or with a history of MSSA/MRSA infection, optimized perioperative glycemic control, smoking cessation, use of preoperative chlorhexidine, depilation using electric clippers, and global assessment of other risk factors such as immunosuppression or presence of previously implanted hardware [40,41].

Superficial

Guidelines for Prevention of SSI distinguish between superficial incisional SSI, deep incisional SSI and organ/space SSI [45]. According to the Centers for Disease Control and Prevention (CDC) criteria, superficial SSIs are defined as involving the skin and subcutaneous tissue of the incision only and have to occur within 30 days of the operation [45]. Symptoms include swelling, redness, tenderness and purulent discharge. Physical exam findings may not be sufficient to differentiate between superficial and deep wound infections. Advanced imaging (MRI, ultrasound) and labs may be necessary in some cases to make the distinction [42]. Diagnostic imaging can help determine implant involvement and labs, such as blood cultures, can help determine systemic spread. If there is purulent discharge from the wound, bacterial cultures should be obtained [42].

Superficial infections may be managed with an oral antibiotic directed at common gram-positive pathogens, such as a first-generation cephalosporin, for 7–10 days [40,41]. MRSA coverage should be added for patients with risk factors or a known history of MRSA infection [42]. Patients should have an outpatient follow-up to assess treatment response. If oral antibiotics fail, evaluation for deep wound infection is recommended [42].

Deep

Deep incisional SSIs are defined as infections that occur within 30 or 90 days of surgery and involve the deep soft tissues of the incision. Patients must have at least one of the following: Pus from the incision, wound dehiscence (spontaneous or deliberately opened by a surgeon), fever, pain or tenderness [45].

Obtaining a thorough clinical history and physical examination is important in recognizing device related infections and differentiating superficial infections from deep infections. In addition to an examination, laboratory testing such as white blood count, erythrocyte sedimentation rate (ESR), C-reactive protein (CRP) and blood cultures should be considered [42]. Diagnostic imaging, such as magnetic resonance imaging (MRI) or computed tomography (CT) scans, should be obtained if deep infections are suspected. MRIs are preferred if presentation is suggestive of osteomyelitis or discitis [38]. If the peripheral nerve stimulator is MRI unsafe, positron emission tomography (PET)–CT may be helpful to confirm discitis/osteomyelitis [42].

In patients who present with systemic signs of infection and/or are unstable, empiric antibiotics for gram-positive organisms should be initiated immediately. For stable patients, empiric antibiotics can be delayed until cultures are obtained [46]. Device/hardware removal is usually necessary to treat deep PNS infections, and infectious disease specialists should be involved in complicated infections to help determine antibiotic selection and treatment duration [47]. Following device removal, if cultures are negative and source control is achieved, 7–10 days of antibiotics may be adequate [42]. In more complicated cases, longer antibiotic courses may be necessary.

Pocket pain

Another biological complication associated with PNS is pain at the site of the implantable pulse generator, referred to as "pocket pain". Given the scarce evidence on PNS pocket pain, most data are inferred from spinal cord stimulators.

Revision surgery has been estimated to occur in as many as 20% of patients with spinal cord stimulators [48]. A common cause of revision surgery is pocket pain, which has been estimated to occur in 1%–19% of patients [49].

Risk factors for the development of pocket pain are unknown. Scar tissues, central sensitization and mechanical traction are possible contributing factors [49]. The effects of IPG size and location on pocket pain have not been studied, and pocket size remains a problem even with smaller IPGs [49].

Management of pocket pain includes first ruling out infection as a cause. Once this is ruled out, conservative management with medication can be considered. If symptoms persist, surgical revision may be necessary.

Surgical management includes placement of the IPG at the same site or in a different location. If the IPG is too superficial, which can be seen with rechargeable systems, a deeper placement can be considered. However, one should maintain the ability to charge the device adequately. If pocket pain is related to clothing discomfort (i.e., IPG under the belt), repositioning the IPG to another site can be considered [49]. Preoperative planning and marking the incision while the patient is upright can help prevent improper placement of the IPG. On rare occasions, a full system explant may be necessary.

Skin erosion

The extrusion of device components through the skin may result from the complex interplay between myriad patient, device and procedural factors, including compromised tissue integrity, chronic disease conditions, significant weight loss, superficial target nerve depth and suboptimal surgical technique [50] While the precise incidence of skin erosion techniques and using modern, purpose-built PNS systems remains unkown, older surgical approaches and lead designs were associated with an incidence as high as 12.5% [51]. The adoption of percutaneous techniques over traditional open methods facilitated by smaller incisions requiring less tissue disruption, has PNS lead placement, markedly reduced th risk [52].

Although rare, skin erosion can involve any of the PNS system's implanted components, including the electrode array, tunneled lead, implanted pulse generator, or anchor [53]. As such, meticulous attention to each step of the surgical plan is necessary. If an anchor system is used, for example, it is imperative to close the wound in multiple layers to reduce the risk of skin erosion [53]. An acute or delayed SSI is one of the feared complications following skin erosion, contributing to increased procedural morbidity and, ultimately, risking explanation of the system and failure of the therapy.

Traditionally, spinal cord stimulator leads were used to stimulate peripheral nerve targets. Owing to the larger diameter of these leads, a higher incidence of skin erosion was seen with their use [52]. With the introduction of PNS-specific leads, skin erosion has become exceedingly rare [31]. For reference, the diameter of the Sprint coiled MicroLead (Fig. 33.2) is 0.2 mm, whereas a cylindrical SCS lead is 1.3 mm in diameter [11]. A retrospective case series analyzing PNS outcomes from 2004 to 2017 with SCS-intended leads reported lead or anchor erosion in six of 72 patients (8.33%). More recent studies with PNS-specific leads from Refs. [13–16,30,54] reported no skin erosions or other serious device-related adverse events. Ongoing vigilance is essential to detecting and accurately reporting this infrequent complication.

The anatomical location of peripheral nerves can also contribute to the risk of hardware erosion. Occipital and craniofacial placement, in particular, have a higher incidence of skin erosion due to the superficial position of the neural targets. Two cases of percutaneous occipital stimulator tip erosion were reported in one series [55]. A larger case series also reported 2 cases of skin erosion in a cohort of 24 craniofacial PNS lead placements[56]. Interestingly, the authors of this study found that modifying the surgical technique to include the use of a silastic anchor, prevented further instances of hardwareerosion [56].

When evaluating for this dreaded complication, it is essential to distinguish skin erosion from skin irritation, as these adverse events may present similarly. The authors of a study investigating lumbar medial branch PNS [54] identified skin irritation as the most common adverse event, often manifesting as redness or pruritus at the site of the waterproof dressing, bandage, or stimulator's hydrogel mounting pad. If irritation persists despite meticulous dermatological care, superficial lead placement should be considered, as it may ultimately result in skin erosion.

Neurological injury

PNS carries inherent risks, as the placement of leads near neural tissue may result in direct neural trauma or compression [57]. Adverse effects can occur due to direct injury or indirectly through secondary mechanisms such as hemorrhage or infection. To mitigate the risk of nerve damage, implanting physicians must possess a comprehensive understanding of the relevant anatomy and remain vigilant for postoperative neuralgia. Due to the susceptibility of critical internal structures during PNS placement, the implementation of high-resolution fluoroscopy or ultrasound is warranted [57].

Although the incidence of nerve injury from PNS therapy is undetermined, it is generally regarded as a rare complication [53]. The initial designs of PNS leads included paddle and cuff leads that encircled the targeted nerve [31,58]. This technique required open surgical dissection, leading to considerable scarring and nerve injury, which restricted early adoption. Although the advent of cylindrical percutaneous leads has significantly reduced this complication rate, it should be acknowledged that no studies directly comparing these two approaches have been conducted [40,41,59,60].

Irrespective of the chosen approach, both techniques carry the risk of neurological injury through a variety of mechanisms. Nerve damage may result from direct surgical trauma during dissection, needle/sheath insertion, or lead placement. Additionally, foreign body or allergic reactions to the leads may result in perineural scarring or fibrosis [40,41]. In line with SCS, surgical site infections also carry the risk of neurological injury. Whereas neurological injury is a well-recognized concern in SCS, there is a lack of evidence of neurological damage specifically linked to percutaneous placement of PNS leads [10].

There is a lack of extensive data on the risk of serious neurological complications from PNS, with the existing literature being assigned a US Preventative Services Task Force evidence heirarchy level II-3 [61] due to its reliance on case reports, small case series, and retrospective analyses. Nonetheless, the available evidence does suggest the risk is low [40,41,62–65]. According to the NACC Safety Guidelines for the Reduction of Severe Neurologic Injury, PNS has not been associated with direct neurologic trauma [40,41]. This is further supported by two large prospective clinical trials, neither of which documented any serious neurological injuries [62,65].

Meticulous perioperative planning and the implementation of risk-mitigating strategies make PNS a valuable tool for the treatment of refractory diseases and reduce the risk of neurological injury. Enhanced patient safety can be achieved by integrating patient feedback during lead placement or employing neural monitoring [40,41]. Treatment options for suspected postoperative neuralgia may include the use of corticosteroids, anticonvulsants, and referral to a neurology specialist [53].

Conclusion

PNS has evolved significantly over the years, transitioning from a technique plagued by high complication rates to a more refined and effective method for managing chronic pain. The development of specialized leads and systems has significantly reduced hardware-related complications such as lead migration and fracture. Despite these advancements, biological complications like infections and neurological injuries remain a concern. Strategies for mitigating these risks include careful patient selection, adherence to infection control guidelines, and innovative device designs that minimize tissue interaction.

The future of PNS holds promise with ongoing innovations in lead design, energy delivery systems, and wearable technologies that enhance patient comfort and device usability. As the field continues to evolve, it is crucial to balance the benefits of PNS with the potential risks, ensuring that advancements in technology are accompanied by rigorous clinical evaluation and patient-centered care. By addressing both hardware-related and biological complications, healthcare providers can optimize the therapeutic efficacy of PNS, offering improved outcomes for patients suffering from chronic pain.

References

[1] Keller T, Krames ES. "On the shoulders of giants": A history of the understandings of pain, leading to the understandings of neuromodulation. Neuromodulation 2009;12(2):77–84.

[2] Shelden CH, Robert HP, James D. Electrical control of facial pain. Am J Surg 1967;114(2):209–12.

[3] Wall PD, Sweet WH. Temporary abolition of pain in man. Science 1967;155(3758):108–9.

[4] Sweet WH. Control of pain by direct electrical stimulation of peripheral nerves. Clin Neurosurg 1976;23:103–11.

[5] Long DM. Electrical stimulation for the control of pain. Arch Surg 1977;112(7):884–8.

[6] Law JD, Swett J, Kirsch WM. Retrospective analysis of 22 patients with chronic pain treated by peripheral nerve stimulation. J Neurosurg 1980;52 (4):482–5.

[7] Weiner RL, Reed KL. Peripheral neurostimulation for control of intractable occipital neuralgia. Neuromodulation 1999;2(3):217–21.

[8] Saper JR, Dodick DW, Silberstein SD, McCarville S, Sun M, Goadsby PJ. Occipital nerve stimulation for the treatment of intractable chronic migraine headache: ONSTIM feasibility study. Cephalalgia 2011;31(3):271–85.

[9] Yaccarino V, Jin MY, Abd-Elsayed A, Kraemer JM, Sehgal N. Peripheral nerve stimulation in painful conditions of the upper extremity: An overview. Biomedicines 2022;10(11):2776.

[10] Xu J, Sun Z, Wu J, Rana M, Garza J, Zhu AC, Chakravarthy KV, Abd-Elsayed A, Rosenquist E, Basi H, Christo P, Cheng J. Peripheral nerve stimulation in pain management: A systematic review. Pain Physician 2021;24(2):E131–52.

[11] Warner NS, Schaefer KK, Eldrige JS, Lamer TJ, Pingree MJ, Bendel MA, Warner MA, Rho RH, Mauck WD. Peripheral nerve stimulation and clinical outcomes: A retrospective case series. Pain Pract 2021;21(4):411–8.

[12] Trescot A. *Curonix, Inc. National peripheral nerve stimulation bioskills course presentation [PowerPoint slide 22]* 2023. [*Chicago, IL*].

[13] Gilligan C, Volschenk W, Russo M, Green M, Gilmore C, Mehta V, Deckers K, De Smedt K, Latif U, Sayed D, Georgius P, Gentile J, Mitchell B, Langhorst M, Huygen F, Baranidharan G, Patel V, Mironer E, Ross E, Carayannopoulos A, Hayek S, Gulve A, Van Buyten JP, Tohmeh A, Fischgrund J, Lad S, Ahadian F, Deer T, Klemme W, Rauck R, Rathmell J, Maislin G, Heemels JP, Eldabe S. Five-year longitudinal follow-up of restorative neurostimulation shows durability of effectiveness in patients with refractory chronic low back pain associated with multifidus muscle dysfunction. Neuromodulation 2024;27(5):930–43.

[14] Hatheway J, Hersel A, Engle M, Gutierrez G, Khemlani V, Kapural L, et al., Comfort Study Group. Clinical study of a micro-implantable pulse generator for the treatment of peripheral neuropathic pain: 12-Month results from the COMFORT-randomized controlled trial. Reg Anesth Pain Med 2026;51(3):278–84. https://doi.org/10.1136/rapm-2024-106099.

[15] Hatheway J, Hersel A, Song J, Engle M, Gutierrez G, Khemlani V, et al. Clinical study of a micro-implantable pulse generator for the treatment of peripheral neuropathic pain: 3-Month and 6-month results from the COMFORT-randomised controlled trial. Reg Anesth Pain Med 2025;50(7):561–7. https://doi.org/10.1136/rapm-2023-105264.

[16] Engle M, Hersel A, Gutierrez G, et al., COMFORT Study Group. Long-term clinical outcomes (24 months) of peripheral nerve stimulation in the treatment of chronic pain - COMFORT RCT. Chronic Pain Manag J 2026;10(01):179. https://doi.org/10.29011/2576-957X.100079.

[17] Wu H, Evazyan T. Permanent peripheral nerve stimulator lead adhesions leading to loss of therapy and difficult extraction: A case report. Pain Med Case Rep 2023;7(4):211–5.

[18] Abd-Elsayed A, D'Souza RS. Peripheral nerve stimulation: The evolution in pain medicine. Biomedicines 2021;10(1):18.

[19] Carnicer-Lombarte A, Chen ST, Malliaras GG, Barone DG. Foreign body reaction to implanted biomaterials and its impact in nerve neuroprosthetics. Front Bioeng Biotechnol 2021;9:622524.

[20] SPR Therapeutics, Inc. *SPRINT Peripheral nerve stimulator system 510(k) premarket notification. US Food and Drug Administration Website*. 2018. https://www.accessdata.fda.gov/cdrh_docs/pdf18/K181422.pdf. Published July 31, 2018. Accessed February 6, 2025.

[21] Hoffmann CM, Coy DS, Moeschler SM, Pingree MJ, Mauck WD. Incidence of temporary peripheral nerve stimulator lead tip retention: A retrospective review of 80 lead placements. Neuromodulation 2023;26(3):690–3.

[22] Ilfeld BM, Plunkett A, Vijjeswarapu AM, Hackworth R, Dhanjal S, Turan A, Cohen SP, Eisenach JC, Griffith S, Hanling S, Sessler DI, Mascha EJ, Yang D, Boggs JW, Wongsarnpigoon A, Gelfand H. Percutaneous peripheral nerve stimulation (neuromodulation) for postoperative pain: A randomized, sham-controlled pilot study. Anesthesiology 2021;135(1):95–110.

[23] Gilmore CA, Kapural L, McGee MJ, Boggs JW. Percutaneous peripheral nerve stimulation (PNS) for the treatment of chronic low back pain provides sustained relief. Neuromodulation 2019;22(5):615–20.

[24] Ilfeld BM, Finneran JJ 4th, Gabriel RA, Said ET, Nguyen PL, Abramson WB, Khatibi B, Sztain JF, Swisher MW, Jaeger P, Covey DC, Meunier MJ, Hentzen ER, Robertson CM. Ultrasound-guided percutaneous peripheral nerve stimulation: Neuromodulation of the suprascapular nerve and brachial plexus for postoperative analgesia following ambulatory rotator cuff repair. A proof-of-concept study. Reg Anesth Pain Med 2019;44(3):310–8.

[25] Shellock FG, Zare A, Ilfeld BM, Chae J, Strother RB. In vitro magnetic resonance imaging evaluation of fragmented, open-coil, percutaneous peripheral nerve stimulation leads. Neuromodulation 2018;21(3):276–83.

[26] Hoffmann C, Fautsch KJ, D'Souza RS. Incidence of lead tip fracture and retention after percutaneous lead implantation for peripheral nerve stimulation with an external pulse generator: A multicenter comparative analysis of 456 lead implants across two lead hardware generations. Neuromodulation 2025;15(25):S1094–7159. 00022-4.

[27] Eldabe S, Buchser E, Duarte RV. Complications of spinal cord stimulation and peripheral nerve stimulation techniques: A review of the literature. Pain Med 2016;17(2):325–36.

[28] Mainstay Medical Limited. *ReActiv8 implantable neuromodulation system summary of safety and effectiveness data. 2020. US Food and Drug Administration website*. https://www.accessdata.fda.gov/cdrh_docs/pdf19/P190021B.pdf. Published May 20, 2020. Accessed February 6, 2025.

[29] Rauck RL, Kapural L, Cohen SP, North JM, Gilmore CA, Zang RH, Boggs JW. Peripheral nerve stimulation for the treatment of postamputation pain–a case report. Pain Pract 2012;12(8):649–55.

[30] Deer TR, Pope JE, Kaplan M. A novel method of neurostimulation of the peripheral nervous system: The stimrouter implantable device. Tech Reg Anesth Pain Manag 2012;16(2):113–7.

[31] Helm S, Shirsat N, Calodney A, Abd-Elsayed A, Kloth D, Soin A, Shah S, Trescot A. Peripheral nerve stimulation for chronic pain: A systematic review of effectiveness and safety. Pain Ther 2021;10(2):985–1002.

[32] Nalu Medical, Inc. *Nalu neurostimulation System 510(k) Premarket Notification. US Food and Drug Administration website*. https://www.accessdata.fda.gov/cdrh_docs/pdf23/K232415.pdf. Published August 21, 2024. Accessed February 6, 2025.

[33] Bioness, Inc. *StimRouter neuromodulation system 510(k) premarket notification. US Food and Drug Administration website*. https://www.accessdata.fda.gov/cdrh_docs/pdf21/K211965.pdf. 2022. Published February 22, 2022. Accessed February 6, 2025.

[34] Curonix. *Freedom Peripheral Nerve Stimulator System 510(k) Premarket Notification. US Food and Drug Administration website*. https://www.accessdata.fda.gov/cdrh_docs/pdf23/K233162.pdf. 2024. Published June 20, 2024. Accessed February 6, 2025.

[35] Elsharkawy H. Curonix, Inc. Regional peripheral nerve stimulation bioskills course presentation [powerpoint slide 19]. 2025.

[36] Choi H, Gaiha R, Moeschler SM, Bendel MA, McCormick ZL, Teramoto M, Rosenow JM, Kielb S, Avram MJ, Walega DR. Factors associated with implantable pulse generator site pain: A multicenter cross-sectional study. Neuromodulation 2021;24(8):1351–6.

[37] van Kroonenburgh I, Tan SKH, Heiden P, Wirths J, Matis G, Seifert H, Visser-Vandewalle V, Andrade P. Incidence and management of hardware-related wound infections in spinal cord, peripheral nerve field, and deep brain stimulation surgery: A single-center study. Stereotact Funct Neurosurg 2024;102(1):13–23.

[38] Bendel MA, O'Brien T, Hoelzer BC, Deer TR, Pittelkow TP, Costandi S, Walega DR, Azer G, Hayek SM, Wang Z, Eldrige JS, Qu W, Rosenow JM, Falowski SM, Neuman SA, Moeschler SM, Wassef C, Kim C, Niazi T, Saifullah T, Yee B, Kim C, Oryhan CL, Warren DT, Lerman I, Mora R, Hanes M, Simopoulos T, Sharma S, Gilligan C, Grace W, Ade T, Mekhail NA, Hunter JP, Choi D, Choi DY. Spinal cord stimulator related infections: Findings from a multicenter retrospective analysis of 2737 implants. Neuromodulation 2017;20(6):553–7.

[39] Yusuf E, Bamps S, Thüer B, Mattheussen J, Ursi JP, Del Biondo E, de Smedt K, Van Paesschen R, Berghmans D, Hofkens K, Van Schaeren J, van Havenbergh T, Van Herendael B. A multidisciplinary infection control bundle to reduce the number of spinal cord stimulator infections. Neuromodulation 2017;20(6):563–6.

[40] Deer TR, Provenzano DA, Hanes M, Pope JE, Thomson SJ, Russo MA, McJunkin T, Saulino M, Raso LJ, Lad SP, Narouze S, Falowski SM, Levy RM, Baranidharan G, Golovac S, Demesmin D, Witt WO, Simpson B, Krames E, Mekhail N. The neurostimulation appropriateness consensus committee (NACC) recommendations for infection prevention and management. Neuromodulation 2017a;20(1):31–50.

[41] Deer TR, Lamer TJ, Pope JE, Falowski SM, Provenzano DA, Slavin K, Golovac S, Arle J, Rosenow JM, Williams K, McRoberts P, Narouze S, Eldabe S, Lad SP, De Andrés JA, Buchser E, Rigoard P, Levy RM, Simpson B, Mekhail N. The neurostimulation appropriateness consensus committee (NACC) safety guidelines for the reduction of severe neurological injury. Neuromodulation 2017b;20(1):15–30.

[42] Esquer Garrigos Z, Farid S, Bendel MA, Sohail MR. Spinal cord stimulator infection: Approach to diagnosis, management, and prevention. Clin Infect Dis 2020;70(12):2727–35.

[43] Ege E, Briggi D, Javed S, Huh A, Huh BK. Risk factors for surgical site infection in advanced neuromodulation pain procedures: A retrospective study. Pain Manag July 2023;13(7):397–404.

[44] Engle MP, Vinh BP, Harun N, Koyyalagunta D. Infectious complications related to intrathecal drug delivery system and spinal cord stimulator system implantations at a comprehensive cancer pain center. Pain Physician 2013;16(3):251–7.

[45] Mangram AJ, Horan TC, Pearson ML, Silver LC, Jarvis WR. Guideline for prevention of surgical site infection, 1999. centers for disease control and prevention (CDC) hospital infection control practices advisory committee. Am J Infect Control 1999;27(2):97–132.

[46] Esquer Garrigos Z, George MP, Khalil S, Vijayvargiya P, Abu Saleh OM, Friedman PA, Steckelberg JM, DeSimone DC, Wilson WR, Baddour LM, Sohail MR. Predictors of bloodstream infection in patients presenting with cardiovascular implantable electronic device pocket infection. Open Forum Infect Dis 2019;6(4):ofz084.

[47] Deer TR, Stewart C. Complications of spinal cord stimulation: identification, treatment, and prevention. Pain Med 2008;9(S1):S93–101.

[48] Bao J, Khazen O, Olmsted ZT, Gechtman G, Shao MM, DiMarzio M, Topp G, Sukul VV, Staudt MD, Pilitsis JG. Treatment strategies for generator pocket pain. Pain Med 2021;22(6):1305–11.

[49] Dietvorst S, Decramer T, Lemmens R, Morlion B, Nuttin B, Theys T. Pocket pain and neuromodulation: Negligible or neglected? Neuromodulation 2017;20(6):600–5.

[50] Uppal P, Wright TB, Dahbour L, Watterworth B, Lee SJ, Gattu K, Stansbury LG, Benoit J. Difficult removal of exposed peripheral nerve stimulator leads: A report of 2 cases. Pain Rep 2021;6(3):e946.

[51] Slavin KV. Peripheral nerve stimulation for neuropathic pain. Neurotherapeutics 2008;5(1):100–6.

[52] McJunkin T, Lynch P, Srejic E. Complications of peripheral nerve stimulation: Open technique, percutaneous technique, and peripheral nerve field stimulation. In: Reducing risks and complications of interventional pain procedures. Philadelphia: Elsevier Saunders; 2012.

[53] Ranson MT, Pope JE. Reducing risks and complications of interventional pain procedures. Philadelphia: Elsevier Saunders; 2012.

[54] Gilmore CA, Desai MJ, Hopkins TJ, Li S, DePalma MJ, Deer TR, Grace W, Burgher AH, Sayal PK, Amirdelfan K, Cohen SP, McGee MJ, Boggs JW. Treatment of chronic axial back pain with 60-day percutaneous medial branch PNS: Primary end point results from a prospective, multicenter study. Pain Pract 2021;21(8):877–89.

[55] Trentman TL, Dodick DW, Zimmerman RS, Birch BD. Percutaneous occipital stimulator lead tip erosion: Report of 2 cases. Pain Physician 2008;11(2):253–6.

[56] Zhou L, Ashkenazi A, Smith JW, Jen N, Deer TR, Zhou C. Long-term clinical outcome of peripheral nerve stimulation for chronic headache and complication prevention. Anesth Pain Med 2016;6(4):e35983.

[57] Strand N, D'Souza RS, Hagedorn JM, Pritzlaff S, Sayed D, Azeem N, Abd-Elsayed A, Escobar A, Huntoon MA, Lam CM, Deer TR. Evidence-based clinical guidelines from the American society of pain and neuroscience for the use of implantable peripheral nerve stimulation in the treatment of chronic pain. J Pain Res 2022;15:2483–504.

[58] Finch P, Price L, Drummond P. High-frequency (10 kHz) electrical stimulation of peripheral nerves for treating chronic pain: A double-blind trial of presence vs absence of stimulation. Neuromodulation 2019;22(5):529–36.

[59] Stanton-Hicks M, Panourias IG, Sakas DE, Slavin KV. The future of peripheral nerve stimulation. Prog Neurol Surg 2011;24:210–7.

[60] Rasskazoff SY, Slavin KV. An update on peripheral nerve stimulation. J Neurosurg Sci 2012;56(4):279–85.

[61] Harris R, Helfand M, Woolf S, et al., Methods Work Group Third US Preventative Services Task Force. Current methods of the US Preventative Services Task Force: A review of the process. Am J Prev Med 2001;20(3 Suppl 1):21–35. https://doi.org/10.1016/s0749-3797(01)00261-6.

[62] Dodick DW, Silberstein SD, Reed KL, Deer TR, Slavin KV, Huh B, Sharan AD, Narouze S, Mogilner AY, Trentman TL, Ordia J, Vaisman J, Goldstein J, Mekhail N. Safety and efficacy of peripheral nerve stimulation of the occipital nerves for the management of chronic migraine: Long-term results from a randomized, multicenter, double-blinded, controlled study. Cephalalgia 2015;35(4):344–58.

[63] Ishizuka K, Oaklander AL, Chiocca EA. A retrospective analysis of reasons for reoperation following initially successful peripheral nerve stimulation. J Neurosurg March 2007;106(3):388–90.

[64] Lee PB, Horazeck C, Nahm FS, Huh BK. Peripheral nerve stimulation for the treatment of chronic intractable headaches: Long-term efficacy and safety study. Pain Physician 2015;18(5):505–16.

[65] Deer T, Pope J, Benyamin R, Vallejo R, Friedman A, Caraway D, Staats P, Grigsby E, Porter McRoberts W, McJunkin T, Shubin R, Vahedifar P, Tavanaiepour D, Levy R, Kapural L, Mekhail N. Prospective, multicenter, randomized, double-blinded, partial crossover study to assess the safety and efficacy of the novel neuromodulation system in the treatment of patients with chronic pain of peripheral nerve origin. Neuromodulation 2016;19(1):91–100.

Section 10

Stimulation of the brain and cranial nerves

Introduction to section 10 stimulation of the brain and cranial nerves

Developments in neuromodulation over the last decade have influenced our specialty's forward momentum. Deep Brain Stimulation (DBS) has evolved from simple targeting to a field driven by profound technological leaps in devices, neuroimaging, and surgical technique. This transformation, led by functional neurosurgery and neurology, hinges on a deepened understanding of neuroanatomy and neurophysiology. The variety of invasive and non-invasive approaches to the brain and cranial nerves compels us as clinicians to address an expanded range of clinical conditions, while recalling the origins and history of the procedure.[1]

Neuromodulation treatment addresses numerous conditions, including pain, movement disorders, epilepsy, and psychiatric, sleep, and respiratory dysfunction. The exquisite, interconnected anatomy of the central nervous system (CNS) offers an unparalleled array of targets, enabling improved outcomes and clinical reach. This complexity dictates the profound implications for addressing chronic conditions via stimulation. Treatment options now span open and stereotactic surgery to deep brain targets, direct nerve stimulation, and less invasive percutaneous, subcutaneous, and noninvasive methods. This section establishes the revolutionary potential to electrically reengineer the CNS.

The heart of this surgical frontier is DBS. We start with its definitive role in movement disorders. DBS is now the gold standard for advanced Parkinson's disease and essential tremor, offering a powerful, adjustable mechanism that restores motor control by normalizing pathological neural oscillations in key subcortical structures.

The utility of DBS must now be recognized as expanding beyond the motor system. Our discussion pivots to compelling, rapidly developing applications in psychological and pain syndromes. By targeting precise circuits in emotional regulation—such as the subgenual cingulate—DBS represents a high-potential, decisive therapeutic avenue for severe, treatment-resistant depression, OCD, and other debilitating psychological disorders. We should not forget that the roots of DBS were in attempts to alleviate intractable chronic pain, and its capacity to directly disrupt ascending nociceptive pathways where pharmacological options have failed.

Shifting to the peripheral nervous system, the cranial nerves are strategic, less-invasive access points for neural modulation. We prioritize Vagal Nerve Stimulation (VNS), which exploits the vagus nerve as a bidirectional superhighway. We discuss the established efficacy of implanted VNS in refractory epilepsy and chronic depression, and the groundbreaking emergence of external, noninvasive VNS. This non-invasive form enhances access to autonomic control, expanding its use from cluster headaches to inflammatory disorders.

1. Gardner J. A history of deep brain stimulation: Technological innovation and the role of clinical assessment tools. Soc Stud Sci 2013;43(5):707–28. https://doi.org/10.1177/0306312713483678. PMCID: PMC3785222.

Finally, we investigate highly specialized applications, such as hypoglossal nerve stimulation as a specific intervention for obstructive sleep apnea. This approach exemplifies the required shift toward targeted neuromodulation to restore life-critical autonomic functions.

As we embrace these advances, we conclude this section with an essential analysis of the Complications of Brain and CNS Stimulation. A comprehensive understanding of potential hardware issues, surgical risks, and ethical considerations is paramount, ensuring practitioners approach these sophisticated therapies with clinical rigor.

There is a decisive role for neuromodulation in establishing a new era of restorative, targeted intervention for brain and cranial nerve targets in both somatic and autonomic disorders. The future demands that we leverage precision neurotechnology to best address conditions addressed through stimulating the central nervous system.

Chapter 34

Deep brain stimulation for movement disorders

Jonathan Bao[1], Danika L. Paulo[2] and Dario J. Englot[1]
[1]Department of Neurosurgery, Vanderbilt University Medical Center, Nashville, TN, United States; [2]Department of Neurosurgery, Henry Ford Hospital, Detroit, MI, United States

Introduction

Deep brain stimulation (DBS) is a surgical procedure that is a cornerstone for the treatment of many movement disorders in which medication may not adequately control symptoms. The DBS system consists of one or two intracranial electrodes connected to a subclavicular implantable pulse generator (IPG) via extension wires. This system supplies electrical current to the brain region and network within the field of current to modulate the abnormal activity within the network that produces movement disorder symptoms. Currently, DBS is FDA approved for the treatment of three common movement disorders: essential tremor (ET), Parkinson's Disease (PD), and dystonia [1–3]. However, ongoing DBS advancements and trials have demonstrated efficacy in the treatment of other neuropsychological disorders including epilepsy, depression and obsessive-compulsive disorder [4,5].

The origins of DBS therapy are intertwined with the development of stereotactic neurosurgery, a technique that uses a three-dimensional coordinate system combined with imaging to precisely and accurately target specific regions of the brain. While targeted lesioning of brain structures had been successfully accomplished in the early 1900s, it was specifically the stereotactic apparatus pioneered by Spiegel and Wycis in 1947 which enabled accurate lesioning of deep brain structures and helped greatly reduce mortality rates [6]. Physicians such as Guiot built off these early devices in the 1950 and 1960s and made significant progress treating medically refractory PD with surgical pallidotomies in hundreds of patients, identifying key structures that could be targeted later with DBS [7]. During these lesioning procedures, several multi-contact electrodes would first be implanted, guided by preoperatively determined coordinates from post-mortem brain atlases. Patients would then undergo intraoperative neurostimulation testing, monitoring for symptom improvement and side-effects prior to ablation [8]. Other neuroscientists during this time began performing neurophysiological recordings similar to modern day intraoperative microelectrode recordings (MER) which helped identify subtle electrophysiological differences between different regions and subcortical layers [9]. These efforts together helped create a coordinate atlas which helped improve lesioning accuracy and limit side-effects. However, the continuous stimulation required for DBS was not truly feasible until the development of battery technology utilized in cardiac pacemakers in the 1950s [10]. Subsequent research efforts expanded upon these developments and by the 1980 and 1990s, DBS was shown to be effective in multiple animal and human-based studies. Following several trials, FDA approvals for essential tremor, Parkinson's Disease, and dystonia were obtained in 1997, 2002, and 2003, respectively.

Since the first implantation, DBS has evolved significantly both in terms of surgical technique and technological advancements. With widespread availability and reliable high-quality resolution of modern CT and MRI, targeting is now patient-specific based on both imaging and intraoperative MER to optimize lead placement [11]. Newer MRI sequences including Fast Gray matter Acquisition T1 Inversion Recovery (FGATIR) have improved imaging capabilities of subcortical structures [12]. Diffusion-weighted MRI sequences have also enabled the development of the field of connectomics which aims to visualize in vivo white matter tracts, shifting focus toward targeting and modulating neural networks as opposed to individual brain regions [13]. Additionally, in light of advanced imaging techniques that enable detailed visualization of deep structures and white matter pathways commonly targeted in DBS, there has been a recent

A Modern Atlas for Implantable Devices of the Spine, Brain, and Nerve. https://doi.org/10.1016/B978-0-443-36528-7.00028-5

rise of performing DBS with the patient asleep. Research demonstrates non-inferiority of asleep DBS relative to awake DBS with possible benefits including reduced procedure duration and patient comfort [14]. In terms of stereotactic systems, the Leksell frame, developed by Lars Leksell in 1948, is still widely used for stereotaxis. However, many newer stereotactic methods have developed which include alternative frame, mini-frame, frameless and robotic-assisted systems, some of which are paired with real-time neuronavigation. Specifically, robot-assisted lead placement is highly versatile and has been successfully performed with nearly submillimeter accuracy and has growing popularity [15]. DBS hardware and technology have also undergone significant improvements in recent years. Rechargeable batteries and improved battery life allow for longer intervals between IPG replacement surgeries. Importantly, directional lead contacts which have segmented contacts and current steering have revolutionized DBS as they allow for simulation fields to be more finely adjusted [16]. DBS devices have also been enhanced with expanded programming capabilities as well as new sensing capabilities that integrate local field potentials to guide therapy. These devices have enabled the development of closed-loop systems which utilize sensing technology to detect alterations in neurophysiology and adjust stimulation parameters in response to these changes.

Key points (four to six bullet points)

- DBS is a multi-stage procedure that requires significant pre-operative planning and screening in coordination with a multidisciplinary team
- DBS is FDA approved for the treatment of Parkinson's Disease, essential tremor, and dystonia refractory to medical treatments
- Patients tolerate DBS well with a low risk profile and experience significant improvements in motor symptoms, disability scores, and quality of life metrics over long periods of time
- Ongoing research and technological advancements are aimed at further personalizing treatment options and improving programming capabilities to minimize side-effects

Relevant anatomy

The primary movement disorder targets for DBS are located within the basal ganglia and thalamus as part of the cortico-striato-thalamocortical circuit which is central for the control and regulation of movement and is disrupted in movement disorders [17,18]. Figure 34.1 highlights these important structures on MRI. The basal ganglia are comprised of subcortical nuclei, including the substantia nigra, subthalamic nucleus (STN), and striatum which contains the caudate, putamen, and globus pallidus (GP). The GP is a pale structure due to high myelination and is subdivided into the globus pallidus externa (GPe) and globus pallidus internus (GPi). The GP can be localized just below the level of the

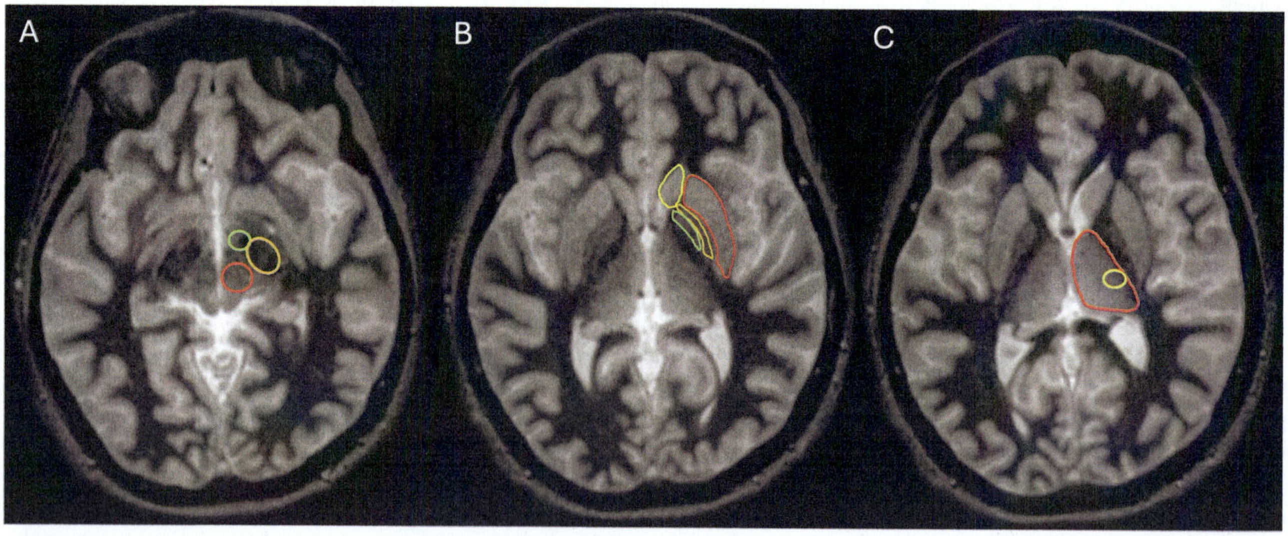

FIGURE 34.1 Relevant anatomy for DBS. These are axial MRI FGATIR sequence slices. A) Red – red nucleus, orange – substantia nigra, green – subthalamic nucleus. B) Red – putamen, orange – globus pallidus externus, green – globus pallidus internus, yellow – caudate. C) Red – thalamus, yellow – ventral intermediate nucleus.

commissural plane, medial to the putamen and lateral to the internal capsule. The GPe and GPi are separated by the medial medullary lamina with the GPe being slightly larger and located more laterally next to the putamen. The STN is a small lens-shaped nucleus which makes up a majority of the subthalamus. The STN is located ventral to the thalamus, medial to the internal capsule, and dorsal to the midbrain and substantia nigra. Within these basal ganglia structures, the STN and GPi are most targeted for treatment.

The thalamus contains multiple subregions, most important to movement disorders being the ventral intermediate (VIM), ventral anterior (VA), and ventrolateral (VL) nuclei. The VIM nucleus is a wedge-shaped nucleus within the thalamus and has been specifically targeted for tremor management. Of these nuclei, the VIM is most targeted for movement disorder treatment. This target lies within the dentatorubrothalamic tract, a white matter tract connecting the primary motor cortex to the cerebellar dentate nucleus via the red nucleus and VIM that is implicated in motor coordination and control [18].

Stereotactic procedures, like DBS, use a Cartesian system of coordinates originating at the midcommissural point, halfway between the anterior commissure and posterior commissure that border the third ventricle, such that X values denote distance from the mid-commissural point in the coronal plane, Y values in the sagittal plane and Z values in the axial plane. Each target can be indirectly targeted using typical coordinates which rely on the region's location relative to known and readily visible structures. Direct targeting relies on detailed visualization of the brain region or white matter tract of interest.

Procedure

Diagnosis

ICD 10 Codes of movement disorder diagnoses for which DBS is indicated include: G20 (Parkinson's disease), G24 (dystonia) and G25 (essential tremor).

Indications

Current movement disorder indications for DBS include medically refractory motor-predominant PD, essential tremor, and primary generalized dystonia. DBS can be used off-label to treat other movement disorders including Tourette syndrome and Huntington's disease, secondary dystonia and dystonic disorders such as Meige syndrome, as well as tremors unrelated to ET or PD including Holmes tremor.

Patient selection

Age, contraindications, maintenance concerns

Ideally, patients with movement disorders should be first evaluated by a neurologist to establish the etiology of the patient's symptoms and confirm a diagnosis. Once formally diagnosed with a movement disorder, patients should be first treated with medical therapy. If they are deemed to be refractory to medical treatment or have a significant side-effect profile that limits further titration of medications and they have predominant and disabling motor symptoms, they should be considered for DBS. Prior to surgical evaluation, patients complete extensive testing including motor and gait testing on and off medication. Preoperative assessments with neuropsychiatrists are routinely performed to assess for cognitive impairment and mood or behavioral disorders which may disqualify patients from surgery. To safely undergo surgery, patients should be in good medical health with optimized medical comorbidities prior to DBS. While there is no age limitation for DBS consideration, careful consideration of surgical risk and potential cognitive implications must be weighed in the elderly population. Studies have demonstrated that DBS is both safe and effective in PD patients 75 and older and opens the door for more laxity in age criteria [19,20]. Following these considerations, a critical step in improving patient outcomes is managing expectations and educating patients on which symptoms are likely to improve (tremor, bradykinesia, rigidity), their expected degree of improvement (70%–80%), and any anticipated side-effects from the surgery or stimulation (paresthesias, dysarthria, ataxia) [21].

DBS can be considered in patients who have idiopathic primary PD with a primary motor component, at least 30% improvement in motor scores on levodopa medication, and disabling side-effects associated with levodopa and all other medical therapies. Patients with significant motor symptoms to their PD including tremor, rigidity, bradykinesia, dyskinesias or motor fluctuations are favorable candidates for DBS. This procedure is contraindicated in patients experiencing symptoms consistent with atypical parkinsonism, PD dementia, or severe psychological symptoms including depression or psychosis. Because of these relatively strict criteria, many patients have had longstanding disease duration and progression prior to surgical referral. However, there have been recent studies which support that early consideration of DBS is also effective and should be considered in select patients [22].

In ET, patients optimal for surgery are those who relay significant disruptions in their daily living and social embarrassment due to their symptoms. Only approximately 50% of patients respond to medications like propranolol or primidone and others experience significant side-effects leading to inability to uptitrate the medication or discontinuation of medication altogether [23,24]. DBS can be considered in these patients with medically refractory essential tremor.

Dystonia is subcategorized into primary dystonia and secondary dystonia. Primary dystonia is defined a disorder in which dystonia is caused in the absence of any structural lesion or neuropathological processes and is often associated with genetic causes [25]. Secondary dystonia on the other hand refers to dystonia with an identifiable neuropathological lesion or cause. DBS is generally most often considered effective for primary dystonia due to significant improvements in symptomology, as opposed to secondary dystonia. DBS can successfully treat secondary dystonia; however, the clinical improvements are generally not as profound and may not be as consistent as with primary dystonia [26]. Similar to the other disorders, dystonia patients should be considered for DBS when refractory to medical treatments including botulin toxin therapy and the symptom severity outweighs the surgical risks.

All DBS patients must be amenable to living with an implanted device and be responsible for following up regularly with their providers for programming sessions and surgical replacements of IPGs.

Training recommendations

To safely and effectively perform DBS, neurosurgeons trained in the United States must complete a 7-year neurosurgical residency program accredited by the Accreditation Council for Graduate Medical Education. Within this timeframe, neurosurgeon trainees must gain exposure to performing a minimum of at least 10 cases to treat a functional movement disorder, although most programs exceed this case requirement. Neurosurgeons choosing to focus on the subspecialty of functional neurosurgery in their practice may choose to pursue a 1-year post-graduate fellowship in stereotactic and functional fellowship programs accredited by the Committee on Accreditation of Subspecialty Training. These programs provide training under board-certified functional neurosurgeons where fellows learn the nuances of a variety of functional procedures including the surgical treatment of movement disorders, epilepsy, pain and psychiatric disorders. Trainees become board certified by the American Board of Neurological Surgeons upon completion of both the written and oral components of the examination, typically completed within 3–5 years of graduation from training.

Technique

While each institution may have variations to the surgical procedure based on the stereotactic system used and surgeon preference, DBS surgery is generally performed in two stages: 1) electrode placement and 2) implantation of extension wires and IPG. Prior to surgery, patients complete a thin-cut MRI and CT of the brain for surgical planning in a planning software program. Care is taken to precisely target the most effective area within the target region, enter within a gyrus and avoid any blood vessels along the trajectory. Electrode implantation can be completed with the patient awake to perform intraoperative testing such as microelectrode recording or test stimulation or can be performed with the patient asleep under general anesthesia. Once in the operating room, the patient is positioned supine or seated, their head is affixed to the stereotactic system and incisions are marked based on the pre-operative plan. The patient's head is prepped and draped in usual sterile fashion and local anesthetic is injected. Incisions are made with a blade and electrocautery to expose the skull. The entry point of the trajectory is again marked, and a burr hole is made with a high-speed drill centered around this entry point. A locking cap to hold the electrode in place is secured around the burr hole. The dura is then opened with a blade and bipolar cautery. A precise mechanical drive is typically used to advance a cannula through the brain to the planned target. At this point, microelectrode recordings can be performed by a neurophysiologist to evaluate local field potentials and multiunit activity within close proximity to the target, with relative increases and decreases in activity signifying entrance into and exit from the target of interest, respectively. It is also at this point that testing stimulation can be performed, with a provider evaluating changes in the patient's motor symptoms and any side effects related to stimulation. Once a final electrode position has been chosen, the electrode is passed down the cannula, the cannula is retreated, and the electrode is secured in place with a locking device. An intraoperative CT scan may be performed to visualize and confirm appropriate electrode placement as shown in Fig. 34.2. The ends of the electrodes are then tunneled to the parietal region of the side the IPG will be placed in stage two. Wounds are then sutured in a multilayer fashion. Operative time for a bilateral electrode placement is approximately 3–5 h.

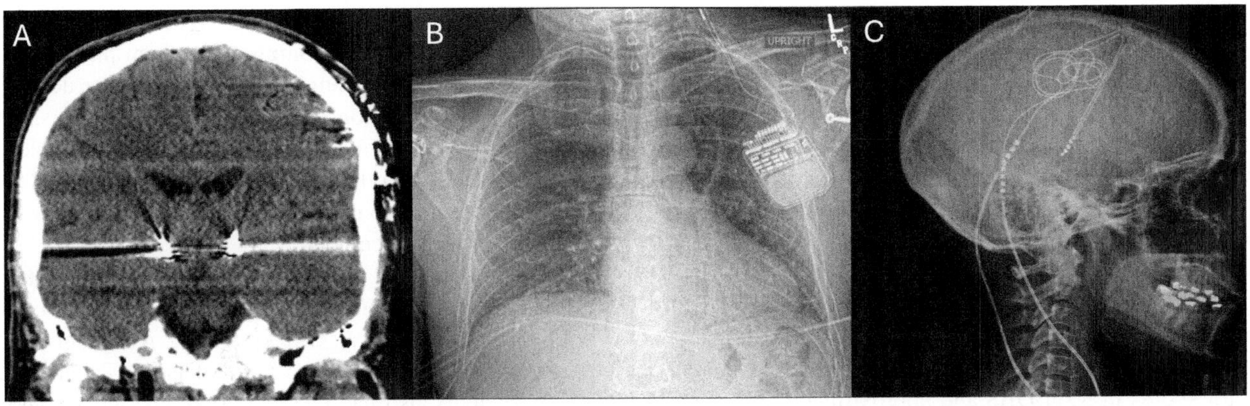

FIGURE 34.2 DBS hardware. A) CT scan demonstrating bilateral leads terminating in the STN. B) Chest X-ray demonstrating IPG device located in a subclavicular pocket connected to distal ends of extension wires. C) Lateral skull X-ray demonstrating bilateral intracranial electrodes and extension wires tunneled postauricularly.

During stage two, extension wires connecting the intracranial electrodes to the subclavicular IPG are implanted. Once under general anesthesia, the patient is laid supine with their head turned away from the side where the wiring will be tunneled and the chest pocket will be created for the device. Incisions are made in the posterior auricular region to locate the distal ends of the intracranial electrodes, and the upper chest wall to create a subcutaneous, suprafascial pocket for the device. A tunneler is passed from the posterior auricular region in the subgaleal plane, over the clavicle, down to the subcutaneous pocket and the extension wires are passed through the tunneler to connect the two sites. The extension wires are connected to the intracranial electrodes and inserted into the IPG which is placed into the pocket. An impedance check is performed by a device representative, confirming impedances within normal range prior to closing all incisions in a multilayer fashion. Figure 34.2 highlights the final placement of these devices. Operative time for stage two is approximately 1–1.5 h.

Post operative considerations

After stage one, patients will generally stay at least one night at the hospital for close monitoring with strict blood pressure control to ensure their pain is adequately controlled on oral medications and that they are able to eat, void and ambulate prior to discharge. Stage two is an outpatient procedure and patients are discharged the same day as surgery. While rare, hemorrhage, infection, peri-lead edema, and acute neurological changes can occur perioperatively with reported rates ranging from 1%–5% [27,28]. Images of these complications are shown in Fig. 34.3. Once both stages are completed, patients are instructed to avoid strenuous activity and lifting more than 8–10lb for approximately 2–4 weeks until the incisions heal. Beyond that timeframe, patients can resume normal activity. The system will generally be turned on and

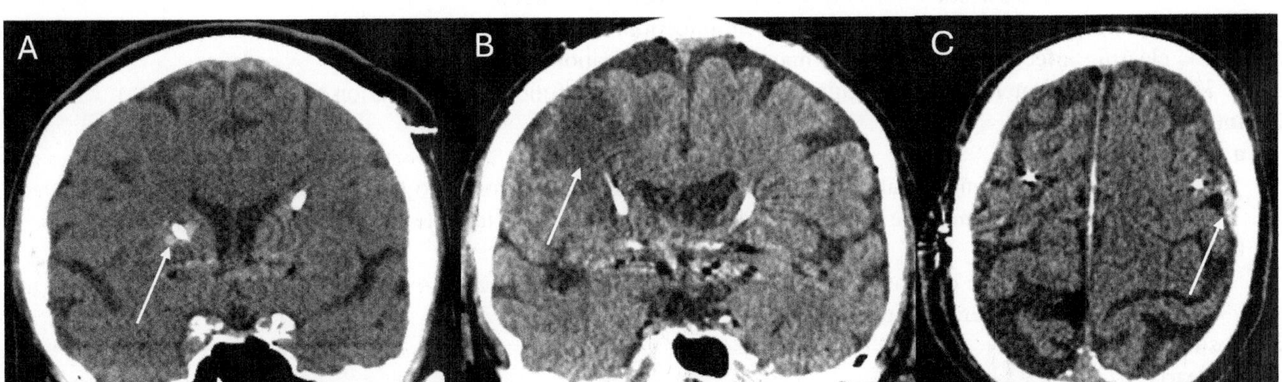

FIGURE 34.3 Complications from DBS. These are non-contrasted CT scans in coronal orientation (A/B) and axial (C) orientations. A) Tract hemorrhage around lead, B) Peri-lead edema, C) Subdural hematoma at site of lead insertion.

programmed approximately 4 weeks after implantation in the outpatient clinic. Prior to device programming, some patients may experience transient improvements in their symptoms which is due to the lesioning effect from placement of the electrodes. However, these effects will subside and patients should continue to their medication until the device is programmed and activated, after which their dosing may be adjusted at the discretion of the neurology providers. Programming sessions with a movement disorder neurology provider occur over several monthly appointments in order to establish the most appropriate settings to maximize symptoms improvement and minimize stimulation-induced side effects. Non-rechargeable IPGs have a battery life of approximately 5–7 years prior to requiring surgical replacement, with rechargeable IPGs lasting approximately 15 years prior to requiring surgical replacement.

Most DBS patients experience significant improvements in motor symptoms and continue to have durable benefits for many years after surgery. For PD, patients treated with DBS had greater improvement in motor scores, quality of life metrics, and fewer side-effects as compared to patients treated with only medicine [29]. One systematic review of all PD studies reported that patients experienced approximately 50% improvement on Unified Parkinson's Disease Rating Scale motor scores in STN DBS and approximately 30% in GPi DBS [30]. Patients also had reduced dopaminergic medicines with STN DBS and significant improvements in depression scores [31]. These effects are durable with one study demonstrating continued clinical improvements and reduction in dopaminergic drugs at 15 years post-implantation [32]. For ET, patients experienced significant improvements in motor symptoms with few side effects which lasted at least six to 7 years post-implantation [33]. Specifically, unilateral DBS demonstrated 53%–63% improvements and bilateral DBS demonstrated greater improvements at 66%–78% in both the Essential Tremor Rating Assessment Scale and Fahn-Tolosa-Marin scale [34]. For dystonia, DBS treatment yielded meaningful improvements in movement symptoms, disability, and overall quality of life metrics for all types of dystonia with improvements of up to 90% on the Global Dystonia Scale [26,35]. However, one meta-analysis demonstrated greater efficacy and less side-effects in primary dystonia as compared to secondary dystonia [26].

Pearls and Pitfalls

1. Preoperative
   a. Pearls:
      i. Patient selection is key as well as setting expectations for the benefits therapy can provide
      ii. Must counsel that this is not a cure – the underlying disorder still exists and is progressive, but stimulation settings can be tailored to address recurrence of symptoms
      iii. Informative pamphlets or packets may be helpful to provide detailed information for patients that they can reference after the pre-operative appointment
      iv. Consider patient lifestyle factors in decision to pursue surgery and target/device selection (discuss goals of surgery, rechargeable vs. non-rechargeable battery, laterality of battery)
      v. Need to have high quality pre-operative imaging for planning, may consider obtaining under anesthesia to limit movement
   b. Pitfalls:
      i. Need thorough evaluations of cognitive status and other medical comorbidities, delay surgery if any concern or further work up needed – it is truly a purely elective procedure
      ii. If patients have a history of prior or recent infection, consider infectious disease consultation given difficulty of clearing infection with a device (may require explanation if severe)
      iii. Avoid antiplatelet or anticoagulant use perioperatively (follow any institution specific guidelines)
2. Intraoperative
   a. Pearls
      i. Intraoperative testing is valuable, but is time consuming and costly so these factors must be weighed
      ii. Patient must be amenable if doing awake surgery and able to tolerate it
   b. Pitfalls:
      i. 1–2 mm can be the difference between good or suboptimal benefit, so if lead is found to be off planned trajectory on intraoperative imaging, consider revising
3. Postoperative
   a. Pearls:
      ii. Obtain post-operative CT head to evaluate for hemorrhage
      iii. Ensure patients have adequate support at home after electrode implantation
      iv. Inform details about proper wound care

   - **v.** Track patient outcomes to ensure effectiveness of surgical and programming method
   - **vi.** Ensure patient regularly follows up at programming visit and when surgical replacement of IPG is needed
   - **b.** Pitfalls
     - **i.** Proper counseling about limiting activity for 2–4 weeks post-operatively
     - **ii.** Proper timing of restarting blood thinning medications (resume 5–7 days post-operation)

4. Scope related
   - **a.** Pearls
     - **i.** Use evidence-based support when counseling as able, particularly for off-label uses
     - **ii.** Stay up to date with new indications and recent literature in order to apply most up to date knowledge to patient care
     - **iii.** Be aware of new devices/technology that could aid in surgery
   - **b.** Pitfalls:
     - **i.** Use caution when considering DBS for uncommon or rarely studied indications
     - **ii.** Counsel patients appropriately with guarded expectations and appropriate assessment of risk

References

[1] Hartmann CJ, et al. An update on best practice of deep brain stimulation in Parkinson's disease. Ther Adv Neurol Disord 2019;12. 1756286419838096.

[2] Iorio-Morin C, Fomenko A, Kalia SK. Deep-brain stimulation for essential tremor and other tremor syndromes: A narrative review of current targets and clinical outcomes. Brain Sci 2020;10(12).

[3] Rodrigues FB, et al. Deep brain stimulation for dystonia. Cochrane Database Syst Rev 2019;1(1). CD012405.

[4] Delaloye S, Holtzheimer PE. Deep brain stimulation in the treatment of depression. Dialogues Clin Neurosci 2014;16(1):83–91.

[5] Mar-Barrutia L, et al. Deep brain stimulation for obsessive-compulsive disorder: A systematic review of worldwide experience after 20 years. World J Psychiatry 2021;11(9):659–80.

[6] Hariz MI, Blomstedt P, Zrinzo L. Deep brain stimulation between 1947 and 1987: The untold story. Neurosurg Focus 2010;29(2):E1.

[7] Guiot G. [Treatment of parkinsonian syndromes by destruction of internal pallidum]. Neurochirurgia 1958;1(1):94–8.

[8] Sem-Jacobsen CW. Depth electrographic stimulation and treatment of patients with Parkinson's disease including neurosurgical technique. Acta Neurol Scand Suppl 1965;13(Pt 1):365–77.

[9] Albe-Fessard D. Electrophysiological methods for the identification of thalamic nuclei. Z Neurol 1973;205(1):15–28.

[10] Cavallieri F, Mulroy E, Moro E. The history of deep brain stimulation. Parkinsonism Relat Disord 2024;121:105980.

[11] Paulo DL, et al. Intraoperative physiology augments atlas-based data in awake deep brain stimulation. J Neurol Neurosurg Psychiatry 2023;95 (1):86–96.

[12] Sudhyadhom A, et al. A high resolution and high contrast MRI for differentiation of subcortical structures for DBS targeting: the Fast Gray Matter Acquisition T1 Inversion Recovery (FGATIR). Neuroimage 2009;47(Suppl. 2):T44–52.

[13] Henderson JM. "Connectomic surgery": diffusion tensor imaging (DTI) tractography as a targeting modality for surgical modulation of neural networks. Front Integr Neurosci 2012;6:15.

[14] Lim ML, et al. Awake versus asleep anesthesia in deep brain stimulation surgery for Parkinson's disease: A systematic review and meta-analysis. Stereotact Funct Neurosurg 2024;102(3):141–55.

[15] Huang Z, et al. Efficacy and safety of robot-assisted deep brain stimulation for Parkinson's disease: A meta-analysis. Front Aging Neurosci 2024;16:1419152.

[16] Timmermann L, et al. Multiple-source current steering in subthalamic nucleus deep brain stimulation for Parkinson's disease (the VANTAGE study): A non-randomised, prospective, multicentre, open-label study. Lancet Neurol 2015;14(7):693–701.

[17] Jahanshahi A, Mai JK, Temel Y. Anatomy of targets for deep brain stimulation. In: Temel Y, et al., editors. Fundamentals and clinics of deep brain stimulation: An interdisciplinary approach. Cham: Springer International Publishing; 2020. p. 15–28.

[18] Middlebrooks EH, et al. Neuroimaging advances in deep brain stimulation: Review of indications, anatomy, and brain connectomics. AJNR Am J Neuroradiol 2020;41(9):1558–68.

[19] Charles PD, et al. Deep brain stimulation in early Parkinson's disease: Enrollment experience from a pilot trial. Parkinsonism Relat Disord 2012;18 (3):268–73.

[20] Jiang C, et al. Short- and long-term efficacy and safety of deep-brain stimulation in Parkinson's disease patients aged 75 years and older. Brain Sci 2022;12(11).

[21] Knoop CD, et al. Bridging the gaps in patient education for DBS surgery in Parkinson's disease2017. Parkinsons Dis; 2017. p. 9360354.

[22] Hacker ML, et al. Deep brain stimulation in early-stage Parkinson disease: Five-year outcomes. Neurology 2020;95(4):e393–401.

[23] Krishnan S, et al. Deep brain stimulation for movement disorders. Neurol India 2018;66(Suppl. ment):S90–101.

[24] Zesiewicz TA, et al. Practice parameter: therapies for essential tremor: Report of the quality standards subcommittee of the American academy of neurology. Neurology 2005;64(12):2008–20.

[25] Tanabe LM, et al. Primary dystonia: Molecules and mechanisms. Nat Rev Neurol 2009;5(11):598–609.

[26] Fan H, et al. Deep brain stimulation treating dystonia: A systematic review of targets, body distributions and etiology classifications. Front Hum Neurosci 2021;15:757579.
[27] Chen T, et al. Complication rates, lengths of stay, and readmission rates in "awake" and "asleep" deep brain simulation. J Neurosurg 2017;127 (2):360–9.
[28] Revell MA. Deep brain stimulation for movement disorders. Nurs Clin North Am 2015;50(4):691–701.
[29] Schuepbach WM, et al. Neurostimulation for Parkinson's disease with early motor complications. N Engl J Med 2013;368(7):610–22.
[30] Lachenmayer ML, et al. Subthalamic and pallidal deep brain stimulation for Parkinson's disease-meta-analysis of outcomes. npj Parkinson's Dis 2021;7(1):77.
[31] Mansouri A, et al. Deep brain stimulation for Parkinson's disease: Meta-analysis of results of randomized trials at varying lengths of follow-up. J Neurosurg 2018;128(4):1199–213.
[32] Bove F, et al. Long-term outcomes (15 Years) after subthalamic nucleus deep brain stimulation in patients with Parkinson disease. Neurology 2021;97(3):e254–62.
[33] Rehncrona S, et al. Long-term efficacy of thalamic deep brain stimulation for tremor: Double-blind assessments. Mov Disord 2003;18(2):163–70.
[34] Dallapiazza RF, et al. Outcomes from stereotactic surgery for essential tremor. J Neurol Neurosurg Psychiatry 2019;90(4):474–82.
[35] Kamel WA, et al. Surgical management for dystonia: Efficacy of deep brain stimulation in the long term. Neurol Int 2021;13(3):371–86.

Chapter 35

Deep brain stimulation—Major depressive disorder and other neuropsychiatric circuit pathologies

Jayunkumar Shah[1], Daniel Cummins[2] and Brian Harris Kopell[3]

[1]Center for Neuromodulation, The Icahn School of Medicine at Mount Sinai, New York, NY, United States; [2]Department of Neurosurgery, The Icahn School of Medicine at Mount Sinai, New York, NY, United States; [3]Center of Neuromodulation, Neurology, Psychiatry, and Neuroscience, The Icahn School of Medicine at Mount Sinai, New York, NY, United States

Introduction

Deep brain stimulation (DBS) is a surgical procedure in which electrodes are placed in specific anatomical targets of the brain to modulate neural networks through electrical stimulation. Before DBS, ablative procedures were the dominant surgical method to address neuropsychiatric conditions. However, these methods are irreversible and static. DBS, by contrast, is reversible and modifiable. One of the unmet needs in medical practice is the treatment of therapy-resistant neuropsychiatric diseases. For example, according to World Health Organization (WHO), approximately 280 million people worldwide and 21 million people in the United States suffer from major depression. Every year, more than 700,000 people die due to suicide, which is the fourth leading cause of death in the 15–29 year age group. Approximately 30% of patients with major depression and 20%–60% of patients with obsessive-compulsive disorder (OCD) are drug-resistant [1]. For the last 20 years, DBS has been explored for treating various drug-resistant neuropsychiatric disorders, with the majority of reported cases being for Major Depressive Disorder (MDD), OCD, and Tourette syndrome.

The first modern use of DBS in neuropsychiatric disorders was reported in 1999 by Nuttin et al. [2] in four patients with severe drug-resistant OCD, with DBS targeted at the anterior limb of internal capsule (ALIC). Three of the four patients had beneficial effects. Ultimately, this work led to the US Food and Drug Administration granting a Humanitarian Device Exemption for DBS for treatment-resistant OCD in 2009 [3]. Since then, multiple case reports and trials have been published for DBS in Treatment-Resistant Depression (TRD), OCD, and Tourette syndrome. A smaller number of case reports have been published using DBS to treat schizophrenia and posttraumatic stress disorder (PTSD). While preliminary, these initial reports provide a robust foundation for future explorations.

Anatomy

While much work has explored the functional anatomy of neuropsychiatric disorders, the largest share of the literature has focused on treatment-resistant depression (TRD). Much of the relevant anatomy for TRD is also shared with other neuropsychiatric conditions, which may be treated by DBS, including OCD and Tourette syndrome. On functional neuroimaging studies, Mayberg and colleagues have found that depression is associated with increased activity in the subcallosal cingulate cortex (SCC) and decreased activity in prefrontal cortex, which reverses during recovery from major depressive episodes [4]. Other authors have confirmed that increased metabolism has been found in cortical regions including the orbitofrontal, anterior insular, and SCC, while decreased metabolism in the dorsolateral prefrontal cortex (DLPFC) during depression [5]. Beyond the involvement of these cortical regions alone in neuropsychiatric conditions, a strong role has been found in connectivity between cortical structures and subcortical structures such as the basal ganglia and thalamus. Modulation of neural loops involving these structures therefore plays a vital role in treating

A Modern Atlas for Implantable Devices of the Spine, Brain, and Nerve. https://doi.org/10.1016/B978-0-443-36528-7.00032-7

neuropsychiatric disorders [6]. The following loops have been identified as playing a prominent role in neuropsychiatric conditions, and have been focuses of DBS for treatment:

(1) *Thalamocortical (TC) and Cortico-striato-thalamo-cortical (CSTC) loops*—As the name suggests, the TC loops are defined by widespread reciprocal connections between the cortex and thalamus. Cortical areas involved in TC loops are deeply involved in modulating sensory, motor and cognitive information, which is transferred to the thalamus and then back to cortical areas [7]. The CSTC loops are a more complex pathway, which further involve the basal ganglia (striatum) as a modulator between cortical and thalamic connections. In the CSTC, striatal structures of the caudate and nucleus accumbens (NAc) act as input, while the globus pallidus interna (GPi) and substantia nigra (SNr) act as output nuclei in a closed-loop manner. Among the CSTC loops, data from functional neuroimaging suggests that the limbic and prefrontal loops are the most important for psychiatric diseases [8].

(2) *Dorsolateral Prefrontal loop*—Dorsolateral prefrontal cortex (DLPFC) and orbitofrontal cortex (OFC) have separate reciprocal projections to the basal ganglia. These structures project to specific thalamic nuclei including the ventral anterior thalamic and dorsomedial thalamic nuclei, which ultimately project back to the DLPFC and OFC. This loop has a predominant role in memory and executive function, and dysfunction leads to loss of insight and inability to suppress negative feelings associated with neuropsychiatric conditions [6].

(3) *Limbic loop*—Medial orbitofrontal cortex and anterior cingulate cortex project to the ventromedial striatum through the anterior limb of the internal capsule and then onto the dorsomedial nucleus of the thalamus. This loop also receives reciprocal connections from thalamus [6].

One lens through which to see the role DBS plays in the treatment of these disorders comes from biophysical and in vitro neurophysiological data on the effects of extracellular electrical stimulation in the brain. As much of the functional anatomy of these disorders involves connections between cortical and subcortical structures, targeting the anatomical connections between regions may explain the efficacy of DBS. Biophysically, the dominant element of the neural structure affected by DBS is the axon/fiber of passage [9]. First order axons can generate axon potentials responsively to DBS-type stimulation on a 1:1 basis [10]. However, ultimately synaptic transmission fails due to neurotransmitter depletion at the downstream synapto-dendritic junctions. DBS, therefore, can be conceptualized as an initiating desynchronization event, removing attractor state dynamics from a circuit entrained in pathological synchronous activity. Ultimately, the true "therapeutic" effects of DBS may require behaviorally (or other therapeutical) reinforced activities to harness the neuroplasticity of the remaining circuits.

Neuropsychiatric disorder indications for DBS

Major depressive disorder

Major depressive disorder (MDD is a common psychiatric illness affecting 6% of the population per year worldwide and may affect one in six adults in their lifetime [11]. The cardinal symptoms are depressed mood and anhedonia. To fit a diagnosis of MDD, a patient must experience the core symptoms plus at least five of the following last at least 2 weeks: increase or decrease in sleep, decreased energy, decreased concentration, executive dysfunction, memory deficit, feeling worthlessness, suicidal thoughts or psychomotor symptoms. The severity of MDD is clinically measured using Hamilton Depression Rating Scale (HDRS) and Montgomery-Asberg Depression Rating Scale (MADRS), wherein an HDRS >23 or MADRDS >34 is considered severe depression.

First line treatments for MDD are medications, psychotherapy or a combination of two. Approximately 30% of patients have refractory symptoms, or treatment-resistant depression (TRD) [12]. There is no consensus definition of TRD. However, the definition adopted by the U.S Food and Drug Administration [13] is failure to respond to at least two antidepressant treatments despite adequate dose, duration and adherence to treatment. This group of patients with TRD may be candidates for DBS therapy. DBS has not yet been approved by the FDA or any other major regulatory agency for the treatment of TRD [14]. Open label studies and meta-analyses have reported positive outcomes in a segment of patients treated with DBS for TRD, but randomized-controlled trials have shown mixed results. Apart from DBS, vagus nerve stimulation (VNS) is an alternative FDA-approved treatment for MDD, which has shown beneficial effect [15].

Patient selection criteria

Predicting with patients with TRD will respond well to DBS has been a clinical challenge in preliminary trials. Usual criteria for inclusion are—(1) Severe MDD (as described above) averaged over 4 weeks period (2) Substantial functional impairment defined by Global Assessment of Functioning Score ≤50 [16] (3) Current episode lasting at least 12 months.

(4) Failure of at least four adequate antidepressant treatments, defined as >3 on antidepressant treatment including documented ECT (Electroconvulsive Therapy) failure or intolerance, and (5) Low risk of suicide [14]. Absolute contraindications for DBS in depression have not been defined. However relative contraindications may include severe anxiety, acute psychotic episode, personality disorders, suicidal ideations and cognitive impairment.

Target

Subgenual cingulate cortex (SCC, Brodmann's area 25) has been the most studied target and was the first target used in humans for depression [17], where four out of six patients had clinical benefit. The second most commonly studied target is VC (Ventral Capsule)/VS (ventral striatum), also called the ventral anterior limb of internal capsule (vALIC). This region includes the Nucleus Accumbens (NAcc) [18]. Other less commonly studied DBS targets for depression are the medial forebrain bundle—superolateral branch [19], lateral habenula, inferior thalamic peduncle, and the bed nucleus of stria terminalis [20–22].

Of note, modern work has demonstrated that patient-specific connectivity may dictate the optimal target for DBS in depression, rather than generalized anatomical regions. When the SCC target was selected based on tractography involving white fibers from forceps minor, cingulum bundle, uncinate fasciculus and frontostriatal fibers, it significantly improves clinical outcome [23]. Several distinct anatomical targets may be interconnected, and modulating activity of one target might influence the entire behavioral circuitry involving affective networks, reward networks, cognitive networks, and somatomotor networks, which are all involved in the pathophysiological basis of depression [14].

Clinical outcome

A meta-analysis by Reddy et al. suggested that the long-term response and remission rates were 48% and 35%, respectively, with time to reach 50% improvement around 23 months, and the anatomical target having no significant effect on outcome [24]. Open trials reported significantly greater improvement than RCTs [24,25]. However few sham-controlled trials do not report improvement over placebo [26,27], possibly due to lack of tractography-based anatomical targeting, patient selection, and study design. An ongoing RCT will better define the clinical outcome and other parameters for DBS in MDD. Use of biomarkers to objectively quantify the depressive state and its implications in programming DBS, as well as its correlation to tractographic analysis, would further improve clinical outcome by redefining the approach to TRD patients with DBS [28].

Obsessive-compulsive disorder (OCD)

OCD is a neuropsychiatric condition characterized by the presence of persistent intrusive thoughts, images or urges (obsessions) that lead to compulsions, repetitive mental or motor acts, or avoidance behaviors, in order to reduce anxiety [29]. Approximately 50% patients with OCD experience onset of symptoms in childhood or adolescence [30]. The prevalence of OCD is 1.8% in children [31] and 1.2% in adults [32]. As described previously, the CSTC loop is the main circuit implicated in OCD, as supported by functional imaging data [5]. The severity of OCD is measured by Yale-Brown Obsessive Compulsive Scale (Y-BOCS) [33], with scores of >34 classified as severe [34].

The standard treatments for OCD are selective serotonin reuptake inhibitors (SSRIs) along with cognitive behavioral therapy (CBT), particularly exposure and response prevention (ERP). Despite best medical management and CBT, approximately only 20% of patients achieve remission after long-term follow up of 10–20 years, which suggests a high disease burden in the population [35]. Deep transcranial magnetic stimulation (dTMS) targeted to the medial prefrontal cortex and anterior cingulate cortex has shown good efficacy in patients who are nonresponders to medications and CBT [36]. A meta-analysis done by Kisley et al. showed partial remission achieved in significant number of patients treated with dTMS compared with a sham control [37]. DBS is a further option in refractory OCD, as studies have consistently reported that approximately 60% of patients can achieve reductions of >35% on Y-BOCS, marking a clinically significant improvement [38].

Patient selection criteria

The criteria set by the FDA for DBS in OCD under a humanitarian device exemption is as follow-age ≥18 years, severe OCD symptoms (Y-BOCS ≥30), symptoms duration of more than 5 years, comorbid depression and anxiety but no other psychiatric disorders or substance abuse, failure to at least three SSRIs (selective serotonin reuptake inhibitors) and CBT, no other neurological disorders such as dementia, nonpregnant, no bleeding disorder or blood thinners, target of stimulation is not destroyed by previous brain surgery and without serious medical illness including cardiovascular diseases, hepatic or renal failure, diabetes mellitus [39]. Most studies have considered disease duration of 5 years and Y-BOCS scale >28 as inclusion criteria, in addition to failure to respond to three medications, an adequate CBT trial (20 sessions), and significantly impaired functioning [40].

Target

The most common anatomical target of DBS for OCD is the anterior limb of the internal capsule (ALIC). The first case of ALIC DBS for OCD was published by Nuttin et al. based on their previous experience with capsulotomy in the same region [2]. ALIC stimulation would modulate the activities of DLPFC, OFC and various basal ganglia and thalamic structures, which in essence affecting the limbic and prefrontal circuits. Nucleus Accumbens (NAc), which is the ventral most part of ALIC, was used as target for OCD by Sturm et al., considering its proximity to the amygdaloid complex and basal ganglia and its connections to thalamus, prefrontal cortex. In their early series, NAc-DBS was associated with good clinical outcomes [41]. Bed nucleus of Stria terminalis (BNST) lies several millimeters posterior to NAc. All of these targets (ALIC, NAc, BNST) are encompassed by the larger region of the ventral capsule/ventral striatum (VC/VS). The STN, GPi and midbrain have also been used as targets of DBS for OCD, with variable outcomes [42]. There has been some suggestion that different anatomical targets may affect different components of OCD. For example, DBS of VC/VS achieves greater mood improvement than STN DBS, while DBS of anteromedial STN may particularly improve cognitive flexibility in OCD [43].

Clinical outcome

A Meta-analysis published by Mar-Barrutia et al. summarized the clinical outcomes of DBS for OCD in both the short term and long term. Clinical response was considered when Y-BOCS score reduced by >35%. Using this criteria, 70.7% patients responded in the long-term versus 60.6% in the short-term [44]. Patients responding to DBS had their maximum symptom reduction in first 12–14 months after implantation [45]. Further, the best response occurred when patients were engaged in simultaneous behavioral therapy. Data suggests three patterns of long-term response: 49.5% had good and sustained response, 26.6% were nonresponders, and 22.4% were partial responders. Most of the adverse effects were transient, with hypomania being the most common psychiatric side effect [44].

Tourette syndrome

Tourette syndrome (TS) is a neuropsychiatric disorder characterized by multiple motor tics plus one or more vocal tics, lasting longer than 1 year. The prevalence of TS is around 1%, and onset is usually around 6–8 years of age with peak of symptoms at 10–12 years. TS is frequently associated with OCD, attention deficit hyperactivity disorder (ADHD) and other psychiatric comorbidities [46].

The tic severity and tic impairment are measured by Yale Global Tic Severity Scale (YGTSS) [47] and its revised version [48], with a score >35 considered severe. The standard treatment of TS is psychosocial and behavior interventions. If tics cause subjective discomfort or social problems and do not respond to behavioral treatment, pharmacological treatment with typical or atypical antipsychotics can be used. Clonidine is the first choice in children [49].

Patient selection criteria

If tics from TS are severe enough to cause functional impairment and are resistant to behavioral and pharmacological measures, surgery can be considered. DBS is typically considered when YGTSS is > 35, disease is present for more than 5 years, and adequate treatment has been trialed including three different classes of medications [50].

Target

The pathophysiological basis for TS is within the previously described CSTC [51]. Meta-analysis studying the effect of DBS on various targets concluded that the four most commonly used DBS targets for TS include the centromedian nucleus–nucleus ventrooralis internus (CM-Voi) and the centromedian nucleus-parafascicular (CM-Pf) complexes of the thalamus, and the posteroventrolateral (pvIGPi) and the anteromedial portion of the globus pallidus internus (amGPi), which all resulted in significant reductions in YGTSS score [52]. GPi targets showed greater reduction in YGTSS score than thalamic targets [52].

Clinical outcome

DBS for TS is effective in appropriately selected patients. A meta-analysis showed that more than 60% of patients had symptom reduction of at least 50% over long-term follow up [52]. The effect of DBS for TS also increases over the duration of chronic therapy. As the studies included in meta-analysis of DBS for TS lack prospective, randomized evidence, future well designed RCTs will give more insight and confirm the efficacy of DBS for TS.

Pre-operative considerations

A multidisciplinary team comprising of a neurosurgeon, psychiatrist and neuropsychologist considers the appropriateness of DBS for the individual patient. The psychiatrist is the first contact for screening a patient and assesses the patient in detail based on severity scales, medication history, noninvasive/invasive procedural treatment history, and supportive therapies. When considered appropriate for surgical intervention, the neuropsychologist assesses cognitive function of all patients. Those with severe decline in function are considered inappropriate for surgery. Finally, the patient will see a neurosurgeon for consultation regarding surgery. At this point, preoperative counseling is done regarding the realistic expectations of the patient from surgery, possible complications, and relevant patient-specific medical and surgical considerations.

Preoperative workup

Apart from routine preoperative medical clearance for surgery, preoperative magnetic resonance imaging (MRI) under general anesthesia (to avoid any movement during MRI) is usually performed a few days before surgery. MRI sequences commonly used to localize the DBS target are fast gray matter acquisition T1 inversion recovery (FGATIR), quantitative susceptibility mapping (QSM), and diffusion weighted images (DWI). Diffusion weighted tractography is used to develop probabilistic or deterministic tractography, to map relevant white matter tracts and their junctions to localize the anatomical target. We prefer to use probabilistic tractography for many neuropsychiatric conditions. In DBS for depression, SCC localization is performed by targeting the junction of the forceps minor, cingulum bundle, uncinate fasciculus, and fronto-striatal fibers, as shown in Fig. 35.1. Recent data published by Figee et al. suggests that based on tractography analysis, stimulating this ALIC target involving fibers from VLPFC, VMPFC and midbrain (medial and lateral) gives significant reduction in Y-BOCS score for OCD patients [53]. We use tractography for ALIC target selection in DBS for OCD at the junction of these white fibers as shown in Fig. 35.2.

Target planning

Once preoperative imaging is obtained as above, the final target, entry point on the scalp, and the trajectory are selected to avoid critical brain structures, and so that maximum electrode contacts remain within the target.

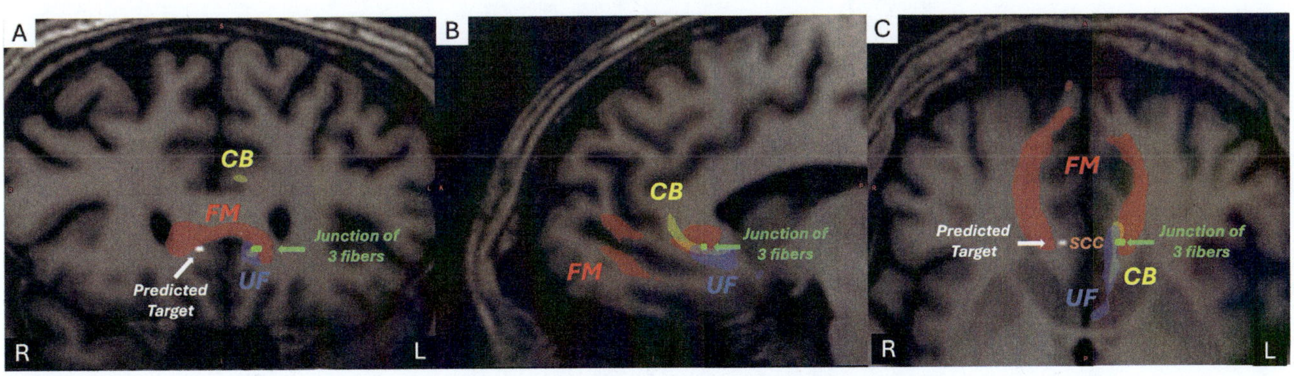

FIGURE 35.1 A, B, C (coronal, sagittal, and axial sections, respectively) show white matter fiber projections on probabilistic tractography analysis of the left hemisphere. Red-forceps minor, yellow-cingulum bundle, and blue-uncinate fasciculus. The predicted SCC target is marked as a green rectangle on the left side, which is the junction of these white matter fiber tracts. The corresponding right SCC target is marked as a small white rectangle in A and C. *CB*, cingulum bundle; *FM*, forceps minor; *SCC*, subcallosal cingulate cortex; *UF*, uncinate fasciculus. *Images provided by Dr Ki Sueng Choi, Associate Professor, Radiology and Neurosurgery, Nash Family Center for Advanced Circuit Therapeutics Biomedical Engineering and Imaging Institute, Icahn School of Medicine at Mount Sinai.*

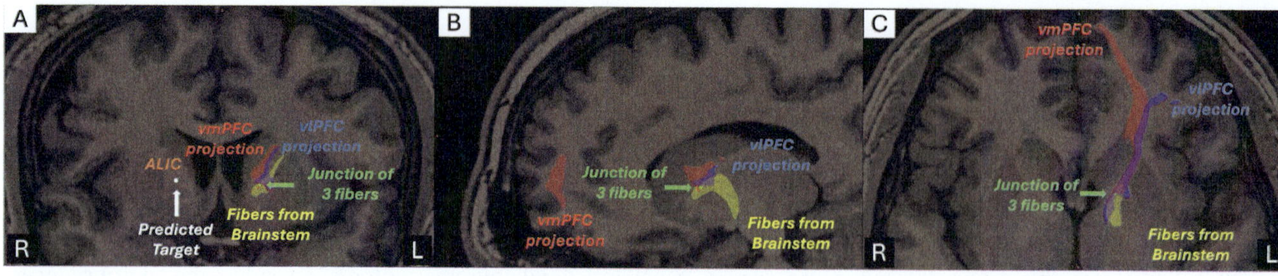

FIGURE 35.2 A, B, C (coronal, sagittal, and axial sections, respectively) show white matter fiber projections on probabilistic tractography analysis of the left hemisphere. Orange fibers-VMPFC projection, blue fibers—VLPFC projection, and yellow fibers-from the brainstem. The ALIC target is marked as a green dot on the left side, which is the junction of these white matter fibers. The corresponding right ALIC target is marked with a white dot in A. *ALIC*, anterior limb of internal capsule; *vlPFC*, ventrolateral prefrontal cortex; *vmPFC*, ventromedial prefrontal cortex. *Images provided by Dr Ki Sueng Choi, Associate Associate Professor, Radiology and Neurosurgery, Nash Family Center for Advanced Circuit Therapeutics Biomedical Engineering and Imaging Institute, Icahn School of Medicine at Mount Sinai.*

Surgical technique

Lead placement surgery can be done using several different operative techniques: (1) O-arm guidance, using an intraoperative CT scan; (2) MRI guidance, using an intraoperative MRI; and (3) ROSA (Robotized operating surgical assistant) guidance, with robot-guided placement. Published literature demonstrates good accuracy with all of these techniques [54–56]. DBS surgery can also be done in stages or as a single procedure. Many surgeons prefer to perform implantation in three stages, with lead placement on the left and right hemispheres performed three to four weeks apart, followed by battery implantation 1 week after. DBS implantation can also be done as a single procedure, with both hemispheres lead placements and battery placement as a single procedure. Data shows conflicting evidence in one strategy being superior over the other [57,58].

Positioning

Under transient sedation and local anesthesia at each pin site, a stereotactic headframe (Fig. 35.3) is rigidly fixed to the patient's skull through pins. Another option involves the use of "frameless" stereotactic systems. Once the frame is applied, the patient is moved to operating table, positioned supine. During the surgery, the operating table is kept in a beach chair position to increase venous return, leading to reduced intracranial pressure reduced likelihood of bleeding.

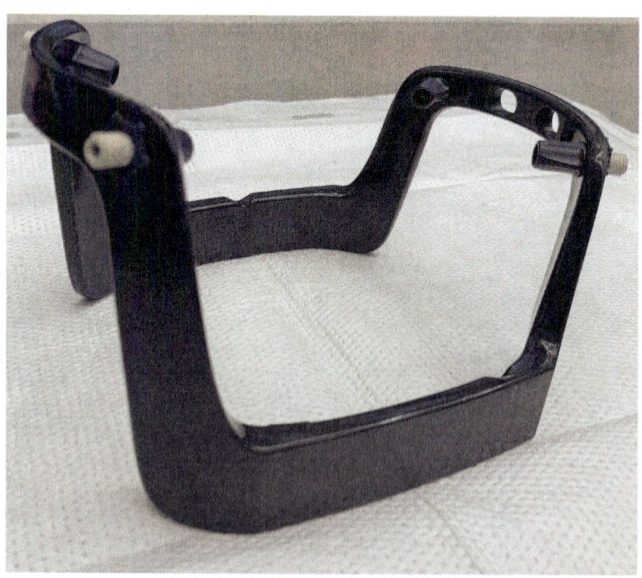

FIGURE 35.3 Leksell vantage stereotactic frame.

Anesthesia considerations

Lead placement surgeries can be performed under moderate sedation, so that patient is awake for intraoperative microelectrode recording and clinical examination, to confirm the lead position accuracy and possible side effects due to stimulation. When the patient is not cooperative or particularly anxious, or if the procedure is done under MRI guidance, general anesthesia is preferred. During the procedure, especially when passing the cannula into the brain, the systolic blood pressure is kept <120 mm Hg. Ceftriaxone and Vancomycin are given as preoperative prophylaxis 30 min before incision.

Equipment

The equipment necessary for DBS placement will be determined by the surgical methodology used. We focus on the O-arm guided system, which necessitates the O-Arm for intraoperative imaging (Fig. 35.4). Initially, the first acquired images from the O-arm are checked for accurate placement of the stereotactic frame with accepted accuracy of less than 0.3 mm. These initial O-Arm images are then fused to the preoperative MRI with previously planned trajectories to obtain the frame-based coordinates for placement using the Medtronic Stealth Station or similar software (Fig. 35.5). Many motorized automatic remote-control operated drives or manually operated drives are available for lead placement. The automatic or manual drive is used to advance the electrodes during DBS placement. Electrodes from Medtronic, Abbott and Boston Scientific having various spacing between contacts (0.5 mm/1.5 mm) are available with rechargeable and nonrechargeable batteries. Several advancements in electrode technology have occurred, such as directional leads that can direct electrical current, and bidirectional leads, which can record local brain activity as well as deliver therapeutic stimulation.

Procedure

Once the target coordinates are obtained intraoperatively, the incision is marked, and prepped and draped in sterile fashion. A burr hole is made through the skull, and the dura is opened to expose the brain. Then the brain cannula is advanced carefully, and a CT scan is obtained using the O-arm to check the catheter position in relation to target and intended trajectory, to assess for any deviation from the preoperative target. If there is any deviation, fine adjustment is done while inserting the DBS lead and again a CT scan is obtained using the O-arm for final lead position. At this point, clinical examination is done with therapeutic stimulation to assess for any side effects and clinical benefits. If this testing is satisfactory, the lead is secured, the burr hole is covered, and an X-ray is obtained to confirm that lead has not moved (Fig. 35.6). The other end of lead is then placed through a subcutaneous tunnel behind the ear for its later access to connect to the battery, which is later implanted in the chest. The usual duration of surgery is approximately 3 hours for a unilateral lead placement surgery.

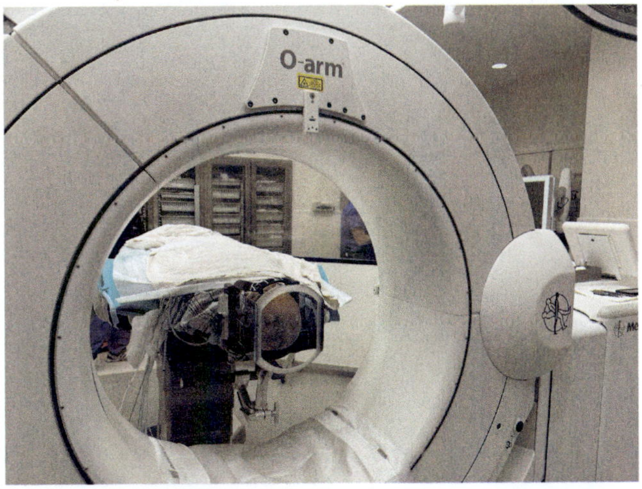

FIGURE 35.4 Medtronic O-arm with patient's head in the gantry.

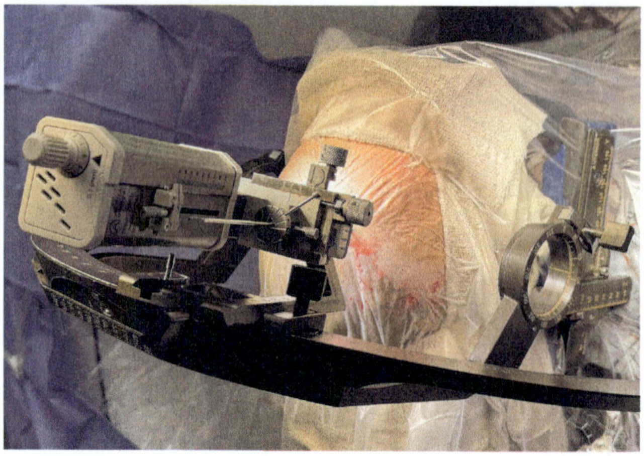

FIGURE 35.5 Leksell stereotactic frame with X,Y,Z coordinates and micromotor drive fixed to patient's head.

Postoperative considerations

As the DBS placement is done using moderate sedation, the patient wakes up relatively quickly, and is then brought to the postoperative anesthesia care unit, where systolic blood pressure is targeted below 130 mm Hg. A CT scan of the head is done to rule out any postoperative hemorrhage. The patient can resume all preoperative medications and goes home the next day. Two doses of intravenous antibiotics are given postoperatively. Patients are instructed to clean the wound every day and apply bacitracin ointment to the incision. At 1 week postoperatively, they undergo a wound check, and suture removal after 2 weeks. Patients are advised not to drink alcohol or drive for 2 weeks after each brain lead implantation, due to risk of seizures. Lifting of weight more than 10 lbs is avoided to prevent development of a hematoma at the implantable pulse generator (IPG) implantation site.

The IPG of the DBS system is typically implanted in the right side of the chest wall, with an incision below the clavicle. An incision at the anterior axillary line can also be used to put the IPG under the pectoralis muscle, which gives a better cosmetic outcome.

The DBS programming starts usually 2 weeks after IPG placement by an experienced psychiatrist familiar with programming. Regular follow up with the psychiatrist occurs with periodic medication and stimulation parameter adjustments, based on clinical improvement and potential side effects. In addition to psychiatric care, neurosurgical follow up occurs at 1, 3 and 12 months postoperatively, and then yearly. After surgery, adjunctive therapies, such as exposure and response prevention (ERP) for OCD, is used to complement the effects of DBS.

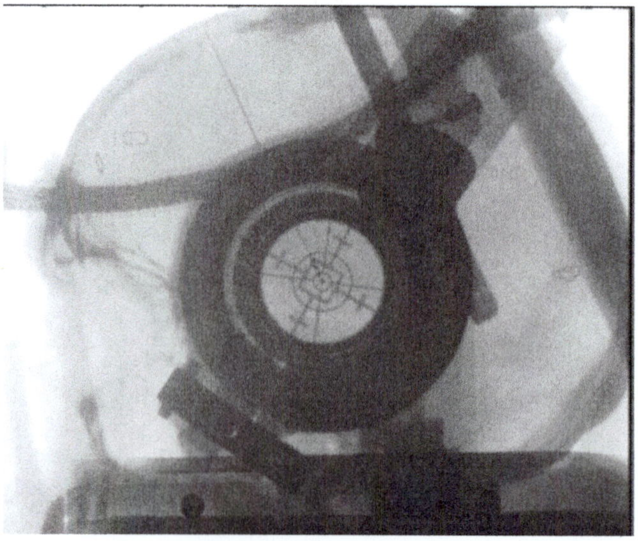

FIGURE 35.6 X-ray image showing tip of the lead position in the center of the arc—confirms its accurate position.

In summary, DBS is a well-established therapy for treatment-resistant OCD, and offers significant promise for management of treatment-resistant depression. With further understanding of the pathophysiological basis of neuropsychiatric conditions, developing imaging techniques, and disease biomarkers, DBS may become an increasingly common therapy for a range of treatment-resistant neuropsychiatric conditions.

Acknowledgments

We are very grateful to Dr. Ki Sueng Choi, Associate Professor, Radiology and Neurosurgery, Nash Family Center for Advanced Circuit Therapeutics, Biomedical Engineering and Imaging Institute, Icahn School of Medicine at Mount Sinai, for providing both tractography images.

References

[1] Zhdanava M, Pilon D, Ghelerter I, et al. The prevalence and national burden of treatment-resistant depression and major depressive disorder in the United States. J Clin Psychiatry 2021;82(2).

[2] Nuttin B, Cosyns P, Demeulemeester H, Gybels J, Meyerson B. Electrical stimulation in anterior limbs of internal capsules in patients with obsessive-compulsive disorder. Lancet 1999;354(9189):1526.

[3] Kahn L, Sutton B, Winston HR, Abosch A, Thompson JA, Davis RA. Deep brain stimulation for obsessive-compulsive disorder: real world experience post-FDA-humanitarian use device approval. s.l. Front Psychiatr 2021;12:568932.

[4] Mayberg HS, Liotti M, Brannan SK, McGinnis S, Mahurin RK, Jerabek PA, Silva JA, Tekell JL, Martin CC, Lancaster JL, Fox PT. Reciprocal limbic-cortical function and negative mood: converging PET findings in depression and normal sadness. Am J Psychiatr May 1999;156(5):675–82.

[5] Dougherty D, Rauch SL. Neuroimaging and neurobiological models of depression. Harv Rev Psychiatr 1997:138–59.

[6] Kopell BH, Greenberg BD. Anatomy and physiology of the basal ganglia: implications for DBS in psychiatry. Neurosci Biobehav Rev 2008;32 (3):408–22.

[7] Shepherd GM, Yamawaki N. Untangling the cortico-thalamo-cortical loop: cellular pieces of a knotty circuit puzzle. s.l. Nat Rev Neurosci 2021;22 (7):389–406.

[8] Rauch SL. Euroimaging and neurocircuitry models pertaining to the neurosurgical treatment of psychiatric disorders. N Neurosurg Clin N Am 2003;14(2):213–23.

[9] Sotiropoulos SN, Steinmetz PN. Assessing the direct effects of deep brain stimulation using embedded axon models. s.l. J Neural Eng 2007;4 (2):107–19.

[10] Anderson RW, Farokhniaee A, Gunalan K, Howell B, McIntyre CC. Action potential initiation, propagation, and cortical invasion in the hyperdirect pathway during subthalamic deep brain stimulation. s.l. Brain Stimul 2018;11(5):1140–50.

[11] Bromet E, Andrade LH, Hwang I, et al. Cross-national epidemiology of DSM-IV major depressive episode. BMC Med 2011;90(9).

[12] Rush AJ, Trivedi MH, Wisniewski SR, Nierenberg AA, Stewart JW, Warden D, Niederehe G, Thase ME, Lavori PW, Lebowitz BD, McGrath PJ, Rosenbaum JF, Sackeim HA, Kupfer DJ, Luther J, Fava M. Acute and longer-term outcomes in depressed outpatients requiring one or several treatment steps: a STAR*D report. Am J Psychiatr 2006;163(11):1905–17.

[13] US Food and Drug Administration. Major depressive disorder: developing drugs for treatment. Silver Spring: US: Food and Drug Administration: Center for Drug Evaluation and Research; 2018.

[14] Johnson KA, Okun MS, Scangos KW, Mayberg HS, de Hemptinne C. Deep brain stimulation for refractory major depressive disorder: a comprehensive review. Mol Psychiatr 2024;29(4):1075–87.

[15] Rush AJ, Sackeim HA, Marangell LB, George MS, Brannan SK, Davis SM, et al. Effects of 12 months of vagus nerve stimulation in treatment-resistant depression: a naturalistic study. Biol Psychiatry 2005:355–63.

[16] Hall RC. Global assessment of functioning: a modified scale. Psychosomatics 1995;36(3):267–75.

[17] Mayberg HS, Lozano AM, Voon V, McNeely HE, Seminowicz D, Hamani C, Schwalb JM, Kennedy SH. Deep brain stimulation for treatment-resistant depression. Neuron 2005;45(5):651–60.

[18] Schlaepfer T, Cohen M, Frick C, et al. Deep brain stimulation to reward circuitry alleviates anhedonia in refractory major depression. Neuropsychopharmacology 2008;33:368–77.

[19] Schlaepfer TE, Bewernick BH, Kayser S, Mädler B, Coenen VA. Rapid effects of deep brain stimulation for treatment-resistant major depression. Biol Psych. 2013;73(12):1204–12.

[20] Sartorius A, Kiening KL, Kirsch P, von Gall CC, Haberkorn U, Unterberg AW, Henn FA, Meyer-Lindenberg A. Remission of major depression under deep brain stimulation of the lateral habenula in a therapy-refractory patient. Biol Psych. 2010;67(2):e9–11.

[21] Jiménez F, Velasco F, Salin-Pascual R, Hernández JA, Velasco M, Criales JL, Nicolini H. A patient with a resistant major depression disorder treated with deep brain stimulation in the inferior thalamic peduncle. Neurosurgery 2005;57(3):585–93.

[22] Fitzgerald PB, Segrave R, Richardson KE, Knox LA, Herring S, Daskalakis ZJ, Bittar RG. A pilot study of bed nucleus of the stria terminalis deep brain stimulation in treatment-resistant depression. Brain Stimul 2018;11(4):921–8.

[23] Riva-Posse P, Choi KS, Holtzheimer PE, Crowell AL, Garlow SJ, Rajendra JK, McIntyre CC, Gross RE, Mayberg HS. A connectomic approach for subcallosal cingulate deep brain stimulation surgery: prospective targeting in treatment-resistant depression. Mol Psychiatr April 2018;23 (4):843–9.

[24] Reddy S, Kabotyanski KE, Hirani S, Liu T, Naqvi Z, Giridharan N, Hasen M, Provenza NR, Banks GP, Mathew SJ, Goodman WK, Sheth SA. Efficacy of deep brain stimulation for treatment-resistant depression: systematic review and meta-analysis. Biol Psychiatry Cogn Neurosci Neuroimaging 2024;9(12):1239–48.
[25] Himes L, et al. Subcallosal cingulate deep brain stimulation for depression: long-term safety and effectiveness outcomes from a pooled analysis of 172 patients. Biol Psychiatry 2024;95(10):S209–10.
[26] Dougherty DD, Rezai AR, Carpenter LL, Howland RH, Bhati MT, O'Reardon JP, Eskandar EN, Baltuch GH, Machado AD, Kondziolka D, Cusin C, Evans KC, Price LH, Jacobs K, Pandya M, Denko T, Tyrka AR, Brelje T, Deckersbach T, Kubu C, Malone Jr DA. A randomized sham-controlled trial of deep brain stimulation of the ventral capsule/ventral striatum for chronic treatment-resistant depression. Biol Psych 2015;78(4):240–8.
[27] Paul EH, Husain MM, Lisanby SH, Taylor SF, Whitworth LA, McClintock S, Slavin KV, Berman J, McKhann GM, Patil PG, Rittberg BR, Abosch A, Pandurangi AK, Holloway KL, et al. Subcallosal cingulate deep brain stimulation for treatment-resistant depression: a multisite, randomised, sham-controlled trial. Lancet Psychiatry 2017;4(11):839–49.
[28] Alagapan S, Choi KS, Heisig S, et al. Cingulate dynamics track depression recovery with deep brain stimulation. Nature 2023:130–8.
[29] Americal Psychiatric Association. Diagnostic and statistical manual of mental disorders. In: Americal psychiatric pub, vols. 5th ed. (DSM-5); 2013.
[30] Fenske JN, Petersen K. Obsessive-compulsive disorder: diagnosis and management. Am Fam Physician 2015;92(10):896–903.
[31] Canals J, Hernández-Martínez C, Cosi S, Voltas N. The epidemiology of obsessive-compulsive disorder in Spanish school children. J Anxiety Disord 2012;26(7):746–52.
[32] Ruscio AM, Stein DJ, Chiu WT, Kessler RC. The epidemiology of obsessive-compulsive disorder in the national comorbidity survey replication. Mol Psychiatr 2010;15(1):53–63.
[33] Goodman WK, Price LH, Rasmussen SA, Mazure C, Fleischmann RL, Hill CL, Heninger GR, Charney DS. The Yale-Brown obsessive compulsive scale. I. Development, use, and reliability. Arch Gen Psychiatry 1989;46(11):1006–11.
[34] Storch EA, De Nadai AS, Conceição do Rosário M, Shavitt RG, Torres AR, Ferrão YA, Miguel EC, Lewin AB, Fontenelle LF. Defining clinical severity in adults with obsessive-compulsive disorder. Compr Psychiatry 2015;63:30–5.
[35] Bloch MH, Green C, Kichuk SA, Dombrowski PA, Wasylink S, Billingslea E, Landeros-Weisenberger A, Kelmendi B, Goodman WK, Leckman JF, Coric V, Pittenger C. Long-term outcome in adults with obsessive-compulsive disorder. Depress Anxiety 2013;30(8):716–22.
[36] Carmi L, Tendler A, Bystritsky A, Hollander E, Blumberger DM, Daskalakis J, Ward H, Lapidus K, Goodman W, Casuto L. Efficacy and safety of deep transcranial magnetic stimulation for obsessive-compulsive disorder: a prospective multicenter randomized double-blind placebo-controlled trial. Am J Psychiatr 2019;176(11):931–8.
[37] Kisely S, Hall K, Siskind D, Frater J, Olson S, Crompton D. Deep brain stimulation for obsessive-compulsive disorder: a systematic review and meta-analysis. Psychol Med 2014;44(16):3533–42.
[38] Alonso P, Cuadras D, Gabriëls L, Denys D, Goodman W, Greenberg BD, Jimenez-Ponce F, Kuhn J, Lenartz D, Mallet L, Nuttin B, Real E, Segalas C, Schuurman R, du Montcel ST, Menchon JM. Deep brain stimulation for obsessive-compulsive disorder: a meta-analysis of treatment outcome and predictors of response. PLoS One 2015;10(7):e0133591.
[39] (fda.gov), Humanitarian device exemption. Humanitarian Device Exemption (HDE). 2009.
[40] Garnaat SL, Greenberg BD, Sibrava NJ, Goodman WK, Mancebo MC, Eisen JL, Rasmussen SA. Who qualifies for deep brain stimulation for OCD? Data from a naturalistic clinical sample. J Neuropsychiatry Clin Neurosci 2014;26(1):81–6.
[41] Sturm V, Lenartz D, Koulousakis A, Treuer H, Herholz K, Klein JC, Klosterkötter J. The nucleus accumbens: a target for deep brain stimulation in obsessive-compulsive- and anxiety-disorders. J Chem Neuroanat December 2003;26(4):293–9.
[42] Raviv N, Staudt MD, Rock AK, MacDonell J, Slyer J, Pilitsis JG. A systematic review of deep brain stimulation targets for obsessive compulsive disorder. Neurosurgery 2020;87(6):1098–110.
[43] Tyagi H, Apergis-Schoute AM, Akram H, Foltynie T, Limousin P, Drummond LM, Fineberg NA, Matthews K, Jahanshahi M, Robbins TW, Sahakian BJ, Zrinzo L, Hariz M, Joyce EM. A randomized trial directly comparing ventral capsule and anteromedial subthalamic nucleus stimulation in obsessive-compulsive disorder: clinical and imaging evidence for dissociable effects. Biol Psychiatry 2019;85(9):726–34.
[44] Mar-Barrutia L, Real E, Segalás C, Bertolín S, Menchón JM, Alonso P. Deep brain stimulation for obsessive-compulsive disorder: a systematic review of worldwide experience after 20 years. World J Psychiatr 2021;11(9):659–80.
[45] Menchón JM, Real E, Alonso P, Aparicio MA, Segalas C, Plans G, Luyten L, Brunfaut E, Matthijs L, Raymakers S, Bervoets C, Higueras A, Katati M, Guerrero J, Hurtado M, Prieto M, Stieglitz LH, Löffelholz G, Walther S, Pollo C, Zurowski B, Tronnier V. A prospective international multi-center study on safety and efficacy of deep brain stimulation for resistant obsessive-compulsive disorder. Mol Psychiatr April 2021;26(4):1234–47.
[46] Robertson MM. Tourette syndrome, associated conditions and the complexities of treatment. Brain 2000;123:425–62.
[47] Leckman JF, Riddle MA, Hardin MT, Ort SI, Swartz KL, Stevenson J, Cohen DJ. The Yale global tic severity scale: initial testing of a clinician-rated scale of tic severity. J Am Acad Child Adolesc Psychiatry 1989;28:566–73.
[48] McGuire JF, Piacentini J, Storch EA, Murphy TK, Ricketts EJ, Woods DW, Walkup JW, Peterson AL, Wilhelm S, Lewin AB, McCracken JT, Leckman JF, Scahill L. A multicenter examination and strategic revisions of the Yale global tic severity scale. Neurology 2018;90(19):e1711–9.
[49] Seideman MF, Seideman TA. A review of the current treatment of tourette syndrome. J Pediatr Pharmacol Therapeut 2020;25(5):401–12.

[50] Schrock LE, Mink JW, Woods DW, Porta M, Servello D, Visser-Vandewalle V, Silburn PA, Foltynie T, Walker HC, Shahed-Jimenez J, Savica R, Klassen BT, Machado AG, Foote KD, Zhang JG, Hu W, Ackermans L, Temel Y, Mari Z, Changizi BK, Lozano A, Auyeung M. Tourette syndrome deep brain stimulation: a review and updated recommendations. Mov Disord April 2015;30(4):448–71.

[51] Priori A, Giannicola G, Rosa M, Marceglia S, Servello D, Sassi M, Porta M. Deep brain electrophysiological recordings provide clues to the pathophysiology of Tourette syndrome. Neurosci Biobehav Rev 2013;37(6):1063–8.

[52] Wehmeyer L, Schüller T, Kiess J, Heiden P, Visser-Vandewalle V, Baldermann JC, Andrade P. Target-specific effects of deep brain stimulation for tourette syndrome: a systematic review and meta-analysis. Front Neurol 2021;12:769275.

[53] Figee M, et al. Precision deep brain stimulation targeting for obsessive-compulsive disorder based on tractography. Biol Psychiatry 2024;95(10): S30.

[54] Rajabian A, Vinke S, Candelario-Mckeown J, Milabo C, Salazar M, Nizam AK, Salloum N, Hyam J, Akram H, Joyce E. Accuracy, precision, and safety of stereotactic, frame-based, intraoperative MRI-guided and MRI-verified deep brain stimulation in 650 consecutive procedures. J Neurosurg 2022;138(6):1702–11.

[55] Liu L, Mariani SG, De Schlichting E, Grand S, Lefranc M, Seigneuret E, Chabardès S. Frameless ROSA robot-assisted lead implantation for deep brain stimulation: technique and accuracy. Oper Neurosurg 2020;19(1):57–64.

[56] Sharma M, Deogaonkar M. Accuracy and safety of targeting using intraoperative "O-arm" during placement of deep brain stimulation electrodes without electrophysiological recordings. J Clin Neurosci 2016;27:80–6.

[57] Peng S, Levine D, Ramirez-Zamora A, Chockalingam A, Feustel PJ, Durphy J, Hanspal E, Novak P, Pilitsis JG. A comparison of unilateral deep brain stimulation (DBS), simultaneous bilateral DBS, and staged bilateral DBS lead accuracies. Neuromodulation 2017;20(5):478–83.

[58] Petraglia FW, Farber SH, Han JL, Verla T, Gallis J, Lokhnygina Y, Parente B, Hickey P, Turner DA, Lad SP. Comparison of bilateral vs. Staged unilateral deep brain stimulation (DBS) in Parkinson's disease in patients under 70 Years of age. Neuromodulation 2016;19(1):31–7.

Chapter 36

Deep brain stimulation: Pain

Inamullah Khan[1] and Rushna Ali[2]

[1]University of Missouri, Columbia, MO, United States; [2]Mayo Clinic, Rochester, MN, United States

Key points

1. Deep Brain Stimulation (DBS) has emerged as a promising neuromodulatory approach for treating intractable pain conditions.
2. While its use in movement disorders is well established, its application in pain management remains less common but increasingly explored.
3. This chapter reviews the historical evolution of DBS for pain, the indications and patient selection criteria, advancements in technology, the mechanisms underlying its efficacy, as well as the complications and limitations associated with its use.
4. We also discuss modern innovations and potential future directions in DBS for pain management.

Introduction

Deep Brain Stimulation (DBS) is a neurosurgical intervention that involves the implantation of electrodes in subcortical target regions to modulate neural activity through controlled electrical impulses [1]. Although DBS has been widely adopted for the treatment of movement disorders such as Parkinson's disease, dystonia, and essential tremor, its application in chronic pain management remains controversial [2,3]. Chronic pain, particularly neuropathic pain, is a debilitating condition defined as pain persisting beyond the typical healing period of 3 months, which is associated with reduced productivity, psychological distress, and increased healthcare costs [4,5]. The Institute of Medicine has identified chronic pain as a major public health concern, with financial burden in the U.S. estimated between $560 to $635 billion annually [6]. In industrialized nations, the prevalence of chronic pain is reported to be approximately 20%–30% of the population [7]. Given the limitations of long-term pharmacological treatment and the risks associated with dependency on opioids, there has been a growing emphasis on alternative or adjunctive therapeutic approaches [8–10].

DBS has been used to manage chronic pain since the 1960s, but regulatory obstacles and inconsistent outcomes have prevented it from becoming a mainstream therapy [3]. Early studies targeted structures such as the periaqueductal gray (PAG), sensory ventrocaudalis thalamic nucleus (Vc), and anterior cingulate cortex (ACC) to modulate pain perception. However, despite promising case reports and small clinical studies, two multicenter trials aimed at obtaining FDA approval failed to meet efficacy criteria, leading to its classification as an off-label procedure in the U.S. [11,12]. Nevertheless, DBS continues to show therapeutic potential in pain syndromes such as poststroke pain, phantom limb pain, brachial plexus injury, failed back surgery syndrome, and pain associated with Parkinson's disease [8,13–15]. Advances in DBS technology, including directional leads, current steering, and adaptive stimulation, have improved targeting precision and individualized therapy. As research progresses, emerging innovations such as functional MRI and tractography for improved targeting, as well as biomarker-driven stimulation and closed-loop programming, may further optimize outcomes, renewing interest in DBS as a viable approach for refractory chronic pain.

This chapter explores the historical evolution of DBS for pain management, from its early use in the 1960s to modern advancements in neuromodulation. We review key indications, including neuropathic pain syndromes, failed back surgery syndrome, and central pain disorders, alongside essential patient selection criteria. Additionally, we discuss technological innovations such as directional leads, current steering, and adaptive stimulation, which have improved precision and efficacy.

A Modern Atlas for Implantable Devices of the Spine, Brain, and Nerve. https://doi.org/10.1016/B978-0-443-36528-7.00041-8

Historical perspective

The application of DBS for pain dates to the 1950 and 1960s, when early research explored electrical stimulation of deep brain structures for analgesic effects. Pioneers such as Heath, Mazars, and Hosobuchi investigated thalamic and PAG/PVG stimulation for pain relief in the 1970s [16–18]. Around the same time, Adams et al. introduced anterior limb of internal capsule (ALIC) DBS for pain, though this target never gained widespread use [19]. Over the years, advancements in imaging, neurophysiology, and device engineering have refined DBS techniques, making them safer and more effective.

In 1977, Richardson et al. introduced periventricular gray (PVG) and periaqueductal gray (PAG) DBS for pain, with Hosobuchi later demonstrating independently that its analgesic effects could be reversed with the opioid antagonist naloxone, suggesting an endogenous opioid-mediated mechanism [18,20]. The success of thalamic and PVG/PAG DBS led to widespread use in the late 1970s, with Medtronic even trademarking the term "DBS" in the context of subcortical stimulation for pain [21]. However, despite its early promise, DBS for pain never received FDA approval due to the lack of controlled trials demonstrating efficacy [12]. While its use persisted in Europe alongside stereotactic ablative procedures, interest in DBS for pain declined in the U.S. over subsequent decades. In recent years, however, there has been renewed interest in DBS for chronic pain, fueled by advancements in neuromodulation and the success of DBS in movement disorders [22–24]. Major limitations for widespread adoption include small sample size of various studies, lack of long-term outcome data, loss of efficacy over time and habituation.

Indications and patient selection

DBS is primarily indicated for severe, refractory pain conditions, including chronic neuropathic pain, central pain syndromes, and facial pain (Table 36.1).

Central post-stroke pain

Central post-stroke pain (CPSP) remains one of the most common and challenging indications for DBS. Patients typically suffer from debilitating neuropathic pain following thalamic or cortical infarcts, which can lead to hemibody or regional pain. A recent systematic review identified CPSP as the leading indication among 228 patients who had a DBS system implanted for pain [8]. Studies have targeted both the PAG/PVG and ventral posterolateral/ventral posteromedial (VPL/VPM) thalamus. However, outcomes have varied. For instance, Rasche et al. found that only 2 of 11 patients with CPSP proceeded to permanent implantation after a trial period of stimulation at PVG and sensory thalamus [10]. On the other hand, Boccard et al. reported up to 40% reduction in visual analog scale (VAS) pain scores for CPSP patients at 1-year

TABLE 36.1 Pain indication for DBS.

Central Poststroke pain (CPSP)	Chronic pain following ischemic or hemorrhagic stroke often affects the extremities.
Phantom limb pain	Pain perceived in an amputated limb; often neuropathic and treatment resistant.
Brachial plexus avulsion	Severe neuropathic pain from traumatic root avulsion of the brachial plexus.
Postspinal cord injury pain.	Deafferentation pain following spinal cord lesion.
Failed back surgery syndrome (FBSS)	Chronic neuropathic back/leg pain persists after spine surgery.
Trigeminal neuropathic facial pain	Intractable unilateral facial pain, including after nerve injury or postsurgical pain.
Peripheral neuropathy or MS-related pain Spinal pathology-related pain Postcordotomy dysesthesia	Chronic pain due to nerve injury or demyelination Includes pain from degenerative disc disease, central pain postmyelopathy, or spinal trauma. Central pain following ablative lesioning of spinal pain pathways.
Anesthesia dolorosa	Pain in areas of sensory loss following nerve ablation or damage.
Complex regional pain syndrome	Severe, burning pain typically develops after injury or surgery; sometimes categorized as CRPS type II.
Chronic pain with catastrophizing	Targeting affective-emotional modulators of chronic pain using ACC or VS/IC DBS.

follow-up in 70% ($n = 16/23$) of patients [25]. A meta-analysis showed that 50% of patients with poststroke pain had a successful trial, and [26] among those who underwent a permanent implant, 58% experienced ongoing pain relief at 1 year, highlighting that a carefully selected subset of patients can derive meaningful benefit from DBS.

Phantom limb pain

Phantom limb pain (PLP) has shown some of the most encouraging responses to DBS. Studies consistently support targeting the sensory thalamus, with or without PAG/PVG costimulation. Pereira et al. reported 90% improvement in VAS pain score at 12 months with VPL stimulation among five patients [27]. Yamamoto et al. studied stimulation of Vc in 18 patients, including 11 with phantom limb pain reporting >60% reduction in VAS scores at long-term follow-up [28]. Abreu et al. reported on 16 patients, including six patients with PLP who underwent VPL stimulation and achieved 53% reduction in their VAS pain scores at 3 years follow up [29]. Boccard et al. reported sustained benefit in 89% of PLP patients ($n = 8/9$) at o 2 year follow-up [25].

Brachial plexus avulsion

Brachial plexus avulsion (BPA) pain has mixed central and peripheral components, and DBS for this indication has yielded mixed results. Pereira et al. trialed seven BPA patients with VPL stimulation, with six patients proceeding to permanent implantation who had 52.7% improvement at 12-month follow-up [27]. Boccard's cohort of BPA patients had lower response rates, with only 3 out of 6 with meaningful benefit during trial stimulation [25]. These differences likely reflect BPA's more complex deafferentation pain mechanisms.

Post–spinal cord injury pain

Spinal cord injury (SCI) related central pain presents a formidable challenge due to diffuse and multi-level pain processing disruptions. Although some patients experience temporary relief, long-term outcomes remain inconsistent. In the study by Frizon et al. DBS for SCI-related pain had lower success rates, ranging from 24.5% to 52% [8]. The targets included PAG/PVG, VPL/VPM and bilateral ACC. In another study, 5 out of 12 patients had a successful trial, and at a mean follow-up time of 3.5 years, only one patient had >50% pain relief with simulation of VPL/PVG [10].

Failed back surgery syndrome

DBS for Failed Back Surgery Syndrome (FBSS) is considered after a patient has field a trial of spinal cord stimulation [9]. In one of the larger studies conducted, 32 of the 39 patients implanted achieved good to excellent pain relief with stimulation of PVG, VPL and ALIC. Overall, this translated to a 74% success rate among all FBSS cases. These outcomes were among the most favorable reported in the series, with DBS demonstrating higher efficacy in FBSS compared to other pain syndromes included in the study [9]. Stimulation of the PVG region, first introduced by Hosobuchi and Richardson, is particularly effective for nociceptive, midline-dominant pain such as that seen in FBSS, especially when spinal cord stimulation is not feasible or has failed [30,31]. A clinical trial is underway to assess the efficacy of subgenual cingulate cortex DBS in FBSS (NCT04085406).

Trigeminal neuropathic facial pain

Trigeminal neuropathic pain, especially anesthesia dolorosa, has been treated using DBS targeting VPM and PAG. Ben-Haim et al. observed dramatic pain reductions in facial pain patients, with VAS scores dropping from 9.0 to 2.6 at 1-year follow-up [32]. Mandat et al. and others confirmed improvements in pain-specific quality of life indices, validating this as a robust DBS indication [33,34]. While rare, DBS has been piloted for neuropathic dental pain using advanced technologies like directional leads. Krüger et al. demonstrated >90% pain relief with precise targeting of VPM and CM thalamic nuclei, suggesting potential for select cases with intractable dental pain [35].

Peripheral neuropathy/radiculopathy and MS-related pain

Peripheral nerve injury with localized but persistent neuropathic symptoms may benefit from DBS, particularly with Vc targeting. Kumar et al. identified six patients with peripheral neuropathy or radiculopathy who underwent stimulation of PVG and sensory thalamus with moderate success in pain relief [9]. Bittar et al. demonstrated 90.5% success in patients who underwent DBS for lumbosacral radiculopathy and 77.8% in patients with lumbar arachnoiditis [26]. Boccard et al. reported meaningful improvements in both pain and quality of life among patients with discogenic and posttraumatic etiologies, supporting DBS in highly selected cases [25]. Levy et al. reported on five patients who were treated for postcordotomy dysesthesia with 60% success rate in alleviation of pain symptoms [2]. Hosobuchi et al. treated three patients with postcordotomy dysesthesia and reported success in all three patients [18].

Cordella et al. studied five multiple sclerosis (MS) patients with refractory trigeminal neuralgia who underwent DBS targeting the posterior hypothalamus. Four patients achieved pain control with DBS and medication, though recurrence in other branches required additional radiofrequency rhizotomies in three cases [36]. The beneficial effects were durable, with follow-up ranging from 1 to 4 years, and only one patient needed minor adjustments for pain recurrence in the first branch [36]. In addition, Hamami et al. reported good long-term benefit for pain control in one out of two patients with MS with DBS targeting of Vc for left-sided extremity pain [37].

Anesthesia dolorosa

Anesthesia dolorosa associated with profound sensory loss and chronic persistent pain, has long been a target for DBS. Outcomes have been variable, with some patients reporting meaningful reductions in pain intensity, particularly when the sensory thalamus is targeted. Patel et al. found PAG stimulation led to 56% pain relief, and CmPF stimulation had 67% responder rate [38]. Levy et al. treated 12 patients with anesthesia dolorosa and showed an initial success rate of 67%, which later dropped to 18% at long-term follow-up [2].

Complex regional pain syndrome

Complex regional pain syndrome (CRPS) has been included in DBS cohorts, albeit rarely. Kumar et al. included two such cases in their series, where one patient (PVG target) continued to have excellent relief at long term, while the other (PVG + Vc) experienced long-term failure [9]. Such results suggest that carefully selected patients might benefit from neuromodulation, although robust data are lacking.

Chronic pain with catastrophization

In recent years, significant attention has shifted toward the affective-motivational aspects of pain, particularly in patients where the sensory-discriminative component is less responsive to conventional targets. Frizon et al. highlighted studies targeting the anterior cingulate cortex (ACC) and VS/ALIC [8]. Boccard et al. demonstrated improvements in quality of life and pain affect, even when intensity measures like VAS did not significantly change [23]. The Cleveland Clinic's double-blind study showed that active VS/ALIC stimulation improved depression, affective pain measures, and overall patient satisfaction [39]. These findings support an emerging paradigm that seeks to modulate not just pain perception but also its emotional salience.

Targets for DBS in pain management

The table summarizes key neuroanatomical targets for deep brain stimulation (DBS) in chronic pain management, correlating each region with its rationale and associated pain syndromes. Historically, the periaqueductal/periventricular gray (PAG/PVG) [8,9,27,32] and sensory thalamic nuclei (VPL/VPM) [8,25,27,32,35] have been primary targets due to their roles in pain modulation, PAG/PVG via descending inhibitory pathways and endogenous opioids, and VPL/VPM via somatotopically organized sensory-discriminative signaling. These targets are commonly used in conditions such as central poststroke pain, phantom limb pain, FBSS, and neuropathic facial pain (Table 36.2).

Recent approaches have expanded to include affective-emotional circuits such as the anterior cingulate cortex (ACC) [23,24], centromedian–parafascicular complex (CM–Pf) [38,40], and ventral striatum (VS)/ALIC [24], particularly in refractory pain where emotional processing is prominent. Dual-targeting strategies, such as combining ACC with thalamic stimulation, and advances in directional leads and dual-frequency programming enhance personalization and efficacy, as reported in multifocal and complex neuropathic syndromes [32,38].

Ultimately, target selection is tailored to the patient characteristics: sensory-dominant pain often warrants thalamic or PAG/PVG stimulation, while affective targets are favored in diffuse or catastrophizing overlay. The evolution toward individualized, network-based DBS is driven by both clinical insights and technological progress (Fig. 36.1).

TABLE 36.2 DBS targets in pain management.

DBS target	Rationale/Mechanism	Typical pain syndromes/ Causes	Target coordinates
Periaqueductal/Periventricular gray (PAG/PVG) [8,9,27,32]	Modulates descending nociceptive pathways; endogenous opioid release	Central poststroke pain, phantom limb pain, FBSS, and facial pain	2–3 mm lateral to the third ventricle at AC-PC 23 mm ventrolateral to the aqueduct at the level of the superior colliculus
Ventral posterolateral/Ventral posteromedial thalamus (VPL/VPMs) [8,25,27,32,35]	Relays sensory-discriminative pain signals to cortex; somatotopic targeting	Central pain (poststroke, SCI), phantom limb pain, and facial/dental pain	8–10 mm posterior and 10–12 mm lateral to MCP VPM: 3–4 mm medial to the internal capsule VPL: 2–3 mm from arm pain, 1–2 mm for leg pain—medial to internal capsule At AC-PC
Centromedian parafascicular complex (CMPf) [38,40]	Modulation of medial/affective pain pathways	Neuropathic pain, deafferentation pain, and complex regional pain	5–7 mm lateral, 8–11 mm posterior, and 0–3 mm inferior to the MCP
Anterior cingulate cortex (ACC) [23,24,41]	Modulation of affective, emotional response to pain	Chronic pain with strong affective/emotional component (refractory neuropathic pain, complex pain syndromes)	20 mm posterior to the anterior tip of the frontal horn 7 mm from midline 1 mm above the roof of the ventricle
Ventral striatum/Anterior limb of internal capsule (VS/ALIC) [24]	Influences affective and motivational aspects of pain	Chronic pain with substantial affective distress	Deep ventral at ALIC 0–1 mm Posterior to the anterior commissure 5–6 mm from the midline
Anterior pulvinar nucleus of thalamus [35]	Sensory integration: potential relay in chronic facial pain	Neuropathic dental pain andfacial pain	12 mm superior, 5–6 mm lateral, and 0–2 mm anterior to the MCP
Dual/Combined Targets [32,38]	Synergistic targeting of sensory (thalamic) and affective (ACC/CMPf) components	Chronic, refractory neuropathic pain and complex pain syndromes	

AC, anterior commissure; MCP, midcommissural point; PC, posterior commissure.

Complications of deep brain stimulation for pain

The clinical use of deep brain stimulation (DBS) for pain is limited by a range of complications that highlight the importance of careful patient selection and ongoing management. Hardware-related issues, such as lead migration, infection, and device malfunction, are the most frequently reported and may necessitate revision surgery. The infection rates are reported at 2.5%–4.2% leading to hardware removal in such cases [8,40].

Neuropsychiatric and neurological adverse effects, though less common, are clinically significant [8]. Mood alterations, emotional blunting, and apathy may occur, especially when affective regions like the anterior cingulate cortex are targeted [23]. Sensory disturbances or paresthesias can arise from off-target stimulation, and rare but serious events like intracranial hemorrhage may occur during electrode placement, though the incidence is less than 1%. Tolerance to stimulation, commonly referred to as habituation or stimulation fatigue, is another limitation, with some patients experiencing a decline in therapeutic benefit over time [2,8]. Moreover, response rates vary widely (20%–70%), and improvements in quality of life are not consistently observed across studies [8,25].

To mitigate risks, preoperative psychiatric screening, test stimulation trials, and rigorous follow-up are recommended. Overall, the safety and efficacy of DBS for pain depend on multidisciplinary care, technical precision, and individualized treatment planning.

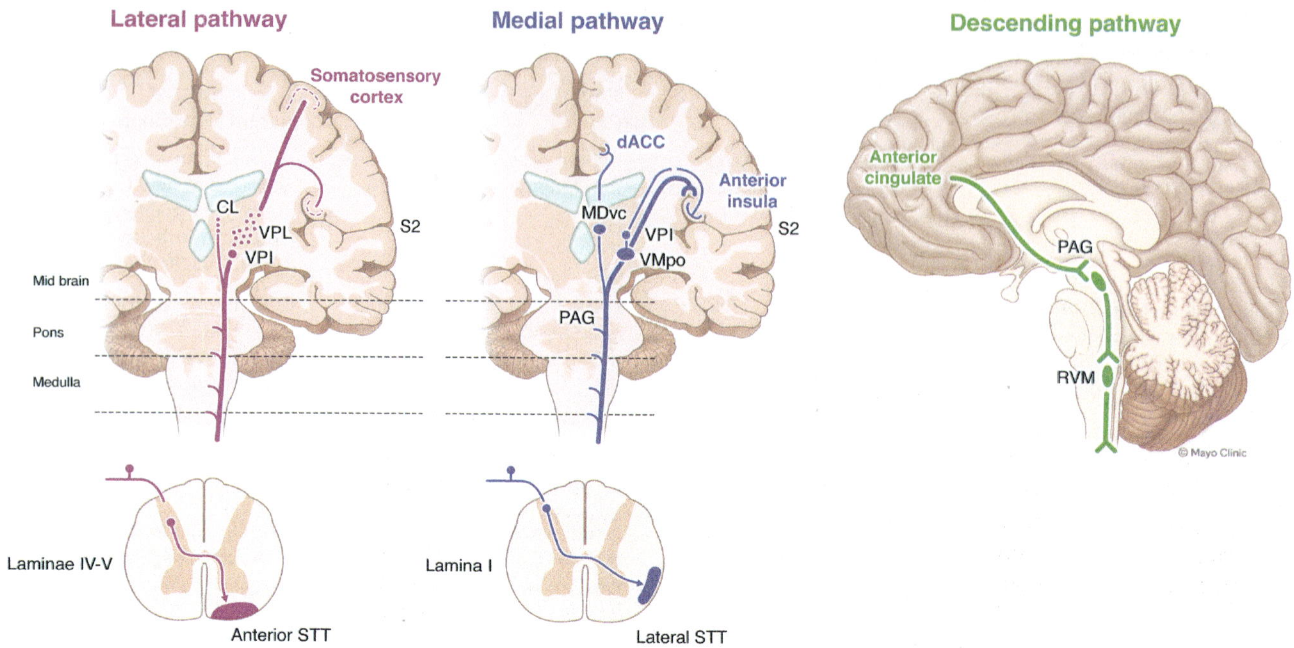

FIGURE 36.1 Shows the three pain pathways targeted in DBS for pain management.

New directions for DBS in pain management

Recent advances in deep brain stimulation for chronic pain reflect a concerted effort to overcome historical limitations and enhance clinical outcomes across diverse pain syndromes.

Expansion of DBS targets and network-level engagement

While traditional targets such as the periaqueductal/periventricular gray (PAG/PVG) and sensory thalamic nuclei remain central to DBS for pain, there is increasing interest in regions involved in the affective-emotional dimensions of pain, particularly the anterior cingulate cortex (ACC) and the VS/ALIC [22,41–44]. Recent studies have explored the feasibility and safety of stimulating both sensory and affective regions, such as the thalamus and ACC, within the same patient to better address the multidimensional nature of chronic neuropathic pain [22,43]. This shift reflects a broader transition toward modulating distributed pain networks rather than isolated regions, incorporating personalized and network-informed approaches to account for interindividual variability in central pain processing [45].

Technological advancements: Closed-loop and imaging-guided DBS

Traditional open-loop DBS systems employ static stimulation parameters, but closed-loop (adaptive) systems are emerging as a promising innovation. These systems use real-time neural recordings, such as local field potentials, to dynamically adjust stimulation in response to physiological indicators of pain [46,47]. Translational research is actively working to identify reliable biomarkers of pain perception and decode both acute and chronic pain states in real-world settings [46,47]. In parallel, advanced neuroimaging techniques, including diffusion tensor imaging (DTI) and functional studies, are being used to guide lead placement and optimize targeting in complex structures like the thalamus, as well as to explain variability in patient response [48,49].

Combined and hybrid stimulation paradigms

Efforts are also underway to design novel stimulation paradigms that allow concurrent modulation of multiple pain circuits. Dual-target or dual-frequency stimulation via a single electrode has been proposed to simultaneously engage both sensory and affective pathways [50]. For instance, combining thalamic or PAG/PVG stimulation with centromedian–parafascicular complex (CM–Pf) stimulation is being investigated to address the full spectrum of pain-related experiences [50].

A growing emphasis on precision medicine is reshaping DBS targeting strategies. Rather than relying solely on anatomical landmarks, contemporary approaches are increasingly informed by individual brain connectivity patterns and network topology [45,49]. This shift acknowledges the complexity and heterogeneity of central pain processing and the need for personalized stimulation strategies to maximize therapeutic benefit.

Conclusion

DBS for pain management has evolved significantly since its initial applications in the mid-20th century. Although early enthusiasm was tempered by regulatory hurdles and inconsistent trial outcomes, the development of advanced technologies such as directional leads, current steering, and adaptive stimulation has renewed interest in DBS as a viable therapy for chronic, refractory pain conditions. Careful patient selection and precise targeting, particularly of structures like the periaqueductal gray (PAG), ventral posterolateral thalamus (VPL), and affective circuits such as the anterior cingulate cortex (ACC), are crucial for achieving meaningful outcomes. While results vary across different pain syndromes, ranging from promising responses in phantom limb pain and failed back surgery syndrome to more modest benefits in spinal cord injury-related pain, DBS remains an important tool for a select group of patients who are refractory to conventional medical treatments. Ongoing innovations in biomarker-driven programming, dual-target strategies, and closed-loop optimisation hold the potential to further refine outcomes and expand indications. As the field progresses, a deeper understanding of both the sensory and emotional dimensions of pain will be essential in tailoring DBS therapy to the individual needs of each patient.

References

[1] Farokhniaee A, McIntyre CC. Theoretical principles of deep brain stimulation induced synaptic suppression. Brain Stimul 2019;12(6):1402–9.

[2] Levy RM, Lamb S, Adams JE. Treatment of chronic pain by deep brain stimulation: long term follow-up and review of the literature. Neurosurgery 1987;21(6):885–93.

[3] Hariz MI, Blomstedt P, Zrinzo L. Deep brain stimulation between 1947 and 1987: the untold story. Neurosurg Focus 2010;29(2):E1.

[4] Hange N, Poudel S, Ozair S, Paul T, Nambakkam M, Shrestha R, et al. Managing chronic neuropathic pain: recent advances and new challenges. Neurol Res Int 2022;2022(1):8336561.

[5] Merskey HE. Classification of chronic pain: descriptions of chronic pain syndromes and definitions of pain terms. Pain 1986;(3):S1–226. PMID: 3461421.

[6] Gaskin DJ, Richard P. The economic costs of pain in the United States. J Pain 2012;13(8):715–24.

[7] Leadley R, Armstrong N, Lee Y, Allen A, Kleijnen J. Chronic diseases in the European Union: the prevalence and health cost implications of chronic pain. J Pain Palliat Care Pharmacother 2012;26(4):310–25.

[8] Frizon LA, Yamamoto EA, Nagel SJ, Simonson MT, Hogue O, Machado AG. Deep brain stimulation for pain in the modern era: a systematic review. Neurosurgery 2020;86(2):191–202.

[9] Kumar K, Toth C, Nath RK. Deep brain stimulation for intractable pain: a 15-year experience. Neurosurgery 1997;40(4):736–47.

[10] Rasche D, Rinaldi PC, Young RF, Tronnier VM. Deep brain stimulation for the treatment of various chronic pain syndromes. Neurosurg Focus 2006;21(6):1–8.

[11] Cruccu G, Aziz T, Garcia-Larrea L, Hansson P, Jensen TS, Lefaucheur JP, et al. EFNS guidelines on neurostimulation therapy for neuropathic pain. Eur J Neurol 2007;14(9):952–70.

[12] Coffey RJ. Deep brain stimulation for chronic pain: results of two multicenter trials and a structured review. Pain Med 2001;2(3):183–92.

[13] Bittar RG, Burn SC, Bain PG, Owen SL, Joint C, Shlugman D, et al. Deep brain stimulation for movement disorders and pain. J Clin Neurosci 2005;12(4):457–63.

[14] Falowski SM. Deep brain stimulation for chronic pain. Curr Pain Headache Rep 2015;19:1–4.

[15] Flouty O, Yamamoto K, Germann J, Harmsen IE, Jung HH, Cheyuo C, et al. Idiopathic Parkinson's disease and chronic pain in the era of deep brain stimulation: a systematic review and meta-analysis. J Neurosurg 2022;137(6):1821–30.

[16] Heath RG, Becker HC, Bersadsky L, Corrigan RM, Epstein AW, Founds WL, et al. Studies in schizophrenia: a multidisciplinary approach to mind-brain relationships. Harvard University Press; 1954.

[17] Mazars G. Stimulations thalamiques intermittentes antalgiques. Note preliminair Rev Neurol. 1973;128:273–9.

[18] Hosobuchi Y, Rossier J, Bloom FE, Guillemin R. Stimulation of human periaqueductal gray for pain relief increases immunoreactive β-endorphin in ventricular fluid. Science 1979;203(4377):279–81.

[19] Adams JE, Hosobuchi Y, Fields HL. Stimulation of internal capsule for relief of chronic pain. J Neurosurg 1974;41(6):740–4.

[20] Richardson DE, Akil H. Pain reduction by electrical brain stimulation in man: Part 1: acute administration in periaqueductal and periventricular sites. J Neurosurg 1977;47(2):178–83.

[21] Coffey RJ. Deep brain stimulation devices: a brief technical history and review. Artif Organs 2009;33(3):208–20.

[22] Leplus A, Lanteri-Minet M, Donnet A, Darmon N, Regis J, Fontaine D. Treatment of chronic refractory pain by combined deep brain stimulation of the anterior cingulum and sensory thalamus (EMOPAIN study): rationale and protocol of a feasibility and safety study. Brain Sci 2022;12(9):1116.

[23] Boccard SGJ, Pereira EAC, Moir L, Van Hartevelt TJ, Kringelbach ML, FitzGerald JJ, et al. Deep brain stimulation of the anterior cingulate cortex: targeting the affective component of chronic pain. Neuroreport 2014;25(2):83–8.

[24] Nüssel M, Zhao Y, Knorr C, Regensburger M, Stadlbauer A, Buchfelder M, et al. Deep brain stimulation, stereotactic radiosurgery and high-intensity focused ultrasound targeting the limbic pain matrix: a comprehensive review. Pain Ther 2022;11(2):459–76.

[25] Boccard SG, Pereira EA, Moir L, Aziz TZ, Green AL. Long-term outcomes of deep brain stimulation for neuropathic pain. Neurosurgery 2013;72(2):221–31.

[26] Bittar RG, Kar-Purkayastha I, Owen SL, Bear RE, Green A, Wang S, et al. Deep brain stimulation for pain relief: a meta-analysis. J Clin Neurosci 2005;12(5):515–9.

[27] Pereira EA, Boccard SG, Linhares P, Chamadoira C, Rosas MJ, Abreu P, et al. Thalamic deep brain stimulation for neuropathic pain after amputation or brachial plexus avulsion. Neurosurg Focus 2013;35(3):E7.

[28] Yamamoto T, Katayama Y, Obuchi T, Kano T, Kobayashi K, Oshima H, et al. Thalamic sensory relay nucleus stimulation for the treatment of peripheral deafferentation pain. Stereotact Funct Neurosurg 2006;84(4):180–3.

[29] Abreu V, Vaz R, Rebelo V, Rosas MJ, Chamadoira C, Gillies MJ, et al. Thalamic deep brain stimulation for neuropathic pain: efficacy at three years' follow-up. Neuromodulation Technol Neural Interf 2017;20(5):504–13.

[30] The current status of analgesic brain stimulation. In: Hosobuchi Y, editor. Advances in stereotactic and functional neurosurgery 4: Proceedings of the 4 th Meeting of the European Society for Stereotactic and Functional Neurosurgery, Paris 1979. Springer; 1980.

[31] Richardson DE, Akil H. Pain reduction by electrical brain stimulation in man: Part 2: chronic self-administration in the periventricular gray matter. J Neurosurg 1977;47(2):184–94.

[32] Ben-Haim S, Mirzadeh Z, Rosenberg WS. Deep brain stimulation for intractable neuropathic facial pain. Neurosurg Focus 2018;45(2):E15.

[33] Mandat V, Zdunek PR, Krolicki B, Szalecki K, Koziara HM, Ciecierski K, et al. Periaqueductal/periventricular gray deep brain stimulation for the treatment of neuropathic facial pain. Front Neurol 2023;14:1239092.

[34] Deep brain stimulation for chronic pain. In: Whitworth LA, Fernández J, Feler CA, editors. Seminars in Neurosurgery. Copyright© 2004 by Thieme Medical Publishers, Inc.; 2004. p. 333 [Seventh Avenue, New …].

[35] Krüger MT, Avecillas-Chasin JM, Heran MK, Naseri Y, Sandhu MK, Polyhronopoulos NE, et al. Directional deep brain stimulation can target the thalamic "sweet spot" for improving neuropathic dental pain. Oper Neurosurg 2021;21(2):81–6.

[36] Cordella R, Franzini A, La Mantia L, Marras C, Erbetta A, Broggi G. Hypothalamic stimulation for trigeminal neuralgia in multiple sclerosis patients: efficacy on the paroxysmal ophthalmic pain. Multiple Scler J 2009;15(11):1322–8.

[37] Hamani C, Schwalb JM, Rezai AR, Dostrovsky JO, Davis KD, Lozano AM. Deep brain stimulation for chronic neuropathic pain: long-term outcome and the incidence of insertional effect. Pain 2006;125(1–2):188–96.

[38] Sims-Williams HP, Javed S, Pickering AE, Patel NK. Characterising the analgesic effect of different targets for deep brain stimulation in trigeminal anaesthesia dolorosa. Stereotact Funct Neurosurg 2016;94(3):174–81.

[39] Lempka SF, Malone Jr DA, Hu B, Baker KB, Wyant A, JGt O, et al. Randomized clinical trial of deep brain stimulation for poststroke pain. Ann Neurol 2017;81(5):653–63.

[40] Abdallat M, Saryyeva A, Blahak C, Wolf ME, Weigel R, Loher TJ, et al. Centromedian–parafascicular and somatosensory thalamic deep brain stimulation for treatment of chronic neuropathic pain: a contemporary series of 40 patients. Biomedicines 2021;9(7):731.

[41] Boccard SG, Prangnell SJ, Pycroft L, Cheeran B, Moir L, Pereira EA, et al. Long-term results of deep brain stimulation of the anterior cingulate cortex for neuropathic pain. World Neurosurg 2017;106:625–37.

[42] Pagano RL, Dale CS, Campos ACP, Hamani C. Translational aspects of deep brain stimulation for chronic pain. Front Pain Res (Lausanne). 2022;3:1084701.

[43] Fontaine D, Leplus A, Donnet A, Darmon N, Balossier A, Giordana B, et al. Safety and feasibility of deep brain stimulation of the anterior cingulate and thalamus in chronic refractory neuropathic pain: a pilot and randomized study. J Headache Pain 2025;26(1):1–11.

[44] Plow EB, Malone DA, Machado A. Deep brain stimulation of the ventral striatum/anterior limb of the internal capsule in thalamic pain syndrome: study protocol for a pilot randomized controlled trial. Trials 2013;14:1–10.

[45] Motzkin JC, Kanungo I, D'Esposito M, Shirvalkar P. Network targets for therapeutic brain stimulation: towards personalized therapy for pain. Front Pain Res 2023;4:1156108.

[46] Shirvalkar P, Veuthey TL, Dawes HE, Chang EF. Closed-loop deep brain stimulation for refractory chronic pain. Front Comput Neurosci 2018;12:18.

[47] Shirvalkar P, Chin G, Dawes H, Starr P, Chang E. Decoding acute and chronic pain state from ambulatory intracranial recordings: towards closed-loop brain stimulation (233). Neurology 2020;94(Suppl. 15):233.

[48] Jones SE, Lempka SF, Gopalakrishnan R, Baker KB, Beall EB, Bhattacharyya P, et al. Functional magnetic resonance imaging correlates of ventral striatal deep brain stimulation for poststroke pain. Neuromodulation 2021;24(2):259–64.

[49] Kim W, Chivukula S, Hauptman J, Pouratian N. Diffusion tensor imaging-based thalamic segmentation in deep brain stimulation for chronic pain conditions. Stereotact Funct Neurosurg 2016;94(4):225–34.

[50] Hollingworth M, Sims-Williams HP, Pickering AE, Barua N, Patel NK. Single electrode deep brain stimulation with dual targeting at dual frequency for the treatment of chronic pain: a case series and review of the literature. Brain Sci 2017;7(1):9.

Chapter 37

Hypoglossal nerve peripheral stimulation (HNS) for sleep apnea

Qing Zhao Ruan[1], Harman Chopra[5], Ahmed Khawer[3], Mustafa Broachwala[2] and Tariq AlFarra[4]

[1]*Warren Alpert Medical School, Brown University, Providence, RI, United States;* [2]*Pain Anesthesia, University of California San Diego, San Diego, CA, United States;* [3]*Department of Physical Medicine and Rehabilitation, Johns Hopkins University School of Medicine, Baltimore, MD, United States;* [4]*Department of Rehabilitation and Human Performance, Icahn School of Medicine at Mount Sinai, New York, NY, United States;* [5]*Department of Pain, Weill Cornell Medicine, New York, NY, United States*

Anatomy, physiology, and pathophysiology

Obstructive sleep apnea

Obstructive sleep apnea (OSA) is a sleep disorder characterized by repetitive episodes of complete or partial upper airway collapse, resulting in sleep fragmentation, intermittent hypoxemia, hypercapnia, and heightened sympathetic activity. Repeat episodes of apnea or hypopnea can manifest as symptoms such as loud, disruptive snoring, gasping or choking during sleep, excessive daytime sleepiness, difficulty concentrating, and reduced libido [1]. Untreated OSA is linked with significant adverse health outcomes, including hypertension, coronary artery disease, arrythmia, heart failure, stroke, and overall increased cardiovascular morbidity and mortality [2]. In North America, the estimated prevalence of OSA ranges from 15% to 30% in males and 10%–15% in females [3].

The diagnosis of OSA is based on a combination of clinical signs and symptoms and is typically confirmed through in-laboratory polysomnogram or home sleep apnea testing. A diagnosis requires the presence of at least five or more obstructive respiratory events per hour of sleep. The American Academy of Sleep Medicine classifies OSA severity using the apnea-hypopnea index (AHI), categorizing it as mild (5–15), moderate (15–30), or severe OSA (AHI>30).

Management of OSA begins with behavior modifications, including weight loss, regular exercise, and avoidance of alcohol and sedatives. These interventions are recommended for and beneficial to OSA patients, however, should be combined with a primary treatment approach. Positional therapy, which encourages sleep postures that minimize airway obstruction, may also be an option for certain individuals. Additionally, custom-made oral appliances such as mandibular advancement devices or tongue advancement devices can also be beneficial for use in mild to moderate OSA [4]. These improve airway patency by advancing the mandible or tongue, reducing obstruction during sleep [5].

Continuous positive airway pressure (CPAP) remains the gold standard of treatment for obstructive sleep apnea [6]. Originally described by Sullivan in 1981 [6], CPAP functions as a pneumatic splint, preventing upper airway collapse by maintaining positive intraluminal pressure. This mechanism reduces intermittent hypoxia, enhances sleep quality, and has been shown to lower blood pressure and decrease the risk of cardiovascular complications [7].

Despite continued advancements in CPAP technology, patient adherence remains a significant challenge, with compliance rates ranging from 30% to 60% [8,9]. One study indicated that between 29% and 83% of patients report <4 h of CPAP use per night [7]. Common barriers to adherence include mask discomfort, claustrophobia, feelings of suffocation, nasal dryness due to inadequate humidity, and the overall inconvenience of using a machine at night. Given that consistent and prolonged CPAP use yields better clinical outcomes, suboptimal adherence significantly diminishes its long-term benefits. Studies suggests that at least 5–6 h of nightly CPAP use is required to achieve meaningful reduction in cardiovascular risk and daytime sleepiness [10]. For patients who fail conservative measures and PAP therapy, surgical treatments may be considered.

A Modern Atlas for Implantable Devices of the Spine, Brain, and Nerve. https://doi.org/10.1016/B978-0-443-36528-7.00049-2

Hypoglossal nerve stimulation (HNS) has emerged as a promising therapeutic alternative for patients with moderate to severe OSA who are intolerant or resistant to CPAP therapy. The goal of hypoglossal nerve stimulation is to activate upper airway musculature during inspiration to prevent airway collapse and improve air flow during sleep [11].

Anatomy of the hypoglossal nerve

The hypoglossal nerve, or cranial nerve XII, originates from the hypoglossal nucleus, situated midline in the posterior paramedian medulla, beneath the floor of the fourth ventricle, within the hypoglossal trigone [12]. The axons project ventrally, traveling lateral to the medial longitudinal fasciculus and medial lemniscus, exiting between the inferior olivary nucleus and the pyramid. The hypoglossal nucleus receives its blood supply through the anterior spinal and vertebral arteries [13]. Within the pre-medullary cistern, the nerve rootlets lie near the vertebral artery. The rootlets fuse forming the hypoglossal nerve and then exit through the hypoglossal canal, inferior to the jugular foramen [12,13]. As it exits the canal, the nerve gives off small dural branches prior to entering the nasopharyngeal carotid space, coursing medial to cranial nerves IX (glossopharyngeal), X (vagus), and XI (spinal accessory), within the carotid sheath. It then travels between the internal carotid artery and the internal jugular vein to the level of the C1 vertebra [12]. At this level, the hypoglossal nerve passes anteriorly, descending alongside the internal and external carotid arteries, before passing between the posterior belly of the digastric muscle near the hyoid bone, entering the digastric triangle. The hypoglossal nerve then separates into muscular or lingual branches that supply the intrinsic muscles and all but one of the extrinsic muscles of the tongue. The extrinsic muscles innervated by the hypoglossal nerve include genioglossus, styloglossus and hyoglossus, while the palatoglossus muscle is innervated by the vagus nerve (CN X). [Fig. 37.1].

The functions of these muscles are as follows: genioglossus draws the tongue root forward, hyoglossus retracts the tongue and depresses the tongue sides, while styloglossus draws the tongue upwards. The intrinsic muscles (superior and

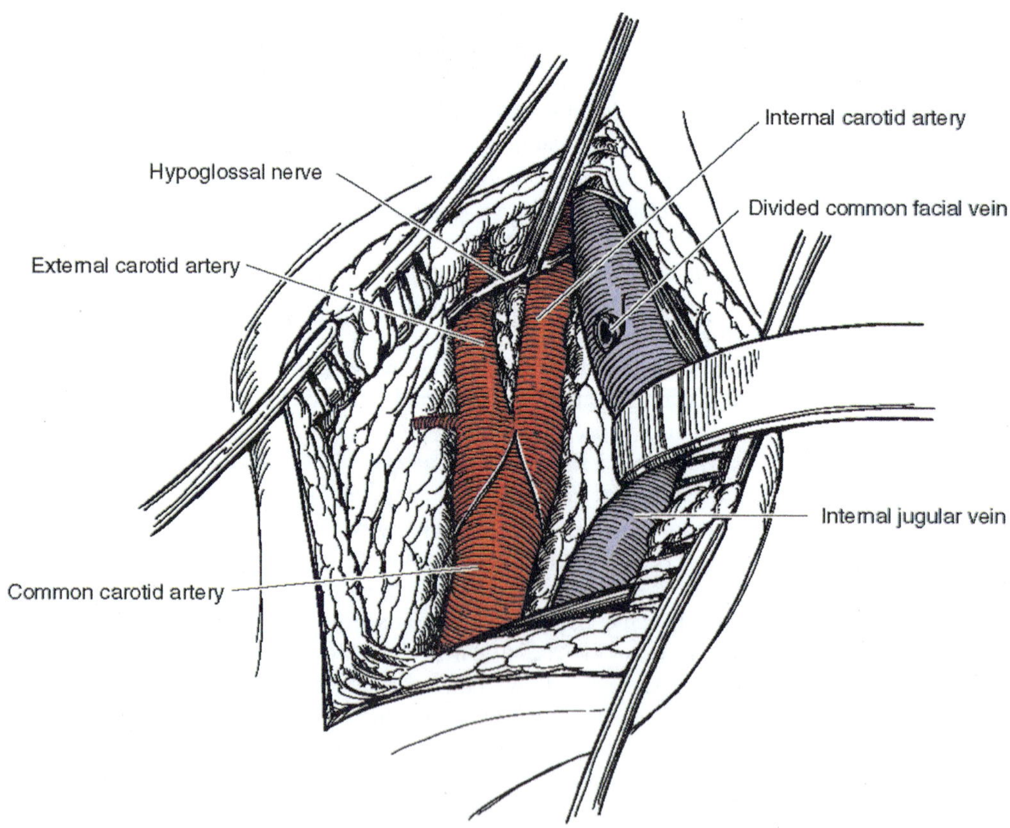

FIGURE 37.1 Anatomical course of the hypoglossal nerve (CN XII) in the cervical region. The hypoglossal nerve is seen emerging from the hypoglossal canal and coursing anteriorly, looping around the occipital artery and traveling deep to the posterior belly of the digastric muscle. It passes lateral to the external carotid artery and medial to the posterior margin of the sternocleidomastoid. The image also highlights nearby structures including the ansa cervicalis, vagus nerve (CN X), spinal accessory nerve (CN XI), and the cervical plexus branches, providing context for the nerve's location and its relationships in the neck.

inferior longitudinales, transversus, and verticalis) function to alter the tongue shape, such as shortening, narrowing, or curving the tongue [14].

Additionally, the hypogolossal nerve has contribution form cervical and spinal nerves. The meningeal branch arises from C1 and C2 nerve roots, while the descending branches from C1, C2 and C3 combine with the ansa cervicalis to innervate the infrahyoid muscles [14].

Hypoglossal nerve stimulation

Upper airway patency is maintained by several muscles, with the genioglossus muscle playing a crucial role [15]. This muscle comprises a substantial portion of the tongue and is innervated by the hypoglossal nerve. During sleep, reduced activation of the genioglossus muscle results in posterior displacement of the tongue, narrowing the airway. This risk is further exacerbated by factors such as obesity and anatomical abnormalities of soft tissue/bony structures [2]. Hypoglossal nerve stimulation mitigates this issue by stimulating and activating branches of the hypoglossal nerve, causing subsequent contraction of the genioglossus muscle, causing tongue stiffness and protrusion. This allows anterior movement of the tongue, effectively widening the airway and preventing its collapse during sleep [Fig. 37.2].

The STAR trial, a multi-center, prospective, single-group cohort study, evaluated the clinical safety and effectiveness of upper airway stimulation in patients with moderate-to-severe OSA over 12 months, revealing 68% decrease in median AHI from 29.3 events per hour to nine events per hour; and decrease in Oxygen Desaturation Index (ODI) by 70% (from 25.4 events per hour to 7.4 events per hour). Additionally, significant improvement in secondary outcomes like sleepiness using the Epworth Sleepiness Scale (ESS), functional sleep outcomes, using the Functional Outcomes of Sleep Questionnaire score (FOSQ), and improved quality of life was also reported [16]. These outcomes were maintained at 5-year follow up, with a mean AHI of 12.4 events per hour, ODI 9.9 events per hour [17].

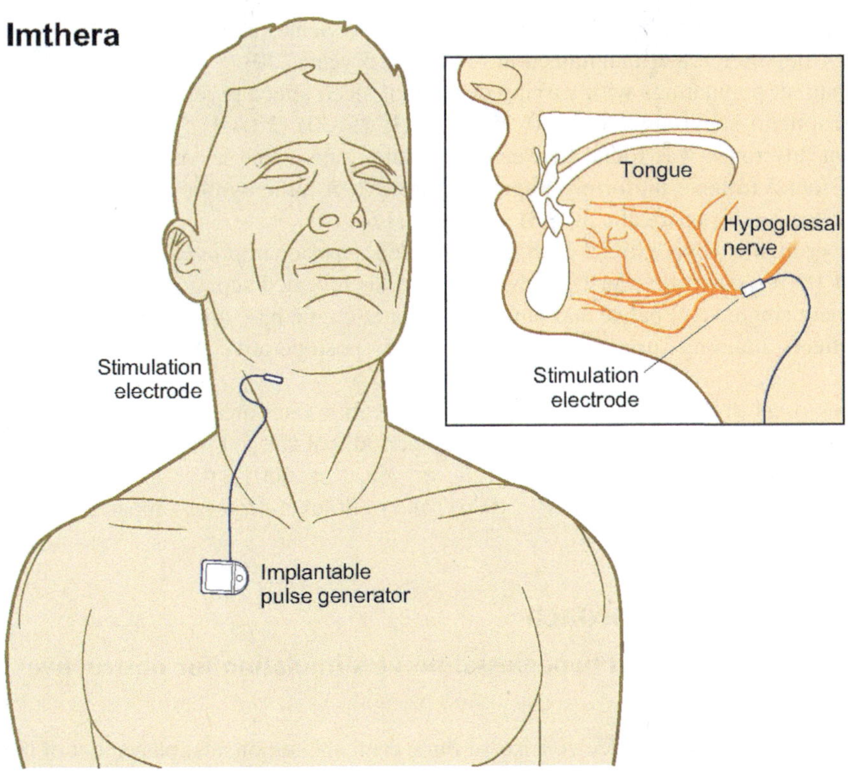

FIGURE 37.2 The hypoglossal nerve stimulation device is composed of two implantable parts. An implantable pulse generator (IPG) and a stimulation lead with a cuff that has six electrodes. It is placed over the principal trunk of the hypoglossal nerve in a more proximal position.

Indications, patient selection, and clinical evidence

Indications and contraindications for hypoglossal PNS

OSA patients considered for PNS must meet criteria for moderate to severe obstructive sleep apnea (OSA) with apnea-hypopnea index (AHI) $\geq$ 15 but $\leq$65 with BMI <35 and minimum age of 22. They must not exhibit concentric airway collapse at the level of the soft palate, and must attempt and failed, or not tolerate the use of positive pressure airway therapies such as continuous positive airway pressure (CPAP) or bi-level positive airway pressure (BiPAP). Intolerance to conventional positive airway therapies is defined by the inability to adopt CPAP or BiPAP for more than five nights per week and for more than 4 h per session. Younger patients (aged 18–21) meeting the above criteria could also be considered for PNS use when traditional surgeries such as adenotonsillectomy are contraindicated or ineffective in the management sleep apnea symptoms [18].

Contraindications for PNS therapy include significant central and mixed apnea making up over one-fourth of total AHI, as well as patients with implantable devices which could interfere with PNS function. The Inspire PNS demonstrates partial MRI compatibility and is therefore MRI conditional under clearly defined circumstances. It is at present controversial whether existing pregnancy or future pregnancy would be compatible with device use [18].

Predictors of therapeutic success

Certain factors have been identified as predictors of success in the treatment of OSA with hypoglossal PNS. Using the ADHERE registry (an active international, multicenter prospective observational database approved by site-specific ethics committees or institutional review boards), Thaler et al. reported that the female gender had 90% increased odds of an improved therapy response measured via AHI compared to the male population [19]. It was also found that each unit reduction in BMI translated to an 8.5% increase in odds of improved AHI response. On the contrary, other baseline characteristics such as age, baseline AHI values, and tongue motion evident from hypoglossal nerve stimulation during PNS implantation did not appear to influence therapeutic success [19].

Clinical evidence

Woodson et al. demonstrated real-world outcomes of hypoglossal PNS implants over 5 years in a multicenter prospective cohort study, demonstrating significant improvement in sleepiness (Epworth Sleepiness Scale) and quality of life. AHI improvement was seen in 75% of the study population and maintained at 63% over 5 years [20].

Bosschieter et al. further dissected outpatient populations with varying degrees of sleep apnea severity based on their recorded AHI before hypoglossal PNS treatment: subgroup 1 (AHI 0–15), 2 (AHI 15–30), 3 (AHI $\geq$30–50), 4 (AHI >50–65), and 5 (AHI >65). No significant difference was found between these subgroups when it comes to treatment success (66.6%). Daytime sleepiness was found to have uniformly improved throughout all subgroups. In conclusion, PNS adoption in sleep apnea was highly effective if pre-treatment AHI was $\geq$15 [17].

When compared against traditional upper airway, hypoglossal PNS demonstrated superior improvement in pre- and postoperative AHI (32 and 10 vs. 33.5 and 15, respectively). Further subgroup analysis revealed superior AHI compared to both traditional surgical techniques, namely single level palate and multilevel palate/tongue base approaches. The PNS group also had a higher percentage of patients attaining surgical success, defined as postoperative AHI<20 with 50% improvement from preoperative state [21].

Given the minimal invasiveness of hypoglossal PNS implantation, surgical complication rates are decreased compared to traditional sleep apnea surgeries. Nord et al. demonstrated that over a 90-day period, palatal and multilevel surgeries pose significantly higher risks for readmission versus PNS implantation (12% vs. 4%, $P < .0001$), with an even higher complication rate in palatal surgeries compared to PNS (21% vs. 2%, $P < .0001$) and multilevel surgery compared to PNS (22% vs. 3%, $P < .0001$) [22].

Technical considerations and procedural approach

Technical considerations and procedural approach in hypoglossal nerve stimulation for obstructive sleep apnea

The implantation of a hypoglossal nerve stimulation (HNS) device consists of three critical components: placement of the stimulation and tunneling of the lead, as well as implantation and positioning of both the implantable pulse generator

(IPG) and respiratory sensing lead. Careful attention to lead positioning, intraoperative monitoring, and imaging guidance is necessary to optimize patient outcomes and minimize complications.

Surgical approach and lead placement

The procedure begins with a submandibular incision at the level of the hyoid bone to expose the hypoglossal nerve. The stimulation lead is positioned around the medial branches of the nerve that control tongue protrusion while avoiding fibers that innervate retraction muscles, which could paradoxically worsen airway obstruction. Electromyographic (EMG) intraoperative monitoring (IONM) is used to confirm selective stimulation of tongue-protruding muscles, ensuring optimal nerve activation while minimizing off-target effects such as dysarthria or tongue fatigue [23].

Imaging is not routinely required for lead placement, as direct visualization of the hypoglossal nerve via careful dissection is typically sufficient. However, ultrasound guidance may be utilized intraoperatively to assist in nerve identification, particularly in patients with variant anatomy or a history of prior neck surgery [24].

Lead tunneling and anchoring

Once the stimulation lead is secured to the hypoglossal nerve, it is tunneled subcutaneously to the pectoral region, where the IPG will be implanted. Tunneling is performed using a long subcutaneous passer, ensuring that the lead is placed without kinking or excessive tension, which could lead to mechanical failure. The IPG is positioned in a subcutaneous pocket within the pectoral region, at a subcutaneous depth of approximately 1 cm, ensuring both stability and patient comfort while preventing erosion or migration [25]. The lead is secured with suture-based anchors at the point of the submandibular incision to prevent lead migration.

The respiratory sensing lead is then placed in the intercostal space, typically between the second and third ribs in the right parasternal region. This placement is critical, as the sensor must detect respiratory effort accurately to synchronize stimulation with the inspiratory phase. The sensing lead is tunneled to the IPG, where it is connected along with the stimulation lead. Improper placement of the sensing lead can lead to desynchronization, reduced efficacy, or the need for reoperation [26].

Outcomes, efficacy, and complications

Clinical outcomes and efficacy

Hypoglossal nerve stimulation (HNS) has demonstrated significant efficacy in reducing the severity of obstructive sleep apnea (OSA), particularly in patients who are intolerant to continuous positive airway pressure (CPAP) therapy. Studies have consistently shown that HNS leads to a 50%–70% reduction in the Apnea-Hypopnea Index (AHI), accompanied by improvements in oxygen desaturation and sleep efficiency. Quality-of-life assessments, including the Epworth Sleepiness Scale (ESS) and the Functional Outcomes of Sleep Questionnaire (FOSQ), have shown significant improvement following HNS therapy, reflecting reduced daytime sleepiness and enhanced overall well-being [27].

Long-term studies indicate that HNS remains effective for at least 5–7 years, with minimal decline in therapeutic benefit. Patients report continued symptom relief, and objective sleep metrics remain stable over time. The implantable pulse generator (IPG) has an expected battery lifespan of 8–11 years, requiring eventual replacement [28].

Comparison with other sleep apnea treatments

While CPAP remains the gold standard for OSA treatment, achieving AHI reductions of 80%–90%, long-term adherence remains a challenge, with compliance rates as low as 50%–60% due to discomfort, mask intolerance, and inconvenience. In contrast, HNS has an adherence rate exceeding 85%, making it a preferred alternative for patients unable to tolerate CPAP [27].

Surgical interventions such as uvulopalatopharyngoplasty (UPPP) and maxillomandibular advancement (MMA) provide alternative treatment options, with varying degrees of success. UPPP has a success rate of approximately 40%–50%, whereas MMA can achieve AHI reductions of 60%–80% but carries significant morbidity. HNS offers a comparable success rate (~60%–70%) with fewer perioperative risks, making it a favorable surgical alternative [27].

Combination therapies, particularly the use of HNS with mandibular advancement devices (MADs), have shown promise in optimizing outcomes for patients with residual AHI. This approach is especially useful in cases of tongue base collapse or retrognathia, where MADs can enhance airway patency [29].

Complications and risk management

Although HNS is generally well tolerated, complications can occur. The most commonly reported issue is lead migration, which occurs in approximately 4%–10% of cases and may necessitate surgical revision. Migration can lead to ineffective stimulation, reduced therapy efficacy, or discomfort. Hardware malfunctions, including IPG failure and lead fracture, are reported in 1%–3% of cases and may require surgical replacement of the affected components [30].

Adverse effects related to stimulation include transient tongue weakness or dysphagia, which affects 3%–5% of patients due to unintended activation of non-targeted hypoglossal nerve branches. These symptoms typically resolve within weeks to months as patients adjust to the stimulation. Voice changes or speech disturbances occur in fewer than 5% of cases but can often be mitigated by adjusting stimulation parameters. Discomfort at the IPG site, particularly if the device is placed too superficially, has also been reported and may require repositioning [31].

In pediatric populations, particularly in adolescents with Down syndrome and OSA, complication rates are comparable to those in adults, though discomfort and sensation-related complaints may be more common. Studies suggest that careful programming and follow-up adjustments can mitigate many of these issues, allowing for continued use of the therapy [32].

Optimizing patient adherence and minimizing complications, careful patient selection, precise intraoperative lead placement, and individualized device programming are essential. Regular follow-ups allow for fine-tuning of stimulation parameters and early identification of any issues requiring intervention. With ongoing advancements in lead design, surgical technique, and device software, the safety and efficacy of HNS are expected to continue improving, further solidifying its role as a leading alternative therapy for OSA [33].

Future directions, research, and emerging innovations

Ongoing research in hypoglossal nerve stimulation (HNS) is focused on expanding patient eligibility, improving device technology, and optimizing long-term outcomes. Current studies are investigating whether higher BMI patients and those with more severe OSA could benefit from HNS, as well as the role of biomarkers in predicting treatment response [34]. In pediatric populations, HNS is showing promising results in children with Down syndrome and persistent OSA, though challenges remain in device programming and adherence [32]. Technological advancements aim to improve battery longevity, miniaturization, and adaptive stimulation algorithms, with emerging machine learning models designed to adjust therapy in real time based on respiratory patterns and sleep stage transitions [35].

Post-implantation optimization remains a key area of focus, with efforts to standardize outcome reporting and improve remote patient monitoring through wearable sensors and smartphone-connected platforms. Artificial intelligence (AI) is also being integrated into OSA diagnostics and HNS therapy planning, providing personalized, data-driven treatment adjustments [36]. As these innovations advance, HNS is expected to become even more effective and widely applicable, offering a more tailored and less invasive alternative to CPAP and traditional OSA surgeries [37].

References

[1] Spicuzza L, Caruso D, Maria G. Obstructive sleep apnoea syndrome and its management. Ther Adv Chronic Dis 2015;6(5). https://doi.org/10.1177/2040622315590318.

[2] Javaheri S, Barbe F, Campos-Rodriguez F, et al. Sleep apnea: Types, mechanisms, and clinical cardiovascular consequences. J Am Coll Cardiol 2017;69(7). https://doi.org/10.1016/j.jacc.2016.11.069.

[3] Young T, Palta M, Dempsey J, Peppard PE, Nieto FJ, Hla KM. Burden of sleep apnea: rationale, design, and major findings of the Wisconsin sleep cohort study. Wis Med J 2009;108(5).

[4] Epstein LJ, Kristo D, Strollo PJ, et al. Clinical guideline for the evaluation, management and long-term care of obstructive sleep apnea in adults. J Clin Sleep Med 2009;5(3). https://doi.org/10.5664/jcsm.27497.

[5] Ferguson KA, Cartwright R, Rogers R, Schmidt-Nowara W. Oral appliances for snoring and obstructive sleep apnea: A review. Sleep 2006;29(2). https://doi.org/10.1093/sleep/29.2.244.

[6] Sullivan CE, Berthon-Jones M, Issa FG, Eves L. Reversal of obstructive sleep apnoea by continuous positive airway pressure applied through the nares. Lancet 1981;317(8225). https://doi.org/10.1016/S0140-6736(81)92140-1.

[7] Bakker JP, Weaver TE, Parthasarathy S, Aloia MS. Adherence to CPAP: What should we Be aiming for, and how can we get there? Chest 2019;155(6). https://doi.org/10.1016/j.chest.2019.01.012.

[8] Rotenberg BW, Murariu D, Pang KP. Trends in CPAP adherence over twenty years of data collection: A flattened curve. J Otolaryngol - Head Neck Surg 2016;45(1). https://doi.org/10.1186/s40463-016-0156-0.

[9] Weaver TE, Sawyer AM. Adherence to continuous positive airway pressure treatment for obstructive sleep apnoea: Implications for future interventions. Indian J Med Res 2010;131(2).

[10] Weaver TE, Grunstein RR. Adherence to continuous positive airway pressure therapy: The challenge to effective treatment. Proc Am Thorac Soc 2008;5(2). https://doi.org/10.1513/pats.200708-119MG.
[11] Mashaqi S, Patel SI, Combs D, et al. The hypoglossal nerve stimulation as a novel therapy for treating obstructive sleep apnea—a literature review. Int J Environ Res Publ Health 2021;18(4). https://doi.org/10.3390/ijerph18041642.
[12] Joseph SC, Loukas M. The hypoglossal nerve. In: Nerves and nerve injuries. 1; 2015. https://doi.org/10.1016/B978-0-12-410390-0.00030-5.
[13] Alves P. Imaging the hypoglossal nerve. Eur J Radiol 2010;74(2). https://doi.org/10.1016/j.ejrad.2009.08.028.
[14] Kim SY, Naqvi IA. Neuroanatomy, cranial nerve12; 2019 *(Hypoglossal)*.
[15] Kuna ST, Sant'ambrogio G. Pathophysiology of upper airway closure during sleep. JAMA, J Am Med Assoc 1991;266(10). https://doi.org/10.1001/jama.1991.03470100076036.
[16] Strollo PJ, Soose RJ, Maurer JT, et al. Upper-airway stimulation for obstructive sleep apnea. N Engl J Med 2014;370(2). https://doi.org/10.1056/nejmoa1308659.
[17] Bosschieter PFN, de Vries N, Mehra R, et al. Similar effect of hypoglossal nerve stimulation for obstructive sleep apnea in 5 disease severity categories. J Clin Sleep Med 2022;18(6):1657–65. https://doi.org/10.5664/jcsm.9956.
[18] Inspire manual.
[19] Thaler E, Schwab R, Maurer J, et al. Results of the ADHERE upper airway stimulation registry and predictors of therapy efficacy. Laryngoscope 2020;130(5):1333–8. https://doi.org/10.1002/lary.28286.
[20] Woodson BT, Strohl KP, Soose RJ, et al. Upper airway stimulation for obstructive sleep apnea: 5-year outcomes. Otolaryngol Head Neck Surg 2018;159(1):194–202. https://doi.org/10.1177/0194599818762383.
[21] Huntley C, Boon M, Tschopp S, et al. Comparison of traditional upper airway surgery and upper airway stimulation for obstructive sleep apnea. Ann Otol Rhinol Laryngol 2021;130(4):370–6. https://doi.org/10.1177/0003489420953178.
[22] Nord R, Fitzpatrick T, DeShazo JP, Reiter ER. Comparison of readmission and complication rates between traditional sleep surgery and hypoglossal nerve stimulation. Laryngoscope Investig Otolaryngol 2022;7(5):1659–66. https://doi.org/10.1002/lio2.883.
[23] Saugel B, Annecke T, Bein B, et al. Intraoperative haemodynamic monitoring and management of adults having non-cardiac surgery: guidelines of the German society of anaesthesiology and intensive care medicine in collaboration with the German association of the scientific medical societies. J Clin Monit Comput 2024;38(5):945–59. https://doi.org/10.1007/s10877-024-01132-7.
[24] Frequin HL, Bot M, Dilai J, et al. Relative contribution of magnetic resonance imaging, microelectrode recordings, and awake test stimulation in final lead placement during deep brain stimulation surgery of the subthalamic nucleus in Parkinson's disease. Stereotact Funct Neurosurg 2020;98(2):118–28. https://doi.org/10.1159/000505710.
[25] Rabi J, Anitescu M. Late extrusion of an implantable pulse generator of a spinal cord stimulator. Pain Physician 2016;19(4):E671–4.
[26] Malhotra A, Grunstein RR, Fietze I, et al. Tirzepatide for the treatment of obstructive sleep apnea and obesity. N Engl J Med 2024;391(13):1193–205. https://doi.org/10.1056/NEJMoa2404881.
[27] Choi JH, Lee JY, Cha J, Kim K, Hong SN, Lee SH. Predictive models of objective oropharyngeal OSA surgery outcomes: Success rate and AHI reduction ratio. PLoS One 2017;12(9):e0185201. https://doi.org/10.1371/journal.pone.0185201.
[28] Mamukashvili-Delau M, Koburger N, Dietrich S, Rummel-Kluge C. Long-term efficacy of internet-based cognitive behavioral therapy self-help programs for adults with depression: systematic review and meta-analysis of randomized controlled trials. JMIR Ment Health 2023;10:e46925. https://doi.org/10.2196/46925.
[29] Qamar Z, Alghamdi AMS, Haydarah NKB, et al. Impact of temporomandibular disorders on oral health-related quality of life: A systematic review and meta-analysis. J Oral Rehabil 2023;50(8):706–14. https://doi.org/10.1111/joor.13472.
[30] Costantino A, Rinaldi V, Moffa A, et al. Hypoglossal nerve stimulation long-term clinical outcomes: a systematic review and meta-analysis. Sleep Breath 2020;24(2):399–411. https://doi.org/10.1007/s11325-019-01923-2.
[31] Steffen A, Heiser C, Galetke W, et al. Hypoglossal nerve stimulation for obstructive sleep apnea: Updated position paper of the German society of oto-rhino-laryngology, head and neck surgery. Eur Arch Otorhinolaryngol 2022;279(1):61–6. https://doi.org/10.1007/s00405-021-06902-6.
[32] Liu P, Kong W, Fang C, Zhu K, Dai X, Meng X. Hypoglossal nerve stimulation in adolescents with down syndrome and obstructive sleep apnea: A systematic review and meta-analysis. Front Neurol 2022;13:1037926. https://doi.org/10.3389/fneur.2022.1037926.
[33] Pascoe M, Wang L, Aylor J, et al. Association of hypoglossal nerve stimulation with improvements in long-term, patient-reported outcomes and comparison with positive airway pressure for patients with obstructive sleep apnea. JAMA Otolaryngol Head Neck Surg 2022;148(1):61–9. https://doi.org/10.1001/jamaoto.2021.2245.
[34] Suurna MV, Jacobowitz O, Chang J, et al. Improving outcomes of hypoglossal nerve stimulation therapy: current practice, future directions, and research gaps. proceedings of the 2019 international sleep surgery society research forum. J Clin Sleep Med 2021;17(12):2477–87. https://doi.org/10.5664/jcsm.9542.
[35] Soose RJ, Faber K, Greenberg H, Boon M, Woodson T, Strollo P. Post-implant care pathway: lessons learned and recommendations after 5 years of clinical implementation of hypoglossal nerve stimulation therapy. Sleep 2021;44(1):S4–10. https://doi.org/10.1093/sleep/zsaa279.
[36] Cederberg KLJ, Hanif U, Peris SV, et al. Proteomic biomarkers of the apnea hypopnea index and obstructive sleep apnea: insights into the pathophysiology of presence, severity, and treatment response. Int J Mol Sci 2022;23(14). https://doi.org/10.3390/ijms23147983.
[37] Nokes B, Cooper J, Cao M. Obstructive sleep apnea: personalizing CPAP alternative therapies to individual physiology. Expert Rev Respir Med 2022;16(8):917–29. https://doi.org/10.1080/17476348.2022.2112669.

Chapter 38

Vagus nerve stimulation: Implanted and noninvasive

Viktoras Palys[1] and Peter S. Staats[2]

[1]*Department of Neurosurgery, University of Arkansas for Medical Sciences, Little Rock, AR, United States;* [2]*The Vagus Nerve Society and National Spine and Pain Centers, Atlantic Beach, FL, United States*

Introduction

Undoubtedly, the vagus nerve is one of the most interesting targets for neuromodulation today. The vagus nerve occupies a singular position in human physiology. As the 10th cranial nerve, it serves as the major parasympathetic conduit between brain and body, influencing autonomic tone, gastrointestinal function, cardiovascular regulation, pain perception, and systemic inflammation. It is also a key modulator of emotional regulation and neural excitability through its projections into limbic structures.

Anatomy of the vagus nerve

The vagus nerve originates from several nuclei in the medulla oblongata and exits the skull through the jugular foramen as it descends into the neck. The first two branches leaving the vagus at the level of the jugular ganglion are the auricular and meningeal branches. The auricular branch of the vagus is the first readily accessible target for stimulation. Next, the vagus nerve courses downward through the cervical region within the carotid sheath, adjacent to the internal jugular vein and common carotid artery. At the cervical region, on average, the vagus lies only 2.4 cm beneath the skin where it is both easily surgically accessible and an easy target for transcutaneous stimulation at the neck [1,2]. Then, it travels down the neck, thorax, and abdomen to innervate various organs. The fibers of the vagus include both afferent and efferent pathways, with roughly 80% being afferent—carrying sensory information from the viscera to the brain. This predominance of afferent fibers underpins the wide-ranging central effects of VNS.

Most incoming sensory information from vagal afferents is initially integrated in the nucleus of the tractus solitarius (NTS) in the medulla. The NTS then relays this information either directly (e.g., by projecting to the reticular formation in the medulla) or indirectly (e.g., by projecting through the parabrachial nucleus and the locus coeruleus (LC) to other brain regions, including the amygdala, hypothalamus, and orbitofrontal cortex). Stimulation of these circuits has been suggested and approved as a therapeutic technique.

Vagus nerve stimulation

Vagus nerve stimulation (VNS) is a therapeutic technique that involves applying intermittent electrical stimulation to the vagus nerve. Vagus nerve stimulation has a long clinical history with its origins dating back to the late 19th century when neurologists like James Corning first explored its potential to treat seizures. Research in the 1980s demonstrated its anticonvulsant effects, leading to the first human implant in 1988 for epilepsy, which was later approved by the FDA in 1997. Since then, its clinical use has expanded to include treatment-resistant depression, stroke rehabilitation, and rheumatoid arthritis, with advancements including the development of noninvasive stimulation methods that are now also approved by FDA.

A Modern Atlas for Implantable Devices of the Spine, Brain, and Nerve. https://doi.org/10.1016/B978-0-443-36528-7.00042-X

Methods of VNS can be broadly organized depending on whether they are invasive or noninvasive and by the segment of the nerve being stimulated, with the cervical (neck) area and the auricular (ear) area being the most common targets.

Implantable vagus nerve stimulation

Implantable VNS employs a lead with two electrical contacts directly on the cervical portion of vagus nerve and a pacemaker-like pulse-generating device implanted subcutaneously, typically in the anterior chest wall (Figs. 38.1 and 38.2). The common VNS paradigm utilizes continuous (open-loop) electrical stimulation with preset pauses. The time ratio "stimulation on/stimulation off" is called duty cycle. These can be complemented by on-demand stimulation in response to sudden heart rate increases above preset threshold (quasi-closed-loop for epilepsies associated with ictal tachycardia) or by a swift external magnet swipe over the pulse-generating device. VNS received European approval in 1994 and US FDA approval in 1997. As an extracranial neuromodulation system, VNS can be combined with other neuromodulation modalities such as responsive neurostimulation (RNS) and deep brain stimulation (DBS) or any other surgical treatment in various combinations. Importantly, implantable VNS does not carry the CNS side effects associated with medications but does carry surgical risks from implantation and nerve injury.

This chapter provides a comprehensive review of the surgical technique, hardware, indications, contraindications, complications, side effects, perioperative management, and common scenarios encountered by healthcare professionals when caring for patients with implanted VNS systems.

Indications

1) VNS is indicated for **focal-onset epilepsy**, even with anatomically defined single epileptogenic foci. As with every epilepsy surgical modality, VNS is reserved for patient with pharmacoresistant epilepsy, which is defined by the International League Against Epilepsy (ILAE) as failure of adequate trials of two tolerated and appropriately chosen and used antiseizure medication schedules (whether as monotherapies or in combination) to achieve sustained seizure freedom. FDA approval recognized VNS as adjunctive therapy for reducing seizure frequency in patients over 4-years-old with focal-onset seizures refractory to antiepileptic medications. Notably, caution is advised when implanting in very young patients, as the lead may pull on the vagus nerve as the child grows, leading to cases of bradycardia that may resolve after lead replacement [3].

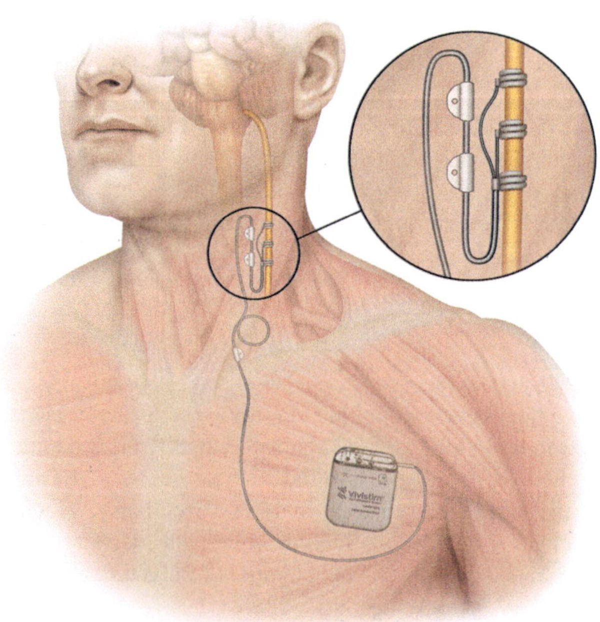

FIGURE 38.1 Schema of VNS system. *Reproduced with permission from MicroTransponder, Inc.*

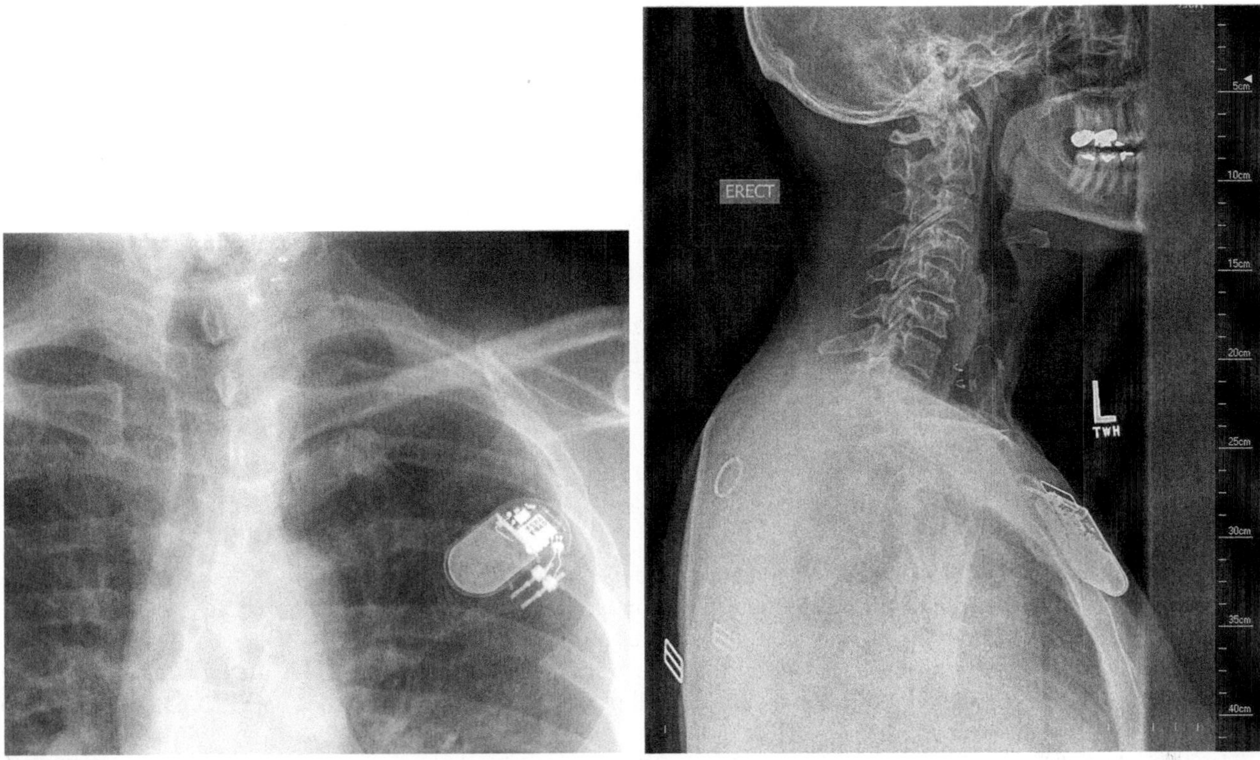

FIGURE 38.2 X-ray views of implanted VNS system—the surgeon was able to implant contacts low on vagus nerve—at C7-T1 level: the left image with LivaNova system; the right image with MicroTransponder system. *The right image is reproduced with permission from MicroTransponder, Inc.*

2) There is evidence supporting the effectiveness of VNS in **generalized epilepsy**, making it one of the treatments for Lennox-Gastaut syndrome. It is crucial to note that the on-label use is limited to focal epilepsy, but off-label use for pharmacoresistant generalized epilepsy has shown significant success with VNS.

3) FDA approval in 2007 extended VNS indications to include adjunctive long-term treatment of chronic or recurrent **depression** for patients 18-years-old or older who are experiencing a major depressive episode not adequately relieved by four or more antidepressant treatments. Importantly, the improvement in mood can be a significant additional benefit for patients suffering from epilepsy or recovering from stroke. Depression prevalence ranges from 13%–37% in patients with epilepsy, with a higher incidence in uncontrolled epilepsy. The antidepressive effect of VNS is independent of its seizure outcome–related benefits.

4) In 2021, FDA added another indication—pairing stimulation of the vagus nerve with rehabilitation therapy to reduce upper extremity motor deficits and improve motor function in **chronic (≥6 months) ischemic stroke** patients with moderate to severe arm impairment. VNS is believed to enhance neuroplasticity [4], as VNS-driven activation of cholinergic, noradrenergic, and serotonergic neurons, combined with intense, task-specific movement training, reorganized motor cortex (neuroplasticity), and reinforced connectivity in spared motor circuits in animal data [5]. Of note, no medications are approved for chronic stroke recovery; thus, rehabilitation is considered the current state-of-the-art treatment for motor deficit due to ischemic stroke.

5) In 2025, FDA approved VNS for the treatment of adults with moderate-to-severe **rheumatoid arthritis** who have had an inadequate response to biologic or targeted synthetic disease-modifying antirheumatic drugs (DMARDs).
Patients should be counseled that VNS is not curative for its current indications and that therapeutic benefits may take months to become evident—or may never occur.

Contraindications

1. VNS is contraindicated in individuals **lacking a vagus nerve** or with history of cervical vagotomy.
2. **Vocal cord paralysis** is a *relative* contraindication, directing the use of the vagus nerve on the opposite side.

3. **Distorted neck anatomy** (history of infection, radiotherapy, radical neck dissection) is another *relative* contraindication, directing the use of the vagus nerve on the opposite side.
4. Individuals who are **not candidates for surgery** under general anesthesia are also excluded for VNS.
   Additional precautions are warranted in pregnancy; chronic pulmonary diseases such as asthma and COPD; obstructive sleep apnea; cardiac bradyarrhythmias or dysfunctional cardiac conduction systems; active peptic ulcer disease; and insulin-dependent diabetes mellitus. Although VNS therapy is FDA-approved for chronic or recurrent depression, one manufacturer (MicroTransponder, Inc.) recommends that patients with moderate or severe depression be observed closely for clinical worsening and suicidality.

Implanted VNS hardware

Implantable components are single-use-only devices and should not be resterilized. Latex is not included in any implantable component.

Leads

LivaNova PLC (London, UK)

LivaNova manufactures VNS systems for the treatment of epilepsy and depression. Currently, the company offers three lead models: VNS Therapy (model 302), PerenniaDURA (model 303), and the latest PerenniaFLEX (model 304). The model 300, which features a dual-pin connector, is no longer in production.

Each lead has three helices: two helices house helical electrodes, one helix is empty and is used for anchoring around the distal (caudal) portion of the nerve. Each helix has a small polyester suture string attached on each end, which is useful for deploying helix around the nerve (Fig. 38.3).

The lead characteristics for the available models include silicone insulation, a connector pin made of 300 series stainless steel, electrodes made of platinum iridium and separated by 8 mm (center to center), lead body conductor made of MP-35N alloy in helical quadfilar (models 302, 304) or trifilar (model 303) configuration, and a connector pin-to-electrode resistance ranging from 120 to 180 Ohms (models 302, 304) or 180–250 Ohms (model 303). Each lead is 43 cm long and is available in two sizes (2.0- and 3.0-mm electrode inner diameter) to ensure optimal electrode fit on nerves with different diameters (Figs. 38.4 and 38.5).

The lead's lifespan is undetermined by the manufacturer. A lead would require replacement if a lead fracture were suspected and accompanied by worsened symptoms, such as increased seizure frequency or intermittent pain along VNS hardware that resolves after VNS has been turned off.

MicroTransponder, Inc. (Austin, TX, USA)

MicroTransponder currently offers a single lead model (Fig. 38.6), similar in design to LivaNova's leads: silicone insulation; a connector pin made of 300-series stainless steel; platinum–iridium electrodes separated by 8 mm (center to

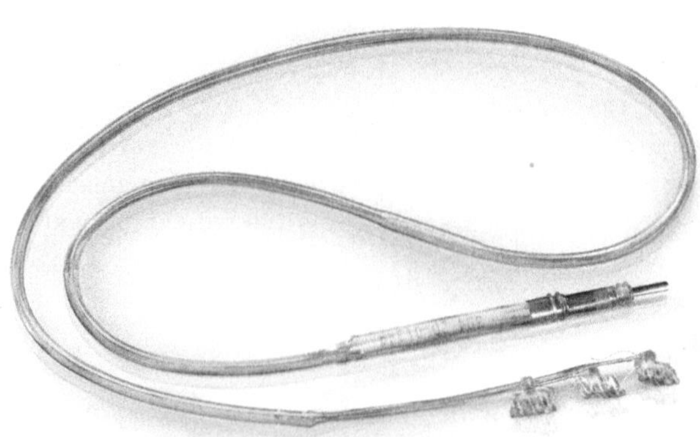

FIGURE 38.3 Photograph of LivaNova VNS lead. *Reproduced with permission from LivaNova PLC.*

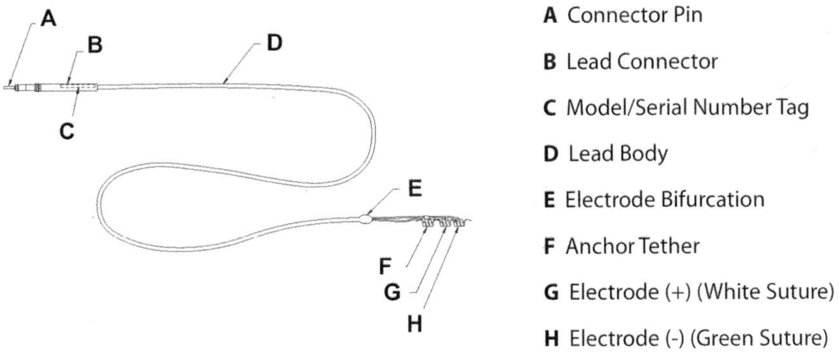

FIGURE 38.4 LivaNova VNS leads (models 302 and 304). *Reproduced with permission from LivaNova PLC.*

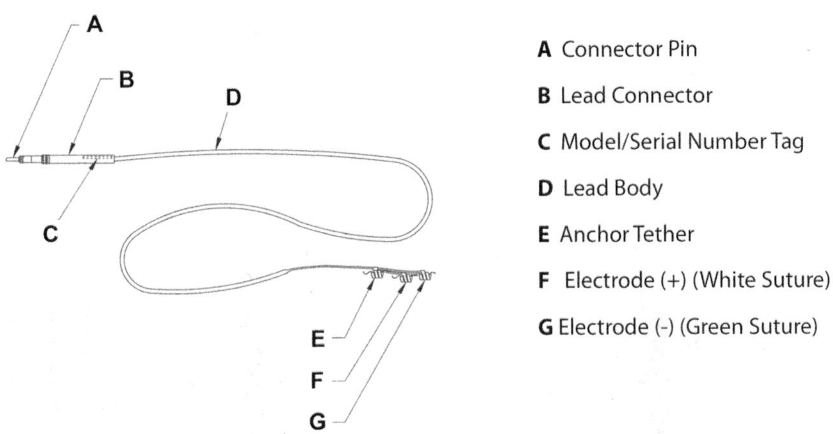

FIGURE 38.5 LivaNova VNS lead (model 303). *Reproduced with permission from LivaNova PLC.*

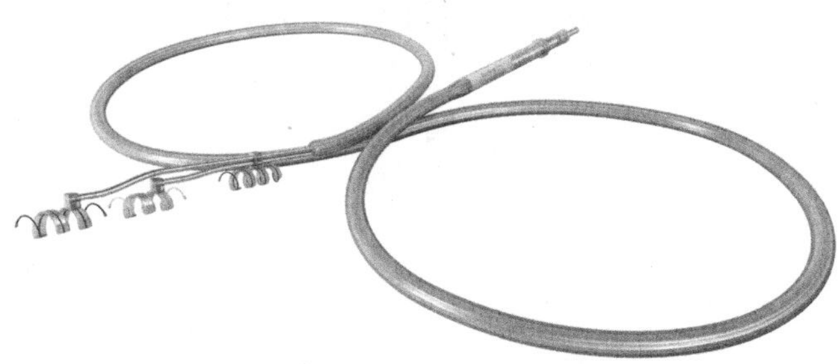

FIGURE 38.6 MicroTransponder VNS lead (model 3000). *Reproduced with permission from MicroTransponder, Inc.*

center); a lead-body conductor of MP-35N alloy in a helical quadfilar configuration; and a connector pin-to-electrode resistance of 100–250 Ohms. The lead is 43 cm long and is available in two sizes (2.0- and 3.0-mm electrode inner diameter) to ensure optimal electrode fit on nerves with different diameters.

Implantable pulse generators

LivaNova PLC

LivaNova VNS implantable pulse generators (IPG) are nonrechargeable and available in two footprint shapes and sizes (Fig. 38.7), each with different charge capacities:

1. Smaller models (103, 104, 1000, 1000D, 8301) feature a charge capacity of 1 Ah (3.3 V battery model 2183 made by Wilson Greatbatch Ltd.).

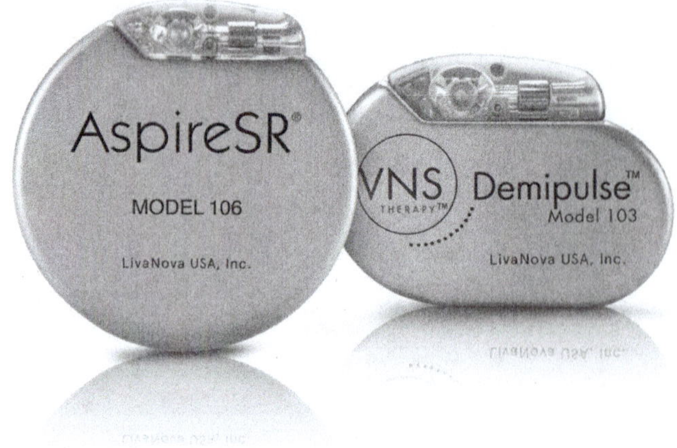

FIGURE 38.7 LivaNova VNS IPGs—shape comparison of larger model (106) and smaller model (103). *Reproduced with permission from LivaNova PLC.*

2. Larger models (102, 102R, 105, 106) offer a higher charge capacity of 1.7 Ah (3.3 V battery model 2075 made by Wilson Greatbatch Ltd.).

Legacy models are 100–105, while models 106 and above are currently manufactured modern models.

Key characteristics of the LivaNova VNS IPG system include a hermetically sealed titanium case with polyurethane (Tecothane TT-1075D-M Thermoplastic) header and stainless-steel lead connector blocks.

The IPG can be identified by X-ray. Of note, the serial number and model number of the IPG are marked on its titanium case, but do not appear on the X-ray. The serial number and model number can be identified by interrogating the IPG with the clinician programmer.

IPGs have a low self-discharge rate of less than 1% per year, ensuring long-term reliability. The batteries are designed to last for approximately 10,000 h of stimulation. The modern IPG models (103 and above) demonstrate consistent performance from 100% to 1%, although clinical observations suggest that patients may experience worsening of seizures when the battery falls below 10%, a phenomenon currently lacking the resolved scientific basis.

Modern heart rate sensing and responding (AutoStim) models

ASPIRE SR (model 106) (Fig. 38.8).

SENTIVA (model 1000) (Fig. 38.9)—this model has additional features:

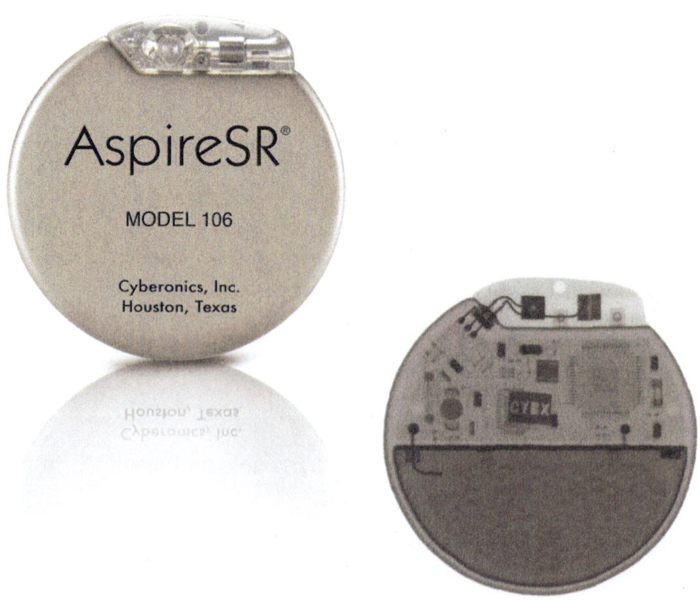

FIGURE 38.8 LivaNova VNS IPG—Aspire SR (model 106) and its X-ray view. *Reproduced with permission from LivaNova PLC.*

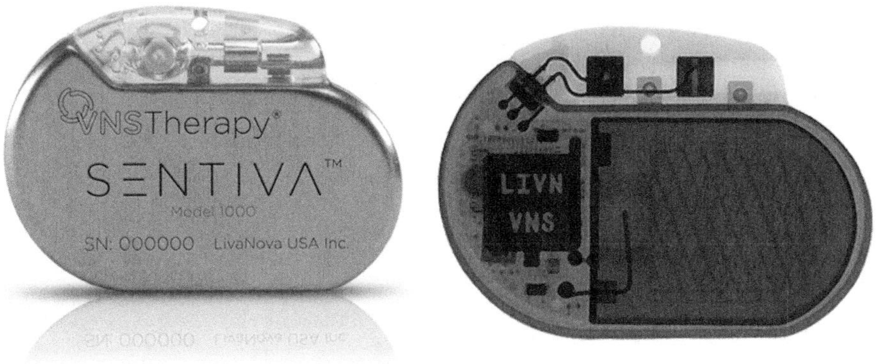

FIGURE 38.9 LivaNova VNS IPG—Sentiva (model 1000) and its X-ray view. *(Reproduced with permission from LivaNova PLC).*

1. Low heart rate detection.
2. Prone position detection.
3. Guided programming + scheduled programming titration schedule—can be programmed during one office visit and delivered while the patient lives their life (e.g., scheduled increase in stimulation current every 2 weeks at the specific time of the day until therapeutic target is reached).
4. Day and night programming—enables two independent sets of parameters to be customized and delivered based on each patient's needs. For example, if a patient experiences diurnal seizure cycles, it may allow for the delivery of a higher dose of stimulation during seizure-prone hours and the conservation of battery charge by using a lower dose of stimulation during other hours.
5. Events and trends—enables to view data at follow-up visits on events that may be associated with seizures.

SENTIVA DUO (model 1000-D) (Fig. 38.10)—dual pin connector design for patients with legacy dual-pin VNS leads still in place.

Model for depression treatment

SYMMETRY (model 8103) (Fig. 38.11)—does not offer AutoStim.

MicroTransponder Inc

MicroTransponder offers a single nonrechargeable IPG model—Vivistim (model 1001) (Fig. 38.12). The Vivistim IPG provides a range of stimulation parameters that is practically similar to LivaNova IPG models, except that Vivistim IPGs allow more granular steps and do not include heart-rate detection. The IPG features a charge capacity of 2.5 Ah (3.3 V battery, model WG 9086, made by Wilson Greatbatch Ltd.; the battery voltage gradually decreases as it nears end of life).

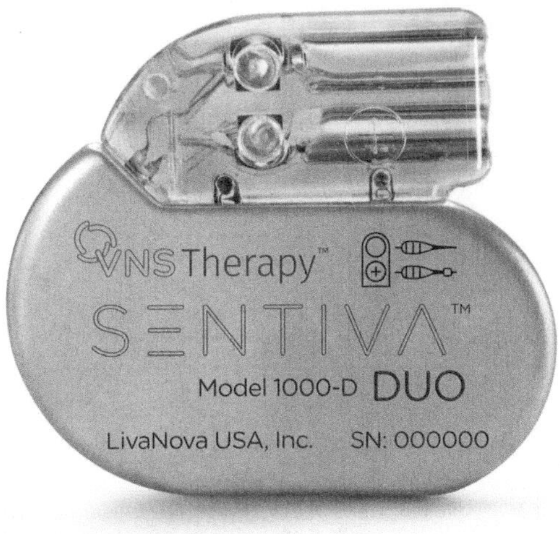

FIGURE 38.10 LivaNova VNS IPG—Sentiva Duo (model 1000-D) with dual pin receptacle. *Reproduced with permission from LivaNova PLC.*

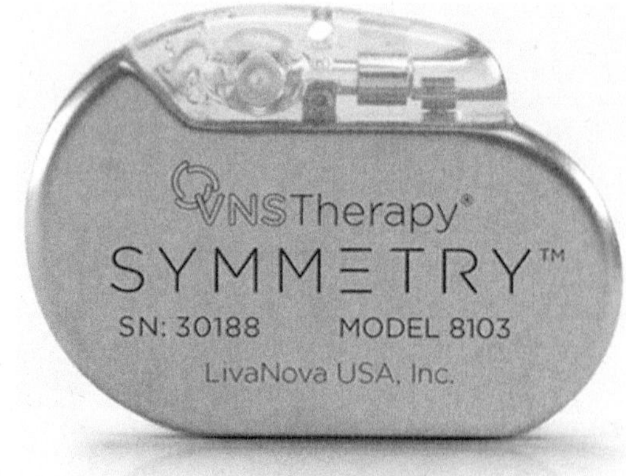

FIGURE 38.11 LivaNova VNS IPG—Symmetry (model 8103). *Reproduced with permission from LivaNova PLC.*

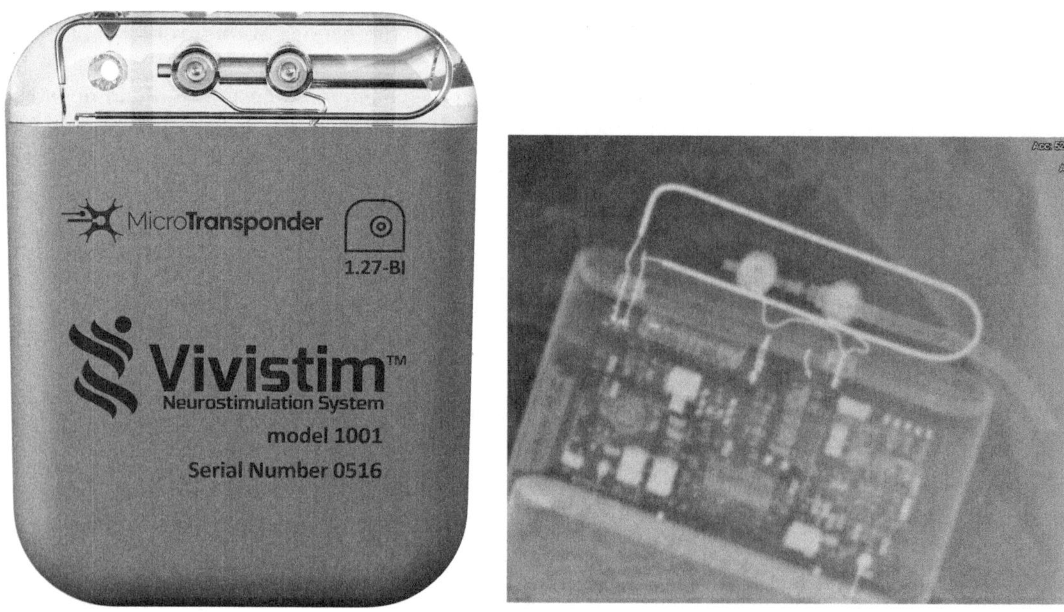

FIGURE 38.12 MicroTransponder VNS IPG—Vivistim (model 1001) and its X-ray view. *Reproduced with permission from MicroTransponder, Inc.*

Surgical noninplantable accessories

For the surgical procedure, a specialized tunneler (Figs. 38.13 and 38.14) is available as an option but, alternatively, a conventional neurosurgical shunt subcutaneous tunneler may be used.

An accessory kit (e.g., LivaNova model #502—Fig. 38.15) is also optional and includes a spare screwdriver (although one screwdriver is included in the package with each IPG), tie-downs, and a 4000 Ohms test resistor (for "Generator Diagnostics," if indicated).

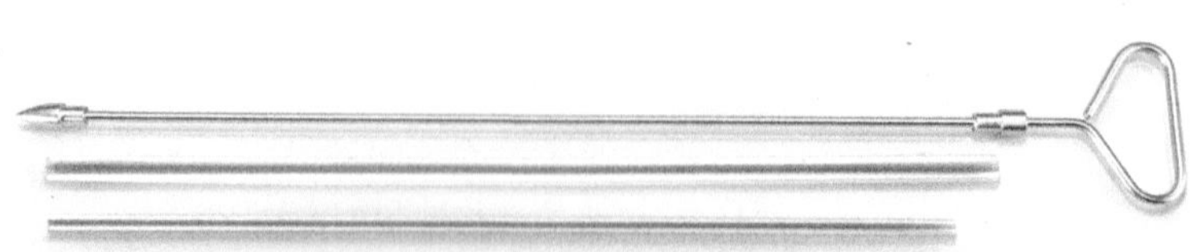

FIGURE 38.13 LivaNova VNS tunneler (model 402). *Reproduced with permission from LivaNova PLC.*

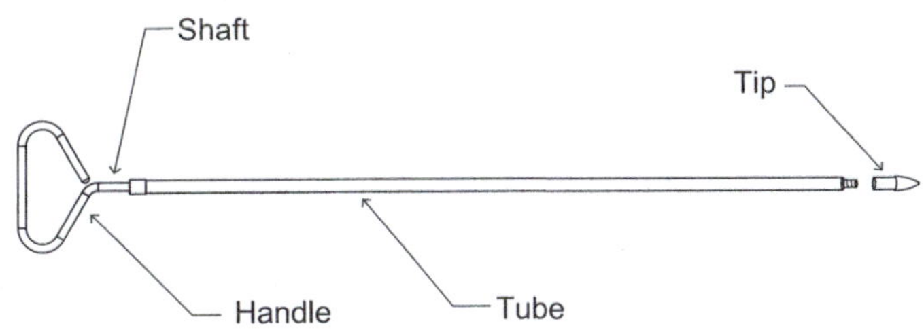

FIGURE 38.14 MicroTransponder VNS tunneler (model 6001). *Reproduced with permission from MicroTransponder, Inc.*

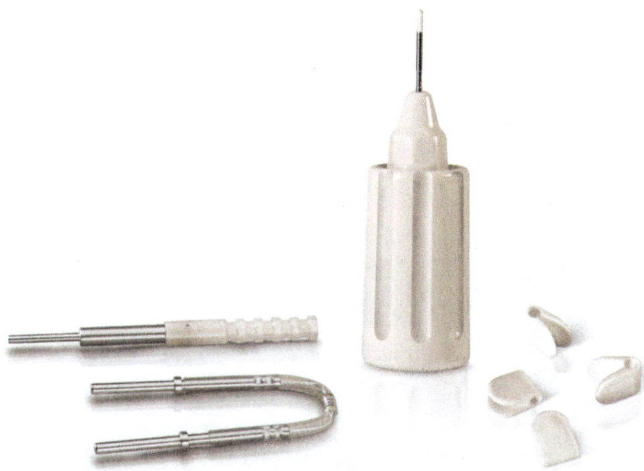

FIGURE 38.15 VNS accessory kit (model 502). *Reproduced with permission from LivaNova PLC.*

Nonsurgical accessories

LivaNova PLC

With each IPG implantation, the patient receives two VNS Therapy magnets (Fig. 38.16), each providing a minimum of 50 G at 1 inch. Magnets can be utilized for on-demand stimulation enhancement or output inhibition, as detailed in the following paragraphs.

The epilepsy care professional is provided with a clinician programmer equipped with a wireless wand (Fig. 38.17) for VNS system interrogation. The wand can be held by the patient but must remain strictly positioned over the IPG site (Fig. 38.18); otherwise, an error message will be issued.

Currently, epilepsy patients lack tools to directly communicate with their implanted VNS device. However, future models may incorporate Bluetooth technology, enabling device access for patients and facilitating remote data access for healthcare providers.

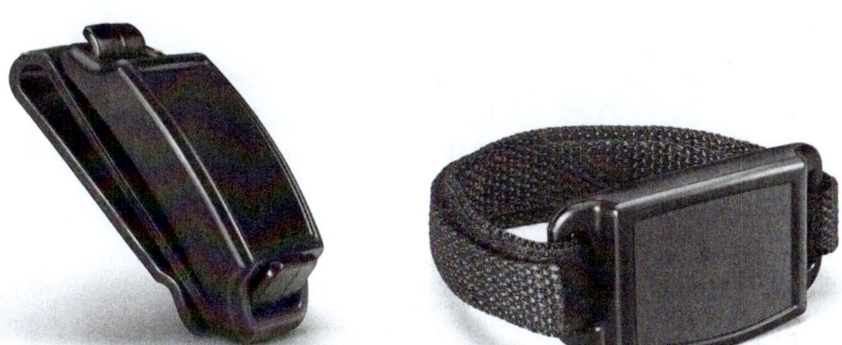

FIGURE 38.16 VNS Therapy magnets (model 220): pager-style (belt clip) and watch-style (wristband). *Reproduced with permission from LivaNova PLC.*

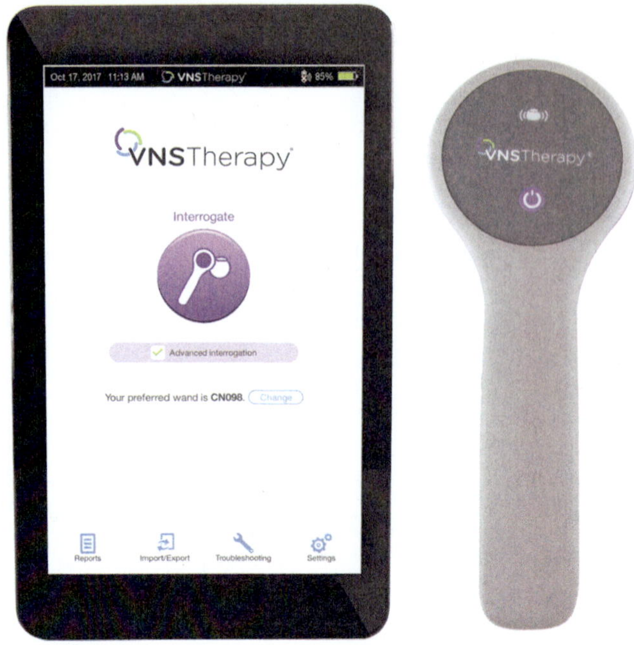

FIGURE 38.17 Clinician programmer unit. *Reproduced with permission from LivaNova PLC.*

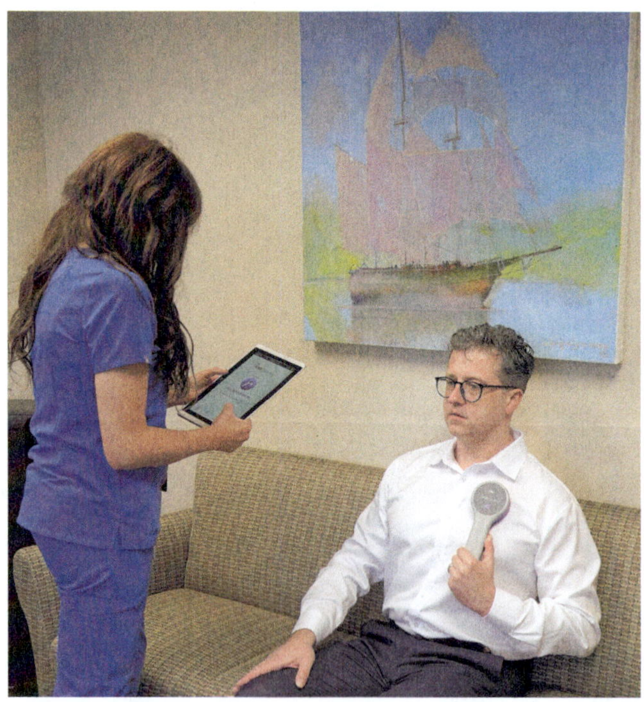

FIGURE 38.18 VNS system interrogation.

MicroTransponder Inc.

Stroke rehabilitation therapists are provided with a laptop running the Stroke Application & Programming Software (SAPS) and a wireless transmitter to communicate with the IPG (Fig. 38.19) at distances up to 1 m. During rehabilitation, the therapist activates VNS (Fig. 38.20) using a remote control (Fig. 38.21)—so-called Vivistim Paired VNS therapy. In-clinic rehabilitation therapy typically lasts 6 weeks, with sessions a few times per week. Of note, vagus nerve stimulation with Paired VNS therapy typically occurs for about 90 min per session, whereas epilepsy VNS therapy typically

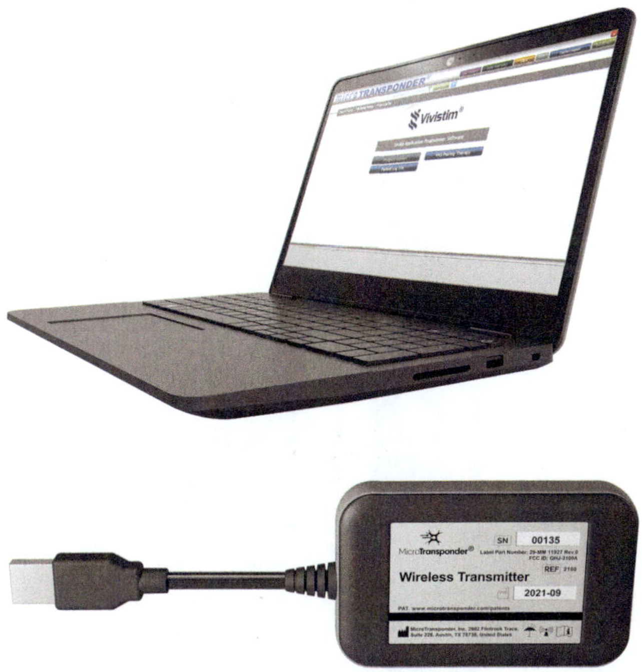

FIGURE 38.19 Vivistim system laptop and wireless transmitter. *Reproduced with permission from MicroTransponder, Inc.*

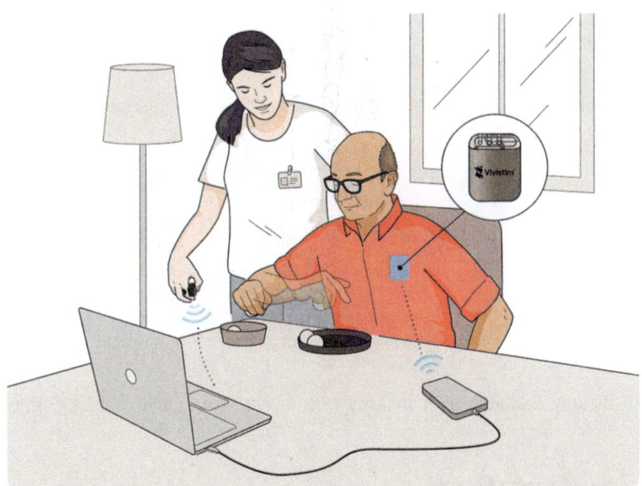

FIGURE 38.20 Vivistim Paired VNS therapy in use during rehabilitation session in clinic. *Reproduced with permission from MicroTransponder, Inc.*

stimulates 24 h a day. For the recommended selection of stimulation parameters, see the "Programming" section in the following.

Depending on the therapy-session setup, during rehabilitation exercises or daily activities, patients or family members can swipe the external magnet (Fig. 38.22) to pair vagus nerve stimulation with intentional movement at home (Fig. 38.23). This activates the IPG to typically deliver stimulation for 30 min. The patient may also secure the magnet over the IPG to stop stimulation if a system malfunction or significant side effects are suspected; holding the magnet over the IPG for at least 30 s stops any stimulation for as long as it remains in place. Of note, the magnet may damage televisions, computer disks, credit cards, and other items affected by strong magnetic fields. At present, stroke patients have no means to directly interface with their implanted MicroTransponder VNS device for interrogation.

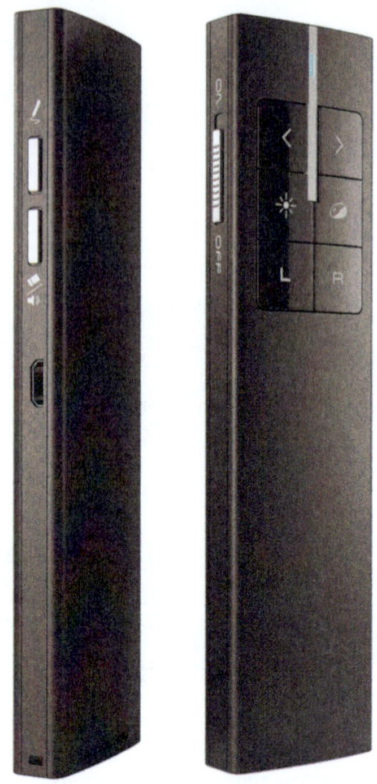

FIGURE 38.21 Vivistim Paired VNS therapy system remote control for therapist's use. *Reproduced with permission from MicroTransponder, Inc.*

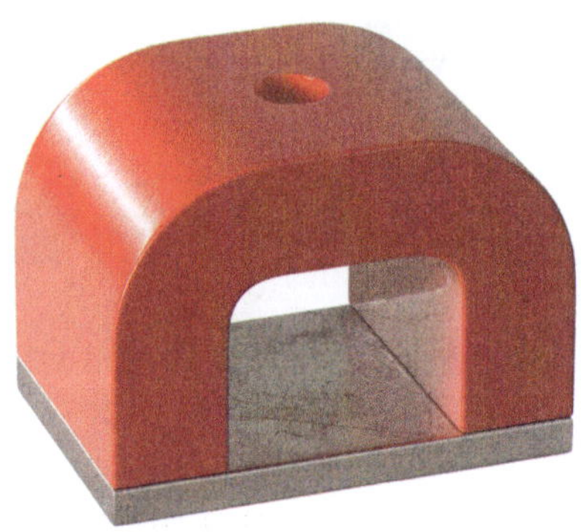

FIGURE 38.22 Vivistim Paired VNS therapy self-activation magnet with a pull force rated at 4.5 kg. *Reproduced with permission from MicroTransponder, Inc.*

De Novo VNS system implantation

Preoperative workup

In the patient consultation process, it is essential to confirm that the patient has a well-established diagnosis of pharmacoresistant epilepsy/depression/ischemic stroke. For example, for epilepsy patients, it is imperative to review the brain MRI, ideally conducted on a $\geq$3 T scanner with an epilepsy protocol, and carefully examine the scalp EEG report. Additionally, inquire about the patient's history of obstructive sleep apnea, as well as their occupation and hobbies that may require a clear voice. Also, assess history of any prior neck surgeries and inquire about cardiological problems. Conduct a thorough physical examination, including auscultation for carotid bruits as carotid artery requires some manipulation during surgery. As part of the process, order an ECG to examine for bradyarrhythmias, such as AV node or bundle branch blocks, as these pose a higher risk of cardiac side effects during VNS stimulation. Ensure effective patient counseling regarding the anticipated side effects of VNS and MRI restrictions as outlined in the following. In addition, counsel about the magnet use on demand, and the need for future IPG replacements but only if VNS effectiveness is documented. It is important to set realistic expectations for therapy outcomes based on published data.

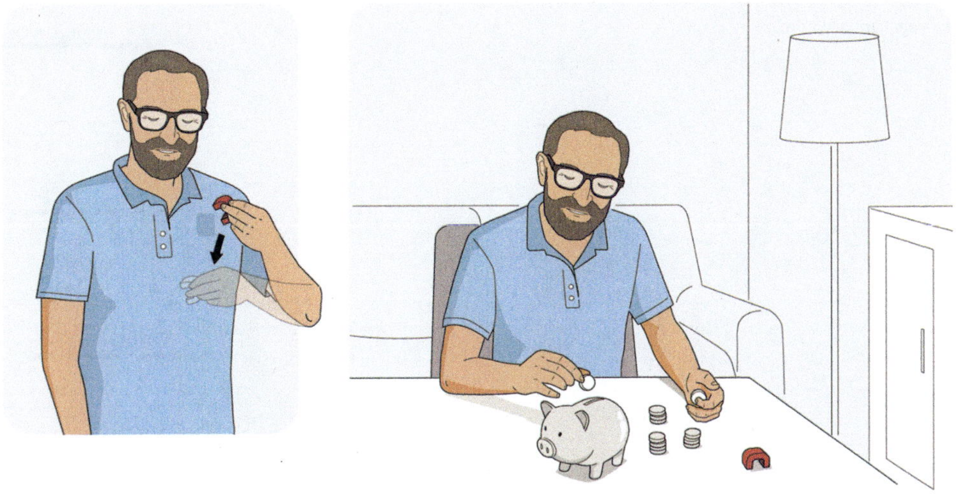

FIGURE 38.23 Vivistim Paired VNS therapy self-activation using magnet swipe at home. *Reproduced with permission from MicroTransponder, Inc.*

Surgical technique

The surgeon aims to place stimulator contacts on the cervical vagus nerve below the point where the superior and inferior cervical cardiac branches diverge from the nerve (Fig. 38.24). Stimulation of either cervical vagus nerve is effective, but the left nerve (Fig. 38.25) is typically chosen due to its lower theoretical likelihood of causing cardiac effects, more detailed in the further section.

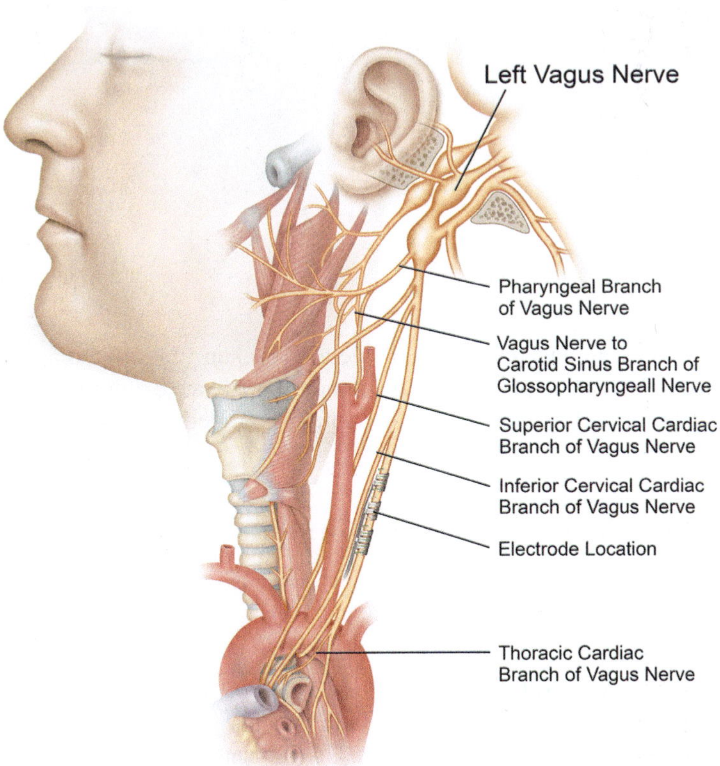

FIGURE 38.24 Outline of relevant neck anatomy. *Reproduced with permission from MicroTransponder, Inc.*

FIGURE 38.25 Schematic of cardiac vagal innervation.

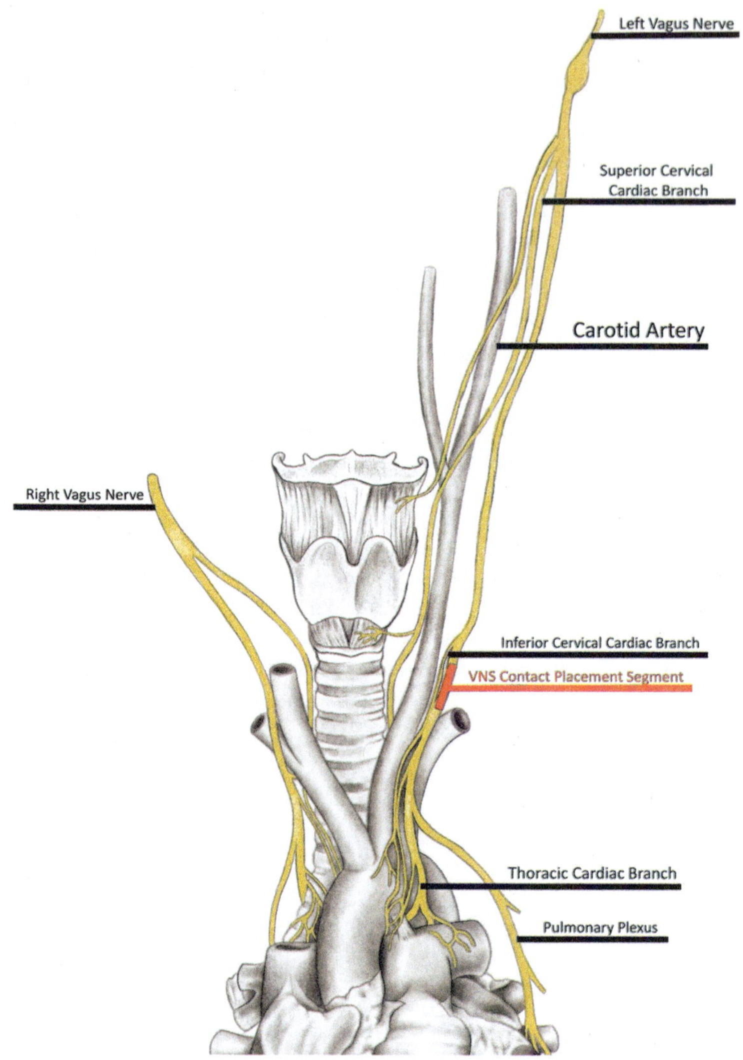

Patient position

During the preanesthesia time out, ensure that a spare VNS lead and IPG are available as a backup.

After the general endotracheal anesthesia is employed, the head is placed on a gel donut in moderate extension with a small roll under the neck to push cervical viscera anteriorly (Fig. 38.26). Head rotation considerations include the following:

1. Keeping the head straight to avoid distorting anterior cervical anatomy.
2. If rotation is necessary, rotate the head to the right. Note that this moves the chin away from surgical access but be cautious as the internal jugular vein tends to overlap the vagus nerve.

The arm position is determined by the planned IPG implantation site:

1. Keep the arms tucked at the sides for classical IPG implantations just below the clavicle.
2. If the IPG incision is planned lateral to the breast, position the ipsilateral arm abducted on the armrest. Some experts prefer making all IPG incisions along the anterior axillary fold, especially for female patients.
3. When patient tampering with the IPG site is a concern, it may be advisable to consider implanting the battery in the back.

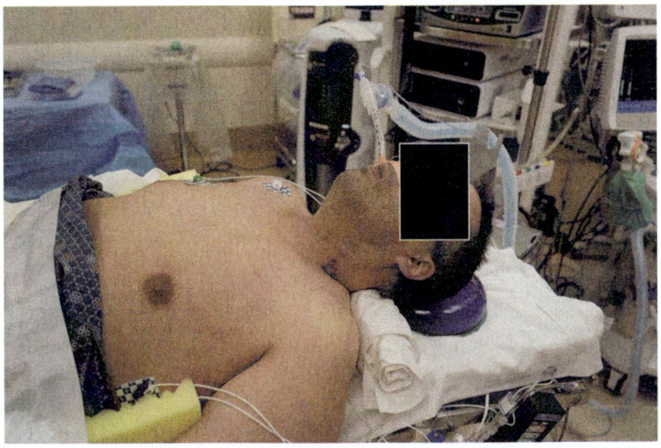

FIGURE 38.26 Patient position.

Marking skin incisions

After the surgical site has been clipped of hair and prepared with povidone–iodine scrub followed by isopropyl alcohol–soaked gauze, the planned skin incisions are outlined using a sterile surgical marking pen (Fig. 38.27).

Cervical skin incision

The goal is to expose left cervical vagus nerve below its cardiac branches. A transverse "collar" incision is marked along a natural skin crease at the level of the palpable cricothyroid membrane (Fig. 38.28), in a similar fashion to a C5-6 anterior cervical discectomy, or even lower if the neck anatomy permits. 3–4 cm length of incision should be centered to where carotid pulse is palpable, generally, with some overlap over medial edge of sternocleidomastoid muscle.

Chest skin incision

Traditionally, the IPG is implanted in a subcutaneous pocket just below the clavicle in the left upper chest.

Try to place the generator at fourth rib or above, which is above the nipple in male patients, to provide the patient with maximum flexibility for MRI postoperatively. To pinpoint the optimal IPG location, palpate the anterior chest wall

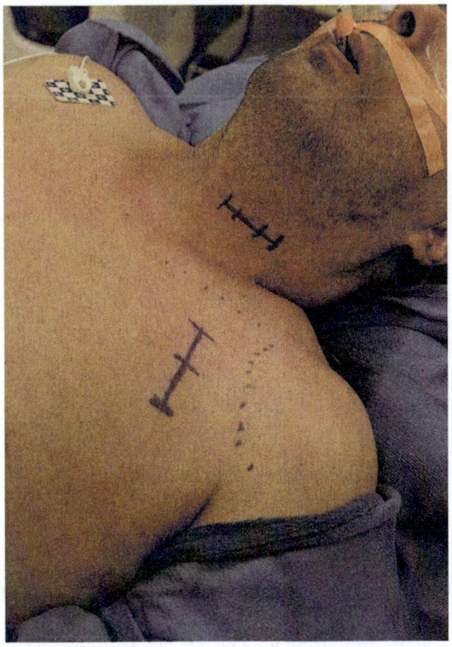

FIGURE 38.27 Skin incisions marked.

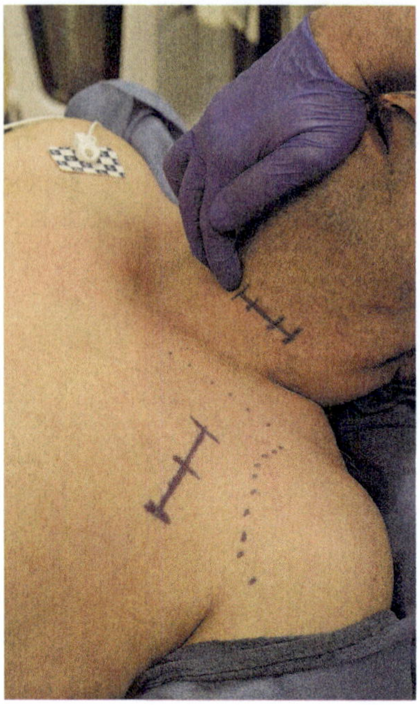

FIGURE 38.28 Palpable cricothyroid membrane.

tissues, identifying an area with sufficient tissue bulk to cover the IPG. This ensures optimal cosmesis and minimizes the risk of skin dehiscence. Ensure the incision is two fingerbreadths away from the clavicle and two fingerbreadths away from the deltopectoral groove (Fig. 38.29) to minimize interference with upper limb movements. The skin incision may be made either perpendicular or parallel to the clavicle, or alternatively along the anterior axillary line when the IPG is to be placed in a subpectoral position (Fig. 38.30).

Cervical dissection

Administer local anesthetic with epinephrine early in the process, preferably during the skin prepping phase. This timing allows the hemostatic effect of epinephrine to begin while the patient is being sterilely draped. Minimize the use of

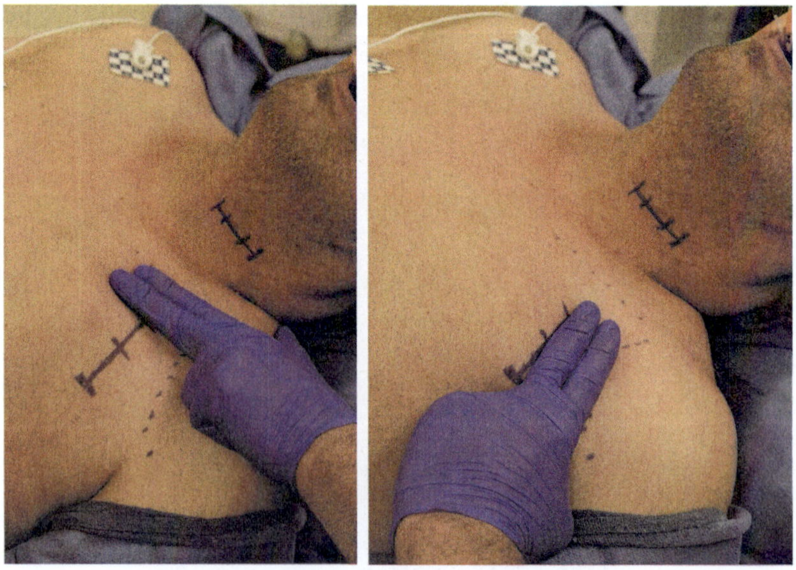

FIGURE 38.29 Incision is two fingerbreadths away from the clavicle and two fingerbreadths away from the deltopectoral groove.

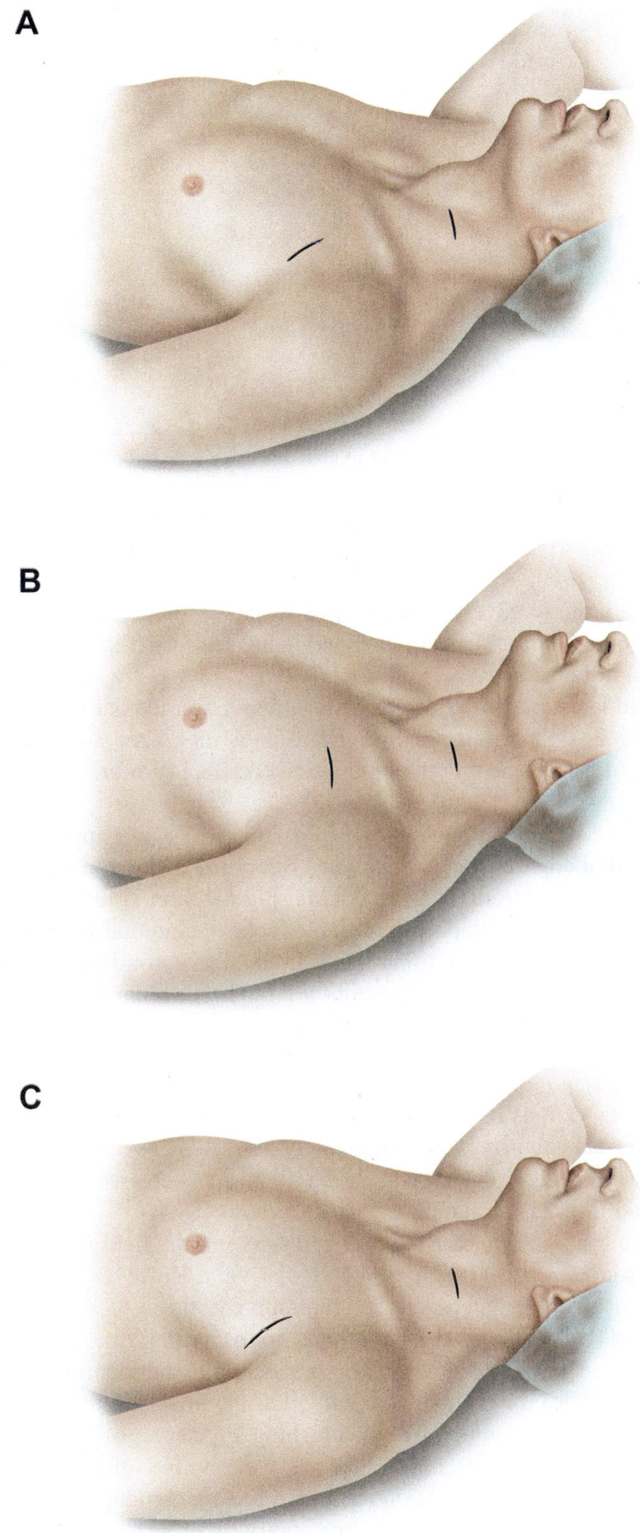

FIGURE 38.30 Incision variations: (a) IPG skin incision perpendicular to the clavicle; (b) IPG skin incision parallel to the clavicle; (c) IPG skin incision along the anterior axillary line. *Reproduced with permission from MicroTransponder, Inc.*

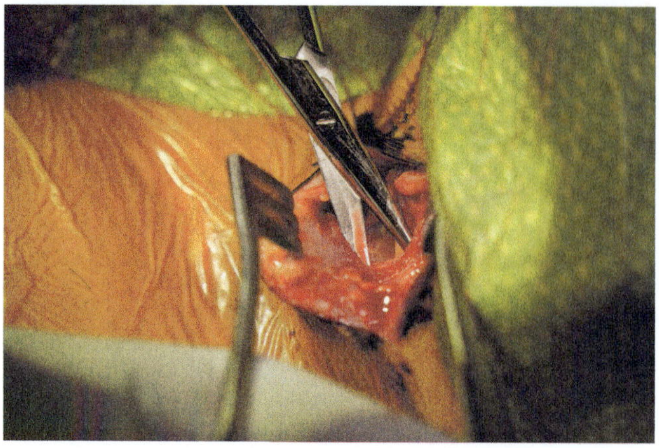

FIGURE 38.31 Cut platysma using scissors.

electrosurgical tools, limiting them to occasional bipolar cautery during dissection. There should be no need for monopolar cautery.

Make the skin incision with a knife (e.g., #10 blade). Upon reaching the platysma, two approaches are available: (1) transect the platysma transversely (parallel to the skin incision) using scissors (Fig. 38.31), or (2) split the platysma along its fibers (perpendicular to the skin incision).

Upon reaching the sternocleidomastoid muscle (Fig. 38.32), dissection is continued in the plane between its medial border and strap muscles (Fig. 38.33). Sternocleidomastoid muscle is mobilized and retracted laterally.

To facilitate access, dissect and retract the omohyoid muscle (Fig. 38.34) inferiorly using a vessel loop or another set of retractors.

Proceed with dissection using a technique analogous to a two-level ACDF approach: advance toward the anterior surface of the spine along the medial edge of the carotid. Then direct the dissection laterally along the anterior aspect of the carotid until the groove between the carotid and the internal jugular vein is identified. Avoid dissecting beneath the sternocleidomastoid muscle. There is no topographical need to expose the internal jugular vein. After opening the carotid sheath, consider leaving some adventitia (edges of the sheath) on the carotid and internal jugular vein to facilitate engagement of the retractor blades. Typically, two retractors are required; blunt Weitlaner retractors are preferred.

Vagus nerve exposure

Using delicate surgical instruments such as toothless Gerald tissue forceps, a right-angle dissector, and Metzenbaum or tenotomy scissors, expose the cervical vagus nerve approximately halfway between the clavicle and mastoid process. This point is below where the superior and inferior cervical cardiac branches separate from the vagus nerve, as stimulating either of these branches may lead to bradycardia and/or asystole.

Identify the main vagus nerve trunk (Fig. 38.35), the largest nerve in the field (Fig. 38.36), classically located in the posterior groove between the carotid artery and the internal jugular vein. However, in a study of 50 cadavers examining vagus syntropy, the left vagus was situated anterior to the common carotid in 68% of cases [6]. Additionally, a thinner nerve—the superior root of the ansa cervicalis (Fig. 38.37)—may loop anteriorly between the internal jugular vein and the carotid artery. Sometimes, a small nerve—the vagus cardiac branch—may be identified medial to the main vagus trunk. Therefore, it may be encountered before the vagus nerve and could be mistaken for it.

During the surgical procedure, exercise caution to avoid crushing any nerve in the forceps; instead, lift and manipulate nerves using their epineurium (Fig. 38.38). Dissect the vagus nerve circumferentially, aiming to expose a 3 cm (1.2 inch) segment—sufficient for the placement of lead helices on the nerve. Ensure meticulous hemostasis by using gelatin sponge (e.g., Gelfoam) with thrombin and avoiding the use of electrocautery on or near the nerve. Be mindful that stretching the nerve or allowing it to dry may lead to temporary swelling, constriction, and subsequent vocal cord dysfunction. Some experts prefer thorough nerve skeletonization, removing all epineurium to minimize tissue impedances (with the goal of <1500 Ohms to conserve VNS battery). However, this approach carries the risk of disturbing vasa nervorum and inducing later nerve fibrosis with increased impedances.

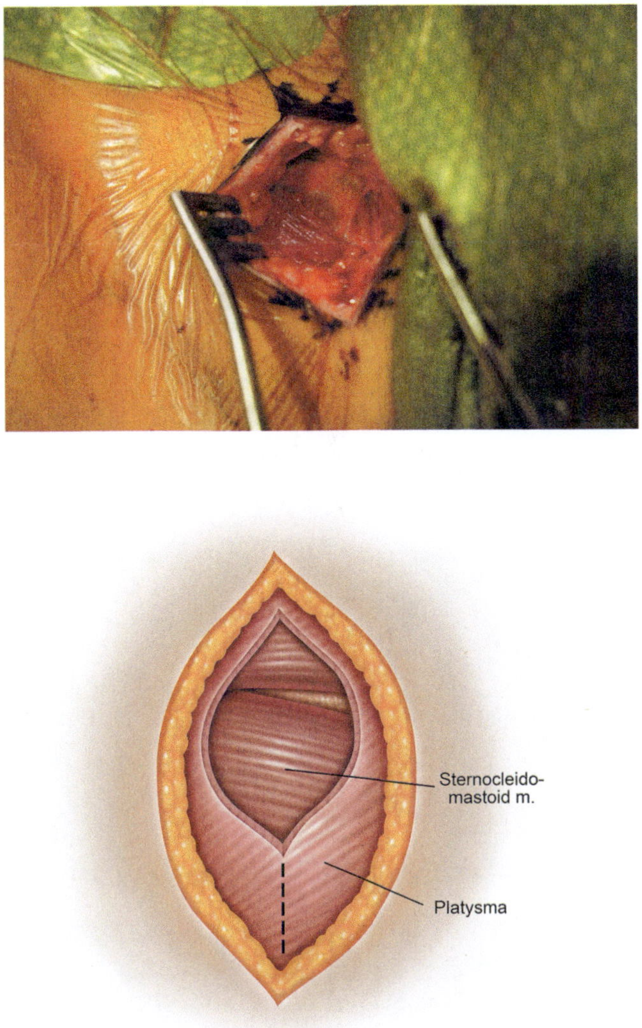

FIGURE 38.32 Sternocleidomastoid muscle exposed. *The schematic figure is reproduced with permission from MicroTransponder, Inc.*

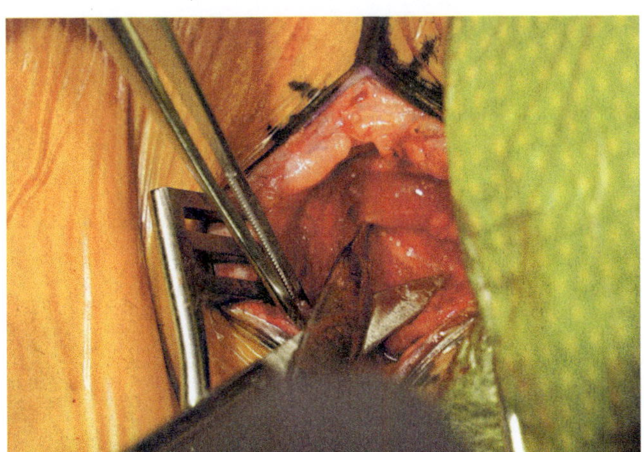

FIGURE 38.33 Dissection in the plane between sternocleidomastoid medial border and strap muscles.

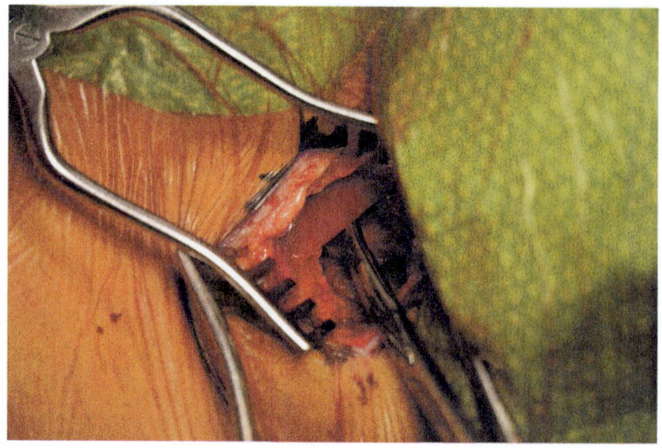

FIGURE 38.34 Omohyoid muscle exposed.

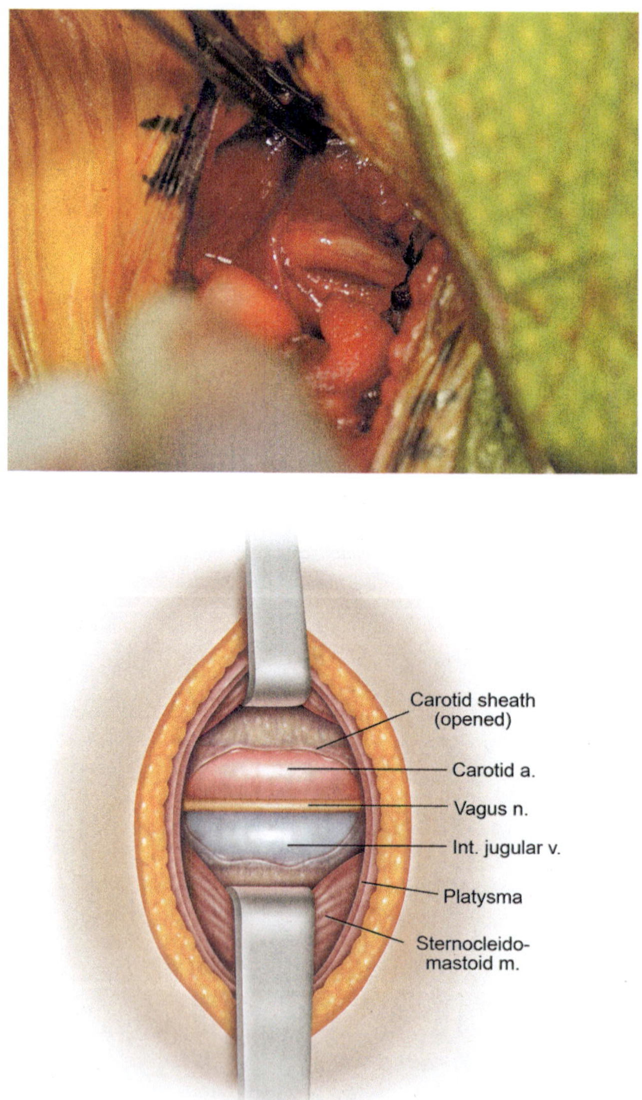

FIGURE 38.35 The main vagus nerve trunk located between the carotid artery and the internal jugular vein. *The schematic figure is reproduced with permission from MicroTransponder, Inc.*

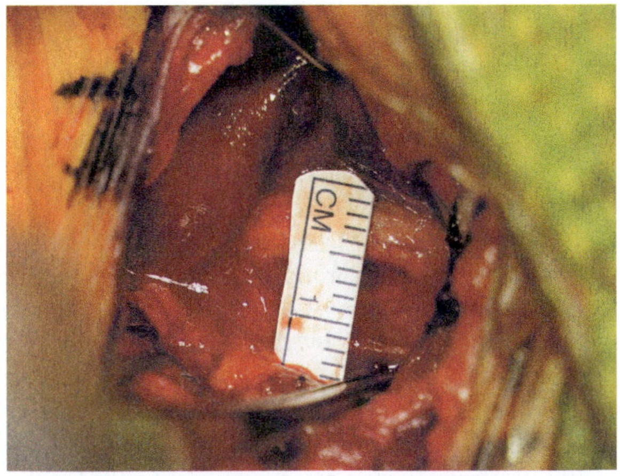

FIGURE 38.36 The diameter of the main vagus nerve trunk.

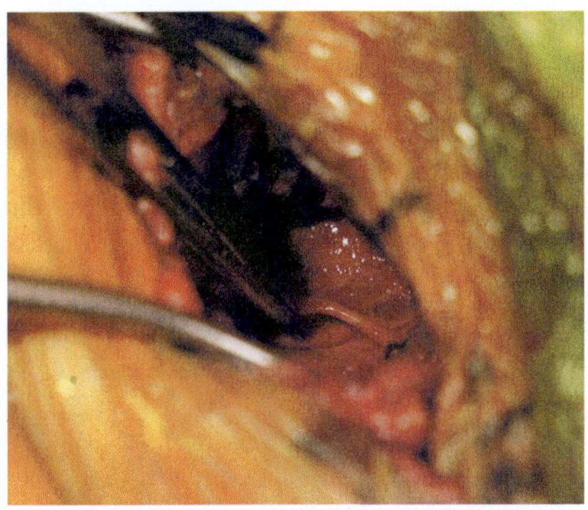

FIGURE 38.37 The root of ansa cervicalis.

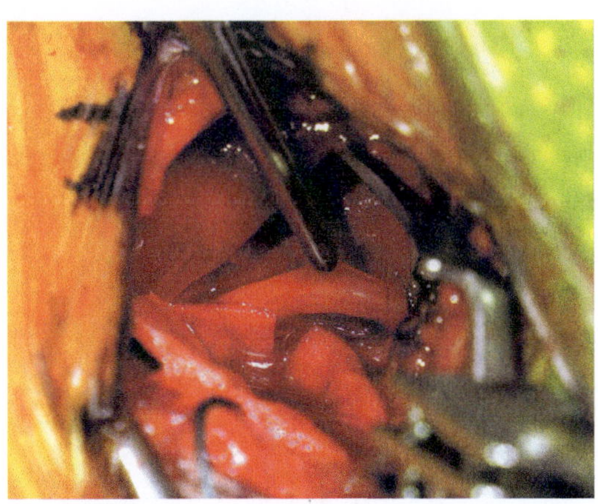

FIGURE 38.38 Manipulate nerves using their epineurium.

Wrapping lead contacts on the nerve

Select the appropriate lead size, with either 2.0- or 3.0-mm electrode inner diameter, ensuring a snug contact fit without constricting the nerve. Generally, a 2.0-mm lead should accommodate most nerves. Open the lead from its package only when ready to implant to avoid exposure to dust or other particulates that may attract to its silicone insulation. Avoid soaking the lead in saline or a similar solution before implantation, as it may cause insulated portions of the connector pin to swell and later become difficult to insert into the IPG receptacle.

Use delicate forceps on the epineurium or soft rubber vessel loops around the nerve to elevate it (Fig. 38.39). If nerve tends to retract dorsally into the groove between the carotid and jugular, surgeon may place a small cottonoid or a 1.0 × 0.5-inch piece of gelatin sponge soaked in thrombin solution underneath the nerve to keep nerve gently elevated anteriorly (Fig. 38.40). The gelatin sponge is preferred by the authors, as it provides a soft, moist, and hemostatic environment. In the event of a small piece of sponge getting caught or trapped between a nerve/instrument/lead helix, it can be easily pulled out, and any microscopic remnant will rapidly absorb in vivo.

Coil two helical electrodes and one helical anchor tether around the nerve. Remember the correct topographical order to maintain correct polarity: the negative electrode (with a green suture embedded in the helical material) goes cranial, and the positive electrode (with white suture) goes caudal (Fig. 38.41). Applying contacts in reverse order may stimulate efferent nerve fibers, potentially leading to gastrointestinal distress.

When placing the helices, there is no preferred chronological order of placement—some experts place the negative electrode first, while others prefer the anchor tether first.

Using forceps, delicately pull each end of the helix using the attached sutures to spread helices open (Fig. 38.42).

After opening helices directly above and parallel to the exposed nerve, turn helices clockwise at a 45-degree angle to the nerve (Fig. 38.43). Position the turn of the electrode helix where the lead wire connects to the metal ribbon onto the nerve (Fig. 38.44). Alternatively, the authors prefer to position the anchor tether helix first (Fig. 38.45).

Utilize fine-tipped forceps to hold the suture ends, manipulating each end of the helix to wrap around the nerve (Figs. 38.46–38.48). This process typically necessitates a coordinated effort involving three or four hands.

The alternative techniques allow for a single-person procedure if surgical assistant is not available:

1. Technique utilizing **a blunt nerve hook**: stretch and rotate the helices as above so that the metal contact sits on the nerve; then release the stretch, allowing the helices to recoil and grasp the nerve. Subsequently, move the nerve hook under the nerve, then hook and rotate to pull the helix around the nerve (Figs. 49 and 50), repeating the process on the other end of the helix.

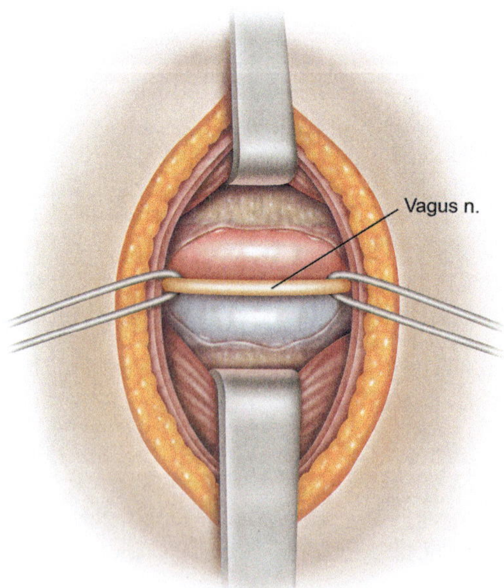

FIGURE 38.39 Vessel loops around the nerve. *Reproduced with permission from MicroTransponder, Inc.*

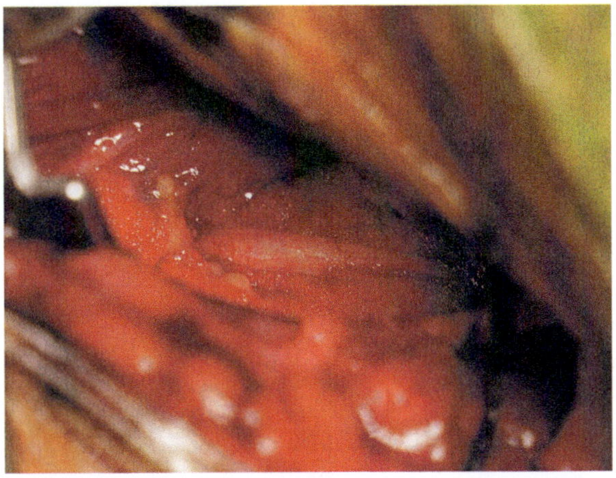

FIGURE 38.40 Gelatin sponge underneath the nerve.

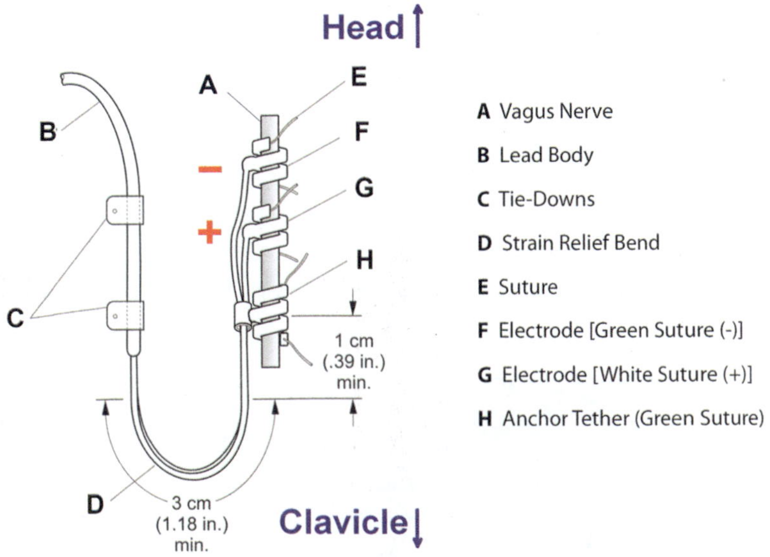

FIGURE 38.41 Helices on the nerve with correct polarity. *(The figure has been adapted from copyrighted material of LivaNova PLC, and is used with permission).*

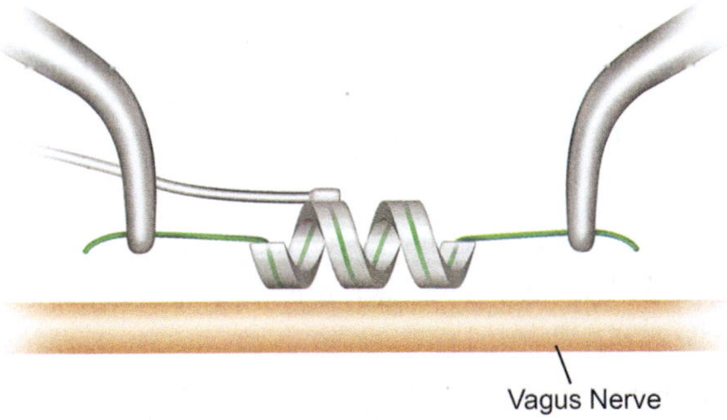

FIGURE 38.42 Pull using the attached sutures to spread the helix. *Reproduced with permission from MicroTransponder, Inc.*

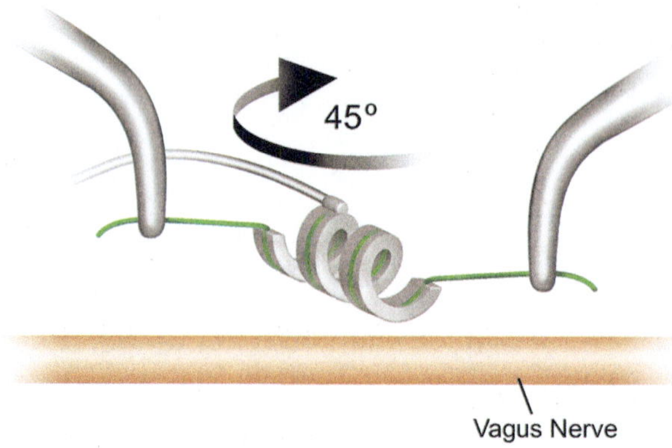

FIGURE 38.43 Turn the helix clockwise at a 45-degree angle to the nerve. *Reproduced with permission from MicroTransponder, Inc.*

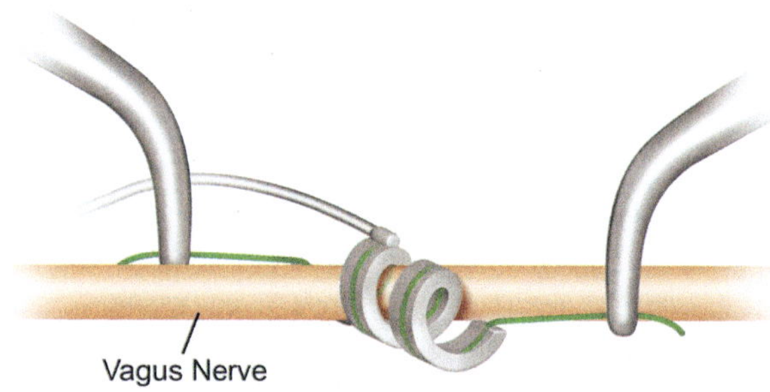

FIGURE 38.44 Position the turn of the helix onto the nerve. *Reproduced with permission from MicroTransponder, Inc.*

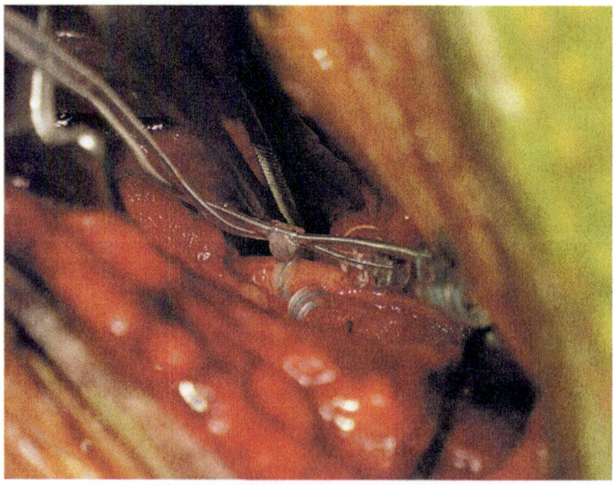

FIGURE 38.45 Position the anchor tether helix.

2. Technique utilizing **a right-angled dissector**: pass the dissector under the nerve, open the dissector jaw, and securely grasp the tip of suture (Fig. 38.51). Pull the dissector back while wrapping the helix around the nerve. Repeat the process on the other end of the helix (Fig. 38.52).

After the first helix is wrapped (Fig. 38.53), slide it along the nerve caudally (or cranially) to bring the next helix into the center of the exposed nerve segment. Repeat the steps above until all three helices are placed onto the nerve (Fig. 38.54). When irrigating surgical wound with the exposed vagus nerve, do not use a cold solution as it may cause temporary bradycardia or other cardiac effects.

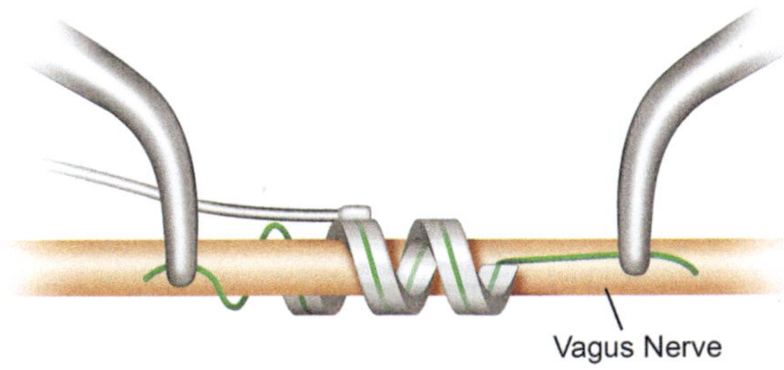

FIGURE 38.46 Utilize fine-tipped forceps to hold the suture ends. *Reproduced with permission from MicroTransponder, Inc.*

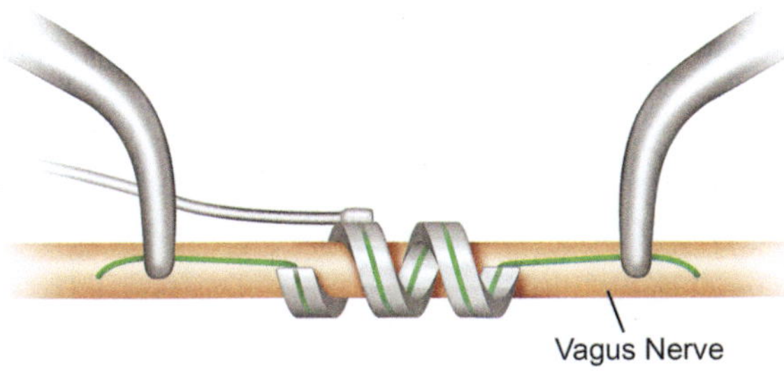

FIGURE 38.47 Wrap helices around the nerve: pass the distal suture portion of the helix under the nerve and back around so that it encircles the nerve. *Reproduced with permission from MicroTransponder, Inc.*

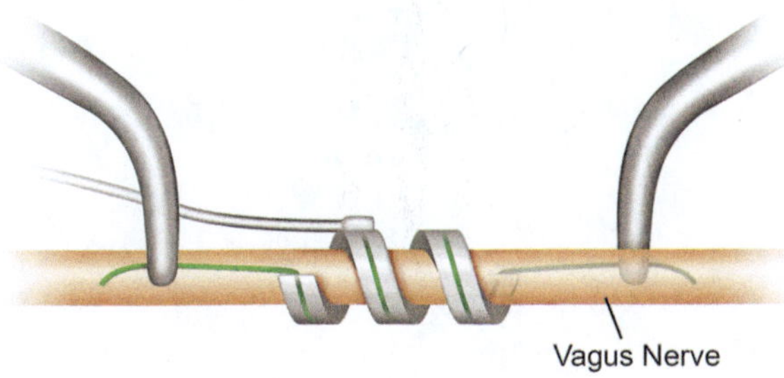

FIGURE 38.48 Wrap helices around the nerve: pass the proximal helix under the nerve and back around so that it encircles the nerve. *Reproduced with permission from MicroTransponder, Inc.*

Creating IPG pocket

Creating the IPG pocket in the chest wall is a brief step, taking only 1–2 min, making it advisable to postpone it until the vagus nerve is fully exposed and helices are placed. After the skin incision is made, conduct a subcutaneous sharp dissection (Fig. 38.55) until reaching the pectoralis fascia (Fig. 38.56). Monopolar electrocautery dissection is also permissible to expedite hemostatic dissection (Fig. 38.57). After reaching the fascia, continue the dissection, including atraumatic blunt finger dissection along the tissue plane (Fig. 38.58), parallel and above the fascia in the direction of the planned IPG pocket. A subcutaneous pocket must be large enough to accommodate the IPG. Additionally, consider creating a short tissue flap in the opposite direction to facilitate skin mobilization for tension-less closure. To prevent IPG communication difficulties, it is advised that the pocket depth should not exceed 2.5 cm beneath the skin. Similarly, implanting the IPG below the muscle is not recommended.

Lead tunneling

It may be optional to perform this step before wrapping lead helix contacts around the nerve to reduce the risk of lead dislodgement during tunneling. Use a tunneler with a bullet-tip end and plastic protective sheath (Fig. 38.59), and tunnel

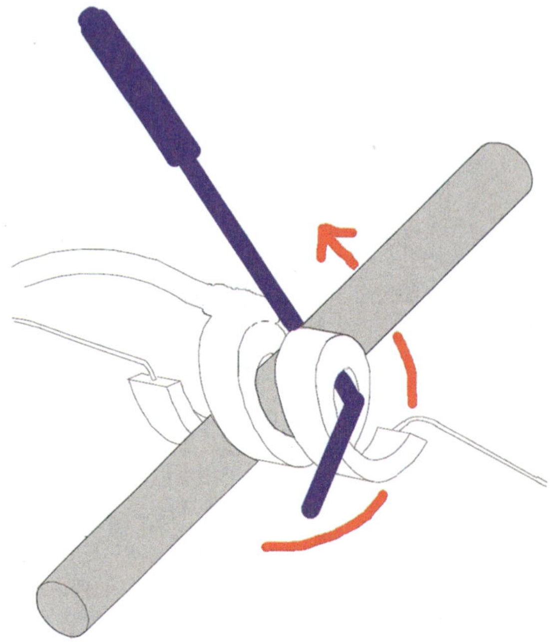

FIGURE 38.49 Technique utilizing a blunt nerve hook (schematic). *The figure has been adapted from copyrighted material of LivaNova PLC, and is used with permission.*

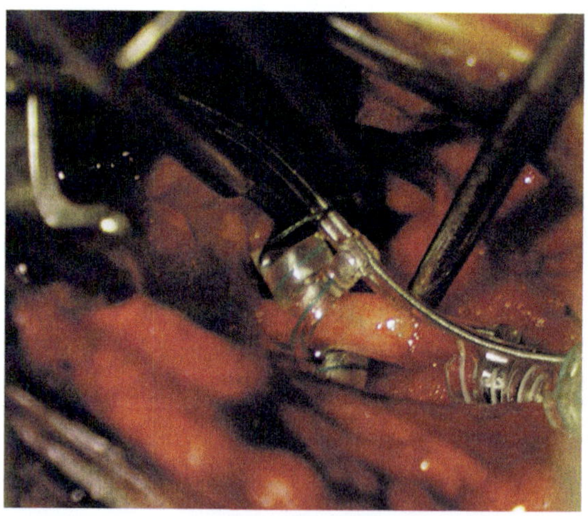

FIGURE 38.50 Technique utilizing a blunt nerve hook.

subcutaneously above clavicle, in a plane just above the sternocleidomastoid muscle (Fig. 38.60). Avoid routing the lead through muscle. Once the bullet tip has passed from one incision to the other, unscrew the bullet and withdraw the metal shaft from the plastic sleeve, leaving the sleeve extended through both incisions. Insert the tip of lead connector into the cervical end of the sleeve (Fig. 38.61) and pull the sleeve toward the chest incision until the lead connector completely exits the chest incision (Fig. 38.62). During the process, support the cervical end of the plastic sleeve, as it tends to migrate dorsally into cervical viscera (Fig. 38.63). It should be noted that some manufacturers recommend tunneling in the opposite direction—from the neck incision toward the chest—to minimize the risk of cervical viscera injury. However, this approach can be technically challenging due to the patient's chin position and limited working space. Authors prefer the chest-to-neck direction and using two protective plastic sleeves—one inside another, as provided by LivaNova: tunnel the large sleeve and then pull the smaller sleeve (with VNS lead connector inside) through it—this method facilitates smooth lead pull through tissues and protects the delicate lead body from stretching trauma (Fig. 38.64).

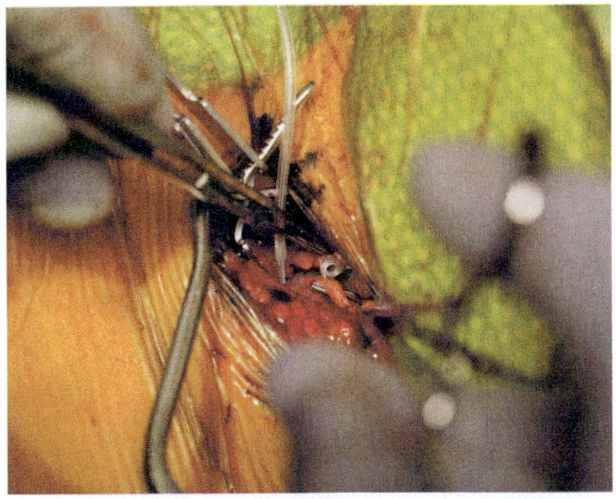

FIGURE 38.51 Grasp the tip of suture with the right-angled dissector under the nerve.

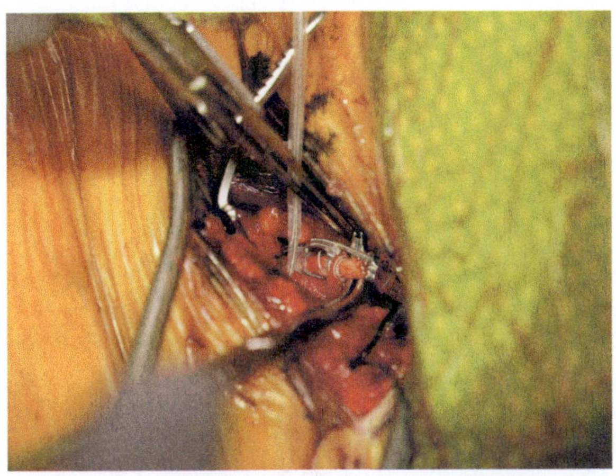

FIGURE 38.52 Repeat the process on the other end of the helix.

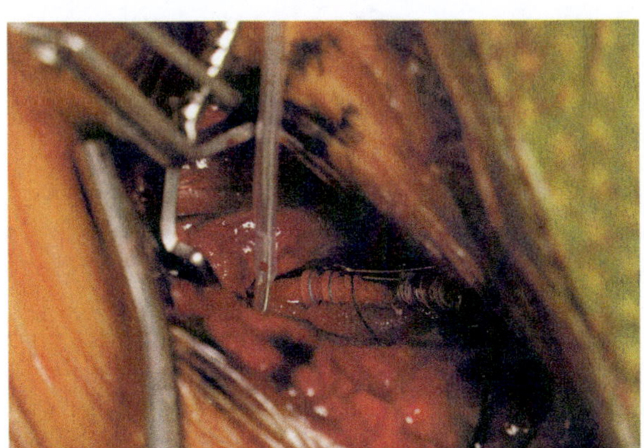

FIGURE 38.53 The first helix is wrapped.

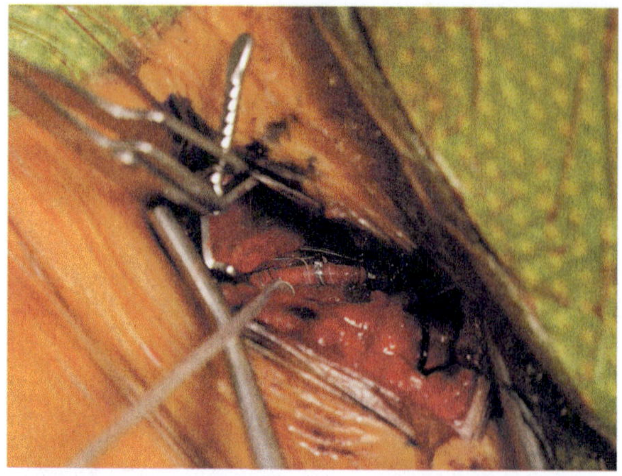

FIGURE 38.54 All helices are wrapped around the nerve.

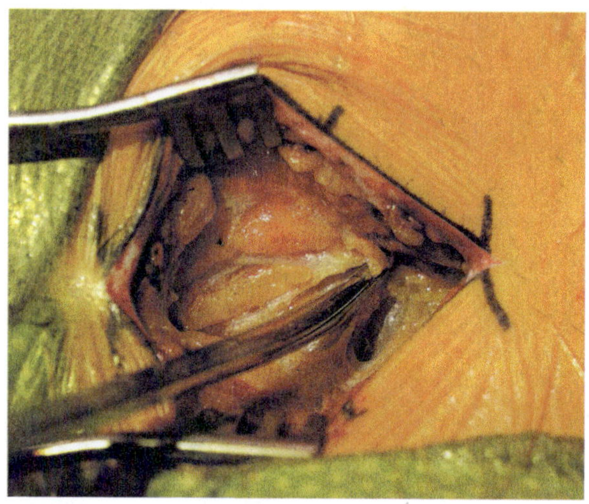

FIGURE 38.55 Sharp dissection using Mmetzenbaum scissors.

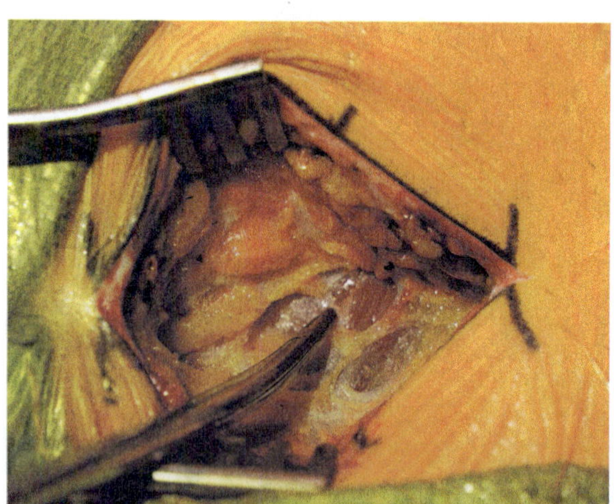

FIGURE 38.56 Dissect until reaching the pectoralis fascia.

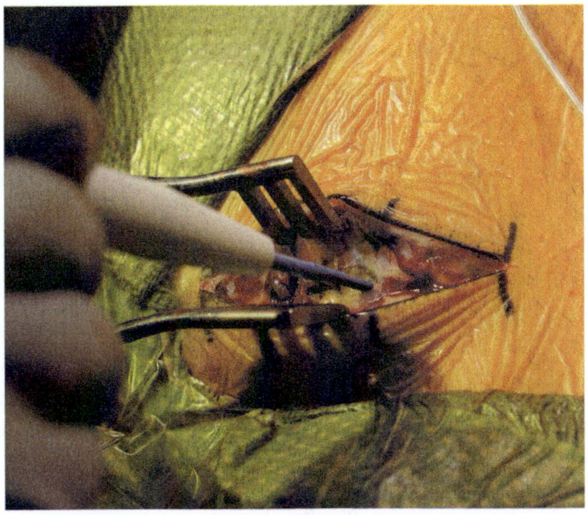

FIGURE 38.57 Monopolar electrocautery dissection.

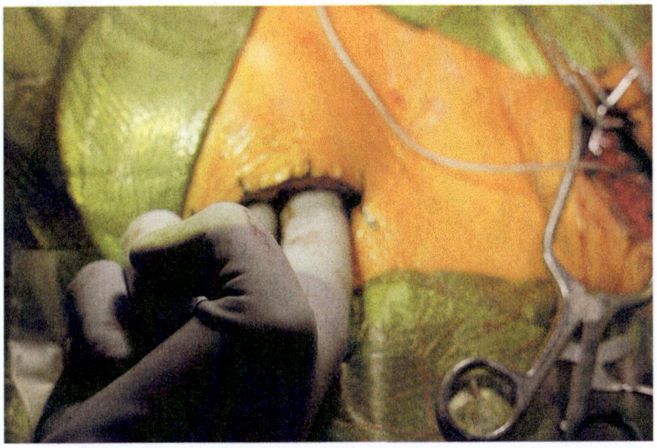

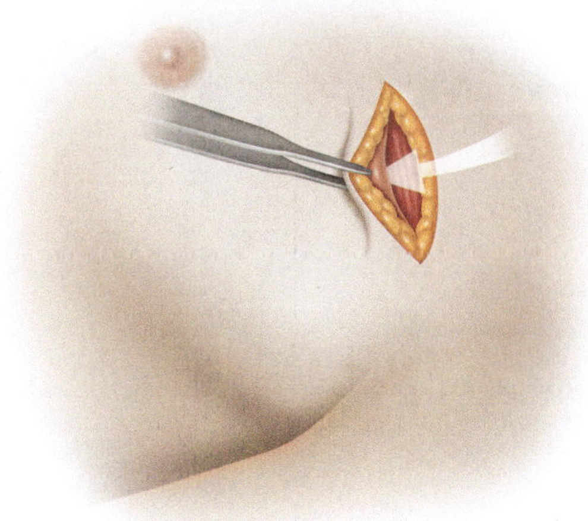

FIGURE 38.58 Atraumatic blunt finger dissection along the tissue plane, just above the pectoralis fascia. *The schematic figure is reproduced with permission from MicroTransponder, Inc.*

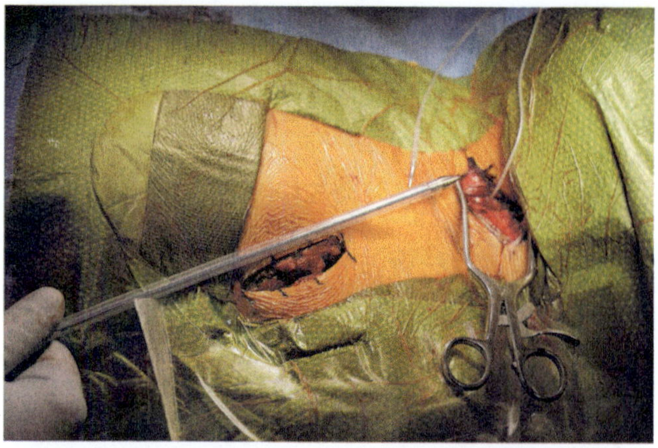

FIGURE 38.59 A tunneler with a bullet-tip end and plastic protective sheath.

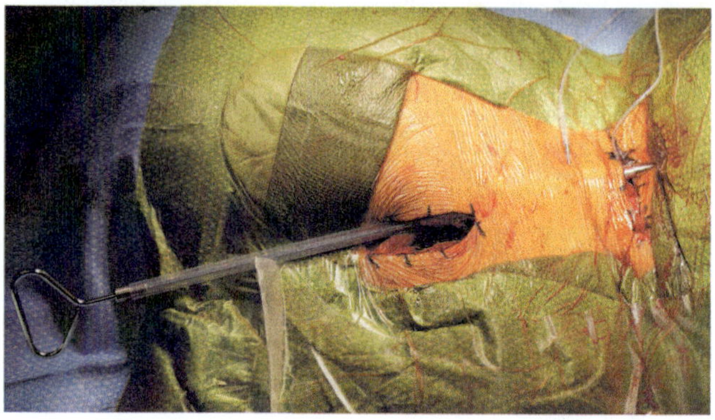

FIGURE 38.60 Tunnel subcutaneously above the clavicle.

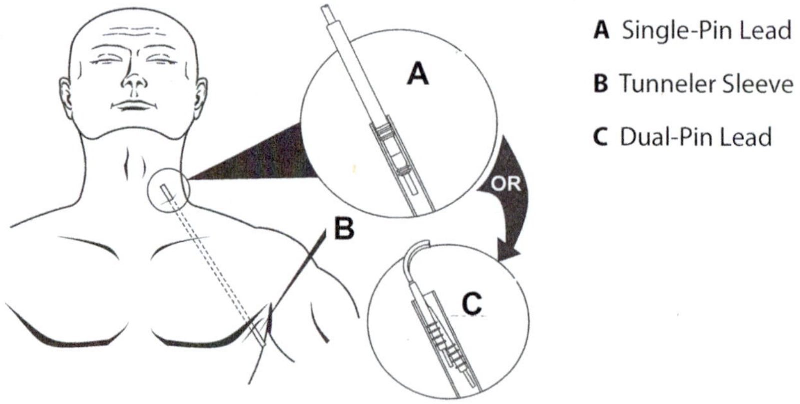

FIGURE 38.61 Insert the tip of lead connector into the cervical end of the sleeve. *Reproduced with permission from LivaNova PLC.*

Strain relief bend and loop

After lead is successfully tunneled, create a strain relief bend (Fig. 38.65), laying it caudally inside the carotid sheath, and a strain relief loop (Fig. 38.66) above the sternocleidomastoid muscle. This design ensures adequate slack and allows for neck movement. Secure the lead in this configuration using two or three radiopaque silicone tie-down anchor tabs (Fig. 38.67) provided in the lead kit. Use braided nonabsorbable suture (e.g., 2–0 silk or coated polyester). The common

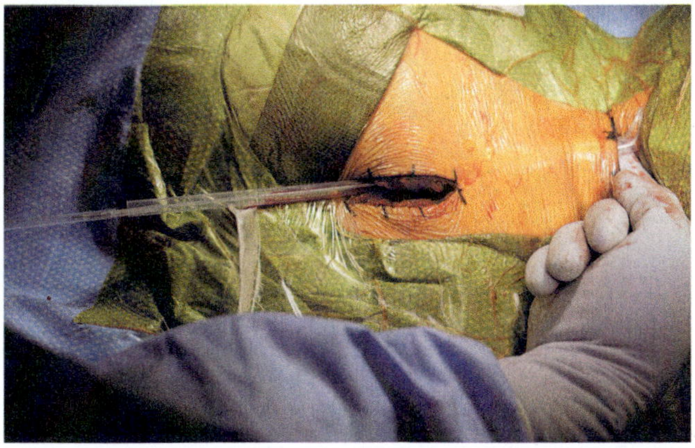

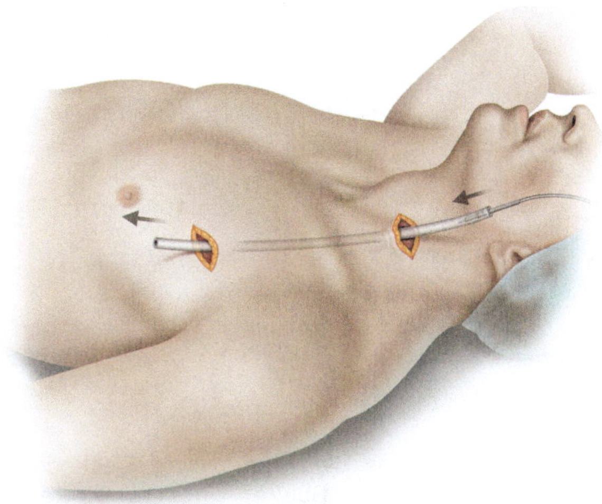

FIGURE 38.62 Pull the sleeve toward the chest incision until the lead connector completely exits the chest incision. *The schematic figure is reproduced with permission from MicroTransponder, Inc.*

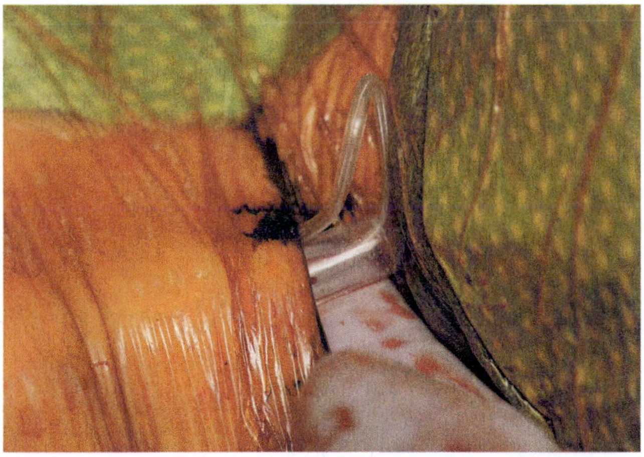

FIGURE 38.63 During the process, support the cervical end of the plastic sleeve.

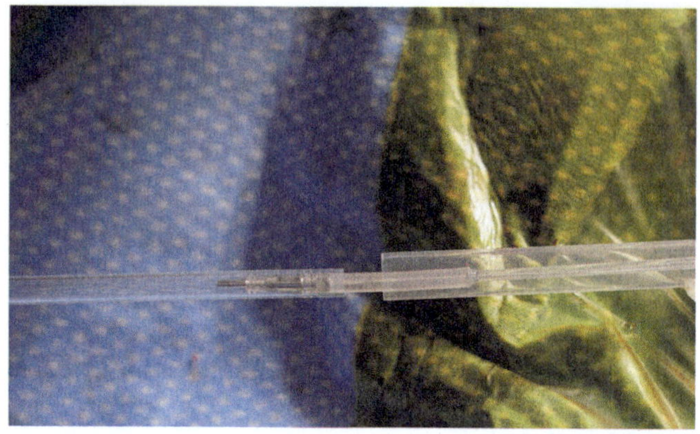

FIGURE 38.64 Two protective plastic sleeves to facilitate a smooth lead pull through tissues.

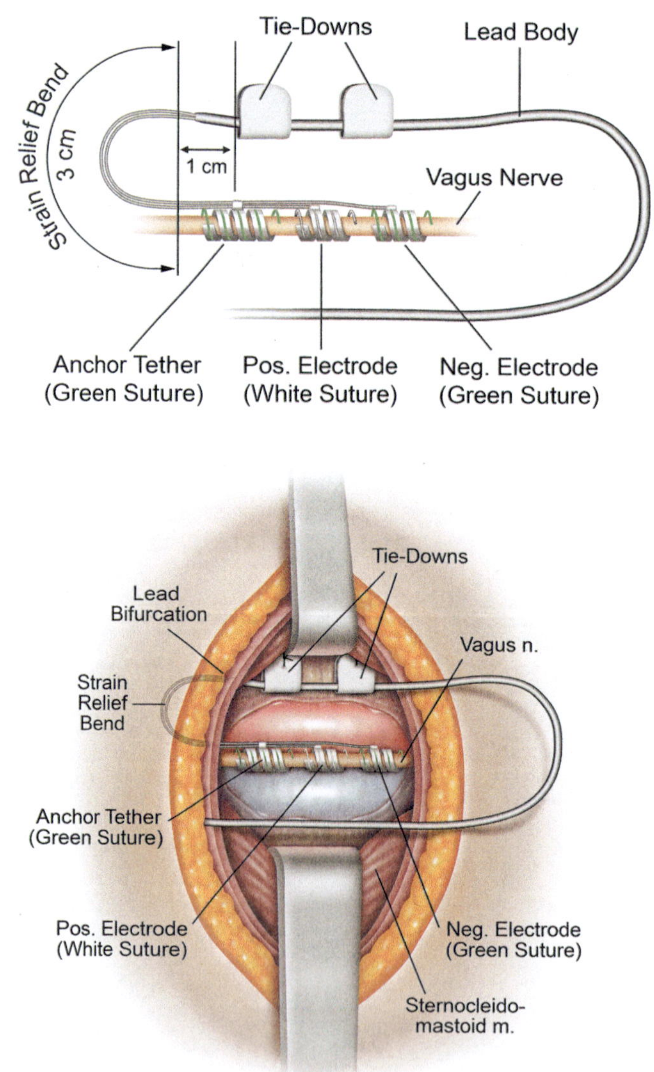

FIGURE 38.65 Strain relief bend. *Reproduced with permission from MicroTransponder, Inc.*

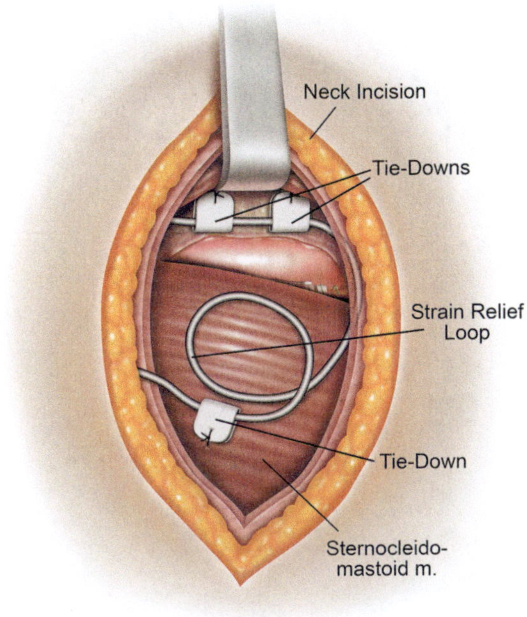

FIGURE 38.66 Strain relief loop. *Reproduced with permission from MicroTransponder, Inc.*

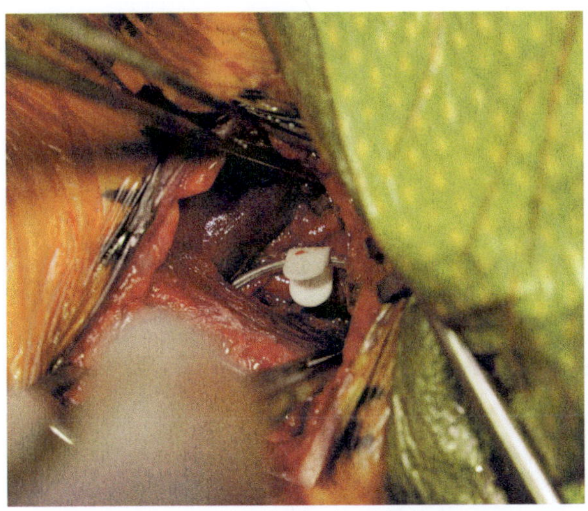

FIGURE 38.67 Silicone tie-down anchor tab.

error to avoid is circling the tab flaps with the suture material. The correct and secure method is to encircle the lead (Fig. 38.68). Aim to suture the lead to fascial tissues and avoid suturing to muscle fascicles. Importantly, avoid placing anchor tabs under the skin to mitigate the risk of erosion; position them at least under the platysma.

Implant IPG

Avoid using electrosurgical equipment after the IPG has been introduced to the sterile field, as exposure to external electric current may damage the IPG. When ready to insert the lead, back out the setscrew slightly (Fig. 38.69). Be careful not to back the setscrew out too far as it can become dislodged and be difficult or impossible to reengage potentially necessitating a new IPG—a costly error. Lead pin is then inserted all the way into IPG receptacle (Fig. 38.70) and then the setscrew is tightened with the hex screwdriver provided (Fig. 38.71). This screwdriver will give way when the appropriate

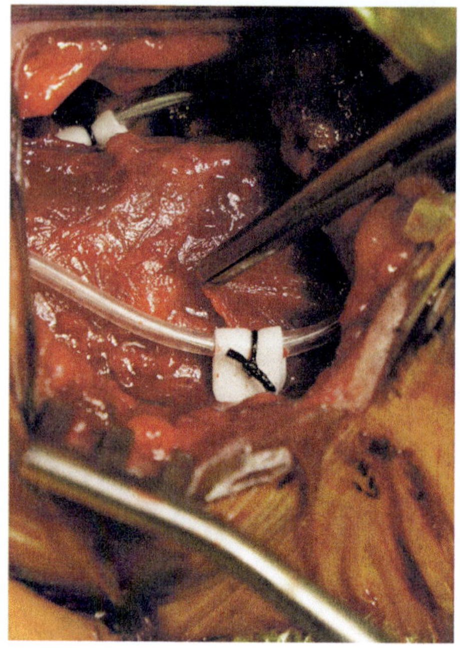

FIGURE 38.68 The correct and secure method is to encircle the lead with the suture material.

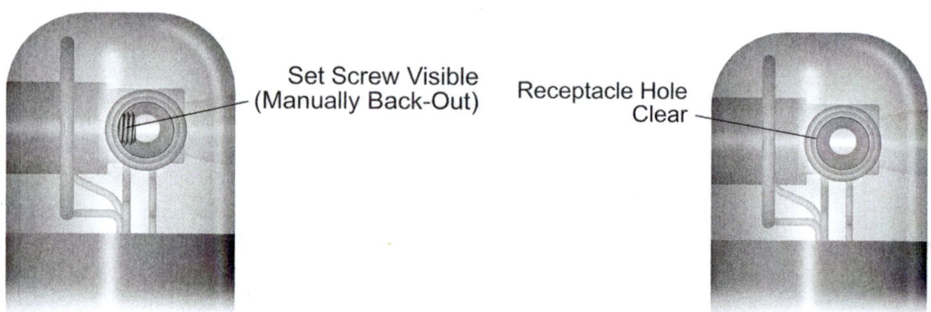

FIGURE 38.69 Back out setscrew slightly until it is no longer visible in the receptacle hole. *Reproduced with permission from MicroTransponder, Inc.*

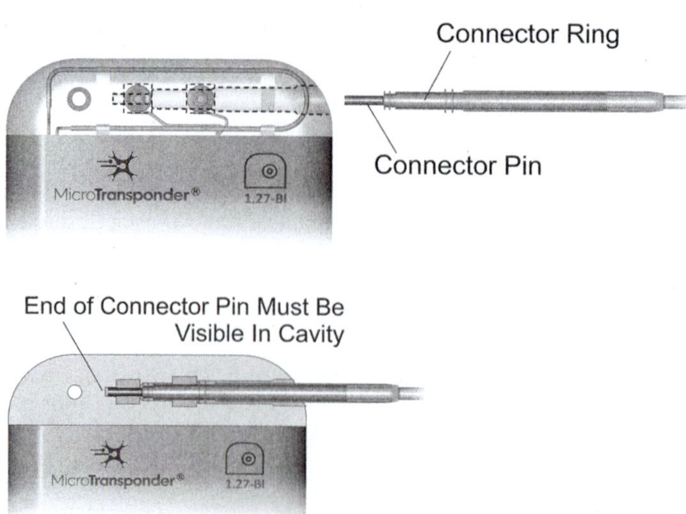

FIGURE 38.70 Lead pin is inserted fully into the IPG receptacle. *Reproduced with permission from MicroTransponder, Inc.*

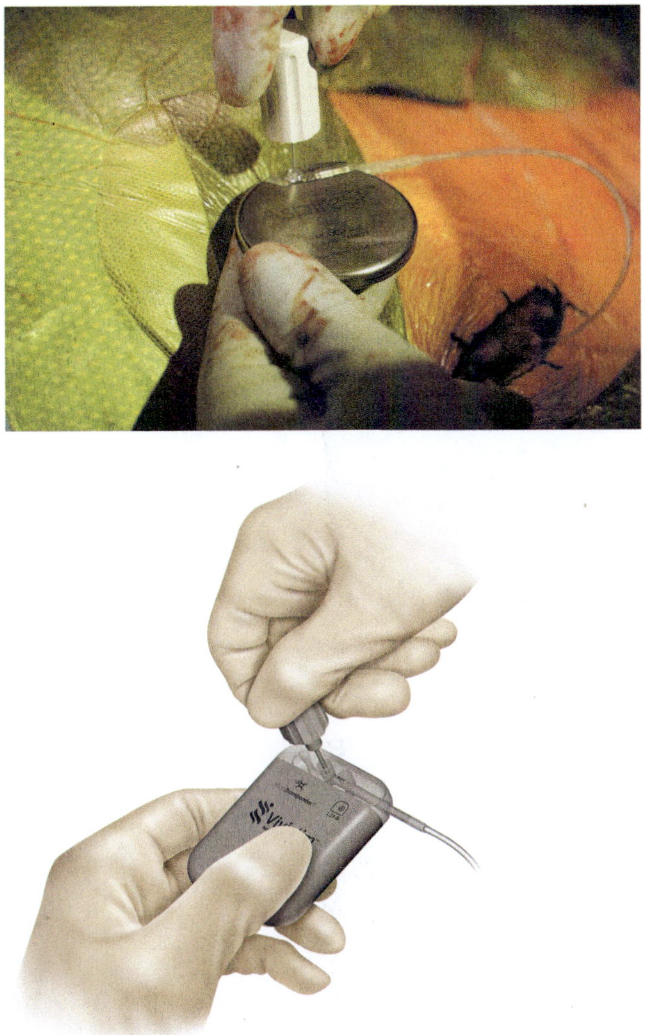

FIGURE 38.71 Setscrew is tightened with the hex screwdriver. *The schematic figure is reproduced with permission from MicroTransponder, Inc.*

torque is reached. Electrical connection between the lead and the IPG is not established until the setscrew is completely tightened with the torque screwdriver.

To ensure proper functioning, place any excess length of lead coiled beside or beneath the IPG. Manufacturers advise against tucking lead slack under the IPG and rather recommend coiling the lead excess next to the IPG (Fig. 38.72) to avoid insulation failure and system malfunction. Manufacturers do not provide any caution if such coiling could induce currents during MRI scanning. It is worth noting that the authors have not observed any complications related to the placement of extra lead coils under the IPG. Definitely, do not place any part of the lead over the IPG as it increases the risk of lead damage during later IPG replacements. The outline of implanted VNS System per manufacturer recommendations is depicted in Fig. 38.73. Additionally, implanting the IPG upside down (i.e., with the label side down) is not recommended but is acceptable, as it does not impact communication with the device.

System Testing

System Testing is a mandatory step following the connection of the lead to the IPG. Introduce the wireless wand to the surgical field inside a sterile clear sleeve and place the wand over the IPG (Fig. 38.74). Of note, MicroTransponder Vivistim system is tested remotely, and the transmitter does not need to be in a sterile sleeve. Activate "System Diagnostics" on a clinician programmer.

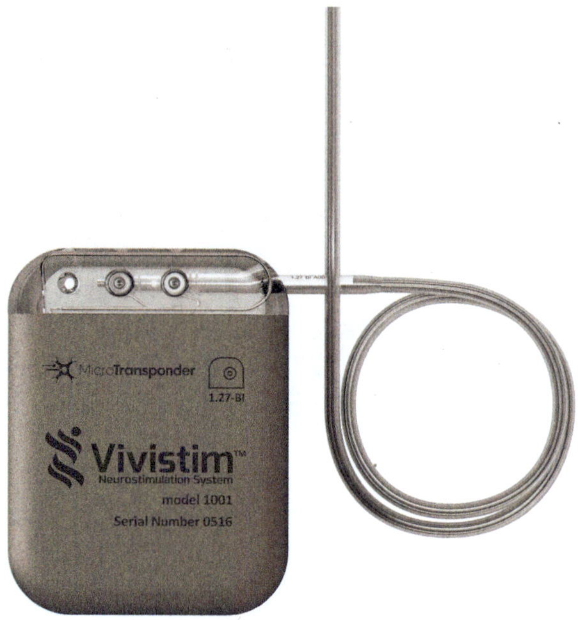

FIGURE 38.72 Lead slack coiled next to the IPG. *Reproduced with permission from MicroTransponder, Inc.*

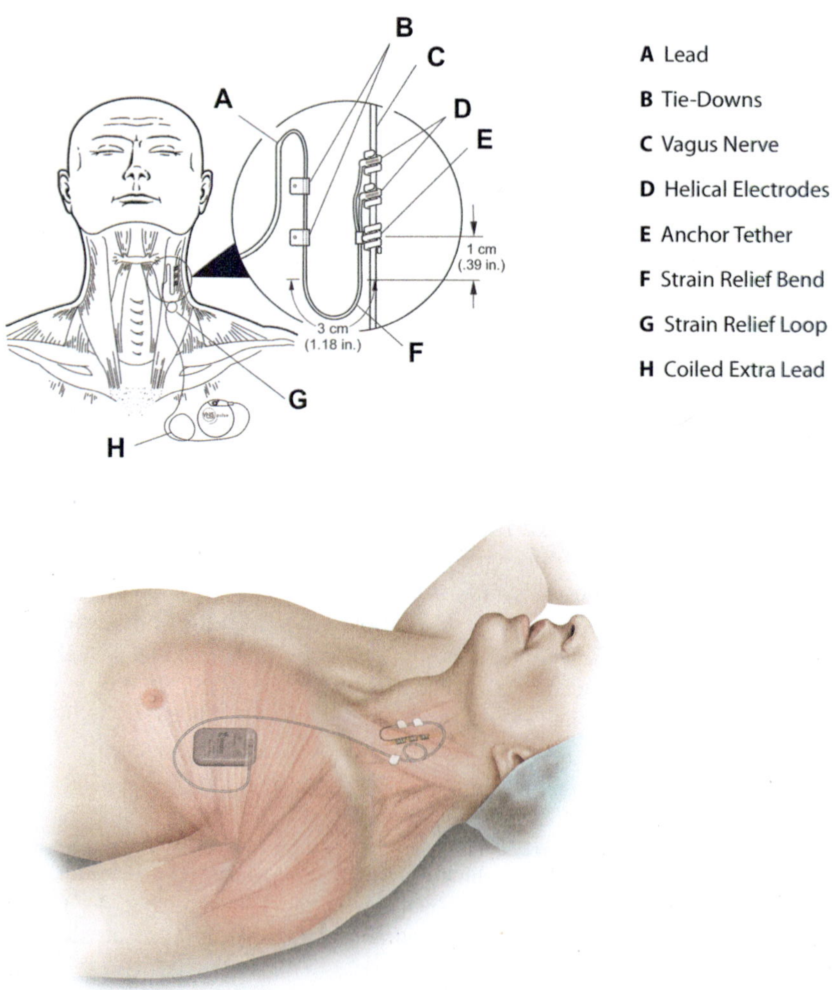

FIGURE 38.73 Outline of implanted VNS system per manufacturer recommendations. *Reproduced with permission from LivaNova PLC and MicroTransponder, Inc.*

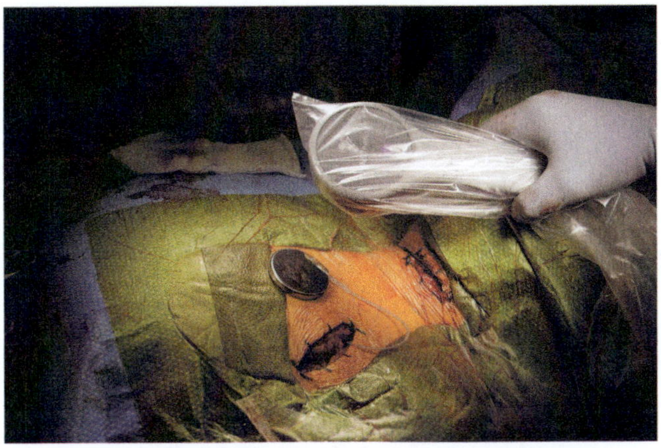

FIGURE 38.74 Place the wireless wand over the IPG.

For legacy LivaNova IPG models 100–102R, the test stimulation was delivered at 1 mA for 14 s.

For LivaNova IPG models 103–106 and 8103, the test stimulation lasts approximately 14 s. When the device is set to 0 mA (new IPGs), it will use 1 mA output current at 20 Hz and 500 μsec. Otherwise, it will use the programmed output current (e.g., 0.75 mA for 5 s if programmed at 0.75 mA with ON time for 5 s, or 2.5 mA for 30 s if programmed at 2.5 mA with ON time for 30 s).

For LivaNova model 1000, the test stimulation uses the programmed output current for approximately 4 s, or at 0.25 mA when the device is set to 0 mA.

Note: Have a setscrew driver ready and watch closely ECG on anesthesia monitor! If the patient goes into severe bradycardia or asystole, quickly disconnect the lead, as the stimulator goes into a test stimulation cycle that won't stop before it is over.

Also, note that the IPG does not need to be in a subcutaneous pocket as impedance is checked between lead contacts ("bipolar montage"). In other words, the impedance is not checked between a contact and the IPG case, which is referred to as the "monopolar montage," a common setup for other neuromodulation devices, such as DBS.

MicroTransponder Vivistim system measures impedance using two pulses at 0.2 mA, 70 μs width.

In case "System Diagnostics" fails, indicated by lead impedance being either "HIGH" or "LOW," try retrieving the pin from the IPG, cleaning the pin surface with a dry, clean gauze, and then reinserting it back into the receptacle. If this maneuver does not resolve impedance abnormalities, proceed with "Generator Diagnostics." This test, performed with the test resistor (Fig. 38.75) included in the IPG packaging or using accessory kit #502, will verify that the IPG is functioning properly, independent of the lead.

When implanting a modern IPG (model ≥106), ensure it senses heart rate. The IPG must be in a subcutaneous pocket to test this (Fig. 38.76). Begin "Verify Heartbeat Detection" using the lowest possible "Sensitivity" ("1" being the least

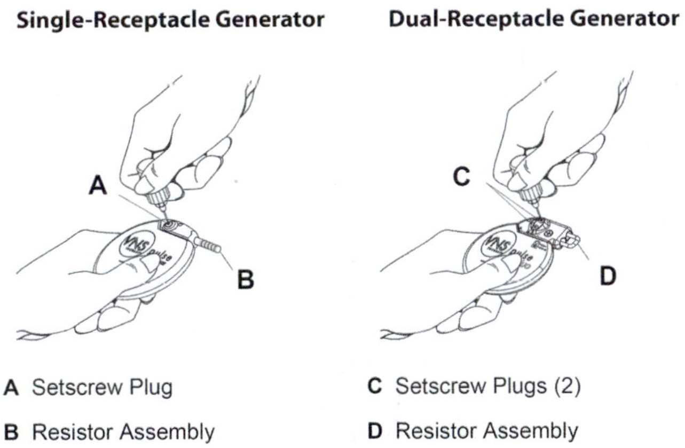

FIGURE 38.75 IPG testing using standard resistor. *Reproduced with permission from LivaNova PLC.*

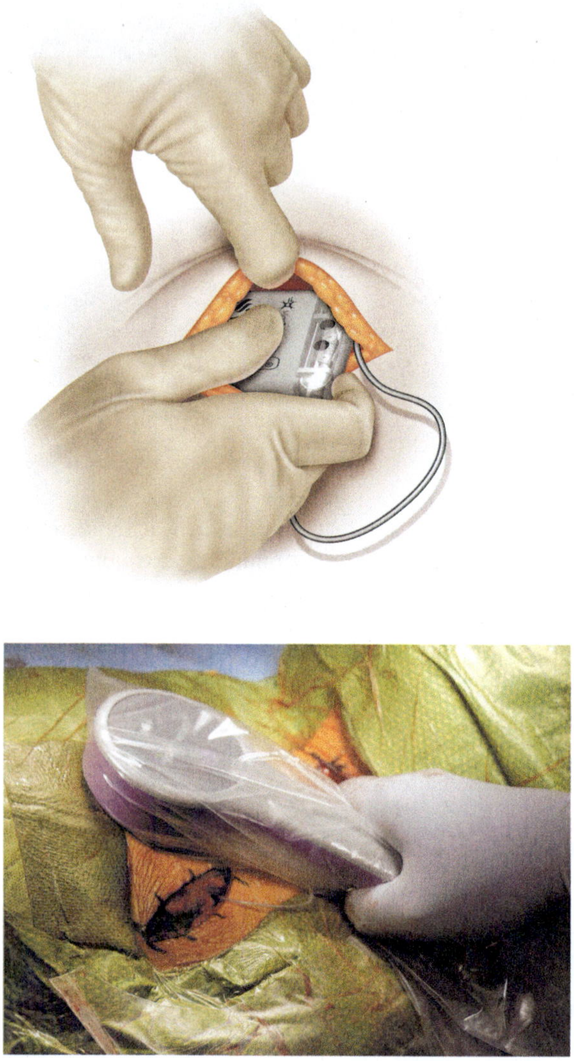

FIGURE 38.76 IPG must be in a subcutaneous pocket to test sensing of heart rate. *The schematic figure is reproduced with permission from MicroTransponder, Inc.*

sensitive and "5" being the most sensitive setting)—and confirm that the device-detected heart rate and pulse-oximetry-detected heart rates match closely. Note that other implanted stimulators, such as DBS, may interfere with the proper heart rate detection.

Closure

Wounds are copiously irrigated. Authors' choice is diluted (<5%) sterile povidone iodine aqueous solution (e.g., betadine, Fig. 38.77) followed by the rinse with a vancomycin-saline solution. Optionally, wounds can be sprinkled with antibiotic (e.g., vancomycin) powder to further reduce the risk of infection. Secure the IPG by placing a braided nonabsorbable suture (e.g., 2–0 silk or coated polyester) through the suture hole and suturing it to the underlying pectoralis fascia (not to muscle) to lower the risk of IPG migration (Fig. 38.78). This step is optional during IPG replacement surgeries when the well-established snug subcutaneous pocket capsule already exists. Note that the IPG has only one hole for anchoring.

Deep interrupted absorbable stitches (e.g., 2–0 polyglactin 910) are used to approximate the bulk of adipose tissue in the chest. For muscle closure in the neck, it is only necessary to approximate the edges of the platysma muscle. The authors prefer to suture skin edges with interrupted inverted (deep dermal) stitches using thinner absorbable sutures (e.g., 3–0 or 4–0 polyglactin 910) in the neck and the chest. If there is an increased risk of skin dehiscence, an additional

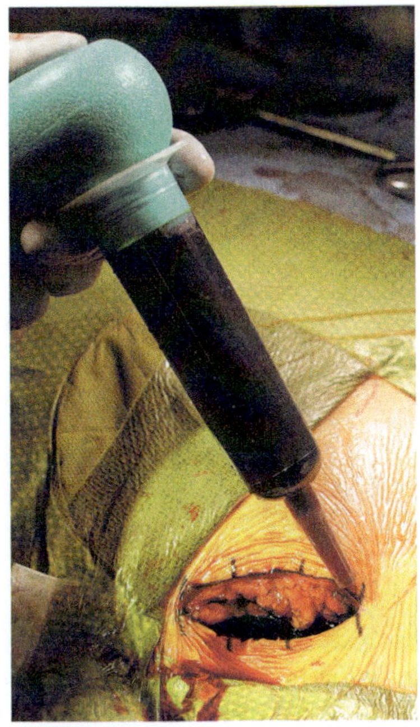

FIGURE 38.77 Betadine irrigation.

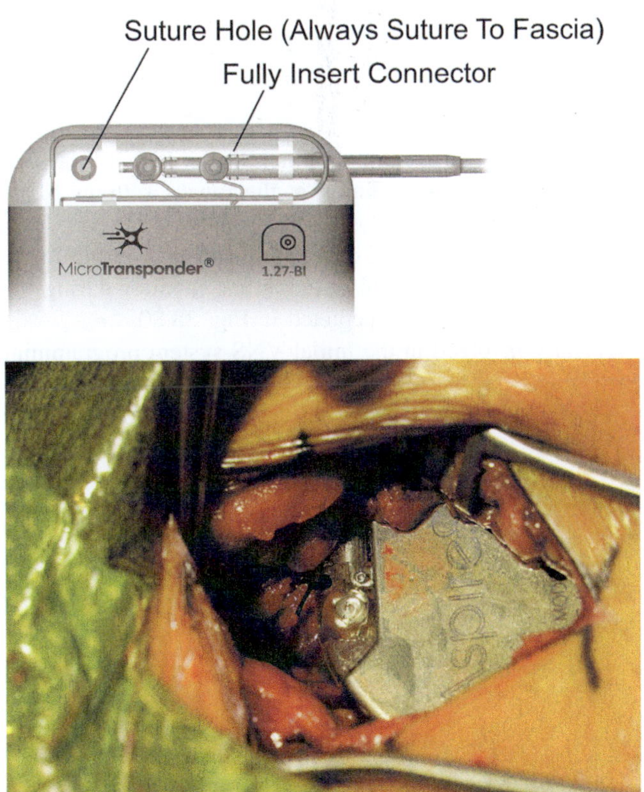

FIGURE 38.78 Secure the IPG to pectoralis fascia. *The schematic figure is reproduced with permission from MicroTransponder, Inc.*

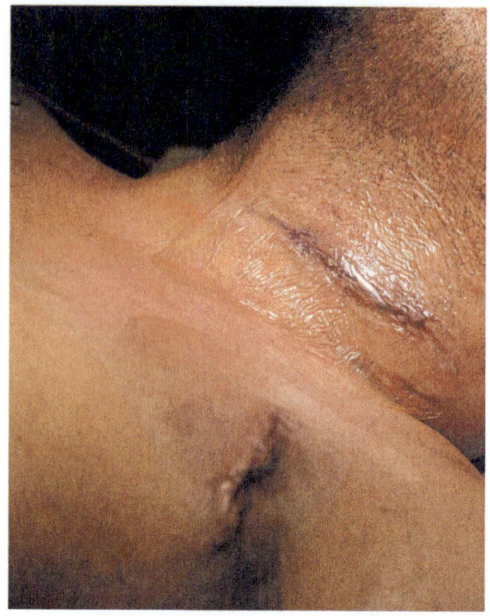

FIGURE 38.79 Sterile impervious dressing.

running absorbable monofilament suture (e.g., 4–0 poliglecaprone 25) can be placed on the epidermis for extra reinforcement. Apply surgical skin adhesive. Once it has completely dried, apply a sterile impervious dressing (e. g., Tegaderm, Fig. 38.79).

Programming

LivaNova—for epilepsy

Historically, the IPG was not programmed to stimulation treatment for at least 14 days after initial implantation surgery. However, the current practice involves starting stimulation at the lowest settings (0.25 mA, leaving other settings to factory default) in the operating or postanesthesia recovery room.

If the patient has experienced a clinically significant change in heart rate during "System Diagnostics" at the time of initial device implantation, the patient should be placed on a cardiac monitor during the initiation of stimulation. It is important to understand the stimulation parameters as depicted in Fig. 38.80.

In summary, the surgeon is typically involved in the initial VNS system programming with the following suggested initial settings:

1. Normal mode:
   1. Output current: 0.25 mA.
   2. Frequency: 20 Hz.
   3. Pulse width: 250 msec.

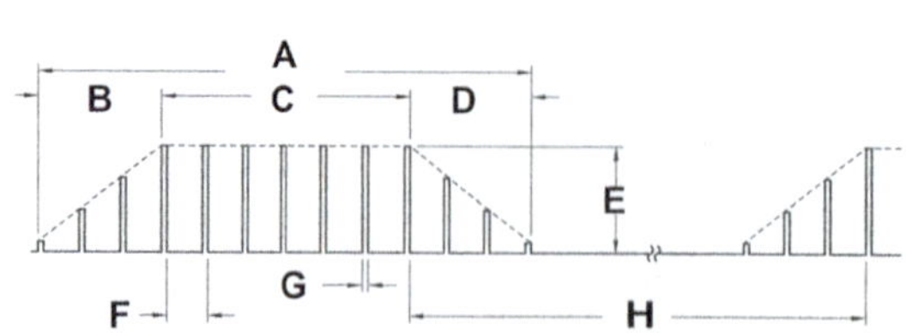

A Stimulation Time
B Ramp Up (2 sec.)
C On Time
D Ramp Down (2 sec.)
E Output Current
F 1/Signal Frequency
G Pulse Width
H Off Time

FIGURE 38.80 VNS stimulation waveform and parameters. *Reproduced with permission from LivaNova PLC.*

   4. On time: 30 s, Off time: 5 min.

2. Magnet mode:

   5. Current: 0.25 mA higher than normal mode output.
   6. Pulse width: 250 msec.
   7. Stim time: 30 s.

3. AutoStim mode:

   8. Current: 0.125 mA higher than normal mode output.
   9. Frequency: 20 Hz.
   10. Pulse width: 250 msec.
   11. Stim time: 30 s.
   12. Use "Sensitivity" established during intraoperative testing.
   13. Heart rate threshold: 50%.

Magnet mode. The patient or caregiver can swipe the magnet over the IPG to provide additional boost stimulation as needed. If the magnet is held over the IPG for longer than just for a routine swipe (e.g., 10 s for LivaNova models 1000/1000-D and 5 s for model 106), the device is turned off and remains off if the magnet is held on. Some patients use creative solutions, such as placing the magnet in a shirt pocket, to keep the magnet on and the VNS off in specific situations, like during marathon running to avoid interference with breathing or for singers to maintain consistent voice without changes.

AutoStim mode (only available in models ≥106). "AutoStim" is a quasi-closed-loop system designed to detect and respond to sudden heart rate increases that might be associated with seizures. Patients with epilepsy involving autonomic centers, exhibiting ictal tachycardia (not common in frontal lobe epilepsy), are potential candidates for AutoStim. Here are key features of AutoStim:

- It monitors the last 5 min of heart rate to establish a baseline.
- Triggers are activated if heart rate increases from baseline to a threshold within 10 s, distinguishing from slower increases during physical exercises.

Considerations

- A programming strategy that relies solely on AutoStim—without chronic stimulation—has drawbacks: continuous stimulation provides long-term neuromodulatory, disease-modifying seizure control; chronic stimulation is likely necessary for depression; and high-current AutoStim can feel like a shock if the vagus nerve is not conditioned by ongoing stimulation.
- Electrical artifacts from other stimulators, like DBS, may affect heart rate detection.
- Notably, sensing heart rate consumes approximately 20% of the battery life (loosely approximating 2 years of battery life), emphasizing the need for careful consideration in choosing AutoStim mode.

A statistic worth noting is that true ictal tachycardia (>100 bpm with at least 55% or 35 bpm increase from baseline) can be detected in 16%–17% seizures, but, using a more liberal threshold of only 20% increase, may increase detection sensitivity to 66% at the expense of seven false detections per hour [7].

When implanting IPG models ≥1000, physicians have the option to activate **low heart rate** and **prone position** detections. These functions are initiated by events that may indicate a seizure, such as a magnet swipe or AutoStim. For the subsequent 7.5 min, the VNS system continuously monitors for two parameters associated with an increased risk of sudden unexpected death in epilepsy (SUDEP): a heart rate falling below a physician-defined threshold and the patient being in a prone position. It is important to note that this function records these events but does not trigger therapeutic stimulation. Beyond serving as a surrogate "SUDEP monitor," current VNS models have limited capacity to gather epilepsy biomarkers.

Following the initial setup of stimulation by a surgeon, an epileptologist conducts further titration of the output current over the next few months. Newer LivaNova models (such as 1000) allow programmed scheduled autotitration—minimizing the need for epileptologist office visits. This significantly enhances patient comfort and eliminates the need for even minimal patient compliance, representing an advancement in patient care. Once the final stimulation parameters are established, ongoing patient compliance is not required. While further guidance on output titration is beyond the scope of this chapter, it is worth mentioning that based on the study by Fahoum et al. the target current is approximately 1.625 mA at 250 μs pulse width. That is, increasing output current beyond 1.625 mA will not further improve seizure control in patients who have already demonstrated response to VNS, although exceptions exist, such as in Dravet or Lenox-Gastaut syndromes. Conversely, increasing output current beyond 1.625 mA is unlikely to convert a nonresponder patient into a responder [8]. Additionally, excessive stimulation—defined by an ON time exceeding the OFF time (duty cycle >50%) in combination with high-frequency stimulation (≥50 Hz)—has produced degenerative nerve damage in laboratory animals.

Electromyography (EMG) of the cricothyroid and thyroarytenoid muscles indicates degeneration of the recurrent laryngeal nerve in 60% of patients after prolonged repetitive stimulation [9].

MicroTransponder—for stroke rehabilitation

The IPG is programmed by the therapist. Stimulation can be initiated through a push button, a computer mouse click, or a brief magnet swipe over the device, depending on the programmed settings. Typical stimulation parameters include 0.8 mA, 30 Hz, 100 μs, with a 0.5-second ON time and a 30-second OFF time (Fig. 38.81). Stimulation is not automatically repeated and must be reinitiated by the therapist, typically every 5–10 s during an in-clinic VNS session lasting 90–120 min. Duty cycles exceeding 50% are inhibited. When operating in magnet mode, stimulation is delivered for a predefined duration—most commonly 30 min—providing 0.5 s of stimulation every 10 s following a magnet swipe over the IPG.

Postoperative regimen

Postoperatively, observation in a hospital for a few hours after surgery is recommended, mainly for watch of neck hematoma that could compromise the airway. Make sure the patient has no vocal cord dysfunction but also educate that intermittent voice hoarseness is expected whenever VNS stimulation is turned on. After discharge, patients are allowed to take a shower anytime, but prolonged soaking the incision is not allowed for 6 weeks. Patients are instructed to remove the dressing at 3 days after surgery, noting that the skin glue will stay on and flake off on its own in a few weeks. In rare cases, a neck brace can be used for the first week to help ensure proper lead stabilization. However, in contrast, most experts encourage gentle range-of-motion neck exercises for 6 weeks to minimize bowstring scar formation along the lead. The epilepsy patient should be reminded that VNS will not result in seizure cessation; thus, they should continue to practice seizure precautions and continue their antiseizure medications. Patients who tend to manipulate the IPG and/or lead through the skin (so called Twiddler's syndrome) or who have significant chest tissue causing significant movement of the IPG may damage or disconnect the lead from the IPG and/or possibly cause damage to the vagus nerve—patients should be warned about such possibility. Similarly, playing certain contact sports (such as boxing) may damage the implanted VNS system. Strong magnets, hair clippers, vibrators, loudspeaker magnets, electronic article surveillance (EAS) system tag deactivators, and other similar electrical or electro-mechanical devices, which may have a strong static or pulsing magnetic field, can cause accidental closure of the internal reed switch, which mimics proprietary magnet action; thus, patients should be cautioned to keep such devices away from the IPG, typically at least 15 cm away. The VNS system is not expected to trigger airport metal detectors or theft-protection devices that are further than about 1.8 m.

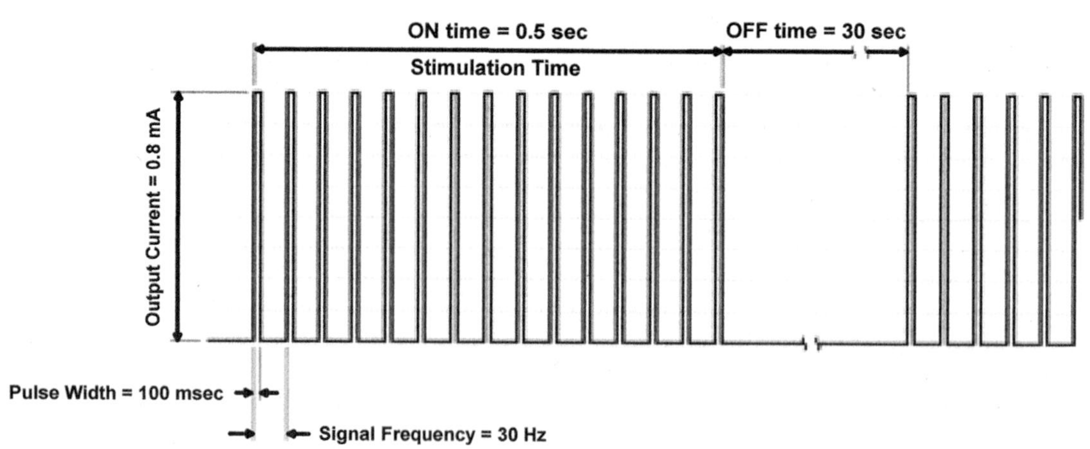

FIGURE 38.81 VNS stimulation waveform and parameters.

Complications

The following complications have been reported:

1. Surgical bed hematoma in the neck can cause airway compromise, necessitating postoperative observation for several hours. In extreme cases, initiation of neck exploration at the bedside may be required.
2. Infection occurs in 3%–8% of cases [9–12]. Early identification is essential, as prompt initiation of antibiotic therapy may prevent the need for device removal. However, in many instances, complete system explantation is required until the infection has resolved. Once infection clearance is achieved, reimplantation of the VNS system may be considered, preferably using an antibiotic-impregnated absorbable pouch within the IPG pocket. It should be noted that infection may result in excessive scar formation, which can make subsequent nerve dissection more challenging.
3. Injury to surrounding structures may lead to vocal cord paralysis, Horner's syndrome, and lower facial muscle paresis, likely due to incisions made too high in the neck.
4. Asystole has been reported exclusively in intraoperative setting and is extremely rare.
5. Hardware failure, including lead fracture and generator malfunction, occurred in approximately 2.7% of patients with a minimum follow-up of 1 year [9].

Side effects of VNS

It is crucial to acknowledge that vagus is a mixed nerve and 20%–40% of its fibers are efferent, contributing to a distinctive profile of anticipated side effects, which can generally be managed through vigilant monitoring, timely intervention, or the expected development of patient tolerance:

1. The nucleus ambiguus of the vagus innervates skeletal laryngeal musculature. Hoarseness or alterations in voice are observed in 30%–50% of cases, potentially posing challenges for certain professions. In addition, dysphagia may occur with active stimulation, and aspiration may result, which are of particular importance for stroke patients.
2. Symptoms resembling airway irritation, such as cough, paresthesia, pain, and dyspnea, can be observed. Fortunately, most patients develop tolerance over time. Of particular concern is the potential for de novo or exacerbated obstructive sleep apnea, especially prevalent with a pulse width of 500 msec. This raises a substantial risk of breathing disorders in overweight patients.
3. The nucleus ambiguus of the vagus sends inhibitory efferents to cardiac conductive system. Asystole has been reported, and instances have been documented more than a year after VNS surgery [13]. While right-sided VNS has been avoided due to preferential connection to the sinoatrial node and risk of causing persistent bradycardia or even asystole, there is evidence for placement of a right-sided lead in patients whose left vagus nerve or implantation area is compromised, or even as a rescue attempt with failure of a left-sided system without other reasonable options. Both left- and right-sided systems may cause pulmonary or cardiac side effects, and patients should be monitored regardless of the side chosen. In the dog model, stimulation of the right vagus nerve caused more cardiac slowing then the left [14]. As left-sided placement is the current indication and conventionally expected, the surgeon should default to the left side if able [15–17].
4. The dorsal nucleus of the vagus may induce gastrointestinal side effects and anorexia.

MRI-conditionality

The LivaNova and MicroTransponder VNS systems are conditionally compatible with 1.5 and 3.0 T MRI. However, specific MRI exclusion zones and coil requirements vary depending on the IPG model and the condition of the lead. Clinicians ordering or performing MRI studies must consult the most recent manufacturer guidelines to avoid potential risks of thermal injury.

MRI restrictions are lifted once the entire VNS system has been explanted, except for cases in which a portion of the lead remains. For LivaNova systems, residual lead segments ≤ 2 cm (Fig. 38.82) are considered MRI-safe, whereas for MicroTransponder leads, it is ≤ 5 cm. The residual lead length can be assessed radiographically. The approximate 2 cm segment corresponds to the distance between the positive and negative electrodes ($\approx$1 cm) plus the additional $\approx$ 1 cm between the positive electrode and the anchor tether, which also typically remains after explantation.

If an implanted lead demonstrates high impedance, if the residual lead segment exceeds 2 cm (or 5 cm for MicroTransponder leads), or if the lead remains intact but is disconnected from the IPG (an abandoned lead), special MRI conditions may apply. During MRI scanning, all VNS outputs must be set to 0 mA. For the MicroTransponder VNS

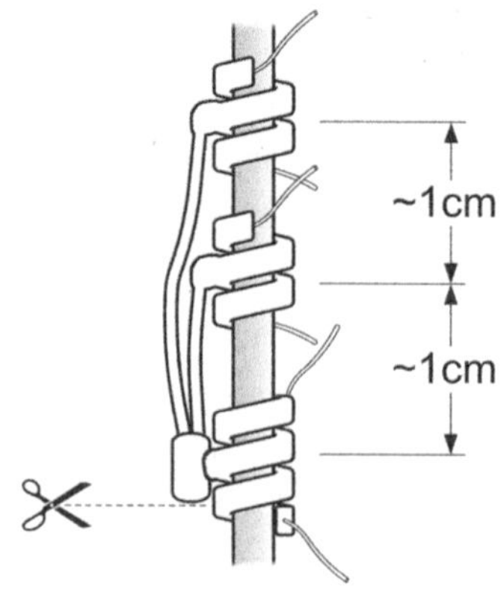

FIGURE 38.82 MRI-safe VNS lead segment (i.e., length ≤2 cm). *Reproduced with permission from LivaNova PLC.*

system, both therapist trigger mode and magnet mode must be set to OFF and subsequently restored to their original settings after the procedure.

Electrosurgery

If a patient with an implanted VNS system is undergoing another surgery, it is permissible to use a monopolar coagulator if it is positioned far from the IPG; however, the exact safe distance is not specified. Ensure the grounding pad is placed strategically to prevent the VNS system from being between the grounding pad and the site where the monopolar coagulator is used. Confirm that the VNS system functions as programmed after electrosurgery.

Diathermy

Do not use shortwave diathermy, microwave diathermy, or therapeutic ultrasound diathermy on patients implanted with a VNS system. Diagnostic ultrasound is not included in this contraindication.

Therapeutic radiation, nuclear imaging

Therapeutic radiation and nuclear imaging may damage the IPG's circuitry, although no definite information on radiation effects is available.

Cardiac defibrillation

The IPG may affect the operation of cardiac pacemakers and implantable defibrillators. Possible effects include sensing problems and inappropriate IPG responses.

External defibrillation may damage the IPG. Attempt to minimize current flowing through the VNS system by positioning defibrillation paddles as far from the IPG as possible and using the lowest clinically appropriate energy output (watt-seconds).

Confirm VNS system function after any internal or external defibrillation.

IPG replacement

Routine VNS system interrogations indicate the battery status, presenting the following labels for LivaNova systems:

1. **"OK"** Signifying a normal operating range, this label indicates that no special attention is required. The battery charge levels for this category include the following:
   - 75%–100%
   - 50%–75%
   - 25%–50%
   - 11%–25%

2. **"Intensified Follow-up Indicator (IFI)"** Signals that the battery has depleted to a level requiring more frequent clinical monitoring. This occurs at the following charge levels:
   - 5%–11% (for models 105 and 106)
   - 8%–18% (for models 103 and 104)
3. **"Near End of Service (NEOS)"** Indicates that the generator should be replaced as soon as possible but battery still maintains 3.3 V.
4. **"End of Service (EOS)"** Warns that the generator is no longer supplying stimulation, and immediate replacement is recommended. The battery starts gradual drop in voltage and generator will eventually lose the ability to communicate with the clinician programmer, and a preoperative impedance check will not be possible.

For *MicroTransponder systems*, the indicators are slightly different:

1. **"Elective Replacement Indicator (ERI)"** flags when there is less than 15% of the battery life is left (likely 9 months or less).
2. **"End of life (EOL)"** flags when there is less than 5% of the battery life remaining and indicates that the IPG will cease to function in the very near future.

The predicted duration between the Beginning of Life (BOL) and the EOL flag is a minimum of 5 years, and the predicted duration between the ERI flag and the EOL flag is a minimum of 3 months at programmed settings of 3.5 mA, 30 Hz, 1000 μs pulse width, 0.5 s pulse train, a separation of 10 s between pulse trains, and a magnet mode duration of 30 min.

For optimal patient care and decision-making regarding VNS system management, consider the following recommendations:

Clinic visit at IFI (Intensified Follow-up Indicator) stage. It is advisable for the surgeon to see the patient in the clinic when the battery indicates IFI. This approach allows sufficient time to order and review updated brain MRIs and EEGs. This is particularly relevant when encountering epilepsy patients with VNS and lesional MRI, such as those where VNS was placed long time ago when modern epilepsy surgical work up was not available or simply patients refused resective surgery. Modern minimally invasive or nondestructive surgical techniques—such as laser interstitial thermal therapy (LITT), responsive neurostimulation (RNS), and deep brain stimulation (DBS)—may be more appealing to patients today.

Avoiding inertia. To prevent inertia in cases where the original VNS showed no efficacy, it is important to refrain from replacing the device simply because the patient has a VNS and the battery is low. Careful consideration and evaluation of efficacy are crucial before proceeding with IPG replacements.

Testing efficacy. If unsure about VNS efficacy, particularly in epilepsy, consider turning down the normal output to 1.0 mA and observing the seizure response. This initiative-taking strategy is preferred over allowing the VNS to expire and then assessing, considering potential liability issues if the patient goes into status epilepticus due to abrupt VNS therapy cessation.

Abandoning dead battery. Leaving a dead IPG implanted is deemed harmless as it will not leak harmful materials.

Patient education. Educate the patient about the ideal timing for battery replacement, emphasizing that it should occur at the NEOS stage. Highlight the risks associated with every surgery, including the potential for infection leading to VNS explantation. Additionally, caution against early battery replacement, as it unnecessarily exposes the patient to surgical risks and increases the overall number of surgeries in their lifetime. Encourage patients to perform daily magnet activation to check stimulation and advise consulting with the physician if stimulation is not felt.

Calculating battery life. Calculating the exact time to NEOS is challenging due to various factors. The LivaNova recommends involving support service to determine the Battery Life Calculated (BLC) based on current interrogation data. Surgeons can also use tables (available on LivaNova website) to calculate intervals from IFI to NEOS.

Scheduled battery replacement. Schedule battery replacement surgery near the predicted NEOS time, and thus, plan frequent clinic visits at IFI stage with either the surgeon or referring neurologist for ongoing monitoring and timely intervention when NEOS flags.

Full information about existing VNS system. The surgeon must personally interrogate VNS system preoperatively. Make sure the impedance, battery level, implanted lead, and IPG models are known preoperatively as the older electrode designs (two pin) will require legacy IPG models for compatibility. If such information is missing and IPG battery is completely depleted, perform X-ray to identify the system. Ensure that the informed consent includes VNS lead revision if indicated.

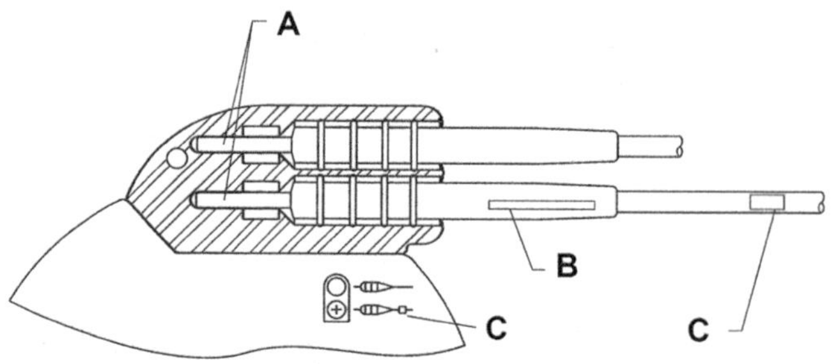

FIGURE 38.83 Dual-pin legacy systems with correct polarity and pin marking. *Reproduced with permission from LivaNova PLC.*

Anesthesia type. IPG replacements are typically done as an outpatient procedure using local anesthesia. Anxious patients may require intravenous sedation, i.e., monitored anesthesia care (MAC). Noncooperative patients require general anesthesia.

Surgical dissection. IPG replacement requires dissection to the IPG pocket, with care being taken not to damage the VNS lead. Thus, electrosurgical dissection at low current may be safer than sharp dissection using scissors and knife.

Dual-pin legacy systems. Ensure that the correct polarity of pins is maintained during IPG replacement (Fig. 38.83). For simplicity, it is recommended to disconnect one pin from old IPG and connect it to the new IPG. Only then, disconnect the second pin from old IPG and connect it to the new IPG.

Disposal. Explanted components may be returned to manufacturer for examination and proper disposal. Do not incinerate the IPG, because it can explode if subjected to incineration or cremation temperatures.

Special considerations related to the replacement of **an IPG battery that has been completely depleted (EOS or EOL)**:

1. Inability to perform preoperative impedance testing (starting with LivaNova model 103, VNS battery conserves some charge for a limited system testing); thus, the patient must be counseled about unknown VNS lead status and that it means the chance of needing to convert a simple IPG replacement surgery under conscious sedation to the surgery with entire system replacement under general anesthesia.
2. Intraoperatively, external extension leads and external batteries for testing lead impedance are not commercially available. Consequently, the assessment of lead impedance during the procedure will require the connection of a new sterile IPG. Furthermore, dual-to-single pin adapters are also not commercially available. Consequently, in cases with legacy dual-pin leads, the assessment of lead impedance will require a dual-receptacle IPG, which will be wasted if a legacy lead needs to be replaced with the modern single-pin lead. Thus, when the legacy dual-pin lead is reasonably suspected to be damaged, it is worth proactively replacing it with the modern single-pin lead or considering other neuromodulatory solutions for epilepsy.
3. Following the surgical procedure, initiate postoperative stimulation at a lower output level to avoid extremely uncomfortable sudden vagus irritation.

Lead revision

Routine interrogations of the VNS system include impedance measurements, providing essential insights into VNS lead integrity. Abnormal impedance readings:

Low lead impedance is defined as $\leq$ 600 Ohms (<250 Ohms for MicroTransponder systems).

Low lead impedance indicates short circuit condition within the lead or a defective IPG.

High lead impedance is defined as $\geq$ 5300 Ohms ($\geq$10,000 Ohms for MicroTransponder systems); high lead impedance does not have a set upper limit where the IPG stops therapy delivery. However, if impedance exceeds 10 kOhm, it likely signifies minimal therapy delivery.

High lead impedance can be caused by any of the following: fibrosis between the nerve and electrode, dry nerve (during surgery), lead fracture, or high battery impedance approaching end of life. However, the most common cause of high impedance is incorrect connection of the IPG and lead.

Workup for abnormal impedances

Of note, although 1000–3000 Ohms may be typical lead impedance at implantation, the impedance may increase to 3000–5000 Ohms during the life of the implant.

When observing abnormal impedance, it is advisable:

1. to look for **historic impedances**, as sudden significant changes strongly suggest lead problems.
2. to review **cervical X-rays**—however, it rarely visualizes VNS lead discontinuities.
3. to correlate abnormal impedance readings with the **patient's clinical status**, considering factors such as an increase in seizure burden/worsening of upper extremity motor deficits, patient perception of erratic/limited/no stimulation, and instances of a short-circuit condition, often characterized by a painful feeling in the neck that cease upon turning off the VNS.
4. LivaNova suggests an experimental, practically seldom used approach involving skin electrodes on the neck, along with **evoked potential monitoring** equipment or an oscilloscope, to analyze the stimulus waveform for electrical discontinuity verification (Fig. 38.84). A differentiated waveform with narrowed pulses or no waveform can confirm a discontinuity.

Surgical management of abnormal impedances

If abnormal impedances persist for an extended period, the patient may not be receiving VNS therapy, necessitating a proactive approach similar to new system implantation:

- During the preoperative phase, carefully examine the ECG for AV node or bundle branch blocks.
- Following the surgical procedure, initiate postoperative stimulation at a lower output level to avoid extremely uncomfortable sudden vagus irritation.

VNS lead revisions are typically done as an outpatient procedure using general anesthesia similar to the de novo VNS system implantations. If during surgery, the problem is not obvious upon inspection, and cleaning lead contacts and reconnecting to IPG does not resolve abnormal impedances, it is advisable to use 4000 Ohms test resistor (such as provided with LivaNova VNS accessory kit, model 502, Fig. 38.15)—this should test the health of IPG. Replacing faulty IPG is an expensive maneuver, thus, always coordinate this with the manufacturer representative to avoid costly errors. If IPG is deemed functioning properly but impedance issues persist, consider replacing the lead. There is no need to explant the entire old lead, as the patient's MRI conditionality will stay unchanged with the presence of the VNS system. The excessive nerve manipulation may cause transient hoarseness.

Explantation of entire VNS system

The decision to explant the entire VNS system is typically limited to specific indications, such as instances of infection, claims of inefficacy, or the necessity for an MRI within an anatomical exclusion zone. Importantly, in cases where VNS shows no efficacy, it is advisable to retain the VNS in situ, as future paradigms may introduce new more effective stimulation protocols.

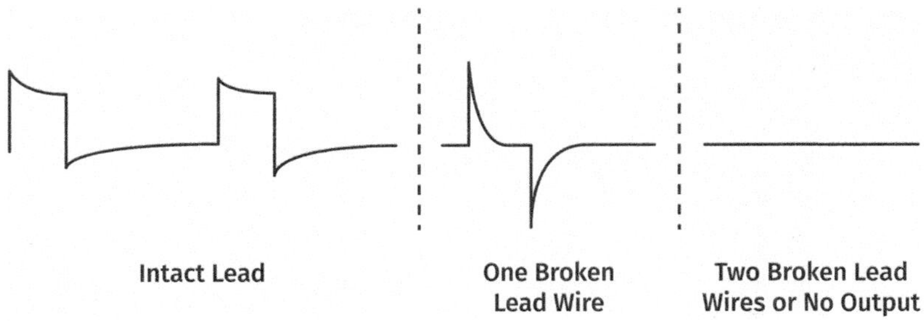

FIGURE 38.84 Stimulus evoked potential waveforms in various conditions. *Reproduced with permission from LivaNova PLC.*

To ensure a tolerable and nondetrimental outcome for seizure control, it is recommended, when conditions permit, to turn off stimulation for several months before VNS explantation.

When performing system explantation, the objective is to remove as much of the lead as safely possible. Ideally, no more than 2 cm of the LivaNova lead (or 5 cm of the MicroTransponder lead) should remain to preserve MRI compatibility within the defined exclusion zone (Fig. 38.74).

Noninvasive vagus nerve stimulation

While VNS is an established treatment, access to VNS has been limited over the first few decades of use due to the invasive and expensive nature of implantable VNS. Consequently, noninvasive transcutaneous VNS (tVNS) has been developed as a less expensive, safe, and easily applicable alternative. This has opened the door for scientists to study the effects of vagal stimulation more closely and has moved this area forward.

TaVNS (transcutaneous auricular vagus nerve stimulation) and CtVNS (transcutaneous cervical vagus nerve stimulation) are two forms of noninvasive vagus nerve stimulation.

Transcutaneous auricular vagus nerve stimulation

In principle, TaVNS is methodologically similar to conventionally administered transcutaneous electrical nerve stimulation (TENS) used to treat musculoskeletal pain disorders. The difference is that TaVNS is delivered to specific anatomical ear targets.

The auricle is innervated by cranial nerves and spinal nerves (Fig. 38.85). Innervations of at least four nerves supply the anterior auricle: the auriculotemporal nerve, the auricular branch of the vagus nerve (ABVN), the lesser occipital nerve, and the greater auricular nerve. The ABVN is the only peripheral branch of the vagus nerve, and this makes it well-

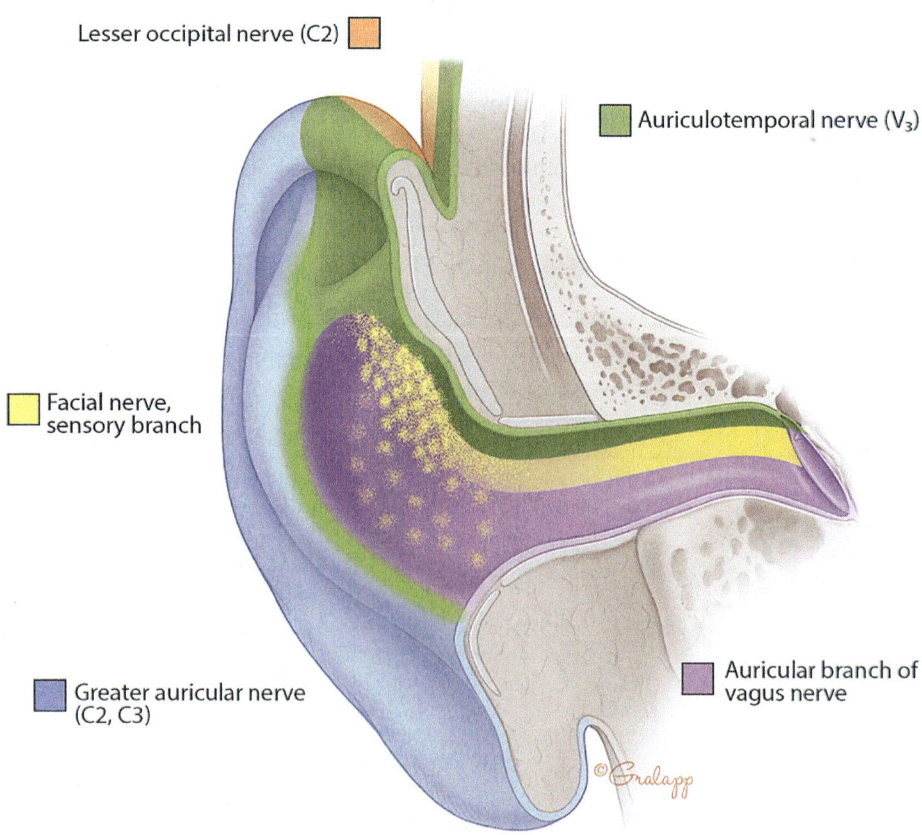

FIGURE 38.85 Auricle skin innervation.

suited for tVNS [18]. It is believed that stimulation of ABVN fibers should produce therapeutic effects that are similar to those of implantable VNS [19]. In fact, functional magnetic resonance imaging (fMRI) of the brain has demonstrated that tVNS can stimulate brain areas consistent with the contemporaneously accepted understanding of central vagal projections [20].

TaVNS is administered through electrodes placed on specific areas of the outer ear, typically the tragus or the cymba conchae, areas of the ear innervated by the ABVN. The earlobe is often used for sham stimulation, as it has minimal ABVN innervation [21]. Stimulation may be applied to the left, right, or both ears. Research has traditionally favored the left ear, primarily due to conventions established during decades of using invasive VNS devices, while some do explore the different effects of right-sided or bilateral stimulation. Selection of the stimulation site appears to be arbitrary, either predetermined by the device employed in the experiment or based on other previous studies [22].

A stimulation unit, which can be part of a device that resembles an ear bud, is used to deliver the electrical current. The device is typically clipped or fitted to specific areas of the ear. The electrodes applied to the surface of the skin are usually titanium since it is a durable and hypoallergenic material, making it a suitable choice for electrodes that have direct and prolonged contact with the skin. These electrodes deliver the electrical current to the vagus nerve endings in the ear. Many devices can be customized through a companion mobile app, allowing the user to adjust the intensity and frequency of the electrical pulses. Electrode design, configuration (monopolar/bipolar), target location, and stimulation parameters vary widely, but most commonly used TaVNS waveform parameters are highly similar to the typical parameters used for the stimulation of the cervical vagus, at a pulse width of 250 μs and frequency of 20 Hz. Many researchers agree that optimal parameters for TaVNS are still being explored. Side effects of TaVNS are minimal, with skin irritation or redness being the most common side effect.

NEMOS (distributed by tVNS Technologies GmbH, previously Cerbomed) is the most widely used commercially available TaVNS device (Fig. 38.86). The device targets the concha of the outer ear and is CE-marked (European Conformity) for the European market for use in the treatment of epilepsy, depression, chronic pain, and anxiety. This device does not yet have FDA clearance for these indications.

It is a handheld, battery-driven device connected to a specialized ear electrode made of titanium/titanium-iridium. Stimulation intensity can be adjusted by the patient, caregiver, or treating physician (increased at steps of 0.1 mA until the perception threshold of the electrical stimulation is reached). Impedance is measured automatically and insufficient electrode contact with the skin evokes an alarm. During stimulation, a series of electrical pulses (pulse width: 250 μs, frequency: 25 Hz, duty cycle: 30 s ON, 30 s OFF, to avoid habituation) are applied to the skin of the concha. Patients are asked to stimulate for a total of 4 h per day [23].

Transcutaneous cervical vagus nerve stimulation

CtVNS is applied to the neck, where the vagus nerve runs closer to the surface and is a similar location to where the electrodes for implantable VNS are positioned (Fig. 38.87). It involves placing electrodes over the skin on the side of the neck, near the sternocleidomastoid muscle, to stimulate the cervical vagal nerve branch [24].

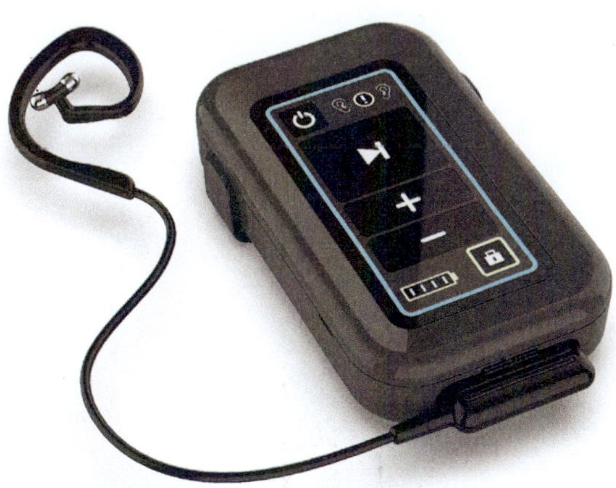

FIGURE 38.86 NEMOS/t-VNS.

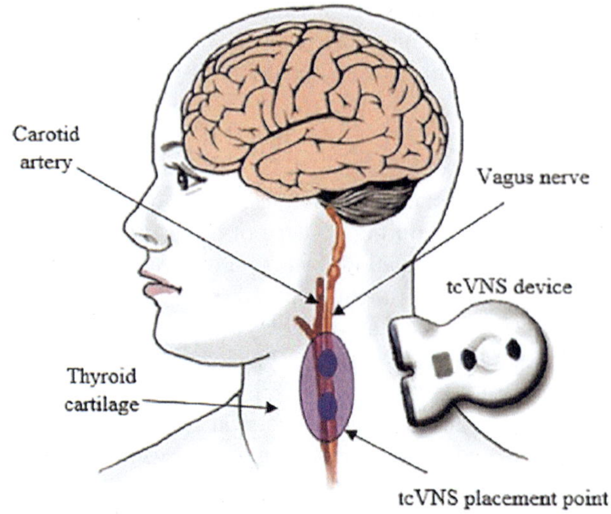

FIGURE 38.87 tcVNS placement point. *From Ref. [25].*

An MRI-derived finite element method model was developed to analyze the cellular components activated with TcVNS. Due to the different types of tissue between the surface electrodes on the skin and the VN, both macroscopic (skin, muscle, fat) and mesoscopic (nerve sheath, cerebrospinal fluid) components were used to predict activation thresholds and electric field changes. It was demonstrated that the overall current requirement to achieve adequate stimulation is influenced by deeper tissues and that tissue conductivity has a direct effect on axon membrane polarization. This model predicted that TcVNS can activate A and B axon fibers, but not C fibers [2].

The most widely commercially available TcVNS device (gammaCore, electroCore, Inc.) in the United States, the gammaCore device, received FDA approval for the treatment of acute cluster headache treatment in 2017, and for acute migraine treatment and adjunctive cluster headache prevention in 2018.

gammaCore Sapphire (noninvasive vagus nerve stimulator) is a hand-held, rechargeable, portable device (Fig. 38.88) consisting of a rechargeable battery, signal-generating and -amplifying electronics, and a control button for the patient to control the signal amplitude. It is intended for single patient use and can deliver multiple stimulations a day. The device provides visible (display) and audible (beep) feedback on the device and stimulation status. A pair of stainless-steel surfaces, which are the skin contact surfaces ("stimulation surfaces"), allow the delivery of a proprietary electrical signal. This signal consists of five 5000 Hz pulses repeated at a rate of 25 Hz for a maximum of 120 s per dose. The waveform of the electric pulses approximates a sine wave with peak voltage limited to ±30 V (24 V when against the skin of the neck) and a maximum output current of 60 mA. The amplitude of the stimulation, depending on the control type, is adjusted by using the thumbwheel or by using buttons located on the device.

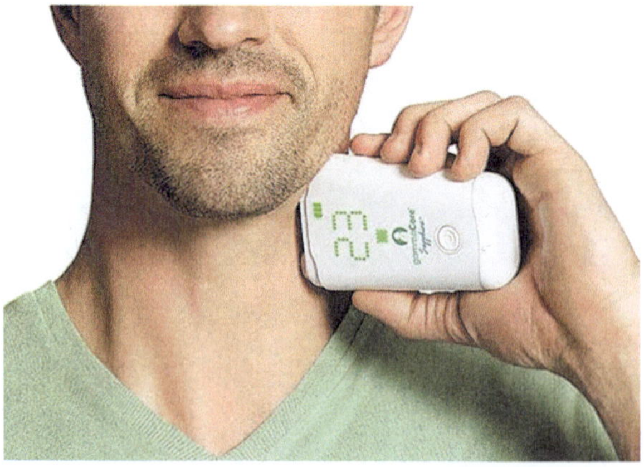

FIGURE 38.88 gammaCore Sapphire.

The patient applies electroCore-approved gel to the stimulation surfaces to maintain an uninterrupted conductive path from the stimulation surfaces to the skin on the neck. Tubes of electroCore-approved gel are provided with each unit. The stimulation surfaces are capped when not in use.

While not appropriate for all indications the ease of use and safety of this approach positions cervical nVNS and auricular VNS as a safe, effective, and durable means of engaging vagal physiology. By analogy to peripheral nerve stimulation, its distant but powerful central effects may represent not a limitation but an advantage.

References

[1] Hammer N, et al. Cervical vagus nerve morphometry and vascularity in the context of nerve stimulation - a cadaveric study. Sci Rep 2018;8:7997.

[2] Mourdoukoutas AP, Truong DQ, Adair DK, Simon BJ, Bikson M. High-resolution multi-scale computational model for non-invasive cervical vagus nerve stimulation. Neuromodulation 2018;21:261–8.

[3] Clark AJ, Kuperma N RA, Auguste KI, Sun PP. Intractable episodic bradycardia resulting from progressive lead traction in an epileptic child with a vagus nerve stimulator: a delayed complication - case report. J Neurosurg Pediatr 2012;9.

[4] Dawson J, et al. Vagus nerve stimulation paired with rehabilitation for upper limb motor function after ischaemic stroke (VNS-REHAB): a randomised, blinded, pivotal, device trial. Lancet 2021;397:1545–53.

[5] Hulsey DR, Shedd CM, Sarker SF, Kilgard MP, Hays SA. Norepinephrine and serotonin are required for vagus nerve stimulation directed cortical plasticity. Exp Neurol 2019;320:112975.

[6] Hojaij F, et al. Syntopy of vagus nerve in the carotid sheath: a dissectional study of 50 cadavers. Laryngoscope Investig Otolaryngol 2019;4.

[7] Boon P, et al. A prospective, multicenter study of cardiac-based seizure detection to activate vagus nerve stimulation. Seizure 2015;32:52–61.

[8] Fahoum F, et al. VNS parameters for clinical response in Epilepsy. Brain Stimul 2022;15.

[9] Smyth MD, Tubbs RS, Bebin EM, Grabb PA, Blount JP. Complications of chronic vagus nerve stimulation for epilepsy in children. J Neurosurg 2003;99.

[10] Patel NC, Edwards MS. Vagal nerve stimulator pocket infections. Pediatr Infect Dis J 2004;23.

[11] Ortler M, Luef G, Kofler A, Bauer G, Twerdy K. Deep wound infection after vagus nerve stimulator implantation: treatment without removal of the device. Epilepsia 2001;42.

[12] Murphy JV, Hornig GW, Schallert GS, Tilton CL. Adverse events in children receiving intermittent left vagal nerve stimulation. Pediatr Neurol 1998;19.

[13] Scott H, Moore A, Paydak H, Hundley K, Palys V. Reproducible asystole following vagal nerve stimulator lead replacement: a case report. BMC Neurol 2022;22.

[14] Rutecki P. Anatomical, physiological, and theoretical basis for the antiepileptic effect of vagus nerve stimulation. Epilepsia 1990;31.

[15] McGregor A, Wheless J, Baumgartner J, Bettis D. Right-sided vagus nerve stimulation as a treatment for refractory epilepsy in humans. Epilepsia 2005;46. https://doi.org/10.1111/j.0013-9580.2005.16404.x. Preprint at.

[16] Spuck S, Nowak G, Renneberg A, Tronnier V, Sperner J. Right-sided vagus nerve stimulation in humans: an effective therapy? Epilepsy Res 2008;82.

[17] Navas M, et al. Treatment of refractory epilepsy in adult patients with right-sided vagus nerve stimulation. Epilepsy Res 2010;90. https://doi.org/10.1016/j.eplepsyres.2010.04.007. Preprint at.

[18] Ueno N, et al. [Innervation of the external ear in humans and the musk shrew]. Nihon Jibiinkoka Gakkai Kaiho 1993;96:212–8.

[19] Bermejo P, et al. Innervation of the human Cavum conchae and auditory canal: anatomical basis for transcutaneous auricular nerve stimulation. BioMed Res Int 2017;2017:7830919.

[20] Frangos E, Ellrich J, Komisaruk BR. Non-invasive access to the vagus nerve central projections via electrical stimulation of the external ear: fMRI evidence in humans. Brain Stimul 2015;8:624–36.

[21] Peuker ET, Filler TJ. The nerve supply of the human auricle. Clin Anat 2002;15:35–7.

[22] Yap JYY, et al. Critical review of transcutaneous vagus nerve stimulation: challenges for translation to clinical practice. Front Neurosci 2020;14:284.

[23] Straube A, Ellrich J, Eren O, Blum B, Ruscheweyh R. Treatment of chronic migraine with transcutaneous stimulation of the auricular branch of the vagal nerve (auricular t-VNS): a randomized, monocentric clinical trial. J Headache Pain 2015;16:543.

[24] Goadsby PJ, Grosberg BM, Mauskop A, Cady R, Simmons KA. Effect of noninvasive vagus nerve stimulation on acute migraine: an open-label pilot study. Cephalalgia 2014;34:986–93.

[25] Choudhary T, et al. Effect of transcutaneous cervical vagus nerve stimulation on declarative and working memory in patients with Posttraumatic Stress Disorder (PTSD): a pilot study. J Affect Disord 2023;339:418–25.

Chapter 39

Complications of brain and cranial nerve stimulation

Steven Falowski[1], Inamullah Khan[2], Manish Ranjan[3] and Rushna Ali[4]

[1]*Neurosurgery, Neurosurgical Associates of Lancaster, Lancaster, PA, United States;* [2]*University of Missouri, Columbia, MO, United States;* [3]*Neurosurgery and Neuroscience, West Virginia University, Morgantown, WV, United States;* [4]*Neurosurgery, Mayo Clinic, Rochester, MN, United States*

Key points

1. Deep Brain Stimulation is a well-established safe and effective procedure.
2. Deep Brain Stimulation is used for movement disorders, chronic pain, epilepsy, and psychiatric illnesses.
3. Common cranial nerve stimulation procedures include vagal nerve stimulation, trigeminal nerve stimulation, occipital nerve stimulation, and hypoglossal nerve stimulation
4. Multidisciplinary team evaluation and care is crucial for right patient selection and optimum treatment outcome.

Introduction

Brain and cranial nerve neuromodulation interventions have become the cornerstone treatments for a variety of neurological and psychiatric disorders [1]. These procedures involve implanting electrodes that deliver electrical impulses to targeted regions of the brain or cranial nerves to alleviate symptoms associated with movement disorders, chronic pain, epilepsy, and psychiatric illnesses [2]. Deep brain stimulation (DBS) has revolutionized the treatment of Parkinson's disease (PD), essential tremor (ET) dystonia, pain, depression, obsessive compulsive disorder (OCD) and epilepsy after receiving Food and Drug Administration (FDA) and Conformité Européene (CE) approval [2–4]. Responsive neurostimulation (RNS) has also been used in the treatment of epilepsy. On the other hand, cranial nerve stimulation (CNS) techniques such as vagus nerve stimulation (VNS), trigeminal nerve stimulation (TNS), Occipital nerve stimulation (ONS) and hypoglossal nerve stimulation (HNS) have shown efficacy in treatment of epilepsy, neurorehabilitation in stroke patients, psychiatric diseases, chronic pain and obstructive sleep apnea (OSA) [5–7].

The delivery of electrical impulses to targeted brain regions or cranial nerves alters the abnormal pattern of neuronal activity associated with the disease state and provides symptomatic improvement. Neuromodulation therapies are generally reserved for patients with refractory conditions who fail to respond to conservative treatments. The field continues to evolve with advancements in electrode design, targeting precision, and adaptive stimulation technologies.

Historical perspective and timeline of advancements

The evolution of brain and cranial nerve stimulation spans several centuries, with landmark discoveries shaping modern neuromodulation. In 153AD, ancient Roman history identifies the use of electric torpedo fish on the forehead of patients by Scribonious Largus for treating headaches [8]. In the late 19th century, pioneering work by Fritsch and Hitzig on cortical electrical stimulation laid the foundation for brain stimulation research [9]. In the 1930s, Wilder Penfield conducted cortical mapping through electrical stimulation, improving our understanding of motor and sensory functions [10]. The 1940s saw the advent of stereotactic surgery by Spiegel and Wycis, providing precise targeting for deep brain structures [11].

A Modern Atlas for Implantable Devices of the Spine, Brain, and Nerve. https://doi.org/10.1016/B978-0-443-36528-7.00045-5

Robert Heath performed early DBS experiments in psychiatric patients, showing that electrical stimulation could influence mood and behavior [12]. The 1970 and 1980s witnessed the introduction of DBS for pain management, followed by its expansion to movement disorders [13]. The FDA approved DBS for essential tremor and Parkinson's disease in 1990s [14,15]. Introduction of directional leads and rechargeable neurostimulators improved stimulation precision and device longevity [16,17]. In the modern era, development of closed-loop and adaptive DBS systems has enabled real-time neural feedback and personalized therapy [18].

In a similar manner, the evolution of cranial nerve stimulation (CNS) dates to 1884 when Dr. James Cornig, studied carotid "electrocompressor" for epilepsy management [19]. The seizure improvement was later found out to be related to vagus nerve stimulation by the fork-like instrument that was used as carotid electrocompressor. In 1938, Bailey and Bremer demonstrated that VNS activated orbitofrontal regions in a feline model, suggesting direct afferent projections to the brain [20]. In 1952, Zanchetti and colleagues further showed that VNS reduced experimentally induced epileptic waveforms, indicating its potential to modulate cortical excitability [20,21]. Modern VNS development began in the 1980s with Jacob Zabara, who created an implantable VNS system that successfully terminated chemically induced seizures in canines [22]. This research led to the first human implant by Penry and Dean in 1990, showing seizure reduction in three out of four patients [23]. Following a pivotal trial in 310 patients, the FDA approved VNS for epilepsy in 1997 [24]. Subsequent approvals expanded its use to treatment-resistant depression in 2005 and morbid obesity in 2015 [25,26].

In addition to its use for facial pain syndromes, Trigeminal nerve stimulation (TNS) also has been shown to induce cerebral vasodilation, modulate metabolism and neurotransmission, and reduce neuroinflammation [27–29]. It also influences the autonomic nervous system, peripheral vasoconstriction, and systemic inflammation. Clinically, TNS was first applied to cluster headaches in 1989 and drug-resistant epilepsy in 2003 [30,31]. It has since been explored for conditions such as depression, post-traumatic stress disorder (PTSD), prolonged disorders of consciousness, and recovery following subarachnoid hemorrhage [32]. FDA-approved indications include migraine, pediatric attention deficit hyperactivity disorder (ADHD), and cognitive dysfunction in mild TBI, MS, and cerebral palsy [33–37]. Preclinical studies highlight its cerebroprotective effects in TBI, hemorrhagic shock, SAH, and ischemic stroke. With its expanding applications, TNS is emerging as a leading neuromodulation therapy, comparable to VNS.

Innovations in brain and cranial nerve stimulation

Advancements in neuromodulation have significantly improved efficacy, safety, and patient outcomes across brain and cranial nerve stimulation applications. One major development is in electrode and lead design, where traditional monopolar electrodes have been replaced by segmented, directional leads that allow precise current steering, thereby enhancing therapeutic effects while minimizing side effects [16,17]. Additionally, closed-loop and adaptive stimulation systems now integrate real-time sensing and machine learning to dynamically adjust stimulation parameters based on neural activity, improving treatment outcomes in conditions such as Parkinson's disease and epilepsy [18,38].

With respect to cranial nerve stimulation, the transition from open to closed-loop VNS has allowed real-time adjustment of stimulation parameters based on physiological signals, improving seizure control and autonomic modulation [39]. Occipital nerve stimulation now features multicontact leads and adaptive programming, improving outcomes in chronic migraine and cluster headaches by refining current delivery to reduce side effects [33,40,41]. Hypoglossal nerve stimulation has adaptive stimulation algorithms improving upper airway patency and sleep quality for OSA [42–44]. These innovations continue to refine CNS applications, broadening therapeutic indications and optimizing patient-centered.

Parallel advancements in surgical techniques have further refined neuromodulation procedures. Image-guidance, integrated tractography and robotic-assisted implantation methods have improved targeting precision, reducing complications such as lead migration, suboptimal placement, and hardware-related failures [45,46]. The integration of artificial intelligence (AI) in neuromodulation is also a rapidly growing field, where AI-driven algorithms are being developed to optimize stimulation settings, predict treatment responses, and enhance closed-loop feedback systems [18,47].

Relevant anatomy

The anatomical targets vary by indication:

Deep Brain Stimulation (DBS) for movement disorders

DBS (CPT code 61,880, 61,885, 61,886, and 61,888) is widely used to treat movement disorders such as Parkinson's disease (ICD 10: G20), essential tremor (ICD 10: G25.0), and dystonia (ICD 10: G24.3), with stimulation targeting specific subcortical structures to modulate abnormal neural circuitry. On-label indications include Parkinson's disease (STN, GPi DBS), essential tremor (VIM DBS), dystonia (STN, GPi DBS).

Subthalamic nucleus (STN)

The STN is a key component of the basal ganglia circuitry, playing a crucial role in motor control through its excitatory influence on the globus pallidus internus (GPi) and substantia nigra pars reticulata (SNr) (Fig. 39.1) [48]. In Parkinson's disease, loss of dopaminergic input from the substantia nigra pars compacta (SNc) leads to overactivity of the STN, resulting in excessive inhibition of the thalamocortical motor pathway and causing bradykinesia and rigidity. DBS of the STN reduces this overactivity, restoring balanced basal ganglia output and improving motor symptoms [14,49].

Globus pallidus internus (GPi)

The GPi is another critical basal ganglio structure that exerts inhibitory control over the thalamus (Fig. 39.1). In dystonia, excessive and prolonged firing of GPi neurons contributes to sustained muscle contractions and abnormal postures. DBS of the GPi reduces this excessive inhibition, alleviating dystonic symptoms and improving motor function [50,51]. GPi DBS is also an effective alternative to STN DBS for Parkinson's disease, particularly in patients who experience significant medication-induced dyskinesias [52].

Ventral intermediate nucleus (VIM) of the thalamus

The VIM is the primary relay center for proprioceptive and cerebellar input to the motor cortex and plays a central role in tremor generation [53]. DBS of the VIM is the preferred target for essential tremor, as it disrupts tremor-related oscillatory activity within the cerebello-thalamo-cortical pathway, leading to significant symptom relief [54–56]. VIM stimulation is also effective in tremor-dominant Parkinson's disease but does not address bradykinesia or rigidity as effectively as STN or GPi DBS [57].

DBS for pain modulation

DBS can be used off-label for the treatment of neuropathic pain syndromes and central pain disorders, including chronic pain syndrome (ICD 10: G89.4), failed back surgery syndrome (ICD 10: M96.1), and trigeminal neuropathic pain (ICD 10: G50.0).

Periaqueductal gray (PAG)

The PAG integrates input from the limbic system and projects to the rostral ventromedial medulla (RVM) and dorsal horn of the spinal cord, where it modulates nociceptive pain transmission [58]. DBS of the PAG activates endogenous opioid pathways and inhibits pain transmission, providing relief in chronic neuropathic pain conditions such as post-stroke pain and phantom limb pain [59,60].

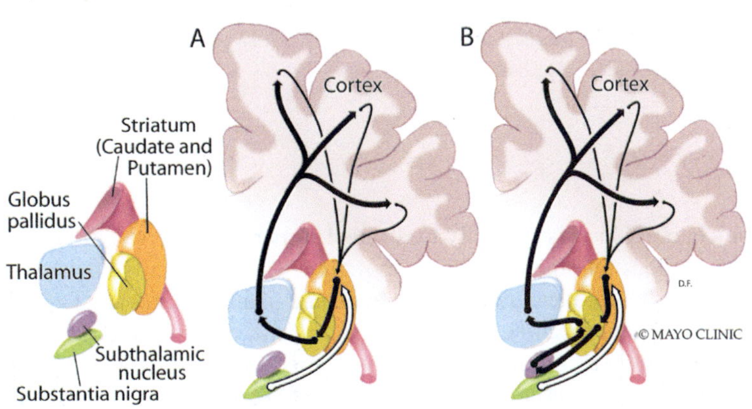

FIGURE 39.1 Basal ganglia circuit.

Ventral posterolateral (VPL) thalamus

The VPL nucleus of the thalamus is a critical relay center for somatosensory and pain processing, receiving input from the spinothalamic and trigeminothalamic pathways before transmitting signals to the primary somatosensory cortex [61]. In patients with central pain syndromes (G 89.0), such as post-stroke pain and thalamic pain syndrome, DBS of the VPL modulates aberrant thalamocortical activity and alters pain perception [62,63]. This effect is thought to occur by disrupting pathological hyperexcitability and synchrony within the pain-processing network.

Several other DBS targets have been explored for pain management. The centromedian-parafascicular (CM-Pf) complex of the thalamus has been studied for neuropathic pain, particularly in patients with post-stroke pain syndrome [64]. The anterior cingulate cortex (ACC), a key region involved in the affective-emotional aspect of pain, has also been a target for chronic pain syndromes, including fibromyalgia and phantom limb pain [65]. Additionally, the posterior hypothalamus has shown efficacy in treating cluster headaches and other refractory facial pain conditions by modulating autonomic and nociceptive pathways [66,67].

Cranial nerve stimulation

Vagus nerve stimulation (VNS) (CPT 64,568)

The vagus nerve originates from the medulla and provides both afferent and efferent autonomic fibers to the brainstem, heart, lungs, and digestive tract [68]. Approximately 80% of vagal fibers are afferent, transmitting sensory information to the nucleus tractus solitarius (NTS), locus coeruleus, and dorsal raphe nucleus, which then modulate activity in widespread cortical and subcortical structures, including the thalamus, amygdala, and prefrontal cortex [69]. VNS is used for epilepsy, depression, increased neuroplasticity and improvement in autonomic dysfunction.

Trigeminal nerve stimulation (TNS) (CPT 64,599)

The trigeminal nerve is the largest cranial nerve and has sensory and motor components. Its ophthalmic (V1) and maxillary (V2) branches provide sensory innervation to the forehead, face, and scalp, while its mandibular (V3) branch carries both sensory and motor fibers [70]. The trigeminal ganglion projects to the trigeminal nucleus, which connects to pain-processing centers such as the thalamus, insula, and cingulate cortex [71]. Majority of the stimulation procedures for trigeminal nerve are for treatment of trigeminal neuralgia/neuropathy; however, there is an increasing list of indications in the literature including epilepsy, depression, and migraine [33–37].

Occipital nerve stimulation (ONS) (CPT 64,553, 64,555)

The greater occipital nerve (GON) and lesser occipital nerve (LON) arises from the C2 and C3 spinal nerve respectively. The occipital nerves provide sensory innervation to the posterior scalp (Fig. 39.2). They communicate with the trigeminal nucleus caudalis (TNC), integrating nociceptive signals from the cervical and trigeminal systems [72]. Dysfunction in this network is implicated in chronic headache disorders and occipital neuralgia [73].

Hypoglossal nerve stimulation (HNS) (CPT 64,582, 64,583, 64,584)

The hypoglossal nerve (cranial nerve XII) arises from the medulla and primarily controls tongue movements. It innervates the genioglossus muscle, which maintains upper airway patency during breathing [43]. In OSA, upper airway collapses during sleep leads to intermittent hypoxia. HNS stimulates the hypoglossal nerve to contract the genioglossus muscle, preventing airway collapse and improving airflow [44].

Procedure

Deep brain stimulation

Deep Brain Stimulation (DBS) is a neurosurgical procedure which is typically performed in two or more stages [74].

The first stage involves the implantation of DBS electrodes into the targeted brain region. The preoperative magnetic resonance imaging (MRI) and computed tomography (CT) scans are integrated into stereotactic planning software. Frame-based or frameless systems can be utilized. The lead implantation can be performed awake with minimal anesthesia or general endotracheal anesthesia. During surgery, microelectrode recording (MER) may be used to map neuronal activity and confirm the optimal target [75]. Once the final electrode position is confirmed, a permanent DBS lead is implanted and secured to the skull.

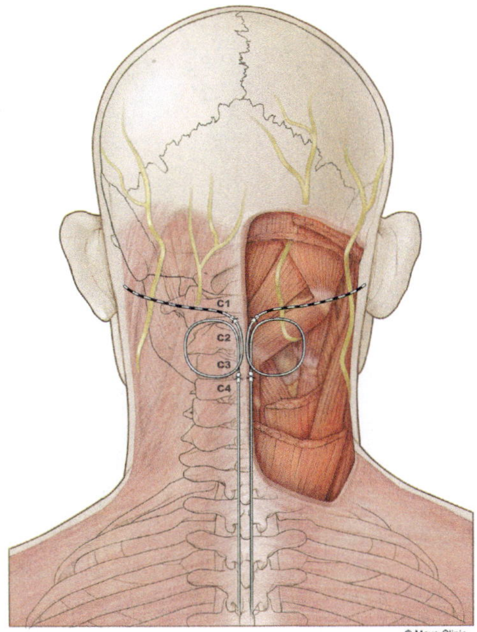

FIGURE 39.2 Occipital nerve and bilateral subcutaneous stimulation leads.

After lead placement, the internal pulse generator (IPG) is implanted in a separate procedure, typically 1–2 weeks later, in the subclavicular area [76].

Cranial nerve stimulation

The procedure involves implanting a neurostimulation device that delivers electrical impulses to specific cranial nerves, such as the vagus nerve, occipital nerve, trigeminal nerve or hypoglossal nerve. While the approach differs slightly for each cranial nerve, the general process includes surgical implantation of leads and an internal pulse generator (IPG), followed by post-operative programming to optimize therapy.

In case of TNS or ONS for pain there are initial trial leads placement which allows the patient to test the efficacy of pain control for 7–10 days [77]. In cases of VNS and HNS the permanent implants are placed in single procedure along with the IPG [78].

Following implantation, the neuromodulation system is programmed using a clinician programmer, with initial settings tailored to the patient's symptoms and side effects. Over time, adjustments are made to optimize therapy. Patients undergo regular follow-ups for battery longevity assessment, software updates, and potential reprogramming to maintain efficacy (Fig. 39.3 and 39.4)

Patient selection considerations

Both DBS and CNS therapies are generally indicated for adults [79,80]. However, in specific cases such as refractory epilepsy and dystonia, pediatric patients may also be considered [81,82]. Multidisciplinary team evaluation is essential to ensure appropriate patient selection.

Contraindications

Patients with significant cognitive decline or advanced dementia are generally excluded, as they may have difficulty complying with post-surgical care or benefit less from stimulation [83]. Patients with active infections or those who are at high risk of infections are contraindicated, as implanting devices under these circumstances could lead to sepsis or chronic device infection. While not an absolute contraindication, patients with active or uncontrolled psychiatric disorders (such as severe depression, psychosis, or mania) may be at higher risk of complications or suboptimal outcomes [84]. Stimulation therapy can sometimes affect mood, and ongoing psychiatric management may be required in such cases.

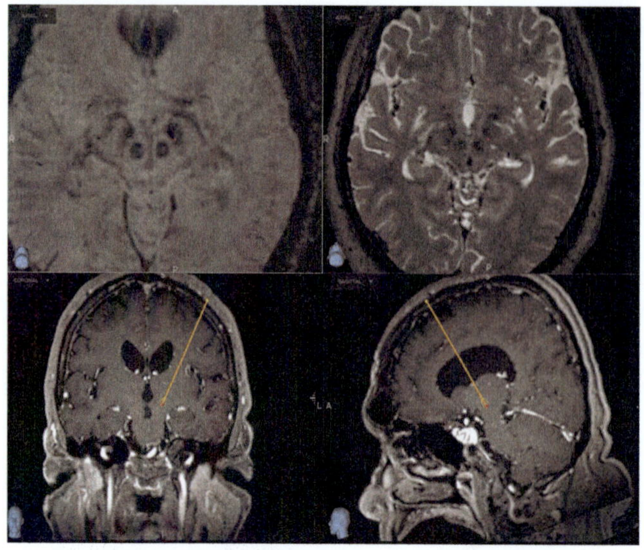

FIGURE 39.3 Showing the Left STN target (red dot) within the left STN on SWI (top left panel) and T2 axial (top right panel) MRI with corresponding trajectory in the bottom panel in coronal (bottom left) and sagittal plane (bottom right).

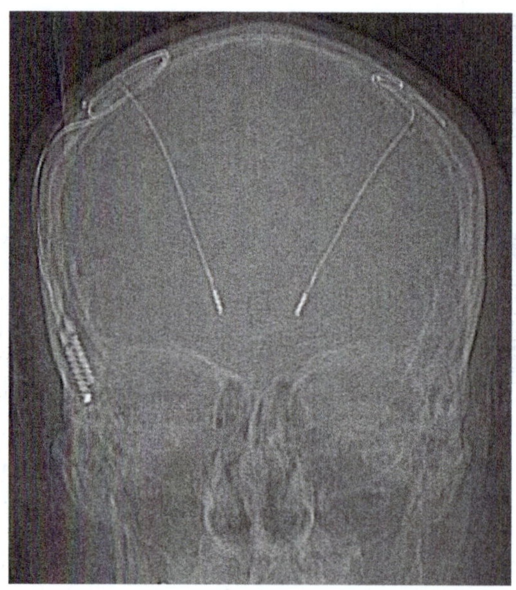

FIGURE 39.4 X-ray tomogram showing post-op bilateral DBS electrode and extension.

Maintenance concerns

Once a patient undergoes DBS or CNS implantation, regular maintenance and monitoring are essential to ensure the device's optimal functioning. Over time, patients may require periodic adjustments to the stimulation settings to optimize symptom management and minimize side effects. These adjustments are typically done during outpatient visits and may involve changes in the frequency, intensity, or duration of the stimulation. The battery life of the internal pulse generator (IPG) varies depending on the type of device, stimulation parameters, and patient activity levels. Most IPGs last between 3 and 5 years, after which the battery needs to be replaced. In rechargeable devices, patients must ensure regular recharging to maintain consistent performance.

Training recommendations

Training in functional neurosurgery and pain neuromodulation is essential for the competence and expertise required in Deep Brain Stimulation (DBS) and cranial nerve stimulation (CNS) procedures. An accredited fellowship with a comprehensive curriculum that includes expertise in stereotactic and functional neurosurgery along with surgical management of chronic pain is typically required. This fellowship provides comprehensive training in preoperative planning, surgical technique, patient selection, and post-operative management specific to for the management of movement disorders, chronic pain management, epilepsy and psychiatric conditions.

The Committee on Advanced Subspecialty Training (CAST) outlines procedural requirements for advanced neurosurgical training [85]. The minimum number of for DBS for any indication and neuromodulation for pain is 20 in each category. Further procedural benchmarks include at least 10 cases of trigeminal neuralgia or hemifacial spasm surgery. These training requirements ensure that neurosurgical fellows develop comprehensive expertise in stereotactic, functional and pain neurosurgery, allowing them to manage complex cases and provide comprehensive care.

Surgical technique

Deep Brain Stimulation (DBS) is typically performed in two stages [74].The first stage involves implantation of the lead. Implanting of the lead takes approximately 2–3 h and is generally performed using moderate intravenous sedation, as well as local anesthesia for the incisions. More recently, general anesthesia has also been utilized. MRI or CT scan imaging is obtained prior to the case. It is then integrated into stereotactic navigation planning software (either frame based or frameless) and used to guide implantation of the electrodes. A representative of the vendor is generally present to supply the necessary product and support the case. The patient is positioned supine with the head elevated. There is the creation of a parasagittal frontal burr hole through a small incision. During surgery, microelectrode recording (MER) may be used to map neuronal activity and confirm the optimal target [75]. Additional test stimulation can be performed to confirm proper placement without unwanted side effects from adjacent structures. Once the final electrode position is confirmed, a permanent DBS lead is implanted and secured to the skull.

The second stage of the procedure, the implantation of the internal pulse generator (IPG), can be performed immediately after lead implantation or more typically 1–2 weeks later, in the subclavicular area [76]. This portion of the surgery is generally 45 min. The patient is placed supine. The leads are tunneled from the head to the subclavicular region to connect to the IPG. A representative of the vendor is generally present to supply the necessary product and also help perform the system check to determine proper impedances.

Potential complications

The risk profile for DBS placement is relatively low. The most significant serious complication that can occur is an intracranial hematoma. This can include bleeding at the cortical insertion site or within the brain along the track of the electrode. The incidence has been quoted from 1% to 4% with most of them being asymptomatic [62,86]. The risk of permanent neurological deficits ranges from 1% to 3.4% [86].

As with any surgical procedure there is the risk of infection. This can be hardware related or intracranial. The incidence ranges from 2% to 13% and generally hardware related [62,86]. Antibiotics alone will resolve most instances, but some cases may require wound debridement, as well as device revision/removal. However, some literature has demonstrated infections rates of 1.9% utilizing techniques to isolate the implants from skin incisions. [87].

There is the risk of further complications throughout the lifespan of the implanted device related to the hardware. The incidence is 7% and can include lead fracture, erosion, lead migration, or generator malfunction [62,86].

Post-operative consideration

Brain and cranial nerve stimulation is one of the very satisfying procedures, both for the treating team as well as the patients and their families. It not only restores the function but also enables patient a better control of the primary disease and active lifestyle. Although, the procedures are helpful to restore the function but it's a process/journey which patients go through along with the treating team.

Recovery and recovery timeline

Unlike many surgical procedures for the brain and cranial nerves, the surgery for the brain and cranial nerve stimulation is associated with relatively faster recovery. Most of the procedure for cranial nerve stimulation is usually done as an outpatient surgery and typically patients go home the very same day of the surgery, whether it is vagus nerve stimulation, trigeminal nerve stimulation or hypoglossal nerve stimulation. For those having brain stimulation, patients typically stay overnight and get discharged the next day. Even outpatient DBS surgery emerged as an alternative with a good outcome [88], though it still needs to be tested in a larger patient population across different centers. Healing phase lasts several weeks; however, the immediate and initial post-operative period is focused on incisional care. Pain management, infection prevention, and monitoring for adverse neurological effects are critical in the early recovery phase [45].

Activity limitation

Post-operative activity limitations are crucial to ensure proper healing and device functionality. Patients are generally advised to avoid strenuous activities and heavy lifting for few weeks following surgery and depending upon the surgery could last about 4–6 weeks.

Efficacy estimates

The efficacy of brain and cranial nerve stimulation depends on the indication and patient-specific factors. DBS and certain cranial nerve stimulation are the standard of care for movement disorders and epilepsy with good outcomes and cost-effectiveness [45,89–93]. Depending upon the primary indication, various scales are used to assess the efficacy. Unified Parkinson's Disease Rating Scale (UPDRS), Burke-Fahn-Marsden Dystonia Rating Scale (BFMDRS), Tremor Research Group Essential Tremor Assessment Scale (TETRAS), Clinical Rating Scale for Tremor (CRST) are the common scales used in movement disorders depending upon the primary indication, while Yale–Brown Obsessive–Compulsive Scale (Y–BOCS) used for OCD. For surgical outcome in epilepsy, Engel classification system is used for seizure outcome assessment.

For DBS in movement disorders efficacy rates range from 50% to 80% in improving motor symptoms [94]. DBS is effective in about 60% of patients with OCD [95,96]. In epilepsy, VNS has been shown to reduce seizure frequency by 50%–100% in approximately 45%–65% of the patients [97], while with long-term treatment with Responsive Neuro-stimulation, the response rate is about 75% with more than one-third of patients having a ≥90% reduction in seizures [98]. Ongoing adjustments to stimulation parameters and rehabilitation with medical optimization are necessary to maximize therapeutic benefits.

Pearls and pitfalls

There is no substitute for selecting the right patient for the right procedure. Patient selection is paramount and often facilitated by a multidisciplinary team consisting of a neurologist, psychiatrist, pain physician, neuropsychologist, social workers and the neurosurgeon. Once the right patient is identified, perioperative evaluation, relevant bloodwork including coagulation profile is necessary for the safe surgery. In diabetic patients, HgbA1C should be evaluated and a value ≤ 7 is ideal; however, the risk and feasibility need to be assessed on an individual case basis. A high-resolution brain MRI with and without contrast is important for target selection and planning a safe surgical trajectory. Some specific sequences are helpful in identifying and selecting specific brain targets, such as FGATIR, PD, GRE/SWI and QSM.

As the brain and cranial nerve stimulation surgery are multidisciplinary, it is of utmost importance that the team members from different expert domains are familiar with the surgical plan and orchestration. Anesthesia team should be informed of the SBP goal of <140 mmHg (preferably <130 mmHg) as well as avoiding or selecting certain medications during the procedure, as that may affect the MER. Besides appropriate targeting, blood-pressure management and limiting of MER track passes should be exercised as best possible to minimize the bleeding risk [99,100]. Closing pericranium and isolating the stimlock/hardware from the skin could help to avoid hardware damage and contamination [101]. Post-operatively, patients are monitored appropriately for adequate pain management, BP monitoring and post-operative imaging. Patient's home meds need to be promptly re-started, especially Parkinson's disease medication which are typically held prior to surgery. Post-operative CT brain is merged with preoperative MRI brain to assess DBS lead location and/or any complication, especially brain hemorrhage and extent of pneumocephalus. Any lead misplacement and deviation need to be noted and appropriately addressed if significant, which may require revision surgery if misplacement or deviation is clinically significant. Post-operative stimulation programming is highly dependent on the electrode location, as well as intraoperative mapping, and hence it is important to communicate with the neurologist or the relevant team.

References

[1] Perlmutter JS, Mink JW. Deep brain stimulation. Annu Rev Neurosci 2006;29:229–57.

[2] Krauss JK, Lipsman N, Aziz T, Boutet A, Brown P, Chang JW, et al. Technology of deep brain stimulation: Current status and future directions. Nat Rev Neurol 2021;17(2):75–87.

[3] Chua MM, Warren AE, Cosgrove GR, Rolston JD. Publication rates and characteristics of clinical trials in deep brain and responsive neurostimulation. Stereotact Funct Neurosurg 2023;101(5):287–300.
[4] Siegfried J, Lippitz B. Bilateral chronic electrostimulation of ventroposterolateral pallidum: A new therapeutic approach for alleviating all parkinsonian symptoms. Neurosurgery 1994;35(6):1126–9.
[5] Adair D, Truong D, Esmaeilpour Z, Gebodh N, Borges H, Ho L, et al. Electrical stimulation of cranial nerves in cognition and disease. Brain Stimul 2020;13(3):717–50.
[6] Howland RH. Vagus nerve stimulation. Curr Behav Neurosci Rep 2014;1(2):64–73.
[7] Mashaqi S, Patel SI, Combs D, Estep L, Helmick S, Machamer J, et al. The hypoglossal nerve stimulation as a novel therapy for treating obstructive sleep apnea-a literature review. Int J Environ Res Public Health 2021;18(4).
[8] Francis J, Dingley J. Electroanaesthesia–from torpedo fish to TENS. Anaesthesia 2015;70(1):93–103.
[9] Fritsch G. The excitable cerebral cortex. Fritsch, G., Hitzig, E. Uber die elektrische Erregbarkeit des Grosshirns. Arch Anat Physiol Wissen. 1870;37:300–32.
[10] Penfield W, Boldrey E. Somatic motor and sensory representation in the cerebral cortex of man as studied by electrical stimulation. Brain 1937;60 (4):389–443.
[11] Spiegel EA, Wycis HT, Marks M, Lee AJ. Stereotaxic apparatus for operations on the human brain. Science. 1947;106(2754):349–50.
[12] Heath RG. Electrical self-stimulation of the brain in man. Am J Psychiatr 1963;120(6):571–7.
[13] Ohye C, Feger J, Albe-Fessard D. Study in awake monkeys of connections between the corpus striatum and pallidum with the substantia nigra and subthalamus. In: Mechanisms in transmission of signals for conscious behaviour. Amsterdam: North-Holland Publ; 1976. p. 45–59.
[14] Benabid AL. Deep brain stimulation for Parkinson's disease. Curr Opin Neurobiol 2003;13(6):696–706.
[15] Benabid AL, Pollak P, Hoffmann D, Gervason C, Hommel M, Perret J, et al. Long-term suppression of tremor by chronic stimulation of the ventral intermediate thalamic nucleus. Lancet 1991;337(8738):403–6.
[16] Steigerwald F, Müller L, Johannes S, Matthies C, Volkmann J. Directional deep brain stimulation of the subthalamic nucleus: A pilot study using a novel neurostimulation device. Mov Disord 2016;31(8):1240–3.
[17] Waln O, Jimenez-Shahed J. Rechargeable deep brain stimulation implantable pulse generators in movement disorders: Patient satisfaction and conversion parameters. Neuromodulation 2014;17(5):425–30.
[18] Arlotti M, Colombo M, Bonfanti A, Mandat T, Lanotte MM, Pirola E, et al. A new implantable closed-loop clinical neural interface: First application in Parkinson's disease. Front Neurosci 2021;15:763235.
[19] Corning JL. Electrization of the sympathetic and pneumogastric nerves, with simultaneous bilateral compression of the carotids. New York Med J 1884. p. 61.
[20] Badran BW, Austelle CW. The future is noninvasive: A brief review of the evolution and clinical utility of vagus nerve stimulation. Focus 2022;20(1):3–7.
[21] Zanchetti A, Wang S, Moruzzi G. The effect of vagal afferent stimulation on the EEG pattern of the cat. Electroencephalogr Clin Neurophysiol 1952;4(3):357–61.
[22] Zabara J. Peripheral control of hypersynchonous discharge in epilepsy. Electroencephalogr Clin Neurophysiol 1985;61:S162.
[23] Penry JK, Dean JC. Prevention of intractable partial seizures by intermittent vagal stimulation in humans: preliminary results. Epilepsia 1990;31 (Suppl. 2):S40–3.
[24] Handforth A, DeGiorgio C, Schachter S, Uthman B, Naritoku D, Tecoma E, et al. Vagus nerve stimulation therapy for partial-onset seizures: a randomized active-control trial. Neurology 1998;51(1):48–55.
[25] O'Reardon JP, Cristancho P, Peshek AD. Vagus nerve stimulation (VNS) and treatment of depression: To the brainstem and beyond. Psychiatry (Edgmont). 2006;3(5):54–63.
[26] de Lartigue G. Role of the vagus nerve in the development and treatment of diet-induced obesity. J Physiol. 2016;594(20):5791–815.
[27] Electrical stimulation of the infraorbital nerve induces diving reflex in a dose-controlled manner. In: Shah KA, Sonti AN, Wu Y-C, Powell K, Doobay M, Narayan RK, et al., editors. 2020 42nd annual international conference of the IEEE engineering in medicine and biology society (EMBC). IEEE; 2020.
[28] Nash C, Powell K, Lynch DG, Hartings JA, Li C. Nonpharmacological modulation of cortical spreading depolarization. Life Sci 2023;327:121833.
[29] Feletti A, Santi GZ, Sammartino F, Bevilacqua M, Cisotto P, Longatti P. Peripheral trigeminal nerve field stimulation: Report of 6 cases. Neurosurg Focus 2013;35(3):E10.
[30] Fanciullacci M, Fusco B, Alessandri M, Campagnolo V, Sicuteri F. Unilateral impairment of pupillary response to trigeminal nerve stimulation in cluster headache. Pain 1989;36(2):185–91.
[31] DeGiorgio CM, Shewmon DA, Whitehurst T. Trigeminal nerve stimulation for epilepsy. Neurology 2003;61(3):421–2.
[32] Powell K, Lin K, Tambo W, Saavedra AP, Sciubba D, Al AY, et al. Trigeminal nerve stimulation: A current state-of-the-art review. Bioelectron Med 2023;9(1):30.
[33] Reed K, Black S, Banta C, Will K. Combined occipital and supraorbital neurostimulation for the treatment of chronic migraine headaches: Initial experience. Cephalalgia 2010;30(3):260–71.
[34] McGough JJ, Sturm A, Cowen J, Tung K, Salgari GC, Leuchter AF, et al. Double-Blind, sham-controlled, pilot study of trigeminal nerve stimulation for attention-deficit/hyperactivity disorder. J Am Acad Child Adolesc Psychiatry 2019;58(4).

[35] Ptito A, Papa L, Gregory K, Folmer RL, Walker WC, Prabhakaran V, et al. A prospective, multicenter study to assess the safety and efficacy of translingual neurostimulation plus physical therapy for the treatment of a chronic balance deficit due to mild-to-moderate traumatic brain injury. Neuromodulation: Technol Neural Interface 2021;24(8):1412–21.

[36] Ignatova T, Kolbin V, Scherbak S, Sarana A, Sokolov AV, Trufanov GE, et al., editors. Translingual neurostimulation in treatment of children with cerebral palsy in the late residual stage. Case study. BIOSIGNALS; 2018.

[37] Neurorehabilitation using the Portable Neuromodulation Stimulator (PoNS (R)) for treating patients with chronic balance deficit due to mild-to-moderate traumatic brain injury (mTBI): A 26-week study. In: Tyler M, Skinner K, Prabhakaran V, editors. Brain injury. Milton Park, Abingdon or14 4rn, Oxon: Taylor and Francis Ltd 2-4 Park Square; 2019.

[38] Little S, Pogosyan A, Neal S, Zavala B, Zrinzo L, Hariz M, et al. Adaptive deep brain stimulation in advanced Parkinson disease. Ann Neurol 2013;74(3):449–57.

[39] Winston GM, Guadix S, Lavieri MT, Uribe-Cardenas R, Kocharian G, Williams N, et al. Closed-loop vagal nerve stimulation for intractable epilepsy: A single-center experience. Seizure 2021;88:95–101.

[40] Magis D, Allena M, Bolla M, De Pasqua V, Remacle JM, Schoenen J. Occipital nerve stimulation for drug-resistant chronic cluster headache: A prospective pilot study. Lancet Neurol 2007;6(4):314–21.

[41] Wilbrink LA, de Coo IF, Doesborg PGG, Mulleners WM, Teernstra OPM, Bartels EC, et al. Safety and efficacy of occipital nerve stimulation for attack prevention in medically intractable chronic cluster headache (ICON): A randomised, double-blind, multicentre, phase 3, electrical dose-controlled trial. Lancet Neurol 2021;20(7):515–25.

[42] Strohl MP, Yamauchi M, Peng Z, Strohl KP. Insights since FDA approval of hypoglossal nerve stimulation for the treatment of obstructive sleep apnea. Curr Sleep Med Rep 2017;3:133–41.

[43] Strollo Jr PJ, Soose RJ, Maurer JT, de Vries N, Cornelius J, Froymovich O, et al. Upper-airway stimulation for obstructive sleep apnea. N Engl J Med 2014;370(2):139–49.

[44] Kent D, Huyett P, Yu P, Roy A, Mehra R, Rundo JV, et al. Comparison of clinical pathways for hypoglossal nerve stimulation management: In-laboratory titration polysomnography vs home-based efficacy sleep testing. J Clin Sleep Med 2023;19(11):1905–12.

[45] Lozano AM, Lipsman N, Bergman H, Brown P, Chabardes S, Chang JW, et al. Deep brain stimulation: current challenges and future directions. Nat Rev Neurol 2019;15(3):148–60.

[46] Furlanetti L, Ellenbogen J, Gimeno H, Ainaga L, Narbad V, Hasegawa H, et al. Targeting accuracy of robot-assisted deep brain stimulation surgery in childhood-onset dystonia: A single-center prospective cohort analysis of 45 consecutive cases. J Neurosurg Pediatr 2021;27(6):677–87.

[47] De Ridder D, Maciaczyk J, Vanneste S. The future of neuromodulation: Smart neuromodulation. Expet Rev Med Dev 2021;18(4):307–17.

[48] Utter AA, Basso MA. The basal ganglia: An overview of circuits and function. Neurosci Biobehav Rev 2008;32(3):333–42.

[49] Deuschl G, Schade-Brittinger C, Krack P, Volkmann J, Schäfer H, Bötzel K, et al. A randomized trial of deep-brain stimulation for Parkinson's disease. N Engl J Med 2006;355(9):896–908.

[50] Vidailhet M, Vercueil L, Houeto JL, Krystkowiak P, Benabid AL, Cornu P, et al. Bilateral deep-brain stimulation of the globus pallidus in primary generalized dystonia. N Engl J Med 2005;352(5):459–67.

[51] Ostrem JL, Starr PA. Treatment of dystonia with deep brain stimulation. Neurotherapeutics 2008;5(2):320–30.

[52] Anderson VC, Burchiel KJ, Hogarth P, Favre J, Hammerstad JP. Pallidal vs subthalamic nucleus deep brain stimulation in Parkinson disease. Arch Neurol 2005;62(4):554–60.

[53] Klein JC, Barbe MT, Seifried C, Baudrexel S, Runge M, Maarouf M, et al. The tremor network targeted by successful VIM deep brain stimulation in humans. Neurology 2012;78(11):787–95.

[54] Vaillancourt DE, Sturman MM, Verhagen Metman L, Bakay RA, Corcos DM. Deep brain stimulation of the VIM thalamic nucleus modifies several features of essential tremor. Neurology 2003;61(7):919–25.

[55] Kumar K, Kelly M, Toth C. Deep brain stimulation of the ventral intermediate nucleus of the thalamus for control of tremors in Parkinson's disease and essential tremor. Stereotact Funct Neurosurg 1999;72(1):47–61.

[56] Yu H, Neimat JS. The treatment of movement disorders by deep brain stimulation. Neurotherapeutics 2008;5(1):26–36.

[57] Chandra V, Hilliard JD, Foote KD. Deep brain stimulation for the treatment of tremor. J Neurol Sci 2022;435:120190.

[58] Loyd DR, Murphy AZ. The role of the periaqueductal gray in the modulation of pain in males and females: Are the anatomy and physiology really that different? Neural Plast 2009;2009:462879.

[59] Hosobuchi Y, Adams JE, Linchitz R. Pain relief by electrical stimulation of the central gray matter in humans and its reversal by naloxone. Science 1977;197(4299):183–6.

[60] Bittar RG, Kar-Purkayastha I, Owen SL, Bear RE, Green A, Wang S, et al. Deep brain stimulation for pain relief: A meta-analysis. J Clin Neurosci 2005;12(5):515–9.

[61] Studtmann C, Ladislav M, Safari M, Khondaker R, Chen Y, Vaughan GA, et al. Ventral posterolateral and ventral posteromedial thalamocortical neurons have distinct physiological properties. J Neurophysiol 2023;130(6):1492–507.

[62] Levy RM, Deer TR, Henderson J. Intracranial neurostimulation for pain control: A review. Pain Physician 2010;13(2):157.

[63] Rasche D, Rinaldi PC, Young RF, Tronnier VM. Deep brain stimulation for the treatment of various chronic pain syndromes. Neurosurg Focus 2006;21(6):1–8.

[64] Nowacki A, Zhang DY, Sarica C, Elias GJ, Bajaj S, Franzini A, et al. Thalamic deep brain stimulation for central poststroke pain syndrome: An international multicenter study. J Neurosurg 2025;1(aop):1–12.

[65] Boccard SGJ, Prangnell SJ, Pycroft L, Cheeran B, Moir L, Pereira EAC, et al. Long-term results of deep brain stimulation of the anterior cingulate cortex for neuropathic pain. World Neurosurg 2017;106:625–37.

[66] Leone M, Franzini A, Cecchini AP, Broggi G, Bussone G. Hypothalamic deep brain stimulation in the treatment of chronic cluster headache. Ther Adv Neurol Disord 2010;3(3):187–95.

[67] Franzini A, Messina G, Cordella R, Marras C, Broggi G. Deep brain stimulation of the posteromedial hypothalamus: Indications, long-term results, and neurophysiological considerations. Neurosurg Focus 2010;29(2):E13.

[68] Kenny BJ, Bordoni B. Neuroanatomy, cranial nerve 10 (vagus nerve). StatPearls. Treasure Island (FL): StatPearls Publishing LLC.; 2025.

[69] Groves DA, Brown VJ. Vagal nerve stimulation: a review of its applications and potential mechanisms that mediate its clinical effects. Neurosci Biobehav Rev 2005;29(3):493–500.

[70] Freddi TAL, Ottaiano AC, Lucio LL, Corrêa DG, Hygino da Cruz Jr LC. The trigeminal nerve: Anatomy and pathology. Semin Ultrasound CT MR 2022;43(5):403–13.

[71] Chiluwal A, Narayan RK, Chaung W, Mehan N, Wang P, Bouton CE, et al. Neuroprotective effects of trigeminal nerve stimulation in severe traumatic brain injury. Sci Rep 2017;7(1):6792.

[72] Goadsby PJ, Knight YE, Hoskin KL. Stimulation of the greater occipital nerve increases metabolic activity in the trigeminal nucleus caudalis and cervical dorsal horn of the cat. Pain 1997;73(1):23–8.

[73] Weiner RL, Reed KL. Peripheral neurostimulation for control of intractable occipital neuralgia. Neuromodulation 1999;2(3):217–21.

[74] Kramer DR, Halpern CH, Buonacore DL, McGill KR, Hurtig HI, Jaggi JL, et al. Best surgical practices: A stepwise approach to the university of Pennsylvania deep brain stimulation protocol. Neurosurg Focus 2010;29(2):E3.

[75] Kinfe TM, Vesper J. The impact of multichannel microelectrode recording (MER) in deep brain stimulation of the basal ganglia. Acta Neurochir Suppl 2013;117:27–33.

[76] Willems YR, van der Gaag NA, Kho KH, Tveiten ØV, Krüger MT, Jakobs M. Choice of implantable pulse generators for deep brain stimulation: An overview of clinical practice. Stereotact Funct Neurosurg 2023;101(2):135–45.

[77] Bina RW, Palsma RS, Weinand ME, Kasoff WS. Peripheral nerve stimulation for refractory trigeminal pain: recent single-institution case series with long-term follow-up and review of the literature. Neuromodulation 2020;23(6):796–804.

[78] Giordano F, Zicca A, Barba C, Guerrini R, Genitori L. Vagus nerve stimulation: Surgical technique of implantation and revision and related morbidity. Epilepsia 2017;58(Suppl. 1):85–90.

[79] Dallapiazza RF, De Vloo P, Fomenko A, Lee DJ, Hamani C, Munhoz RP, et al. Considerations for patient and target selection in deep brain stimulation surgery for Parkinson's disease. Exon Publications; 2018. p. 145–60.

[80] DeGiorgio CM, Soss J, Cook IA, Markovic D, Gornbein J, Murray D, et al. Randomized controlled trial of trigeminal nerve stimulation for drug-resistant epilepsy. Neurology 2013;80(9):786–91.

[81] Gelineau-Morel R, Kruer MC, Garris JF, Abu Libdeh A, Barbosa DAN, Coffman KA, et al. Deep brain stimulation for pediatric dystonia: A review of the literature and suggested programming algorithm. J Child Neurol 2022;37(10–11):813–24.

[82] Jain P, Arya R. Vagus nerve stimulation and seizure outcomes in pediatric refractory epilepsy: Systematic review and meta-analysis. Neurology 2021;96(22):1041–51.

[83] Block CK, Patel M, Risk BB, Staikova E, Loring D, Esper CD, et al. Patients with cognitive impairment in Parkinson's disease benefit from deep brain stimulation: A case-control study. Mov Disord Clin Pract 2023;10(3):382–91.

[84] Fleury V, Vingerhoets F, Horvath J, Pollak P, Burkhard P. Deep brain stimulation for movement disorders: Indications, results and complications. Rev Med Suisse 2015;11(472):4–7. 962.

[85] Shlobin NA, Graffeo CS, Dornbos DL, Mukherjee D, Sivakumar W, Johnson J. The Committee on advanced subspecialty training-accredited postgraduate neurosurgery fellowship application experience: A national survey. J Neurosurg 2023;138(4):1124–31.

[86] Parmar VK, Gee L, Smith H, Pilitsis JG. Supraspinal stimulation for treatment of refractory pain. Clin Neurol Neurosurg 2014;123:155–63.

[87] Falowski S, Cher- Ooi Y, Smith A, Verhargen L, Bakay R. An evaluation of hardware and surgical complications with deep brain stimulation based on diagnosis and lead location. Stereotact Funct Neurosurg 2012;90(3):173–80. https://doi.org/10.1159/000338254. Epub 2012 Jun 5. PMID: 22678355.

[88] Thakur V, Kessler B, Khan MB, Hodge JO, Brandmeir NJ. Outpatient deep brain stimulation surgery is a safe alternative to inpatient admission. Oper Neurosurg 2023;25(1):66–71. https://doi.org/10.1227/ons.0000000000000683.

[89] Chan HY, Wijnen BFM, Majoie M, Evers S, Hiligsmann M. Economic evaluation of deep brain stimulation compared with vagus nerve stimulation and usual care for patients with refractory epilepsy: A lifetime decision analytic model. Epilepsia 2022;63(3):641–51. https://doi.org/10.1111/epi.17158.

[90] Dams J, Siebert U, Bornschein B, Volkmann J, Deuschl G, Oertel WH, Dodel R, Reese JP. Cost-effectiveness of deep brain stimulation in patients with Parkinson's disease. Mov Disord 2013;28(6):763–71. https://doi.org/10.1002/mds.25407.

[91] Honey CR, Ranjan M. Deep brain stimulation for Parkinson's disease—A review. Eur Neurol Rev 2012;08:12.

[92] Najera RA, Kabotyanski KE, McLaughlin NC, Gregory ST, Anand A, Shofty B, Provenza NR, Storch EA, Goodman WK, Sheth SA. Cost-effectiveness analysis of deep brain stimulation versus treatment as usual for treatment-resistant obsessive-compulsive disorder. J Neurosurg 2025:1–10. https://doi.org/10.3171/2024.7.JNS232642.

[93] Ngan Kee N, Foster E, Marquina C, Tan A, Pang SST, O'Brien TJ, Kwan P, Jackson GD, Chen Z, Ademi Z. Systematic review of cost-effectiveness analysis for surgical and neurostimulation treatments for drug-resistant epilepsy in adults. Neurology 2023;100(18):e1866–77. https://doi.org/10.1212/WNL.0000000000207137.

[94] Larson PS. Deep brain stimulation for movement disorders. Neurotherapeutics 2014;11(3):465–74. https://doi.org/10.1007/s13311-014-0274-1.
[95] Greenberg BD, Gabriels LA, Malone Jr DA, Rezai AR, Friehs GM, Okun MS, Shapira NA, Foote KD, Cosyns PR, Kubu CS, Malloy PF, Salloway SP, Giftakis JE, Rise MT, Machado AG, Baker KB, Stypulkowski PH, Goodman WK, Rasmussen SA, Nuttin BJ. Deep brain stimulation of the ventral internal capsule/ventral striatum for obsessive-compulsive disorder: Worldwide experience. Mol Psychiatry 2010;15(1):64–79. https://doi.org/10.1038/mp.2008.55.
[96] Ranjan M, Mahoney 3rd JJ, Rezai AR. Neurosurgical neuromodulation therapy for psychiatric disorders. Neurotherapeutics 2024;21(3):e00366. https://doi.org/10.1016/j.neurot.2024.e00366.
[97] Toffa DH, Touma L, El Meskine T, Bouthillier A, Nguyen DK. Learnings from 30 years of reported efficacy and safety of vagus nerve stimulation (VNS) for epilepsy treatment: A critical review. Seizure 2020;83:104–23. https://doi.org/10.1016/j.seizure.2020.09.027.
[98] Nair DR, Laxer KD, Weber PB, Murro AM, Park YD, Barkley GL, Smith BJ, Gwinn RP, Doherty MJ, Noe KH, Zimmerman RS, Bergey GK, Anderson WS, Heck C, Liu CY, Lee RW, Sadler T, Duckrow RB, Hirsch LJ, Study RNSSL. Nine-year prospective efficacy and safety of brain-responsive neurostimulation for focal epilepsy. Neurology 2020;95(9):e1244–56. https://doi.org/10.1212/WNL.0000000000010154.
[99] Cheyuo C, Vetkas A, Sarica C, Kalia SK, Hodaie M, Lozano AM. Comprehensive characterization of intracranial hemorrhage in deep brain stimulation: A systematic review of literature from 1987 to 2023. J Neurosurg 2024;141(2):381–93. https://doi.org/10.3171/2024.1.JNS232385.
[100] Rasiah NP, Maheshwary R, Kwon CS, Bloomstein JD, Girgis F. Complications of deep brain stimulation for Parkinson disease and relationship between micro-electrode tracks and hemorrhage: Systematic review and meta-analysis. World Neurosurg 2023;171:e8–23. https://doi.org/10.1016/j.wneu.2022.10.034.
[101] Falowski SM, Ooi YC, Bakay RA. Long-term evaluation of changes in operative technique and hardware-related complications with deep brain stimulation. Neuromodulation 2015;18(8):670–7. https://doi.org/10.1111/ner.12335.

Section 11

External brain devices

Introduction to section 11 external brain devices

Konstantin V. Slavin[1, 2]

[1]*Department of Neurosurgery, University of Illinois at Chicago, Chicago, IL, United States;* [2]*Neurology Section, Jesse Brown Veterans Administration Medical Center, Chicago, IL, United States*

In the universe of neuromodulation, the modalities are divided based on the underlying principle (electrical, chemical, acoustic, thermal, etc.), targeted substrates (central, including the brain and spinal cord, or peripheral, such as the nerve roots, ganglia, plexuses, and nerves), and, perhaps, most notably, the degree of invasiveness, as neuromodulation can be delivered via fully implantable devices (that have an internal power supply), implanted but externally powered ones (when the system has an implanted receiver while the power source is outside the body), partially implanted systems (when an implanted electrode, waveguide, or a catheter is connected to an external device), or fully external contraptions.

Obviously, there are pros and cons for each of these approaches, and those have to do not only with clinical efficacy and procedural safety, but also with patients' convenience, the ability to reach the desired target, and, to a large extent, the reproducibility and consistency of the clinical effects. And while the fully implanted or partially implanted devices tend to be associated with lower power consumption, the proximity of the device to the intended target, achieved by surgical implantation, is inevitably linked to the inherent risks of implantation.

This situation, understandably, makes external devices much more attractive to the treatment recipients. When given a choice, most patients would prefer less invasive options, and therefore, at least in our surgical practice, trying an approach that delivers treatment without a need of an implant is considered a desired recommendation, if not a requisite for proceeding with an implanted device.

There are many examples of external brain neuromodulation devices. Most of them are based on electrical or magnetic stimulation while others use infrared light or ultrasonic energy, and by reaching the specific part of the brain, be that the more superficial cortical targets or the deeper subcortical structures, such as white matter tracts or the thalamus/basal ganglia, external brain neuromodulation has been successfully used to treat psychiatric conditions, chronic pain, movement disorders, poststroke paralysis, and other illnesses.

Even more external neuromodulation targets are located in the periphery, starting from the trigeminal branches in one's forehead or vagus nerves in the earlobe and all the way to the peripheral nerves in the wrists and ankles. Here, the devices may be considered "wearables"—a household name that includes smart watches and oxygenation monitors—making them even more acceptable for millions of potential users.

The important aspect that makes this technology more relevant for the neuromodulation practitioners that specialize in implanting neuromodulation devices is that the external neuromodulation devices may serve not only as an alternative to the more familiar implanted technology, but also as an initial step in the treatment algorithm or even as a screening tool for subsequent surgically placed systems. Therefore, the awareness of noninvasive neuromodulation options and understanding their roles in the development of individually tailored treatment plans is essential for everyone who offers neuromodulatory treatments to their patients.

Chapter 40

External devices for pain and depression

Matthew Slitzky[1], Christopher L. Robinson[2] and Michael E. Schatman[3,4]

[1]*Burke Rehabilitation Hospital, Montefiore Health System, White Plains, NY, United States;* [2]*Department of Anesthesiology, Perioperative & Pain Medicine, Harvard Medical School, Brigham & Women's Hospital, Boston, MA, United States;* [3]*Department of Anesthesiology, Perioperative Care, and Pain Medicine, NYU Grossman School of Medicine, New York, NY, United States;* [4]*Department of Population Health-Division of Medical Ethics, NYU Grossman School of Medicine, New York, NY, United States*

Introduction

For the treatment of pain and depression, a multidisciplinary and multimodal approach is a necessary, useful strategy to help those suffering with these comorbid conditions [1]. Among such treatments that can be employed are external devices, which are utilized to reduce pain and may improve mood. Use of such extrinsic physical modalities dates back as far as 3500 B C E. For example, the Edwin Smith Papyrus made countless references to cold-water immersion as a practice to treat myriad conditions, including pain, and ancient Greeks similarly used cold-water as a therapy to improve mood [2]. Since antiquity, innovation and technology have provided practitioners with an expansive toolkit of external devices that are used today as primary and adjuvant treatments for pain and depression. This chapter will explore said devices.

External noninvasive peripheral nerve stimulation

External noninvasive peripheral nerve stimulation is a noninvasive form of neuromodulation that localizes and targets specific peripheral nerves in the treatment of pain and chronic pain syndromes [3]. Neuromodulation can be defined as the process by which central, peripheral, or autonomic neural activity and information processing are altered [4,5]. This is often accomplished via electrical means that result in the release of neurotransmitters, neuropeptides, or other signaling molecules to accomplish this change [4,5]. Currently, neuromodulation is used for the treatment of many diseases, including movement disorders, epilepsy, psychiatric disorders such as depression, anxiety, and obsessive-compulsive disorder, and chronic pain [5]. Modern neuromodulation began in the early 1950s and 1960s, with reports of deep brain stimulation and spinal cord stimulators being used for intractable pain [4]. Melzack and Wall's gate control theory of pain in 1965 was supremely influential and sparked major evolution in neuromodulation, which helped lead to major advancements, such as spinal cord stimulators [4]. Subsequently, neuromodulation technologies have progressively demonstrated their ability to alleviate symptoms of many different neurological disorders, particularly those that involve refractory pain [4]. However, spinal cord stimulators, dorsal root ganglion stimulators, and classic peripheral nerve stimulators are internal, as opposed to external noninvasive devices that are completely external while providing electrical current via a nerve-mapping probe that is placed on the skin and connected to a power source [6]. This electrical current is applied to the peripheral nerves to treat pain via preferential activation of myelinated fibers [6]. This preferential activation induces long-term depression of synaptic efficacy, leading to a decrease in pain [6]. Currently, external noninvasive peripheral nerve stimulation is being studied and used for conditions similar to classic neuromodulatory devices, those being neuropathic pain (ICD-10 M79.2), complex regional pain syndrome (ICD-10 G90), and pain secondary to peripheral nerve injury (ICD-10 S14.4XXA, S24.4XXA, S13.4XXA) [6]. When examining the effect of these devices for these conditions, studies have suggest that they provide significant short-term pain relief, with some patients also exhibiting improvements in quality of life and function [6]. In a study examining long-term outcomes, it was revealed that a majority of participants had a greater than 50% reduction in pain, a duration of beneficial treatments lasting more than 12 h, and had improvement in their daily function, as well as decreased pain medication use. Impressively, all participants

A Modern Atlas for Implantable Devices of the Spine, Brain, and Nerve. https://doi.org/10.1016/B978-0-443-36528-7.00051-0

enrolled in this study reported a reduction in frequency of pain flare-ups during device use [7]. Pitfalls involved in this treatment modality include the need for accurate determination of the nerve needing to be stimulated to treat the participants' pain, as well as skin irritation, which may be expected in persons who have a sensitivity to aqueous gel or electrode pads [8]. While generally being well tolerated, contraindications of this modality are not well outlined and may include implanted devices active skin infections and implanted electronic devices proximal to stimulations sites. Additional contraindications may include areas of the body in which a participant has poor sensation, and pregnancy due to potential risks to the infant [7]. External noninvasive peripheral nerve stimulation is a promising tool for pain management that offers significant benefits in select patient populations, although further research is needed to refine its applications, understand its efficacy, and establish its role relative to other neuromodulation techniques.

Transcutaneous electrical nerve stimulation

Use of electrical currents to treat pain has a long and storied history dating to approximately 60 AD, when Roman physician Scribonius Largus proposed using an "electric fish" for pain management [9]. From this principal, transcutaneous electrical nerve stimulation (TENS) emerged as an external device that delivers electrical stimuli activating large diameter afferent fibers which activates descending inhibitory systems, resulting in a reduction in pain [10]. As blockage of neuronal activity in the periaqueductal gray, rostral ventromedial medulla, and spinal cord can inhibit analgesic effects, meaning TENS provides part of its analgesia by acting through these pathways [10]. In addition, studies of individuals with fibromyalgia have demonstrated that TENS can restore central pain modulation, which is a measure of central inhibition [10]. Therefore, TENS potentially results in a reduction in pain via both peripheral and central mechanisms [10].

TENs units are widely used today, in part, because in most countries, TENS equipment and support accessories are available without prescription, the costs and follow-up clinical support for TENS are inexpensive, treatment can be self-administered without concern for any type of toxicities, and it has the potential to offer symptomatic relief of pain throughout the day [11]. The appeal of TENS units is further bolstered by their mechanism of analgesia allowing their indication in the aid of the treatment of numerous ailments such as acute postoperative pain (ICD-10 G89.18), acute nonpostoperative pain (ICD-10 G89.1), low back pain (ICD-10 M54.5), osteoarthritis pain (ICD-10 M19.0), diabetic peripheral neuropathy (ICD-10 E13.40), fibromyalgia (ICD-10 M79.7), and neuropathic pain (ICD-10 M79.2) from conditions such as spinal cord injury [9].

There are three distinct modes of TENS currently employed to treat pain syndromes [9]. Intense TENS functions as a "counterirritant." This form of TENS focuses in on small-diameter, high-threshold cutaneous afferents (A-δ), deploying high frequencies and intensities for brief intervals [12]. Acupuncture-like TENS (AL-TENS) is more oriented tor hyperstimulation and is at times employed for patients unresponsive to conventional TENS [9]. It uses titration to low frequency, higher intensity, and extended pulse width, targeting small-diameter, high-threshold peripheral afferents (A-δ) [9]. Lastly, conventional TENS utilizes a high-frequency, low-intensity, and short pulse duration approach to selectively stimulate large-diameter, low-threshold, nonnoxious afferents (A-β) [9]. This form of TENs has a niche in treating dermatomal pain distributions [9].

Regardless of the form of TENS being used for treatment, three important factors come into play for determining TENS' efficacy: tolerance to repeated TENS, intensity of the stimulation, and electrode placement [10]. When TENS is repeatedly applied, it can result in analgesic tolerance, thus reducing treatment effects. However, this can be mitigated by modulation of TENS parameters, such as pulse frequency and pulse intensity [10]. Proper intensity is the second crucial pillar, as research has outlined the importance of proper intensity to ensure effective treatment, with inadequate intensities representing one of the primary factors attributed to conflicting reports of TENS efficacy [10]. Lastly, electrode site placement is critical, as application of TENS at the proper acupoints reduces nociception more effectively than when applied over nonacupoint sites when experimentally measuring pain and pain thresholds to heat and pressure in normal subjects well as in patient populations [10].

TENS is used to treat a wide range of conditions, with the literature supporting its effectiveness for various pain syndromes. For example, while studies have consistently demonstrated significant pain reductions, as high as 36% in postoperative pain, it is less clear for other conditions [10]. Systematic reviews and meta-analyses have yielded conflicting results for the efficacy of TENS for low back pain, varying from not recommended, inconclusive, and effective for providing analgesia [10]. Aside from treating the pain conditions discussed, TENS has also demonstrated efficacy in the treatment of depression in those with fibromyalgia and older adults with mild cognitive impairment [13,14]. For example, one study performed on institutionalized elderly adults determined that 6 weeks of TENs applied for 30 min daily 5 times a week resulted in a significant decrease in Beck Depression Inventory scores [15]. A clear positive impact on depression is unfortunately not evidenced in all populations, as a systematic review examining the impact of TENs on depression in participants with chronic low back pain identified little to no difference in benefits between TENs and TENs with-medication versus the same medication alone [16].

Although TENS therapy is commonly used, it is important to remember that certain pitfalls and contraindications exist. First and foremost, TENS functions as a treatment and not a cure and should therefore only be offered as a tool for symptomatic pain relief [9]. In operating these devices, it is crucial to read the manufacturer's instruction booklet, as each brand or unit might have slight differences in recommendations [10]. Treatment sessions occur at the patient's convenience. However, they should not occur during the operation of heavy machinery, driving, bathing, showering, or swimming [10]. TENS units should also be powered off prior to applying the pads. Also, due to potential complications, individuals with pacemakers, epilepsy, or pregnant persons in labor are generally advised against TENS use [10]. Theoretical risks extend to transdermal drug delivery systems and dermatologic concerns, as well, urging a cautious approach [10]. In some patients, side effects such as nausea and presyncope can occur, and although participants as young as 4 years of age can tolerate TENS, those with cognitive impairment may not be able to comprehend instructions [17]. These devices may be used while a person is sleeping, although this is provided that the device has a timer, allowing it to automatically switch off [17].

Biofeedback

Biofeedback instruments are external devices that can be employed to treat pain and depression. They measure physiological activity such as brainwaves, heart function, breathing, muscle activity, and skin temperature, and in real time accurately provide feedback and information to the user [18]. This can be described as operant conditioning of physiological activity, whereby the users learn to self-regulate their own physiological processes with the help of the feedback provided by the device. There are various aims that biofeedback can target, such as developing a greater sense of awareness or control of physiological processes and thus consciously reducing muscle tension [18].

Based on the parameters being measured, biofeedback can be divided into two major groups: biomechanical and physiologic [19]. Biomechanical techniques assess body activity and movement using either basic inertial sensors or advanced video motion sensors. Several modalities are used to measure physiological activity [19]. One of the most common is muscle activity, which is assessed through electromyography [19]. Other methods include monitoring cardiac activity via heart rate and heart rate variability, measuring breathing activity through respiratory rate and depth, and evaluating electrodermal activity using skin conductance [19].

Biofeedback devices are commonly used tools showcased by a recent in—person survey of health— and illness-related experiences. The study revealed that in the United States alone, approximately 38% of adults and 12% of children are using some form of a biofeedback device for general healthcare and wellness or in the treatment of a pathology [20]. Although initially introduced into physical therapy more than 50 years ago as an effective management technique for neuromuscular disorders, biofeedback is used to treat numerous disorders today [19]. These disorders include, but are not limited to, pain conditions, such as chronic pain (ICD-10 G89.2) and headache (ICD-10 R51.9), as well as other conditions including depressive disorders (ICD-10 F32.0), posttraumatic stress disorder (ICD-10 F43.1), and fibromyalgia (ICD-10 M79.7) [20].

Biofeedback can be useful in the treatment of these disorders as a stand-alone, alternative, or an adjunctive therapy and can be particularly useful for individuals who are intolerant of medication or for whom pharmacological treatment may be contraindicated [20]. While the efficacy of biofeedback is inconsistent among the plethora of conditions it is used to treat, studies have consistently demonstrated that biofeedback treatment can lead to improvements in various pain-related outcomes, both in the short and long terms [21]. A metaanalysis revealed a significant small-to-medium effect size for pain intensity reduction when using biofeedback devices that appeared to be stable with a significant small-to-large effect size over an average follow-up phase of 8 months [21]. Similar positive results have been evidenced in relation to mood, revealing a moderate positive effect size in reducing depression (Hedges' $g = 0.40$), as well as improving cognitive coping skills (Hedges' $g = 0.57$) [21]. In controlled studies, these effects remained stable at follow-up, and moderator analyses have suggested that a greater proportion of biofeedback in treatment to be more effective for reducing depression [21].

A recent innovation in biofeedback is the use of virtual reality (VR) to provide cues that are multimodal, so that perceptive and cognitive functions are involved in the treatment motivating the participant to remain attentive and engaged. This approach is simple and easy to understand and helps avoid overloading the patient with information [22]. Biofeedback delivered via VR is already beginning to yield promising results, demonstrating a reduction in both pain and anxiety in participants with musculoskeletal disorders such as rheumatoid arthritis, systemic lupus erythematosus, osteoarthritis, and fibromyalgia [23].

Although biofeedback can be an efficacious tool for treating myriad conditions, including pain and depression, there are pitfalls to consider [19]. Successful biofeedback training requires a significant amount of motivation and participation by the participant [19]. Furthermore, the individual must be able to communicate and comprehend and follow through with the treatment's instructions. Certain biofeedback modalities are more beneficial for certain diseases than others [19]. For example, electromyographic biofeedback is more commonly used for musculoskeletal conditions, while real-time ultrasound biofeedback is more often applied for pelvic floor dysfunction [19]. In the treatment of headaches, blood volume pulse feedback has been demonstrated to have the strongest evidence for reducing headache severity and frequency [19]. Biofeedback does not have any absolute contraindications and therefore may be used for any age population. It has generally been accepted as a safe treatment [19].

However, as previously discussed, the participant must be able to play an active participatory role, so it may not be an apt treatment if the patient cannot comprehend and follow commands [19]. It is also not appropriate in cases of complete paralysis [19]. Biofeedback should not be used as the sole treatment for severe hypertension, given the risks associated with the condition, and the cases of acute psychiatric patients should be considered with caution [19].

Interferential current therapy

Interferential current therapy devices are simple, noninvasive external treatments used in clinical practice for pain management [24]. This therapy uses medium-frequency alternating currents with the intention to deliver currents to deeper tissues [24]. Developed by Dr Hans Nemec in the early 1950s in Vienna, the aim of crossing two medium-frequency alternating currents was to utilize the concept that the skin offers little ohmic resistance to the passage of medium frequencies, unlike direct currents and low frequencies, which encounter very high ohmic resistance [24]. To illustrate with an example, one of the alternating currents may be a fixed frequency at 4000 Hz, while the other frequency alternating current could be set between 4000 and 4250 Hz [24]. These two medium-frequency currents cause interference within the tissues and produce an amplitude-modulated low beat frequency, which is the difference between the values of the two currents applied [24]. This interference results in analgesia via multiple proposed mechanisms. The first mechanism is the previously described gate control theory of pain, regarding which it has been suggested that an interferential current frequency of 100 Hz can activate the large-diameter, low-threshold nerve fibers, thus inhibiting signals from pain signal carrying nerve fibers [24]. This modality also takes advantage of physiological blockage, also known as Wedensky inhibition, whereby C and Aδ fibers may not conduct nociceptive impulses following frequency stimuli greater than approximately 15 and 40 Hz, respectively [24]. Finally, similar to TENS, it has been proposed to take advantage of the descending pain suppression pathway involving endogenous opioids released from periaqueductal gray matter and the rostral ventral medulla, which serve an important function in the control of nociceptive messages from primary afferent nerves [24].

When utilizing these devices, there are many potential parameters. Each has a wide variety of options that can be adjusted or altered, including the carrier frequency, amplitude-modulated frequency, sweep frequency, sweep mode or swing pattern, application type (bipolar or quadripolar application) as well as application time and intensity [24]. Most therapists and users of interferential current therapy devices select their settings via trial and error, and given the wide variety of parameters, it is reasonable to assume that certain programs may be more effective for treating a particular cause of pain than others [24]. Currently, interferential current therapy devices are being used in the treatment of a multitude of pain conditions with significant benefit, including neck pain (ICD-10 M54.2), acute and chronic low back pain (ICD-10 M54.5), knee osteoarthritis (ICD-10 M17.0), and postoperative knee pain (ICD-10 G89.28) [25]. In fact, it has been determined that the majority of interferential current therapy parameters do not seem to affect their analgesic efficacy, with the exception of carrier frequencies of 1 or 4 kHz, which appear to enhance analgesic effects more than higher, more comfortable carrier frequencies [24]. Beyond these pain generating ailments, interferential current therapy has also been demonstrated to be an effective adjunct in the treatment of depression (ICD-10 F33.0) and anxiety (ICD-10 F40.0). This therapy has resulted in significant improvement in these symptoms when interferential current stimulation is performed in addition to exercise, based on Goldberg Depression Scale and Personal Psychological Apprehension Scale scores, when compared to therapeutic exercise alone [26].

Despite the successful implementation of these devices for pain and depression, there are potential pitfalls associated with this modality. As previously discussed, interferential current therapy provides its users with the ability to customize several parameters, and as a result, studies assessing its efficacy used different treatment protocols, which may have resulted in moderate-to-high heterogeneity of some results [27]. More research is required to formulate a standard treatment plan [27]. Therefore, it is important to recognize that certain settings may be more or less beneficial for individual patients depending on their anatomy and the condition aiming to be treated. For safety purposes, stimulation to the head and neck should be avoided for individuals with seizure histories, as well as stimulation to the anterior neck, carotid sinus, eyes, and reproductive organs [28]. Beyond these considerations, contraindications include patients with tumor, fever, acute inflammation, cardiac pacemaker, pregnant individuals, and participants with an aversion to electrical current therapy [13,14,24]. Irrespective, interferential current therapy appears to be an effective tool providing a customizable therapy utilizing alternating current to treat both pain and depression.

Transcranial magnetic stimulation

Repetitive transcranial magnetic stimulation is a treatment modality in which brief magnetic pulses are applied, leading to cortical stimulation [29]. These pulses are generated in an external and noninvasive fashion, as they do not require craniotomy or seizure induction to stimulate nerve cells [29]. Transcranial magnetic stimulation interconverts electrical and magnetic energy to induce electromagnetic phenomena via a coil placed on the scalp, and an effective pulsatile magnetic field depolarizing cortical neurons is generated for a brief period of time [29]. This magnetic field is approximately 1.5 T, roughly equivalent to the strength of magnetic resonance imaging, and the levels of excitability of neuronal stimulation can be regulated either by high or low frequency [29].

From a historical perspective, the current use of electromagnetic induction for transcranial stimulation dates to the United Kingdom in 1985 [30]. At that time, Barker and his associated invented the initial form of transcranial magnetic stimulation [30]. Additionally, Barker empirically demonstrated the influence of magnetic stimulation on the motor cortex of the human brain during the same year [30]. However, the original tools were slow when recharging and repetitive stimulation, a common modality used today, could substantially raise the coil's temperature [30].

Currently, transcranial magnetic stimulation is divided into three subtypes, based on the protocol being utilized, and is being used for both diagnostic and therapeutic applications [31]. Single-pulse transcranial magnetic stimulation occurs via stimulation of the motor cortex and electromyographical monitoring of muscle activation in the contralateral limb [31]. This protocol, along with electromyography, is useful in presurgical planning for corticospinal tract mapping [31]. The paired-pulse protocol is delivered over the motor cortex and is used to measure the cortical excitation to inhibition ratio. Two pulses are delivered consecutively at a fixed interstimulus interval to reveal the regional inhibitory or excitatory signaling strength [31]. Lastly, in the treatment of psychiatric and pain disorders, the repetitive protocol is often used [31]. In this protocol, magnetic pulses are delivered for 5–10 s and turned off for the following 30–60 s due to the risk of seizures and to prevent overheating [31]. Repetitive transcranial magnetic stimulation produces repetitive stimulations that increase synaptic plasticity, causing greater duration of effect, even after stimulation ceases. This stimulation has been demonstrated to produce therapeutic potential in the treatment of obsessive compulsive disorder (ICD10-F42), posttraumatic stress disorder (ICD-10 F43), Tourette disorder (ICD-10 F95.2), treatment-resistant depression (ICD-10 F33.3), chronic pain syndrome (ICD-10 G89.4), bipolar disorder (ICD-10 F31), and movement disorders (ICD-10 G25.8) [29]. When utilizing this modality for pharmacoresistant depression, the left dorsolateral prefrontal cortex is stimulated at a frequency of 10–20 Hz daily for 4–6 weeks [31]. This treatment has been determined to be effective, as a randomized, double-blind, sham-controlled, cross-over study produced a statistically significant decrease in depressive symptoms on the Hamilton Depression Rating Scale. Further, a metaanalysis examining the effect on depression revealed a mean percentage reduction on depression rating scale scores ranging between 25% and 76% [32,33].

Although more recent to the realm of pain management, repetitive transcranial magnetic stimulation is already being used with success in empirical investigations to treat many pain generating syndromes including central poststroke pain, central pain due to spinal cord injury, fibromyalgia, headache, orofacial pain, phantom limb pain, low back pain, myofascial pain syndrome, pelvic pain, and complex regional pain syndrome [3]. Despite being an effective and generally well-tolerated therapy, it is important to be aware of risk of seizure induction, which is typically <0.01% per session, although in epileptic patients, the risk is higher but remains below 3% per session [31]. More benign complications include local pain, primarily headache or neck pain, and transient tinnitus. Hyperacusis may also occur due to the loud clicks during the sessions, making hearing protection essential. These adverse effects are typically short-lived and very mild [31]. Given the known decrease in seizure threshold, repetitive transcranial magnetic stimulation is contraindicated in epilepsy, as well as preexisting neurological disease, in adolescents, during change in medication regimen, and substance use [31]. Metallic/electronic implants or cochlear implants that are in close contact with electrical coils, previous severe head trauma or neurosurgical intervention in the past, an active brain tumor, and intracranial hypertension are absolute contraindications [31,34]. Despite these contraindications, repetitive transcranial magnetic stimulation appears to be an external and noninvasive, evidence-based neuromodulatory therapy with significant potential to aid in the treatment of depression and pain disorders.

Transcutaneous auricular vagus nerve stimulation

Transcutaneous auricular vagus nerve stimulation devices are external and noninvasive forms of classic vagus nerve stimulation used to treat pain and depression [35]. They utilize a surface electrode to apply an electrical stimulus over the skin of the outer ear, which targets afferent fibers of the auricular branch of the nerve [36]. This leads to activation of the ipsilateral nucleus of tractus solitarius through the vagal projections in the brainstem and forebrain, resulting in enhanced autonomic balance and function in various autonomic, neurological, psychiatric, and rheumatologic disorders, among others [35,36]. Classical vagus nerve stimulation began in the late 18th century when Dr James Corning employed its use to decrease cerebral blood flow, which at the time, physicians believed would help control seizures in epileptic patients [37]. The modality was rediscovered in the late 1980s as a potential tool to aid in the treatment of refractory epilepsy [38]. As vagus nerve stimulation requires a surgical procedure, can have side effects, and can be expensive and not readily available, transcutaneous auricular vagus nerve stimulation was developed approximately 20 years ago as a noninvasive, less expensive, and easily applicable alternative [35,38]. There are two subsets for transcutaneous auricular vagus nerve stimulation, motor-activated auricular stimulation, and respiratory-gated nerve stimulation [39]. Motor-activated auricular vagus nerve stimulation pairs transcutaneous auricular vagus nerve stimulation with motor activity, which has been determined to be a potential neurorehabilitation tool and a facilitator of motor learning in neonates [39]. This technique is also being investigated in the use of adult poststroke rehabilitation [39]. Respiratory-gated auricular vagal afferent nerve stimulation is based on the concept that inhalation induces transient inhibition of vagus nerve activity. Currently, this form of vagus nerve stimulation is being investigated and has demonstrated promise in the management of treatment-resistant depression (ICD-10 F33.8) and pain disorders. This modality has been particularly effective in aiding in the management of pain in disorders of the autoimmune system including, rheumatoid arthritis (ICD-10 M06.9), systemic sclerosis (ICD-10 M34.9), systemic lupus erythematosus (ICD-10M32.9), and fibromyalgia (ICD-10 M79.7), as well as other syndromes, such as migraine headache (ICD-10 G43) and osteoarthritis (ICD-10 M19.0) [39–41]. Regarding its effect on depression, studies have demonstrated that transcutaneous auricular vagus nerve stimulation results in a modulatory effect on the brain circuitries that regulate response to negative stress and is associated with significant acute reduction of depression and anxiety, improving baseline mood and invigoration in engagement with everyday tasks [42,43]. A major side effect to consider is potential laryngotracheal dysfunction that is related to the stimulation of the inferior recurrent laryngeal nerve [44]. However, this is less common in transcutaneous nerve stimulation as compared to more classic vagus nerve stimulation modalities [44]. Contraindications include any current or past history of cardiovascular disorders, facial or ear pain, recent ear trauma, and metal implants above the level of the neck [45]. Transcutaneous auricular vagus nerve stimulation provides a promising, noninvasive and external alternative to traditional vagus nerve stimulation, offering potential therapeutic benefits for a range of neurological-, psychiatric-, and pain-related conditions. Its significant potential as an accessible and cost-effective neuromodulation technique should not be understated.

Cranial electrotherapy stimulation

Cranial electrotherapy stimulation is another external and noninvasive neuromodulatory technique used in treating several disorders including pain, insomnia, anxiety, and depression. This modality involves delivering a low-electrical current via a pair of electrodes, which are attached to bilateral anatomical positions around the head, to acutely modulate central and peripheral nervous system activity [46]. While the exact physiological, neurochemical, and metabolic mechanisms underlying its effects are currently unknown, computational modeling suggests that electrical current administered with these devices at the earlobes can reach cortical and subcortical regions at very low intensities associated with subthreshold neuromodulatory effects [46]. Another theory suggests that cranial electrotherapy stimulation modulates brain stem, limbic, and cortical regions and to increase relative parasympathetic to sympathetic drive in the autonomic nervous system [46].

Cranial electrotherapy stimulation evolved from the concept of "electrosleep," which was first investigated in the beginning of the 20th century, with most of the early investigation taking place in Russia [47]. Beginning in the 1960s, the concept of cranial electrotherapy stimulation became of greater interest in the United States as an insomnia treatment powered by the relaxing effect of the current stimulation [47]. Following an initial spark in research interest in the 1970s and early 1980s, published research entered a quiescent phase, but then resumed and accelerated beginning in 2005 [47]. Currently, this tool is being investigated for conditions including anxiety (ICD-10 F41.9), depression (ICD-10 F32.A), headache (ICD-10 R51.9), fibromyalgia (ICD-10 M79.7), complex regional pain syndrome (ICD-10 G90), and chronic pain (ICD-10 G89.2) of the musculoskeletal system [47,48]. Its effect on chronic pain syndromes is well documented, with studies suggesting a significant and durable decrease in chronic pain among participants with an expansive range of pain-related disorders [48,49]. In the treatment of psychiatric disorders, cranial electrotherapy has been determined to be a powerful instrument for reducing anxiety symptoms, with moderate effect size in patients with both primary and secondary anxiety [50]. Its effect on depression has been equally significant, creating significant decreases in depression, as well as in feelings of anger and tension as measured on the Profile of Mood States Scale [51]. Repeated stimulation led to a cumulative effect associated with a decrease of symptoms of depression including somatization, interpersonal sensitivity, obsessive or compulsive thoughts, excessive worry, hostility, fearfulness, alcohol and substance use, and paranoia [52].

When examining the risk profile for this modality, it was virtually negligible, with mild and self-limiting episodes of vertigo, cervicogenic headaches when the current was too high, and skin irritation, which occurred at the electrode site, reported in fewer than 1% of patients [52]. Another crucial aspect to consider is that studies involving cranial electrotherapy stimulation were often using it as an adjunctive therapy to more conventional therapies, which should be taken into account when considering its effectiveness [52]. Similar to the previously discussed devices, contraindications include pregnancy and those with implanted metal medical devices, such as pacemakers [53]. Cranial electrotherapy stimulation appears to be an effective and well-tolerated noninvasive external therapy for pain and psychiatric disorders. As research continues to expand, it may play an increasingly valuable role in integrative treatment approaches.

Conclusion

Noninvasive, external devices including TENS, biofeedback, external noninvasive peripheral nerve stimulation, interferential current therapy, repetitive transcranial magnetic stimulation, transcutaneous auricular vagus nerve stimulation, and cranial electrotherapy stimulations have the potential to become valuable tools in treating pain and depression. Each presents its own unique benefits and operates through diverse mechanisms, such as modulating central and peripheral pathways, stimulating neurochemical release, and altering autonomic function to enhance patient outcomes in pain management and mental health treatment. Crucially these therapies should ultimately provide viable nonpharmacologic and noninvasive treatments that provide substantial benefits. As research into pain and depression management continues to advance, these modalities hold great promise for expanding therapeutic options and improving quality of life.

References

[1] Borys C, Lutz J, Strauss B, Altmann U. Effectiveness of a multimodal therapy for patients with chronic low back pain regarding pre-admission healthcare utilization. PLoS One 2015;10(11):e0143139. https://doi.org/10.1371/JOURNAL.PONE.0143139.

[2] Allan R, Malone J, Alexander J, et al. Cold for centuries: a brief history of cryotherapies to improve health, injury and post-exercise recovery. Eur J Appl Physiol 2022;122(5):1153. https://doi.org/10.1007/S00421-022-04915-5.

[3] Yang S, Chang MC. Effect of repetitive transcranial magnetic stimulation on pain management: a systematic narrative review. Front Neurol 2020;11:114. https://doi.org/10.3389/FNEUR.2020.00114.

[4] Sivanesan E, North RB, Russo MA, et al. A definition of neuromodulation and classification of implantable electrical modulation for chronic pain. Neuromodulation 2024;27(1):1–12. https://doi.org/10.1016/J.NEUROM.2023.10.004. Technology at the Neural Interface.

[5] Anderson RU. Focal neuromuscular therapies for chronic pelvic pain syndromes in women. In: Female Urology: Text with DVD; 2008. p. 905–15. https://doi.org/10.1016/B978-1-4160-2339-5.50140-3.

[6] Johnson S, Ayling H, Sharma M, Goebel A. External noninvasive peripheral nerve stimulation treatment of neuropathic pain: a prospective audit. Neuromodulation 2015;18(5):384–91. https://doi.org/10.1111/NER.12244. Technology at the Neural Interface.

[7] Johnson S, Goebel A. Long-term treatment of chronic neuropathic pain using external noninvasive external peripheral nerve stimulation in five patients. Neuromodulation 2016;19(8):893–6. https://doi.org/10.1111/ner.12365.

[8] Johnson S, Goebel A, Richey R, Holmes E, Hughes D. A randomised, patient-assessor blinded, sham-controlled trial of external non-invasive peripheral nerve stimulation for chronic neuropathic pain following peripheral nerve injury (EN-PENS trial): study protocol for a randomised controlled trial. Trials 2016;17(1):574. https://doi.org/10.1186/S13063-016-1709-2.

[9] Aiyer R, Johnson E, Poli J. Transcutaneous electrical nerve stimulation. In: Anesthesiology In-Training Exam Review: Regional Anesthesia and Chronic Pain; 2024. p. 347–50. https://doi.org/10.1007/978-3-030-87266-3_66.

[10] Vance CGT, Dailey DL, Rakel BA, Sluka KA. Using TENS for pain control: the state of the evidence. Pain Manag 2014;4(3):197. https://doi.org/10.2217/PMT.14.13.

[11] Johnson MI, Paley CA, Jones G, Mulvey MR, Wittkopf PG. Efficacy and safety of transcutaneous electrical nerve stimulation (TENS) for acute and chronic pain in adults: a systematic review and meta-analysis of 381 studies (the meta-TENS study). BMJ Open 2022;12(2):e051073. https://doi.org/10.1136/BMJOPEN-2021-051073.

[12] Liebano RE, Rakel B, Vance CGT, Walsh DM, Sluka KA. An investigation of the development of analgesic tolerance to transcutaneous electrical nerve stimulation (TENS) in humans. Pain 2010;152(2):335. https://doi.org/10.1016/J.PAIN.2010.10.040.

[13] Mark IJ, Leica SC, Peter GH, Gareth J, Carole AP. Transcutaneous electrical nerve stimulation (TENS) for fibromyalgia in adults. Cochrane Database Syst Rev 2017;10(10):250–2. https://doi.org/10.1002/14651858.CD012172.PUB2.

[14] Luijpen MW, Swaab DF, Sergeant JA, Scherder EJA. Effects of transcutaneous electrical nerve stimulation (TENS) on self-efficacy and mood in elderly with mild cognitive impairment. Neurorehabilitation Neural Repair 2004;18(3):166–75. https://doi.org/10.1177/0888439004268785.

[15] Cameron MH, Lonergan E, Lee H. Transcutaneous electrical nerve stimulation (TENS) for dementia. Cochrane Database Syst Rev 2003;2003(3): CD004032. https://doi.org/10.1002/14651858.CD004032.

[16] Verville L, Hincapié CA, Southerst D, et al. Systematic review to inform a World health Organization (WHO) clinical practice guideline: benefits and harms of transcutaneous electrical nerve stimulation (TENS) for chronic primary low back pain in adults. J Occup Rehabil 2023;33(4):651. https://doi.org/10.1007/S10926-023-10121-7.

[17] Johnson PM. Transcutaneous electrical nerve stimulation: mechanisms, clinical application and evidence. Rev Pain 2007;1(1):7. https://doi.org/10.1177/204946370700100103.

[18] Lazaridou A, Paschali M, Vilsmark ES, Edwards RR. Biofeedback EMG alternative therapy for chronic low back pain: study protocol of a pilot randomized controlled trial. Contemp Clin Trials 2022;121. https://doi.org/10.1016/J.CCT.2022.106888.

[19] Van Puyvelde M, Pattyn N. Biofeedback. In: Handbook of Mental Performance: Lessons from High Performance Domains; 2023. p. 169–97. https://doi.org/10.4324/9781003378969-11.

[20] Frank DL, Khorshid L, Kiffer JF, Moravec CS, McKee MG. Biofeedback in medicine: who, when, why and how? Ment Health Fam Med 2010;7(2):85. https://pmc.ncbi.nlm.nih.gov/articles/PMC2939454/. [Accessed 29 January 2025].

[21] Sielski R, Rief W, Glombiewski JA. Efficacy of biofeedback in chronic back pain: a meta-analysis. Int J Behav Med 2017;24(1):25–41. https://doi.org/10.1007/S12529-016-9572-9.

[22] Huang H, Wolf SL, He J. Recent developments in biofeedback for neuromotor rehabilitation. J NeuroEng Rehabil 2006;3(1):11. https://doi.org/10.1186/1743-0003-3-11.

[23] Venuturupalli RS, Chu T, Vicari M, Kumar A, Fortune N, Spielberg B. Virtual reality–based biofeedback and guided meditation in rheumatology: a pilot study. ACR Open Rheumatol 2019;1(10):667. https://doi.org/10.1002/ACR2.11092.

[24] Rampazo ÉP, Liebano RE. Analgesic effects of interferential current therapy: a narrative review. Medicina 2022;58(1):141. https://doi.org/10.3390/MEDICINA58010141.

[25] Almeida CC de, da SVZM, Júnior GC, Liebano RE, Durigan JLQ. Transcutaneous electrical nerve stimulation and interferential current demonstrate similar effects in relieving acute and chronic pain: a systematic review with meta-analysis. Braz J Phys Ther 2018;22(5):347. https://doi.org/10.1016/J.BJPT.2017.12.005.

[26] Albornoz-Cabello M, Pérez-Mármol JM, Barrios Quinta CJ, Matarán-Peñarrocha GA, Castro-Sánchez AM, de la Cruz Olivares B. Effect of adding interferential current stimulation to exercise on outcomes in primary care patients with chronic neck pain: a randomized controlled trial. Clin Rehabil 2019;33(9):1458–67. https://doi.org/10.1177/0269215519844554.

[27] Chen HL, Yang FA, Lee TH, Liou TH, Escorpizo R, Chen HC. Effectiveness of interferential current therapy in patients with knee osteoarthritis: a systematic review and meta-analysis of randomized controlled trials. Sci Rep 2022;12(1):9694. https://doi.org/10.1038/S41598-022-13478-6.

[28] Albornoz-Cabello M, Sanchez-Santos JA, Melero-Suarez R, Heredia-Rizo AM, Espejo-Antunez L. Effects of adding interferential therapy electro-massage to usual care after surgery in subacromial pain syndrome: a randomized clinical trial. J Clin Med 2019;8(2). https://doi.org/10.3390/JCM8020175.

[29] Rizvi S, Khan AM. Use of transcranial magnetic stimulation for depression. Cureus 2019;11(5):e4736. https://doi.org/10.7759/CUREUS.4736.

[30] Noohi S, Amirsalari S. History, studies and specific uses of repetitive transcranial magnetic stimulation (rTMS) in treating epilepsy. Iran J Child Neurol 2016;10(1):1. https://pmc.ncbi.nlm.nih.gov/articles/PMC4815479/. [Accessed 2 February 2025].

[31] Tergau F, Steinhoff BJ. Repetitive transcranial magnetic stimulation. Textbook of Epilepsy Surgery 2023:1208–19. https://doi.org/10.2165/00023210-200317060-00002.

[32] Akpinar K, Kalkan Oğuzhanoğlu N, Toker Uğurlu T. Efficacy of transcranial magnetic stimulation in treatment-resistant depression. Turk J Med Sci 2022;52(4):1344–54. https://doi.org/10.55730/1300-0144.5441.

[33] Sonmez AI, Camsari DD, Nandakumar AL, et al. Accelerated TMS for depression: a systematic review and meta-analysis. Psychiatry Res 2018;273:770. https://doi.org/10.1016/J.PSYCHRES.2018.12.041.

[34] Attal N, Poindessous-Jazat F, De Chauvigny E, et al. Repetitive transcranial magnetic stimulation for neuropathic pain: a randomized multicentre sham-controlled trial. Brain 2021;144(11):3328–39. https://doi.org/10.1093/BRAIN/AWAB208.

[35] Hilz MJ. Transcutaneous vagus nerve stimulation - a brief introduction and overview. Auton Neurosci 2022;243. https://doi.org/10.1016/J.AUTNEU.2022.103038.

[36] Costa V, Gianlorenço AC, Andrade MF, et al. Transcutaneous vagus nerve stimulation effects on chronic pain: systematic review and meta-analysis. Pain Rep 2024;9(5):e1171. https://doi.org/10.1097/PR9.0000000000001171.

[37] Lanska DJJL. Corning and vagal nerve stimulation for seizures in the 1880s. Neurology 2002;58(3):452–9. https://doi.org/10.1212/WNL.58.3.452.

[38] Badran BW, Austelle CW. The future is noninvasive: a brief review of the evolution and clinical utility of vagus nerve stimulation. Focus 2022;20(1):3. https://doi.org/10.1176/APPI.FOCUS.20210023. Journal of Life Long Learning in Psychiatry.

[39] Amar AP, Levy ML, Liu CY, Apuzzc MLJ. Vagus nerve stimulator. Proc IEEE 2023;96(7):1142–51. https://doi.org/10.1109/JPROC.2008.922569.

[40] Bellocchi C, Carandina A, Della Torre A, et al. Transcutaneous auricular branch vagal nerve stimulation as a non-invasive add-on therapeutic approach for pain in systemic sclerosis. RMD Open 2023;9(3):e003265. https://doi.org/10.1136/RMDOPEN-2023-003265.

[41] Tavares-Figueiredo I, Pers YM, Duflos C, et al. Effect of transcutaneous auricular vagus nerve stimulation in chronic low back pain: a pilot study. J Clin Med 2024;13(24):7601. https://doi.org/10.3390/JCM13247601/S1.

[42] Garcia RG, Cohen JE, Stanford AD, et al. Respiratory-gated auricular vagal afferent nerve stimulation (RAVANS) modulates brain response to stress in major depression. J Psychiatr Res 2021;142:188–97. https://doi.org/10.1016/J.JPSYCHIRES.2021.07.048.

[43] Ferstl M, Teckentrup V, Lin WM, et al. Non-invasive vagus nerve stimulation boosts mood recovery after effort exertion. Psychol Med 2021;52 (14):3029. https://doi.org/10.1017/S0033291720005073.

[44] Toffa DH, Touma L, El Meskine T, Bouthillier A, Nguyen DK. Learnings from 30 years of reported efficacy and safety of vagus nerve stimulation (VNS) for epilepsy treatment: a critical review. Seizure 2020;83:104–23. https://doi.org/10.1016/J.SEIZURE.2020.09.027.

[45] Badran BW, Yu AB, Adair D, et al. Laboratory administration of transcutaneous auricular vagus nerve stimulation (taVNS): technique, targeting, and considerations. J Vis Exp 2019;2019(143). https://doi.org/10.3791/58984.

[46] Brunyé TT, Patterson JE, Wooten T, Hussey EK. A critical review of cranial electrotherapy stimulation for neuromodulation in clinical and non-clinical samples. Front Hum Neurosci 2021;15:625321. https://doi.org/10.3389/FNHUM.2021.625321.

[47] Shekelle P, Cook I, Miake-Lye IM, Mak S, Booth MS, Shanman R, Beroes JM. The effectiveness and risks of cranial electrical stimulation for the treatment of pain, depression, anxiety, PTSD, and insomnia. Syst Rev 2018. https://pubmed.ncbi.nlm.nih.gov/29630193/. [Accessed 5 February 2025]. PMID 29630193.

[48] Manag JHPP. Cumulative response from cranial electrotherapy stimulation (CES) for chronic pain. HolubecPract Pain Manag 2009;9(9):80–3. https://www.alpha-med.co.il/html5/Web/9415/20.pdf. [Accessed 5 February 2025].

[49] Gabis L, Shklar B, Baruch YK, Raz R, Gabis E, Geva D. Pain reduction using transcranial electrostimulation: a double blind "active placebo" controlled trial. J Rehabil Med 2009;41(4):256–61. https://doi.org/10.2340/16501977-0315.

[50] Ching PY, Hsu TW, Chen GW, Pan CC, Chu CS, Chou PH. Efficacy and tolerability of cranial electrotherapy stimulation in the treatment of anxiety: a systemic review and meta-analysis. Front Psychiatr 2022;13. https://doi.org/10.3389/FPSYT.2022.899040.

[51] Chang WD, Tsou YA, Chen YY, Hung BL. Cranial electrotherapy stimulation to improve the physiology and psychology response, response-ability, and sleep efficiency in athletes with poor sleep quality. Int J Environ Res Publ Health 2022;19(4):1946. https://doi.org/10.3390/IJERPH19041946.

[52] Price L, Briley J, Haltiwanger S, Hitching R. A meta-analysis of cranial electrotherapy stimulation in the treatment of depression. J Psychiatr Res 2021;135:119–34. https://doi.org/10.1016/J.JPSYCHIRES.2020.12.043.

[53] Chu CS, Chang CH, Pan CC, et al. Effect of cranial electrotherapy stimulation as an add-on therapy on late-life generalized anxiety disorder: an open-label study. J Formos Med Assoc 2024;123(7):781–7. https://doi.org/10.1016/J.JFMA.2023.12.002.

Chapter 41

External peripheral nerve devices

Marshall D. Bedder[1], Leonardo Kapural[2, 3] and Michael Flamm[4]

[1]*Wellstar/MCG Department of Psychiatry and Health Behavior, Chief of Pain Medicine, VA Augusta Health System, Addiction Medicine Fellowship Program, Augusta, GA, United States;* [2]*Carolinas Pain Institute, Winston-Salem, NC, United States;* [3]*Atrium Heath, Wake Forest Baptist Pain Center-Premier, Winston Salem, NC, United States;* [4]*Interventional Pain Physician, VA Harbor Health System, Rusk Institute of NYU Langone Health, New York, NY, United States*

Introduction

a. Scope of Procedure
b. Brief Historical Perspective
c. Brief Procedure Innovation
d. Brief Most Relevant Advancements

Traditional Spine surgery has long been moving from conventional open procedures to outpatient minimally invasive spine surgery [1]. The general trends we are seeing in pain medicine is for more minimally invasive pain procedures being utilized even before traditional surgical procedures [2]. The next evolution in true neuromodulation techniques is the application of non-invasive, non-implantable therapies. The two modern magnetically generated waveform technologies discussed in this Textbook both started and were derived from the same device and principles in 1982 by Polson [3]. One evolved into transcranial or repetitive transcranial magnetic stimulation (TMS/rTMS). The other developed later into what today is called magnetic peripheral nerve stimulation (mPNS), to differentiate itself from electrical nerve stimulation. Magnetic Peripheral Nerve Stimulation is FDA-cleared to treat chronic and intractable post-traumatic, post-surgical pain, and chronic painful diabetic neuropathy (PDN) in the lower extremities. Each individual type of device is underpinned by strong science, data and patient experience behind it. They can be administered to patients who are not appropriate candidates for traditional invasive therapies, in the case of mPNS, due to weight restrictions, blood glucose dysregulation or from personal preference for a nonprocedural/surgical approach. mPNS opens the ability to treat pain and especially neuropathic pain without resorting to invasive implantable surgical techniques. Both techniques show remarkably safe patient side effects profiles which will be further elucidated.

Mechanism of action

The waveforms in each therapy differ with repetitive TMS (rTMS) delivered in trains lasting a couple of minutes and is commonly used to suppress neuropsychiatric symptom. The usual protocols use a frequency of 10–20 Hz used daily for 4–6 weeks. In contrast, mPNS uses a patent protected, ultra-low frequency with a biphasic wave with a period of 290 μs delivered over 13.3 min for a total of 400 pulses. The protocol involves a total of six treatments within the first month followed by monthly maintenance treatments. The low-frequency pulses aim to induce action potentials and neuronal activity in ascending and descending pathways of the peripheral and central nervous system [4].

mPNS treatment is a painless procedure, making it a more attractive option for those with hypersensitivity. This analgesia is due to the physics of induced fields and the differential recruitment of nerve fibers within a bundle. mPNS recruitment is proportional to the inverse square of the fiber diameter [5] A typical fiber diameter ratio of A-beta (sensory) to A-delta (pain) fibers is 3:1, resulting in a recruitment ratio of 9:1. In contrast, to other therapies like electrical PNS (ePNS) and transcutaneous electrical nerve stimulation (TENS) recruit A-beta fibers in proportion to the inverse of the

A Modern Atlas for Implantable Devices of the Spine, Brain, and Nerve. https://doi.org/10.1016/B978-0-443-36528-7.00044-3

fiber diameter, a 3:1 ratio [6]. This results in a higher proportion of undesirable A-delta recruitment, reducing the beneficial A-beta recruitment as the field intensity is reduced based on the patient's pain tolerance.

The type of field generated by mPNS is drastically different than electrical fields generated along linear electrodes. Figure 41.1 HERE. A magnetic field has greater penetration and spread than the diffuse non focused electrical field. Figure 41.2.

Another important MOA in magnetic fields is their ability to induce an initial neuronal blockade [7,8]. This sensory blockade produces immediate results in approximately 60%–75% of patients, even those who have suffered with neuropathic pain for decades [9]. It appears to further enhance the peripheral reconditioning of the central nervous system.

Shared decision making and consent is an important part of medical ethics, and fundamental to good medical practice. It is gaining more importance as another valid factor in patient care. Even if another therapy is more effective, a patients preference overweighs the providers preference. The patient may have multiple reasons for wanting a noninvasive option as opposed to an invasive or implantable option. The identification of the main contributing pain mechanism and the integration of the patients' view on their condition, including beliefs, preferences, concerns and expectations, are key in the personalized clinical management of pain [1].

Real world pilot trial

The VA Augusta real world pilot study using the latest iteration of the Axon Therapy™ device was published in 2023 [9]. Figure 41.3 HERE. This study took all comers with neuropathic pain with no inclusion or exclusion criteria. Patients had a mix of postoperative, posttraumatic and other neuropathic conditions including painful diabetic neuropathy (PDN). Twenty-four patients with predominantly neuropathic post-traumatic or postoperative pain were treated as per protocol and followed for 3 months. At 1 month, there was a 3.8 average reduction in pre-pain scores using a visual analogue scale (VAS), and that relief was generally durable measured out to 3 months. Two-thirds of patients, deemed responders, showed an 87% reduction in pain. Opioid reduction was seen in 58.3% of responders as well.

The Safety and efficacy of Axon Therapy (SEAT Study) 2024, utilizing magnetic peripheral nerve stimulation (mPNS) for treatment of neuropathic pain was the first RCT, multi-site clinical trial to compare long-term safety and efficacy of mPNS in patients with chronic, intractable, post-traumatic or post-surgical neuropathic pain to comprehensive Conventional Medical Management (CMM) [10]. A total of 65 patients were followed for 3 months, 71% of subjects were considered responders (>50% pain relief) in the mPNS + CMM group versus 13% of subjects in the CMM group. The mPNS + CMM group had a mean reduction in VAS scores at Day 90 of 3.8 points (>50% reduction), while CMM showed less than a one-point (0.7 point) mean reduction or ~10% reduction ($P < .0001$). The EQ-5D-3L score increased in the mPNS + CMM study group, whereas the CMM group showed no improvement in EQ-5D-3L at Day 90. PGIC responder rates were 80.6% and 4.3% at Day 90 for mPNS + CMM and CMM groups, respectively. Data has been analyzed for 1 year and excellent and improving durability has been shown. This data is now in process of publication.

FIGURE 41.1 Magnetic waveform.

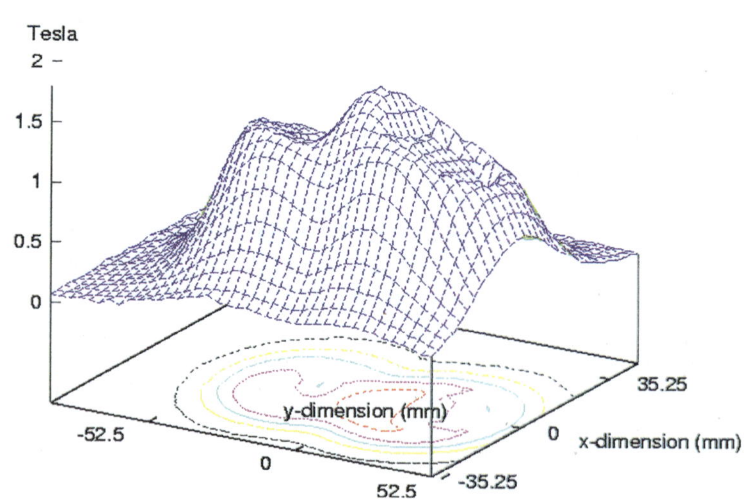

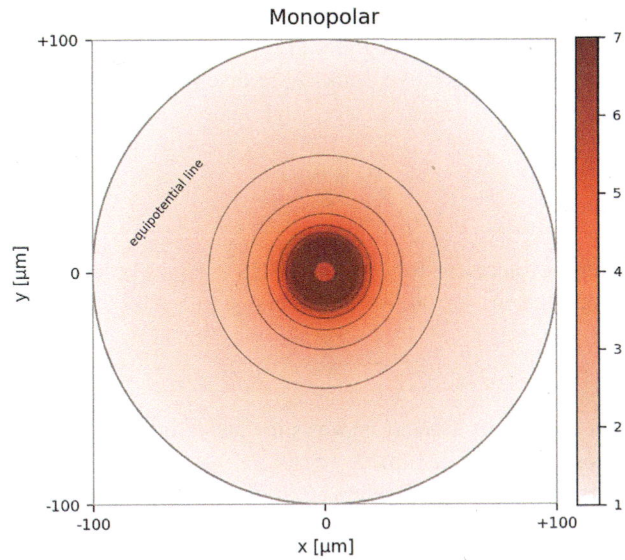

FIGURE 41.2 Monopolar electric waveform.

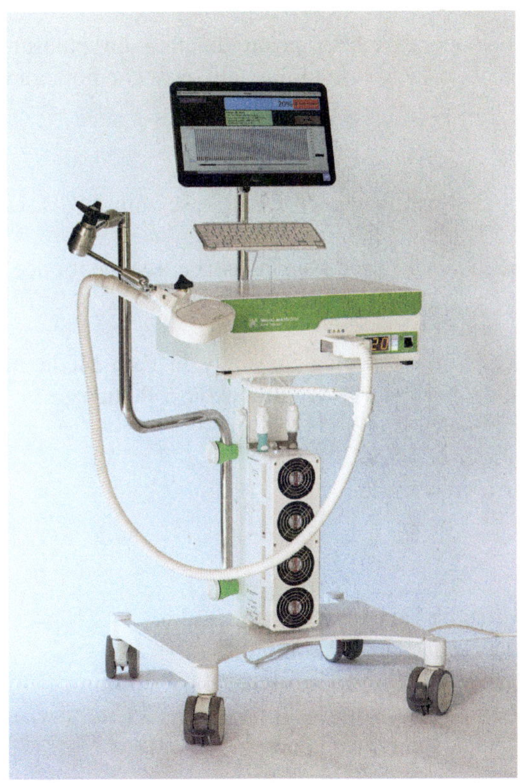

FIGURE 41.3 Axon magnetic peripheral nerve stimulator device.

A third study has been completed looking at Magnetic Therapy for Diabetic Neuropathy[in press]. This was an RCT, multi-site crossover sham study looking at mPNS plus conventional medical management (CMM) or Sham pus CMM. The high pain responder rate at 90 days (FAS 70.0%; PP 81.4%) and pain reduction (FAS 75.7%; PP 75.5%) are statistically significant. These findings are similar to the recently published Safety and Efficacy of Axon Therapy (SEAT) study. The conclusions suggest mPNS should be considered early in the chronic PDN treatment algorithm, directly after

CMM and before any invasive procedures. This study resulted in the FDA clearance of Axon Therapy mPNS for PDN. It also reinforced its inclusion in the ASPN guideline for PDN [11].

Off label: OAB, Osteoarthritis, acute postoperative pain, acute disc herniation pain.

Key points

1. Alternative to invasive procedures
2. Painless
3. Outcomes as good or better than the literature for PNS and SCS
4. No significant adverse events reported in over 4000 treatments

Relevant anatomy

a. Peripheral nerve anatomy. Most commonly treated nerves/sites are femoral, sciatic, saphenous, tibial, medial nerve, greater occipital, pericapsular nerve group (for hip)
b. Editor's note: Reference appropriate Anatomy Chapters

Procedure

a. Painful Diabetic Neuropathy (with ICD 10 Codes)
b. Indications
- **a.** On label: Chronic intractable postoperative pain, posttraumatic pain, painful diabetic neuropathy
- **b.** Off label: Acute perioperative pain, osteoarthritic joint pain, post chemotherapy pain, overactive bladder (S3), lumbar and cervical disc herniations.

c. Patient Selection Considerations
- **a.** 18–85 years old
- **b.** Contraindications: Do not place coil over shrapnel. Do not use with AICD. Do not use within 4 cm of Pacemaker. Do not use on head.
- **c.** Maintenance concerns. Most patients will need a maintenance treatment once per month. Many go 2–3 months between treatments

d. Training Recommendations
- **a.** ACGME Fellowship and or Residency Training Specialty in Pain Medicine, PM&R, Neurology, Surgical specialties such as Plastics, Vascular, Neurosurgery, Orthopedics, Podiatry.
- **b.** Suggested Case Volume for Competence: 10
- **c.** Proctoring Recommendation: First two cases
- **d.** Case Peer Review: 3 cases per review cycle

Technique

a. Patient positioning (see Fig. 41.4 for the Quick Reference Guide).
b. Anesthesia considerations: no sedation/anesthesia required.
c. Procedure time estimate: 13.33 min per therapy. Therefore, allow 30 min per total time per case.
d. Relevant vendor support: Initial training and sign off for Providers administering therapy.
e. Procedure: See Fig. 41.4 for the Quick Reference Guide.

Post therapy considerations

a. No "recovery" period
b. Efficacy Estimates of up to 80% responder rates
c. Activity Limitations: None
d. Maintenance Considerations: Most patient will need a monthly treatment for maintenance of effects.

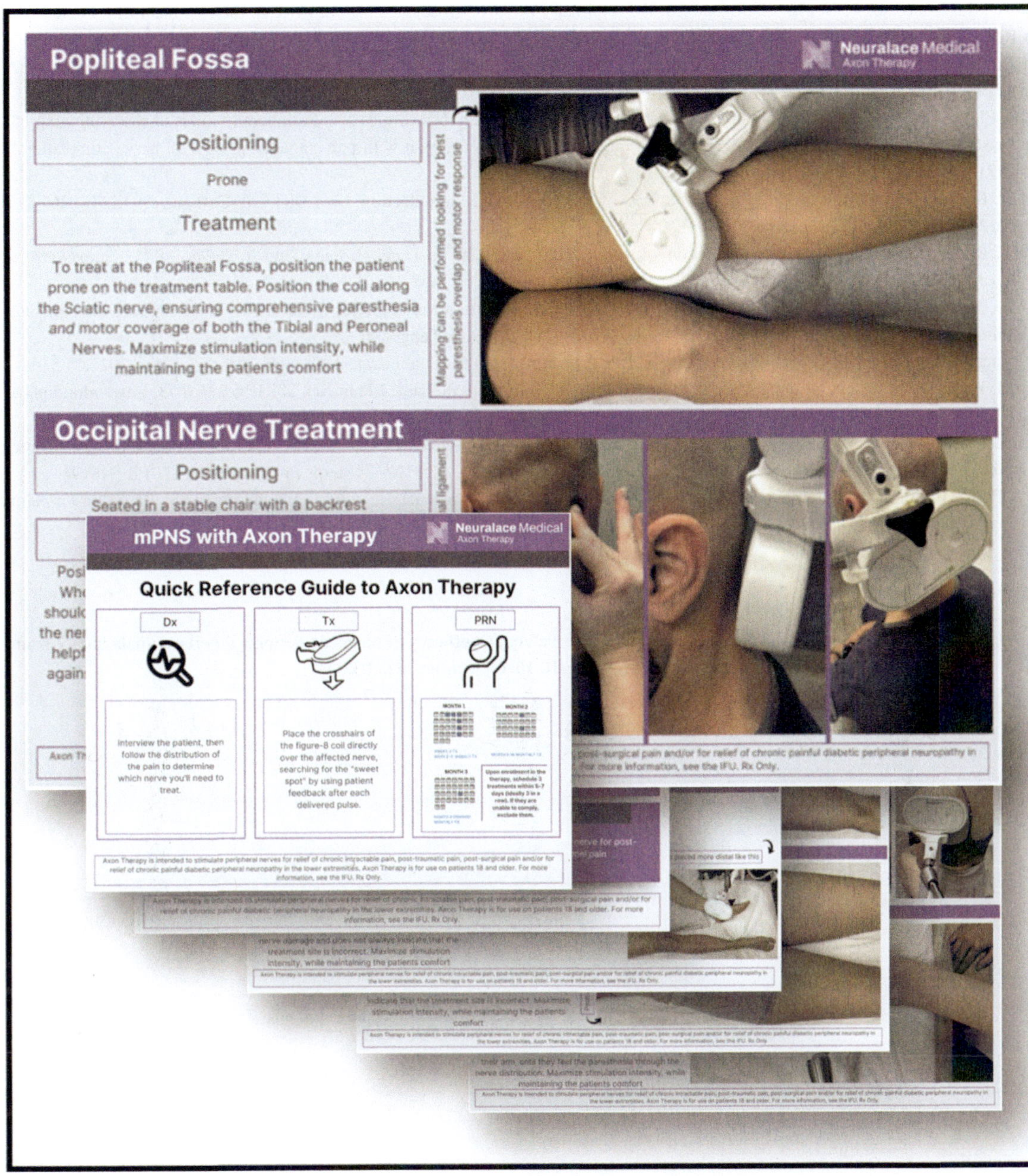

FIGURE 41.4 Provider quick reference guide for coil placement.

Pearls and Pitfalls

a. Preprocedure: Proper patient selection of patients with known peripheral neuropathies
b. Intraprocedure: Monitor for any movement of coil and gently reposition for maximal effect
c. Postoprocedure: There will often be immediate effects from mPNS, but having the patient wait and move the affected body part will show an increased effect within 5 min.

References

[1] Basil GW, Wang MY. Trends in outpatient minimally invasive spine surgery. J Spine Surg 2019;5(1):S108–14. https://doi.org/10.21037/jss.2019.04.17.

[2] Cahana A, Mavrocordatos P, Geurts JW, Groen GJ. Do minimally invasive procedures have a place in the treatment of chronic low back pain? Expert Rev Neurother 2004;4(3):479–90. https://doi.org/10.1586/14737175.4.3.479.
[3] Polson MJR, Barker AT, Freeston IL. Stimulation of nerve trunks with time varying magnetic fields. Med Biol Eng Comput 1982;20:243–4. https://doi.org/10.1007/BF02441362.
[4] Deer TR, Eldabe S, Falowski SM, Huntoon MA, Staats PS, Cassar IR, Crosby ND, Boggs JW. Peripherally induced reconditioning of the central nervous system: A proposed mechanistic theory for sustained relief of chronic pain with percutaneous peripheral nerve stimulation. J Pain Res 2021;14:721–36. https://doi.org/10.2147/JPR.S297091.
[5] Basser PJ, Roth BJ. Stimulation of a myelinated nerve axon by electromagnetic induction. Med Biol Eng Comput 1991;29(3):261–8. https://doi.org/10.1007/BF02446708.
[6] McNeal DR. Analysis of a model for excitation of myelinated nerve. IEEE Trans Biomed Eng 1976;23:329–37. https://doi.org/10.1109/tbme.1976.324593.
[7] Jones MG, Rogers ER, Harris JP, et al. Neuromodulation using ultra low frequency current waveform reversibly blocks axonal conduction and chronic pain. Sci Transl Med 2021;13(608). https://doi.org/10.1126/scitranslmed.abg9890.
[8] Ye H, Dima M, Hall V, et al. Cellular mechanisms underlying carry-over effects after magnetic stimulation. Sci Rep 2024;14:5167.
[9] Bedder M, Parker L. Magnetic peripheral nerve stimulation (mPNS) for chronic pain. J Pain Res 2023;16:2365–73. https://doi.org/10.2147/JPR.S409331.
[10] Kapural L, Patel J, Rosenberg JC, Li S, Amirdelfan K, Bedder M. Safety and efficacy of axon therapy (SEAT study), utilizing magnetic peripheral nerve stimulation (mPNS) for treatment of neuropathic pain. J Pain Res 2024;17:3167–74. https://doi.org/10.2147/JPR.S481944.
[11] Sayed d, Deer TR, et al. A systematic guideline by the ASPN workgroup on the evidence, education, and treatment algorithm for painful diabetic neuropathy: sweet. J Pain Res 2024;17:1461–501.

Further reading

[1] Brown L, Gage M, Cordner H, Kapural L, Rosenberg J, Bedder M. Safety and efficacy of magnetic peripheral nerve stimulation for painful diabetic neuropathy. Neuromodulation 2025;28(8):1366–73. https://doi.org/10.1016/j.neurom.2025.03.074.

Section 12

Intrathecal drug delivery

Introduction to section 12 intrathecal drug delivery

Intrathecal therapy (IT), also known as intrathecal drug delivery (IDD), is a targeted treatment modality that has been available since the 1980s for managing chronic, severe, and refractory pain—both cancer-related and non-cancer in origin. By delivering medication directly into the cerebrospinal fluid (CSF), IDD bypasses systemic circulation, allowing for significantly lower doses of medication to achieve potent analgesia with fewer systemic side effects. While commonly employed in the United States for pain management, internationally, IDD has been more broadly utilized to manage conditions such as severe spasticity and movement disorders, reflecting regional differences in training, resource allocation, and regulatory approval pathways.

In contrast to other implantable pain therapies, such as spinal cord stimulation (SCS)—which follows well-defined, algorithm-driven programming protocols—IDD is a highly individualized treatment that requires intensive management by a skilled and knowledgeable healthcare team. The responsibility for ongoing care, including drug selection, dosage adjustments, and device maintenance, falls largely on the implanting physician and their extended care team. As such, successful implementation of IDD demands a nuanced understanding of pharmacokinetics, pharmacodynamics, and the physicochemical properties of the medications within the intrathecal space.

Key clinical decisions—such as the choice of medication or combination therapy, drug concentration, rate and method of infusion, catheter tip location (both longitudinally along the spinal axis and circumferentially around the cord), and site of pump reservoir placement—must be tailored to the individual patient. Additionally, trialing strategies (catheter vs. single shot, location of medication (intrathecal, epidural, or oral), inpatient vs. outpatient) are not explicitly standardized, requiring clinicians to use experience-based judgment. To guide practitioners, the Polyanalgesic Consensus Conference (PACC) has developed a comprehensive and regularly updated framework to synthesize current evidence and expert opinion into best practices for IDD use.

Despite its proven clinical efficacy and long-term cost-effectiveness—often exceeding that of SCS—IDD is seeing a decline in utilization. Contributing factors include the limited pipeline of new intrathecal medications, lack of exposure to IDD during ACGME-accredited pain medicine fellowships, and a stagnation in high-quality, prospective clinical trials relative to other neuromodulation therapies. As a result, IDD remains underrepresented in contemporary pain management strategies, despite its value in treating patients with complex and intractable pain.

Revitalizing the use of IDD in modern pain practice requires a two-pronged approach: simplifying the delivery model for both patients and providers, and advocating for renewed investment in on-label medication approvals, formulation innovation, and data-driven research. The therapy's future hinges on the ability of the pain management community to re-engage with the modality and integrate it as a core part of the therapeutic armamentarium.

Intrathecal drug delivery remains one of the most satisfying and low-burden therapies for chronic pain—providing meaningful, sustained relief for patients who may have exhausted other options. For clinicians already familiar with this modality, this section aims to reinvigorate your interest by presenting updated concepts and techniques. For those new to IDD, it offers a foundation in a time-tested, effective therapy that deserves strong consideration in any comprehensive pain management practice.

Chapter 42

Intrathecal drug delivery: Patient selection

Edward Podgorski, III [1], Ramneek Dhillon[2], Tolga Suvar[3] and Ahmed Khawer[4]

[1]Hawthorne Oncology Pain Experts (HOPE), Tampa, FL, United States; [2]Evolve Restorative Center, Santa Rosa, CA, United States; [3]Rush University, Chicago, IL, United States; [4]Johns Hopkins University, Baltimore, MD, United States

Indications

Intrathecal drug delivery (IDD) is a well-established method for managing chronic pain and spasticity through targeted administration of analgesic and antispasmodic agents into the intrathecal space. The implantation of an intrathecal drug delivery system requires meticulous surgical technique to ensure optimal placement and function while minimizing complications. Appropriate patient selection, guided by a thorough assessment of disease etiology, prior treatment response, and risk–benefit analysis, is essential for optimizing outcomes.

Cancer pain

Cancer pain, particularly when refractory to systemic opioids and adjuvant analgesics, is one of the most well-established indications for IDD. Malignant pain often involves a combination of nociceptive and neuropathic components, requiring multimodal analgesia. The Polyanalgesic Consensus Conference (PACC) guidelines recommend intrathecal opioid therapy, often in combination with adjuvants such as clonidine or bupivacaine, for patients with intolerable opioid side effects or inadequate pain relief despite escalating systemic doses [1]. Studies have demonstrated that intrathecal opioids, particularly morphine and hydromorphone, provide significant pain relief with reduced sedation and gastrointestinal side effects compared with oral or intravenous administration [2]. Equally as important, catheter location to ensure the delivery of medication to the posterior elements of the spinal cord as well as the level of catheter placement will require an appreciation for the type of cancer and the location of effected dermatomes.

Chronic nonmalignant pain

Patients with chronic nonmalignant pain (CNMP) refractory to conservative management, including high-dose oral opioids, may benefit from IDD. Conditions such as failed back surgery syndrome (FBSS), complex regional pain syndrome (CRPS), and postherpetic neuralgia have been shown to respond favorably to targeted intrathecal analgesia [3]. The use of intrathecal ziconotide, a nonopioid calcium channel blocker, has been particularly effective in opioid-resistant neuropathic pain [4]. Additionally, the ability to titrate medications precisely within the CSF improves therapeutic outcomes and minimizes opioid-induced hyperalgesia.

Severe spasticity

Patients with spasticity secondary to conditions such as spinal cord injury (SCI), multiple sclerosis (MS), stroke, and cerebral palsy frequently experience significant functional impairment and pain. Intrathecal baclofen (ITB) therapy is a well-established treatment for severe spasticity unresponsive to oral medications or physical therapy. Studies have demonstrated that ITB significantly improves muscle tone, pain, and functional independence in appropriately selected

A Modern Atlas for Implantable Devices of the Spine, Brain, and Nerve. https://doi.org/10.1016/B978-0-443-36528-7.00036-4

patients [5]. Notably, ITB therapy requires careful patient selection due to the potential for withdrawal symptoms, overdose, and catheter-related complications.

Appropriate patient selection, guided by a thorough assessment of disease etiology, prior treatment response, and risk–benefit analysis, is essential for optimizing outcomes. As research advances, the integration of novel agents and targeted drug delivery protocols continues to expand the therapeutic potential of IDD in pain and spasticity management.

Comorbid conditions

Psychologic assessment

The interplay between pain and psychological wellbeing is well recognized and plays a critical role in the success of long-term outcomes of patients receiving implantable devices [6]. Psychological screening data in patients being considered for intrathecal drug delivery systems is limited, but data in patients receiving spinal cord stimulator implants has shown a strong correlation between poor outcomes and patients with unrecognized or undertreated psychological conditions. Factors have been identified as predictors of poor outcomes, and screening tools have been developed to assist implanters with choosing the appropriate candidates [7–9]. As a result, consensus for preimplantation psychological assessment for chronic pain indications has remained consistent with grade B, evidence level IB, and moderate level of certainly that an assessment should be performed and maintained throughout treatment. In contrast, psychological screening in cancer patients is not required (grade B, level II, low level of certainty). However, updated guidelines do highlight that treatment and assessment do remain an important tool in cancer patients if time allows. This is especially true in patients with preexisting conditions or when concerns exist that the patient has an undiagnosed or undertreated psychological condition [10]. Finally, it should not be understated that reduction in pain with implantable devices can have a profound and positive impact on psychological wellbeing.

Pulmonary

Conditions that effect the respiratory system should be considered when choosing intrathecal drugs, during initial dosing, when adjusting medications, and in patients concurrently using central nervous system depressants [7,11]. Opioid medications are the main driver of this risk, with drugs that are more hydrophilic increasing overall risk. While opioid-tolerant patients have a decreased risk of respiratory depression, caution is always warranted and mitigation strategies include starting with lower doses, titrating slowly, and considering implantation in the inpatient setting in high-risk patients. In contrast to opioid-based intrathecal therapy, ziconotide does not carry an increased risk of respiratory depression [12,13].

Cardiac

In patients with cardiac comorbidities, special attention should be given to medications that impact blood pressure and cardiac function, specifically clonidine and bupivacaine. Clonidine is known to cause hypotension at lower doses and hypertension at higher doses. It is also important to note that abrupt cessation of clonidine can cause profound rebound hypertension [13–15]. High risks patients include those with low baseline blood pressure, when a catheter tip is located in close proximity to the cardiac accelerator fibers (T4-6), and when bolus devices are utilized [16]. It is also important to note that opioids can cause hypotension and contribute to cardiac risk. Risk mitigation strategies are similar to those for patients with pulmonary comorbidities.

Renal and hepatic

Diseases that cause renal or hepatic dysfunction can impact excretion and metabolism of drugs, respectively. However, the intrathecal route allows for a significant reduction in serum drug levels, reducing this impact when compared with systemic medications [17]. The one exception to this benefit is ziconotide, which is known to cause both asymptomatic and symptomatic increases in creatine kinase (CK). This is especially true in patients with baseline renal dysfunction. Baseline CK analysis, recurrent CK analysis, and special attention to signs and symptoms of elevated CK levels (e.g., muscle weakness or soreness) are advised.

Endocrine

Diabetes, specifically the risk of inadequate wound healing and infection, is the primary endocrine consideration when utilizing intrathecal drug delivery systems. Despite proposed Hba1c cutoffs, data suggests that Hba1c alone is not sufficient to estimate wound healing and surgical site infection risk. Both long-term and perioperative glycemic control are important considerations to reduce these risks, with some data suggesting that the emphasis should be placed on the perioperative period [18]. Although the optimal glucose range has not been established, a target of 140–180 mg/dL has been suggested [19,20].

Coagulopathies and white blood cells

Patients on antiplatelet or anticoagulant medications, with hypocoagulable states, and cancer patients require appropriate management and mitigation strategies to reduce the risk bleeding and neurological complications. For antiplatelet and anticoagulant medications, strict adherence to the American Society of Regional Anesthesia guidelines remains standard practice [21]. Patients with hypocoagulable states (i.e., hemophilia, factor V Leiden mutations, etc.) require collaboration with hematology and consideration of presurgical treatment strategies. Cancer patients have an increased risk of thromboembolism, and shared decision-making surrounding the risk of anticoagulant discontinuation is recommended. While bridging with low-molecular-weight heparin is an option, this strategy has shown to increase the risk of perioperative bleeding [22].

White blood cell, platelet, and neutrophil counts are also critical considerations with respect to bleeding, wound healing, and infectious risk. Evidence-based guidelines for each of these cell lines do not exist, but thresholds have been proposed, and data has supported their use. A platelet count of <80,000/uL has been proposed as the lowest acceptable cutoff for catheter insertion, but data does demonstrate an increased risk in mortality and morbidity for patients with platelet cell counts <100,000/uL [23]. Platelet transfusions can assist with the correction of thrombocytopenia preoperatively, but need to be weighed against the risks of transfusion. Leukopenia and neutropenia are defined as < 4000/uL and <1500/uL, respectively, and a neutrophil cutoff of <500/ul has been proposed and is associated with a decreased risk of infection [24]. In cancer patients with low WBC counts, granulocyte-stimulating factors (e.g., filgrastim) can be considered. It is also important to monitor post-chemo WBC trends and to understand that peak nadirs typically occur 7–10 days post-treatment.

Pretrial and implant medications

Due to the rapid expansion of intrathecal drug delivery (IDD) and IDD systems for chronic painful conditions, including cancer- and non–cancer-related pain in the 1990s, medication guidance was needed. Considering that intrathecal polypharmacy with a variety of concentrations and formulations were commonplace, the International Neuromodulation Society (INS) developed a series of Polyanalgesic Consensus Conferences (PACC) guidelines in 1999 [7]. To avoid risks such as pump failures, dosing errors, and potential safety issues from the use of non–FDA-approved medications, it is crucial that the decision-making should be guided by both labeling in the jurisdiction of practice and by evidence and guidance in the PACC guidelines (Table 42.1) [7,25].

Trialing methods fall into four categories: single-shot intrathecal bolus injection, multiple intrathecal bolus injections, continuous intrathecal infusion, and continuous epidural infusion [7]. Based on medication choice and lipid solubility, a trialing strategy can be determined. Hydrophilic opioids such as morphine, hydromorphone, and baclofen diffuse in the

TABLE 42.1 Polyanalgesic Consensus Conference evidence and recommendations on intrathecal therapy [26].

Statement	Evidence level	Recommendation grade	Consensus strength
Intrathecal therapy should be utilized for active cancer-related pain.	I for opioids; I for ziconotide	A	Strong
Intrathecal therapy should be utilized for non–cancer-related pain.	III-2 for opioids; II-3 for opioids in combination with bupivacaine; I for ziconotide	B	Strong

TABLE 42.2 Starting infusion dosage ranges for single medications intended for long-term intrathecal delivery recommended by PACC 2017.

Drug	Dose
Morphine	0.1–0.5 mg/day
Hydromorphone	0.01–0.15 mg/day
Ziconotide	0.5–2.4 mcg/day
Fentanyl	25–75 mcg/day
Bupivacaine	0.5–6 mg/day[a]
Clonidine	20–100 mcd/day
Sufentanil	10–20 mcg/day

Opioid doses listed here are for patients who are opioid naive. Patients with cancer pain on high systemic doses of opioids who are transitioned to IDD should receive intrathecal opioids at approximately 50%–75% of the conversion doses from systemic opioids.
[a]*This is the only change from the PACC 2017 recommendations.*

CSF father away from the administration site and may be conducted with a single shot bolus [27]. Lipophilic opioids such as fentanyl, sufentanil, and bupivacaine do not diffuse widely from the catheter tip and can be conducted through continuous intrathecal or epidural infusions [28]. Lastly, ziconotide has a relatively restricted dural distribution and must be administered intrathecally with serial single-shot boluses [29,30]. Per recommendations by the PACC, a trial should be considered before initiating IT drug delivery for noncancer pain; however, it is not a necessity for cancer pain [31].

When initiating intrathecal therapy, the patient's response and tolerability from the trial can help provide some guidance to the initial starting dose, which can be found in Table 42.2. However, these initial starting doses are for opioid naïve patients. For patients with oncologic diseases, initial morphine dosage may sometimes be higher. A retrospective study by Sindt et al. proposed an initial intrathecal dose titration in patients with cancer using a 100:1 oral to intrathecal morphine conversion ratios, which was safe and well tolerated [32]. Once the pump has been implanted with the appropriate medication and dosage, it will still need to be adjusted over the course of several weeks to optimize dosing.

An important point to keep in mind is that patients with chronic noncancer pain being considered for IDD with opioids should be weaned off other systemic opioids or to the lowest possible dose and preferably weaned off benzodiazepines [29]. When opioids are being used, there is always concern for opioid dose escalation in both cancer- and non–cancer-related pain due to tolerance and diminishing analgesic response. Due to the PACC guidelines, a combination of opioid with bupivacaine, regardless of when the local anesthetic is added, appears to blunt opioid dose escalation and might be beneficial from the outset of IDD [29]. Clonidine as an adjunct is also recommended for both nociceptive and neuropathic pain management with intrathecal infusion [33]. Since tolerance and diminished response is not uncommon, opioid rotation should be considered with the discontinuation of the old opioid and the initiation of a new one. Lastly, the concept of microdosed (low-dose) IDD in combination with systemic opioid reduction or elimination may be useful in treating mechanical axial back pain [29].

Psychological assessment

Psychological factors play a critical role in pain perception by influencing how individuals process, interpret, and respond to pain stimuli. Psychiatric comorbidities, maladaptive coping strategies, or unrealistic treatment expectations can often hinder treatment success [34]. This underscores the necessity of integrating comprehensive psychological assessment as part of interdisciplinary assessments for patients being considered for intrathecal therapy.

The impact of psychosocial factors on surgical outcomes is now well established, leading to widespread endorsement of presurgical psychological evaluations. Psychological assessments, while may not necessarily predict procedural outcomes, are instrumental in guiding individualized treatment plans and optimizing patient preparedness for implantation [35]. Identifying high-risk individuals early can help prevent unnecessary invasive procedures and enable timely interventions to optimize outcomes. Additionally, these evaluations provide valuable insights into a patient's mental state, coping mechanisms, and potential psychological barriers, facilitating informed patient selection enhancing treatment success [34].

Psychological factors, such as somatization, depression, anxiety, and maladaptive coping strategies, are associated with poor interventional outcomes [36]. Schizophrenia with psychosis, major mood disorders, personality disorders, suicidality, and active substance abuse have generally been considered contraindicated for implantation therapy [34,37,38]. The general consensus has been to exclude these patients [39]. Identifying modifiable psychological conditions such as anxiety and depression is crucial, as they can exacerbate pain perception and impair coping abilities. However, when properly managed, they can enhance patient preparation and help set realistic expectations [34,40]. Depression has been consistently associated with poor trial and long-term outcomes [41,42]. However, it has been also shown that depression can be a consequence of chronic pain and can actually improve with implantation therapy [43]. Further, a study evaluating changes in Minnesota Multiphasic Personality Inventory (MMPI) profiles pre- and post-intraspinal opioid therapy found that patients with mildly elevated MMPI experienced greater pain improvement after 4 years of IT therapy, compared with those with more normal MMPI results [44].

Pain psychologists should be introduced early in the interdisciplinary treatment process as key contributors to patient care. A pretrial or preimplant psychological consultation for patients being consulted for intrathecal therapy is recommended [37]. Psychology appointments may occur at multiple stages of the treatment course, including the presurgical evaluation, during the stimulation trial and at scheduled postimplantation follow-up. These evaluations can help monitor pain progression and facilitate the continued implementation of targeted behavioral strategies to enhance functional outcomes [45].

The first part of a psychological evaluation is a clinical interview, allowing for an in-depth assessment of the patient's psychiatric history, coping mechanisms, social support system, and treatment expectations. Psychological testing can enhance the evaluation process by providing objective data to complement clinical assessments. Common standardized tools include the Beck Depression Inventory-II, the Minnesota Multiphasic Personality Inventory (MMPI), the Milton Clinical Multiaxial Inventory III (MCMI-III), the Symptom Check List 90-R (SCL-90-R), and the Pain Catastrophizing Scale [46–48]. This data combined with clinical evaluation can determine the patient's suitability for implantation.

Given the high prevalence of psychiatric conditions among chronic pain patients, patient selection remains a challenge. Targeted psychological and behavioral interventions can mitigate these factors, improving patient prognosis, and ensuring adequate support for patients pre- and postimplantation [37]. A comprehensive evaluation, incorporating structured interviews, standardized testing, and ongoing psychological care, refines patient selection and maximizes treatment success [46].

References

[1] Deer TR, Pope JE, Hayek SM, et al. The Polyanalgesic Consensus Conference (PACC): recommendations for intrathecal drug delivery. Neuromodulation 2017;20(2):96–132.

[2] Smith TJ, Staats PS, Deer T, et al. Randomized clinical trial of an implantable drug delivery system compared with comprehensive medical management for refractory cancer pain: impact on pain, drug-related toxicity, and survival. J Clin Oncol 2005;23(22):4040–9.

[3] Pope JE, Deer TR, Amirdelfan K. Intrathecal therapy for chronic pain: a review of morphine and ziconotide as first-line options. Pain Med 2020;21(4):723–35.

[4] Wallace MS, Rauck RL, Fisher R, et al. Intrathecal ziconotide for severe chronic pain: safety and efficacy in patients with refractory pain. J Pain Symptom Manag 2006;31(4):393–406.

[5] Penn RD, Savoy SM, Corcos D, et al. Intrathecal baclofen for severe spinal spasticity. N Engl J Med 1989;320(23):1517–21.

[6] Sydora BC, Whelan LJ, Abelseth B, et al. Identification of presurgical risk factors for the development of chronic postsurgical pain in adults: a comprehensive umbrella review. J Pain Res 2024;17:2511–30. https://doi.org/10.2147/jpr.S466731.

[7] Deer TR, Hayek SM, Grider JS, et al. The Polyanalgesic Consensus Conference (PACC)®: intrathecal drug delivery guidance on safety and therapy optimization when treating chronic noncancer pain. Neuromodulation October 2024;27(7):1107–39. https://doi.org/10.1016/j.neurom.2024.03.003.

[8] Prabhala T, Kumar V, Gruenthal E, et al. Use of a psychological evaluation tool as a predictor of spinal cord stimulation outcomes. Neuromodulation February 2019;22(2):194–9. https://doi.org/10.1111/ner.12884.

[9] Thomson S, Huygen F, Prangnell S, et al. Appropriate referral and selection of patients with chronic pain for spinal cord stimulation: European consensus recommendations and e-health tool. Eur J Pain July 2020;24(6):1169–81. https://doi.org/10.1002/ejp.1562.

[10] Deer TR, Hayek SM, Grider JS, et al. The Polyanalgesic Consensus Conference (PACC)®: Updates on clinical pharmacology and comorbidity management in intrathecal drug delivery for cancer pain. Neuromodulation Sep 2025.

[11] Deer TR, Pope JE, Hayek SM, et al. The Polyanalgesic Consensus Conference (PACC): recommendations for intrathecal drug delivery: guidance for improving safety and mitigating risks. Neuromodulation February 2017;20(2):155–76. https://doi.org/10.1111/ner.12579.

[12] Deer TR, Pope JE, Hanes MC, McDowell GC. Intrathecal therapy for chronic pain: a review of morphine and ziconotide as firstline options. Pain Med April 1, 2019;20(4):784–98. https://doi.org/10.1093/pm/pny132.

[13] Kroin JS, McCarthy RJ, Penn RD, Lubenow TJ, Ivankovich AD. Continuous intrathecal clonidine and tizanidine in conscious dogs: analgesic and hemodynamic effects. Anesth Analg March 2003;96(3):776–82. https://doi.org/10.1213/01.Ane.0000048087.57487.0c.

[14] Filos KS, Goudas LC, Patroni O, Polyzou V. Hemodynamic and analgesic profile after intrathecal clonidine in humans. A dose-response study. Anesthesiology September 1994;81(3):591–601. https://doi.org/10.1097/00000542-199409000-00011. Discussion 27A-28A.

[15] Lee HM, Ruggoo V, Graudins A. Intrathecal clonidine pump failure causing acute withdrawal syndrome with 'stress-induced' cardiomyopathy. J Med Toxicol March 2016;12(1):134–8. https://doi.org/10.1007/s13181-015-0505-9.

[16] Yaksh TL, Fisher CJ, Hockman TM, Wiese AJ. Current and future issues in the development of spinal agents for the management of pain. Curr Neuropharmacol 2017;15(2):232–59. https://doi.org/10.2174/1570159x14666160307145542.

[17] Brogan SE, Sindt JE, Jackman CM, White J, Wilding V, Okifuji A. Prospective association of serum opioid levels and clinical outcomes in patients with cancer pain treated with intrathecal opioid therapy. Anesth Analg April 2020;130(4):1035–44. https://doi.org/10.1213/ane.0000000000004276.

[18] Hagedorn JM, Bendel MA, Hoelzer BC, Aiyer R, Caraway D. Preoperative hemoglobin A1c and perioperative blood glucose in patients with diabetes mellitus undergoing spinal cord stimulation surgery: a literature review of surgical site infection risk. Pain Pract January 2023;23 (1):83–93. https://doi.org/10.1111/papr.13145.

[19] Dogra P, Anastasopoulou C, Jialal I. Diabetic perioperative management. *StatPearls*. StatPearls Publishing LLC.; 2025.

[20] Raju TA, Torjman MC, Goldberg ME. Perioperative blood glucose monitoring in the general surgical population. J Diabetes Sci Technol November 1, 2009;3(6):1282–7. https://doi.org/10.1177/193229680900300607.

[21] Narouze S, Benzon HT, Provenzano D, et al. Interventional spine and pain procedures in patients on antiplatelet and anticoagulant medications (Second Edition): guidelines from the American Society of Regional Anesthesia and Pain Medicine, the European Society of Regional Anaesthesia and Pain Therapy, the American Academy of Pain Medicine, the International Neuromodulation Society, the North American Neuromodulation Society, and the World Institute of Pain. Reg Anesth Pain Med April 2018;43(3):225–62. https://doi.org/10.1097/aap.0000000000000700.

[22] Marquez J, Togami JC, Dant CR, Herrera A, Marshik P, Burnett AE. Peri-procedural antithrombotic management: time to burn the bridge? J Thromb Thrombolysis April 2018;45(3):337–44. https://doi.org/10.1007/s11239-018-1616-3.

[23] Glance LG, Blumberg N, Eaton MP, et al. Preoperative thrombocytopenia and postoperative outcomes after noncardiac surgery. Anesthesiology January 2014;120(1):62–75. https://doi.org/10.1097/ALN.0b013e3182a4441f.

[24] Sindt JE, Larsen SD, Dalley AP, Collier WH, Brogan SE. The rate of infectious complications after intrathecal drug delivery system implant for cancer-related pain is low despite frequent concurrent anticancer treatment or Leukopenia. Anesth Analg July 2020;131(1):280–7. https://doi.org/10.1213/ane.0000000000004639.

[25] US FDA. Use caution with implanted pumps for intrathecal administration of medi- cines for pain management: FDA safety communication. November 14, 2018. p. 2–5.

[26] Deer TR, Pope J, Hayek S. The Polyanalgesic Consensus Conference (PACC) recom- mendations on intrathecal drug infusion systems best practices and guidelines. Neuromodulation 2017;20(4):405–6. https://doi.org/10.1111/ner.12618. https://pubmed.ncbi.nlm.nih.gov/28042904/.

[27] Kroin JS, Ali A, York M, Penn RD. The distribution of medication along the spinal canal after chronic intrathecal administration. Neurosurgery 1993;33:226–30 [discussion 30].

[28] Ummenhofer WC, Arends RH, Shen DD, Bernards CM. Comparative spinal dis- tribution and clearance kinetics of intrathecally administered morphine, fentanyl, alfentanil, and sufentanil. Anesthesiology 2000;92:739–53.

[29] Deer TR, Hayek SM, Pope JE, et al. The Polyanalgesic Consensus Conference (PACC®) recommendations for trialing of intrathecal drug delivery infusion therapy. Neuromodulation 2017;20:133–54. https://doi.org/10.1111/ner.12543.

[30] Mohammed SI, Eldabe S, Simpson KH, et al. Bolus intrathecal injection of zico- notide (Prialt(R)) to evaluate the option of continuous administration via an implanted intrathecal drug delivery (ITDD) system: a pilot study. Neuromodulation 2013;16:576–81 [discussion 582].

[31] Deer TR, Hayek S, Pope JE, Lamer TJ, Hamza M, Grider JS, Rosen SM, Narouze S, Perruchoud C, Thomson S, Russo M, Grigsby E, Doleys DM, Jacobs MS, Saulino M, Christo P, Kim P, Huntoon EM, Krames E, Mekhail N. The Polyanalgesic Consensus Conference (PACC): recom- mendations for trialing of intrathecal drug delivery infusion therapy. Neuromodulation 2017. https://doi.org/10.1111/ner.12543. E-pub ahead of print.

[32] Sindt JE, Odell DW, Tariq R, Presson AP, Zhang C, Brogan SE. Initial intrathecal dose titration and predictors of early dose escalation in patients with cancer using a 100 : 1 oral to intrathecal morphine conversion ratio. Neuromodulation 2021;24:1157–66.

[33] Deer TR, Pope JE, Hayek S, Lamer TJ, Veizi IE, Erdek M, Wallace MS, Grider JS, Levy RM, Prager J, Rosen SM, Saulino M, Yaksh TL, De Andres JA, Abejon Gonzalez D, Vesper J, Schu S, Simpson B, Mekhail N. The Polyanalgesic Consensus Conference (PACC): recommendations for intrathecal drug delivery: guidance for improving safety and mitigating risks. Neuromodulation 2017. https://doi.org/10.1111/ner.12579. E-pub ahead of print.

[34] Deer T, Masone RJ. Selection of spinal cord stimulation candidates for the treatment of chronic pain. Pain Med 2008;9(Suppl. 1). https://doi.org/10.1111/j.1526-4637.2008.00443.x.

[35] Doleys DM. Preparing patients for implantable technologies. In: Psychological approaches to pain management: a practitioner's Handbook. 2nd ed. 2002.

[36] Celestin J, Edwards RR, Jamison RN. Pretreatment psychosocial variables as predictors of outcomes following lumbar surgery and spinal cord stimulation: a systematic review and literature synthesis. Pain Med 2009;10(4). https://doi.org/10.1111/j.1526-4637.2009.00632.x.

[37] Deer TR, Smith HS, Cousins M, et al. Consensus guidelines for the selection and implantation of patients with noncancer pain for intrathecal drug delivery. Pain Physician 2010;13(3). https://doi.org/10.36076/ppj.2010/13/e175.

[38] Campbell CM, Jamison RN, Edwards RR. Psychological screening/phenotyping as predictors for spinal cord stimulation. Curr Pain Headache Rep 2013;17(1). https://doi.org/10.1007/s11916-012-0307-6.

[39] Nelson DV, Kennington M, Novy DM, Squitieri P. Psychological selection criteria for implantable spinal cord stimulators. Pain Forum 1996;5(2). https://doi.org/10.1016/s1082-3174(96)80042-0.

[40] Sparkes E, Duarte RV, Mann S, Lawrenc TR, Raphael JH. Analysis of psychological characteristics impacting spinal cord stimulation treatment outcomes: a prospective cohort assessment. Pain Physician 2015;18(3). https://doi.org/10.36076/ppj.2015/18/e369.

[41] Olson KA, Bedder MD, Anderson VC, Burchiel KJ, Villanueva MR. Psychological variables associated with outcome of spinal cord stimulation trials. Neuromodulation 1998;1(1). https://doi.org/10.1111/j.1525-1403.1998.tb00025.x.

[42] Shanthanna H, Eldabe S, Provenzano DA, et al. Evidence-based consensus guidelines on patient selection and trial stimulation for spinal cord stimulation therapy for chronic non-cancer pain. Reg Anesth Pain Med 2023;48(6). https://doi.org/10.1136/rapm-2022-104097.

[43] Fishbain DA, Cutler R, Rosomoff HL, Rosomoff RS. Chronic pain-associated depression: antecedent or consequence of chronic pain? A review. Clin J Pain 1997;13. https://doi.org/10.1097/00002508-199706000-00006.

[44] Doleys DM, Brown J. MMPI profile as an outcome "predictor" in the treatment of noncancer pain patients utilizing intraspinal opioid therapy. Neuromodulation 2001;4(3). https://doi.org/10.1046/j.1525-1403.2001.00093.x.

[45] Van Dorsten B. Psychological considerations in preparing patients for implantation procedures. Pain Med 2006;7(Suppl. 1). https://doi.org/10.1111/j.1526-4637.2006.00122.x.

[46] Prager J, Jacobs M. Evaluation of patients for implantable pain modalities: medical and behavioral assessment. Clin J Pain 2001;17(3). https://doi.org/10.1097/00002508-200109000-00004.

[47] Blackburn DR, Romers CC, Copeland LA, et al. Presurgical psychological assessments as correlates of effectiveness of spinal cord stimulation for chronic pain reduction. Neuromodulation 2016;19(4). https://doi.org/10.1111/ner.12431.

[48] Fama CA, Chen N, Prusik J, et al. The use of preoperative psychological evaluations to predict spinal cord stimulation success: our experience and a review of the literature. Neuromodulation 2016;19(4). https://doi.org/10.1111/ner.12434.

Chapter 43

Implant methods of intrathecal drug delivery

Tolga Suvar[1], Edward Podgorski, III[2], Michael Danko[3], Ramneek Dhillon[4], Adelaide Viguri[5] and Jonathan Paris[6]

[1]*Rush University, Chicago, IL, United States;* [2]*Hawthorne Oncology Pain Experts (HOPE), Tampa, FL, United States;* [3]*Premier Pain Treatment Institute, Loveland, OH, United States;* [4]*Evolve Restorative Center, Santa Rosa, CA, United States;* [5]*Regenerative Pain & Spine, Chicago, IL, United States;* [6]*Center for Pain Management at Stony Brook Medicine, Stony Brook, NY, United States*

Preoperative considerations

Successful ITDD implantation begins with thorough preoperative planning, which includes patient selection, medication trialing, and risk assessment. Ideal candidates for intrathecal therapy are those with refractory chronic pain, cancer pain, or spasticity who have failed conservative treatment modalities [1]. A trial period using an externalized intrathecal catheter or single-shot intrathecal injection helps determine efficacy and tolerability before committing to permanent implantation [2]. For those patients with cancer-related pain, a trial is not mandated, and the physician can proceed to implantation.

Imaging studies, including MRI or CT scans, should be reviewed to identify any anatomical variations, spinal pathology, or previous surgeries that could influence catheter placement [3]. A multidisciplinary approach involving pain specialists, neurosurgeons, and physical therapists can help optimize patient outcomes. Additionally, patients should be counseled on the risks and benefits of ITDD, including potential complications such as infection, cerebrospinal fluid (CSF) leaks, catheter migration, and pump malfunction [4]. As with neuromodulation, reviewing anticoagulation parameters per American Society of Regional Anesthesia and Pain Medicine (ASRA) guidelines and coagulation profile should always be reviewed prior to proceeding with ITDD implantation.

Positioning, prepping, and draping

Proper patient positioning is crucial to facilitate accurate and safe implantation of the ITDD system. The patient is typically placed in a lateral or prone position on a radiolucent table to allow for fluoroscopic guidance [5]. The positioning of the patient is prudent for where the ITDD implantation will take place. For example, abdominal placement will most likely warrant lateral positioning, and if the patient prefers posterior implantation, the patient will be in the prone position. A bolster may be placed under the abdomen to reduce lumbar lordosis and improve access to the intrathecal space. An axillary roll is neuroprotective and prevents brachial plexus injury during the surgery.

The surgical site, including the lower back and flank region, is prepped with a broad-spectrum antiseptic solution such as chlorhexidine or povidone-iodine. A wide sterile drape is applied to maintain aseptic technique and reduce the risk of surgical site infections [6]. Preprocedural planning will take place by reviewing CT or MRI imaging, and the skin is marked for optimal catheter entry at the appropriate intervertebral level, typically between L3 and L5, ensuring direct access to the intrathecal space.

Needle placement

Accurate needle placement is fundamental to the success of ITDD implantation. Under fluoroscopic guidance, a Tuohy needle is introduced into the intrathecal space at the predetermined lumbar level [7]. A loss-of-resistance technique is used

A Modern Atlas for Implantable Devices of the Spine, Brain, and Nerve. https://doi.org/10.1016/B978-0-443-36528-7.00017-0

to confirm entry into the subarachnoid space, followed by aspiration of CSF to verify correct placement. The needle trajectory should be adjusted as necessary to ensure optimal catheter positioning and minimize the risk of complications such as dural puncture at unintended levels.

Once the intrathecal space is accessed, the intrathecal catheter is carefully threaded through the needle to the desired spinal level, typically targeting the midthoracic region for pain management or the cervical region for spasticity control [6]. Fluoroscopy is used to confirm catheter placement, ensuring that the tip is positioned posteriorly and appropriately to deliver the intended medication effectively. The needle is then withdrawn, and the catheter is tunneled subcutaneously to connect with the implanted pump, which is secured in a subcutaneous pocket, usually in the abdominal wall.

Following implantation, a thorough assessment of catheter function is performed, including aspiration of CSF and test dosing to confirm medication delivery. Patients are closely monitored for immediate postoperative complications, and a structured follow-up plan is established to ensure long-term efficacy and device functionality [3].

Catheter placement

Catheter tip placement is the most important factor in achieving adequate pain relief postimplant [8]. For this reason, consensus remains strong (grade A, level IB) that the catheter should be placed at the dermatomal level that best matches the painful area being treated [1,9]. For chronic pain indications, published tables serve as a reference for the appropriate catheter tip location [10]. For cancer patients, both sympathetically mediated pain and disease progression should factor into catheter tip location, and implanters should err on the side of a higher catheter tip placement if necessary. The importance of posterior catheter tip placement has recently been debated, but due to limited drug distribution, posteriorly located pain receptors, and a trend toward lower doses with time, a posterior approach is favored [11,12].

Posterior placement of the catheter tip is the initial goal when advancing the catheter and is performed under lateral fluoroscopy. Optimal placement of the Tuohy needle, including appropriate angle and adequate distance below the conus, is the first step in achieving posterior placement. The anterior dura can be used to the implanter's mechanical advantage by allowing the catheter tip to bounce posteriorly off the dura prior to reaching the level of the conus. Early posterior placement of the catheter allows for a higher chance of the catheter tip remaining posterior and allows the implanter to focus on achieving dermatomal placement and midline position of the catheter tip. Cephalad advancement should occur under AP fluoroscopy and be met with minimal resistance. Any resistance or neurologic response from the patient should be further evaluated, and careful catheter tip repositioning should be considered. While intrathecal catheters are not specifically designed for steerability, rotation of the catheter at the needle hub or at the stylet hub can produce torque and assist with guidance of the catheter tip to the midline position. A slight bend can also be placed in the distal stylet tip to assist with steering, but caution should be taken as this manipulation can increase the risk of neural trauma.

Once the catheter tip is at the target location, the stylet is removed. Free flow of CSF should be observed, and a myelogram with compatible contrast should show intrathecal spread of contrast, minimal resistance, and both cephalad and caudad flow. Until the spinal catheter is connected to the pump segment, it is advisable to clamp the catheter to minimize CSF loss. Catheter tip location should be closely observed when performing the remaining steps of the procedure to avoid migration from the target level. It is also important to note that purse string placement, anchoring, connecting pin placement, tunneling and pump suturing are all possible areas of catheter compromise and should be performed with caution.

Catheter anchoring

It is important to properly anchor the catheter to prevent rare, however, potentially serious complications of cranial or rostral catheter migration [13]. Once the catheter tip is located at the desired level, a nonabsorbable suture should be used to fashion a purse-string suture into the lumbar paraspinal fascia around the needle barrel entry point, thus minimizing leakage of CSF and preventing catheter movement [14,15]. After the needle and stylet are removed, check for CSF flow [15]. The proper purse-string suture or closure is performed by taking equidistant bites of fascia around the catheter, making sure entry and exit points are adjacent to each other in a circular fashion until the two free ends come together, whereby pulling the fascia together will reduce the defect, making sure not to tighten the suture so much that CSF flow is compromised. A knot is then placed to join the two ends. It is important to ensure the catheter is secured into the fascia and not fat or muscle [16]. Muscle contraction can cause catheter migration if the catheter is improperly secured to the muscle. Catheter migration is the most common complication aside from infection, and the occurrence of migration is associated with failure to anchor the catheter to the underlying fascia [17]. Anchors come in various shapes, sometimes two pieces, but more commonly they are biwing shaped.

If using the widely used Medtronic ITDD system, insert the catheter tip through a metal casing where the biwing anchor is preloaded onto the anchor dispenser, until the end of the catheter passes through the opposite end. Insert the tip of the anchor while loaded onto the dispenser into the fascia. Contrary to the way a thumb against the plunger of a syringe moves toward the patient while injecting, the anchor dispenser device holds the anchor snug into the fascia with the operator's thumb held against the end, while the index and middle fingers pull the plunger toward the stationary thumb [13]. Hold the anchor tip buried into the fascia with forceps for added stability when deploying the anchor, keeping in mind not to compress the anchor and catheter too hard with the forceps. Using 0 or 2–0 silk or Ethibond (braided polyester, nonabsorbable suture), secure the anchor by tying the islet in each wing to the lumbodorsal fascia [17]. Place an additional suture around the neck and into the groove of the anchor to further adhere it to the fascia [18]. It is crucial to place the anchor as close as possible to where the catheter enters the fascia so that possible migration is avoided. After each step, CSF flow must be checked to ensure there is no kinking of the catheter.

Catheter tunneling

Once securely anchoring the catheter to the fascia, the catheter can be tunneled from the lumbar area to the abdominal pocket. The most frequently used location for intrathecal pump implantation is the left flank, requiring the patient to be placed in the lateral decubitus position with the left side up [13]. A malleable hollow tunneling device is used to bluntly dissect through the subcutaneous fat, maintaining equal depth as it passes laterally. The tunneling device is passed from the posterior incision to the pocket if using a two-piece catheter and from the pocket to the posterior incision when using a one-piece catheter [14]. It is important to maintain the same depth as you are tunneling through the plane; too superficial a plane can lead to erosion or decubitus over time, while going too deep can cause injuries to internal organs [13]. One author suggests it may be easier to pass the tunneling device from the smaller posterior incision to the larger pocket incision, and in most patients, tunneling can be done in a single pass, while in very obese patients, it may be necessary to use two passes with a midaxillary small incision in between [18]. Use your dominant hand to drive the tunneling device and your nondominant hand to feel the tip while it passes, ensuring it stays below the dermal layers [18–21]. Once the tunneling device has reached the opposite side, the stylet can be removed, and the catheter can be fed into the pocket where it can be connected to the pump.

Pocket formation

Creating a subcutaneous pocket to harbor the drug delivery device utilized in intrathecal drug delivery (ITDD) is a vital step in the implantation process. This part of the procedure involves five key components outlined in Table 43.1. In the preparation of pocket creation, follow Polyanalgesic Consensus Conference (PACC) guidelines and identify the optimal location for pump site implantation [1].

To ensure the safe and effective placement of the device, demarcate the skin of the lower abdomen or another area of the body where the device may be accessed and concealed under clothing [25]. For a lower abdomen pocket site, identify

TABLE 43.1 The five key components to successful pocket creation in ITDD [22–24].

Pocket site selection	Demarcate the intended pump implantation site in the lower abdomen quadrant above the iliac crest or in the lower buttocks, medial and inferior to the greater trochanter.
Local anaesthetization	Utilize a generous amount of local anesthesia to anaesthetize the skin over this area. Safe doses: Lidocaine: 4 mg/kg to 4.5 mg/kg; Lidocaine with epinephrine: 7 mg/kg; Bupivacaine: 175 mg in a single dose or a maximum of 400 mg per 24 h.
Pocket dissection	Use a No. 11 or 15 blade to make an incision 2.5 cm deep and 8 cm lengthwise down to the underlying subcutaneous fat layer. Employ a combination of sharp and blunt dissection in which all four of your fingers can fit in the pocket.
Pocket-size confirmation	Insert the pump into the pocket. Widen and deepen the pocket accordingly to permit closure without tension.
Pocket hemostasis and irrigation	Verify hemostasis at incision sites to prevent postoperative hematoma formation. Irrigate with an antibiotic solution to reduce the risk of postoperative infection.

a location superior to the patient's iliac crest and inferior to the umbilicus. If the patient's lower abdomen is not a viable location due to prior surgery or anatomic variation, a location in the upper quadrant of the lower buttocks, approximately medial and inferior to the greater trochanter, is a reasonable second option [22].

After following these provisions, continue on to the local anaesthetization phase. During this step, inject a generous amount of local anesthesia with lidocaine, lidocaine with epinephrine, or bupivacaine. The exact dosage should be based on the patient's size, the location of the pocket, and the surgeon's preference [26]. The safe dose for lidocaine is 4 mg/kg to 4.5 mg/kg; lidocaine with epinephrine is 7 mg/kg; and bupivacaine is 175 mg in a single dose or a maximum of 400 mg per 24 h [27]. If needed, sedation can also be added at this point.

After anaesthetization, begin dissecting out the pocket. Make an approximately 8 cm lengthwise incision to the underlying subcutaneous fat layer [26]. Take care to follow the natural lines of the skin, also known as Langer's lines, to mitigate scarring and promote optimal healing. The incision is then deepened to open a larger subcutaneous pocket, where the ITDD device will subsequently be placed. An incision with a depth of approximately 2.5 cm at the chosen site is appropriate [22]. A depth greater than 2.5 cm may not reliably permit telemetry and add difficulty to pump refilling. Blunt dissection utilizing the second digit can then be employed to carve out the remaining pocket. Generally, if all four digits can fit into the pocket, the pocket should be large enough for closure without tension [28].

Next, confirm the pocket size by trialing ITDD device insertion. Adjust the width and depth of the pocket accordingly. It is important to tailor the pocket and ensure a tight fit around the ITDD device to prevent complications such as infection, seroma, or device migration [27].

The final step is pocket hemostasis and irrigation. Ensure hemostasis of the incision site to prevent postoperative hematoma. Irrigate the pocket with antibiotic solution to reduce the risk of infection [23].

Connecting and securing the pump

After tunneling the catheter subcutaneously to adjoin the pump, the catheter can be trimmed so that an excess of 5–10 cm lies beyond the catheter entry point within the pump pocket, ensuring sufficient length exists for a stress relief loop in the posterior midline incision and pump pocket [19,29]. Using 0–0 silk, place at least three sutures into the suture loops of the pump, anchoring it to the fascia. Placing fewer than three sutures can place the pump at risk for flipping over. These can be loosely secured to adjacent surgical towels with hemostats, which will later be secured once all connections are complete. After confirming the tunneled catheter has free-flowing CSF, connect the tip of the catheter to the proximal catheter attachment via a collet (think "collar" or segmented sleeve that unites both ends). Make the final connection by taking the hub on the opposite end of the catheter attachment and snapping it onto the catheter port of the pump, which should rotate without resistance. With the provided needle in the kit, access the catheter side port and confirm that CSF can be gently aspirated, ensuring flow to the pump [19]. Take the excess catheter slack and coil it behind the pump, avoiding entanglement with the sutures and potential kinking of the catheter [13,14]. As the pump is lowered down into the pocket, make sure the reservoir fill port is facing outward with the tapered end of the catheter side port oriented medially [15]. Positioning the catheter side port medially, where the overlying soft tissue is usually thicker, mitigates against skin erosion over the pump, especially in thinner patients [19]. Once you are satisfied with the pump position and can confirm the coiled catheter is secured behind the pump, well away from the pump ports, you may tie the three sutures to secure the pump to the underlying fascia and begin your closure [21,30].

Wound closure

Wound closure is a critical step in the surgical process of implanting devices for intrathecal drug delivery (ITDD). It is essential to follow PACC guidelines to ensure proper wound closure to prevent infection, promote healing, and secure the implanted device in place [1].

The process involves three-layer suturing of the subcutaneous pocket at each incision site utilizing various techniques depending on the wound closure goal. Sutures are grouped by several different characteristics. The main factors to classify suture types include absorbable versus nonabsorbable, synthetic versus natural, and monofilament versus multifilament (Fig. 43.1). Each type of suture should be carefully considered to optimize wound closure after ITDD implantation [31].

The first step in the wound closure of an ITDD is to approximate the deep subcutaneous tissues using absorbable sutures. Absorbable sutures are those that lose most of their tensile strength over a few weeks to several months. Synthetic absorbable options, such as Monocryl, Vicryl, and PDS II, are recommended and are commonly utilized to provide temporary support while the tissues heal. These synthetic materials are designed to be absorbed by the body by hydrolysis,

- Absorbable vs. non-absorbable
- Synthetic vs. natural
- Monofilament vs. multifilament

FIGURE 43.1 The main factors to consider while classifying and choosing ideal suture types for ITDD wound closure.

which results in minimal tissue inflammation. Natural materials should be avoided as they are degraded by proteolysis and result in relatively higher amounts of tissue inflammation [32].

After the deep subcutaneous fascial layers are sutured, finish the subcutaneous wound closure with subcuticular sutures. Similar to that of deep wound closure, Vicryl or Monocryl is commonly used. These sutures demonstrate various relative advantages and disadvantages with comparable rates of complications. Vicryl has advantages given its multifilament structure. As such, it is considered to be more secure and easier to handle due to a lower tendency to return to its original shape. Meanwhile, Monocryl is less likely to form a hypertrophic scar than Vicryl due to its monofilament structure. Thus, either suture material choice is reasonable [33].

For the superficial skin closure, nonabsorbable synthetic sutures, such as Ethilon and Prolene, are recommended to provide long-term support with minimal tissue reactivity. The sutures ensure the wound remains securely closed during the healing process. Natural nonabsorbable sutures, such as surgical silk, should be avoided due to higher rates of infection and inflammation compared to synthetic alternatives [34].

The final step involves solidifying the wound with adhesives such as surgical glue and dressing the superficial wound with sterile steri-strips. After wound closure, a postclosure assessment should be performed. Assess for the presence, type and volume of exudate. This includes serous, serosanguineous, or purulent exudate. Assess the wound margins for tunneling, undermining, fibrotic changes or dehiscence. Verify there are no signs of infection such as malodorous scent, warmth, tenderness, or delayed healing (Tables 43.2 and 43.3).

Postoperative care

The postoperative course for patients following implantation of an intrathecal drug delivery system shares many similarities with other commonly performed medical device-related surgeries. However, there are important considerations unique to intrathecal pumps that can be encountered in that time period. These can be categorized as surgery-specific, device-related, and medication-related considerations.

Intrathecal pump implantation is a neuraxial procedure. In the immediate postoperative period, the surgeon must be vigilant for bleeding complications and infectious complications. New onset neurological deficits within the first several hours following surgery may be indicative of an epidural hematoma [35]. Surgical site infections typically occur during the first 3 months following surgery [36]. These can include superficial incisional infections, deep incisional infections that commonly compromise the device, and epidural abscesses. The presence of an infection in the postoperative period will commonly necessitate removal of the device components. The onset of a postdural puncture headache (PDPH) is common after intrathecal pump placement. Neuman et al. reported a 23% incidence of PDPH amongst 285 patients evaluated over a 20-year period [37]. The majority of patients reporting PDPH symptoms can be successfully treated conservatively; however, an epidural blood patch procedure can be considered for patients with persistent symptoms. The need for surgical exploration for primary dural repair is rare.

TABLE 43.2 Absorbable sutures.

I	II	III
Synthetic	Monocryl Vicryl PDS II	Monofilament Multifilament Monofilament
Natural	Chromic gut Plain gut	Monofilament Monofilament

Column I, absorbable synthetic versus natural; *Column II*, examples of absorbable synthetic and natural sutures; *Column III*, absorbable suture examples monofilament versus multifilament; *Monocryl*, poliglecaprone 25; *PDS II*, polydioxanone; *Vicryl*, polyglactin 910.

TABLE 43.3 Nonabsorbable sutures.

I	II	III
Synthetic	Ethanol Prolene	Monofilament Monofilament
Natural	Surgical cotton Surgical silk Surgical steel	Multifilament Multifilament Mono- or multifilament

Column I, nonabsorbable synthetic versus natural; *Column II,* examples of nonabsorbable synthetic and natural sutures; *Column III,* nonabsorbable suture examples monofilament versus multifilament; *Ethilon,* nylon; *Prolene,* polypropylene.

Device-specific considerations can be subdivided into factors related to the two main components of an intrathecal drug delivery system (IDDS), the catheter and the pump. Goel et al. have estimated that catheter complications account for 25% of adverse events following IDDS surgery [37,38]. Potential catheter-related complications include migration, occlusion, kinking, catheter shearing, and disconnection from the pump or extension piece [18,35]. Intrathecal catheter tip granuloma formation is believed to most commonly be associated with increasing drug concentrations over the course of therapy and would be an exceedingly rare complication during the immediate postoperative period. Due to the risk of catheter migration, patients should be strongly advised to abide by postoperative activity restrictions. Consideration can be given to lumbosacral orthosis utilization to prevent excessive bending and twisting activities. Cerebrospinal fluid (CSF) leak is another potential complication related to catheter placement. Seroma is a common complication related to the pump. If clinically relevant, glucose testing can help differentiate between CSF and third-space fluid. Usage of an abdominal binder for 6 weeks following intrathecal pump implantations and pump replacements is recommended. Compression and conservative management are generally recommended for seroma management. Drainage of symptomatic seromas is a therapeutic option, but does introduce the risk of infection. As such, prevention with compression is the best treatment [35].

The three primary medication-related considerations during the postoperative period are when therapy is initiated, initial dosing recommendations, and medication side effects. The two most common times for initiation of intrathecal therapy are immediately after surgery or 10–14 days postoperatively. When therapy is initiated immediately, the medication is placed inside the pump reservoir during the surgical procedure. Alternatively, the intrathecal pump may be implanted with sterile water or saline remaining in the reservoir. Then, a pump refill procedure is performed approximately 10–14 days after surgery, with therapy initiated at that time. The 2017 PACC publication (Table 43.4) provides guidance for starting dosages for the medications commonly initiated for pump therapy. Adverse events related to intrathecal opioid medication include pruritus, nausea, vomiting, urinary retention, peripheral edema, and respiratory depression. Intrathecal ziconotide may cause nausea, nystagmus, dizziness, ataxia, agitation, hallucination, and sedation [1]. The risk for respiratory depression with intrathecal opioids appears to be dose-dependent, as data indicate that respiratory depression has not been observed with starting Morphine dosages less than 200 μg per day [23,39]. Patient reports

TABLE 43.4 Recommended starting dosage ranges of intrathecal medications for long-term therapy delivery.

Drug	Recommendation of starting dose[a]
Morphine	0.1–0.5 mg/day
Hydromorphone	0.01–0.15 mg/day
Ziconotide	0.5–1.2 mcg/day (to 2.4 mcg/day per product labeling)
Fentanyl	25–75 mcg/day
Bupivacaine	0.01–4 mg/day
Clonidine	20–100 mcg/day
Sufentanil	10–20 mcg/day

[a]*Starting doses of continuous intrathecal delivery should be half of the trial dose for opioid-based medications.*
Table from 2017 Polyanalgesic Consensus Conference: Recommendations on Intrathecal Drug Infusion Systems Best Practices and Guidelines.

of urinary retention should be addressed in a timely manner through dose adjustment, medication rotation, or therapy discontinuation to avoid serious complications such as bladder rupture. Foley catheter placement also increases the risk of urinary tract infection. Peripheral edema typically has an onset within the first few weeks of therapy. The mechanism for opioid-induced edema is not well understood; however, it is postulated that hydrophilic opioids may stimulate posterior pituitary secretion of vasopressin, resulting in water retention and urinary retention [35]. Treatment of opioid-induced lower extremity edema includes conservative treatment with compression, diuretics, and opioid dose reduction. If symptoms persist, opioid rotation is likely necessary.

References

[1] Deer TR, Pope JE, Hayek SM, et al. The polyanalgesic consensus conference (PACC): recommendations for intrathecal drug delivery. Neuromodulation Technol Neural Interf 2017;20(2):96–132.

[2] Pope JE, Deer TR, Falowski S. Clinical trials in neuromodulation: a comprehensive review of literature. Neuromodulation 2014;17(3):191–9.

[3] Penn RD, Paice JA. Chronic intrathecal morphine for intractable pain. J Neurosurg 2018;59(5):933–7.

[4] Hayek SM, Hanes MC, Pope JE, et al. Intrathecal therapy for cancer and non-cancer pain. Pain Med 2011;12(4):755–68.

[5] Deer TR, Pope JE, Falowski S, et al. The neuromodulation appropriateness consensus committee on best practices for intrathecal drug delivery. Neuromodulation Technol Neural Interf 2019;22(6):675–95.

[6] Smith HS, Deer TR, Wallace MS. The role of intrathecal therapy in the treatment of chronic pain. Pain Med 2020;21(1):26–34.

[7] Wallace MS, Rauck RL, Fisher R, et al. Intrathecal drug delivery for pain: safety and efficacy of trialing methods. Neuromodulation 2015;18 (8):735–41.

[8] Cohen SP, Dragovich A. Intrathecal analgesia. Anesthesiol Clin December 2007;25(4):863–82. https://doi.org/10.1016/j.anclin.2007.07.001.

[9] Deer TR, Hayek SM, Grider JS, et al. The polyanalgesic consensus conference (PACC): intrathecal drug delivery guidance on safety and therapy optimization when treating chronic noncancer pain. Neuromodulation October 2024;27(7):1107–39. https://doi.org/10.1016/j.neurom.2024.03.003.

[10] Chen GH, Spiegel MA, Magram YC, et al. Evaluation of fixed intrathecal bupivacaine infusion doses in the oncologic population. Neuromodulation October 2020;23(7):984–90. https://doi.org/10.1111/ner.13161.

[11] Brogan SE, Odell DW, Sindt JE, et al. Dorsal versus ventral intrathecal catheter tip location and effect on dose escalation and opioid use in patients with cancer pain. Neuromodulation August 2023;26(6):1233–9. https://doi.org/10.1016/j.neurom.2022.02.230.

[12] Podgorski EP G, Cain C, Weaver T. Targeted drug delivery: dorsal receptors mean dorsal catheter tip placement is critical. 2023. p. S97.

[13] Abd-Elsayed A, Abejón González D, Abad Salom C. Intrathecal pump implant. In: Abd-Elsayed A, editor. Neuromodulation techniques for the spine. Elsevier; 2024. p. 194–210. Chap. 23.

[14] Bagnall D. The use of spinal cord stimulation and intrathecal drug delivery in the treatment of low back-related pain. Phys Med Rehabil Clin November 2010;21(4):851–8. https://doi.org/10.1016/j.pmr.2010.06.004.

[15] Walkowski, Singla AK, Vivian DG, editors. Pain procedures in clinical practice. 3rd ed. Hanley & Belfus; 2011. p. 483–506.

[16] Belverud S, Mogilner A, Schulder M. Intrathecal pumps. Neurotherapeutics 2008;5(1):107–14.

[17] Ethans K. Intrathecal baclofen therapy: indications, pharmacology, surgical implant, and efficacy. Acta Neurochir Suppl 2007;97(1):155–62.

[18] Follett KA, et al. A prospective study of catheter-related complications of intrathecal drug delivery systems. J Pain Symptom Manag 2000;19 (3):209–15.

[19] Beall DP, Munk PL, DePalma MJ, Davis T, Amirdelfan K, Hunter CW. Intrathecal pump drug delivery. In: Medical radiology; 2022. p. 192–200.

[20] Furnish T, Peters Hamsher C, Wallace MS. Intrathecal drug delivery. In: Practical management of pain. Elsevier; 2023. p. 963–79. Chapter 72.

[21] Van Zundert J, Rauck R. Intrathecal drug delivery in the management of chronic pain. Best Pract Res Clin Anaesthesiol 2023;37(2):157–69.

[22] Bottros MM, Christo PJ. Current perspectives on intrathecal drug delivery. J Pain Res 2014;7:615–26. https://doi.org/10.2147/JPR.S37591.

[23] Prager J, Deer T, Levy R, Bruel B, Buchser E, Caraway D, Cousins M, Jacobs M, McGlothlen G, Rauck R, Staats P, Stearns L. Best practices for intrathecal drug delivery for pain. Neuromodulation 2014;17(4):354–72. https://doi.org/10.1111/ner.12146.

[24] Ver DA, Vranken JH, Puylaert M, Hayek S, Mikhail N, Van Zundert J. Intrathecal drug administration in chronic pain syndromes. Pain Pract 2014;14(5):461–76. https://doi.org/10.1111/papr.12111.

[25] Stearns LM, Abd-Elsayed A, Perruchoud C, et al. Intrathecal drug delivery systems for cancer pain: an analysis of a prospective, multicenter product surveillance registry. Anesth Analg 2020;130(2):289–97. https://doi.org/10.1213/ANE.0000000000004425.

[26] Deer TR, Smith HS, Cousins M, et al. Consensus guidelines for the selection and implantation of patients with noncancer pain for intrathecal drug delivery. Pain Physician 2010;13(3):E175–213. https://doi.org/10.36076/ppj.2010/13/e175.

[27] Harsh V, Viswanathan A. Surgical/radiological interventions for cancer pain. Curr Pain Headache Rep 2013;17:331. https://doi.org/10.1007/s11916-013-0331-1.

[28] Hamza M, Doleys D, Wells M, et al. Prospective study of 3-year follow-up of low-dose intrathecal opioids in the management of chronic nonmalignant pain. Pain Med 2012;13(10):1304–613. https://doi.org/10.1111/j.1526-4637.2012.01451.

[29] National Center for Biotechnology Information. Intrathecal drug delivery: a practical guide. In: Bookshelf; 2019. https://www.ncbi.nlm.nih.gov/books/NBK538237/.

[30] Medtronic. SynchroMed II 8637 programmable implant manual. Medtronic; 2022.

[31] Li L, Shao Q, He W, et al. Close orthopedic surgery skin incision with combination of barbed sutures and running subcuticular suturing technique for less dermal tension concentration: a finite element analysis. J Orthop Surg Res 2023;18(1):333. https://doi.org/10.1186/s13018-023-03755-z.

[32] Lloyd JD, Marque MJ 3rd, Kacprowicz RF. Closure techniques. Emerg Med Clin 2007;25(1):73–81. https://doi.org/10.1016/j.emc.2007.01.002.

[33] Niessen FB, Spauwen PH, Kon M. The role of suture material in hypertrophic scar formation: Monocryl vs. Vicryl-rapide. Ann Plast Surg 1997;39(3):254–60. https://doi.org/10.1097/00000637-199709000-00006.

[34] Selvi F, Cakarer S, Can T, Kirli Topcu Sİ, Palancioglu A, Keskin B, Bilgic B, Yaltirik M, Keskin C. Effects of different suture materials on tissue healing. J Istanbul Univ Fac Dent 2016;50(1):35–42. https://doi.org/10.17096/jiufd.79438.

[35] Deer, et al. The polyanalgesic consensus conference (PACC): recommendations for intrathecal drug delivery: guidance for improving safety and mitigating risks. Neuromodulation 2017;20:155–76.

[36] Fluckiger, et al. Device-related complications of long-term drug therapy via implanted pumps. Spinal Cord 2008;46:639–43.

[37] Neuman SA, Eldrige JS, Qu W, Freeman ED, Hoelzer BC. Post dural puncture headache following intrathecal drug delivery system placement. Pain Physician 2013;16(2):101–7.

[38] Goel, et al. Adverse events and complications associated with intrathecal delivery systems: insights from the manufacturer and user facility device experience (MAUDE) database. Neuromodulation 2021;24(7):1181–9.

[39] Hatheway, et al. Embrace TDD primary objective results: clinical success rate with low dose intrathecal morphine monotherapy (LDITM). Neuromodulation 2022;25(8):S9.

Chapter 44

Drug selection and dosing strategies of intrathecal delivery

Jay S. Grider[1], Christopher J. Mallard[2], Hamzah Adel Ramawad[4], Jonathan Paris[5], Daniel Wang[3] and Adelaide Viguri[6]

[1]*Div Interventional Pain, UofL Health, Louisville, KY, United States;* [2]*University of Kentucky, Lexington, KY, United States;* [3]*University of Miami Miller School of Medicine/Health System, Miami, FL, United States;* [4]*Center for Pain Medicine & Surgery Center, Fargo, ND, United States;* [5]*Center for Pain Management at Stony Brook Medicine, Stony Brook, NY, United States;* [6]*Regenerative Pain & Spine, Chicago, IL, United States*

Introduction

Intrathecal drug delivery (ITDD) is an accepted modality of neuromodulation in the advanced treatment of patients with chronic spinal, neuropathic, and appendicular skeletal pain. A deep understanding of the pharmacology pharmacokinetics and treatment nuances for each of the medications available for intrathecal drug delivery are the key to excellent outcomes for patients. In this chapter we will create a broad overview of the latest information regarding opiates, local anesthetics, ziconotide, and baclofen in the treatment of chronic spinal pain and spasticity. In addition adjuvant medications such as clonidine will be reviewed. The treatment options are constantly evolving and the interested reader is directed toward the Poly Analgesic Consensus Committee guidelines (PACC) as they are updated every 2 to 3 years.

Initial drug selection: opioids

Utilizing opioids for intrathecal drug delivery (ITDD) is a well-established method for managing chronic pain, particularly when other treatments have failed. It allows for targeted delivery to the spinal cord. This enables the reduction of systemic side effects in addition to relatively lower doses compared to oral or parenteral administration. Intrathecal opioids further allows for more effective pain control for patients with refractory pain conditions [1,2]. Adverse effects include respiratory depression, nausea, vomiting, pruritus, and urinary retention; risk of inflammatory masses/granulomas especially with chronic morphine infusion; and device-related complications including catheter or pump malfunction and infection [3–5].

The choice between hydrophilic and lipophilic opioids is crucial due to their differing pharmacokinetic properties and clinical implications.

Hydrophilic opioids

Hydrophilic opioids such as morphine and hydromorphone can have a slower onset and longer duration of action due to their limited ability to cross lipid membranes. This effect results in a more localized response within the cerebrospinal fluid (CSF) and a broader spread within the intrathecal space. Morphine, for instance, is often used for continuous infusion due to its prolonged action and extensive receptor binding in the dorsal horn of the spinal cord. Hydrophilic opioids are preferred for continuous infusion rather than single-shot administration because their prolonged action can provide sustained analgesia with fewer fluctuations in pain control [1,6].

Lipophilic opioids

Lipophilic opioids such as fentanyl and sufentanil have a rapid onset and shorter duration of action due to their ability to quickly cross lipid membranes and enter systemic circulation. This results in a more localized and intense analgesic effect

A Modern Atlas for Implantable Devices of the Spine, Brain, and Nerve. https://doi.org/10.1016/B978-0-443-36528-7.00003-0

but with a limited spread within the CSF. Lipophilic opioids are often used for single-shot administration due to their rapid onset, making them suitable for acute pain management. However, their rapid clearance and potential for early supraspinal side effects limit their use in continuous infusion [6].

Monitoring after trials

Patients undergoing ITDD trials should be closely monitored for efficacy and adverse effects. When given initially, hospitalization is often recommended to observe for signs of respiratory depression, hypotension, and other acute side effects. Continuous monitoring of pain relief, functional improvement, and side effects is essential. Adjustments to the dosage or opioid selection may be necessary based on the patient's response and tolerance [7].

The choice between hydrophilic and lipophilic opioids for ITDD depends on the clinical scenario and different factors including duration of action and intended effect. Hydrophilic opioids are preferred for continuous infusion due to their prolonged effect, while lipophilic opioids are suitable for single-shot administration due to their rapid onset. Careful monitoring and dose adjustments are crucial to optimize therapeutic outcomes and minimize complications.

Initial drug selection implantation: other drugs (third and fourth line combinations from PACC guidelines for initial dosing)

The Polyanalgesic Consensus Conference (PACC) guidelines provide a structured approach for the selection and combination of intrathecal drugs for pain management. For third-line drug combinations, the PACC guidelines recommend the following [8–10]:

- Morphine with bupivacaine: This combination leverages the synergistic effects of an opioid with a local anesthetic to enhance pain relief and reduce opioid dosage requirements.
- Hydromorphone with bupivacaine: Similar to morphine-bupivacaine, this combination is used for patients who may not tolerate morphine or require an alternative opioid.
- Fentanyl with bupivacaine: This combination is used for patients needing a more lipophilic opioid (and thus rapid onset/faster clearance) with a local anesthetic for enhanced analgesia

For fourth-line drug combinations, the PACC guidelines recommend the following [8–10]:

- Morphine with clonidine: Clonidine, an alpha-2 adrenergic agonist, is added to enhance analgesic effects and provide additional pain relief, particularly in neuropathic pain.
- Hydromorphone with clonidine: This combination is used for patients who require an alternative to morphine and benefit from the addition of clonidine.
- Fentanyl with clonidine: This combination is used for patients who need a lipophilic opioid (and thus rapid onset/faster clearance) with the added benefits of clonidine.

The PACC guidelines emphasize that these combinations are considered after first and second-line therapies have failed. The choice of combination depends on the patient's specific pain characteristics, previous response to intrathecal therapy, and potential side effects. As always, monitoring for efficacy and adverse effects is critical to optimize therapeutic outcomes and minimize complications [8–10].

Dose titration in continuous flow

Continuous flow is the most common initial protocol for intrathecal drug delivery. The continuous infusion method is a specific daily dose delivered via continuous flow or repeated microboluses over a 24-hour period. It has been recommended for non-cancer pain that dosing adjustments begin with increments somewhere between 10% and 25% every 1 to 2 weeks to evaluate symptom relief and side effects. If the pain remains uncontrolled after 4-5 adjustments, medication rotation or combination therapy may be required. Regarding cancer-related pain, more aggressive titration schedules are adopted due to the urgency of symptom control, with adjustments occurring every few days [9]. While continuous flow strategies remain standard, the specific drug, concentration, and delivery rate should be tailored to each patient [9].

Application of PTM to continuous flow

Patient Therapy Manager (PTM) technology has been increasingly integrated into continuous flow intrathecal therapy to allow for patient-activated analgesia. PTM enhances pain management by enabling patients to administer additional doses during pain flares while maintaining a baseline infusion rate. PTM bolus doses can be administered at intervals programmed to prevent overdose, or side effects ensuring patient safety. Ilias and Todoroff found that satisfaction and acceptance of the PTM was >80% with physicians and patients reporting individualized treatment with better analgesia, and increased independence in a study optimizing pain control with implantable pumps [9].

Opioids and PTM use

When integrated with PTM, the intrathecal opioids provide patients with the flexibility to address episodic pain exacerbations. However, the cumulative effects of PTM boluses, especially in patients already receiving continuous opioid infusions, require careful monitoring to prevent respiratory depression, sedation, and other opioid-related side effects [3].

Combination therapy: opioids and bupivacaine

The addition of bupivacaine, an amide local anesthetic, to intrathecal opioids can enhance pain relief by addressing both nociceptive and neuropathic components of chronic pain. Bolus doses containing opioid-bupivacaine combinations can potentially provide broader pain relief. It has been shown that the opioid-bupivacaine therapy can attenuate opioid tolerance and dose-related adverse effects. However, due to the additive effects of these medications cumulative side effects must be managed with careful dosing adjustments and patient education [11,12].

Combination therapy: opioids and clonidine

Clonidine, an alpha-2 adrenergic agonist, is often combined with opioids in intrathecal therapy to improve analgesia and reduce opioid requirements. PTM boluses containing opioid-clonidine combinations are effective for managing episodic pain flares. However, clonidine's additive effects on blood pressure and sedation must be considered. At excessive doses clonidine can lead to bradycardia, hypotension and sedation [9].

Ziconotide monotherapy and combination therapy

Ziconotide is the only non-opioid intrathecal medication approved for chronic pain by the Food and Drug Administration (FDA). Ziconotide acts by blocking presynaptic N-type calcium channels in the dorsal horn of the spinal cord, which can reduce pain in opioid tolerant patients. PTM use with ziconotide enables patients to self-administer boluses during acute pain episodes. However, given ziconotide's steep dose-response curve, narrow therapeutic index, and side effect profile, PTM dosing requires cautious titration to avoid side effects like dizziness, nausea, and confusion.

Combination therapy with ziconotide and other agents can improve efficacy but demands close attention to cumulative dosing effects of the combined medications. Case studies have highlighted the effectiveness of PTM ziconotide in reducing emergency visits and managing episodic neuropathic pain [13].

Continuous flow is typically the most common initial protocol for intrathecal drug delivery by providing a specific daily over a 24-hour period. PTM technology, when applied to continuous flow systems, enhances intrathecal therapy by providing individualized patient-controlled analgesia. Whether used with opioids alone, ziconotide alone, or combination therapies, PTM use has been shown to improve patient satisfaction and outcomes. When using either continuous dosing or PTM strategies ongoing close monitoring and tailored dosing regimens remain key to balancing efficacy, side effects and safety.

Evidence for combination therapy

Literature has shown that the addition of bupivacaine to opioids intrathecally blunts opioid dose escalation while also improving analgesia. The (PACC) strongly support the use of bupivacaine as the most common adjuvant to opioids, with combination therapy recommended early in the treatment algorithm for chronic pain patients.

Another advantage of opioid/bupivacaine therapy is its ability to attenuate opioid tolerance and dose-related adverse effects. By allowing for lower opioid doses, this combination minimizes the risk of opioid-induced hyperalgesia, granuloma formation, and other complications associated with chronic high-dose opioid therapy [9].

Kumar et al. has shown that adding bupivacaine to opioid therapy in patients with mixed nociceptive and neuropathic pain not only restored pain control but also improved activity levels and quality of life metrics [11,12]. Hayek et al.'s data further supports the opioid-sparing effects of this combination. In patients receiving intrathecal opioid therapy, the addition of bupivacaine resulted in a significantly lower rate of opioid dose escalation over 6 and 12 months. Specifically, the rate of dose increase was markedly lower in the opioid + bupivacaine cohort compared to the opioid-only group. Also, patients in opioid + bupivacaine cohort were more likely to achieve 30% or greater pain relief than those in the opioid only group [11].

Conditions responding to combination therapy

The combination of opioid and bupivacaine can be used in diffuse or localized nociceptive and neuropathic pain states in cancer and non-cancer pain. Catheter location can be important for those with localized pain to enhance segmental analgesia by targeting specific spinal segments involved in pain transmission [9].

For example, it has been demonstrated that in patients with lumbar post-laminectomy syndrome, the addition of bupivacaine to opioids provided significant pain relief while reducing the incidence of opioid-related side effects. It has also been reported improved analgesia in cancer patients with mixed nociceptive and neuropathic pain when bupivacaine was added to morphine. Importantly, this combination therapy also slowed the progression of intrathecal morphine dose escalation during periods of stable analgesia [9].

The combination of opioids and bupivacaine represents an approach to targeted intrathecal drug delivery, in patients with chronic pain syndromes that involve both nociceptive and neuropathic components. Literature has shown that the combination of opioid and bupivacaine provides superior pain relief than opioid alone in multiple pain states. Other advantages to the combination include reduced opioid dose escalation, reduced risk of opioid induced hyperalgesia, and enhanced quality of life.

Baclofen

Initial drug selection trialing for baclofen in intrathecal drug delivery

Intrathecal baclofen (ITB) therapy is widely utilized for the management of severe spasticity that is unresponsive to oral spasmolytic medications or focal treatment. The selection and dosing strategies for baclofen trialing are crucial steps that ensure the optimal efficacy and safety of the treatment. To adopt the best practices for baclofen trialing, follow the Polyanalgesic Consensus Conference (PACC) guidelines and tailor the approach to the patient's needs [14,15].

Dosing strategies for baclofen trialing

The initial phase of ITB trialing involves prudent titration to obtain the minimum effective dose that provides symptom relief without causing adverse effects. The standard practice begins with a test dose administered intrathecally as a bolus, often through a lumbar puncture, to determine the patient's responsiveness to the drug. The standard initial test dose is generally 50 mcg. In certain circumstances, such as in small children or patients who rely on spasticity for mobility, 25 mcg is used. If there is an inadequate response, it is important to distinguish the etiology of the spasticity prior to titrating. For spinal cord-origin spasticity, increase the dose by 10%–30%. For cerebral-origin spasticity, increase the dose by 5%–15%. This incremental approach adjusted to the patient's diagnosis helps to minimize the risk of overdose and allows for close monitoring of the patient's response. During trialing, the patient is observed for 4–8 h to assess efficacy. The screening dose that provides a positive response during the first 24 h is then doubled and administered via an implantable pump with an intrathecal catheter [14–19].

Determining efficacy for baclofen trialing

Determining the efficacy of baclofen trialing involves both objective and subjective assessments. Objective measures, as highlighted in Table 44.1, include clinical scales, biomechanics, and other methods which can be applied to evaluate the clinical benefits of ITB therapy. Subjective measures, such as reports given by the patient and caregiver, also provide valuable insights into the improvements in quality of life and symptom relief. By combining these objective measures and subjective reports, an informed decision can be made about the effectiveness of the baclofen trial and the appropriate dosage for ongoing treatment [19].

Others

Besides the FDA approved medications, the PACC recommends other opioid medications, such as hydromorphone, fentanyl, and sufentanil, and the nonopioids bupivacaine and clonidine, used alone or in combination, for intrathecal (IT)

TABLE 44.1 Objective spasticity measurement methods [6].

Clinical scales	Ashworth scale Modified Ashworth scale
Biomechanics	Pendulum test Isokinetic dynamometers
Neurophysiological-electrophysiological methods	H Response H/M ratio F response, F/M ratio
Walking analysis methods	Dynamic EMG Kinematic and kinetic registration
Other	Ultrasound elastography Myotonometry

administration. Adjuvants for IT medication include midazolam, ketamine, octreotide. Recommended doses for intrathecal bolus trailing and starting dosage ranges for long-term therapy delivery are outlined in Tables 44.2 and 44.3, respectively [9].

Baclofen dosing and drug considerations

When initiating intrathecal baclofen (ITB) therapy, careful consideration must be given to the dosing to ensure effective management of spasticity. The initial dose is typically determined through the screening trial as outlined earlier in this chapter. Some considerations include the patient's baseline spasticity utilizing measures mentioned in Table 44.1, body weight, and response to the test dose. Following a successful trial, the implantation of an intrathecal pump is scheduled and the settings for infusion are set. At this point, the starting dose is often set at the lowest effective dose identified during the trial, and it is gradually titrated based on the patient's clinical response and any adverse effects. Spasticity originating from the spinal cord usually requires 300–800 μg of baclofen daily. Meanwhile, patients with spasticity of cerebral origin typically experience adequate pain relief on daily doses that range from 90 to 703 μg [18].

Once an effective ITB dosing strategy is achieved, regular follow-up and dose adjustments are essential to maintain optimal control of spasticity. Consider adjusting the infusion mode if the patient is experiencing tolerance to the current continuous ITB dosing. Pulsatile bolus dosing, also known as flex dosing, can be classified into variable and regular schedules. This mode of infusion should be considered for more severe cases of primary dystonia that were unresponsive to simple continuous ITB therapy. Thus, it is critical to consistently monitor and adjust baclofen dosing and infusion modes to optimize care for the patient [14,16,18].

TABLE 44.2 PACC recommended doses for intrathecal bolus trialing [9].

Drug	Recommended dose for trialing[a]
Morphine	0.1–0.5 mg
Hydromorphone	0.025–0.1 mg
Ziconotide	1–5 mcg
Fentanyl	15–75 mcg
Bupivacaine	0.5–2.5 mg
Clonidine	5–20 mcg
Sufentanil	5–20 mcg

[a]Starting doses of medication in the opioid-naive patient for outpatient bolus delivery do not exceed 0.15 mg of morphine, 0.04 mg hydromorphone, or 25 mcg fentanyl.

TABLE 44.3 PACC recommended starting dosage ranges of intrathecal medications for long-term therapy delivery [9].

Drug	Recommendation of starting dose[a]
Morphine	0.1–0.5 mg/day
Hydromorphone	0.01–0.15 mg/day
Ziconotide	0.5–1.2 mcg/day (to 2.4 mcg/day per product labeling)
Fentanyl	25–75 mcg/day
Bupivacaine	0.01–4 mg/day
Clonidine	20–100 mcg/day
Sufentanil	10–20 mcg/day

[a]Starting doses of continuous intrathecal delivery should be half of the trial dose for opioid-based medications.

1. Drug Rotation and Drug Holiday

Intrathecal drug delivery (ITDD) systems offer significant benefits for managing chronic pain and spasticity, but long-term use can lead to tolerance, reduced efficacy, and potential side effects. Tolerance is defined as a declining effect during a stable dose of a drug, requiring a dose increase to produce the same previously obtained effect. The hypothesis of the pharmacodynamic mechanism behind tolerance in intrathecal therapy is reduction of the total number of receptors or receptor desensitization. To avert tolerance, drug rotation and drug holidays are given. Different strategies are utilized for opioids (morphine, hydromorphone, fentanyl, sufentanil, methadone), baclofen, and ziconotide [14,20,21].

Baclofen

ITB, similar to IT opioids, can lead to tolerance or tachyphylaxis. However, drug holidays are the more advocated strategy to treat ITB tolerance, along with modulating the infusion mode to pulsatile bolus delivery. The drug holiday period is generally 2–8 weeks. During this time, baclofen is tapered off and most commonly replaced with IT morphine. Other antispasmodic agents, such as tizanidine or diazepam, can be deployed parenterally during a drug rotation to prevent the risk of baclofen withdrawal symptoms. As a result, hospital admissions are mandatory during an ITB drug holiday. In addition, physical therapy and non-pharmacological interventions such as hydrotherapy can be pursued during this period to reduce spasticity pain [9,22,23].

Ziconotide

Ziconotide, unlike opioids and baclofen, does not lead to tolerance. This makes it a valuable option in IT drug rotation strategies. However, its use can be limited by side effects like dizziness, nausea, and cognitive changes. In such cases, temporarily discontinuing ziconotide in a drug holiday can help alleviate these adverse effects. During this period, patients might be managed with other intrathecal medications or oral analgesics. Reintroducing ziconotide at a lower dose or in combination with other agents can help maintain pain control while minimizing side effects [9,24].

Monodose opioids

When considering intrathecal drug delivery, the simplest approach is to utilize monodose opioids in the form of either morphine, hydromorphone, fentanyl, or, in rare cases, sufentanil. Although only morphine is FDA-approved for use in the intrathecal space, all of these medications have been reported in the literature with demonstrated efficacy and safety [9]. Morphine and hydromorphone, being hydrophilic, have advantages in the intrathecal space, as their spread can be facilitated by both infusion and diffusion. On the other hand, fentanyl and sufentanil, due to their lipophilicity, tend to be confined to the region around the intrathecal catheter tip [9].

Regarding intrathecal drug delivery, inferences can be drawn from virtually all published studies concerning monodose opioids. The studies by Grider et al. and Hamza and colleagues outlined the efficacy of monodose opioids using a low-dose approach for treating mechanical or axial low back pain [25,26]. In both studies, the goal was to eliminate or reduce systemic opioids prior to the introduction of IT opioids. This resulted in, stable and effective pain relief with doses as low as 1 mg or less.

The demographics in the Grider study showed no significant age or diagnosis differences, meaning that spinal stenosis, persistent pain after lumbar surgery, and degenerative disc disease all responded well to monodose opioid therapy [25]. However, it should be noted that mixed mechanical and neuropathic pain syndromes, as well as pure neuropathic pain syndromes, were less responsive to monodose opioids than pure mechanical back pain. This suggests that monodose opioid therapy is more effective for axial and possibly appendicular skeletal pain, while neuropathic pain may not respond as well to opioids alone. While the Hamza study did not focus on demographics, it demonstrated sustained efficacy of monodose opioid therapy over a 36-month prospective period [26].

As previously mentioned, when considering monodose opioid therapy, catheter tip placement and the location of pain are critical to ensuring adequate coverage of spinal targets with pharmacologic treatment.

Safety concerns

There are safety concerns that must be addressed when initiating monodose opioid therapy, as outlined by Coffey and colleagues [27]. Ethical drug delivery combined with opioid prescribing should be approached with caution [27]. It has been suggested that doses above 750 μg of intrathecal morphine may pose a risk when combined with oral opioid therapy. This could occur when continuing previously prescribed systemic opioid therapy or in the context of postoperative pain management after intrathecal drug delivery system placement. In either case, caution must be exercised when combining intrathecal opioids with systemic opioids [27]. In the author's experience, it is possible to manage intrathecal drug delivery system placement without prescribing postoperative opioids [25]. The Coffey study suggested that the risk is higher in opioid-naive patients than in those with some degree of opioid tolerance.

The initiation of opioid therapy in a monodose approach is outlined in Table 44.1, from the Poly-analgesic Consensus Committee Guidelines. Note that most opioids are administered in the lowest reported doses, with the understanding that titration in the days and weeks following implantation can be done safely. Patients should be reassured that if they have not been on high doses of systemic opioids, efficacy can often be achieved with lower microgram doses, making titration a relatively rapid process.

Reestablishing efficacy in maintenance therapy

In pioneering work by Anderson and Burchiel, it was first demonstrated that dosing stability is often achieved for several months to years after initial opioid titration [28]. This efficacy is typically maintained over an extended period (months to years). If, after a prolonged period of efficacy, there is a sudden loss of effectiveness, the algorithm outlined in the 2024 PACC guidelines can be followed [9]. If there is pain with infusion, an MRI should be obtained to check for the presence of a granuloma. A catheter side-port study should be conducted to ensure all connections are intact and that there are no hidden breaks in the catheter. Dye should be visible on fluoroscopy or CT imaging to confirm continuity in the intrathecal space. If the system is intact, attention should turn to the possibility of opioid tolerance or lack of efficacy of the pharmacologic agent.

It has been suggested that a rapid mid-therapy trial should be performed, where increases in dose are made in short intervals (e.g., weekly). In this scenario, a patient would be seen weekly or every 10 days, with a 10% increase in dose each time. If no improvement in efficacy is seen, or if only minimal improvement occurs during this rapid titration, rotating to another medication should be considered. It is important to remember that cross-tolerance to opioids is incomplete, so rotating to a different medication may help reestablish efficacy. Based on our experience and consensus opinion in the PACC, it is not uncommon to rotate back to the initial medication after several years, resulting in the reestablishment of efficacy [9].

Conclusion

Given the rapidity with which studies are published which change our thinking concerning the pharmacologic nature and pharmacokinetics of intrathecal drug delivery the interested reader is directed toward the PACC guidelines which are updated every 2 to 3 years. It is clear that intrathecal drug delivery, with three randomized controlled trials evaluating ziconotide and two large observational studies for intrathecal opiate and local anesthetic there established efficacy over the past 2 decades [9]. It will be interesting to see what other pharmacologic agents and therapeutic regimens are introduced in the coming years for this exciting field of drug delivery and study in the treatment of chronic benign pain, cancer pain and spasticity.

References

[1] Aman MM, Mahmoud A, Deer T, et al. The American Society of Pain and Neuroscience (ASPN) best practices and guidelines for the interventional management of cancer-associated pain. J Pain Res 2021;14:2139–64. https://doi.org/10.2147/JPR.S315585.

[2] Smyth C, Ahmadzai N, Wentzell J, et al. Intrathecal analgesia for chronic refractory pain: current and future prospects. Drugs 2015;75 (17):1957–80. https://doi.org/10.1007/s40265-015-0471-1.

[3] Sayed D, Grider J, Strand N, et al. The American Society of Pain and Neuroscience (ASPN) evidence-based clinical guideline of interventional treatments for low back pain. J Pain Res 2022;15:3729–832. https://doi.org/10.2147/JPR.S386879.

[4] Chalil A, Staudt MD, Harland TA, et al. A safety review of approved intrathecal analgesics for chronic pain management. Expet Opin Drug Saf 2021;20(4):439–51. https://doi.org/10.1080/14740338.2021.1889513.

[5] Allen JW, Horais KA, Tozier NA, Yaksh TL. Opiate pharmacology of intrathecal granulomas. Anesthesiology 2006;105(3):590–8. https://doi.org/10.1097/00000542-200609000-00025.

[6] Bujedo BM. Spinal opioid bioavailability in postoperative pain. Pain Pract 2014;14(4):350–64. https://doi.org/10.1111/papr.12099.

[7] Infumorph (morphine sulfate) injection, solution [package insert]. DailyMed. Hikma Pharmaceuticals USA Inc. Revised: December 2025. Accessed 2024.

[8] Hassenbusch SJ, Portenoy RK, Cousins M, et al. Polyanalgesic consensus conference 2003: an update on the management of pain by intraspinal drug delivery– report of an expert panel. J Pain Symptom Manag 2004;27(6):540–63. https://doi.org/10.1016/j.jpainsymman.2004.03.001.

[9] Deer TR, Hayek SM, Grider JS, et al. The polyanalgesic consensus conference (PACC)®: updates on clinical pharmacology and comorbidity management in intrathecal drug delivery for cancer pain. Neuromodulation 2025;28(7):1029–53. https://doi.org/10.1016/j.neurom.2024.08.006.

[10] Karri J, Singh M, Modi DJ, et al. Combination intrathecal drug therapy strategies for pain management. Pain Physician 2021;24(8):549–69.

[11] Hayek SM, McEwan MT, Veizi E, DeLozier SJ, Pogrebetskaya M. Effects of bupivacaine on opioid patient-controlled intrathecal analgesia in chronic pain patients implanted with drug delivery systems. Pain Med 2021;22(1):22–33. https://doi.org/10.1093/pm/pnaa076.

[12] Veizi IE, Hayek SM, Narouze S, Pope JE, Mekhail N. Combination of intrathecal opioids with bupivacaine attenuates opioid dose escalation in chronic noncancer pain patients. Pain Med 2011;12(10):1481–9. https://doi.org/10.1111/j.1526-4637.2011.01232.x.

[13] McDowell GC, Pope JE. Intrathecal ziconotide: dosing and administration strategies in patients with refractory chronic pain. Neuromodulation 2016;19(5):522–32. https://doi.org/10.1111/ner.12392.

[14] Deer TR, Prager J, Levy R, Burton A, Buchser E, Caraway D, et al. Polyanalgesic Consensus Conference–2012: recommendations on trialing for intrathecal (intraspinal) drug delivery: report of an interdisciplinary expert panel. Neuromodulation 2012;15:420–35.

[15] Ethans K. Intrathecal baclofen therapy: indications, pharmacology, surgical implant, and efficacy. In: Sakas DE, Simpson BA, Krames ES, editors. Operative neuromodulation. Acta neurochirurgica supplements, 97/1. Vienna: Springer; 2007. https://doi.org/10.1007/978-3-211-33079-1_21.

[16] Boster AL, Bennett SE, Bilsky GS, Gudesblatt M, Koelbel SF, McManus M, Saulino M. Best practices for intrathecal baclofen therapy: screening test. Neuromodulation 2016;19(6):616–22. https://doi.org/10.1111/ner.12437.

[17] Shah N, Di Napoli R, Padalia D. Implantable intrathecal drug delivery system. In: StatPearls. Treasure Island (FL): StatPearls Publishing; 2025. https://www.ncbi.nlm.nih.gov/books/NBK538237.

[18] Ghanavatian S, Derian A. Baclofen. In: StatPearls. Treasure Island (FL): StatPearls Publishing; 2025. https://www.ncbi.nlm.nih.gov/books/NBK526037/.

[19] Balci BP. Spasticity measurement. Noro Psikiyatr Ars 2018;55(Suppl. 1):S49–53. https://doi.org/10.29399/npa.23339.

[20] Dumas EO, Pollack GM. Opioid tolerance development: a pharmacokinetic/pharmacodynamic perspective. AAPS J 2008;10(4):537–51. https://doi.org/10.1208/s12248-008-9056-1.

[21] Stevens CW, Yaksh TL. Potency of infused spinal antinociceptive agents is inversely related to magnitude of tolerance after continuous infusion. J Pharmacol Exp Therapeut 1989;250:1–8.

[22] Heetla H, Staal M, van Laar T. Tolerance to continuous intrathecal baclofen infusion can be reversed by pulsatile bolus infusion. Spinal Cord 2010;48:483–6. https://doi.org/10.1038/sc.2009.156.

[23] Boster AL, et al. Best practices for intrathecal baclofen therapy: dosing and long-term management. Neuromodulation 2016;19(6):623–31.

[24] Matis G, De Negri P, Dupoiron D, Likar R, Zuidema X, Rasche D. Intrathecal pain management with ziconotide: time for consensus? Brain Behav 2021;11(Suppl. 1):e02055. https://doi.org/10.1002/brb3.2055.

[25] Grider JS, Etscheidt MA, Harned ME, Lee J, Smith B, Lamar C, Bux A. Trialing and maintenance dosing using a low-dose intrathecal opioid method for chronic nonmalignant pain: a prospective 36-month study. Neuromodulation 2016;19(2):206–19. https://doi.org/10.1111/ner.12352.

[26] Hamza M, Doleys D, Wells M, Weisbein J, Hoff J, Martin M, Soteropoulos C, Barreto J, Deschner S, Ketchum J. Prospective study of 3-year follow-up of low-dose intrathecal opioids in the management of chronic nonmalignant pain. Pain Med 2012;13(10):1304–13. https://doi.org/10.1111/j.1526-4637.2012.01451.x.

[27] Coffey RJ, Owens ML, Broste SK, Dubois MY, Ferrante FM, Schultz DM, Stearns LJ, Turner MS. Mortality associated with implantation and management of intrathecal opioid drug infusion systems to treat noncancer pain. Anesthesiology 2009;111(4):881–91.

[28] Anderson VC, PhD B, Kim JMD. A prospective study of long-term intrathecal morphine in the management of chronic nonmalignant pain. Neurosurgery 1999;44(2):289–300.

Further reading

[1] Dominguez E, Sahinler B, Bassam D, Day M, Lou L, Racz G, et al. Predictive value of intrathecal narcotic trials for long-term therapy with implantable drug administration systems in chronic non-cancer pain patients. Pain Pract 2002;2:315–25.
[2] Horn TS, Yablon SA, Stokic DS. Effect of intrathecal baclofen bolus injection on temporospatial gait characteristics in patients with acquired brain injury. Arch Phys Med Rehabil 2005;86:1127–33.
[3] Dahm P, Nitescu P, Appelgren L, Curelaru I. Efficacy and technical complications of long-term continuous intraspinal infusions of opioid and/or bupivacaine in refractory nonmalignant pain: a comparison between the epidural and the intrathecal approach with externalized or implanted catheters and infusion pumps. Clin J Pain 1998;14:4–16.

Chapter 45

Complications of intrathecal drug delivery

Gladstone C. McDowell, II [1], Jacqueline Weisbein[2], Harjot S. Bhandal[3], Daniel Wang[4] and Mark N. Malinowski[5]

[1]*Targeted Care Solutions, Columbus, OH, United States;* [2]*Napa Valley Orthopaedic Medical Group, Napa, CA, United States;* [3]*MarinHealth, Larkspur, CA, United States;* [4]*University of Miami Miller School of Medicine/Health System, Miami, FL, United States;* [5]*Ohio Health Hospital System, Columbus, OH, United States*

Intrathecal catheter problems are relatively infrequent but are the most common source of intrathecal drug delivery system malfunction.

The open or percutaneous placement of an intrathecal catheter carries significant risk and requires adherence to specific surgical techniques, use of fluoroscopic guidance, and vigilance. Whether the patient is in the lateral decubitus or prone position the recommended technique for needle placement is through a paramedian approach, ipsilateral to pocket placement, advancing the Tuohy needle under fluoroscopic guidance preferably below the level of the termination of the spinal cord [1].

The recommended insertion levels are at the L2-3 or L3-4 level, unless previous surgery, anatomical abnormalities, or other extenuating circumstances require placement above this. A shallow angle and strict attention to the position of the needle is important [1,2] (Fig. 45.1). Some authors recommend puncturing the dura with the bevel in the vertical position to theoretically separate the fibers, rather than transect them, and then rotate the bevel superiorly and immediately pass the intrathecal catheter under fluoroscopic guidance into the posterior intrathecal space whenever possible. This approach minimizes the risks of neural injury and catheter kinking. The catheter tip is advanced to the desired level paying close attention to patient response for complaints of paresthesias, or evidence of movement during catheter passage.

In patients under general anesthesia muscle relaxants should be avoided and spinal cord monitoring is recommended [2].

Potential risks during insertion of intrathecal catheter

Neurologic injury

Damage to the spinal cord or nerve roots are among the most feared complications during intrathecal pump implantation. Misplacement of the intrathecal catheter to an intramedullary position in the spinal cord is a rare but severe complication [3].

Lack of attention to the position of the Touhy needle and passage of the catheter centrally or anteriorly within the intrathecal space may be implicated. There may be a higher risk of this going undetected intraoperatively in patients under general anesthesia using paralytic or muscle relaxant agents. The lack of cerebrospinal fluid draining from the catheter should raise immediate concerns and warrant fluoroscopic review and catheter evaluation.

Initial troubleshooting involves performing a catheter study with direct aspiration of CSF. The inability to easily aspirate is suggestive of catheter malposition or occlusion and the injection of aspirated fluid, or contrast, should be avoided and catheter replacement considered. If full aspiration is successful a water-soluble radiographic contrast medium such as Omnipaque may be injected and fluoroscopy used to observe flow from the catheter tip in the AP and lateral projections (Figs. 45.2 and 45.3). This examination may identify catheter position with contrast visible within and adjacent to the catheter or confirm migration from original catheter placement.

A Modern Atlas for Implantable Devices of the Spine, Brain, and Nerve. https://doi.org/10.1016/B978-0-443-36528-7.00021-2

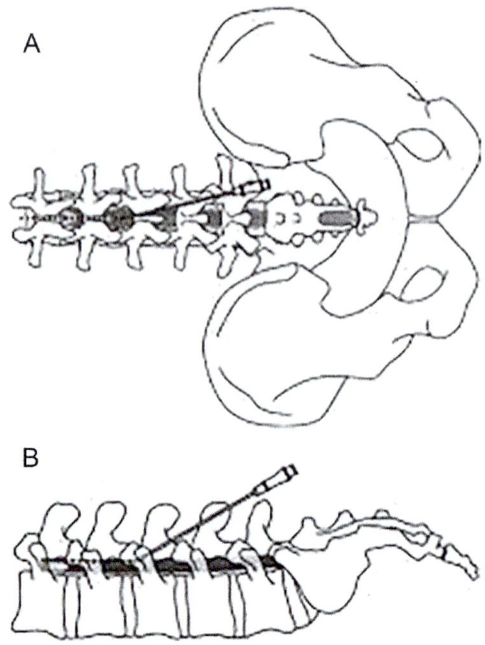

FIGURE 45.1 An illustration showing the recommended paramedian approach to the intrathecal space. AP and lateral views of the lumbar spine and pelvis. *Adapted from Ref. [1].*

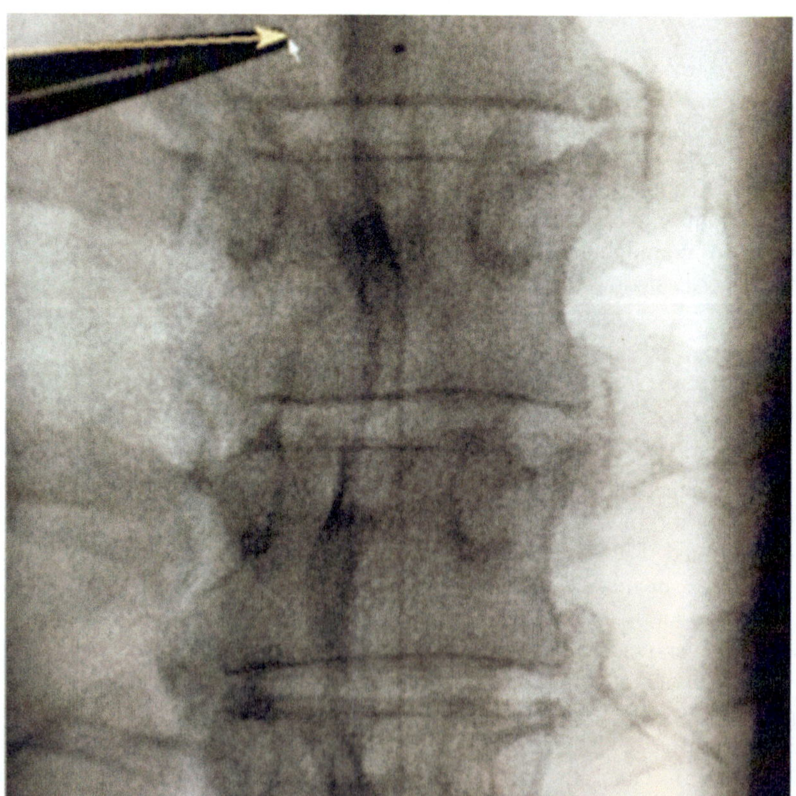

FIGURE 45.2 AP and lateral images confirming catheter position with contrast study. *Images courtesy of Gladstone C. McDowell II MD.*

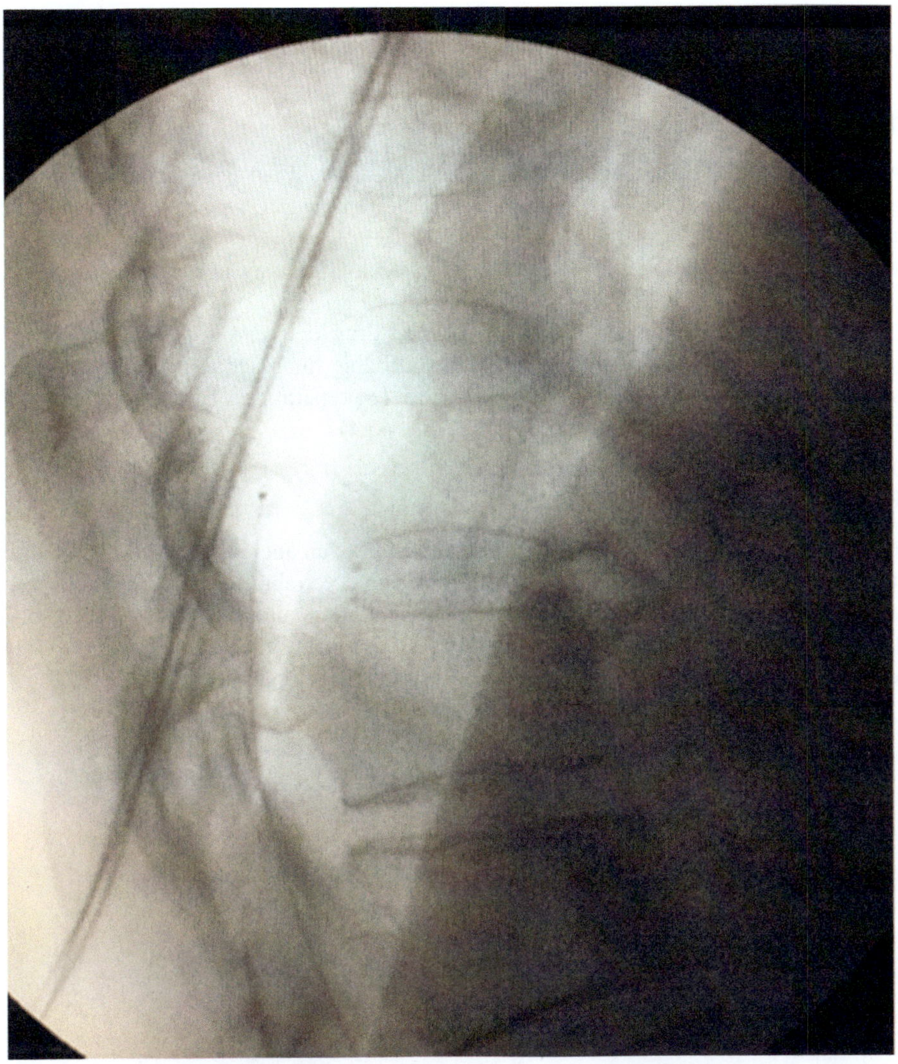

FIGURE 45.3 *Images courtesy of Gladstone C. McDowell II MD.*

Intraperitoneal injury

The risk of peritoneal entry and bowel perforation is rare and may occur during the tunneling procedure with the highest risk during passage to the abdominal pocket location. Tunneling is accomplished by passing the flexible tunneling device between the lumbar incision and superficial pump pocket incision through the subcutaneous adipose tissue of the flank. The tunneling device is usually bent to accommodate the curve of the abdomen and properly passed with intermittent palpation by the nondominant hand to ensure subcutaneous location.

There are a few reports of delayed discovery of intraperitoneal catheter placement with trans-colonic penetration requiring open surgical repair [4].

Attention to position of the tunneling rod, with continuous confirmation of the subcutaneous position through palpation by the nondominant hand, will minimize risk of intraperitoneal passage.

Catheter shearing

Once the intrathecal catheter is in position it is recommended to remove the Touhy needle first, while holding the catheter, and then remove the stylet. Due to the relatively high coefficient of friction between the catheter and its internal stylet, attempting to retract the catheter or stylet through the needle (in the fascia) may risk accordioning the catheter against needle edge resulting in perforation, or total shearing off a portion of the catheter. Should this occur, do not attempt to remove the retained catheter (if not visible) and instead place a purse string to reduce CSF leakage and then repeat paramedian needle access on the contralateral side, or at a different vertebral level.

Cerebrospinal fluid leak at catheter insertion site

Placement of a nonabsorbable purse-string suture through the lumbar dorsal fascia is recommended before removal of the needle and then tightened gently around the catheter, after needle removal, to reduce the likelihood of a CSF leak with hygroma formation [1].

There are reports that smaller needles and this purse string technique may not actually prevent postdural puncture headache.

The incidence of postural puncture headaches after targeted drug delivery implant is approximately 1.8% and if indicated may be treated with epidural blood patch procedures utilizing fluoroscopy below the level of the catheter entry [5]. Refractory cases have been treated with epidural fibrin glue (a preparation of pooled human plasma obtained from plasmapheresis) injection performed under fluoroscopy [6] (Fig. 45.4).

Catheter migration and dislodgement

Placement of an anchor is manufacturer-recommended. The omission of an anchor is tempting to shortened surgical times, but may result in catheter dislodgement and migration from the desired vertebral level, with postoperative development of a hygroma, and increased risk of infection [1]. The initial fascia anchoring suture(s) should also be placed before removal of the Tuohy needle to minimize the risk of catheter damage while placing the needle.

An AP and lateral X-ray images should be obtained to document final catheter position.

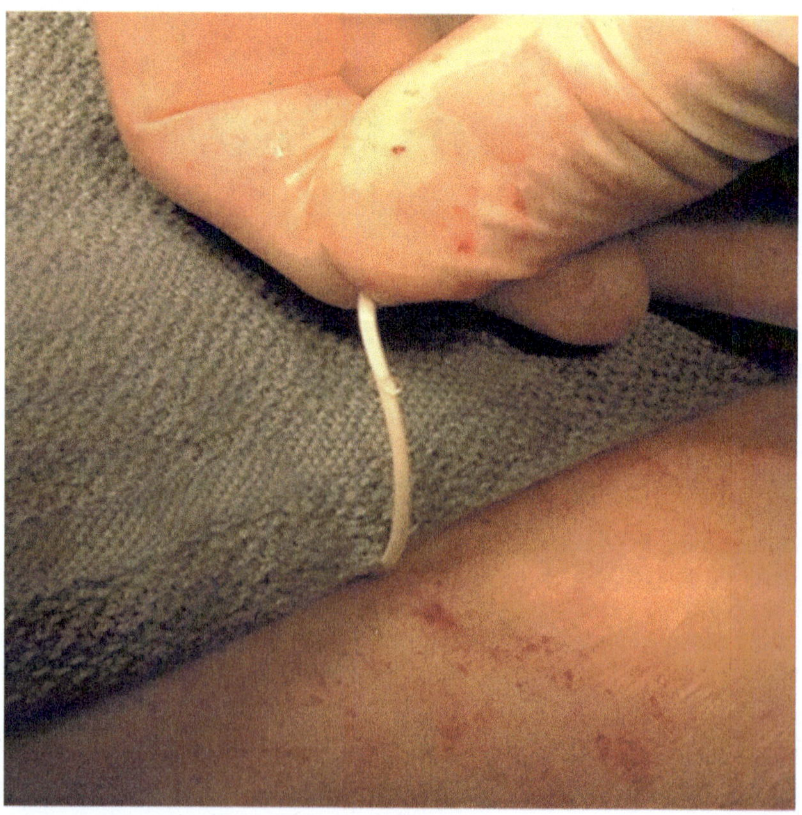

FIGURE 45.4 Evaluation of swelling at lumbar catheter insertion site through catheter access study identified subcutaneous contrast collection. Exploration identified catheter fracture proximal to anchor. *Image courtesy of Eric Grigsby, Napa, CA.*

Epidural hemorrhage

The risk of epidural hemorrhage during placement of the intrathecal catheter is minimal 0.3% in the Maude study and mitigated by stopping preoperative anticoagulants, NSAIDS and supplements [5,7,8] and fluoroscopic guidance during intraspinal access procedure.

Infection

Surgical site infections are described as the second most reported healthcare related infections. The CDC reviewed national data that indicate an increase in the standardized infection ratio you know the surgical categories examined between 2021 and 2022 sharing a 4% increase.

The cost of hospital acquired surgical site infections is estimated to be 28,219 costing the national healthcare budget an estimated $3.3 billion a year [9].

Surgical site infections following intrathecal pump implants typically occur within the first 30–60 days postoperatively. There are reports of infections occurring at later dates, but these are uncommon.

The American Society of Regional Anesthesia and Pain Medicine released new guidelines in 2025.

The rate of SSI is significantly higher among patients with diabetes mellitus with a hemoglobin A1C greater than 7% and perioperative glucose greater than or equal to 200 mg/dL [10].

Tobacco abuse, immunosuppression not related to malignancy, and malnutrition may place patients at higher risk. Patients being treated for cancer are especially susceptible to infections as they are often immunocompromised from the disease or cytotoxic agents.

The risk of infection leading to meningitis is the most devastating and can be mitigated by adherence to preoperative patient screening, bacteriostatic preoperative scrubs and strict adherence to intraoperative sterile surgical technique.

Complications of intrathecal drug delivery pump implantation

Infection

Infections are one of the most prevalent complications following intrathecal pump implantation. Analysis of the Manufacturer and User Facility Device Experience (MAUDE) database has shown that infection and erosion account for approximately 15.7% of reported adverse events [11]. The risk of infection is often related to factors such as improper aseptic technique, patient comorbidities, or hematogenous spread. Clinical presentations range from localized erythema and wound dehiscence to systemic sepsis (Fig. 45.5). Infections may necessitate systemic antibiotic therapy, wound debridement, or complete explantation of the device. Preventative measures include strict sterile techniques during implantation and the use of prophylactic antibiotics [12].

Infection due to patient self-attempted access

A serious but preventable cause of infection occurs when patients attempt to access the pump themselves using nonsterile tools. Unauthorized access efforts, such as attempting to refill or manipulate the pump with household objects or unsterilized needles, can introduce bacterial contamination directly into the device pocket or catheter system (Fig. 45.6). This may lead to localized abscess formation, systemic sepsis, or even pump malfunction due to fluid contamination. Patients who engage in self-access attempts often present with signs of infection, including localized pain, swelling, erythema, fever, and purulent drainage at the pump site. In some cases, these infections necessitate device removal and aggressive antimicrobial therapy. Prevention strategies include thorough patient education on the risks of nonsterile self-access, regular follow-up to address concerns about medication availability, and psychological or addiction support for patients who may be struggling with dependence or fear of withdrawal.

Wound dehiscence

Wound dehiscence, or the separation of surgical wound edges, is another potential complication following intrathecal pump implantation. Dehiscence can result from poor wound healing, infection, excessive tension on the surgical site, or repeated mechanical stress from patient movement. Studies indicate that patients with diabetes, obesity, or chronic steroid use are at increased risk for this complication [13].

Early signs of wound dehiscence include increased drainage, localized pain, and widening of the surgical site (Figs. 45.7 and 45.8). If left untreated, dehiscence can lead to pump or catheter exposure, further increasing the risk of infection

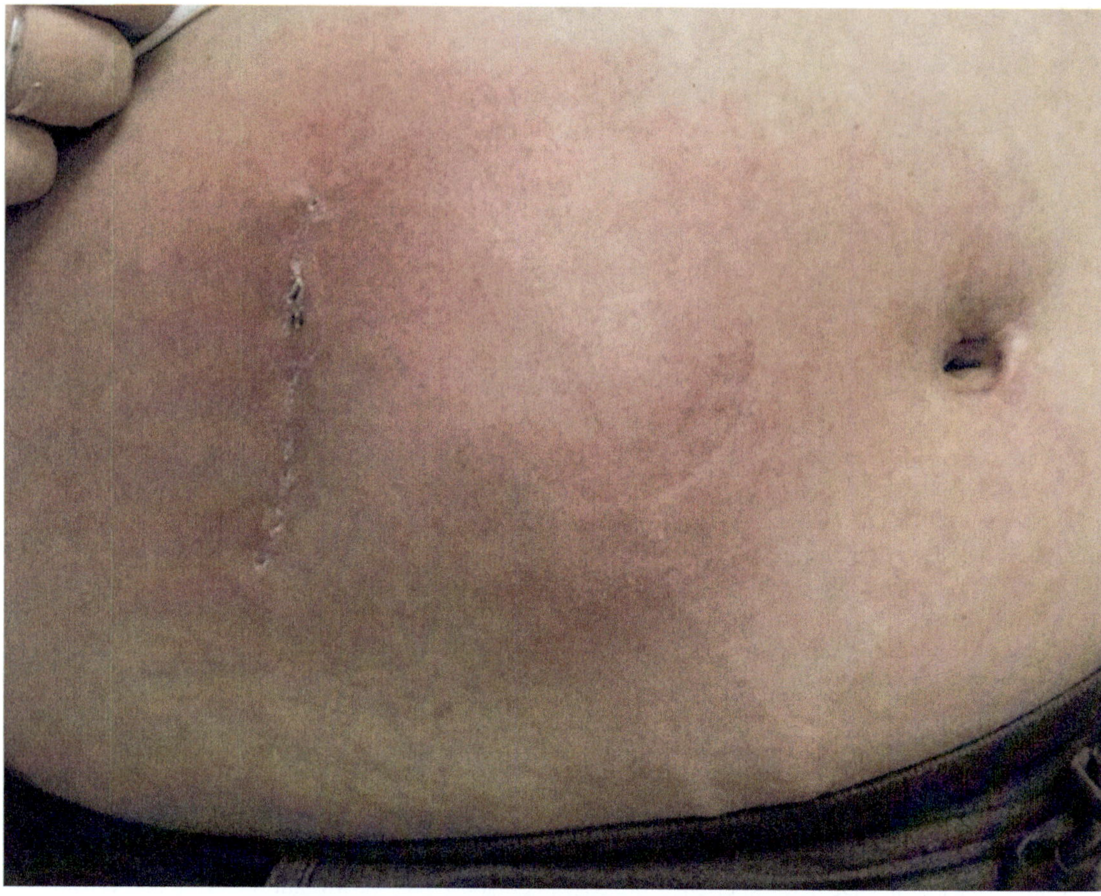

FIGURE 45.5 Pump abscess after implantation. *Image courtesy of Jacqueline Weisbein, DO.*

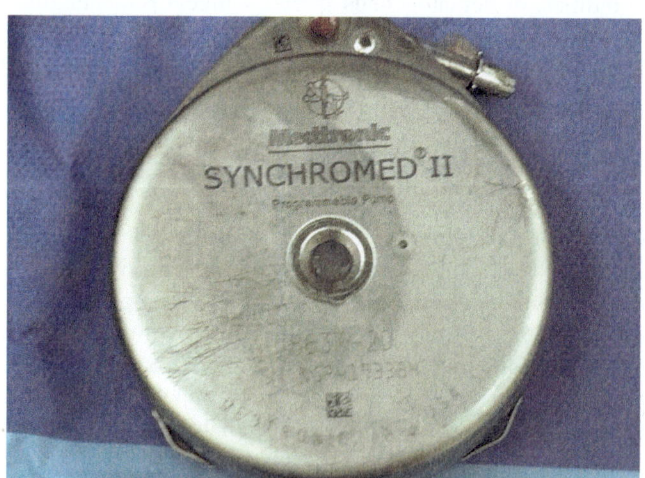

FIGURE 45.6 Patient self-attempted pump access with scratches near refill port. *Image courtesy of Jacqueline Weisbein, DO.*

and requiring surgical revision. Management strategies include wound reinforcement, antibiotic therapy for secondary infection, and in severe cases, surgical reclosure or explantation.

Movement (rotation/flipping)

Pump displacement, including rotation or flipping within the subcutaneous pocket, is another significant concern. This issue can interfere with reservoir refilling, leading to dosing errors and potential medication withdrawal syndromes [14].

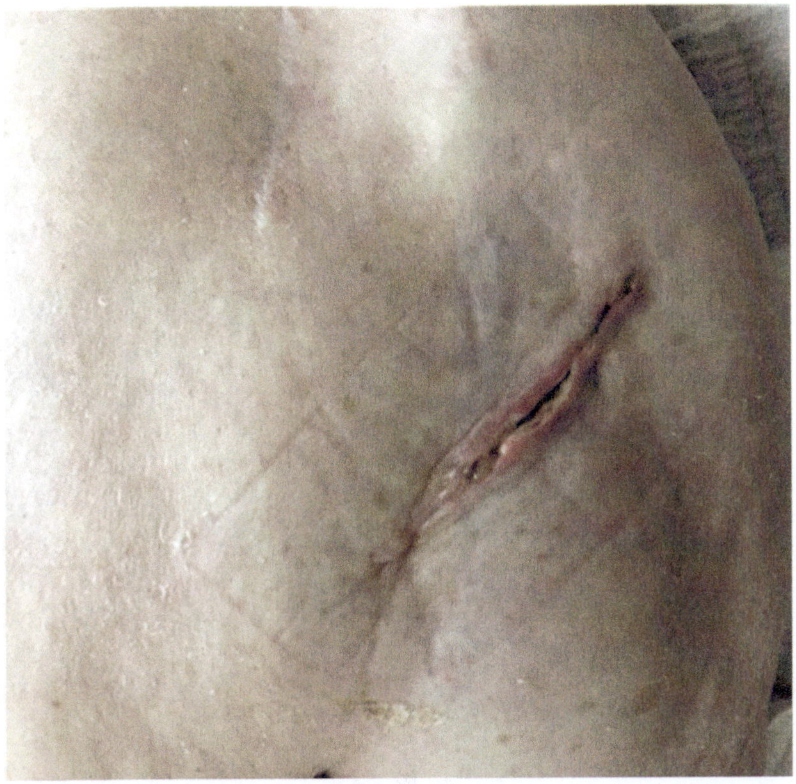

FIGURE 45.7 Early wound separation. *Image courtesy of Jacqueline Weisbein, DO.*

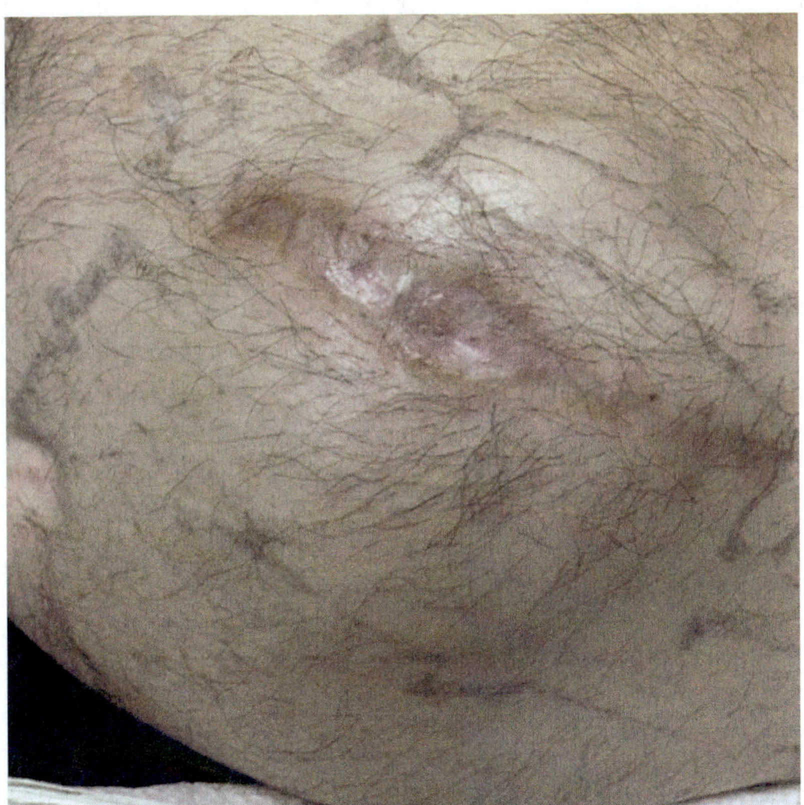

FIGURE 45.8 Delayed incomplete fascial healing-abd. *Image courtesy of Jacqueline Weisbein, DO.*

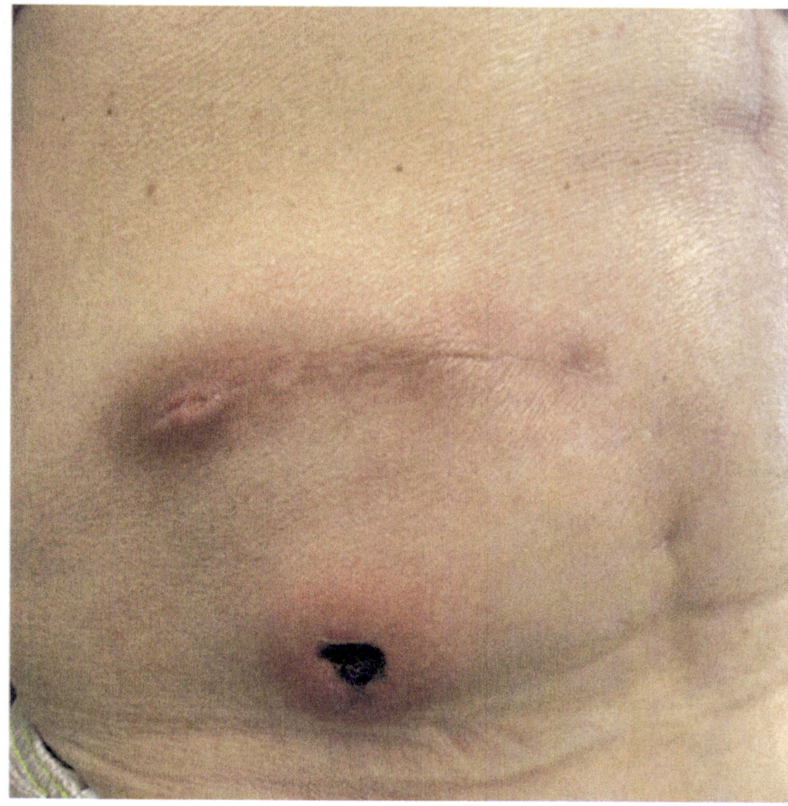

FIGURE 45.9 Posterior lower lumbar pump placement in a patient who contracted COVID several weeks after implantation, requiring intubation in ICU for several weeks, and was not rotated in bed. *Image courtesy of Gladstone C. McDowell II MD.*

Improper anchoring of the pump during implantation, excessive patient movement, or insufficient pocket size may contribute to this complication.

Patients with pump flipping, or rotation, may present with difficulties in refilling the reservoir, localized discomfort, or palpable hardware irregularities. Preventative strategies involve securing the pump with appropriate suture fixation and ensuring a well-formed subcutaneous pocket.

Erosion

Device erosion occurs when the pump or catheter migrates superficially, leading to skin breakdown over the implanted hardware. Prolonged pressure on the overlying skin (Figs. 45.9 and 45.10), poor tissue integrity, and prior infections can increase the risk of erosion. In cases where erosion exposes the pump, there is a high risk of secondary infection and device failure [13].

Treatment of erosion typically requires device removal, surgical repair of the affected area, and, in some cases, reimplantation at an alternate site. Prevention involves ensuring adequate soft tissue coverage and avoiding excess tension or superficial placement of the pump.

Impingement on adjacent structures

Intrathecal pump placement may result in impingement on adjacent anatomical structures, leading to pain, discomfort, or functional impairment. Potential sites of impingement include the iliac crest, ribs, abdominal organs, or neural structures, depending on the implantation site (Fig. 45.11). Incorrect pump positioning or improper pocket formation may contribute to this issue. Patients experiencing impingement may report localized tenderness, reduced mobility, or neurological symptoms. Imaging studies, such as ultrasound or MRI, can assist in diagnosing mechanical compression. Surgical revision or repositioning of the pump may be required in severe cases [11].

Intrathecal drug delivery infusion issues

Section pending from coauthors discussed with Barbara Makinster.

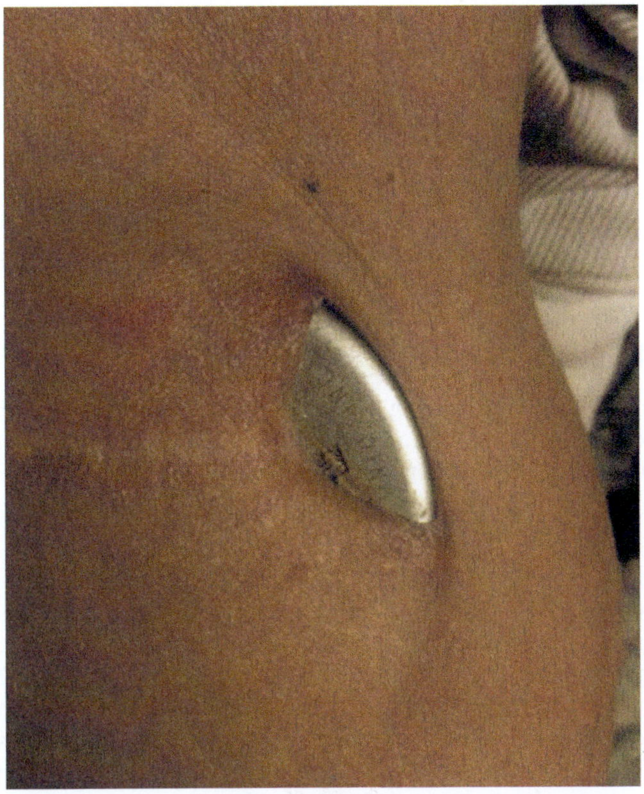

FIGURE 45.10 Abdominal position pump extrusion in wheelchair-bound patient who chronically leans to one side. *Image courtesy of Gladstone C McDowell II MD.*

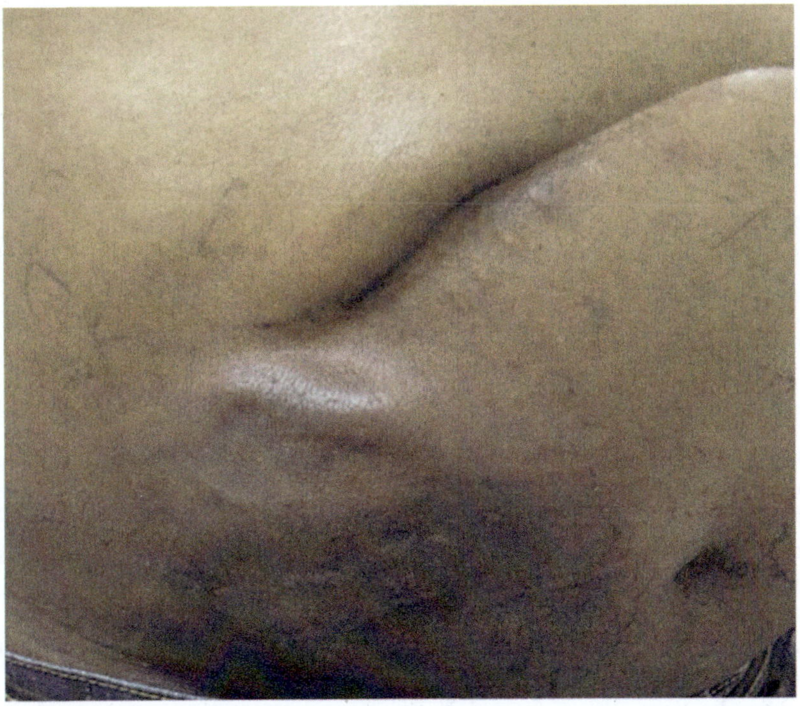

FIGURE 45.11 Pump impinging on anterior iliac crest. *Image courtesy of Jacqueline Weisbein, DO.*

Intrathecal drug delivery system catheter complications: Delayed-onset issues after surgical implantation

Epidemiology

Delayed catheter related complications (DCRC) may occur with an added incidence of 10%–20% of those patients receiving intrathecal drug delivery systems (IDDS). Factors that have been implicated in catheter complications include catheter types, surgical techniques and patient specific risks. Manifestations of these complications may be detected early by discrepancies in reservoir residual volume expected versus calculated, or maybe obvious in late findings such as patient overdose, patient withdrawal symptoms for neurological deficits [10,15].

Etiology and pathophysiology

There are several potential findings when evaluating for catheter complication. These include, but are not limited to, catheter migration or dislodgement, catheter kinking or occlusion, granuloma formation at the catheter tip, catheter fracture/disconnection/maceration, Late onset infectious complications, and catheter tip adhesion or fibrosis [12,15–17].

Catheter migration or dislodgement

Over time, movement of the catheter because of normal spinal motion, patient biomechanical overactivity or improper anchoring can lead to dislodgement or dislocation of the catheter tip from initial placement. Most commonly, patients present with reduced or loss of therapeutic efficacy, breakthrough pain or return of spasticity over time. Radiography or computed tomography (CT) myelography is often used to evaluate catheter tip position. The catheter tip may be found dislodged from its original position such as retraction into the epidural space or subcutaneous tissues or may be found more cephalad than the original position due to catheter stretch. Management of these cases most often require surgical intervention. If catheter stretch has occurred, then surgical replacement altogether must occur. Catheter dislodgement may further be evaluated by catheter dye study whereby myelographically appropriate contrast solution is injected through the catheter access port. This must be preceded by aspiration of catheter contents to not inadvertently provide a bolus of medication to the patient intrathecally. When catheter replacement occurs, standard of care requires exact measurement of catheter implanted to properly determine exact dosing through intrathecal drug delivery reservoir software programming [5,17,18].

Catheter kinking or occlusion

Kinking or occlusion of the catheter often occurs because of fibrosis or anatomical shifts or because of aberrant placement of the catheter at high motion junctions whereby the catheter is subject to anatomy of the spine both above and below its position. Most commonly, loss of therapeutic efficacy, waxing and waning therapeutic benefit, or even drug withdrawal effects may be noted on clinical presentation. Diagnosis of occlusion of the catheter is most often performed by intrathecal catheter dye study under fluoroscopic imaging to include aspiration of catheter contents to include cerebral spinal fluid. In addition, catheter flushing may benefit and mitigate the situation but most reliably, surgical correction is necessary [5,18] (Fig. 45.12).

Granuloma formation at the catheter tip

Granulomas are sterile inflammatory masses that may develop near the tip of an intrathecal catheter, primarily in response to chronic exposure of lower volume concentrated intrathecal opioid administration [19]. While granulomas are rare in patients receiving intrathecal baclofen therapy [20], their formation may be linked to higher drug concentrations [19].

In addition, mechanical localized irritation may also contribute. Patients may present with clinical signs and symptoms of compressive pathology of the neurological tissues such as the spinal cord and/or surrounding nerve roots. Patients may present with signs of neurological deficit, weakness, radiculopathy or cauda equina-like symptoms. A hallmark symptom is worsening pain despite increasing medication doses, as the granuloma obstructs drug distribution within the intrathecal space. These masses typically develop between the spinal cord and dura mater, most commonly in the thoracic region.

MRI imaging with contrast is definitive for visualization of granulomatous masses at the tip of the catheter (Fig. 45.13). Clinical mitigation involves preemption of the formation of granuloma by the usage of low concentrations of intrathecal drug delivery medications. When formed, drug concentration reduction, catheter repositioning or surgical decompression may be needed in severe cases [12,16–18] (Fig. 45.14).

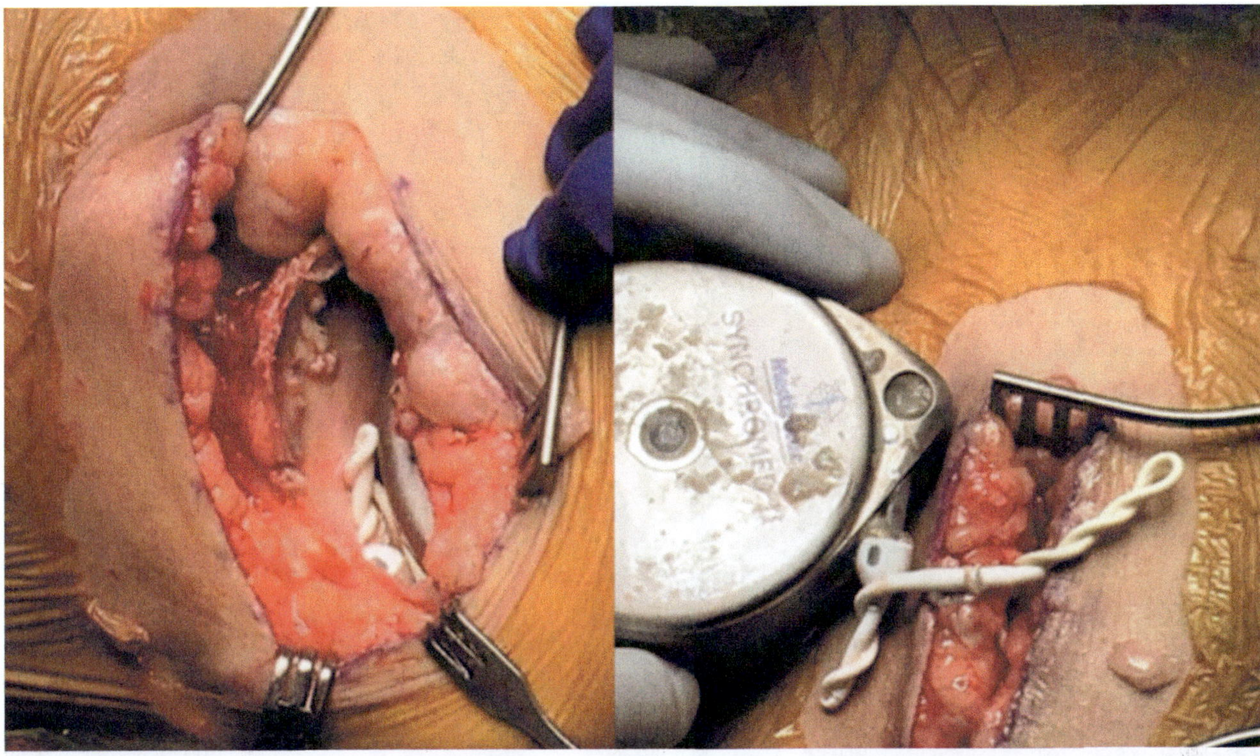

FIGURE 45.12 Significant twisting of catheter with inability to aspirate on catheter access study necessitating open exploration and repair. *Image courtesy of Lawrence Poree MD.*

Management strategies include relocating the catheter to a different spinal level or discontinuing the opioid infusion, as the granuloma may resolve spontaneously [19]. If no neurological deficits are present, the intrathecal opioid should be replaced with sterile normal saline [21]. Surgical removal of the granuloma is reserved for cases with significant neurological impairment.

Catheter fracture or disconnection

CSF leaks may result from catheter-pump disconnection, catheter-catheter disconnection, or catheter fracture or damage. Catheters are subject to fractures because of repeated stress such that may occur between repeated flexion or extension between bony processes resulting in a nutcracker like compression of the catheter. The catheter may fracture altogether resulting in dislodgement into the spinal fluid as a free-floating object or may result in catheter maceration without complete fracture, and subsequent leakage of medication in the extradural space. Disconnection of the catheter may also occur distally at the site of the pump due to improper surgical technique [17]. This is particularly relevant for older systems with sutured catheter-pump connections, as the suture itself may sever the connection, leading to a CSF leak. A significant CSF leak can cause withdrawal symptoms, though minor leaks rarely do. If a patient undergoing IDDS therapy presents with severe post-dural puncture headache (PDPH), catheter-related abnormalities must be ruled out [22]. CSF leaks should also be considered when CSF cannot be aspirated from the pump port or when it accumulates around the pump.

In cases of older reservoir, catheters may have required surgical cerclage of the catheter to the reservoir, and unreliable suture technique the result in disconnection. In all cases, surgical intervention is necessary, and reimplantation of a new catheter is required for continuing effective therapy [5,10]. Although catheter design has improved over the years, physicians must remain knowledgeable about managing these potential complications.

Minor leaks and mild PDPH can often be managed conservatively with fluids, over-the-counter analgesics, caffeine, and rest. However, severe CSF leaks can lead to intracranial hypovolemia and, in some cases, subdural hematoma, necessitating emergency intervention. In cases of significant symptoms, treatment options may include an epidural blood patch, surgical repair of the dural defect, catheter replacement, or placement of additional sutures near the catheter entry site [22].

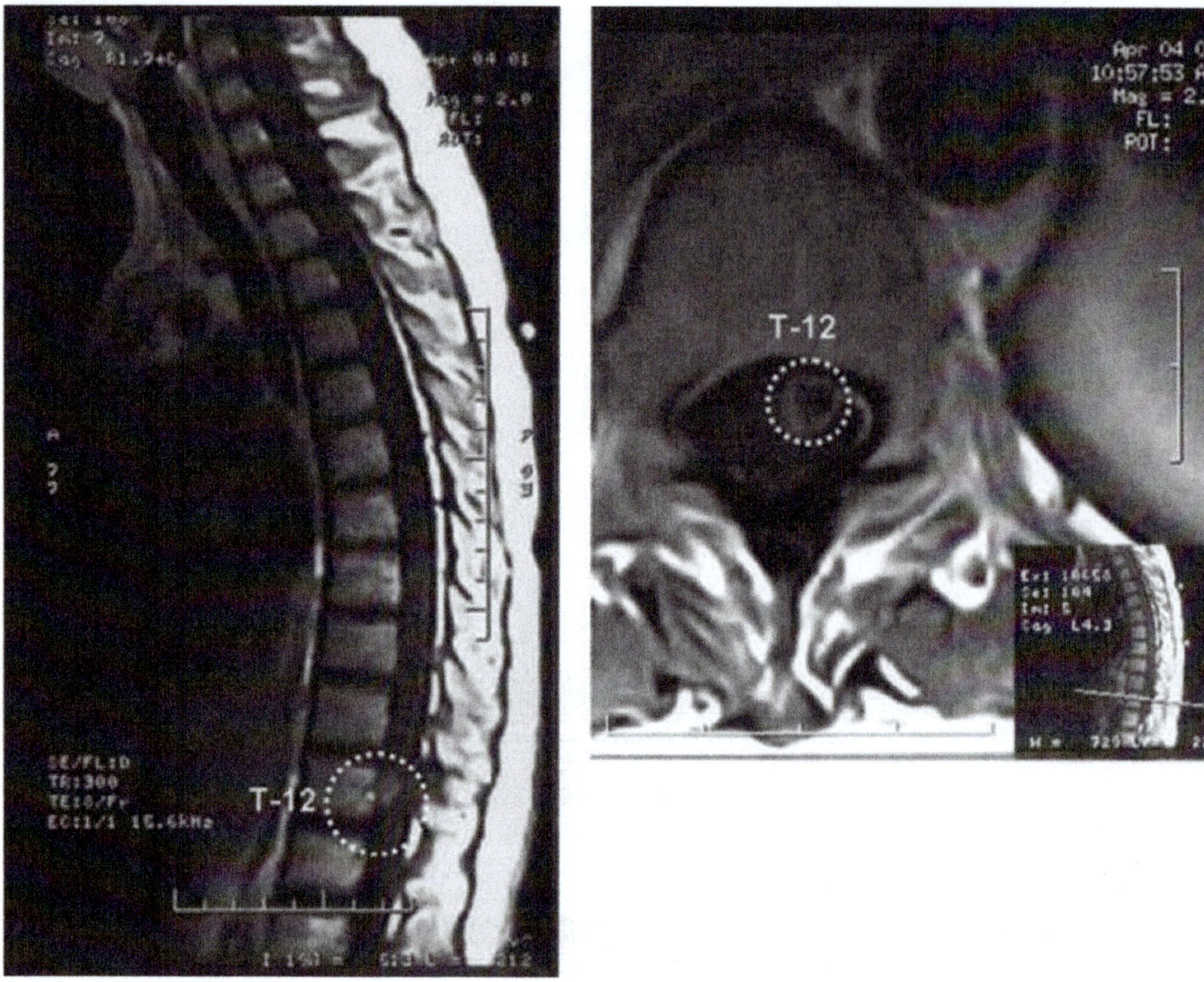

FIGURE 45.13 MRI demonstrating granuloma formation.

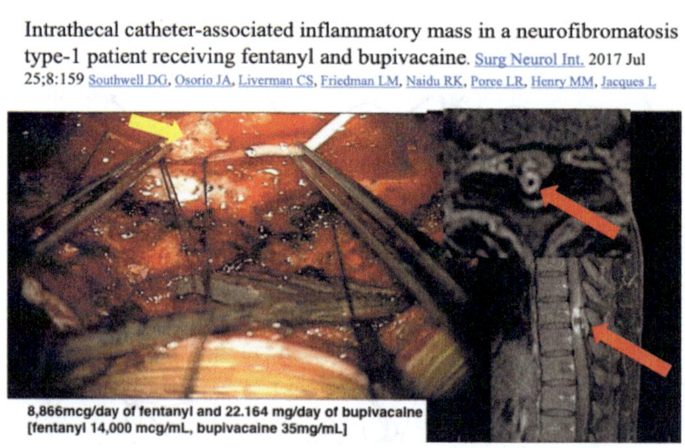

FIGURE 45.14 Granuloma involving intrathecal catheter confirmed on open exploration. *Image courtesy of Lawrence Poree MD.*

Delayed catheter complications often result in reduced medication delivery into the intrathecal space, leading to a gradual return of symptoms or, in cases of abrupt catheter failure, withdrawal. If intrathecal drug delivery is suddenly interrupted, symptoms can emerge within several hours to 48 h, varying based on the specific medication. Baclofen withdrawal is particularly concerning, as it can be life-threatening and, in rare cases, fatal [23]. However, ziconotide is an exception, as it can be discontinued abruptly without withdrawal effects [10]. Overdose events are typically caused by incorrect pump programming or pump failure, but catheter disconnection or loosening of a connection can also result in overdose from local absorption. Management of overdose requires supportive treatment with close monitoring, often in a hospital or intensive care unit setting [10]. Intravenous naloxone is necessary for opioid overdoses.

Timely diagnosis is crucial, as catheter-related interruptions can present with a variety of symptoms that may lead to misdiagnosis and delays in treatment—potentially with life-threatening consequences. A thorough clinical evaluation, including patient history and symptom assessment, is essential for diagnosis. Imaging studies such as X-ray and fluoroscopy are the primary diagnostic tools in acute settings, as they can identify common catheter issues, including migration, fracture, occlusion due to kinking, and disconnection [24]. Additional imaging modalities, such as contrast dye studies through the pump's access port, CT myelography, MRI, and 111In-DTPA scintigraphy, may also be utilized [17]. Although radioisotope studies can detect catheter malfunction, they are neither as timely nor as specific as catheter contrast studies.

A catheter contrast study involves accessing the catheter access port (CAP) with a sterile needle under fluoroscopy. The first step is to aspirate the CAP and confirm the return of at least 2 mL of cerebrospinal fluid (CSF) [17]. If no CSF is aspirated, the procedure must be halted to prevent an injection overdose, which could occur if the highly concentrated catheter contents are inadvertently flushed into the intrathecal space. If fluid aspiration is successful, low volumes of contrast material is injected, and fluoroscopy is used to assess catheter integrity, detect leaks, and confirm proper intrathecal distribution of the contrast material [17].

Infectious complications

Infectious complications are known to be late onset and can be a result of hematogenous spread or device contamination or because of localized infections. Patients experience fever, localized pain and erythema over the interest SQL drug delivery reservoir pocket site, signs and symptoms of meningitis or global pleocytosis of the cerebral spinal fluid. Blood cultures, analysis of the CSF and high-fidelity imaging is needed to rule out abscess formation. Parenteral antibiotics and device removal is necessary in all cases [5,16,25].

Catheter tip adhesions and fibrosis

Scar formation at the catheter tip because of chronic inflammation that does not result necessarily in granuloma formation. Gradual loss of therapeutic benefit without clear mechanical failure is often seen. Intrathecal catheter dye studies with myelographically appropriate contrast solution demonstrates restricted flow under direct visualization. In almost all cases, catheter repositioning or surgical removal is necessary [5].

Prevention and risk mitigation of catheter complications

Risk stratification and mitigation of complications is necessary in all cases for the benefit of good clinical practice and patient care. Iatrogenic causes must be understood before implant, and surgeons must be adept at catheter anchoring, strategizing catheter entry points into the CSF and tunneling techniques. Knowledge of the concentration and flow rates of intrathecal drug delivery solutions is crucial to avoid unnecessary localized irritation. Regular monitoring and patient assessment are necessary at appropriate intervals to ensure accurate drug delivery therapy. Device innovations such as catheters with kink resistance and appropriate flexibility are important for complication prevention [10].

Patient outcomes are significantly impacted by delayed identification of catheter complications. Providers must be vigilant in early identification and assessment, and strategies to intervene on catheter complications must be well thought out. Early collaboration among interventional and surgical specialties as well as radiology is paramount for optimal patient care.

Pocket fill complication and management

Pocket fill complications in intrathecal drug delivery (ITDD) systems occur when the drug intended for the intrathecal space is inadvertently injected into the subcutaneous pocket surrounding the pump. This may lead to unintended and adverse effects, including inadequate pain control and drug overdose. The American Society of Pain and Neuroscience (ASPN) provides guidelines for the avoidance and management of these complications (Figs. 45.15–45.17).

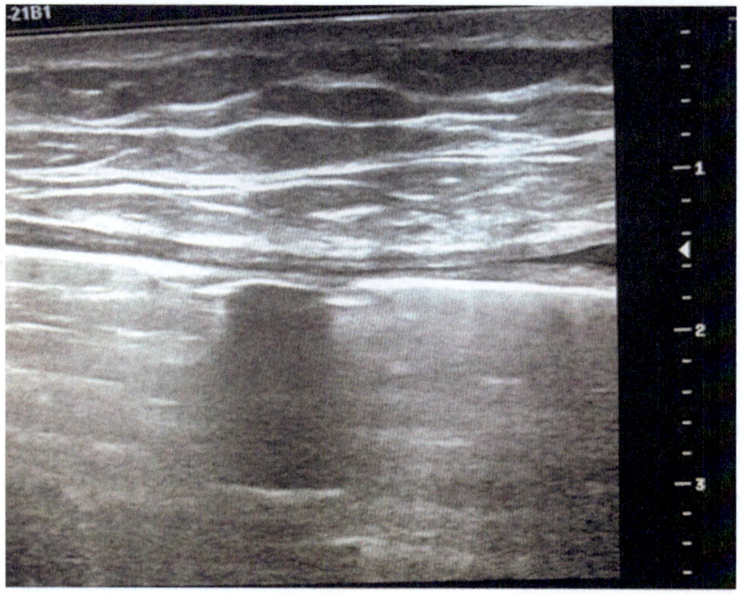

FIGURE 45.15 Normal ultrasound image of the pump refill port showing no significant fluid (hypoechoic finding) above or around the pump at approximately 1.5 cm. *Image courtesy of Gladstone C McDowell II MD.*

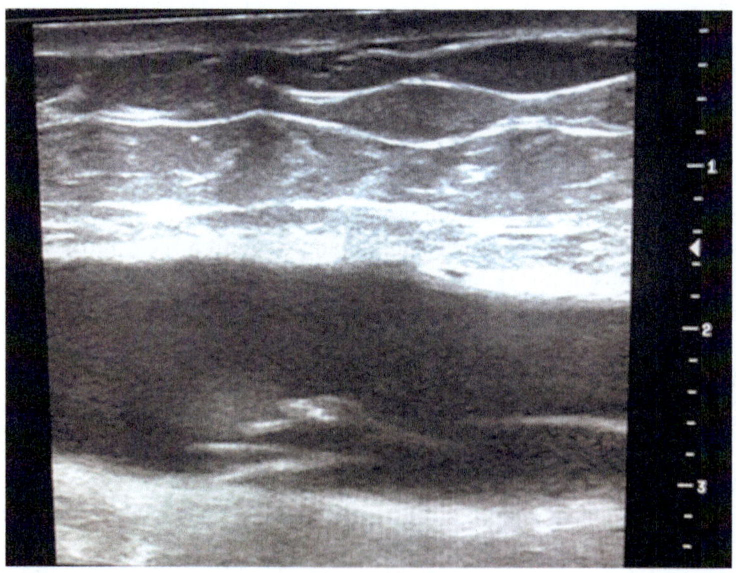

FIGURE 45.16 Image of fluid collection between 1.8 and 3 cm similar to an image seen with a pocket-fill (hypoechoic finding) above the pump. *Image courtesy of Gladstone C McDowell II MD.*

Avoidance strategies

1. Proper Training and Technique: Ensuring that healthcare providers are well-trained in the refill procedure is crucial. Thus, it is critical to adhere to strict aseptic techniques and proper handling of the pump and catheter during refills to prevent pocket fills [26].
2. Use of Imaging: Utilizing fluoroscopy or ultrasound guidance during the refill procedure can help confirm the correct placement of the needle into the pump reservoir. This ultimately helps reduce the risk of pocket fills [27].
3. Volume Discrepancy Monitoring: Monitoring the volume discrepancy between the injected drug volume and the volume measured inside the pump reservoir can help identify potential pocket fills. A significant volume discrepancy should prompt further investigation [27].

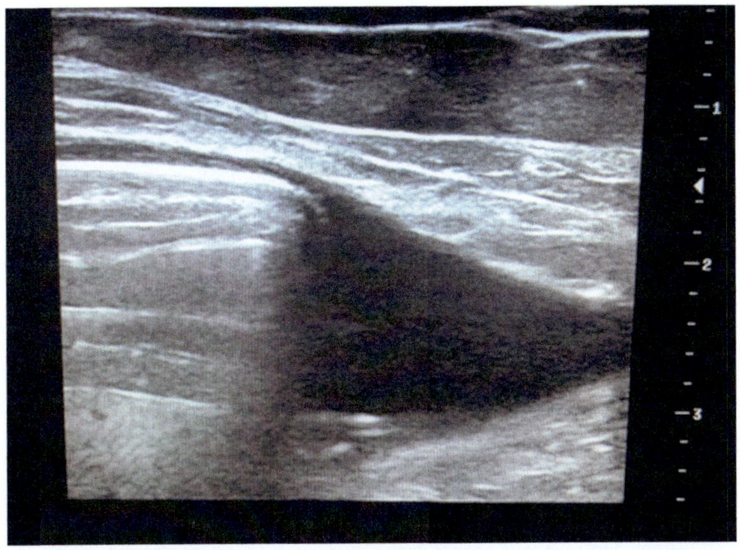

FIGURE 45.17 Image of fluid collection between 1.5 and 3 cm similar to an image seen with a pocket-fill (hypoechoic finding) above and lateral to the pump. *Image courtesy of Gladstone C McDowell II MD.*

4. Patient Positioning: The patient should be in a comfortable and stable position to minimize movement. This proper patient positioning during the refill procedure can help ensure accurate needle placement [26].

Management strategies

1. Immediate Response: If a pocket fill is suspected, immediate action is required.
   Symptoms of overdose, such as respiratory depression, sedation, and hypotension, should be closely monitored. Hospitalization and supportive care may be necessary to manage these symptoms [26,27].
2. Aspiration: In cases where a pocket fill is confirmed, aspiration of the subcutaneous pocket may be performed to remove the excess drug. This helps mitigate the risk of systemic toxicity [5].
3. Patient Education: Educating patients about the signs and symptoms of drug overdose and the importance of seeking immediate medical attention if they experience these symptoms is essential. This can help ensure timely intervention and reduce the risk of serious complications [26,27].
4. Regular Follow-Up: Regular follow-up appointments are necessary to monitor the patient's response to the intrathecal therapy and to check for any signs of complications.
   Adjustments to the dosage or opioid selection may be necessary based on the patient's response and tolerance [27].

Monitoring after trials

Patients undergoing ITDD trials should be closely monitored for efficacy and adverse effects (Fig. 45.18). Initial hospitalization is recommended to observe for signs of respiratory depression, hypotension, and other acute side effects. Continuous monitoring of pain relief, functional improvement, and side effects is essential. Adjustments to the dosage or opioid selection may be necessary based on the patient's response and tolerance [26,27].

In summary, pocket fill complications in ITDD can be serious but are preventable with proper training, technique, and monitoring. Immediate management and patient education are crucial to mitigate risks and ensure patient safety. The ASPN guidelines provide a comprehensive framework for the avoidance and management of these complications, emphasizing the importance of proper technique, imaging guidance, and patient education [5,26].

Pump motor stalls in intrathecal drug delivery systems

A pump motor stall implicitly stalls the delivery, or fails to provide delivery, of the pharmacotherapeutic to the intrathecal space resulting in adverse outcomes.

EMERGENCY ACTION CARD

Inadvertent Soft-Tissue Injection While Refilling an Implanted Drug Delivery Device Reservoir

Johnson ML, Visser EJ, Goucke CR

1 **STOP the injection.** Aspirate tissues if possible (e.g. pocket or seroma).

2 **CALL FOR HELP.** Consider activating the hospital's emergency team.

3 **Check 'ABC'** — ensure airway, breathing, and circulation.

4 Establish **intravenous access**, high-flow oxygen, set up **monitoring**.

5 **Urgent advanced resuscitation** if required.

6 Confirm **type and dose of injected drugs** and consider the possible effects and time course.

7 **Check the IDDD** — consider test aspiration of the reservoir and switching off.

8 **Resuscitation, supportive care, critical care monitoring.**

9 **Outline of specific treatments:**

Opioids	**Naloxone**, respiratory support; manage conscious state.
Clonidine	Invasive blood pressure monitoring, advanced cardiovascular (pharmacological) support; manage conscious state.
Bupivacaine	**Intralipid® 20%** therapy.
Baclofen	*a.* 'Overdose': supportive care. *b.* 'Under-dose' (withdrawal from IT baclofen): **baclofen, benzodiazepines, dantrolene.**
Ziconotide	Supportive care, critical care monitoring.

10 **Transfer patient to a high dependency or intensive care facility urgently.**

For clinical use only · Verify all drug dosages against current formulary · Not a substitute for clinical judgment

FIGURE 45.18 Suggested emergency checklist if a pocket fill occurs.

Motor stalls in drug delivery therapy can lead to serious complications, leading to underdelivery, overdelivery, or complete failure of drug administration [28–30].

Pump stalls occur because of either mechanical, electrical or potentially software related nuances, and when identified require immediate attention and intervention [28–30]. Under-delivery of medication from motor stalls may lead to inadequate symptom control of pain or spasticity.

Opioid withdrawal with resultant increased pain and manifestation of moderate to severe withdrawal syndrome, while bothersome, is not usually life-threatening. Baclofen withdrawal on the other hand is potentially life-threatening with symptoms and signs to include high fever, seizures, hallucinations, muscle rigidity, and autonomic instability [29,31].

Overdelivery of medication may occur if the motor stalls and suddenly resumes at an inappropriate rate causing an overdose of medication, with resultant toxicity (e.g., respiratory depression with opioids, hypotension with baclofen). Pump electronics designed for wireless communication may be impacted by electromagnetic interference (EMI) from an MRI scan. Some SynchroMed II pumps may switch into a state in which the pump is waiting for communication (telemetry mode). In rare cases where this occurred in combination with a pump alarm, the pump would remain stalled until interrogated. Labeling for SynchroMed pumps requires interrogation of the pump after MRI to ensure the pump has resumed normal operation, [DS1] and telemetry mode was designed out of the more recent SynchroMed III pump [39] (Fig. 45.19).

The Medtronic SynchroMed II pump has a history of motor stalls [28]. In November 2012, Medtronic issued a safety notice highlighting an increased risk of permanent motor stalls associated with the use of unapproved drug formulations in SynchroMed pumps [32]. The notice emphasized that using such formulations could lead to motor corrosion and subsequent pump failure. A published response by a coalition of experience pump implanters/managers indicated that not all patients respond to monotherapy with FDA approved analgesics, and combination drug therapy is not only necessary, but common practice, in attempts to effectively managing intractable pain [33].

In June 2013, Medtronic identified potential electrical short circuits within the SynchroMed II pumps, which could result in motor stalls and loss of therapy [30]. Although the reported occurrence rate was less than 1% at 7 years post-implant, the issue prompted an urgent medical device correction. Design changes to the SynchroMed II pump models were implemented to reduce the likelihood of non-recoverable motor stalls. Modified gear wheel material and encapsulated feedthroughs were implemented in 2016. Applied diamond-like coating to address gear shaft wear was implemented in 2017. Pumps manufactured before this change were recalled to mitigate the risk of motor stall caused by this specific issue. All SynchroMed pumps currently in use contain the three design changes [40].

There is no motor to stall with the Prometra I and II pumps, but there is a theoretical risk of the valves remaining open after exposure to the MRI scan magnetic field, which has been addressed through a flow-activation valve in the Prometra II model. There is no motor to stall with the Prometra I and II pumps, but there is a pumping mechanism that relies on a series of electrically controlled valves. With Prometra I, these valves could fail open during MRI resulting in uncontrolled flow of drug out of the pump. A flow-activated valve was added in Prometra II to reduce the risk of uncontrolled drug flow. Labeling for both Prometra I and Prometra II systems identifies the risk of the valves remaining open after exposure to the MRI scan magnetic field and guides the user to ensure drug is removed prior to scan [30,34].

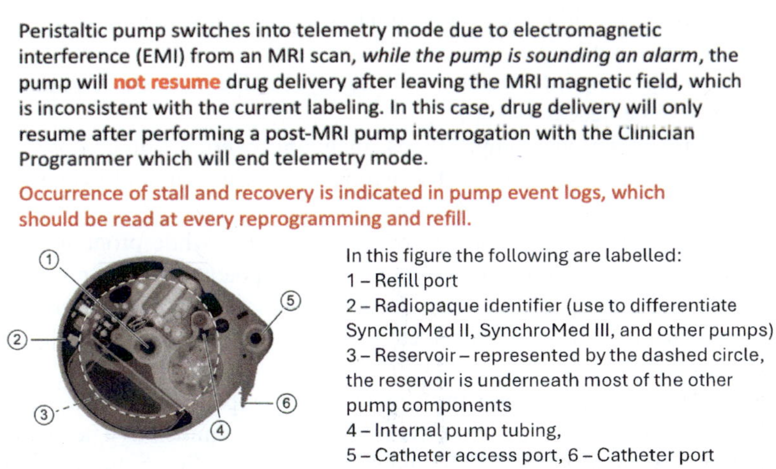

FIGURE 45.19 *SynchroMed III Implant Manual. https://www.medtronic.com/content/dam/emanuals/neuro/M029641C_a_001_view.pdf.*

Causes of motor stalls

- Mechanical obstruction-A common cause of a pause, or complete stall, is a result of mechanical obstruction that occurs within the pump housing or catheter system. This may be due to catheter kinking, a defined blockage or damage within the pump mechanism. As a result, the catheter or the reservoir may become occluded by particulates, drug crystallization resulting in the impediment of flow and subsequent stall [29].
- Battery capacity-Within the housing of the intrathecal drug delivery system there is finite energy capacity within batteries to drive the system. Like any other battery, the capacity is finite, and the energy may be depleted reducing its ability to deliver intrathecal medication accurately especially when it is close end of life. When higher speeds are needed, insufficient energy may lead to stall [29,31].
- Software malfunction-Intrinsic to any medical device that interfaces with programmability options resides software that is complex and critical to function of the device. Software issues can interfere with the system and the accuracy of the motor in relationship to other components of the system leading to failure. Malfunctions may also occur during initialization or part of routine operation and can occur in the form of a sudden error or malfunction [35].

Pump internal catheter issues

The Silastic catheter is an important component in the accurate delivery of medication to the patient. Its length, plasticity and caliber are critical to accuracy of delivery. If there is occlusion or mechanical disruption of the catheter, the upstream motor may not be function appropriately leading to stall [36].

Motor aging and malfunction

Traditional wear and tear of any mechanical motor may occur over time. Degradation of mechanical components may lead to failure despite normal usage. Similarly, the pump motor may need to be replaced over prolonged use [37].

Clinical consequences of motor stalls

Serious adverse outcomes may occur because of pump load or stalls. In the case of interruption of medication delivery, withdrawal syndromes to include fatal withdrawal may occur either directly or lead to secondary fatal outcomes. Sudden opioid withdrawal may lead to medical instability, elevated high blood pressure and cardiac events or stroke for example. Withdrawal of medications used to control spasticity may result in severe hyper-spasticity, hyperpyrexia, muscle break down, renal failure and subsequent acid base imbalances that may lead to fatal outcome. Critically, prompt identification of the need for intervention is paramount. Surgical solutions may be needed and carry intrinsic risk in addition to risks associated with anesthesia in a potentially unstable patient [29–31].

Prevention and management

The prevention of motor stalls involves routine monitoring and maintenance protocols within the clinical setting. Pump diagnostics, programming review, and residual reservoir volumes assessments may be early indicators and helpful with early diagnosis of potential complication [35].

Troubleshooting of the device by pump interrogation, catheter dye studies with aspiration of the catheter, or ultimately catheter or pump replacement may be necessary [36].

Programming errors can result in serious complications, including overdose, underdose, or withdrawal symptoms. Human errors such as incorrect drug concentration entry, wrong drug selection, and inappropriate dose scaling during refills are common causes of these complications [10,19,38].

One critical mistake involves entering the incorrect drug concentration while programming the device. If the concentration is higher than expected, the patient may receive an overdose, potentially leading to life-threatening respiratory depression. Conversely, if the concentration is lower than intended, the patient may experience inadequate pain relief and withdrawal symptoms. Misconfiguring the infusion parameters—including the basal rate, bolus dose, or patient-controlled dose—can also lead to similar complications.

Careful calculations are essential when introducing a bolus dose or patient-controlled dose in patients previously receiving only a simple continuous infusion. The bolus dose is typically determined as a percentage of the total daily dose, with the Polyanalgesic Consensus Conference (PACC) guidelines recommending boluses within a range of 5%–20% of the total daily dose, depending on the patient's needs [10,19]. Additionally, setting appropriate lock-out intervals is crucial; an interval that is too short increases the risk of overdose, whereas an interval that is too long may lead to inadequate pain control.

Clinicians should also be aware of potential errors related to dose scaling during refills. If a patient's medication dose was previously increased, but the refill is programmed using the older, lower dose, withdrawal symptoms can develop. Similarly, changes to the medication in the pump reservoir—such as switching drug formulations or adding adjunct medications—can introduce errors if the pump is not properly primed. IDDS devices require thorough priming to eliminate air bubbles and ensure accurate medication delivery. If the priming volume is skipped or incorrectly set, the patient may experience a delayed onset of action or unpredictable drug effects, which can compromise pain management and safety [2]'.

To minimize these risks, clinicians and their teams should implement a structured checklist for every pump refill or programming session. This checklist should include verification of all essential parameters, such as drug name, drug concentration, infusion rate and reservoir volume. Additionally, the built-in safety checks on the programmer should be used consistently. Any warnings or alarms must be carefully investigated rather than ignored. Thorough staff training on potential programming issues is also critical, ensuring that every team member is proficient in identifying and preventing errors.

Finally, patients should be closely monitored after programming sessions for signs of overdose or withdrawal, allowing for timely intervention if complications arise. By adopting these safety measures, clinicians can enhance the reliability of IDDS therapy and improve patient outcomes.

Reservoir volume discrepancy (RVD) in targeted drug delivery systems refers to a mismatch between the expected and actual drug volume within the reservoir. This discrepancy can have serious clinical implications for pain management and spasticity control.

A volume discrepancy may lead clinicians to misattribute worsening symptoms to disease progression, rather than a drug delivery issue.

Causes of **R**eservoir **V**olume **D**iscrepancy include:

(a) Human Errors with inaccurate priming, or improper documentation during refills or misinterpretation or error in reading expected volume versus actual volume [38].
(b) Device-related Issues such as pump motor stall, software errors, or incorrect infusion rate settings [29,30,35].
(c) Catheter-related Issues: Kinking, disconnection, occlusion, or leakage [19,30].
(d) Pharmacological factors such as drug stability as some drugs may crystallize, or degrade over time [30].
(e) Unexpected drug absorption with interaction with reservoir materials leading to drug loss.

Detection and corrective actions must include regularly checking pump logs for unexpected volume changes. We recommend a "two-person-read-back system "confirming correct medication programming and infusion rates, and double-checking documentation and fill techniques to ensure accuracy. We suggest verifying proper priming during initial pump filling.

Imaging and contrast studies may be necessary to check for catheter integrity and to rule out occlusions or leakage.

If persistent discrepancies exist, consider replacing the catheter or pump. Attention to addressing known manufacturer alerts or recalls related to pump function is crucial.

Conclusion

Although intrathecal drug delivery systems provide significant clinical benefits, adverse events such as infection, movement, erosion, and impingement remain considerable concerns. Careful patient selection, proper surgical technique, and vigilant postoperative monitoring can mitigate these complications and improve patient outcomes. The Polyanalgesic Consensus Conference (PACC) publications of evidence-based guidelines on intrathecal drug delivery are a valuable resource [10]. Continued research and refinement of implantation techniques are essential to minimizing the risks associated with IDDS therapy.

References

[1] Follett KA, Burchiel K, Deer T, Dupen S, Prager J, et al. Prevention of intrathecal drug delivery catheter-related complications. Neuromodulation 2003;6(1):32–41.
[2] Staats PS. Complications of intrathecal therapy. Pain Med May 2008;9(Suppl. 1):S102–7. https://doi.org/10.1111/j.1526-4637.2008.00445.x.
[3] Slavin KV. Intramedullary placement of intrathecal catheter. Report of a rare complication of intrathecal therapy. Neuromodulation Technol Neural Interf 2006;9:94–9.

[4] Deibert CP, Gandhoke GS, Forsythe RM, Moossy JJ. Surgical site infection 18 Months following intrathecal pump placement secondary to an asymptomatic bowel injury. Pain Pract 2015;15:E69–71.

[5] Goel V, Yang Y, Kanwar S, et al. Adverse events and complications associated with intrathecal drug delivery systems: insights from the manufacturer and user facility device experience (MAUDE) database. Neuromodulation 2021;24:1181–9.

[6] Crul BJ, Gerritse BM, van Dongen RT, Schoonderwaldt HC. Epidural fibrin glue injection stops persistent postdural puncture headache. Anesthesiology 1999;91:576–7.

[7] Narouze S, Benzon HT, Provenzano D, et al. Interventional spine and pain procedures in patients on antiplatelet and anticoagulant medications (second edition): guidelines from the American society of regional anesthesia and pain medicine, the European society of regional anaesthesia and pain therapy, the American academy of pain medicine, the international neuromodulation society, the North American neuromodulation society, and the world institute of pain. Reg Anesth Pain Med 2018;43(3):225–62.

[8] Deer TR, Narouze S, Provenzano DA, et al. The Neurostimulation Appropriateness Consensus Committee (NACC): recommendations on bleeding and coagulation management in neurostimulation devices. Neuromodulation 2017;20(1):51–62.

[9] Ban KA, Minei JP, Laronga C, et al. American college of surgeons and surgical infection society: surgical site infection guidelines, 2016 update. J Am Coll Surg 2017;224(1):59–74.

[10] Deer TR, Hayek SM, Grider JS, Hagedorn JM, McDowell II GC, Kim P, Levy RM. The polyanalgesic consensus conference (PACC): intrathecal drug delivery guidance on safety and therapy optimization when treating chronic noncancer pain. Neuromodulation Technol Neural Interf 2024;27.

[11] Adverse events and complications associated with intrathecal drug delivery systems: analysis of the manufacturer and user facility device experience database 2018–2019. PMC9034464.

[12] Engle MP, Vinh BP, Harun N, Koyyalagunta D. Infectious complications related to intrathecal drug delivery system and spinal cord stimulator system implantations at a comprehensive cancer pain center. Pain Phys 2013;16(3):251.

[13] Gerges T, Mavropoulos A, Levin D, Dao T, Acquadro M. A rare intrathecal pump complication caused by prolonged intrathecal pump pocket seroma. Cureus 2023;15(11):e37954.

[14] Uncovering the rate and risk factors of intrathecal baclofen pump complications: a retrospective cohort study. Neurosurg Focus 2024;56(6):E12.

[15] Kamran S, Wright BD. Complications of intrathecal drug delivery systems. Neuromodulation Technol Neural Interf 2001;4(3):111–6.

[16] Follett KA, Naumann CP. A prospective study of catheter-related complications of intrathecal drug delivery systems. J Pain Symptom Manag 2000;19(3):209–15.

[17] Delhaas EM, Huygen FJPM. Complications associated with intrathecal drug delivery systems. BJA Educ 2020;20(2):51–7.

[18] Hitt JM, de Leon-Casasola OA. Complications of intrathecal drug delivery systems. Tech Reg Anesth Pain Manag 2011;15(4):162–6.

[19] Deer TR, Pope JE, Hayek SM. The Polyanalgesic Consensus Conference (PACC): recommendations for intrathecal drug delivery: guidance for improving safety and mitigating risks. Neuromodulation 2017;20:155–76. https://doi.org/10.1111/ner.12579.

[20] Deer TR, Raso LJ, Coffey RJ, Allen JW. Intrathecal baclofen and catheter tip inflammatory mass lesions (granulomas): a reevaluation of case reports and imaging findings in light of experimental, clinicopathological, and radiological evidence. Pain Med 2008;9:391–5. https://doi.org/10.1111/j.1526-4637.2008.00468.x.

[21] Allen JW, Horais KA, Tozier NA, et al. Time course and role of morphine dose and concentration in intrathecal granuloma formation in dogs: a combined magnetic resonance imaging and histopathology investigation. Anesthesiology 2006;105:581–9. https://doi.org/10.1097/00000542-200609000-00024.

[22] Capozza MA, Triarico S, Mastrangelo S, Attinà G, Maurizi P, Ruggiero A. Narrative review of intrathecal drug delivery (IDD): indications, devices and potential complications. Ann Transl Med January 2021;9(2):186. https://doi.org/10.21037/atm-20-3814.

[23] Green LB, Nelson VS. Death after acute withdrawal of intrathecal baclofen: case report and literature review. Arch Phys Med Rehabil 1999;80(12):1600–4. https://doi.org/10.1016/S0003-9993(99)90337-4.

[24] Awaad Y, Rizk T, Siddiqui I, Roosen N, McIntosh K, Waines GM. Complications of intrathecal baclofen pump: prevention and cure. ISRN Neurol 2012;2012:575168. https://doi.org/10.5402/2012/575168.

[25] Engle AM, Malinowski DO MN, Hagedorn JM, Deer TR. Complications of intrathecal drug delivery systems and drugs used. In: Complications of pain-relieving procedures: an illustrated guide; 2022. p. 421–38.

[26] Aman MM, Mahmoud A, Deer T, et al. The American society of pain and neuroscience (ASPN) best practices and guidelines for the interventional management of cancer- associated pain. J Pain Res 2021;14:2139–64. https://doi.org/10.2147/JPR.S315585.

[27] Sayed D, Grider J, Strand N, et al. The American society of pain and neuroscience (ASPN) evidence-based clinical guideline of interventional treatments for low back pain. J Pain Res 2022;15:3729–832. https://doi.org/10.2147/JPR.S386879.

[28] Galica R, Hayek SM, Veizi IE, Lawrence MM, Khalil AA, McEwan MT. Sudden intrathecal drug delivery device motor stalls: a case series. Reg Anesth Pain Med 2016;41(2):135–9.

[29] Chavez M, Smith J, Miller R. Mechanical and technical issues in intrathecal drug delivery systems. J Neurosurg 2016;124(1):110–6.

[30] Galica R, Jones BA, Hayek SM. Managing and minimizing risk of device failure. In: Yaksh T, Hayek S, editors. Neuraxial therapeutics. Cham: Springer; 2023. https://doi.org/10.1007/978-3-031-39558-1_43.

[31] Boudes E, Riviere G, Collet B. Device-related complications in intrathecal drug delivery systems: a comprehensive review. J Pain Manag 2020;35(6):1293–301.

[32] Medtronic I. Use of Unapproved Drugs with the SynchroMed Implantable Infusion Pump. 2012. https://www.medtronic.com/content/dam/medtronic-com/professional/documents/product-advisories/tdd/app-drug-summary.pdf?bypassIM=true.

[33] Deer T, Kim P, Pope J, Hayek S, McDowell G, et al. Physician guidance on the use of off-labeled drugs in intrathecal drug delivery systems of chronic pain. Neuromodulation October 2019;22(7):765–8. https://doi.org/10.1111/ner.12961.

[34] Flowonix Medical I. Prometra II Programmable Pump Manual. 2020. http://wwwflowonixcom/sites/default/files/PL-31790-00 - Prometra II Pro grammable Pump IFU (Flowonix - US Commercial)pdf2015.

[35] Jensen MP, et al. Software malfunctions in intrathecal drug delivery systems: a case series. Neuromodulation 2018;21(1):34–9.

[36] Lange JP, Nguyen TK, Miller M. Catheter-related issues in intrathecal drug delivery systems: a clinical overview. Pain Phys 2017;20(2):87–95.

[37] Noon K, Poree L, Ike K, Jones RCW. Intrathecal pump malfunction: flipped, expired, stalled, and malfunctioned valves and rotors. In: Challenging cases and complication management in pain medicine. Springer; 2018. p. 181–7. https://doi.org/10.1007/978-3-319-60072-7_29.

[38] Kirkendall ES, Timmons K, Huth H, Walsh K, Melton K. Human-based errors involving smart infusion pumps: a catalog of error types and prevention strategies. Drug Saf November 2020;43(11):1073–87. https://doi.org/10.1007/s40264-020-00986-5.

Further reading

[1] Deer TR, Lamer TJ, Pope JE, et al. The Neurostimulation Appropriateness Consensus Committee (NACC) safety guidelines for the reduction of severe neurological injury. Neuromodulation 2017;20(1):15–30.

Index

Note: Page numbers followed by *f* indicate figures and *t* indicate tables.

A

D

F

G

H

I

J

L

M

P

Q

R

S

T

U

V

9780443365287